2nd Edition

HARRISON'S™

GASTROENTEROLOGY
AND HEPATOLOGY

Derived from Harrison's Principles of Internal Medicine, 18th Edition

Editors

DAN L. LONGO, MD

Professor of Medicine, Harvard Medical School;
Senior Physician, Brigham and Women's Hospital;
Deputy Editor, New England Journal of Medicine,
Boston, Massachusetts

DENNIS L. KASPER, MD

William Ellery Channing Professor of Medicine,
Professor of Microbiology and Molecular Genetics,
Harvard Medical School; Director, Channing Laboratory,
Department of Medicine, Brigham and Women's Hospital,
Boston, Massachusetts

J. LARRY JAMESON, MD, PhD

Robert G. Dunlop Professor of Medicine;
Dean, University of Pennsylvania School of Medicine;
Executive Vice-President of the University of Pennsylvania
for the Health System, Philadelphia, Pennsylvania

ANTHONY S. FAUCI, MD

Chief, Laboratory of Immunoregulation;
Director, National Institute of Allergy and Infectious Diseases,
National Institutes of Health, Bethesda, Maryland

STEPHEN L. HAUSER, MD

Robert A. Fishman Distinguished Professor and
Chairman, Department of Neurology,
University of California, San Francisco,
San Francisco, California

JOSEPH LOSCALZO, MD, PhD

Hersey Professor of the Theory and Practice of Medicine,
Harvard Medical School; Chairman, Department of Medicine;
Physician-in-Chief, Brigham and Women's Hospital,
Boston, Massachusetts

2nd Edition

HARRISON'S™
GASTROENTEROLOGY
AND HEPATOLOGY

EDITORS

Dan L. Longo, MD

Professor of Medicine, Harvard Medical School;
Senior Physician, Brigham and Women's Hospital;
Deputy Editor, New England Journal of Medicine
Boston, Massachusetts

Anthony S. Fauci, MD

Chief, Laboratory of Immunoregulation;
Director, National Institute of Allergy and Infectious
Diseases, National Institutes of Health
Bethesda, Maryland

ASSOCIATE EDITOR

Carol A. Langford, MD, MHS

Harold C. Schott Chair
Associate Professor of Medicine
Cleveland Clinic, Cleveland, Ohio

New York   Chicago   San Francisco   Lisbon   London   Madrid   Mexico City
Milan   New Delhi   San Juan   Seoul   Singapore   Sydney   Toronto

Harrison's Gastroenterology and Hepatology, Second Edition

1 2 3 4 5 6 7 8 9 0   CTP/CTP   18 17 16 15 14 13

ISBN 978-0-07-181488-1
MHID 0-07-181488-4

This book was set in Bembo by Cenveo Publisher Services. The editors were James F. Shanahan and Kim J. Davis. The production supervisor was Catherine H. Saggese. Project management was provided by Sandhya Gola of Cenveo® Publisher Services. The cover design was by Thomas DePierro. Cover illustration, villi in the small intestine mucosa, © Visuals Unlimited/Corbis.

China Translation & Printing Services Ltd. was the printer and binder.

Library of Congress Cataloging-in-Publication Data

Harrison's gastroenterology and hepatology / editors, Dan L. Longo, Anthony S. Fauci ; associate editor, Carol A. Langford. — 2nd ed.
    p. ; cm.
    Gastroenterology and hepatology
    Includes index.
    This book is aimed at bringing together the chapters of the current and 18th edition of Harrison's Principles of Internal Medicine related to gastroenterology and hepatology in a conveniently sized book for a focused study of this medical subspecialty.
    ISBN 978-0-07-181488-1 (pbk. : alk. paper)
    ISBN 0-07-181488-4 (pbk. : alk. paper)
I. Longo, Dan L. (Dan Louis), 1949-   II. Fauci, Anthony S., 1940-   III. Langford, Carol A.   IV. Harrison, Tinsley Randolph, 1900-1978.   V. Harrison's principles of internal medicine.   VI. Title: Gastroenterology and hepatology.
    [DNLM: 1. Gastrointestinal Diseases.   2. Liver Diseases.   WI 140]
616.3'3—dc23
                                                                    2012039733

CONTENTS

Numbers in brackets refer to the chapter(s) written or co-written by the contributor.

John C. Atherton, MD, FRCP
Nottingham Digestive Diseases Centre Biomedical Research Unit (NDDC BRU), University of Nottingham and Nottingham University Hospitals NHS Trust, Nottingham, United Kingdom [26]

Evelyn Attia, MD
Professor of Clinical Psychiatry, Columbia College of Physicians and Surgeons; Weill Cornell Medical College, New York, New York [59]

Bruce R. Bacon, MD
James F. King, MD Endowed Chair in Gastroenterology; Professor of Internal Medicine, St. Louis University Liver Center, St. Louis University School of Medicine, St. Louis, Missouri [42, 44]

Peter A. Banks, MD
Professor of Medicine, Harvard Medical School; Senior Physician, Division of Gastroenterology, Brigham and Women's Hospital, Boston, Massachusetts [47, 48]

Miriam J. Baron, MD
Assistant Professor of Medicine, Harvard Medical School; Associate Physician, Brigham and Women's Hospital, Boston, Massachusetts [25]

Robert C. Basner, MD
Professor of Clinical Medicine, Division of Pulmonary, Allergy, and Critical Care Medicine, Columbia University College of Physicians and Surgeons, New York, New York [Appendix]

Jean Bergounioux, MD, PhD
Pediatric Intensive Care Unit, Hôpital Necker-Enfants Malades, Paris, France [28]

Atul K. Bhan, MBBS, MD
Professor of Pathology, Harvard Medical School; Director of Immunopathology, Department of Pathology, Massachusetts General Hospital, Boston, Massachusetts [43]

Henry J. Binder, MD
Professor Emeritus of Medicine; Senior Research Scientist, Yale University, New Haven, Connecticut [15, 16]

Bruce R. Bistrian, MD, PhD
Professor of Medicine, Harvard Medical School; Chief, Clinical Nutrition, Beth Israel Deaconess Medical Center, Boston, Massachusetts [56]

Martin J. Blaser, MD
Frederick H. King Professor of Internal Medicine; Chair, Department of Medicine; Professor of Microbiology, New York University School of Medicine, New York, New York [26, 29]

Richard S. Blumberg, MD
Chief, Division of Gastroenterology, Brigham and Women's Hospital, Boston, Massachusetts [17]

Cynthia D. Brown, MD
Assistant Professor of Medicine, Division of Pulmonary and Critical Care Medicine, University of Virginia, Charlottesville, Virginia [Review and Self-Assessment]

Stephen B. Calderwood, MD
Morton Swartz MD Academy Professor of Medicine (Microbiology and Molecular Genetics), Harvard Medical School; Chief, Division of Infectious Diseases, Massachusetts General Hospital, Boston, Massachusetts [23]

Michael Camilleri, MD
Atherton and Winifred W. Bean Professor; Professor of Medicine and Physiology, Mayo Clinic College of Medicine, Rochester, Minnesota [6]

Brian I. Carr, MD, PhD, FRCP
Professor of Oncology and Hepatology, IRCCS De Bellis Medical Research Institute, Castellana Grotte, Italy [50]

Irene Chong, MRCP, FRCR
Clinical Research Fellow, Royal Marsden NHS Foundation Trust, London and Sutton, United Kingdom [51]

Raymond T. Chung, MD
Associate Professor of Medicine, Harvard Medical School; Director of Hepatology; Vice Chief, Gastrointestinal Unit, Massachusetts General Hospital, Boston, Massachusetts [46]

Darwin L. Conwell, MD
Associate Professor of Medicine, Harvard Medical School; Associate Physician, Division of Gastroenterology, Brigham and Women's Hospital, Boston, Massachusetts [47, 48]

Kathleen E. Corey, MD, MPH
Clinical and Research Fellow, Harvard Medical School; Fellow, Gastrointestinal Unit, Massachusetts General Hospital, Boston, Massachusetts [9]

David Cunningham, MD, FRCP
Professor of Cancer Medicine, Royal Marsden NHS Foundation Trust, London and Sutton, United Kingdom [51]

John Del Valle, MD
Professor and Senior Associate Chair of Medicine, Department of Internal Medicine, University of Michigan School of Medicine, Ann Arbor, Michigan [14]

Jules L. Dienstag, MD
Carl W. Walter Professor of Medicine and Dean for Medical Education, Harvard Medical School; Physician, Gastrointestinal Unit, Department of Medicine, Massachusetts General Hospital, Boston, Massachusetts [38-40, 43, 46]

David F. Driscoll, PhD
Associate Professor of Medicine, University of Massachusetts Medical School, Worcester, Massachusetts [56]

Samuel C. Durso, MD, MBA
Mason F. Lord Professor of Medicine; Director, Division of Geriatric Medicine and Gerontology, Johns Hopkins University School of Medicine, Baltimore, Maryland [2, 3]

Johanna Dwyer, DSc, RD
Professor of Medicine (Nutrition), Friedman School of Nutrition Science and Policy, Tufts University School of Medicine; Director, Frances Stern Nutrition Center, Tufts Medical Center, Boston, Massachusetts [53]

Robert H. Eckel, MD
Professor of Medicine, Division of Endocrinology, Metabolism and Diabetes, Division of Cardiology; Professor of Physiology and Biophysics, Charles A. Boettcher, II Chair in Atherosclerosis, University of Colorado School of Medicine, Anschutz Medical Campus, Director Lipid Clinic, University of Colorado Hospital, Aurora, Colorado [60]

Andrew J. Einstein, MD, PhD
Assistant Professor of Clinical Medicine, Columbia University College of Physicians and Surgeons; Department of Medicine, Division of Cardiology, Department of Radiology, Columbia University Medical Center and New York-Presbyterian Hospital, New York, New York [Appendix]

Jeffrey S. Flier, MD
Caroline Shields Walker Professor of Medicine and Dean, Harvard Medical School, Boston, Massachusetts [57]

Lawrence S. Friedman, MD
Professor of Medicine, Harvard Medical School; Professor of Medicine, Tufts University School of Medicine; Assistant Chief of Medicine, Massachusetts General Hospital, Boston, Massachusetts; Chair, Department of Medicine, Newton-Wellesley Hospital, Newton, Massachusetts [9]

Sonia Friedman, MD
Assistant Professor of Medicine, Harvard Medical School, Boston, Massachusetts [17]

Susan L. Gearhart, MD
Assistant Professor of Colorectal Surgery and Oncology, The Johns Hopkins University School of Medicine, Baltimore, Maryland [19, 20]

Dale N. Gerding, MD
Professor of Medicine, Loyola University Chicago Stritch School of Medicine; Associate Chief of Staff for Research and Development, Edward Hines, Jr. VA Hospital, Hines, Illinois [24]

Marc G. Ghany, MD, MHSc
Staff Physician, Liver Diseases Branch, National Institute of Diabetes and Digestive and Kidney Diseases, National Institutes of Health, Bethesda, Maryland [35]

Roger I. Glass, MD, PhD
Director, Fogarty International Center, Bethesda, Maryland [31]

Norton J. Greenberger, MD
Clinical Professor of Medicine, Harvard Medical School; Senior Physician, Division of Gastroenterology, Brigham and Women's Hospital, Boston, Massachusetts [45, 47, 48]

William L. Hasler, MD
Professor of Internal Medicine, Division of Gastroenterology, University of Michigan Health System, Ann Arbor, Michigan [5, 11]

Douglas C. Heimburger, MD, MS
Professor of Medicine; Associate Director for Education and Training, Vanderbilt Institute for Global Health, Vanderbilt University School of Medicine, Nashville, Tennessee [55]

Anna R. Hemnes, MD
Assistant Professor, Division of Allergy, Pulmonary, and Critical Care Medicine, Vanderbilt University Medical Center, Nashville, Tennessee [Review and Self-Assessment]

Ikuo Hirano, MD
Professor of Medicine, Division of Gastroenterology and Hepatology, Department of Medicine, Northwestern University Feinberg School of Medicine, Chicago, Illinois [4, 13]

Jay H. Hoofnagle, MD
Director, Liver Diseases Research Branch, National Institute of Diabetes, Digestive and Kidney Diseases, National Institutes of Health, Bethesda, Maryland [35]

J. Larry Jameson, MD, PhD
Robert G. Dunlop Professor of Medicine; Dean, University of Pennsylvania School of Medicine; Executive Vice President of the University of Pennsylvania for the Health System, Philadelphia, Pennsylvania [10]

Robert T. Jensen, MD
Digestive Diseases Branch, National Institute of Diabetes; Digestive and Kidney Diseases, National Institutes of Health, Bethesda, Maryland [52]

Stuart Johnson, MD
Associate Professor of Medicine, Loyola University Chicago Stritch School of Medicine; Staff Physician, Edward Hines, Jr. VA Hospital, Hines, Illinois [24]

Peter J. Kahrilas, MD
Gilbert H. Marquardt Professor in Medicine, Division of Gastroenterology, Department of Medicine, Northwestern University Feinberg School of Medicine, Chicago, Illinois [4, 13]

Marshall M. Kaplan, MD
Professor of Medicine, Tufts University School of Medicine, Boston, Massachusetts [8, 36]

Dennis L. Kasper, MD, MA (Hon)
William Ellery Channing Professor of Medicine and Professor of Microbiology and Molecular Genetics, Harvard Medical School; Director, Channing Laboratory, Department of Medicine, Brigham and Women's Hospital, Boston, Massachusetts [25]

Alexander Kratz, MD, PhD, MPH
Associate Professor of Pathology and Cell Biology, Columbia University College of Physicians and Surgeons; Director, Core Laboratory, Columbia University Medical Center, New York, New York [Appendix]

Robert F. Kushner, MD, MS
Professor of Medicine, Northwestern University Feinberg School of Medicine, Chicago, Illinois [58]

Loren Laine, MD
Professor of Medicine, University of Southern California Keck School of Medicine, Los Angeles, California [7]

Regina C. LaRocque, MD
Assistant Professor of Medicine, Harvard Medical School; Assistant Physician, Massachusetts General Hospital, Boston, Massachusetts [23]

Mark E. Mailliard, MD
Frederick F. Paustian Professor; Chief, Division of Gastroenterology and Hepatology, Department of Internal Medicine, University of Nebraska College of Medicine, Omaha, Nebraska [41]

Eleftheria Maratos-Flier, MD
Associate Professor of Medicine, Harvard Medical School; Division of Endocrinology, Beth Israel Deaconess Medical Center, Boston, Massachusetts [57]

Robert J. Mayer, MD
Stephen B. Kay Family Professor of Medicine, Harvard Medical School, Boston, Massachusetts [49]

Samuel I. Miller, MD
Professor of Genome Sciences, Medicine, and Microbiology, University of Washington, Seattle, Washington [27]

Joseph A. Murray, MD
Professor of Medicine, Departments of Internal Medicine and Immunology, Mayo Clinic, Rochester, Minnesota [6]

Thomas B. Nutman, MD
Head, Helminth Immunology Section; Head, Clinical Parasitology Unit, Laboratory of Parasitic Diseases, National Institutes of Health, Bethesda, Maryland [34]

Chung Owyang, MD
H. Marvin Pollard Professor of Internal Medicine; Chief, Division of Gastroenterology, University of Michigan Health System, Ann Arbor, Michigan [11, 18]

Umesh D. Parashar, MBBS, MPH
Lead, Viral Gastroenteritis Epidemiology Team, Division of Viral Diseases, National Center for Immunization and Respiratory Diseases, Centers for Disease Control and Prevention, Atlanta, Georgia [31]

Gustav Paumgartner, MD
Professor Emeritus of Medicine, University of Munich, Munich, Germany [45]

David A. Pegues, MD
Hospital Epidemiologist, David Geffen School of Medicine, University of California, Los Angeles, Los Angeles, California [27]

Michael A. Pesce, PhD
Professor Emeritus of Pathology and Cell Biology, Columbia University College of Physicians and Surgeons; Columbia University Medical Center, New York, New York [Appendix]

Daniel S. Pratt, MD
Assistant Professor of Medicine, Harvard Medical School; Massachusetts General Hospital, Boston, Massachusetts [8, 36]

Russell G. Robertson, MD
Vice President for Medical Affairs, Rosalind Franklin University of Medicine and Science; Dean, Chicago Medical School, Chicago, Illinois [10]

Robert M. Russell, MD
Professor Emeritus of Medicine and Nutrition, Tufts University, Boston, Massachusetts; Office of Dietary Supplements, National Institutes of Health, Bethesda, Maryland [54]

Edward T. Ryan, MD, DTM&H
Associate Professor of Medicine, Harvard Medical School; Associate Professor of Immunology and Infectious Diseases, Harvard School of Public Health; Director, Tropical and Geographic Medicine, Massachusetts General Hospital, Boston, Massachusetts [23, 30]

Philippe Sansonetti, MD, MS
Professor, Collège de France; Institut Pasteur, Paris, France [28]

William Silen, MD
Johnson and Johnson Professor Emeritus of Surgery, Harvard Medical School, Auburndale, Massachusetts [1, 21, 22]

Michael F. Sorrell, MD
Robert L. Grissom Professor of Medicine, University of Nebraska Medical Center, Omaha, Nebraska [41]

Samuel L. Stanley, Jr., MD
President, Stony Brook University, Stony Brook, New York [32]

Paolo M. Suter, MD, MS
Professor, Clinic and Policlinic of Internal Medicine, University Hospital, Zurich, Switzerland [54]

Mark Topazian, MD
Professor of Medicine, Mayo Clinic, Rochester, Minnesota [12]

Matthew K. Waldor, MD, PhD
Edward H. Kass Professor of Medicine, Channing Laboratory, Brigham and Women's Hospital; Harvard Medical School and Howard Hughes Medical Institute, Boston, Massachusetts [30]

B. Timothy Walsh, MD
Professor, Department of Psychiatry, College of Physicians and Surgeons, Columbia University; New York State Psychiatric Institute, New York, New York [59]

Peter F. Weller, MD
Chief, Infectious Disease Division; Chief, Allergy and Inflammation Division, Beth Israel Deaconess Medical Center, Boston, Massachusetts [33, 34]

Charles M. Wiener, MD
Dean/CEO Perdana University Graduate School of Medicine, Selangor, Malaysia; Professor of Medicine and Physiology, Johns Hopkins University School of Medicine, Baltimore, Maryland [Review and Self-Assessment]

Allan W. Wolkoff, MD
Professor of Medicine and Anatomy and Structural Biology; Associate Chair of Medicine for Research; Chief, Division of Gastroenterology and Liver Diseases, Albert Einstein College of Medicine and Montefiore Medical Center, Bronx, New York [37]

Louis Michel Wong Kee Song, MD
Associate Professor, Division of Gastroenterology and Hepatology, Mayo Clinic, Rochester, Minnesota [12]

Bechien U. Wu, MD
Instructor of Medicine, Harvard Medical School; Associate Physician, Division of Gastroenterology, Brigham and Women's Hospital, Boston, Massachusetts [48]

Janet A. Yellowitz, DMD, MPH
Associate Professor; Director, Geriatric Dentistry, University of Maryland Dental School, Baltimore, Maryland [3]

PREFACE

Harrison's Principles of Internal Medicine (HPIM) has long been a major source of information related to the principles and practice of medicine for many practitioners and trainees. Yet, in its aim to cover the broad spectrum of medicine, the book has become more than 3000 pages in length and is pushing the envelope of "portability." *HPIM* has spawned several offspring tailored to diverse uses for sources of medical information. The entire book plus a large cache of supplemental visual and textual information are available as *Harrison's Online*, a component of McGraw-Hill's Access Medicine offering. In addition, the 18th edition of *HPIM* is now available on iPad. A condensed version of *HPIM*, called *Harrison's Manual of Medicine,* has been published in print format suitable for carrying in a white coat pocket and in several electronic formats (PDA, Blackberry, iPhone). A companion to *HPIM* that serves as a study guide for standardized tests in medicine, *HPIM Self-Assessment and Board Review*, is an effective teaching tool that highlights important areas of medicine discussed in *HPIM*. All of these products retain the broad spectrum of topics presented in the *HPIM* "mother book" in variable degrees of depth.

In 2006, for the first time, the Editors of *HPIM* experimented with extracting portions of *HPIM* that were focused on a specific subspecialty of internal medicine. The products of that effort, *Harrison's Endocrinology, Harrison's Rheumatology,* and *Harrison's Neurology,* were very well-received by audiences keenly interested in the respective subspecialties of internal medicine. Accordingly, we extended the concept of sectional publication 2009 with the publication of books in other internal medicine subspecialties including *Harrison's Gastroenterology and Hepatology* based on the 17th edition of *HPIM*. These volumes, too, appeared to serve the needs of many readers. Therefore, we are continuing the publication of books with a subspecialty focus.

According to a report from the National Institute of Diabetes and Digestive and Kidney Diseases, for every 100 residents of the United States, there were 35 ambulatory care contacts and 5 overnight hospital stays at which a digestive disease diagnosis was noted. In 2004, digestive diseases accounted for more than 236,000 deaths. Thus, training in the disciplines of gastroenterology and hepatology are essential to any primary care physician or general internist and even to practitioners of other internal medicine subspecialties.

This book is aimed at bringing together the chapters of the current and 18th edition of *HPIM* related to gastroenterology and hepatology in a conveniently sized book for a focused study of this medical subspecialty. The book is organized into 60 chapters and eleven sections: (I) Cardinal Manifestations of Gastrointestinal Disease; (II) Evaluation of the Patient with Alimentary Tract Symptoms; (III) Disorders of the Alimentary Tract; (IV) Infections of the Alimentary Tract; (V) Evaluation of the Patient with Liver Disease; (VI) Disorders of the Liver and Biliary Tree; (VII) Liver Transplantation; (VIII) Disorders of the Pancreas; (IX) Neoplastic Diseases of the Gastrointestinal System; (X) Nutrition; and (XI) Obesity and Eating Disorders.

The information presented here is contributed by physician/authors who have personally made notable advances in the fields of their expertise. The chapters reflect authoritative analyses by individuals who have been active participants in the extraordinary surge of new information on genetics, cell biology, pathophysiology, and treatment that has characterized all of medicine in the last 20 years. In addition to the didactic value of the chapters, a section of test questions, answers, and an explanation of the correct answers is provided to facilitate learning and assist the reader in preparing for standardized examinations.

Gastroenterology and hepatology, like many other areas of medicine, are changing rapidly. Novel technologies of imaging, development of new drugs, and the application of molecular pathogenesis information to detect disease early and prevent disease in people at risk are just a few of the advances that have made an impact on the practice of gastroenterology. Physicians are now applying endoscopic techniques in ways that were once unimaginable including performing operations successfully without an incision; operations that once required major surgery with attendant morbidity and expense. The pace of discovery demands that physicians undertake nearly continuous self-education. It is our hope that this book will help physicians in this process.

We are grateful to Kim Davis and James Shanahan at McGraw-Hill for their help in producing this book.

We thank Chung Owyang, MD, from the University of Michigan, Jay Hoofnagle, MD, from the National Institutes of Health, and Dennis Kasper, MD, from Harvard Medical School, for helpful discussions in shaping the content of this volume.

Dan L. Longo, MD
Anthony S. Fauci, MD

NOTICE

Medicine is an ever-changing science. As new research and clinical experience broaden our knowledge, changes in treatment and drug therapy are required. The authors and the publisher of this work have checked with sources believed to be reliable in their efforts to provide information that is complete and generally in accord with the standards accepted at the time of publication. However, in view of the possibility of human error or changes in medical sciences, neither the authors nor the publisher nor any other party who has been involved in the preparation or publication of this work warrants that the information contained herein is in every respect accurate or complete, and they disclaim all responsibility for any errors or omissions or for the results obtained from use of the information contained in this work. Readers are encouraged to confirm the information contained herein with other sources. For example and in particular, readers are advised to check the product information sheet included in the package of each drug they plan to administer to be certain that the information contained in this work is accurate and that changes have not been made in the recommended dose or in the contraindications for administration. This recommendation is of particular importance in connection with new or infrequently used drugs.

Review and self-assessment questions and answers were taken from Wiener CM, Brown CD, Hemnes AR (eds). *Harrison's Self-Assessment and Board Review,* 18th ed. New York, McGraw-Hill, 2012, ISBN 978-0-07-177195-5.

The global icons call greater attention to key epidemiologic and clinical differences in the practice of medicine throughout the world.

The genetic icons identify a clinical issue with an explicit genetic relationship.

SECTION I

CARDINAL MANIFESTATIONS OF GASTROINTESTINAL DISEASE

CHAPTER 1
ABDOMINAL PAIN

William Silen

The correct interpretation of acute abdominal pain is challenging. Few other clinical situations demand greater judgment, because the most catastrophic of events may be forecast by the subtlest of symptoms and signs. A meticulously executed, detailed history and physical examination are of the greatest importance. The etiologic classification in **Table 1-1**, although not complete, forms a useful basis for the evaluation of patients with abdominal pain.

The diagnosis of "acute or surgical abdomen" is not an acceptable one because of its often misleading and erroneous connotation. The most obvious of "acute abdomens" may not require operative intervention, and the mildest of abdominal pains may herald an urgently correctable lesion. Any patient with abdominal pain of recent onset requires early and thorough evaluation and accurate diagnosis.

SOME MECHANISMS OF PAIN ORIGINATING IN THE ABDOMEN

Inflammation of the parietal peritoneum

The pain of parietal peritoneal inflammation is steady and aching in character and is located directly over the inflamed area, its exact reference being possible because it is transmitted by somatic nerves supplying the parietal peritoneum. The intensity of the pain is dependent on the type and amount of material to which the peritoneal surfaces are exposed in a given time period. For example, the sudden release into the peritoneal cavity of a small quantity of *sterile* acid gastric juice causes much more pain than the same amount of grossly contaminated neutral feces. Enzymatically active pancreatic juice incites more pain and inflammation than does the same amount of sterile bile containing no potent enzymes. Blood and urine are often so bland as to go undetected if their contact with the peritoneum has not been sudden and massive. In the case of bacterial contamination, such as in pelvic inflammatory disease, the pain is frequently of low intensity early in the illness until bacterial multiplication has caused the elaboration of irritating substances.

The rate at which the irritating material is applied to the peritoneum is important. Perforated peptic ulcer may be associated with entirely different clinical pictures dependent only on the rapidity with which the gastric juice enters the peritoneal cavity.

The pain of peritoneal inflammation is invariably accentuated by pressure or changes in tension of the peritoneum, whether produced by palpation or by movement, as in coughing or sneezing. The patient with peritonitis lies quietly in bed, preferring to avoid motion, in contrast to the patient with colic, who may writhe incessantly.

Another characteristic feature of peritoneal irritation is tonic reflex spasm of the abdominal musculature, localized to the involved body segment. The intensity of the tonic muscle spasm accompanying peritoneal inflammation is dependent on the location of the inflammatory process, the rate at which it develops, and the integrity of the nervous system. Spasm over a perforated retrocecal appendix or perforated ulcer into the lesser peritoneal sac may be minimal or absent because of the protective effect of overlying viscera. A slowly developing process often greatly attenuates the degree of muscle spasm. Catastrophic abdominal emergencies such as a perforated ulcer may be associated with minimal or no detectable pain or muscle spasm in obtunded, seriously ill, debilitated elderly patients or in psychotic patients.

Obstruction of hollow viscera

The pain of obstruction of hollow abdominal viscera is classically described as intermittent, or colicky. Yet the lack of a truly cramping character should not be misleading, because distention of a hollow viscus may

TABLE 1-1

SOME IMPORTANT CAUSES OF ABDOMINAL PAIN

Pain Originating in the Abdomen

Parietal peritoneal inflammation	Vascular disturbances
Bacterial contamination	Embolism or thrombosis
Perforated appendix or other perforated viscus	Vascular rupture
Pelvic inflammatory disease	Pressure or torsional occlusion
Chemical irritation	Sickle cell anemia
Perforated ulcer	Abdominal wall
Pancreatitis	Distortion or traction of mesentery
Mittelschmerz	Trauma or infection of muscles
Mechanical obstruction of hollow viscera	Distention of visceral surfaces, e.g., by hemorrhage
Obstruction of the small or large intestine	Hepatic or renal capsules
Obstruction of the biliary tree	Inflammation of a viscus
Obstruction of the ureter	Appendicitis
	Typhoid fever
	Typhlitis

Pain Referred from Extraabdominal Source

Cardiothoracic	Pleurodynia
Acute myocardial infarction	Pneumothorax
Myocarditis, endocarditis, pericarditis	Empyema
Congestive heart failure	Esophageal disease, spasm, rupture, inflammation
Pneumonia	Genitalia
Pulmonary embolus	Torsion of the testis

Metabolic Causes

Diabetes	Acute adrenal insufficiency
Uremia	Familial Mediterranean fever
Hyperlipidemia	Porphyria
Hyperparathyroidism	C′1 esterase inhibitor deficiency (angioneurotic edema)

Neurologic/Psychiatric Causes

Herpes zoster	Spinal cord or nerve root compression
Tabes dorsalis	Functional disorders
Causalgia	Psychiatric disorders
Radiculitis from infection or arthritis	

Toxic Causes

Lead poisoning
Insect or animal envenomations
Black widow spiders
Snake bites

Uncertain Mechanisms

Narcotic withdrawal
Heat stroke

produce steady pain with only very occasional exacerbations. It is not nearly as well localized as the pain of parietal peritoneal inflammation.

The colicky pain of obstruction of the small intestine is usually periumbilical or supraumbilical and is poorly localized. As the intestine becomes progressively dilated with loss of muscular tone, the colicky nature of the pain may diminish. With superimposed strangulating obstruction, pain may spread to the lower lumbar region if there is traction on the root of the mesentery.

The colicky pain of colonic obstruction is of lesser intensity than that of the small intestine and is often located in the infraumbilical area. Lumbar radiation of pain is common in colonic obstruction.

Sudden distention of the biliary tree produces a steady rather than colicky type of pain; hence, the term *biliary colic* is misleading. Acute distention of the gallbladder usually causes pain in the right upper quadrant with radiation to the right posterior region of the thorax or to the tip of the right scapula, but is not uncommonly midline. Distention of the common bile duct is often associated with pain in the epigastrium radiating to the upper part of the lumbar region. Considerable variation is common, however, so that differentiation between these may be impossible. The typical subscapular pain or lumbar radiation is frequently absent. Gradual dilatation of the biliary tree, as in carcinoma of the head of the pancreas, may cause no pain or only a mild aching sensation in the epigastrium or right upper quadrant. The pain of distention of the pancreatic ducts is similar to that described for distention of the common bile duct but, in addition, is very frequently accentuated by recumbency and relieved by the upright position.

Obstruction of the urinary bladder results in dull suprapubic pain, usually low in intensity. Restlessness without specific complaint of pain may be the only sign of a distended bladder in an obtunded patient. In contrast, acute obstruction of the intravesicular portion of the ureter is characterized by severe suprapubic and flank pain that radiates to the penis, scrotum, or inner aspect of the upper thigh. Obstruction of the ureteropelvic junction is felt as pain in the costovertebral angle, whereas obstruction of the remainder of the ureter is associated with flank pain that often extends into the same side of the abdomen.

Vascular disturbances

A frequent misconception, despite abundant experience to the contrary, is that pain associated with intraabdominal vascular disturbances is sudden and catastrophic in nature. The pain of embolism or thrombosis of the superior mesenteric artery or that of impending rupture of an abdominal aortic aneurysm certainly may be severe and diffuse. Yet, just as frequently, the patient with occlusion of the superior mesenteric artery has only mild continuous or cramping diffuse pain for 2 or 3 days before vascular collapse or findings of peritoneal inflammation appear. The early, seemingly insignificant discomfort is caused by hyperperistalsis rather than peritoneal inflammation. Indeed, absence of tenderness and rigidity in the presence of continuous, diffuse pain in a patient likely to have vascular disease is quite characteristic of occlusion of the superior mesenteric artery. Abdominal pain with radiation to the sacral region, flank, or genitalia should always signal the possible presence of a rupturing abdominal aortic aneurysm. This pain may persist over a period of several days before rupture and collapse occur.

Abdominal wall

Pain arising from the abdominal wall is usually constant and aching. Movement, prolonged standing, and pressure accentuate the discomfort and muscle spasm. In the case of hematoma of the rectus sheath, now most frequently encountered in association with anticoagulant therapy, a mass may be present in the lower quadrants of the abdomen. Simultaneous involvement of muscles in other parts of the body usually serves to differentiate myositis of the abdominal wall from an intraabdominal process that might cause pain in the same region.

REFERRED PAIN IN ABDOMINAL DISEASES

Pain referred to the abdomen from the thorax, spine, or genitalia may prove a vexing diagnostic problem, because diseases of the upper part of the abdominal cavity such as acute cholecystitis or perforated ulcer are frequently associated with intrathoracic complications. A most important, yet often forgotten, dictum is that the possibility of intrathoracic disease must be considered in every patient with abdominal pain, especially if the pain is in the upper part of the abdomen. Systematic questioning and examination directed toward detecting myocardial or pulmonary infarction, pneumonia, pericarditis, or esophageal disease (the intrathoracic diseases that most often masquerade as abdominal emergencies) will often provide sufficient clues to establish the proper diagnosis. Diaphragmatic pleuritis resulting from pneumonia or pulmonary infarction may cause pain in the right upper quadrant and pain in the supraclavicular area, the latter radiation to be distinguished from the referred subscapular pain caused by acute distention of the extrahepatic biliary tree. The ultimate decision as to the origin of abdominal pain may require deliberate and planned observation over a period of several hours, during which repeated questioning and examination will provide the diagnosis or suggest the appropriate studies.

Referred pain of thoracic origin is often accompanied by splinting of the involved hemithorax with respiratory lag and decrease in excursion more marked than that seen in the presence of intraabdominal disease. In addition, apparent abdominal muscle spasm caused by referred pain will diminish during the inspiratory phase of respiration, whereas it is persistent throughout both respiratory phases if it is of abdominal origin. Palpation over the area of referred pain in the abdomen also does not usually accentuate the pain and in many instances actually seems to relieve it. Thoracic disease and abdominal disease frequently coexist and may be difficult or impossible to differentiate. For example, the patient with known biliary tract disease often has epigastric pain during myocardial infarction, or biliary colic may be referred to the precordium or left shoulder in a patient who has suffered previously from angina pectoris.

Referred pain from the spine, which usually involves compression or irritation of nerve roots, is characteristically intensified by certain motions such as cough, sneeze, or strain and is associated with hyperesthesia over the involved dermatomes. Pain referred to the abdomen from the testes or seminal vesicles is generally accentuated by the slightest pressure on either of these organs. The abdominal discomfort is of dull, aching character and is poorly localized.

METABOLIC ABDOMINAL CRISES

Pain of metabolic origin may simulate almost any other type of intraabdominal disease. Several mechanisms may be at work. In certain instances, such as hyperlipidemia, the metabolic disease itself may be accompanied by an intraabdominal process such as pancreatitis, which can lead to unnecessary laparotomy unless recognized. C′1 esterase deficiency associated with angioneurotic edema is often associated with episodes of severe abdominal pain. Whenever the cause of abdominal pain is obscure, a metabolic origin always must be considered. Abdominal pain is also the hallmark of familial Mediterranean fever.

The problem of differential diagnosis is often not readily resolved. The pain of porphyria and of lead colic is usually difficult to distinguish from that of intestinal obstruction, because severe hyperperistalsis is a prominent feature of both. The pain of uremia or diabetes is nonspecific, and the pain and tenderness frequently shift in location and intensity. Diabetic acidosis may be precipitated by acute appendicitis or intestinal obstruction, so if prompt resolution of the abdominal pain does not result from correction of the metabolic abnormalities, an underlying organic problem should be suspected. Black widow spider bites produce intense pain and rigidity of the abdominal muscles and back, an area infrequently involved in intraabdominal disease.

NEUROGENIC CAUSES

Causalgic pain may occur in diseases that injure sensory nerves. It has a burning character and is usually limited to the distribution of a given peripheral nerve. Normal stimuli such as touch or change in temperature may be transformed into this type of pain, which is frequently present in a patient at rest. The demonstration of irregularly spaced cutaneous pain spots may be the only indication of an old nerve lesion underlying causalgic pain. Even though the pain may be precipitated by gentle palpation, rigidity of the abdominal muscles is absent, and the respirations are not disturbed. Distention of the abdomen is uncommon, and the pain has no relationship to the intake of food.

Pain arising from spinal nerves or roots comes and goes suddenly and is of a lancinating type. It may be caused by herpes zoster, impingement by arthritis, tumors, herniated nucleus pulposus, diabetes, or syphilis. It is not associated with food intake,

abdominal distention, or changes in respiration. Severe muscle spasm, as in the gastric crises of tabes dorsalis, is common but is either relieved or is not accentuated by abdominal palpation. The pain is made worse by movement of the spine and is usually confined to a few dermatomes. Hyperesthesia is very common.

Pain due to functional causes conforms to none of the aforementioned patterns. Mechanism is hard to define. Irritable bowel syndrome (IBS) is a functional gastrointestinal disorder characterized by abdominal pain and altered bowel habits. The diagnosis is made on the basis of clinical criteria (Chap. 18) and after exclusion of demonstrable structural abnormalities. The episodes of abdominal pain are often brought on by stress, and the pain varies considerably in type and location. Nausea and vomiting are rare. Localized tenderness and muscle spasm are inconsistent or absent. The causes of IBS or related functional disorders are not known.

APPROACH TO THE PATIENT | Abdominal Pain

Few abdominal conditions require such urgent operative intervention that an orderly approach need be abandoned, no matter how ill the patient. Only those patients with exsanguinating intraabdominal hemorrhage (e.g., ruptured aneurysm) must be rushed to the operating room immediately, but in such instances only a few minutes are required to assess the critical nature of the problem. Under these circumstances, all obstacles must be swept aside, adequate venous access for fluid replacement obtained, and the operation begun. Many patients of this type have died in the radiology department or the emergency room while awaiting such unnecessary examinations as electrocardiograms or CT scans. *There are no contraindications to operation when massive intraabdominal hemorrhage is present.* Fortunately, this situation is relatively rare. These comments do not pertain to gastrointestinal hemorrhage, which can often be managed by other means (Chap. 7).

Nothing will supplant an orderly, painstakingly *detailed history*, which is far more valuable than any laboratory or radiographic examination. This kind of history is laborious and time-consuming, making it not especially popular, even though a reasonably accurate diagnosis can be made on the basis of the history alone in the majority of cases. Computer-aided diagnosis of abdominal pain provides no advantage over clinical assessment alone. In cases of *acute* abdominal pain, a diagnosis is readily established in most instances, whereas success is not so frequent in patients with *chronic* pain. IBS is one of the most common causes of abdominal pain and must always be kept in mind (Chap. 18). The location of the pain can assist in narrowing the differential diagnosis (Table 1-2); however,

TABLE 1-2

DIFFERENTIAL DIAGNOSES OF ABDOMINAL PAIN BY LOCATION

Right Upper Quadrant	Epigastric	Left Upper Quadrant
Cholecystitis	Peptic ulcer disease	Splenic infarct
Cholangitis	Gastritis	Splenic rupture
Pancreatitis	GERD	Splenic abscess
Pneumonia/empyema	Pancreatitis	Gastritis
Pleurisy/pleurodynia	Myocardial infarction	Gastric ulcer
Subdiaphragmatic abscess	Pericarditis	Pancreatitis
Hepatitis	Ruptured aortic aneurysm	Subdiaphragmatic abscess
Budd-Chiari syndrome	Esophagitis	

Right Lower Quadrant	Periumbilical	Left Lower Quadrant
Appendicitis	Early appendicitis	Diverticulitis
Salpingitis	Gastroenteritis	Salpingitis
Inguinal hernia	Bowel obstruction	Inguinal hernia
Ectopic pregnancy	Ruptured aortic aneurysm	Ectopic pregnancy
Nephrolithiasis		Nephrolithiasis
Inflammatory bowel disease		Irritable bowel syndrome
Mesenteric lymphadenitis		Inflammatory bowel disease
Typhlitis		

Diffuse Nonlocalized Pain		
Gastroenteritis	Malaria	
Mesenteric ischemia	Familial Mediterranean fever	
Bowel obstruction	Metabolic diseases	
Irritable bowel syndrome	Psychiatric disease	
Peritonitis		
Diabetes		

Abbreviation: GERD, gastroesophageal reflux disease.

the *chronological sequence of events* in the patient's history is often more important than emphasis on the location of pain. If the examiner is sufficiently open-minded and unhurried, asks the proper questions, and listens, the patient will usually provide the diagnosis. Careful attention should be paid to the extraabdominal regions that may be responsible for abdominal pain. An accurate menstrual history in a female patient is essential. Narcotics or analgesics should *not* be withheld until a definitive diagnosis or a definitive plan has been formulated; obfuscation of the diagnosis by adequate analgesia is unlikely.

In the examination, simple critical inspection of the patient, e.g., of facies, position in bed, and respiratory activity, provides valuable clues. The amount of information to be gleaned is directly proportional to the *gentleness* and thoroughness of the examiner. Once a patient with peritoneal inflammation has been examined brusquely, accurate assessment by the next examiner becomes almost impossible. Eliciting rebound tenderness by sudden release of a deeply palpating hand in a patient with suspected peritonitis is cruel and unnecessary. The same information can be obtained by gentle percussion of the abdomen (rebound tenderness on a miniature scale), a maneuver that can be far more precise

and localizing. Asking the patient to cough will elicit true rebound tenderness without the need for placing a hand on the abdomen. Furthermore, the forceful demonstration of rebound tenderness will startle and induce protective spasm in a nervous or worried patient in whom true rebound tenderness is not present. A palpable gall-bladder will be missed if palpation is so brusque that voluntary muscle spasm becomes superimposed on involuntary muscular rigidity.

As with history taking, sufficient time should be spent in the examination. Abdominal signs may be minimal but nevertheless, if accompanied by consistent symptoms, may be exceptionally meaningful. Abdominal signs may be virtually or totally absent in cases of pelvic peritonitis, so careful *pelvic and rectal examinations are mandatory in every patient with abdominal pain*. Tenderness on pelvic or rectal examination in the absence of other abdominal signs can be caused by operative indications such as perforated appendicitis, diverticulitis, twisted ovarian cyst, and many others.

Much attention has been paid to the presence or absence of peristaltic sounds, their quality, and their frequency. Auscultation of the abdomen is one of the least revealing aspects of the physical examination of a patient with abdominal pain. Catastrophes such as strangulating small intestinal obstruction or perforated appendicitis may occur in the presence of normal peristaltic sounds. Conversely, when the proximal part of the intestine above an obstruction becomes markedly distended and edematous, peristaltic sounds may lose the characteristics of borborygmi and become weak or absent, even when peritonitis is not present. It is usually the severe chemical peritonitis of sudden onset that is associated with the truly silent abdomen. Assessment of the patient's state of hydration is important.

Laboratory examinations may be valuable in assessing the patient with abdominal pain, yet, with few exceptions, they rarely establish a diagnosis. Leukocytosis should never be the single deciding factor as to whether or not operation is indicated. A white blood cell count >20,000/μL may be observed with perforation of a viscus, but pancreatitis, acute cholecystitis, pelvic inflammatory disease, and intestinal infarction may be associated with marked leukocytosis. A normal white blood cell count is not rare in cases of perforation of abdominal viscera. The diagnosis of anemia may be more helpful than the white blood cell count, especially when combined with the history.

The urinalysis may reveal the state of hydration or rule out severe renal disease, diabetes, or urinary infection. Blood urea nitrogen, glucose, and serum bilirubin levels may be helpful. Serum amylase levels may be increased by many diseases other than pancreatitis, e.g., perforated ulcer, strangulating intestinal obstruction, and acute cholecystitis; thus, elevations of serum amylase do not rule out the need for an operation. The determination of the serum lipase may have greater accuracy than that of the serum amylase.

Plain and upright or lateral decubitus radiographs of the abdomen may be of value in cases of intestinal obstruction, perforated ulcer, and a variety of other conditions. They are usually unnecessary in patients with acute appendicitis or strangulated external hernias. In rare instances, barium or water-soluble contrast study of the upper part of the gastrointestinal tract may demonstrate partial intestinal obstruction that may elude diagnosis by other means. If there is any question of obstruction of the colon, oral administration of barium sulfate should be avoided. On the other hand, in cases of suspected colonic obstruction (without perforation), contrast enema may be diagnostic.

In the absence of trauma, peritoneal lavage has been replaced as a diagnostic tool by ultrasound, CT, and laparoscopy. Ultrasonography has proved to be useful in detecting an enlarged gallbladder or pancreas, the presence of gallstones, an enlarged ovary, or a tubal pregnancy. Laparoscopy is especially helpful in diagnosing pelvic conditions, such as ovarian cysts, tubal pregnancies, salpingitis, and acute appendicitis. Radioisotopic hepatobiliary iminodiacetic acid scans (HIDAs) may help differentiate acute cholecystitis from acute pancreatitis. A CT scan may demonstrate an enlarged pancreas, ruptured spleen, or thickened colonic or appendiceal wall and streaking of the mesocolon or mesoappendix characteristic of diverticulitis or appendicitis.

Sometimes, even under the best circumstances with all available aids and with the greatest of clinical skill, a definitive diagnosis cannot be established at the time of the initial examination. Nevertheless, despite lack of a clear anatomic diagnosis, it may be abundantly clear to an experienced and thoughtful physician and surgeon that on clinical grounds alone operation is indicated. Should that decision be questionable, watchful waiting with repeated questioning and examination will often elucidate the true nature of the illness and indicate the proper course of action.

CHAPTER 2

ORAL MANIFESTATIONS OF DISEASE

Samuel C. Durso

As primary care physicians and consultants, internists are often asked to evaluate patients with disease of the oral soft tissues, teeth, and pharynx. Knowledge of the oral milieu and its unique structures is necessary to guide preventive services and recognize oral manifestations of local or systemic disease (Chap. 3). Furthermore, internists frequently collaborate with dentists in the care of patients who have a variety of medical conditions that affect oral health or who undergo dental procedures that increase their risk of medical complications.

DISEASES OF THE TEETH AND PERIODONTAL STRUCTURES

TOOTH AND PERIODONTAL STRUCTURE

Tooth formation begins during the sixth week of embryonic life and continues through the first 17 years of age. Tooth development begins in utero and continues until after the tooth erupts. Normally, all 20 deciduous teeth have erupted by age 3 and have been shed by age 13. Permanent teeth, eventually totaling 2, begin to erupt by age 6 and have completely erupted by age 14, though third molars (wisdom teeth) may erupt later.

The erupted tooth consists of the visible crown covered with enamel and the root submerged below the gum line and covered with bonelike cementum. *Dentin*, a material that is denser than bone and exquisitely sensitive to pain, forms the majority of the tooth substance. Dentin surrounds a core of myxomatous *pulp* containing the vascular and nerve supply. The tooth is held firmly in the alveolar socket by the *periodontium*, supporting structures that consist of the gingivae, alveolar bone, cementum, and periodontal ligament. The periodontal ligament tenaciously binds the tooth's cementum to the alveolar bone. Above this ligament is a collar of attached gingiva just below the crown. A few millimeters of unattached or free gingiva (1–3 mm) overlap the base of the crown, forming a shallow sulcus along the gum-tooth margin.

Dental caries, pulpal and periapical disease, and complications

Dental caries begin asymptomatically as a destructive process of the hard surface of the tooth. *Streptococcus mutans*, principally, along with other bacteria colonize the organic buffering film on the tooth surface to produce *plaque*. If not removed by brushing or the natural cleaning action of saliva and oral soft tissues, bacterial acids demineralize the enamel. Fissures and pits on the occlusion surfaces are the most frequent sites of decay. Surfaces adjacent to tooth restorations and exposed roots are also vulnerable, particularly as teeth are retained in an aging population. Over time, dental caries extend to the underlying dentin, leading to cavitation of the enamel and, ultimately, penetration to the tooth pulp, producing *acute pulpitis*. At this early stage, when the pulp infection is limited, the tooth becomes sensitive to percussion and hot or cold, and pain resolves immediately when the irritating stimulus is removed. Should the infection spread throughout the pulp, *irreversible pulpitis* occurs, leading to pulp necrosis. At this late stage, pain is severe and has a sharp or throbbing visceral quality that may be worse when the patient lies down. Once pulp necrosis is complete, pain may be constant or intermittent, but cold sensitivity is lost.

Treatment of caries involves removal of the softened and infected hard tissue; sealing the exposed dentin; and restoration of the tooth structure with silver amalgam, composite resin, gold, or porcelain. Once irreversible pulpitis occurs, root canal therapy is necessary, and the contents of the pulp chamber and root canals are removed, followed by thorough cleaning, antisepsis, and filling with an inert material. Alternatively, the tooth may be extracted.

Pulpal infection, if it does not egress through the decayed enamel, leads to *periapical abscess* formation, which produces pain on chewing. If the infection is mild and chronic, a *periapical granuloma* or eventually a *periapical cyst* forms, either of which produces radiolucency at the root apex. When unchecked, a periapical abscess can erode into the alveolar bone producing osteomyelitis, penetrate and drain through the gingivae (parulis or gumboil), or track along deep fascial planes, producing a virulent cellulitis (Ludwig's angina) involving the submandibular space and floor of the mouth. Elderly patients, those with diabetes mellitus, and patients taking glucocorticoids may experience little or no pain and fever as these complications develop.

Periodontal disease

Periodontal disease accounts for more tooth loss than caries, particularly in the elderly. Like dental caries, chronic infection of the gingiva and anchoring structures of the tooth begins with formation of bacterial plaque. The process begins invisibly above the gum line and in the gingival sulcus. Plaque, including mineralized plaque (calculus), is preventable by appropriate dental hygiene, including periodic professional cleaning. Left undisturbed, chronic inflammation ensues and produces a painless hyperemia of the free and attached gingivae (*gingivitis*) that typically bleeds with brushing. If ignored, severe *periodontitis* occurs, leading to deepening of the physiologic sulcus and destruction of the periodontal ligament. Pockets develop around the teeth and become filled with pus and debris. As the periodontium is destroyed, teeth loosen and exfoliate. Eventually, there is resorption of the alveolar bone. A role for the chronic inflammation resulting from chronic periodontal disease in promoting coronary heart disease and stroke has been proposed. Epidemiologic studies demonstrate a moderate but significant association between chronic periodontal inflammation and atherogenesis, though a causal role remains unproven.

Acute and aggressive forms of periodontal disease are less common than the chronic forms described earlier. However, if the host is stressed or exposed to a new pathogen, rapidly progressive and destructive disease of the periodontal tissue can occur. A virulent example is *acute necrotizing ulcerative gingivitis* (ANUG) or *Vincent's infection*. Stress, poor oral hygiene, and tobacco and alcohol use are risk factors. The presentation includes sudden gingival inflammation, ulceration, bleeding, interdental gingival necrosis, and fetid halitosis. *Localized juvenile periodontitis*, seen in adolescents, is particularly destructive and appears to be associated with impaired neutrophil chemotaxis. *AIDS-related periodontitis* resembles ANUG in some patients or a more destructive form of adult chronic periodontitis in others. It may also produce a gangrene-like destructive process of the oral soft tissues and bone that resembles *noma*, seen in severely malnourished children in developing nations.

Prevention of tooth decay and periodontal infection

Despite the reduced prevalence of dental caries and periodontal disease in the United States due in large part to water fluoridation and improved dental care, respectively, both diseases constitute a major public health problem worldwide and for certain groups. The internist should promote preventive dental care and hygiene as part of health maintenance. Special populations at high risk for dental caries and periodontal disease include those with xerostomia, diabetics, alcoholics, tobacco users, those with Down's syndrome, and those with gingival hyperplasia. Furthermore, patients lacking dental-care access (low socioeconomic status) and those with reduced ability to provide self-care (e.g., nursing home residents and those with dementia or upper-extremity disability) suffer at a disproportionate rate. It is important to provide counseling regarding regular dental hygiene and professional cleaning, use of fluoride-containing toothpaste, professional fluoride treatments, and use of electric toothbrushes for patients with limited dexterity and to give instruction to caregivers for those unable to perform self-care. Internists caring for international students studying in the United States should be aware of the high prevalence of dental decay in this population. Cost, fear of dental care, and language and cultural differences may create barriers that prevent some from seeking preventive dental services.

Developmental and systemic disease affecting the teeth and periodontium

Malocclusion is the most common developmental problem, which, in addition to a problem with cosmesis, can interfere with mastication unless corrected through orthodontic techniques. Impacted third molars are common and occasionally become infected. Acquired prognathism due to *acromegaly* may also lead to malocclusion, as may deformity of the maxilla and mandible due to *Paget's disease* of the bone. Delayed tooth eruption, receding chin, and a protruding tongue are occasional features of *cretinism* and *hypopituitarism*. Congenital syphilis produces tapering, notched (Hutchinson's) incisors and finely nodular (mulberry) molar crowns.

Enamel hypoplasia results in crown defects ranging from pits to deep fissures of primary or permanent teeth. Intrauterine infection (syphilis, rubella), vitamin deficiency (A, C, or D), disorders of calcium metabolism (malabsorption, vitamin D–resistant rickets, hypoparathyroidism), prematurity, high fever, or rare inherited defects (*amelogenesis imperfecta*) are all causes. Tetracycline, given in sufficiently high doses during the first 8 years, may produce enamel hypoplasia and discoloration. Exposure to endogenous pigments can discolor developing teeth: *erythroblastosis fetalis* (green or bluish-black), congenital liver disease (green or yellow-brown), and porphyria (red or brown that fluoresces with ultraviolet light). *Mottled enamel* occurs if excessive fluoride is ingested during development. Worn enamel is seen with age, bruxism, or excessive acid exposure (e.g., chronic gastric reflux or bulimia).

Premature tooth loss resulting from periodontitis is seen with cyclic neutropenia, Papillon-Lefèvre syndrome, Chédiak-Higashi syndrome, and leukemia. Rapid focal tooth loosening is most often due to infection, but rarer causes include Langerhans cell histiocytosis, Ewing's sarcoma, osteosarcoma, or Burkitt's lymphoma. Early loss of primary teeth is a feature of *hypophosphatasia*, a rare inborn error of metabolism.

Pregnancy may produce severe gingivitis and localized *pyogenic granulomas*. Severe periodontal disease occurs with Down's syndrome and diabetes mellitus. *Gingival hyperplasia* may be caused by phenytoin, calcium channel blockers (e.g., nifedipine), and cyclosporine. *Idiopathic familial gingival fibromatosis* and several syndrome-related disorders appear similar. Removal of the medication often reverses the drug-induced form, though surgery may be needed to control both. *Linear gingival erythema* is variably seen in patients with advanced HIV infection and probably represents immune deficiency and decreased neutrophil activity. Diffuse or focal gingival swelling may be a feature of early or late acute myelomonocytic leukemia (AMML) as well as of other lymphoproliferative disorders. A rare, but pathognomonic, sign of Wegener's granulomatosis is a red-purplish, granular gingivitis (strawberry gums).

DISEASES OF THE ORAL MUCOSA

Infection

Most oral mucosal diseases involve microorganisms (Table 2-1).

Pigmented lesions

See Table 2-2.

Dermatologic diseases

See Tables 2-1, 2-2, and 2-3.

Diseases of the tongue

See Table 2-4.

HIV disease and AIDS

See Tables 2-1, 2-2, 2-3, and 2-5.

Ulcers

Ulceration is the most common oral mucosal lesion. Although there are many causes, the host and pattern of lesions, including the presence of systemic features, narrow the differential diagnosis (Table 2-1). Most acute ulcers are painful and self-limited. Recurrent aphthous ulcers and herpes simplex infection constitute the majority. Persistent and deep aphthous ulcers can be idiopathic or seen with HIV/AIDS. Aphthous lesions are often the presenting symptom in *Behçet's syndrome*. Similar-appearing, though less painful, lesions may occur with reactive arthritis (formerly known as Reiter's syndrome), and aphthous ulcers are occasionally present during phases of discoid or *systemic lupus erythematosus*. Aphthous-like ulcers are seen in Crohn's disease (Chap. 17), but unlike the common aphthous variety, they may exhibit granulomatous inflammation histologically. Recurrent aphthae in some patients with *celiac disease* have been reported to remit with elimination of gluten.

Of major concern are chronic, relatively painless ulcers and mixed red/white patches (erythroplakia and leukoplakia) of more than 2 weeks' duration. Squamous cell carcinoma and premalignant dysplasia should be considered early and a diagnostic biopsy obtained. The importance is underscored because early-stage malignancy is vastly more treatable than late-stage disease. High-risk sites include the lower lip, floor of the mouth, ventral and lateral tongue, and soft palate–tonsillar pillar complex. Significant risk factors for oral cancer in Western countries include sun exposure (lower lip) and tobacco and alcohol use. In India and some other Asian countries, smokeless tobacco mixed with betel nut, slaked lime, and spices is a common cause of oral cancer. Less common etiologies include syphilis and Plummer-Vinson syndrome (iron deficiency).

Rarer causes of chronic oral ulcer such as tuberculosis, fungal infection, granulomatosis with polyangiitis (Wegener's), and midline granuloma may look identical to carcinoma. Making the correct diagnosis depends on recognizing other clinical features and biopsy of the lesion. The syphilitic chancre is typically painless and therefore easily missed. Regional lymphadenopathy is invariably present. Confirmation is achieved using appropriate bacterial and serologic tests.

Disorders of mucosal fragility often produce painful oral ulcers that fail to heal within 2 weeks. *Mucous membrane pemphigoid* and *pemphigus vulgaris* are the major acquired disorders. While clinical features are often distinctive, immunohistochemical examination should be

TABLE 2-1

VESICULAR, BULLOUS, OR ULCERATIVE LESIONS OF THE ORAL MUCOSA

CONDITION	USUAL LOCATION	CLINICAL FEATURES	COURSE
Viral Diseases			
Primary acute herpetic gingivostomatitis [herpes simplex virus (HSV) type 1, rarely type 2]	Lip and oral mucosa (buccal, gingival, lingual mucosa)	Labial vesicles that rupture and crust, and intraoral vesicles that quickly ulcerate; extremely painful; acute gingivitis, fever, malaise, foul odor, and cervical lymphadenopathy; occurs primarily in infants, children, and young adults	Heals spontaneously in 10–14 days. Unless secondarily infected, lesions lasting >3 weeks are not due to primary HSV infection
Recurrent herpes labialis	Mucocutaneous junction of lip, perioral skin	Eruption of groups of vesicles that may coalesce, then rupture and crust; painful to pressure or spicy foods	Lasts about 1 week, but condition may be prolonged if secondarily infected. If severe, topical or oral antiviral may reduce healing time
Recurrent intraoral herpes simplex	Palate and gingiva	Small vesicles on keratinized epithelium that rupture and coalesce; painful	Heals spontaneously in about 1 week. If severe, topical or oral antiviral may reduce healing time.
Chickenpox (varicella-zoster virus)	Gingiva and oral mucosa	Skin lesions may be accompanied by small vesicles on oral mucosa that rupture to form shallow ulcers; may coalesce to form large bullous lesions that ulcerate; mucosa may have generalized erythema	Lesions heal spontaneously within 2 weeks
Herpes zoster (reactivation of varicella-zoster virus)	Cheek, tongue, gingiva, or palate	Unilateral vesicular eruptions and ulceration in linear pattern following sensory distribution of trigeminal nerve or one of its branches	Gradual healing without scarring unless secondarily infected; postherpetic neuralgia is common. Oral acyclovir, famciclovir, or valacyclovir reduce healing time and postherpetic neuralgia
Infectious mononucleosis (Epstein-Barr virus)	Oral mucosa	Fatigue, sore throat, malaise, fever, and cervical lymphadenopathy; numerous small ulcers usually appear several days before lymphadenopathy; gingival bleeding and multiple petechiae at junction of hard and soft palates	Oral lesions disappear during convalescence; no treatment though glucocorticoids indicated if tonsillar swelling compromises airway
Herpangina (coxsackievirus A; also possibly coxsackie B and echovirus)	Oral mucosa, pharynx, tongue	Sudden onset of fever, sore throat, and oropharyngeal vesicles, usually in children under 4 years, during summer months; diffuse pharyngeal congestion and vesicles (1–2 mm), grayish-white surrounded by red areola; vesicles enlarge and ulcerate	Incubation period 2–9 days; fever for 1–4 days; recovery uneventful
Hand, foot, and mouth disease (coxsackievirus A16 most common)	Oral mucosa, pharynx, palms, and soles	Fever, malaise, headache with oropharyngeal vesicles that become painful, shallow ulcers; highly infectious; usually affects children under age 10	Incubation period 2–18 days; lesions heal spontaneously in 2–4 weeks
Primary HIV infection	Gingiva, palate, and pharynx	Acute gingivitis and oropharyngeal ulceration, associated with febrile illness resembling mononucleosis and including lymphadenopathy	Followed by HIV seroconversion, asymptomatic HIV infection, and usually ultimately by HIV disease

(continued)

TABLE 2-1

VESICULAR, BULLOUS, OR ULCERATIVE LESIONS OF THE ORAL MUCOSA (*CONTINUED*)

CONDITION	USUAL LOCATION	CLINICAL FEATURES	COURSE
Bacterial or Fungal Diseases			
Acute necrotizing ulcerative gingivitis ("trench mouth," Vincent's infection)	Gingiva	Painful, bleeding gingiva character-ized by necrosis and ulceration of gingival papillae and margins plus lymphadenopathy and foul odor	Debridement and diluted (1:3) peroxide lavage provide relief within 24 h; antibiotics in acutely ill patients; relapse may occur
Prenatal (congenital) syphilis	Palate, jaws, tongue, and teeth	Gummatous involvement of palate, jaws, and facial bones; Hutchinson's incisors, mulberry molars, glossitis, mucous patches, and fissures on corner of mouth	Tooth deformities in perma-nent dentition irreversible
Primary syphilis (chancre)	Lesion appears where organism enters body; may occur on lips, tongue, or tonsillar area	Small papule developing rapidly into a large, painless ulcer with indurated border; unilateral lymph-adenopathy; chancre and lymph nodes containing spirochetes; serologic tests positive by third to fourth weeks	Healing of chancre in 1–2 months, followed by secondary syphilis in 6–8 weeks
Secondary syphilis	Oral mucosa frequently involved with mucous patches, primarily on palate, also at com-missures of mouth	Maculopapular lesions of oral mucosa, 5–10 mm in diameter with central ulceration covered by grayish membrane; eruptions occurring on various mucosal surfaces and skin accompanied by fever, malaise, and sore throat	Lesions may persist from sev-eral weeks to a year
Tertiary syphilis	Palate and tongue	Gummatous infiltration of palate or tongue followed by ulceration and fibrosis; atrophy of tongue papil-lae produces characteristic bald tongue and glossitis	Gumma may destroy palate, causing complete perforation
Gonorrhea	Lesions may occur in mouth at site of inocu-lation or secondarily by hematogenous spread from a primary focus elsewhere	Most pharyngeal infection is asymp-tomatic; may produce burning or itching sensation; oropharynx and tonsils may be ulcerated and ery-thematous; saliva viscous and fetid	More difficult to eradicate than urogenital infection, though pharyngitis usually resolves with appropriate antimicrobial treatment
Tuberculosis	Tongue, tonsillar area, soft palate	A painless, solitary, 1–5 cm, irregu-lar ulcer covered with a persistent exudate; ulcer has a firm under-mined border	Autoinoculation from pulmo-nary infection usual; lesions resolve with appropriate antimicrobial therapy
Cervicofacial actinomycosis	Swellings in region of face, neck, and floor of mouth	Infection may be associated with an extraction, jaw fracture, or eruption of molar tooth; in acute form resembles an acute pyogenic abscess, but contains yellow "sulfur granules" (gram-positive mycelia and their hyphae)	Typically, swelling is hard and grows painlessly; multiple abscesses with draining tracts develop; penicillin first choice; surgery usually necessary
Histoplasmosis	Any area of the mouth, particularly tongue, gingiva, or palate	Nodular, verrucous, or granuloma-tous lesions; ulcers are indurated and painful; usual source hema-togenous or pulmonary, but may be primary	Systemic antifungal therapy necessary to treat
Candidiasis (Table 2-3)			

(continued)

TABLE 2-1

13

CHAPTER 2 Oral Manifestations of Disease

VESICULAR, BULLOUS, OR ULCERATIVE LESIONS OF THE ORAL MUCOSA (CONTINUED)

CONDITION	USUAL LOCATION	CLINICAL FEATURES	COURSE
Dermatologic Diseases			
Mucous membrane pemphigoid	Typically produces marked gingival erythema and ulceration; other areas of oral cavity, esophagus, and vagina may be affected	Painful, grayish-white collapsed vesicles or bullae of full-thickness epithelium with peripheral erythematous zone; gingival lesions desquamate, leaving ulcerated area	Protracted course with remissions and exacerbations; involvement of different sites occurs slowly; glucocorticoids may temporarily reduce symptoms but do not control the disease
Erythema multiforme (EM) minor and major (Stevens Johnson syndrome)	Primarily the oral mucosa and the skin of hands and feet	Intraoral ruptured bullae surrounded by an inflammatory area; lips may show hemorrhagic crusts; the "iris," or "target," lesion on the skin is pathognomonic; patient may have severe signs of toxicity	Onset very rapid; usually idiopathic, but may be associated with trigger such as drug reaction; condition may last 3–6 weeks; mortality with EM major 5–15% if untreated
Pemphigus vulgaris	Oral mucosa and skin; sites of mechanical trauma (soft/hard palate, frenulum, lips, buccal mucosa)	Usually (>70%) presents with oral lesions; fragile, ruptured bullae and ulcerated oral areas; mostly in older adults	With repeated occurrence of bullae, toxicity may lead to cachexia, infection, and death within 2 years; often controllable with oral glucocorticoids
Lichen planus	Oral mucosa and skin	White striae in mouth; purplish nodules on skin at sites of friction; occasionally causes oral mucosal ulcers and erosive gingivitis	White striae alone usually asymptomatic; erosive lesions often difficult to treat, but may respond to glucocorticoids
Other Conditions			
Recurrent aphthous ulcers	Usually on nonkeratinized oral mucosa (buccal and labial mucosa, floor of mouth, soft palate, lateral and ventral tongue)	Single or clusters of painful ulcers with surrounding erythematous border; lesions may be 1–2 mm in diameter in crops (herpetiform), 1–5 mm (minor), or 5–15 mm (major)	Lesions heal in 1–2 weeks but may recur monthly or several times a year; protective barrier with orabase and topical steroids give symptomatic relief; systemic glucocorticoids may be needed in severe cases
Behçet's syndrome	Oral mucosa, eyes, genitalia, gut, and CNS	Multiple aphthous ulcers in mouth; inflammatory ocular changes, ulcerative lesions on genitalia; inflammatory bowel disease and CNS disease	Oral lesions often first manifestation; persist several weeks and heal without scarring
Traumatic ulcers	Anywhere on oral mucosa; dentures frequently responsible for ulcers in vestibule	Localized, discrete ulcerated lesions with red border; produced by accidental biting of mucosa, penetration by a foreign object, or chronic irritation by a denture	Lesions usually heal in 7–10 days when irritant is removed, unless secondarily infected
Squamous cell carcinoma	Any area in the mouth, most commonly on lower lip, tongue, and floor of mouth	Ulcer with elevated, indurated border; failure to heal, pain not prominent; lesions tend to arise in areas of erythro/leukoplakia or in smooth atrophic tongue	Invades and destroys underlying tissues; frequently metastasizes to regional lymph nodes

(continued)

TABLE 2-1

VESICULAR, BULLOUS, OR ULCERATIVE LESIONS OF THE ORAL MUCOSA (*CONTINUED*)

CONDITION	USUAL LOCATION	CLINICAL FEATURES	COURSE
Acute myeloid leukemia (usually monocytic)	Gingiva	Gingival swelling and superficial ulceration followed by hyperplasia of gingiva with extensive necrosis and hemorrhage; deep ulcers may occur elsewhere on the mucosa complicated by secondary infection	Usually responds to systemic treatment of leukemia; occasionally requires local radiation therapy
Lymphoma	Gingiva, tongue, palate and tonsillar area	Elevated, ulcerated area that may proliferate rapidly, giving the appearance of traumatic inflammation	Fatal if untreated; may indicate underlying HIV infection
Chemical or thermal burns	Any area in mouth	White slough due to contact with corrosive agents (e.g., aspirin, hot cheese) applied locally; removal of slough leaves raw, painful surface	Lesion heals in several weeks if not secondarily infected

Abbreviation: CNS, central nervous system.

TABLE 2-2

PIGMENTED LESIONS OF THE ORAL MUCOSA

CONDITION	USUAL LOCATION	CLINICAL FEATURES	COURSE
Oral melanotic macule	Any area of the mouth	Discrete or diffuse localized, brown to black macule	Remains indefinitely; no growth
Diffuse melanin pigmentation	Any area of the mouth	Diffuse pale to dark-brown pigmentation; may be physiologic ("racial") or due to smoking	Remains indefinitely
Nevi	Any area of the mouth	Discrete, localized, brown to black pigmentation	Remains indefinitely
Malignant melanoma	Any area of the mouth	Can be flat and diffuse, painless, brown to black, or can be raised and nodular	Expands and invades early; metastasis leads to death
Addison's disease	Any area of the mouth, but mostly buccal mucosa	Blotches or spots of bluish-black to dark-brown pigmentation occurring early in the disease, accompanied by diffuse pigmentation of skin; other symptoms of adrenal insufficiency	Condition controlled by adrenal steroid replacement
Peutz-Jeghers syndrome	Any area of the mouth	Dark-brown spots on lips, buccal mucosa, with characteristic distribution of pigment around lips, nose, eyes, and on hands; concomitant intestinal polyposis	Oral pigmented lesions remain indefinitely; gastrointestinal polyps may become malignant
Drug ingestion (neuroleptics, oral contraceptives, minocycline, zidovudine, quinine derivatives)	Any area of the mouth	Brown, black, or gray areas of pigmentation	Gradually disappears following cessation of drug
Amalgam tattoo	Gingiva and alveolar mucosa	Small blue-black pigmented areas associated with embedded amalgam particles in soft tissues; these may show up on radiographs as radiopaque particles in some cases	Remains indefinitely

(continued)

TABLE 2-2

PIGMENTED LESIONS OF THE ORAL MUCOSA (*CONTINUED*)

CONDITION	USUAL LOCATION	CLINICAL FEATURES	COURSE
Heavy metal pigmentation (bismuth, mercury, lead)	Gingival margin	Thin blue-black pigmented line along gingival margin; rarely seen except for children exposed to lead-based paint	Indicative of systemic absorption; no significance for oral health
Black hairy tongue	Dorsum of tongue	Elongation of filiform papillae of tongue, which become stained by coffee, tea, tobacco, or pigmented bacteria	Improves within 1–2 weeks with gentle brushing of tongue or discontinuation of antibiotic if due to bacterial overgrowth
Fordyce "spots"	Buccal and labial mucosa	Numerous small yellowish spots just beneath mucosal surface; no symptoms; due to hyperplasia of sebaceous glands	Benign; remains without apparent change
Kaposi's sarcoma	Palate most common, but may occur in any other site	Red or blue plaques of variable size and shape; often enlarge, become nodular and may ulcerate	Usually indicative of HIV infection or non-Hodgkin's lymphoma; rarely fatal, but may require treatment for comfort or cosmesis
Mucous retention cysts	Buccal and labial mucosa	Bluish-clear fluid-filled cyst due to extravasated mucous from injured minor salivary gland	Benign; painless unless traumatized; may be removed surgically

TABLE 2-3

WHITE LESIONS OF ORAL MUCOSA

CONDITION	USUAL LOCATION	CLINICAL FEATURES	COURSE
Lichen planus	Buccal mucosa, tongue, gingiva, and lips; skin	Striae, white plaques, red areas, ulcers in mouth; purplish papules on skin; may be asymptomatic, sore, or painful; lichenoid drug reactions may look similar	Protracted; responds to topical glucocorticoids
White sponge nevus	Oral mucosa, vagina, anal mucosa	Painless white thickening of epithelium; adolescent/early adult onset; familial	Benign and permanent
Smoker's leukoplakia and smokeless tobacco lesions	Any area of oral mucosa, sometimes related to location of habit	White patch that may become firm, rough, or red-fissured and ulcerated; may become sore and painful but usually painless	May or may not resolve with cessation of habit; 2% develop squamous cell carcinoma; early biopsy essential
Erythroplakia with or without white patches	Floor of mouth common in men; tongue and buccal mucosa in women	Velvety, reddish plaque; occasionally mixed with white patches or smooth red areas	High risk of squamous cell cancer; early biopsy essential
Candidiasis	Any area in mouth	*Pseudomembranous type* ("thrush"): creamy white curdlike patches that reveal a raw, bleeding surface when scraped; found in sick infants, debilitated elderly patients receiving high doses of glucocorticoids or broad-spectrum antibiotics, or in patients with AIDS	Responds favorably to antifungal therapy and correction of predisposing causes where possible

(continued)

TABLE 2-3

WHITE LESIONS OF ORAL MUCOSA (*CONTINUED*)			
CONDITION	USUAL LOCATION	CLINICAL FEATURES	COURSE
		Erythematous type: flat, red, sometimes sore areas in same groups of patients	Course same as for pseudo-membranous type
		Candidal leukoplakia: nonremovable white thickening of epithelium due to *Candida*	Responds to prolonged antifungal therapy
		Angular cheilitis: sore fissures at corner of mouth	Responds to topical antifungal therapy
Hairy leukoplakia	Usually lateral tongue, rarely elsewhere on oral mucosa	White areas ranging from small and flat to extensive accentuation of vertical folds; found in HIV carriers in all risk groups for AIDS	Due to EBV; responds to high-dose acyclovir but recurs; rarely causes discomfort unless secondarily infected with *Candida*
Warts (papillomavirus)	Anywhere on skin and oral mucosa	Single or multiple papillary lesions, with thick, white keratinized surfaces containing many pointed projections; cauliflower lesions covered with normal-colored mucosa or multiple pink or pale bumps (focal epithelial hyperplasia)	Lesions grow rapidly and spread; consider squamous cell carcinoma and rule out with biopsy; excision or laser therapy; may regress in HIV-infected patients on anti-retroviral therapy

Abbreviation: EBV, Epstein-Barr virus.

TABLE 2-4

ALTERATIONS OF THE TONGUE	
TYPE OF CHANGE	CLINICAL FEATURES
Size or Morphology Changes	
Macroglossia	Enlarged tongue that may be part of a syndrome found in developmental conditions such as Down's syndrome, Simpson-Golabi-Behmel syndrome, or Beckwith-Wiedemann syndrome may be due to tumor (hemangioma or lymphangioma), metabolic disease (such as primary amyloidosis), or endocrine disturbance (such as acromegaly or cretinism)
Fissured ("scrotal") tongue	Dorsal surface and sides of tongue covered by painless shallow or deep fissures that may collect debris and become irritated
Median rhomboid glossitis	Congenital abnormality of tongue with ovoid, denuded area in median posterior portion of the tongue; may be associated with candidiasis and may respond to antifungals
Color Changes	
"Geographic" tongue (benign migratory glossitis)	Asymptomatic inflammatory condition of the tongue, with rapid loss and regrowth of filiform papillae, leading to appearance of denuded red patches "wandering" across the surface of the tongue
Hairy tongue	Elongation of filiform papillae of the medial dorsal surface area due to failure of keratin layer of the papillae to desquamate normally; brownish-black coloration may be due to staining by tobacco, food, or chromogenic organisms
"Strawberry" and "raspberry" tongue	Appearance of tongue during scarlet fever due to the hypertrophy of fungiform papillae plus changes in the filiform papillae
"Bald" tongue	Atrophy may be associated with xerostomia, pernicious anemia, iron-deficiency anemia, pellagra, or syphilis; may be accompanied by painful burning sensation; may be an expression of erythematous candidiasis and respond to antifungals

TABLE 2-5

ORAL LESIONS ASSOCIATED WITH HIV INFECTION

LESION MORPHOLOGY	ETIOLOGIES
Papules, nodules, plaques	Candidiasis (hyperplastic and pseudomembranous)[a] Condyloma acuminatum (human papillomavirus infection) Squamous cell carcinoma (preinvasive and invasive) Non-Hodgkin's lymphoma[a] Hairy leukoplakia[a]
Ulcers	Recurrent aphthous ulcers[a] Angular cheilitis Squamous cell carcinoma Acute necrotizing ulcerative gingivitis[a] Necrotizing ulcerative periodontitis[a] Necrotizing ulcerative stomatitis Non-Hodgkin's lymphoma[a] Viral infection (herpes simplex, herpes zoster, cytomegalovirus) *Mycobacterium tuberculosis, Mycobacterium avium-intracellulare* Fungal infection (histoplasmosis, cryptococcosis, candidiasis, geotrichosis, aspergillosis) Bacterial infection (*Escherichia coli, Enterobacter cloacae, Klebsiella pneumoniae, Pseudomonas aeruginosa*) Drug reactions (single or multiple ulcers)
Pigmented lesions	Kaposi's sarcoma[a] Bacillary angiomatosis (skin and visceral lesions more common than oral) Zidovudine pigmentation (skin, nails, and occasionally oral mucosa) Addison's disease
Miscellaneous	Linear gingival erythema[a]

[a]Strongly associated with HIV infection.

performed for diagnosis and to distinguish these entities from *lichen planus* and drug reactions.

Hematologic and nutritional disease

Internists are more likely to encounter patients with acquired, rather than congenital, bleeding disorders. Bleeding after minor trauma should stop after 15 min and within an hour of tooth extraction if local pressure is applied. More prolonged bleeding, if not due to continued injury or rupture of a large vessel, should lead to investigation for a clotting abnormality. In addition to bleeding, petechiae and ecchymoses are prone to occur at the line of vibration between the soft and hard palates in patients with platelet dysfunction or thrombocytopenia.

All forms of leukemia, but particularly acute myelomonocyticleukemia, can produce gingival bleeding, ulcers, and gingival enlargement. Oral ulcers are a feature of agranulocytosis, and ulcers and mucositis are often severe complications of chemotherapy and radiation therapy for hematologic and other malignancies. Plummer-Vinson syndrome (iron deficiency, angular stomatitis, glossitis, and dysphagia) raises the risk of oral squamous cell cancer and esophageal cancer at the postcricoidal tissue web. Atrophic papillae and a red,

burning tongue may occur with pernicious anemia. B-group vitamin deficiencies produce many of these same symptoms as well as oral ulceration and cheilosis. Swollen, bleeding gums, ulcers, and loosening of the teeth are a consequence of scurvy.

NONDENTAL CAUSES OF ORAL PAIN

Most, but not all, oral pain emanates from inflamed or injured tooth pulp or periodontal tissues. Nonodontogenic causes may be overlooked. In most instances, toothache is predictable and proportional to the stimulus applied, and an identifiable condition (e.g., caries, abscess) is found. Local anesthesia eliminates pain originating from dental or periodontal structures, but not referred pains. The most common nondental origin is myofascial pain referred from muscles of mastication, which become tender and ache with increased use. Many sufferers exhibit bruxism (the grinding of teeth, often during sleep) that is secondary to stress and anxiety. *Temporomandibular disorder* is closely related. It affects both sexes with a higher prevalence in women. Features include pain, limited mandibular movement, and temporomandibular joint sounds. The etiologies are complex, and malocclusion does not play the primary role once attributed to it. *Osteoarthritis* is a common cause of masticatory pain. Anti-inflammatory medication, jaw rest, soft foods, and heat provide relief. The temporomandibular joint is involved in 50% of patients with *rheumatoid arthritis* and is usually a late feature of severe disease. Bilateral preauricular pain, particularly in the morning, limits range of motion.

Migrainous neuralgia may be localized to the mouth. Episodes of pain and remission without identifiable cause and absence of relief with local anesthesia are important clues. *Trigeminal neuralgia* (*tic douloureux*) may involve the entire branch or part of the mandibular or maxillary branches of the fifth cranial nerve and produce pain in one or a few teeth. Pain may occur spontaneously or may be triggered by touching the lip or gingiva, brushing the teeth, or chewing. *Glossopharyngeal neuralgia* produces similar acute neuropathic symptoms in the distribution of the ninth cranial nerve. Swallowing, sneezing, coughing, or pressure on the tragus of the ear triggers pain that is felt in the base of the tongue, pharynx, and soft palate and may be referred to the temporomandibular joint. *Neuritis* involving the maxillary and mandibular divisions of the trigeminal nerve (e.g., maxillary sinusitis, neuroma, and leukemic infiltrate) is distinguished from ordinary toothache by the neuropathic quality of the pain. Occasionally, *phantom pain* follows tooth extraction. Often the earliest symptom of Bell's palsy in the day or so before facial weakness develops is pain and hyperalgesia behind the ear and side of the face. Likewise, similar symptoms may precede visible lesions of herpes zoster infecting the seventh nerve (Ramsey-Hunt syndrome) or trigeminal nerve. *Postherpetic neuralgia* may follow either condition. *Coronary ischemia* may produce pain exclusively in the face and jaw and, like typical angina pectoris, is usually reproducible with increased myocardial demand. Aching in several upper molar or premolar teeth that is unrelieved by anesthetizing the teeth may point to *maxillary sinusitis*.

Giant cell arteritis is notorious for producing headache, but it may also produce facial pain or sore throat without headache. Jaw and tongue claudication with chewing or talking is relatively common. Tongue infarction is rare. Patients with subacute thyroiditis often experience pain referred to the face or jaw before the tender thyroid gland and transient hyperthyroidism are appreciated.

Burning mouth syndrome (glossodynia) is present in the absence of an identifiable cause (e.g., vitamin B_{12} deficiency, iron deficiency, diabetes mellitus, low-grade *Candida* infection, food sensitivity, or subtle xerostomia) and predominantly affects postmenopausal women. The etiology may be neuropathic. Clonazepam, alpha-lipoic acid, and cognitive behavioral therapy have benefited

some. Some cases associated with ACE inhibitors have remitted when the drug was discontinued.

DISEASES OF THE SALIVARY GLANDS

Saliva is essential to oral health. Its absence leads to tooth decay and loss. Its major components, water and mucin, serve as a cleansing solvent and lubricating fluid. In addition, it contains antimicrobial factors (e.g., lysozyme, lactoperoxidase, secretory IgA), epidermal growth factor, minerals, and buffering systems. The major salivary glands secrete intermittently in response to autonomic stimulation, which is high during a meal but low otherwise. Hundreds of minor glands in the lips and cheeks secrete mucus continuously. Consequently, oral function becomes impaired when salivary function is reduced. Dry mouth (xerostomia) is perceived when salivary flow is reduced by 50%. The most common etiology is medication, especially drugs with anticholinergic properties, but also alpha and beta blockers, calcium channel blockers, and diuretics. Other causes include Sjögren's syndrome, chronic parotitis, salivary duct obstruction, diabetes mellitus, HIV/AIDS, and radiation therapy that includes the salivary glands in the field (Hodgkin's disease and head and neck cancer). Management involves eliminating or limiting drying medications, preventive dental care, and supplementing oral liquid. Sugarless mints or chewing gum may stimulate salivary secretion if dysfunction is mild. When sufficient exocrine tissue remains, pilocarpine or cevimeline has been shown to increase secretions. Commercial saliva substitutes or gels relieve dryness but must be supplemented with fluoride applications to prevent caries.

Sialolithiasis presents most often as painful swelling but in some instances as just swelling or pain. Conservative therapy consists of local heat, massage, and hydration. Promotion of salivary secretion with mints or lemon drops may flush out small stones. Antibiotic treatment is necessary when bacterial infection in suspected. In adults, *acute bacterial parotitis* is typically unilateral and most commonly affects postoperative, dehydrated, and debilitated patients. *Staphylococcus aureus* including methicillin-resistant forms and anaerobic bacteria are the most common pathogens. Chronic bacterial sialadenitis results from lowered salivary secretion and recurrent bacterial infection. When suspected bacterial infection is not responsive to therapy, the differential diagnosis should be expanded to include benign and malignant neoplasms, lymphoproliferative disorders, Sjögren's syndrome, sarcoidosis, tuberculosis, lymphadenitis, actinomycosis, and granulomatosis with polyangiitis (Wegener's). Bilateral nontender parotid enlargement occurs with diabetes mellitus, cirrhosis, bulimia, HIV/AIDS, and drugs (e.g., iodide, propylthiouracil).

Pleomorphic adenoma comprises two-thirds of all salivary neoplasms. The parotid is the principal salivary gland affected, and the tumor presents as a firm, slow-growing mass. Though benign, recurrence is common if resection is incomplete. Malignant tumors such as mucoepidermoid carcinoma, adenoid cystic carcinoma, and adenocarcinoma tend to grow relatively fast, depending upon grade. They may ulcerate and invade nerves, producing numbness and facial paralysis. Surgical resection is the primary treatment. Radiation therapy (particularly neutron-beam therapy) is used when surgery is not feasible, and it is used post-resection for certain histologic types with a high risk of recurrence. Malignant salivary gland tumors have a 5-year survival rate of about 68%.

DENTAL CARE OF MEDICALLY COMPLEX PATIENTS

Routine dental care (e.g., extraction, scaling and cleaning, tooth restoration, and root canal) is remarkably safe. The most common concerns regarding care of dental patients with medical disease are fear of excessive bleeding for patients on anticoagulants, infection of the heart valves and prosthetic devices from hematogenous seeding of oral flora, and cardiovascular complications resulting from vasopressors used with local anesthetics during dental treatment. Experience confirms that the risks of any of these complications are very low.

Patients undergoing tooth extraction or alveolar and gingival surgery rarely experience uncontrolled bleeding when warfarin anticoagulation is maintained within the therapeutic range currently recommended for prevention of venous thrombosis, atrial fibrillation, or mechanical heart valve. Embolic complications and death, however, have been reported during subtherapeutic anticoagulation. Therapeutic anticoagulation should be confirmed before and continued through the procedure. Likewise, low-dose aspirin (e.g., 81–325 mg) can be safely continued. For patients on aspirin and another antiplatelet medication (e.g., clopidogrel), the decision to continue the second antiplatelet medication should be based on individual consideration of the risks of thrombosis and bleeding.

Patients at risk for bacterial endocarditis should maintain optimal oral hygiene, including flossing, and have regular professional cleaning. Currently, guidelines recommend that prophylactic antibiotics be restricted to those patients at high risk of bacterial endocarditis who undergo dental and oral procedures that involve significant manipulation of gingival or periapical tissue or penetration of the oral mucosa. If unexpected bleeding occurs, antibiotics given within 2 h following the procedure provide effective prophylaxis.

Hematogenous bacterial seeding from oral infection can undoubtedly produce late prosthetic joint infection and therefore requires removal of the infected tissue (e.g., drainage, extraction, root canal) and appropriate antibiotic therapy. However, evidence that late prosthetic joint infection occurs following routine dental procedures is lacking. For this reason, antibiotic prophylaxis is not recommended before dental surgery in patients with orthopedic pins, screws, and plates. It is, however, advised within the first 2 years after joint replacement for patients who have inflammatory arthropathies, immunosuppression, type 1 diabetes mellitus, previous prosthetic joint infection, hemophilia, or malnourishment.

Concern often arises regarding the use of vasoconstrictors in patients with hypertension and heart disease. Vasoconstrictors enhance the depth and duration of local anesthesia, thus reducing the anesthetic dose and potential toxicity. If intravascular injection is avoided, 2% lidocaine with 1:100,000 epinephrine (limited to a total of 0.036 mg epinephrine) can be used safely in those with controlled hypertension and stable coronary heart disease, arrhythmia, or congestive heart failure. Precaution should be taken with patients taking tricyclic antidepressants and nonselective beta blockers because these drugs may potentiate the effect of epinephrine.

Elective dental treatments should be postponed for at least 1 month after myocardial infarction, after which the risk of reinfarction is low provided the patient is medically stable (e.g., stable rhythm, stable angina, and free of heart failure). Patients who have suffered a stroke should have elective dental care deferred for 6 months. In both situations, effective stress reduction requires good pain control, including the use of the minimal amount of vasoconstrictor necessary to provide good hemostasis and local anesthesia.

Bisphosphonate therapy is associated with *osteonecrosis* of the jaw. However, the risk with oral bisphosphonate therapy is very low. Most patients affected have received high-dose aminobisphosphonate therapy for multiple myeloma or metastatic breast cancer and have undergone tooth extraction or dental surgery. Intraoral lesions appear as exposed yellow-white hard bone involving the mandible or maxilla. Two-thirds are painful. Screening tests for determining risk of osteonecrosis are unreliable. Patients slated for aminobisphosphonate therapy should receive preventive dental care that reduces the risk of infection and need for future dentoalveolar surgery.

HALITOSIS

Halitosis typically emanates from the oral cavity or nasal passages. Volatile sulfur compounds resulting from bacterial decay of food and cellular debris account for the malodor. Periodontal disease, caries, acute forms of gingivitis, poorly fitting dentures, oral abscess, and tongue coating are usual causes. Treatment includes correcting poor hygiene, treating infection, and tongue brushing. Xerostomia can produce and exacerbate halitosis. Pockets of decay in the tonsillar crypts, esophageal diverticulum, esophageal stasis (e.g., achalasia, stricture), sinusitis, and lung abscess account for some instances. A few systemic diseases produce distinctive odors: renal failure (ammoniacal), hepatic (fishy), and ketoacidosis (fruity). *Helicobacter pylori* gastritis can also produce ammoniac breath. If no odor is detectable, then pseudohalitosis or even halitophobia must be considered. These conditions represent varying degrees of psychiatric illness.

AGING AND ORAL HEALTH

While tooth loss and dental disease are not normal consequences of aging, a complex array of structural and functional changes occurs with age that can affect oral health. Subtle changes in tooth structure (e.g., diminished pulp space and volume, sclerosis of dentinal tubules, and altered proportions of nerve and vascular pulp content) result in diminished or altered pain sensitivity, reduced reparative capacity, and increased tooth brittleness. In addition, age-associated fatty replacement of salivary acini may reduce physiologic reserve, thus increasing the risk of xerostomia.

Poor oral hygiene often results when vision fails or when patients lose manual dexterity and upper-extremity flexibility. This is particularly common for nursing home residents and must be emphasized because regular oral cleaning and dental care have been shown to reduce the incidence of pneumonia and mortality in this population. Other risks for dental decay include limited lifetime fluoride exposure and preference by some older adults for intensely sweet foods when taste and olfaction wane. These factors occur in an increasing proportion of persons over age 75 who retain teeth that have extensive restorations and exposed roots. Without assiduous care, decay can become quite advanced yet remain asymptomatic. Consequently, much or the entire tooth can be destroyed before the process is detected.

Periodontal disease, a leading cause of tooth loss, is indicated by loss of alveolar bone height. Over 90% of Americans have some degree of periodontal disease by age 50. Healthy adults who have not experienced significant alveolar bone loss by the sixth decade do not typically develop significant worsening with advancing age.

Complete edentulousness with advanced age, though less common than in previous decades, is still present in approximately 50% of Americans age ≥85. Speech, mastication, and facial contours are dramatically affected. Edentulousness may also worsen obstructive sleep apnea, particularly in those without symptoms while wearing dentures. Dentures can improve speech articulation and restore diminished facial contours. Mastication is restored less predictably, and those expecting dentures to improve oral intake are often disappointed. Dentures require periodic adjustment to accommodate inevitable remodeling that leads to a diminished volume of the alveolar ridge. Pain can result from friction or traumatic lesions produced by loose dentures. Poor fit and poor oral hygiene may permit candidiasis to develop. This may be asymptomatic or painful and is indicated by erythematous smooth or granular tissue conforming to an area covered by the appliance.

CHAPTER 3

ATLAS OF ORAL MANIFESTATIONS OF DISEASE

Samuel C. Durso ■ Janet A. Yellowitz

The health status of the oral cavity is linked to cardio-vascular disease, diabetes, and other systemic illnesses. Thus, examining the oral cavity for signs of disease is a key part of the physical exam. This chapter presents numerous outstanding clinical photographs (Figs. 3–1 to 3–27) illustrating many of the conditions discussed in Chap. 2, Oral Manifestations of Disease. Conditions affecting the teeth, periodontal tissues, and oral mucosa are all represented.

FIGURE 3-2
Oral lichen planus.

FIGURE 3-1
Gingival overgrowth secondary to calcium channel blocker use.

FIGURE 3-3
Erosive lichen planus.

FIGURE 3-4
Stevens-Johnson syndrome—reaction to nevirapine.

A

FIGURE 3-5
Erythematosus candidiasis under a denture (i.e., the patient should be treated for this fungal infection).

B

FIGURE 3-7
Angular cheilitis.

FIGURE 3-6
Severe periodontitis.

FIGURE 3-8
Sublingual leukoplakia.

A

B

FIGURE 3-9
A. Epulis (gingival hypertrophy) under denture. *B.* Epulis fissuratum.

FIGURE 3-10
Traumatic lesion inside of cheek.

FIGURE 3-11
Oral leukoplakia, subtype homogenous leukoplakia.

FIGURE 3-12
Oral carcinoma.

FIGURE 3-13
Healthy mouth.

FIGURE 3-14
Geographic tongue.

FIGURE 3-15
Moderate gingivitis.

FIGURE 3-16
Gingival recession.

FIGURE 3-17
Heavy calculus and gingival inflammation.

FIGURE 3-18
Severe gingival inflammation and heavy calculus.

FIGURE 3-19
Root cavity in presence of severe periodontal disease.

FIGURE 3-20
Ulcer on lateral border of tongue—potential carcinoma.

FIGURE 3-23
Salivary stone.

FIGURE 3-21
Osteonecrosis.

A   *B*

FIGURE 3-24
A. Calculus. *B.* Teeth cleaned.

FIGURE 3-22
Severe periodontal disease, missing tooth, very mobile teeth.

FIGURE 3-25
Traumatic ulcer.

FIGURE 3-26
Fissured tongue.

FIGURE 3-27
White coated tongue—likely candidiasis.

ACKNOWLEDGMENT

Dr. Jane Atkinson was a co-author of this chapter in the 17th edition of Harrison's Principles of Internal Medicine. Some of the materials have been carried over into the 18th edition.

CHAPTER 4
DYSPHAGIA

Ikuo Hirano ■ Peter J. Kahrilas

Dysphagia—difficulty with swallowing—refers to problems with the transit of food or liquid from the mouth to the hypopharynx or through the esophagus. Severe dysphagia can compromise nutrition, cause aspiration, and reduce quality of life. Additional terminology pertaining to swallowing dysfunction is as follows. *Aphagia* denotes complete esophageal obstruction, most commonly encountered in the acute setting of a food bolus or foreign body impaction. *Odynophagia* refers to painful swallowing, typically resulting from mucosal ulceration within the oropharynx or esophagus. It commonly is accompanied by dysphagia, but the converse is not true. *Globus pharyngeus* is a foreign body sensation localized in the neck that does not interfere with swallowing and sometimes is relieved by swallowing. *Transfer dysphagia* frequently results in nasal regurgitation and pulmonary aspiration during swallowing and is characteristic of oropharyngeal dysphagia. *Phagophobia* (fear of swallowing) and *refusal to swallow* may be psychogenic or related to anticipatory anxiety about food bolus obstruction, odynophagia, or aspiration.

PHYSIOLOGY OF SWALLOWING

Swallowing begins with a voluntary (oral) phase that includes preparation during which food is masticated and mixed with saliva. This is followed by a transfer phase during which the bolus is pushed into the pharynx by the tongue. Bolus entry into the hypopharynx initiates the pharyngeal swallow response, which is centrally mediated and involves a complex series of actions, the net result of which is to propel food through the pharynx into the esophagus while preventing its entry into the airway. To accomplish this, the larynx is elevated and pulled forward, actions that also facilitate upper esophageal sphincter (UES) opening. Tongue pulsion then propels the bolus through the UES, followed by a peristaltic contraction that clears residue from the pharynx and through the esophagus. The lower esophageal sphincter (LES) relaxes as the food enters the esophagus and remains relaxed until the peristaltic contraction has delivered the bolus into the stomach. Peristaltic contractions elicited in response to a swallow are called *primary peristalsis* and involve sequenced inhibition followed by contraction of the musculature along the entire length of the esophagus. The inhibition that precedes the peristaltic contraction is called *deglutitive inhibition*. Local distention of the esophagus anywhere along its length, as may occur with gastroesophageal reflux, activates *secondary peristalsis* that begins at the point of distention and proceeds distally. Tertiary esophageal contractions are nonperistaltic, disordered esophageal contractions that may be observed to occur spontaneously during fluoroscopic observation.

The musculature of the oral cavity, pharynx, UES, and cervical esophagus is striated and directly innervated by lower motor neurons carried in cranial nerves **(Fig. 4-1)**. Oral cavity muscles are innervated by the fifth (trigeminal) and seventh (facial) cranial nerves; the tongue, by the twelfth (hypoglossal) cranial nerve. Pharyngeal muscles are innervated by the ninth (glossopharyngeal) and tenth (vagus) cranial nerves.

Physiologically, the UES consists of the cricopharyngeus muscle, the adjacent inferior pharyngeal constrictor, and the proximal portion of the cervical esophagus. UES innervation is derived from the vagus nerve, whereas the innervation to the musculature acting on the UES to facilitate its opening during swallowing comes from the fifth, seventh, and twelfth cranial nerves. The UES remains closed at rest owing to both its inherent elastic properties and neurogenically mediated contraction of the cricopharyngeus muscle. UES opening during swallowing involves both cessation of vagal excitation to the cricopharyngeus and simultaneous contraction of the suprahyoid and geniohyoid muscles that pull open the

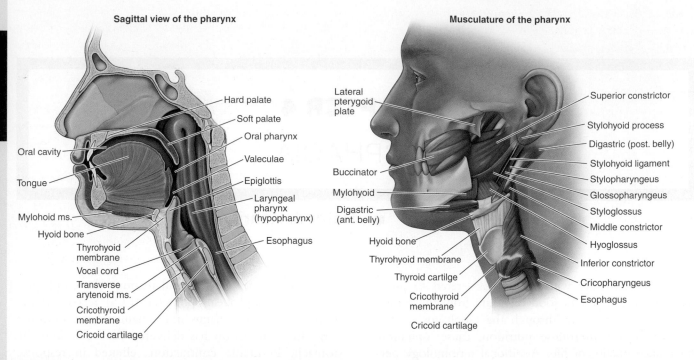

Sagittal view of the pharynx

Musculature of the pharynx

FIGURE 4-1

Sagittal and diagrammatic views of the musculature involved in enacting oropharyngeal swallowing. Note the dominance of the tongue in the sagittal view and the intimate relationship between the entrance to the larynx (airway) and the esophagus. In the resting configuration illustrated, the esophageal inlet is closed. This is transiently reconfigured such that the esophageal inlet is open and the laryngeal inlet closed during swallowing. (*Adapted from PJ Kahrilas, in DW Gelfand and JE Richter [eds]: Dysphagia: Diagnosis and Treatment. New York: Igaku-Shoin Medical Publishers, 1989, pp. 11–28.*)

UES in conjunction with the upward and forward displacement of the larynx.

The neuromuscular apparatus for peristalsis is distinct in proximal and distal parts of the esophagus. The cervical esophagus, like the pharyngeal musculature, consists of striated muscle and is directly innervated by lower motor neurons of the vagus nerve. Peristalsis in the proximal esophagus is governed by the sequential activation of the vagal motor neurons in the nucleus ambiguus. In contrast, the distal esophagus and LES are composed of smooth muscle and are controlled by excitatory and inhibitory neurons within the esophageal myenteric plexus. Medullary preganglionic neurons from the dorsal motor nucleus of the vagus trigger peristalsis via these ganglionic neurons during primary peristalsis. Neurotransmitters of the excitatory ganglionic neurons are acetylcholine and substance P; those of the inhibitory neurons are vasoactive intestinal peptide and nitric oxide. Peristalsis results from the patterned activation of inhibitory followed by excitatory ganglionic neurons, with progressive dominance of the inhibitory neurons distally. Similarly, LES relaxation occurs with the onset of deglutitive inhibition and persists until the peristaltic sequence is complete. At rest, the LES is contracted because of excitatory ganglionic stimulation and its intrinsic myogenic tone, a property that distinguishes it from the adjacent esophagus. The function of the LES is supplemented by the surrounding muscle of the right diaphragmatic crus, which acts as an external sphincter during inspiration, cough, or abdominal straining.

PATHOPHYSIOLOGY OF DYSPHAGIA

Dysphagia can be subclassified both by location and by the circumstances in which it occurs. With respect to location, distinct considerations apply to oral, pharyngeal, or esophageal dysphagia. Normal transport of an ingested bolus depends on the consistency and size of the bolus, the caliber of the lumen, the integrity of peristaltic contraction, and deglutitive inhibition of both the UES and the LES. Dysphagia caused by an oversized bolus or a narrow lumen is called *structural dysphagia*, whereas dysphagia due to abnormalities of peristalsis or impaired sphincter relaxation after swallowing is called *propulsive* or *motor dysphagia*. More than one mechanism may be operative in a patient with dysphagia. Scleroderma commonly presents with absent peristalsis as well as a weakened LES that predisposes patients to peptic stricture formation. Likewise, radiation therapy for head and neck cancer may compound the functional deficits in the oropharyngeal swallow attributable to the tumor and cause cervical esophageal stenosis.

Oral and pharyngeal (oropharyngeal) dysphagia

Oral-phase dysphagia is associated with poor bolus formation and control so that food has prolonged retention within the oral cavity and may seep out of the mouth. Drooling and difficulty in initiating swallowing are other characteristic signs. Poor bolus control also may lead to premature spillage of food into the hypopharynx with resultant aspiration into the trachea or regurgitation into the nasal cavity. Pharyngeal-phase dysphagia is associated with retention of food in the pharynx due to poor tongue or pharyngeal propulsion or obstruction at the UES. Signs and symptoms of concomitant hoarseness or cranial nerve dysfunction may be associated with oropharyngeal dysphagia.

Oropharyngeal dysphagia may be due to neurologic, muscular, structural, iatrogenic, infectious, and metabolic causes. Iatrogenic, neurologic, and structural pathologies are most common. Iatrogenic causes include surgery and radiation, often in the setting of head and neck cancer. Neurogenic dysphagia resulting from cerebrovascular accidents, Parkinson's disease, and amyotrophic lateral sclerosis is a major source of morbidity related to aspiration and malnutrition. Medullary nuclei directly innervate the oropharynx. Lateralization of pharyngeal dysphagia implies either a structural pharyngeal lesion or a neurologic process that selectively targeted the ipsilateral brainstem nuclei or cranial nerve. Advances in functional brain imaging have elucidated an important role of the cerebral cortex in swallow function and dysphagia. Asymmetry in the cortical representation of the pharynx provides an explanation for the dysphagia that occurs as a consequence of unilateral cortical cerebrovascular accidents.

Oropharyngeal structural lesions causing dysphagia include Zenker's diverticulum, cricopharyngeal bar, and neoplasia. Zenker's diverticulum typically is encountered in elderly patients, with an estimated prevalence between 1:1000 and 1:10,000. In addition to dysphagia, patients may present with regurgitation of particulate food debris, aspiration, and halitosis. The pathogenesis is related to stenosis of the cricopharyngeus that causes diminished opening of the UES and results in increased hypopharyngeal pressure during swallowing with development of a pulsion diverticulum immediately above the cricopharyngeus in a region of potential weakness known as Killian's dehiscence. A cricopharyngeal bar, appearing as a prominent indentation behind the lower third of the cricoid cartilage, is related to Zenker's diverticulum in that it involves limited distensibility of the cricopharyngeus and can lead to the formation of a Zenker's diverticulum. However, a cricopharyngeal bar

is a common radiographic finding, and most patients with transient cricopharyngeal bars are asymptomatic, making it important to rule out alternative etiologies of dysphagia before treatment. Furthermore, cricopharyngeal bars may be secondary to other neuromuscular disorders.

Since the pharyngeal phase of swallowing occurs in less than a second, rapid-sequence fluoroscopy is necessary to evaluate for functional abnormalities. Adequate fluoroscopic examination requires that the patient be conscious and cooperative. The study incorporates recordings of swallow sequences during ingestion of food and liquids of varying consistencies. The pharynx is examined to detect bolus retention, regurgitation into the nose, or aspiration into the trachea. Timing and integrity of pharyngeal contraction and opening of the UES with a swallow are analyzed to assess both aspiration risk and the potential for swallow therapy. Structural abnormalities of the oropharynx, especially those which may require biopsies, also should be assessed by direct laryngoscopic examination.

Esophageal dysphagia

The adult esophagus measures 18–26 cm in length and is anatomically divided into the cervical esophagus, extending from the pharyngoesophageal junction to the suprasternal notch, and the thoracic esophagus, which continues to the diaphragmatic hiatus. When distended, the esophageal lumen has internal dimensions of about 2 cm in the anteroposterior plane and 3 cm in the lateral plane. Solid food dysphagia becomes common when the lumen is narrowed to <13 mm but also can occur with larger diameters in the setting of poorly masticated food or motor dysfunction. Circumferential lesions are more likely to cause dysphagia than are lesions that involve only a partial circumference of the esophageal wall. The most common structural causes of dysphagia are Schatzki's rings, eosinophilic esophagitis, and peptic strictures. Dysphagia also occurs in the setting of gastroesophageal reflux disease without a stricture, perhaps on the basis of altered esophageal sensation, distensibility, or motor function.

Propulsive disorders leading to esophageal dysphagia result from abnormalities of peristalsis and/or deglutitive inhibition, potentially affecting the cervical or thoracic esophagus. Since striated muscle pathology usually involves both the oropharynx and the cervical esophagus, the clinical manifestations usually are dominated by oropharyngeal dysphagia. Diseases affecting smooth muscle involve both the thoracic esophagus and the LES. A dominant manifestation of this, absent peristalsis, refers to either the complete absence of swallow-induced contraction or the presence of nonperistaltic, disordered contractions. Absent peristalsis and failure of deglutitive LES relaxation are the defining features of achalasia. In diffuse esophageal spasm (DES), LES function is normal, with the disordered motility restricted to the esophageal body. Absent peristalsis combined with severe weakness of the LES is a nonspecific pattern commonly found in patients with scleroderma.

APPROACH TO THE PATIENT   Dysphagia

Figure 4-2 shows an algorithm for the approach to a patient with dysphagia.

HISTORY The patient history is extremely valuable in making a presumptive diagnosis or at least substantially restricting the differential diagnoses in most patients. Key elements of the history are the localization of dysphagia, the circumstances in which dysphagia is experienced, other symptoms associated with dysphagia, and progression. Dysphagia that localizes to the suprasternal notch may indicate either an oropharyngeal or an esophageal etiology as distal dysphagia is referred proximally about 30% of the time. Dysphagia that localizes to the chest is esophageal in origin. Nasal regurgitation and tracheobronchial aspiration with swallowing are hallmarks of oropharyngeal

dysphagia or a tracheoesophageal fistula. The presence of hoarseness may be another important diagnostic clue. When hoarseness precedes dysphagia, the primary lesion is usually laryngeal; hoarseness that occurs after the development of dysphagia may result from compromise of the recurrent laryngeal nerve by a malignancy. The type of food causing dysphagia is a crucial detail. Intermittent dysphagia that occurs only with solid food implies structural dysphagia, whereas constant dysphagia with both liquids and solids strongly suggests a motor abnormality. Two caveats to this pattern are that despite having a motor abnormality, patients with scleroderma generally develop mild dysphagia for solids only and, somewhat paradoxically, that patients with oropharyngeal dysphagia often have greater difficulty managing liquids than solids. Dysphagia that is progressive over the course of weeks to months raises concern for neoplasia. Episodic dysphagia to solids that is unchanged over years indicates a benign disease process such as a Schatzki's ring or eosinophilic esophagitis. Food impaction with a prolonged inability to pass an ingested bolus even with ingestion of liquid is typical of a structural dysphagia. Chest pain frequently accompanies dysphagia whether

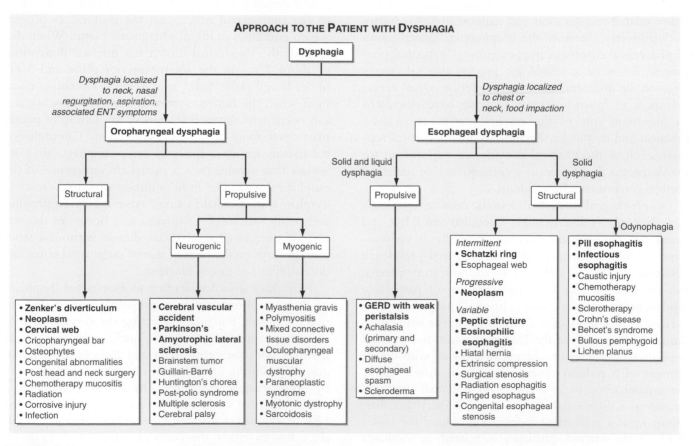

FIGURE 4-2

Aproach to the patient with dysphagia. Etiologies in bold print are the most common. ENT, ear, nose, and throat; GERD, gastroesophageal reflux disease.

it is related to motor disorders, structural disorders, or reflux disease. A prolonged history of heartburn preceding the onset of dysphagia is suggestive of peptic stricture and, less commonly, esophageal adenocarcinoma. A history of prolonged nasogastric intubation, esophageal or head and neck surgery, ingestion of caustic agents or pills, previous radiation or chemotherapy, or associated mucocutaneous diseases may help isolate the cause of dysphagia. With accompanying odynophagia, which usually is indicative of ulceration, infectious or pill-induced esophagitis should be suspected. In patients with AIDS or other immunocompromised states, esophagitis due to opportunistic infections such as *Candida*, herpes simplex virus, or cytomegalovirus and to tumors such as Kaposi's sarcoma and lymphoma should be considered. A strong history of atopy increases concerns for eosinophilic esophagitis.

PHYSICAL EXAMINATION Physical examination is important in the evaluation of oral and pharyngeal dysphagia because dysphagia is usually only one of many manifestations of a more global disease process. Signs of bulbar or pseudobulbar palsy, including dysarthria, dysphonia, ptosis, tongue atrophy, and hyperactive jaw jerk, in addition to evidence of generalized neuromuscular disease, should be elicited. The neck should be examined for thyromegaly. A careful inspection of the mouth and pharynx should disclose lesions that may interfere with passage of food. Physical examination is less helpful in the evaluation of esophageal dysphagia as most relevant pathology is restricted to the esophagus. The notable exception is skin disease. Changes in the skin may suggest a diagnosis of scleroderma or mucocutaneous diseases such as pemphigoid and epidermolysis bullosa, all of which can involve the esophagus.

DIAGNOSTIC PROCEDURES Although most instances of dysphagia are attributable to benign disease processes, dysphagia is also a cardinal symptom of several malignancies, making it an important symptom to evaluate. Even when not attributable to malignancy, dysphagia is usually a manifestation of an identifiable and treatable disease entity, making its evaluation beneficial to the patient and gratifying to the practitioner. The specific diagnostic algorithm to pursue is guided by the details of the history. If oral or pharyngeal dysphagia is suspected, a fluoroscopic swallow study, usually done by a swallow therapist, is the procedure of choice. Otolaryngoscopic and neurologic evaluation also can be important, depending on the circumstances. For suspected esophageal dysphagia, endoscopy is the single most useful test. Endoscopy allows better visualization of mucosal lesions than does barium radiography and also allows one to obtain mucosal biopsies. Furthermore, therapeutic intervention with esophageal dilatation can be done as part of the procedure if it is deemed necessary. Of note, the emergence of eosinophilic esophagitis as a common cause of dysphagia in adults has led to the recommendation that esophageal mucosal biopsies be obtained routinely in the evaluation of unexplained dysphagia even if no endoscopic lesions are evident. For cases of suspected esophageal motility disorders, esophagogastroscopy is still the primary examination as neoplastic and inflammatory conditions can secondarily produce patterns of either achalasia or esophageal spasm. Esophageal manometry is done if dysphagia is not adequately explained by endoscopy or to confirm the diagnosis of a suspected esophageal motor disorder. Barium radiography can provide useful adjunctive information in cases of subtle or complex esophageal strictures, esophageal diverticula, or paraesophageal herniation. In specific cases, CT examination and endoscopic ultrasonography may be useful.

TREATMENT Treatment of dysphagia depends on both the locus and the specific etiology. Oropharyngeal dysphagia most commonly results from functional deficits caused by neurologic disorders. In such circumstances, the treatment focuses on utilizing postures or maneuvers devised to reduce pharyngeal residue and enhance airway protection learned under the direction of a trained swallow therapist. Aspiration risk may be reduced by altering the consistency of ingested food and liquid. Dysphagia resulting from a cerebrovascular accident usually, but not always, spontaneously improves within the first few weeks after the event. More severe and persistent cases may require gastrostomy and enteral feeding. Patients with myasthenia gravis and polymyositis may respond to medical treatment of the primary neuromuscular disease. Surgical intervention with cricopharyngeal myotomy is usually not helpful, with the exception of specific disorders such as the idiopathic cricopharyngeal bar, Zenker's diverticulum, and oculopharyngeal muscular dystrophy. Chronic neurologic disorders such as Parkinson's disease and amyotrophic lateral sclerosis may manifest with severe oropharyngeal dysphagia. Feeding by a nasogastric tube or an endoscopically placed gastrostomy tube may be considered for nutritional support; however, these maneuvers do not provide protection against aspiration of salivary secretions or refluxed gastric contents.

Treatment of esophageal dysphagia is covered in detail in Chap. 13. The majority of causes of esophageal dysphagia are effectively managed by means of esophageal dilatation using bougie or balloon dilators. Cancer and achalasia are often managed surgically, although endoscopic techniques are available for both palliation and primary therapy, respectively. Infectious etiologies respond to antimicrobial medications or treatment of the underlying immunosuppressive state. Finally, eosinophilic esophagitis has emerged as an important cause of dysphagia that is amenable to treatment by elimination of dietary allergens or topical glucocorticoids.

CHAPTER 5
NAUSEA, VOMITING, AND INDIGESTION

William L. Hasler

Nausea is the subjective feeling of a need to vomit. *Vomiting* (emesis) is the oral expulsion of gastrointestinal contents resulting from contractions of gut and thoracoabdominal wall musculature. Vomiting is contrasted with *regurgitation*, the effortless passage of gastric contents into the mouth. *Rumination* is the repeated regurgitation of stomach contents, which may be rechewed and reswallowed. In contrast to vomiting, these phenomena often exhibit volitional control. *Indigestion* is a nonspecific term that encompasses a variety of upper abdominal complaints including nausea, vomiting, heartburn, regurgitation, and dyspepsia (the presence of symptoms thought to originate in the gastroduodenal region). Some individuals with dyspepsia report predominantly epigastric burning, gnawing discomfort, or pain. Others with dyspepsia experience a constellation of symptoms including postprandial fullness, early satiety (an inability to complete a meal due to premature fullness), bloating, eructation (belching), and anorexia.

NAUSEA AND VOMITING

MECHANISMS

Vomiting is coordinated by the brainstem and is effected by responses in the gut, pharynx, and thoracoabdominal wall. The mechanisms underlying nausea are poorly understood but likely involve the cerebral cortex, because nausea requires conscious perception. This is supported by electroencephalographic studies showing activation of temporofrontal regions during nausea.

Coordination of emesis

Brainstem nuclei—including the nucleus tractus solitarius; dorsal vagal and phrenic nuclei; medullary nuclei that regulate respiration; and nuclei that control pharyngeal, facial, and tongue movements—coordinate the initiation of emesis. Neurotransmitters involved in this coordination are uncertain, but neurokinin NK_1, serotonin 5-HT_3, and vasopressin pathways may participate.

Somatic and visceral muscles exhibit stereotypic responses during emesis. Inspiratory thoracic and abdominal wall muscles contract, producing high intrathoracic and intraabdominal pressures that facilitate expulsion of gastric contents. The gastric cardia herniates across the diaphragm and the larynx moves upward to promote oral propulsion of the vomitus. Under normal conditions, distally migrating gut contractions are regulated by an electrical phenomenon, the slow wave, which cycles at 3 cycles/min in the stomach and 11 cycles/min in the duodenum. With emesis, there is slow-wave abolition and initiation of orally propagating spikes that evoke retrograde contractions that assist in oral expulsion of intestinal contents.

Activators of emesis

Emetic stimuli act at several sites. Emesis provoked by unpleasant thoughts or smells originates in the cerebral cortex, whereas cranial nerves mediate vomiting after gag reflex activation. Motion sickness and inner ear disorders act on the labyrinthine apparatus, whereas gastric irritants and cytotoxic agents such as cisplatin stimulate gastroduodenal vagal afferent nerves. Nongastric visceral afferents are activated by intestinal and colonic obstruction and mesenteric ischemia. The area postrema, a medullary nucleus, responds to bloodborne emetic stimuli and is termed the *chemoreceptor trigger zone*. Many emetogenic drugs act on the area postrema, as do bacterial toxins and metabolic factors produced during uremia, hypoxia, and ketoacidosis.

Neurotransmitters that mediate induction of vomiting are selective for these anatomic sites. Labyrinthine disorders stimulate vestibular muscarinic M_1 and histaminergic H_1 receptors, whereas vagal afferent stimuli activate serotonin 5-HT_3 receptors. The area postrema

32

is richly served by nerves acting on 5-HT$_3$, M$_1$, H$_1$, and dopamine D$_2$ subtypes. Transmitters in the cerebral cortex are poorly understood, although cannabinoid CB$_1$ pathways may participate. Optimal pharmacologic therapy of vomiting requires understanding of these pathways.

DIFFERENTIAL DIAGNOSIS

Nausea and vomiting are caused by conditions within and outside the gut as well as by drugs and circulating toxins (Table 5-1).

Intraperitoneal disorders

Visceral obstruction and inflammation of hollow and solid viscera may produce vomiting. Gastric obstruction results from ulcer disease and malignancy, while small-bowel and colonic obstruction occur because of adhesions, benign or malignant tumors, volvulus, intussusception, or inflammatory diseases such as Crohn's disease. The superior mesenteric artery syndrome, occurring after weight loss or prolonged bed rest, results when the duodenum is compressed by the overlying superior mesenteric artery. Abdominal irradiation impairs intestinal motor function and induces strictures. Biliary colic causes nausea via action on visceral afferent nerves. Vomiting with pancreatitis, cholecystitis, and appendicitis is due to visceral irritation and induction of

ileus. Enteric infections with viruses or bacteria such as *Staphylococcus aureus* and *Bacillus cereus* commonly cause vomiting, especially in children. Opportunistic infections such as cytomegalovirus or herpes simplex virus induce emesis in immunocompromised individuals.

Disordered gut sensorimotor function commonly causes nausea and vomiting. *Gastroparesis* is defined as a delay in gastric emptying of food and occurs after vagotomy, with pancreatic adenocarcinoma, with mesenteric vascular insufficiency, or in systemic diseases such as diabetes, scleroderma, and amyloidosis. The most common form of disease, idiopathic gastroparesis, occurs in the absence of systemic illness and may follow a viral prodrome, suggesting an infectious etiology. Intestinal pseudoobstruction is characterized by disrupted intestinal and colonic motor activity and leads to retention of food residue and secretions; bacterial overgrowth; nutrient malabsorption; and symptoms of nausea, vomiting, bloating, pain, and altered defecation. *Intestinal pseudoobstruction* may be idiopathic or inherited as a familial visceral myopathy or neuropathy, or it may result from systemic disease or as a paraneoplastic complication of a malignancy such as small cell lung carcinoma. Patients with gastroesophageal reflux may report nausea and vomiting, as do some individuals with irritable bowel syndrome (IBS).

Other functional disorders without organic abnormalities have been characterized in adults. *Chronic idiopathic nausea* is defined as nausea without vomiting

TABLE 5-1

CAUSES OF NAUSEA AND VOMITING		
INTRAPERITONEAL	**EXTRAPERITONEAL**	**MEDICATIONS/METABOLIC DISORDERS**
Obstructing disorders	Cardiopulmonary disease	Drugs
Pyloric obstruction	Cardiomyopathy	Cancer chemotherapy
Small bowel obstruction	Myocardial infarction	Antibiotics
Colonic obstruction	Labyrinthine disease	Cardiac antiarrhythmics
Superior mesenteric artery syndrome	Motion sickness	Digoxin
Enteric infections	Labyrinthitis	Oral hypoglycemics
Viral	Malignancy	Oral contraceptives
Bacterial	Intracerebral disorders	Endocrine/metabolic disease
Inflammatory diseases	Malignancy	Pregnancy
Cholecystitis	Hemorrhage	Uremia
Pancreatitis	Abscess	Ketoacidosis
Appendicitis	Hydrocephalus	Thyroid and parathyroid disease
Hepatitis	Psychiatric illness	Adrenal insufficiency
Altered sensorimotor function	Anorexia and bulimia nervosa	Toxins
Gastroparesis	Depression	Liver failure
Intestinal pseudoobstruction	Postoperative vomiting	Ethanol
Gastroesophageal reflux		
Chronic idiopathic nausea		
Functional vomiting		
Cyclic vomiting syndrome		
Biliary colic		
Abdominal irradiation		

occurring several times weekly, whereas *functional vomiting* is defined as one or more vomiting episodes weekly in the absence of an eating disorder or psychiatric disease. *Cyclic vomiting syndrome* is a rare disorder of unknown etiology that produces periodic discrete episodes of relentless nausea and vomiting. The syndrome shows a strong association with migraine headaches, suggesting that some cases may be migraine variants. Cyclic vomiting is most common in children, although adult cases have been described in association with rapid gastric emptying and with chronic cannabis use.

Extraperitoneal disorders

Myocardial infarction and congestive heart failure may cause nausea and vomiting. Postoperative emesis occurs after 25% of surgeries, most commonly laparotomy and orthopedic surgery, and is more prevalent in women. Increased intracranial pressure from tumors, bleeding, abscess, or obstruction to cerebrospinal fluid outflow produces prominent vomiting with or without nausea. Motion sickness, labyrinthitis, and Ménière's disease evoke emesis via labyrinthine pathways. Patients with psychiatric illnesses including anorexia nervosa, bulimia nervosa, anxiety, and depression may report significant nausea that may be associated with delayed gastric emptying.

Medications and metabolic disorders

Drugs evoke vomiting by action on the stomach (analgesics, erythromycin) or area postrema (digoxin, opiates, anti–Parkinsonian drugs). Emetogenic agents include antibiotics, cardiac antiarrhythmics, antihypertensives, oral hypoglycemics, and contraceptives. Cancer chemotherapy causes vomiting that is acute (within hours of administration), delayed (after 1 or more days), or anticipatory. Acute emesis resulting from highly emetogenic agents such as cisplatin is mediated by 5-HT$_3$ pathways, whereas delayed emesis is 5-HT$_3$-independent. Anticipatory nausea often responds better to anxiolytic therapy than to antiemetics.

Several metabolic disorders elicit nausea and vomiting. Pregnancy is the most prevalent endocrinologic cause of nausea, which affects 70% of women in the first trimester. Hyperemesis gravidarum is a severe form of nausea of pregnancy that can produce significant fluid loss and electrolyte disturbances. Uremia, ketoacidosis, and adrenal insufficiency, as well as parathyroid and thyroid disease, are other metabolic causes of emesis.

Circulating toxins evoke emesis via effects on the area postrema. Endogenous toxins are generated in fulminant liver failure, whereas exogenous enterotoxins may be produced by enteric bacterial infection. Ethanol intoxication is a common toxic etiology of nausea and vomiting.

APPROACH TO THE PATIENT Nausea and Vomiting

HISTORY AND PHYSICAL EXAMINATION The history helps define the etiology of unexplained nausea and vomiting. Drugs, toxins, and gastrointestinal infections commonly cause acute symptoms, whereas established illnesses evoke chronic complaints. Pyloric obstruction and gastroparesis produce vomiting within 1 h of eating, whereas emesis from intestinal obstruction occurs later. In severe cases of gastroparesis, the vomitus may contain food residue ingested hours or days previously. Hematemesis raises suspicion of an ulcer, malignancy, or Mallory-Weiss tear, whereas feculent emesis is noted with distal intestinal or colonic obstruction. Bilious vomiting excludes gastric obstruction, while emesis of undigested food is consistent with a Zenker's diverticulum or achalasia. Relief of abdominal pain by emesis characterizes intestinal obstruction, whereas vomiting has no effect on pancreatitis or cholecystitis pain. Pronounced weight loss raises concern about malignancy or obstruction. Fevers suggest inflammation; an intracranial source is considered if there are headaches or visual field changes. Vertigo or tinnitus indicates labyrinthine disease.

The physical examination complements information from the history. Orthostatic hypotension and reduced skin turgor indicate intravascular fluid loss. Pulmonary abnormalities raise concern for aspiration of vomitus. Abdominal auscultation may reveal absent bowel sounds with ileus. High-pitched rushes suggest bowel obstruction, while a succussion splash upon abrupt lateral movement of the patient is found with gastroparesis or pyloric obstruction. Tenderness or involuntary guarding raises suspicion of inflammation, whereas fecal blood suggests mucosal injury from ulcer, ischemia, or tumor. Neurologic disease presents with papilledema, visual field loss, or focal neural abnormalities. Neoplasm is suggested by palpation of masses or adenopathy.

DIAGNOSTIC TESTING For intractable symptoms or an elusive diagnosis, selected screening tests can direct clinical care. Electrolyte replacement is indicated for hypokalemia or metabolic alkalosis. Detection of iron-deficiency anemia mandates a search for mucosal injury. Pancreaticobiliary disease is indicated by abnormal pancreatic or liver biochemistries, whereas endocrinologic, rheumatologic, or paraneoplastic etiologies are suggested by hormone or serologic abnormalities. If bowel obstruction is suspected, supine and upright abdominal radiographs may show intestinal air-fluid levels with reduced colonic air. Ileus is characterized by diffusely dilated air-filled bowel loops.

Anatomic studies may be indicated if initial testing is nondiagnostic. Upper endoscopy detects ulcers or malignancy, while small-bowel barium radiography diagnoses partial intestinal obstruction. Colonoscopy or contrast enema radiography can detect colonic obstruction. Ultrasound or CT defines intraperitoneal inflammatory processes, while CT or MRI of the head can delineate intracranial disease. Advances in CT and MRI enterography have improved definition of bowel inflammation, as in Crohn's disease. Mesenteric angiography, CT, or MRI is useful for suspected ischemia.

Gastrointestinal motility testing may detect a motor disorder that contributes to symptoms when anatomic abnormalities are absent. Gastroparesis commonly is diagnosed using gastric scintigraphy, by which emptying of a radiolabeled meal is measured. Isotopic breath tests and wireless motility capsule methods have been validated and may become important alternatives to scintigraphy to define gastroparesis. The diagnosis of intestinal pseudoobstruction often is suggested by abnormal barium transit and luminal dilation on small-bowel contrast radiography. Delayed small-bowel transit also may be detected by wireless capsule techniques. Small-intestinal manometry can confirm the diagnosis and further characterize the motor abnormality as neuropathic or myopathic based on contractile patterns. Such investigation can obviate the need for open intestinal biopsy to evaluate for smooth muscle or neuronal degeneration.

TREATMENT   Nausea and Vomiting

GENERAL PRINCIPLES Therapy of vomiting is tailored to correcting medically or surgically remediable abnormalities if possible. Hospitalization is considered for severe dehydration, especially if oral fluid replenishment cannot be sustained. Once oral intake is tolerated, nutrients are restarted with liquids that are low in fat, as lipids delay gastric emptying. Foods high in indigestible residues are avoided because these also prolong gastric retention.

ANTIEMETIC MEDICATIONS The most commonly used antiemetic agents act on sites in the central nervous system (Table 5-2). Antihistamines such as meclizine and dimenhydrinate and anticholinergic drugs like scopolamine act on labyrinthine pathways and are useful in motion sickness and inner ear disorders. Dopamine D_2 antagonists treat emesis evoked by area postrema stimuli and are useful for medication, toxic, and metabolic etiologies. Dopamine antagonists freely cross the blood-brain barrier and cause anxiety, dystonic reactions, hyperprolactinemic effects (galactorrhea and sexual dysfunction), and irreversible tardive dyskinesia.

Other drug classes exhibit antiemetic properties. Serotonin 5-HT$_3$ antagonists such as ondansetron

and granisetron exhibit utility in postoperative vomiting, after radiation therapy, and for preventing cancer chemotherapy–induced emesis. The usefulness of 5-HT$_3$ antagonists for other causes of emesis is less well established. Low-dose tricyclic antidepressant agents provide symptomatic benefit in patients with chronic idiopathic nausea and functional vomiting as well as in diabetic patients with nausea and vomiting whose disease is of long standing. Other antidepressants such as mirtazapine also may exhibit antiemetic effects.

GASTROINTESTINAL MOTOR STIMULANTS
Drugs that stimulate gastric emptying are indicated for gastroparesis (Table 5-2). Metoclopramide, a combined 5-HT$_4$ agonist and D_2 antagonist, exhibits efficacy in gastroparesis, but antidopaminergic side effects, particularly tardive dyskinesia, limit its use in <25% of patients. Erythromycin, a macrolide antibiotic, increases gastroduodenal motility by action on receptors for motilin, an endogenous stimulant of fasting motor activity. Intravenous erythromycin is useful for inpatients with refractory gastroparesis; however, oral forms also have some utility. Domperidone, a D_2 antagonist not available in the United States, exhibits prokinetic and antiemetic effects but does not cross into most other brain regions; thus, anxiety and dystonic reactions are rare. The main side effects of domperidone relate to induction of hyperprolactinemia via effects on pituitary regions served by a porous blood-brain barrier.

Refractory upper gut motility disorders pose significant challenges. Liquid suspensions of prokinetic drugs may be beneficial, because liquids empty from the stomach more rapidly than pills do. Metoclopramide can be administered subcutaneously in patients unresponsive to oral drugs. Intestinal pseudoobstruction may respond to the somatostatin analogue octreotide, which induces propagative small intestinal motor complexes. Acetylcholinesterase inhibitors such as pyridostigmine are anecdotally observed to benefit some patients with small bowel dysmotility. Pyloric injections of botulinum toxin are reported in uncontrolled studies to benefit patients with gastroparesis. Placement of a feeding jejunostomy reduces hospitalizations and improves overall health in some patients with drug-refractory gastroparesis. Surgical options are limited for unresponsive cases, but postvagotomy gastroparesis may improve with near-total resection of the stomach. Implanted gastric electrical stimulators may reduce symptoms, enhance nutrition, improve quality of life, and decrease health care expenditures in medication-refractory gastroparesis, although small controlled trials report only modest benefits with this method.

SELECTED CLINICAL SETTINGS Some cancer chemotherapeutic agents such as cisplatin are intensely emetogenic. Given prophylactically, 5-HT$_3$ antagonists

TABLE 5-2

TREATMENT OF NAUSEA AND VOMITING

TREATMENT	MECHANISM	EXAMPLES	CLINICAL INDICATIONS
Antiemetic agents	Antihistaminergic	Dimenhydrinate, meclizine	Motion sickness, inner ear disease
	Anticholinergic	Scopolamine	Motion sickness, inner ear disease
	Antidopaminergic	Prochlorperazine, thiethylperazine	Medication-, toxin-, or metabolic-induced emesis
	$5\text{-}HT_3$ antagonist	Ondansetron, granisetron	Chemotherapy- and radiation-induced emesis, postoperative emesis
	NK_1 antagonist	Aprepitant	Chemotherapy-induced nausea and vomiting
	Tricyclic antidepressant	Amitriptyline, nortriptyline	Chronic idiopathic nausea, functional vomiting, cyclic vomiting syndrome, ?gastroparesis
	Other antidepressant	Mirtazapine	?Functional vomiting, ?gastroparesis
Prokinetic agents	$5\text{-}HT_4$ agonist and antidopaminergic	Metoclopramide	Gastroparesis
	Motilin agonist	Erythromycin	Gastroparesis, ?intestinal pseudoobstruction
	Peripheral antidopaminergic	Domperidone	Gastroparesis
	Somatostatin analogue	Octreotide	Intestinal pseudoobstruction
	Acetylcholinesterase inhibitor	Pyridostigmine	?Small intestinal dysmotility /pseudoobstruction
Special settings	Benzodiazepines	Lorazepam	Anticipatory nausea and vomiting with chemotherapy
	Glucocorticoids	Methylprednisolone, dexamethasone	Chemotherapy-induced emesis
	Cannabinoids	Tetrahydrocannabinol	Chemotherapy-induced emesis

Abbreviation: ?, indication is uncertain.

prevent chemotherapy-induced acute vomiting in most cases (Table 5-2). Optimal antiemetic effects often are obtained with a $5\text{-}HT_3$ antagonist combined with a glucocorticoid. Benzodiazepines such as lorazepam are useful to reduce anticipatory nausea and vomiting. Therapy of delayed emesis 1–5 days after chemotherapy is less successful. Neurokinin NK_1 antagonists (e.g., aprepitant) exhibit antiemetic and antinausea effects during both the acute and delayed periods after chemotherapy. Cannabinoids such as tetrahydrocannabinol, long advocated for cancer-associated emesis, produce significant side effects and exhibit no more efficacy than antidopaminergic agents. Most antiemetic regimens produce greater reductions in vomiting than in nausea.

The clinician should exercise caution in managing the pregnant patient with nausea. Studies of the teratogenic effects of available antiemetic agents provide conflicting results. Few controlled trials have been performed in nausea of pregnancy, although antihistamines such as meclizine and antidopaminergics such as prochlorperazine demonstrate efficacy greater than placebo. Some obstetricians offer alternative therapies such as pyridoxine, acupressure, or ginger.

Controlling emesis in cyclic vomiting syndrome is a challenge. In many patients, prophylaxis with tricyclic antidepressants, cyproheptadine, or β-adrenoceptor antagonists can reduce the frequency of attacks. Intravenous $5\text{-}HT_3$ antagonists combined with the sedating effects of a benzodiazepine such as lorazepam are a mainstay of treatment of acute symptom flares. Small studies report benefits with antimigraine therapies, including the serotonin $5\text{-}HT_1$ agonist sumatriptan, as well as selected anticonvulsant drugs such as zonisamide and levetiracetam.

INDIGESTION

MECHANISMS

The most common causes of indigestion are gastroesophageal reflux and functional dyspepsia. Other cases are a consequence of a more serious organic illness.

Gastroesophageal reflux

Gastroesophageal reflux can result from a variety of physiologic defects. Reduced lower esophageal sphincter (LES) tone is an important cause of reflux in scleroderma and pregnancy; it may also be a factor in patients without other systemic conditions. Many individuals exhibit frequent transient LES relaxations during which acid or nonacidic fluid bathes the esophagus. Overeating and aerophagia can transiently override the barrier function of the LES, whereas impaired esophageal body motility and reduced salivary secretion prolong fluid exposure. The role of hiatal hernias is controversial—although most reflux patients exhibit hiatal hernias, most individuals with hiatal hernias do not have excess heartburn.

Gastric motor dysfunction

Disturbed gastric motility is purported to cause gastroesophageal reflux in some cases of indigestion. Delayed gastric emptying is also found in 25–50% of functional dyspeptics. The relation of these defects to symptom induction is uncertain; studies show poor correlation between symptom severity and degrees of motor dysfunction. Impaired gastric fundus relaxation after eating may underlie selected dyspeptic symptoms like bloating, nausea, and early satiety.

Visceral afferent hypersensitivity

Disturbed gastric sensory function is proposed as a pathogenic factor in functional dyspepsia. Visceral afferent hypersensitivity was first demonstrated in patients with IBS who had heightened perception of rectal balloon inflation without changes in rectal compliance. Similarly, dyspeptic patients experience discomfort with fundic distention to lower pressures than healthy controls. Some patients with heartburn exhibit no increase in reflux of acid or nonacidic fluid. These individuals with functional heartburn are believed to have heightened perception of normal esophageal pH and volume.

Other factors

Helicobacter pylori has a clear etiologic role in peptic ulcer disease, but ulcers cause a minority of cases of dyspepsia. *H. pylori* is considered to be a minor factor in the genesis of functional dyspepsia. In contrast, functional dyspepsia is associated with a reduced sense of physical and mental well-being and is exacerbated by stress, suggesting important roles for psychological factors. Analgesics cause dyspepsia, while nitrates, calcium channel blockers, theophylline, and progesterone promote gastroesophageal reflux. Other stimuli that induce reflux include ethanol, tobacco, and caffeine via LES relaxation. Genetic factors may promote development of reflux.

DIFFERENTIAL DIAGNOSIS
Gastroesophageal reflux disease

Gastroesophageal reflux disease (GERD) is prevalent in Western society. Heartburn is reported once monthly by 40% of Americans and daily by 7–10%. Most cases of heartburn occur because of excess acid reflux, although reflux of non acidic fluid may produce similar symptoms. Alkaline reflux esophagitis produces GERD-like symptoms most often in patients who have had surgery for peptic ulcer disease. Approximately 10% of patients with heartburn of a functional nature exhibit normal degrees of esophageal acid exposure and no increase in nonacidic reflux.

Functional dyspepsia

Nearly 25% of the populace has dyspepsia at least 6 times yearly, but only 10–20% of these individuals present to physicians. Functional dyspepsia, the cause of symptoms in 60% of dyspeptic patients, is defined as ≥3 months of bothersome postprandial fullness, early satiety, or epigastric pain or burning with symptom onset at least 6 months before diagnosis in the absence of organic cause. Most cases follow a benign course, but some patients with *H. pylori* infection or on nonsteroidal anti-inflammatory drugs (NSAIDs) develop ulcers. As with idiopathic gastroparesis, some cases of functional dyspepsia result from prior gastrointestinal infection.

Ulcer disease

In most cases of GERD, there is no destruction of the esophagus. However, 5% of patients develop esophageal ulcers, and some form strictures. Symptoms do not reliably distinguish nonerosive from erosive or ulcerative esophagitis. Some 15–25% of cases of dyspepsia stem from ulcers of the stomach or duodenum. The most common causes of ulcer disease are gastric infection with *H. pylori* and use of NSAIDs. Other rare causes of gastroduodenal ulcer include Crohn's disease (Chap. 17) and Zollinger-Ellison syndrome (Chap. 14), a condition resulting from gastrin overproduction by an endocrine tumor.

Malignancy

Dyspeptic patients often seek care because of fear of cancer. However, <2% of cases result from gastroesophageal malignancy. Esophageal squamous cell carcinoma occurs most often in those with histories of tobacco or ethanol intake. Other risk factors include prior caustic ingestion, achalasia, and the hereditary disorder tylosis. Esophageal adenocarcinoma usually complicates long-standing acid reflux. Between 8 and 20% of GERD patients exhibit intestinal metaplasia of the esophagus, termed *Barrett's metaplasia*. This condition predisposes to esophageal adenocarcinoma (Chap. 49). Gastric malignancies include adenocarcinoma, which is prevalent in certain Asian societies, and lymphoma.

Other causes

Opportunistic fungal or viral esophageal infections may produce heartburn or chest discomfort but more often cause odynophagia. Other causes of esophageal inflammation include eosinophilic esophagitis and pill esophagitis. Biliary colic is in the differential diagnosis of dyspepsia, but most patients with true biliary colic report discrete episodes of right upper quadrant or epigastric pain rather than chronic burning discomfort, nausea, and bloating. Intestinal lactase deficiency produces gas, bloating, discomfort, and diarrhea after lactose ingestion. Lactase deficiency occurs in 15–25% of whites of northern European descent but is more common in blacks and Asians. Intolerance of other carbohydrates (e.g., fructose, sorbitol) produces similar symptoms. Small-intestinal bacterial overgrowth may produce dyspepsia, often with bowel dysfunction, distention, and malabsorption. Eosinophilic infiltration of the duodenal mucosa is described in some cases of dyspepsia. Pancreatic disease (chronic pancreatitis and malignancy), hepatocellular carcinoma, celiac disease, Ménétrier's disease, infiltrative diseases (sarcoidosis and eosinophilic gastroenteritis), mesenteric ischemia, thyroid and parathyroid disease, and abdominal wall strain cause dyspepsia. Extraperitoneal etiologies of indigestion include congestive heart failure and tuberculosis. Investigation is ongoing into genetic markers that predispose to developing functional dyspepsia.

APPROACH TO THE PATIENT | **Indigestion**

HISTORY AND PHYSICAL EXAMINATION

Care of the patient with indigestion requires a thorough interview. GERD classically produces heartburn, a substernal warmth in the epigastrium that moves toward the neck. Heartburn often is exacerbated by meals and may awaken the patient. Associated symptoms include regurgitation of acid or nonacidic fluid and water brash, the reflex release of salty salivary secretions into the mouth. Atypical symptoms include pharyngitis, asthma, cough, bronchitis, hoarseness, and chest pain that mimics angina. Some patients with acid reflux on esophageal pH testing do not report heartburn, but note abdominal pain or other symptoms.

Some patients with dyspepsia report a predominance of epigastric pain or burning that is intermittent and not generalized or localized to other regions. Others experience a postprandial distress syndrome characterized by fullness occurring after normal-sized meals and early satiety that prevents completion of regular meals, with associated bloating, belching, or nausea. Functional dyspepsia overlaps with other functional disorders such as IBS.

The physical exam with GERD and functional dyspepsia usually is normal. In atypical GERD, pharyngeal erythema and wheezing may be noted. Recurrent acid regurgitation may cause poor dentition. Functional dyspeptics may report epigastric tenderness or distention.

Discrimination between functional and organic causes of indigestion mandates exclusion of selected historic and examination features. Odynophagia suggests esophageal infection, while dysphagia is worrisome for a benign or malignant esophageal blockage. Other alarming features include unexplained weight loss, recurrent vomiting, occult or gross gastrointestinal bleeding, jaundice, a palpable mass or adenopathy, and a family history of gastrointestinal malignancy.

DIAGNOSTIC TESTING Because indigestion is prevalent and most cases result from GERD or functional dyspepsia, a general principle is to perform only limited and directed diagnostic testing of selected individuals.

Once alarm factors are excluded (Table 5-3), patients with typical GERD do not need further evaluation and are treated empirically. Upper endoscopy is indicated to exclude mucosal injury in cases with atypical symptoms, symptoms unresponsive to acid suppressing drugs, or alarm factors. For heartburn >5 years in duration, especially in patients >50 years old, endoscopy is recommended to screen for Barrett's metaplasia. However, the clinical benefits and cost-effectiveness of this approach have not been validated in controlled studies. Ambulatory esophageal pH testing using a catheter method or an implanted esophageal capsule device is considered for drug-refractory symptoms and atypical symptoms like unexplained chest pain. Esophageal manometry most commonly is ordered when surgical treatment of GERD is considered. A low LES pressure may predict failure of drug therapy and helps select patients who may require surgery. Demonstration of disordered esophageal body peristalsis may affect the decision to operate or modify the type

TABLE 5-3

ALARM SYMPTOMS IN GERD
Odynophagia
Unexplained weight loss
Recurrent vomiting
Occult or gross gastrointestinal bleeding
Jaundice
Palpable mass or adenopathy
Family history of gastrointestinal malignancy

of operation chosen. High-resolution manometric methods improve characterization of ineffective esophageal propulsion, which may contribute to impaired esophageal acid clearance in some GERD patients. Manometry with provocative testing may clarify the diagnosis in patients with atypical symptoms. Blind perfusion of saline and then acid into the esophagus, known as the *Bernstein test*, can delineate whether unexplained chest discomfort results from acid reflux. Nonacidic reflux may be suggested by nuclear medicine reflux scanning or detected by combined esophageal impedance-pH testing, which increases the diagnostic yield by 15% versus pH testing alone. Ambulatory measurement of esophageal bilirubin levels facilitates diagnosis of alkaline reflux.

Upper endoscopy is performed as the initial diagnostic test in patients with unexplained dyspepsia who are >55 years old or who have alarm factors because of the elevated risks of malignancy and ulcer in these groups. The management approach to patients <55 years old without alarm factors is dependent on the local prevalence of *H. pylori* infection. For individuals in regions with low *H. pylori* prevalence (<10%), a 4-week trial of an acid-suppressing medication such as a proton pump inhibitor is recommended. If this fails, a "test and treat" approach is most commonly applied. *H. pylori* status is determined with urea breath testing, stool antigen measurement, or blood serology testing. Those who are *H. pylori* positive are given therapy to eradicate the infection. If symptoms resolve on either regimen, no further intervention is required. For patients in areas with high *H. pylori* prevalence (>10%), an initial test and treat approach is advocated, with a subsequent trial of an acid-suppressing regimen offered for those in whom *H. pylori* treatment fails or for those who are negative for the infection. In each of these patient subsets, upper endoscopy is reserved for those whose symptoms fail to respond to therapy.

Further testing is indicated if other factors are present. If bleeding is reported, a blood count is obtained to exclude anemia. Thyroid chemistries or calcium levels screen for metabolic disease, whereas serologies may suggest celiac disease. For possible pancreaticobiliary causes, pancreatic and liver chemistries are obtained. If abnormalities are found, ultrasound or CT may give important information. Gastric emptying measurement is considered to exclude gastroparesis in patients whose dyspeptic symptoms resemble postprandial distress when drug therapy fails. Gastric scintigraphy also assesses for gastroparesis in patients with GERD, especially if surgical intervention is being considered. Breath testing after carbohydrate ingestion may detect lactase deficiency, intolerance to other carbohydrates, or small-intestinal bacterial overgrowth.

TREATMENT General Principles

For mild indigestion, reassurance that a careful evaluation revealed no serious organic disease may be the only intervention needed. Drugs that cause gastroesophageal reflux or dyspepsia should be stopped, if possible. Patients with GERD should limit ethanol, caffeine, chocolate, and tobacco use because of their effects on the LES. Other measures in GERD include ingesting a low-fat diet, avoiding snacks before bedtime, and elevating the head of the bed.

Specific therapies for organic disease should be offered when possible. Surgery is appropriate in disorders like biliary colic, while diet changes are indicated for lactase deficiency or celiac disease. Some illnesses such as peptic ulcer disease may be cured by specific medical regimens. However, because most indigestion is caused by GERD or functional dyspepsia, medications that reduce gastric acid, modulate motility, or blunt gastric sensitivity are indicated.

ACID-SUPPRESSING OR -NEUTRALIZING MEDICATIONS Drugs that reduce or neutralize gastric acid are often prescribed for GERD. Histamine H_2 antagonists such as cimetidine, ranitidine, famotidine, and nizatidine are useful in mild to moderate GERD. For severe symptoms or for many cases of erosive or ulcerative esophagitis, proton pump inhibitors such as omeprazole, lansoprazole, rabeprazole, pantoprazole, esomeprazole, or dexlansoprazole are needed. These drugs, which inhibit gastric H^+, K^+-ATPase, are more potent than H_2 antagonists. Up to one-third of GERD patients do not respond to proton pump inhibitors; one-third of these patients have nonacidic reflux while 10% have persistent acid-related disease. Acid suppressants may be taken continuously or on demand depending on symptom severity. Infrequent potential complications of long-term proton pump inhibitors may include infection, small intestinal bacterial overgrowth, nutrient deficiency (vitamin B_{12}, iron, calcium), bone demineralization, and impaired medication absorption (e.g. clopidogrel). Many patients started on a proton pump inhibitor can be stepped down to an H_2 antagonist. Combining a proton pump inhibitor with an H_2 antagonist is provided for some refractory cases.

Acid-suppressing drugs are also effective in appropriately selected patients with functional dyspepsia. Meta-analysis of eight controlled trials calculated a risk ratio of 0.86, with a 95% confidence interval of 0.78–0.95, favoring proton pump inhibitor therapy over placebo. The benefits of less potent acid-reducing therapies such as H_2 antagonists are unproven.

Liquid antacids are useful for short-term control of mild GERD but are less effective for severe disease unless given at high doses that elicit side effects (diarrhea and constipation with magnesium- and aluminum-containing agents, respectively). Alginic acid in combination with antacids may form a floating barrier to acid reflux in individuals with upright symptoms. Sucralfate is a salt of aluminum hydroxide and sucrose octasulfate that buffers acid and binds pepsin and bile salts. Its efficacy in GERD is felt to be comparable to that of H$_2$ antagonists.

HELICOBACTER PYLORI ERADICATION

H. pylori eradication is clearly indicated only for peptic ulcer and mucosa-associated lymphoid tissue gastric lymphoma. The utility of eradication therapy in functional dyspepsia is less well established, but <15% of cases relate to this infection. Meta-analysis of 13 controlled trials calculated a risk ratio of 0.91, with a 95% confidence interval of 0.87–0.96, favoring *H. pylori* eradication therapy over placebo. Several drug combinations show efficacy in eliminating the infection (Chap. 14); most include 10–14 days of a proton pump inhibitor or bismuth subsalicylate in concert with two antibiotics. *H. pylori* infection is associated with reduced prevalence of GERD, especially in the elderly. However, eradication of the infection does not worsen GERD symptoms. To date, no consensus recommendations regarding *H. pylori* eradication in GERD patients have been offered.

AGENTS THAT MODIFY GASTROINTESTINAL MOTOR ACTIVITY

Motor stimulants (also known as prokinetics) such as metoclopramide, erythromycin, and domperidone have limited utility in GERD. Several studies have evaluated the effectiveness of motor-stimulating drugs in functional dyspepsia; however, convincing evidence of their benefits has not been found. Some clinicians suggest that patients with symptoms resembling postprandial distress may respond preferentially to prokinetic drugs. The γ-aminobutyric acid B (GABA-B) agonist baclofen reduces esophageal exposure to acid and non acidic fluids by inhibiting transient LES relaxations; this drug is proposed for refractory acid and non acid reflux.

OTHER OPTIONS

Antireflux surgery (fundoplication) is most often offered to GERD patients who are young and may require lifelong therapy, have typical heartburn and regurgitation, and are responsive to proton pump inhibitors. Surgery also is effective for some cases of non acidic reflux. Individuals who may respond less well to operative therapy include those with atypical symptoms and those who have esophageal body motor disturbances. Fundoplications are performed laparoscopically when possible and include the Nissen and Toupet procedures in which the proximal stomach is partly or completely wrapped around the distal esophagus to increase LES pressure. Dysphagia, gas-bloat syndrome, and gastroparesis may be long-term complications of these procedures. The utility and safety of endoscopic therapies for increasing the barrier function of the gastroesophageal junction, including radiofrequency energy delivery and gastroplication, have not been fully investigated for patients with refractory GERD.

Some patients with functional heartburn and functional dyspepsia refractory to standard therapies may respond to low-dose antidepressants in tricyclic and other classes. Their mechanism of action is unknown but may involve blunting of visceral pain processing in the brain. Gas and bloating are among the most troubling symptoms in some patients with indigestion and can be difficult to treat. Dietary exclusion of gas-producing foods such as legumes and use of simethicone or activated charcoal provide benefits in some cases. Therapies that modify gut flora, including antibiotics and probiotic preparations containing active bacterial cultures, are useful for cases of bacterial overgrowth and functional lower gastrointestinal disorders, but their utility in functional dyspepsia is unproven. Psychological treatments may be offered for refractory functional dyspepsia, but no convincing data suggest their efficacy.

CHAPTER 6

DIARRHEA AND CONSTIPATION

Michael Camilleri ■ Joseph A. Murray

Diarrhea and constipation are exceedingly common and, together, exact an enormous toll in terms of mortality, morbidity, social inconvenience, loss of work productivity, and consumption of medical resources. Worldwide, >1 billion individuals suffer one or more episodes of acute diarrhea each year. Among the 100 million persons affected annually by acute diarrhea in the United States, nearly half must restrict activities, 10% consult physicians, ~250,000 require hospitalization, and ~5000 die (primarily the elderly). The annual economic burden to society may exceed $20 billion. Acute infectious diarrhea remains one of the most common causes of mortality in developing countries, particularly among children, accounting for 2–3 million deaths per year. Constipation, by contrast, is rarely associated with mortality and is exceedingly common in developed countries, leading to frequent self-medication and, in a third of those, to medical consultation. Population statistics on chronic diarrhea and constipation are more uncertain, perhaps due to variable definitions and reporting, but the frequency of these conditions is also high. United States population surveys put prevalence rates for chronic diarrhea at 2–7% and for chronic constipation at 12–19%, with women being affected twice as often as men. Diarrhea and constipation are among the most common patient complaints faced by internists and primary care physicians, and they account for nearly 50% of referrals to gastroenterologists.

Although diarrhea and constipation may present as mere nuisance symptoms at one extreme, they can be severe or life-threatening at the other. Even mild symptoms may signal a serious underlying gastrointestinal lesion, such as colorectal cancer, or systemic disorder, such as thyroid disease. Given the heterogeneous causes and potential severity of these common complaints, it is imperative for clinicians to appreciate the pathophysiology, etiologic classification, diagnostic strategies, and principles of management of diarrhea and constipation, so that rational and cost-effective care can be delivered.

NORMAL PHYSIOLOGY

While the primary function of the small intestine is the digestion and assimilation of nutrients from food, the small intestine and colon together perform important functions that regulate the secretion and absorption of water and electrolytes, the storage and subsequent transport of intraluminal contents aborally, and the salvage of some nutrients after bacterial metabolism of carbohydrate that are not absorbed in the small intestine. The main motor functions are summarized in **Table 6-1**. Alterations in fluid and electrolyte handling contribute significantly to diarrhea. Alterations in motor and sensory functions of the colon result in highly prevalent syndromes such as irritable bowel syndrome (IBS), chronic diarrhea, and chronic constipation.

NEURAL CONTROL

The small intestine and colon have intrinsic and extrinsic innervation. The *intrinsic innervation*, also called the

TABLE 6-1

NORMAL GASTROINTESTINAL MOTILITY: FUNCTIONS AT DIFFERENT ANATOMIC LEVELS
Stomach and small bowel
Synchronized MMC in fasting
Accommodation, trituration, mixing, transit
Stomach ~3 h
Small bowel ~3 h
Ileal reservoir empties boluses
Colon: irregular mixing, fermentation, absorption, transit
Ascending, transverse: reservoirs
Descending: conduit
Sigmoid/rectum: volitional reservoir

Abbreviation: MMC, migrating motor complex.

enteric nervous system, comprises myenteric, submucosal, and mucosal neuronal layers. The function of these layers is modulated by interneurons through the actions of neurotransmitter amines or peptides, including acetylcholine, vasoactive intestinal peptide (VIP), opioids, norepinephrine, serotonin, adenosine triphosphate (ATP), and nitric oxide (NO). The myenteric plexus regulates smooth-muscle function, and the submucosal plexus affects secretion, absorption, and mucosal blood flow.

The *extrinsic innervations* of the small intestine and colon are part of the autonomic nervous system and also modulate motor and secretory functions. The parasympathetic nerves convey visceral sensory and excitatory pathways to the colon. Parasympathetic fibers via the vagus nerve reach the small intestine and proximal colon along the branches of the superior mesenteric artery. The distal colon is supplied by sacral parasympathetic nerves (S_{2-4}) via the pelvic plexus; these fibers course through the wall of the colon as ascending intracolonic fibers as far as, and in some instances including, the proximal colon. The chief excitatory neurotransmitters controlling motor function are acetylcholine and the tachykinins, such as substance P. The sympathetic nerve supply modulates motor functions and reaches the small intestine and colon alongside their arterial vessels. Sympathetic input to the gut is generally excitatory to sphincters and inhibitory to nonsphincteric muscle. Visceral afferents convey sensation from the gut to the central nervous system (CNS); initially, they course along sympathetic fibers, but as they approach the spinal cord they separate, have cell bodies in the dorsal root ganglion, and enter the dorsal horn of the spinal cord. Afferent signals are conveyed to the brain along the lateral spinothalamic tract and the nociceptive dorsal column pathway and are then projected beyond the thalamus and brainstem to the insula and cerebral cortex to be perceived. Other afferent fibers synapse in the prevertebral ganglia and reflexly modulate intestinal motility.

INTESTINAL FLUID ABSORPTION AND SECRETION

On an average day, 9 L of fluid enter the gastrointestinal (GI) tract, ~1 L of residual fluid reaches the colon, and the stool excretion of fluid constitutes about 0.2 L/d. The colon has a large capacitance and functional reserve and may recover up to four times its usual volume of 0.8 L/d, provided the rate of flow permits reabsorption to occur. Thus, the colon can partially compensate for excess fluid delivery to the colon because of intestinal absorptive or secretory disorders.

In the colon, sodium absorption is predominantly electrogenic, and uptake takes place at the apical membrane; it is compensated for by the export functions of the basolateral sodium pump. A variety of neural and non-neural mediators regulate colonic fluid and electrolyte balance, including cholinergic, adrenergic, and serotonergic mediators. Angiotensin and aldosterone also influence colonic absorption, reflecting the common embryologic development of the distal colonic epithelium and the renal tubules.

SMALL-INTESTINAL MOTILITY

During fasting, the motility of the small intestine is characterized by a cyclical event called the migrating motor complex (MMC), which serves to clear nondigestible residue from the small intestine (the intestinal "housekeeper"). This organized, propagated series of contractions last, on average, 4 min, occur every 60–90 min, and usually involve the entire small intestine. After food ingestion, the small intestine produces irregular, mixing contractions of relatively low amplitude, except in the distal ileum where more powerful contractions occur intermittently and empty the ileum by bolus transfers.

ILEOCOLONIC STORAGE AND SALVAGE

The distal ileum acts as a reservoir, emptying intermittently by bolus movements. This action allows time for salvage of fluids, electrolytes, and nutrients. Segmentation by haustra compartmentalizes the colon and facilitates mixing, retention of residue, and formation of solid stools. There is increased appreciation of the intimate interaction between the colonic function and the luminal ecology. The resident bacteria in the colon are necessary for the digestion of unabsorbed carbohydrates that reach the colon even in health, thereby providing a vital source of nutrients to the mucosa. Normal colonic flora also keeps pathogens at bay by a variety of mechanisms. In health, the ascending and transverse regions of colon function as reservoirs (average transit, 15 h), and the descending colon acts as a conduit (average transit, 3 h). The colon is efficient at conserving sodium and water, a function that is particularly important in sodium-depleted patients in whom the small intestine alone is unable to maintain sodium balance. Diarrhea or constipation may result from alteration in the reservoir function of the proximal colon or the propulsive function of the left colon. Constipation may also result from disturbances of the rectal or sigmoid reservoir, typically as a result of dysfunction of the pelvic floor, the anal sphincters, or the coordination of defecation.

COLONIC MOTILITY AND TONE

The small intestinal MMC only rarely continues into the colon. However, short duration or phasic contractions mix colonic contents, and high-amplitude

(>75 mmHg) propagated contractions (HAPCs) are sometimes associated with mass movements through the colon and normally occur approximately five times per day, usually on awakening in the morning and post-prandially. Increased frequency of HAPCs may result in diarrhea or urgency. The predominant phasic contractions in the colon are irregular and nonpropagated and serve a "mixing" function.

Colonic tone refers to the background contractility upon which phasic contractile activity (typically contractions lasting <15 s) is superimposed. It is an important cofactor in the colon's capacitance (volume accommodation) and sensation.

COLONIC MOTILITY AFTER MEAL INGESTION

After meal ingestion, colonic phasic and tonic contractility increase for a period of ~2 h. The initial phase (~10 min) is mediated by the vagus nerve in response to mechanical distention of the stomach. The subsequent response of the colon requires caloric stimulation and is mediated at least in part by hormones (e.g., gastrin and serotonin).

DEFECATION

Tonic contraction of the puborectalis muscle, which forms a sling around the rectoanal junction, is important to maintain continence; during defecation, sacral parasympathetic nerves relax this muscle, facilitating the straightening of the rectoanal angle (**Fig. 6-1**).

Distention of the rectum results in transient relaxation of the internal anal sphincter via intrinsic and reflex sympathetic innervation. As sigmoid and rectal contractions increase the pressure within the rectum, the rectosigmoid angle opens by >15°. Voluntary relaxation of the external anal sphincter (striated muscle innervated by the pudendal nerve) in response to the sensation produced by distention permits the evacuation of feces; this evacuation process can be augmented by an increase in intraabdominal pressure created by the Valsalva maneuver. Defecation can also be delayed voluntarily by contraction of the external anal sphincter.

DIARRHEA

DEFINITION

Diarrhea is loosely defined as passage of abnormally liquid or unformed stools at an increased frequency. For adults on a typical Western diet, stool weight >200 g/d can generally be considered diarrheal. Diarrhea may be further defined as *acute* if <2 weeks, *persistent* if 2–4 weeks, and *chronic* if >4 weeks in duration.

Two common conditions, usually associated with the passage of stool totaling <200 g/d, must be distinguished from diarrhea, because diagnostic and therapeutic algorithms differ. *Pseudodiarrhea*, or the frequent passage of small volumes of stool, is often associated with rectal urgency and accompanies IBS or proctitis. *Fecal incontinence* is the involuntary discharge of rectal contents and is most often caused by neuromuscular

FIGURE 6-1

Sagittal view of the anorectum (A) at rest and (B) during straining to defecate. Continence is maintained by normal rectal sensation and tonic contraction of the internal anal sphincter and the puborectalis muscle, which wraps around the anorectum, maintaining an anorectal angle between 80° and 110°. During defecation, the pelvic floor muscles (including the puborectalis) relax, allowing the anorectal angle to straighten by at least 15°, and the perineum descends by 1–3.5 cm. The external anal sphincter also relaxes and reduces pressure on the anal canal. (*Reproduced with permission from A Lembo, M Camilleri: N Engl J Med 349:1360, 2003.*)

disorders or structural anorectal problems. Diarrhea and urgency, especially if severe, may aggravate or cause incontinence. Pseudodiarrhea and fecal incontinence occur at prevalence rates comparable to or higher than that of chronic diarrhea and should always be considered in patients complaining of "diarrhea." Overflow diarrhea may occur in nursing home patients due to fecal impaction that is readily detectable by rectal examination. A careful history and physical examination generally allow these conditions to be discriminated from true diarrhea.

ACUTE DIARRHEA

More than 90% of cases of acute diarrhea are caused by infectious agents; these cases are often accompanied by vomiting, fever, and abdominal pain. The remaining 10% or so are caused by medications, toxic ingestions, ischemia, and other conditions.

Infectious agents

Most infectious diarrheas are acquired by fecal-oral transmission or, more commonly, via ingestion of food or water contaminated with pathogens from human or animal feces. In the immunocompetent person, the resident fecal microflora, containing >500 taxonomically distinct species, are rarely the source of diarrhea and may actually play a role in suppressing the growth of ingested pathogens. Disturbances of flora by antibiotics can lead to diarrhea by reducing the digestive function or by allowing the overgrowth of pathogens, such as *Clostridium difficile* (Chap. 24). Acute infection or injury occurs when the ingested agent overwhelms or bypasses the host's mucosal immune and nonimmune (gastric acid, digestive enzymes, mucus secretion, peristalsis, and suppressive resident flora) defenses. Established clinical associations with specific enteropathogens may offer diagnostic clues.

In the United States, five high-risk groups are recognized:

1. *Travelers.* Nearly 40% of tourists to endemic regions of Latin America, Africa, and Asia develop so-called traveler's diarrhea, most commonly due to enterotoxigenic or enteroaggregative *Escherichia coli* as well as to *Campylobacter, Shigella, Aeromonas,* norovirus, *Coronavirus,* and *Salmonella.* Visitors to Russia (especially St. Petersburg) may have increased risk of *Giardia*-associated diarrhea; visitors to Nepal may acquire *Cyclospora.* Campers, backpackers, and swimmers in wilderness areas may become infected with *Giardia.* Cruise ships may be affected by outbreaks of gastroenteritis caused by agents such as norovirus.

2. *Consumers of certain foods.* Diarrhea closely following food consumption at a picnic, banquet, or restaurant

may suggest infection with *Salmonella, Campylobacter,* or *Shigella* from chicken; enterohemorrhagic *E. coli* (O157:H7) from undercooked hamburger; *Bacillus cereus* from fried rice or other reheated food; *Staphylococcus aureus* or *Salmonella* from mayonnaise or creams; *Salmonella* from eggs; *Listeria* from uncooked foods or soft cheeses; and *Vibrio* species, *Salmonella,* or acute hepatitis A from seafood, especially if raw.

3. *Immunodeficient persons.* Individuals at risk for diarrhea include those with either primary immunodeficiency (e.g., IgA deficiency, common variable hypogammaglobulinemia, chronic granulomatous disease) or the much more common secondary immunodeficiency states (e.g., AIDS, senescence, pharmacologic suppression). Common enteric pathogens often cause a more severe and protracted diarrheal illness, and, particularly in persons with AIDS, opportunistic infections, such as by *Mycobacterium* species, certain viruses (cytomegalovirus, adenovirus, and herpes simplex), and protozoa (*Cryptosporidium, Isospora belli,* Microsporida, and *Blastocystis hominis*) may also play a role. In patients with AIDS, agents transmitted venereally per rectum (e.g., *Neisseria gonorrhoeae, Treponema pallidum, Chlamydia*) may contribute to proctocolitis. Persons with hemochromatosis are especially prone to invasive, even fatal, enteric infections with *Vibrio* species and *Yersinia* infections and should avoid raw fish.

4. *Daycare attendees and their family members.* Infections with *Shigella, Giardia, Cryptosporidium,* rotavirus, and other agents are very common and should be considered.

5. *Institutionalized persons.* Infectious diarrhea is one of the most frequent categories of nosocomial infections in many hospitals and long-term care facilities; the causes are a variety of microorganisms but most commonly *C. difficile.* *C. difficile* can affect those with no history of antibiotic use and may be acquired in the community.

The pathophysiology underlying acute diarrhea by infectious agents produces specific clinical features that may also be helpful in diagnosis (Table 6-2). Profuse, watery diarrhea secondary to small-bowel hypersecretion occurs with ingestion of preformed bacterial toxins, enterotoxin-producing bacteria, and enteroadherent pathogens. Diarrhea associated with marked vomiting and minimal or no fever may occur abruptly within a few hours after ingestion of the former two types; vomiting is usually less, abdominal cramping or bloating is greater, and fever is higher with the latter. Cytotoxin-producing and invasive microorganisms all cause high fever and abdominal pain. Invasive bacteria and *Entamoeba histolytica* often cause bloody diarrhea (referred to as *dysentery*). *Yersinia* invades the terminal ileal and proximal colon mucosa and may cause

TABLE 6-2

ASSOCIATION BETWEEN PATHOBIOLOGY OF CAUSATIVE AGENTS AND CLINICAL FEATURES IN ACUTE INFECTIOUS DIARRHEA

PATHOBIOLOGY/AGENTS	INCUBATION PERIOD	VOMITING	ABDOMINAL PAIN	FEVER	DIARRHEA
Toxin producers					
Preformed toxin					
Bacillus cereus, Staphylococcus aureus,	1–8 h	3–4+	1–2+	0–1+	3–4+, watery
Clostridium perfringens	8–24 h				
Enterotoxin					
Vibrio cholerae, enterotoxigenic Escherichia coli, Klebsiella pneumoniae, Aeromonas species	8–72 h	2–4+	1–2+	0–1+	3–4+, watery
Enteroadherent					
Enteropathogenic and enteroadherent E. coli, Giardia organisms, cryptosporidiosis, helminths	1–8 d	0–1+	1–3+	0–2+	1–2+, watery, mushy
Cytotoxin producers					
C. difficile	1–3 d	0–1+	3–4+	1–2+	1–3+, usually watery, occasionally bloody
Hemorrhagic E. coli	12–72 h	0–1+	3–4+	1–2+	1–3+, initially watery, quickly bloody
Invasive organisms					
Minimal inflammation					
Rotavirus and norovirus	1–3 d	1–3+	2–3+	3–4+	1–3+, watery
Variable inflammation					
Salmonella, Campylobacter, and Aeromonas species, Vibrio parahae-molyticus, Yersinia	12 h–11 d	0–3+	2–4+	3–4+	1–4+, watery or bloody
Severe inflammation					
Shigella species, enteroinvasive E. coli, Entamoeba histolytica	12 h–8 d	0–1+	3–4+	3–4+	1–2+, bloody

Source: Adapted from DW Powell, in T Yamada (ed): *Textbook of Gastroenterology and Hepatology*, 4th ed. Philadelphia, Lippincott Williams & Wilkins, 2003.

especially severe abdominal pain with tenderness mimicking acute appendicitis.

Finally, infectious diarrhea may be associated with systemic manifestations. Reactive arthritis (formerly known as Reiter's syndrome), arthritis, urethritis, and conjunctivitis may accompany or follow infections by *Salmonella*, *Campylobacter*, *Shigella*, and *Yersinia*. Yersiniosis may also lead to an autoimmune-type thyroiditis, pericarditis, and glomerulonephritis. Both enterohemorrhagic *E. coli* (O157:H7) and *Shigella* can lead to the *hemolytic-uremic syndrome* with an attendant high mortality rate. The syndrome of postinfectious IBS has now been recognized as a complication of infectious diarrhea. Acute diarrhea can also be a major symptom of several systemic infections including *viral hepatitis*, *listeriosis*, *legionellosis*, and *toxic shock syndrome*.

Other causes

Side effects from medications are probably the most common noninfectious causes of acute diarrhea, and etiology may be suggested by a temporal association between use and symptom onset. Although innumerable medications may produce diarrhea, some of the more frequently incriminated include antibiotics, cardiac antidysrhythmics, antihypertensives, nonsteroidal anti-inflammatory drugs (NSAIDs), certain antidepressants, chemotherapeutic agents, bronchodilators, antacids, and laxatives. Occlusive or nonocclusive *ischemic colitis* typically occurs in persons >50 years; often presents as acute lower abdominal pain preceding watery, then bloody diarrhea; and generally results in acute inflammatory changes in the sigmoid or left colon while sparing the rectum. Acute diarrhea may accompany colonic *diverticulitis* and *graft-versus-host disease*. Acute diarrhea, often associated with systemic compromise, can follow ingestion of toxins including organophosphate insecticides; amanita and other mushrooms; arsenic; and preformed environmental toxins in seafood, such as ciguatera and scombroid. Acute anaphylaxis to food ingestion can have a similar presentation. Conditions causing chronic diarrhea can also be confused with acute diarrhea early in their course. This confusion may occur with inflammatory bowel disease (IBD) and some of the other inflammatory chronic diarrheas that may have an abrupt rather than insidious onset and exhibit features that mimic infection.

APPROACH TO THE PATIENT | **Acute Diarrhea**

The decision to evaluate acute diarrhea depends on its severity and duration and on various host factors (Fig. 6-2). Most episodes of acute diarrhea are mild and self-limited and do not justify the cost and potential morbidity rate of diagnostic or pharmacologic interventions. Indications for evaluation include profuse diarrhea with dehydration, grossly bloody stools, fever ≥38.5°C (≥101°F), duration >48 h without improvement, recent antibiotic use, new community outbreaks, associated severe abdominal pain in patients >50 years, and elderly (≥70 years) or immunocompromised patients. In some cases of moderately severe febrile diarrhea associated with fecal leukocytes (or increased fecal levels of

the leukocyte proteins) or with gross blood, a diagnostic evaluation might be avoided in favor of an empirical antibiotic trial discussed later.

The cornerstone of diagnosis in those suspected of severe acute infectious diarrhea is microbiologic analysis of the stool. Workup includes cultures for bacterial and viral pathogens, direct inspection for ova and parasites, and immunoassays for certain bacterial toxins (*C. difficile*), viral antigens (rotavirus), and protozoal antigens (*Giardia*, *E. histolytica*). The aforementioned clinical and epidemiologic associations may assist in focusing the evaluation. If a particular pathogen or set of possible pathogens is so implicated, then either the whole panel of routine studies may not be necessary or, in some instances, special cultures may be appropriate as for enterohemorrhagic and other types of *E. coli*, *Vibrio* species, and *Yersinia*. Molecular diagnosis of pathogens in stool can be made by identification of unique DNA sequences; and evolving microarray technologies could lead to a more rapid, sensitive, specific, and cost-effective diagnostic approach in the future.

Persistent diarrhea is commonly due to *Giardia* (Chap. 32), but additional causative organisms that should be considered include *C. difficile* (especially if antibiotics had been administered), *E. histolytica*, *Cryptosporidium*, *Campylobacter*, and others. If stool studies are unrevealing, flexible sigmoidoscopy with biopsies and upper endoscopy with duodenal aspirates and biopsies may be indicated. Brainerd diarrhea is an increasingly recognized entity characterized by an abrupt-onset diarrhea that persists for at least 4 weeks, but may last 1–3 years, and is thought to be of infectious origin. It may be associated with subtle inflammation of the distal small intestine or proximal colon.

Structural examination by sigmoidoscopy, colonoscopy, or abdominal CT scanning (or other imaging approaches) may be appropriate in patients with uncharacterized persistent diarrhea to exclude IBD or as an initial approach in patients with suspected noninfectious acute diarrhea such as might be caused by ischemic colitis, diverticulitis, or partial bowel obstruction.

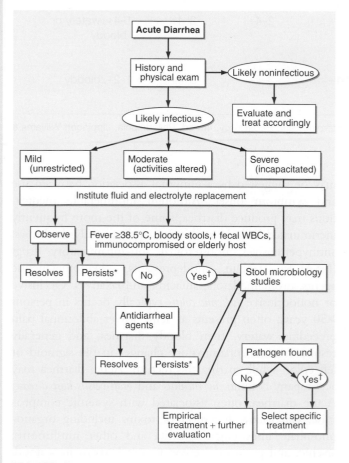

FIGURE 6-2
Algorithm for the management of acute diarrhea. Consider empirical Rx before evaluation with (*) metronidazole and with (†) quinolone. WBCs, white blood cells.

TREATMENT | **Acute Diarrhea**

Fluid and electrolyte replacement are of central importance to all forms of acute diarrhea. Fluid replacement alone may suffice for mild cases. Oral sugar-electrolyte solutions (sport drinks or designed formulations) should be instituted promptly with severe diarrhea to limit dehydration, which is the major cause of death. Profoundly dehydrated patients, especially infants and the elderly, require IV rehydration.

In moderately severe nonfebrile and nonbloody diarrhea, antimotility and antisecretory agents such as loperamide can be useful adjuncts to control symptoms. Such agents should be avoided with febrile dysentery, which may be exacerbated or prolonged by them. Bismuth subsalicylate may reduce symptoms of vomiting and diarrhea but should not be used to treat immunocompromised patients or those with renal impairment because of the risk of bismuth encephalopathy.

Judicious use of antibiotics is appropriate in selected instances of acute diarrhea and may reduce its severity and duration (Fig. 6-2). Many physicians treat moderately to severely ill patients with febrile dysentery empirically without diagnostic evaluation using a quinolone, such as ciprofloxacin (500 mg bid for 3–5 days). Empirical treatment can also be considered for suspected giardiasis with metronidazole (250 mg qid for 7 days). Selection of antibiotics and dosage regimens are otherwise dictated by specific pathogens, geographic patterns of resistance, and conditions found (Chaps. 23 and 27). Antibiotic coverage is indicated, whether or not a causative organism is discovered, in patients who are immunocompromised, have mechanical heart valves or recent vascular grafts, or are elderly. Bismuth subsalicylate

may reduce the frequency of traveler's diarrhea. Antibiotic prophylaxis is only indicated for certain patients traveling to high-risk countries in whom the likelihood or seriousness of acquired diarrhea would be especially high, including those with immunocompromise, IBD, hemochromatosis, or gastric achlorhydria. Use of ciprofloxacin or rifaximin may reduce bacterial diarrhea in such travelers by 90%, though rifaximin is not suitable for invasive disease, but rather as treatment for uncomplicated traveler's diarrhea. Finally, physicians should be vigilant to identify if an outbreak of diarrheal illness is occurring and to alert the public health authorities promptly. This may reduce the ultimate size of the affected population.

CHRONIC DIARRHEA

Diarrhea lasting >4 weeks warrants evaluation to exclude serious underlying pathology. In contrast to acute diarrhea, most of the causes of chronic diarrhea are noninfectious. The classification of chronic diarrhea by pathophysiologic mechanism facilitates a rational approach to management, though many diseases cause diarrhea by more than one mechanism (Table 6-3).

TABLE 6-3

MAJOR CAUSES OF CHRONIC DIARRHEA ACCORDING TO PREDOMINANT PATHOPHYSIOLOGIC MECHANISM

Secretory causes
Exogenous stimulant laxatives
Chronic ethanol ingestion
Other drugs and toxins
Endogenous laxatives (dihydroxy bile acids)
Idiopathic secretory diarrhea
Certain bacterial infections
Bowel resection, disease, or fistula (↓ absorption)
Partial bowel obstruction or fecal impaction
Hormone-producing tumors (carcinoid, VIPoma, medullary cancer of thyroid, mastocytosis, gastrinoma, colorectal villous adenoma)
Addison's disease
Congenital electrolyte absorption defects

Osmotic causes
Osmotic laxatives (Mg^{2+}, PO_4^{-3}, SO_4^{-2})
Lactase and other disaccharide deficiencies
Nonabsorbable carbohydrates (sorbitol, lactulose, polyethylene glycol)

Steatorrheal causes
Intraluminal maldigestion (pancreatic exocrine insufficiency, bacterial overgrowth, bariatric surgery, liver disease)
Mucosal malabsorption (celiac sprue, Whipple's disease, infections, abetalipoproteinemia, ischemia)
Postmucosal obstruction (1° or 2° lymphatic obstruction)

Inflammatory causes
Idiopathic inflammatory bowel disease (Crohn's, chronic ulcerative colitis)
Lymphocytic and collagenous colitis
Immune-related mucosal disease (1° or 2° immunodeficiencies, food allergy, eosinophilic gastroenteritis, graft-vs-host disease)
Infections (invasive bacteria, viruses, and parasites, Brainerd diarrhea)
Radiation injury
Gastrointestinal malignancies

Dysmotile causes
Irritable bowel syndrome (including postinfectious IBS)
Visceral neuromyopathies
Hyperthyroidism
Drugs (prokinetic agents)
Postvagotomy

Factitial causes
Munchausen
Eating disorders

Iatrogenic causes
Cholecystectomy
Ileal resection
Bariatric surgery
Vagotomy, fundoplication

Secretory causes

Secretory diarrheas are due to derangements in fluid and electrolyte transport across the enterocolonic mucosa. They are characterized clinically by watery, large-volume fecal outputs that are typically painless and persist with fasting. Because there is no malabsorbed solute, stool osmolality is accounted for by normal endogenous electrolytes with no fecal osmotic gap.

Medications

Side effects from regular ingestion of drugs and toxins are the most common secretory causes of chronic diarrhea. Hundreds of prescription and over-the-counter medications (see "Acute Diarrhea, Other Causes") may produce diarrhea. Surreptitious or habitual use of stimulant laxatives [e.g., senna, cascara, bisacodyl, ricinoleic acid (castor oil)] must also be considered. Chronic ethanol consumption may cause a secretory-type diarrhea due to enterocyte injury with impaired sodium and water absorption as well as rapid transit and other alterations. Inadvertent ingestion of certain environmental toxins (e.g., arsenic) may lead to chronic rather than acute forms of diarrhea. Certain bacterial infections may occasionally persist and be associated with a secretory-type diarrhea.

Bowel resection, mucosal disease, or enterocolic fistula

These conditions may result in a secretory-type diarrhea because of inadequate surface for reabsorption of secreted fluids and electrolytes. Unlike other secretory diarrheas, this subset of conditions tends to worsen with eating. With disease (e.g., Crohn's ileitis) or resection of <100 cm of terminal ileum, dihydroxy bile acids may escape absorption and stimulate colonic secretion (chol-orrheic diarrhea). This mechanism may contribute to so-called *idiopathic secretory diarrhea*, in which bile acids are functionally malabsorbed from a normal-appearing terminal ileum. This *idiopathic bile acid malabsorption* may account for an average of 40% of unexplained chronic diarrhea. Reduced negative feedback regulation of bile acid synthesis by fibroblast growth factor 19 produced by enterocytes results in a degree of bile-acid synthesis that exceeds the normal capacity for ileal reabsorption, producing bile acid diarrhea.

Partial bowel obstruction, ostomy stricture, or fecal impaction may paradoxically lead to increased fecal output due to fluid hypersecretion.

Hormones

Although uncommon, the classic examples of secretory diarrhea are those mediated by hormones. *Metastatic gastrointestinal carcinoid tumors* or, rarely, *primary bronchial carcinoids* may produce watery diarrhea alone or as part of the carcinoid syndrome that comprises episodic flushing, wheezing, dyspnea, and right-sided valvular heart disease. Diarrhea is due to the release into the circulation of potent intestinal secretagogues including serotonin, histamine, prostaglandins, and various kinins. Pellagra-like skin lesions may rarely occur as the result of serotonin overproduction with niacin depletion. *Gastrinoma*, one of the most common neuroendocrine tumors, most typically presents with refractory peptic ulcers, but diarrhea occurs in up to one-third of cases and may be the only clinical manifestation in 10%. While other secretagogues released with gastrin may play a role, the diarrhea most often results from fat mal-digestion owing to pancreatic enzyme inactivation by low intraduodenal pH. The watery diarrhea hypokalemia achlorhydria syndrome, also called *pancreatic cholera*, is due to a non-β cell pancreatic adenoma, referred to as a *VIPoma*, that secretes VIP and a host of other peptide hormones including pancreatic polypeptide, secretin, gastrin, gastrin-inhibitory polypeptide (also called glucose-dependent insulinotropic peptide), neurotensin, calcitonin, and prostaglandins. The secretory diarrhea is often massive with stool volumes >3 L/d; daily volumes as high as 20 L have been reported. Life-threatening dehydration; neuromuscular dysfunction from associated hypokalemia, hypomagnesemia, or hypercalcemia; flushing; and hyperglycemia may accompany a VIPoma. *Medullary carcinoma of the thyroid* may present with watery diarrhea caused by calcitonin, other secretory peptides, or prostaglandins. Prominent diarrhea is often associated with metastatic disease and poor prognosis. *Systemic mastocytosis*, which may be associated with the skin lesion urticaria pigmentosa, may cause diarrhea that is either secretory and mediated by histamine or inflammatory due to intestinal infiltration by mast cells. Large *colorectal villous adenomas* may rarely be associated with a secretory diarrhea that may cause hypokalemia, can be inhibited by NSAIDs, and are apparently mediated by prostaglandins.

Congenital defects in ion absorption

Rarely, defects in specific carriers associated with ion absorption cause watery diarrhea from birth. These disorders include defective Cl^-/HCO_3^- exchange (*congenital chloridorrhea*) with alkalosis (which results from a mutated *DRA* [down-regulated in adenoma] gene) and defective Na^+/H^+ exchange (*congenital sodium diarrhea*), which results from a mutation in the *NHE3* (sodium-hydrogen exchanger) gene and results in acidosis.

Some hormone deficiencies may be associated with watery diarrhea, such as occurs with adrenocortical insufficiency (Addison's disease) that may be accompanied by skin hyperpigmentation.

Osmotic causes

Osmotic diarrhea occurs when ingested, poorly absorbable, osmotically active solutes draw enough fluid into the lumen to exceed the reabsorptive capacity of the colon. Fecal water output increases in proportion to such a solute load. Osmotic diarrhea characteristically ceases with fasting or with discontinuation of the causative agent.

Osmotic laxatives

Ingestion of magnesium-containing antacids, health supplements, or laxatives may induce osmotic diarrhea typified by a stool osmotic gap (>50 mosmol/L): serum osmolarity (typically 290 mosmol/kg) − [2 × (fecal sodium + potassium concentration)]. Measurement of fecal osmolarity is no longer recommended because, even when measured immediately after evacuation, it may be erroneous because carbohydrates are metabolized by colonic bacteria, causing an increase in osmolarity.

Carbohydrate malabsorption

Carbohydrate malabsorption due to acquired or congenital defects in brush-border disaccharidases and other enzymes leads to osmotic diarrhea with a low pH. One of the most common causes of chronic diarrhea in adults is *lactase deficiency*, which affects three-fourths of non-whites worldwide and 5–30% of persons in the United States; the total lactose load at any one time influences the symptoms experienced. Most patients learn to avoid milk products without requiring treatment with enzyme supplements. Some sugars, such as sorbitol, lactulose, or fructose, are frequently malabsorbed, and diarrhea ensues with ingestion of medications, gum, or candies sweetened with these poorly or incompletely absorbed sugars.

Steatorrheal causes

Fat malabsorption may lead to greasy, foul-smelling, difficult-to-flush diarrhea often associated with weight loss and nutritional deficiencies due to concomitant malabsorption of amino acids and vitamins. Increased fecal output is caused by the osmotic effects of fatty acids, especially after bacterial hydroxylation, and, to a lesser extent, by the neutral fat. Quantitatively, steatorrhea is defined as stool fat exceeding the normal 7 g/d; rapid-transit diarrhea may result in fecal fat up to 14 g/d; daily fecal fat averages 15–25 g with small intestinal diseases and is often >32 g with pancreatic exocrine insufficiency. Intraluminal maldigestion, mucosal malabsorption, or lymphatic obstruction may produce steatorrhea.

Intraluminal maldigestion

This condition most commonly results from pancreatic exocrine insufficiency, which occurs when >90% of pancreatic secretory function is lost. *Chronic pancreatitis*, usually a sequel of ethanol abuse, most frequently causes pancreatic insufficiency. Other causes include *cystic fibrosis*; *pancreatic duct obstruction*; and, rarely, *somatostatinoma*. Bacterial overgrowth in the small intestine may

deconjugate bile acids and alter micelle formation, impairing fat digestion; it occurs with stasis from a blind-loop, small-bowel diverticulum or dysmotility and is especially likely in the elderly. Finally, cirrhosis or biliary obstruction may lead to mild steatorrhea due to deficient intraluminal bile acid concentration.

Mucosal malabsorption

Mucosal malabsorption occurs from a variety of enteropathies, but it most commonly occurs from *celiac disease*. This gluten-sensitive enteropathy affects all ages and is characterized by villous atrophy and crypt hyperplasia in the proximal small bowel and can present with fatty diarrhea associated with multiple nutritional deficiencies of varying severity. Celiac disease is much more frequent than previously thought; it affects ~1% of the population, frequently presents without steatorrhea, can mimic IBS, and has many other GI and extraintestinal manifestations. *Tropical sprue* may produce a similar histologic and clinical syndrome but occurs in residents of or travelers to tropical climates; abrupt onset and response to antibiotics suggest an infectious etiology. *Whipple's disease*, due to the bacillus *Tropheryma whipplei* and histiocytic infiltration of the small-bowel mucosa, is a less common cause of steatorrhea that most typically occurs in young or middle-aged men; it is frequently associated with arthralgias, fever, lymphadenopathy, and extreme fatigue, and it may affect the CNS and endocardium. A similar clinical and histologic picture results from *Mycobacterium avium-intracellulare* infection in patients with AIDS. *Abetalipoproteinemia* is a rare defect of chylomicron formation and fat malabsorption in children, associated with acanthocytic erythrocytes, ataxia, and retinitis pigmentosa. Several other conditions may cause mucosal malabsorption including infections, especially with protozoa such as *Giardia*; numerous medications (e.g., colchicine, cholestyramine, neomycin); amyloidosis; and chronic ischemia.

Postmucosal lymphatic obstruction

The pathophysiology of this condition, which is due to the rare *congenital intestinal lymphangiectasia* or to *acquired lymphatic obstruction* secondary to trauma, tumor, cardiac disease, or infection, leads to the unique constellation of fat malabsorption with enteric losses of protein (often causing edema) and lymphocytopenia. Carbohydrate and amino acid absorption is preserved.

Inflammatory causes

Inflammatory diarrheas are generally accompanied by pain, fever, bleeding, or other manifestations of inflammation. The mechanism of diarrhea may not only be exudation but, depending on lesion site, may include fat malabsorption, disrupted fluid/electrolyte absorption, and hypersecretion or hypermotility from release of cytokines and other inflammatory mediators. The unifying feature on stool analysis is the presence of leukocytes or leukocyte-derived proteins such as calprotectin. With severe inflammation, exudative protein loss can lead to anasarca (generalized edema). Any middle-aged or older person with chronic inflammatory-type diarrhea, especially with blood, should be carefully evaluated to exclude a colorectal tumor.

Idiopathic inflammatory bowel disease

The illnesses in this category, which include *Crohn's disease* and *chronic ulcerative colitis*, are among the most common organic causes of chronic diarrhea in adults and range in severity from mild to fulminant and life-threatening. They may be associated with uveitis, polyarthralgias, cholestatic liver disease (primary sclerosing cholangitis), and skin lesions (erythema nodosum, pyoderma gangrenosum). *Microscopic colitis*, including both lymphocytic and *collagenous colitis*, is an increasingly recognized cause of chronic watery diarrhea, especially in middle-aged women and those on NSAIDs, statins, proton pump inhibitors (PPIs), and selective serotonin reuptake inhibitors (SSRIs); biopsy of a normal-appearing colon is required for histologic diagnosis. It may coexist with symptoms suggesting IBS or with celiac sprue. It typically responds well to anti–inflammatory drugs (e.g., bismuth), to the opioid agonist loperamide, or to budesonide.

Primary or secondary forms of immunodeficiency

Immunodeficiency may lead to prolonged infectious diarrhea. With selective IgA deficiency or common variable *hypogammaglobulinemia*, diarrhea is particularly prevalent and often the result of giardiasis, bacterial overgrowth, or sprue.

Eosinophilic gastroenteritis

Eosinophil infiltration of the mucosa, muscularis, or serosa at any level of the GI tract may cause diarrhea, pain, vomiting, or ascites. Affected patients often have an atopic history, Charcot-Leyden crystals due to extruded eosinophil contents may be seen on microscopic inspection of stool, and peripheral eosinophilia is present in 50–75% of patients. While hypersensitivity to certain foods occurs in adults, true food allergy causing chronic diarrhea is rare.

Other causes

Chronic inflammatory diarrhea may be caused by *radiation enterocolitis*, *chronic graft-versus-host disease*, *Behçet's syndrome*, and *Cronkhite-Canada syndrome*, among others.

Dysmotility causes

Rapid transit may accompany many diarrheas as a secondary or contributing phenomenon, but primary dysmotility is an unusual etiology of true diarrhea. Stool features often suggest a secretory diarrhea, but mild steatorrhea of up to 14 g of fat per day can be produced by maldigestion from rapid transit alone. *Hyperthyroidism, carcinoid syndrome,* and certain drugs (e.g., prostaglandins, prokinetic agents) may produce hypermotility with resultant diarrhea. Primary visceral neuromyopathies or idiopathic acquired intestinal pseudoobstruction may lead to stasis with secondary bacterial overgrowth causing diarrhea. *Diabetic diarrhea,* often accompanied by peripheral and generalized autonomic neuropathies, may occur in part because of intestinal dysmotility.

The exceedingly common IBS (10% point prevalence, 1–2% per year incidence) is characterized by disturbed intestinal and colonic motor and sensory responses to various stimuli. Symptoms of stool frequency typically cease at night, alternate with periods of constipation, are accompanied by abdominal pain relieved with defecation, and rarely result in weight loss.

Factitial causes

Factitial diarrhea accounts for up to 15% of unexplained diarrheas referred to tertiary care centers. Either as a form of *Munchausen syndrome* (deception or self-injury for secondary gain) or *eating disorders*, some patients covertly self-administer laxatives alone or in combination with other medications (e.g., diuretics) or surreptitiously add water or urine to stool sent for analysis. Such patients are typically women, often with histories of psychiatric illness, and disproportionately from careers in health care. Hypotension and hypokalemia are common co-presenting features. The evaluation of such patients may be difficult: contamination of the stool with water or urine is suggested by very low or high stool osmolarity, respectively. Such patients often deny this possibility when confronted, but they do benefit from psychiatric counseling when they acknowledge their behavior.

APPROACH TO THE PATIENT   **Chronic Diarrhea**

The laboratory tools available to evaluate the very common problem of chronic diarrhea are extensive, and many are costly and invasive. As such, the diagnostic evaluation must be rationally directed by a careful history and physical examination (Fig. 6-3A). When this strategy is unrevealing, simple triage tests are often warranted to direct the choice of more complex investigations (Fig. 6-3B). The history, physical examination (Table 6-4), and routine blood studies should attempt to characterize the mechanism of diarrhea, identify diagnostically helpful associations, and assess the patient's fluid/electrolyte and nutritional status. Patients should be questioned about the onset, duration, pattern, aggravating (especially diet) and

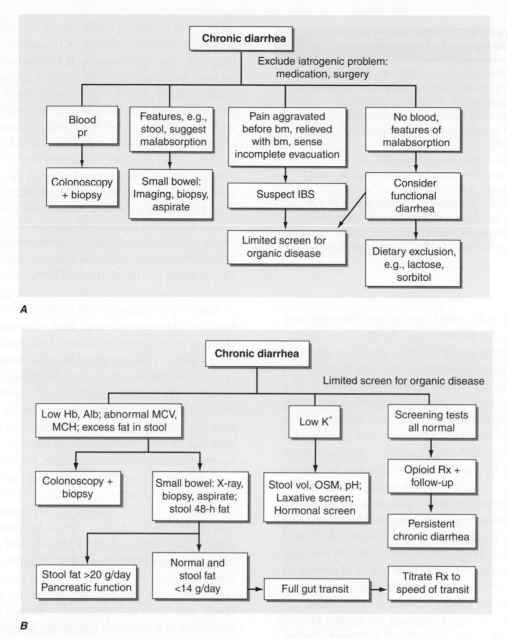

FIGURE 6-3

Chronic diarrhea. A. Initial management based on accompanying symptoms or features. **B.** Evaluation based on findings from a limited age-appropriate screen for organic disease. pr, per rectum; bm, bowel movement; IBS, irritable bowel syndrome; Hb, hemoglobin; Alb, albumin; MCV, mean corpuscular volume; MCH, mean corpuscular hemoglobin; OSM, osmolality. (*Reprinted from M Camilleri: Clin Gastroenterol Hepatol 2:198, 2004.*)

relieving factors, and stool characteristics of their diarrhea. The presence or absence of fecal incontinence, fever, weight loss, pain, certain exposures (travel, medications, contacts with diarrhea), and common extraintestinal manifestations (skin changes, arthralgias, oral aphthous ulcers) should be noted. A family history of IBD or sprue may indicate those possibilities. Physical findings may offer clues such as a thyroid mass, wheezing, heart murmurs, edema, hepatomegaly, abdominal masses, lymphadenopathy, mucocutaneous abnormalities, perianal fistulas, or anal sphincter laxity. Peripheral blood leukocytosis, elevated sedimentation rate, or C-reactive protein suggests inflammation; anemia reflects blood loss or nutritional deficiencies; or eosinophilia may occur with parasitoses, neoplasia, collagen-vascular disease, allergy, or eosinophilic gastroenteritis. Blood chemistries may demonstrate electrolyte, hepatic, or other metabolic disturbances. Measuring tissue transglutaminase antibodies may help detect celiac disease.

TABLE 6-4

PHYSICAL EXAMINATION IN PATIENTS WITH CHRONIC DIARRHEA

1. Are there general features to suggest malabsorption or inflammatory bowel disease (IBD) such as anemia, dermatitis herpetiformis, edema, or clubbing?
2. Are there features to suggest underlying autonomic neuropathy or collagen-vascular disease in the pupils, orthostasis, skin, hands, or joints?
3. Is there an abdominal mass or tenderness?
4. Are there any abnormalities of rectal mucosa, rectal defects, or altered anal sphincter functions?
5. Are there any mucocutaneous manifestations of systemic disease such as dermatitis herpetiformis (celiac disease), erythema nodosum (ulcerative colitis), flushing (carcinoid), or oral ulcers for IBD or celiac disease?

A therapeutic trial is often appropriate, definitive, and highly cost effective when a specific diagnosis is suggested on the initial physician encounter. For example, chronic watery diarrhea, which ceases with fasting in an otherwise healthy young adult, may justify a trial of a lactose-restricted diet; bloating and diarrhea persisting since a mountain backpacking trip may warrant a trial of metronidazole for likely giardiasis; and postprandial diarrhea persisting following resection of terminal ileum might be due to bile acid malabsorption and be treated with cholestyramine or colesevelam before further evaluation. Persistent symptoms require additional investigation.

Certain diagnoses may be suggested on the initial encounter (e.g., idiopathic IBD); however, additional focused evaluations may be necessary to confirm the diagnosis and characterize the severity or extent of disease so that treatment can be best guided. Patients suspected of having IBS should be initially evaluated with flexible sigmoidoscopy with colorectal biopsies; those with normal findings might be reassured and, as indicated, treated empirically with antispasmodics, antidiarrheals, bulk agents, anxiolytics, or antidepressants. Any patient who presents with chronic diarrhea and hematochezia should be evaluated with stool microbiologic studies and colonoscopy.

In an estimated two-thirds of cases, the cause for chronic diarrhea remains unclear after the initial encounter, and further testing is required. Quantitative stool collection and analyses can yield important objective data that may establish a diagnosis or characterize the type of diarrhea as a triage for focused additional studies (Fig. 6-3B). If stool weight is >200 g/d, additional stool analyses should be performed that might include electrolyte concentration, pH, occult blood testing, leukocyte inspection (or leukocyte protein assay), fat quantitation, and laxative screens.

For secretory diarrheas (watery, normal osmotic gap), possible medication-related side effects or surreptitious laxative use should be reconsidered. Microbiologic studies should be done including fecal bacterial cultures (including media for *Aeromonas* and *Pleisiomonas*), inspection for ova and parasites, and *Giardia* antigen assay (the most sensitive test for giardiasis). Small-bowel bacterial overgrowth can be excluded by intestinal aspirates with quantitative cultures or with glucose or lactulose breath tests involving measurement of breath hydrogen, methane, or other metabolite (e.g., $^{14}CO_2$). However, interpretation of these breath tests may be confounded by disturbances of intestinal transit. Upper endoscopy and colonoscopy with biopsies and small-bowel barium x-rays are helpful to rule out structural or occult inflammatory disease. When suggested by history or other findings, screens for peptide hormones should be pursued (e.g., serum gastrin, VIP, calcitonin, and thyroid hormone/thyroid-stimulating hormone, or urinary 5-hydroxyindolacetic acid, and histamine).

Further evaluation of osmotic diarrhea should include tests for lactose intolerance and magnesium ingestion, the two most common causes. Low fecal pH suggests carbohydrate malabsorption; lactose malabsorption can be confirmed by lactose breath testing or by a therapeutic trial with lactose exclusion and observation of the effect of lactose challenge (e.g., a liter of milk). Lactase determination on small-bowel biopsy is not generally available. If fecal magnesium or laxative levels are elevated, inadvertent or surreptitious ingestion should be considered and psychiatric help should be sought.

For those with proven fatty diarrhea, endoscopy with small-bowel biopsy (including aspiration for *Giardia* and quantitative cultures) should be performed; if this procedure is unrevealing, a small-bowel radiograph is often an appropriate next step. If small-bowel studies are negative or if pancreatic disease is suspected, pancreatic exocrine insufficiency should be excluded with direct tests, such as the secretin-cholecystokinin stimulation test or a variation that could be performed endoscopically. In general, indirect tests such as assay of fecal elastase or chymotrypsin activity or a bentiromide test have fallen out of favor because of low sensitivity and specificity.

Chronic inflammatory-type diarrheas should be suspected by the presence of blood or leukocytes in the stool. Such findings warrant stool cultures; inspection for ova and parasites; *C. difficile* toxin assay; colonoscopy with biopsies; and, if indicated, small-bowel contrast studies.

TREATMENT ▶ Chronic Diarrhea

Treatment of chronic diarrhea depends on the specific etiology and may be curative, suppressive, or empirical. If the cause can be eradicated, treatment is curative as with resection of a colorectal cancer, antibiotic administration for Whipple's disease or tropical sprue, or discontinuation of a drug. For many chronic conditions, diarrhea can be controlled by suppression of the underlying mechanism. Examples include elimination of dietary lactose for lactase deficiency or gluten for celiac sprue, use of glucocorticoids or other anti-inflammatory agents for idiopathic IBDs, adsorptive agents such as cholestyramine for ileal bile acid malabsorption, proton pump inhibitors such as omeprazole for the gastric hypersecretion of gastrinomas, somatostatin analogues such as octreotide for malignant carcinoid syndrome, prostaglandin inhibitors such as indomethacin for medullary carcinoma of the thyroid, and pancreatic enzyme replacement for pancreatic insufficiency. When the specific cause or mechanism of chronic diarrhea evades diagnosis, empirical therapy may be beneficial. Mild opiates, such as diphenoxylate or loperamide, are often helpful in mild or moderate watery diarrhea. For those with more severe diarrhea, codeine or tincture of opium may be beneficial. Such antimotility agents should be avoided with severe IBD, because toxic megacolon may be precipitated. Clonidine, an α_2-adrenergic agonist, may allow control of diabetic diarrhea. For all patients with chronic diarrhea, fluid and electrolyte repletion is an important component of management (see "Acute Diarrhea," discussed earlier). Replacement of fat-soluble vitamins may also be necessary in patients with chronic steatorrhea.

CONSTIPATION

DEFINITION

Constipation is a common complaint in clinical practice and usually refers to persistent, difficult, infrequent, or seemingly incomplete defecation. Because of the wide range of normal bowel habits, constipation is difficult to define precisely. Most persons have at least three bowel movements per week; however, low stool frequency alone is not the sole criterion for the diagnosis of constipation. Many constipated patients have a normal frequency of defecation but complain of excessive straining, hard stools, lower abdominal fullness, or a sense of incomplete evacuation. The individual patient's symptoms must be analyzed in detail to ascertain what is meant by "constipation" or "difficulty" with defecation.

Stool form and consistency are well correlated with the time elapsed from the preceding defecation. Hard, pellety stools occur with slow transit, while loose, watery stools are associated with rapid transit. Both small pellety or very large stools are more difficult to expel than normal stools.

The perception of hard stools or excessive straining is more difficult to assess objectively, and the need for enemas or digital disimpaction is a clinically useful way to corroborate the patient's perceptions of difficult defecation.

Psychosocial or cultural factors may also be important. A person whose parents attached great importance to daily defecation will become greatly concerned when he or she misses a daily bowel movement; some children withhold stool to gain attention or because of fear of pain from anal irritation; and some adults habitually ignore or delay the call to have a bowel movement.

CAUSES

Pathophysiologically, chronic constipation generally results from inadequate fiber or fluid intake or from disordered colonic transit or anorectal function. These result from neurogastroenterologic disturbance, certain drugs, advancing age, or in association with a large number of systemic diseases that affect the GI tract (Table 6-5). Constipation of recent onset may be a symptom of significant organic disease such as tumor or stricture. In *idiopathic constipation*, a subset of patients exhibit delayed emptying of the ascending and

TABLE 6-5

CAUSES OF CONSTIPATION IN ADULTS

TYPES OF CONSTIPATION AND CAUSES	EXAMPLES
Recent onset	
Colonic obstruction	Neoplasm; stricture: ischemic, diverticular, inflammatory
Anal sphincter spasm	Anal fissure, painful hemorrhoids
Medications	
Chronic	
Irritable bowel syndrome	Constipation-predominant, alternating
Medications	Ca^{2+} blockers, antidepressants
Colonic pseudoobstruction	Slow-transit constipation, megacolon (rare Hirschsprung's, Chagas' diseases)
Disorders of rectal evacuation	Pelvic floor dysfunction; anismus; descending perineum syndrome; rectal mucosal prolapse; rectocele
Endocrinopathies	Hypothyroidism, hypercalcemia, pregnancy
Psychiatric disorders	Depression, eating disorders, drugs
Neurologic disease	Parkinsonism, multiple sclerosis, spinal cord injury
Generalized muscle disease	Progressive systemic sclerosis

transverse colon with prolongation of transit (often in the proximal colon) and a reduced frequency of propulsive HAPCs. *Outlet obstruction to defecation* (also called *evacuation disorders*) may cause delayed colonic transit, which is usually corrected by biofeedback retraining of the disordered defecation. Constipation of any cause may be exacerbated by hospitalization or chronic illnesses that lead to physical or mental impairment and result in inactivity or physical immobility.

APPROACH TO THE PATIENT   Constipation

A careful history should explore the patient's symptoms and confirm whether he or she is indeed constipated based on frequency (e.g., fewer than three bowel movements per week), consistency (lumpy/hard), excessive straining, prolonged defecation time, or need to support the perineum or digitate the anorectum. In the vast majority of cases (probably >90%), there is no underlying cause (e.g., cancer, depression, or hypothyroidism), and constipation responds to ample hydration, exercise, and supplementation of dietary fiber (15–25 g/d). A good diet and medication history and attention to psychosocial issues are key. Physical examination and, particularly, a rectal examination should exclude fecal impaction and most of the important diseases that present with constipation and possibly indicate features suggesting an evacuation disorder (e.g., high anal sphincter tone).

The presence of weight loss, rectal bleeding, or anemia with constipation mandates either flexible sigmoidoscopy plus barium enema or colonoscopy alone, particularly in patients >40 years, to exclude structural diseases such as cancer or strictures. Colonoscopy alone is most cost-effective in this setting because it provides an opportunity to biopsy mucosal lesions, perform polypectomy, or dilate strictures. Barium enema has advantages over colonoscopy in the patient with isolated constipation because it is less costly and identifies colonic dilation and all significant mucosal lesions or strictures that are likely to present with constipation. Melanosis coli, or pigmentation of the colon mucosa, indicates the use of anthraquinone laxatives such as cascara or senna; however, this is usually apparent from a careful history. An unexpected disorder such as megacolon or cathartic colon may also be detected by colonic radiographs. Measurement of serum calcium, potassium, and thyroid-stimulating hormone levels will identify rare patients with metabolic disorders.

Patients with more troublesome constipation may not respond to fiber alone and may be helped by a bowel-training regimen: taking an osmotic laxative (lactulose, sorbitol, polyethylene glycol) and evacuating

FIGURE 6-4
Algorithm for the management of constipation.

with enema or glycerine suppository as needed. After breakfast, a distraction-free 15–20 min on the toilet without straining is encouraged. Excessive straining may lead to development of hemorrhoids, and, if there is weakness of the pelvic floor or injury to the pudendal nerve, may result in obstructed defecation from descending perineum syndrome several years later. Those few who do not benefit from the simple measures delineated above or require long-term treatment with potent laxatives, with the attendant risk of developing laxative abuse syndrome, are assumed to have severe or intractable constipation and should have further investigation (Fig. 6-4). Novel agents that induce secretion (e.g., lubiprostone, a chloride channel activator) are also available.

INVESTIGATION OF SEVERE CONSTIPATION

A small minority (probably <5%) of patients have severe or "intractable" constipation. These are the patients most likely to be seen by gastroenterologists or in referral centers. Further observation of the patient may occasionally reveal a previously unrecognized cause, such as an evacuation disorder, laxative abuse, malingering, or psychological disorder. In these patients, evaluations of the physiologic function of the colon and pelvic floor and of psychological status aid in the rational choice of treatment. Even among these highly selected patients with severe constipation, a cause can be identified in only about two-thirds of tertiary referral patients (discussed later).

Measurement of colonic transit

Radiopaque marker transit tests are easy, repeatable, generally safe, inexpensive, reliable, and highly applicable in evaluating constipated patients in clinical practice. Several validated methods are very simple. For example, radiopaque markers are ingested; an abdominal flat film taken 5 days later should indicate passage of 80% of the markers out of the colon without the use of laxatives or enemas. This test does not provide useful information about the transit profile of the stomach and small bowel.

Radioscintigraphy with a delayed-release capsule containing radiolabeled particles has been used to noninvasively characterize normal, accelerated, or delayed colonic function over 24–48 h with low radiation exposure. This approach simultaneously assesses gastric, small bowel (which may be important in ~20% of patients with delayed colonic transit because they reflect a more generalized GI motility disorder), and colonic transit. The disadvantages are the greater cost and the need for specific materials prepared in a nuclear medicine laboratory.

Anorectal and pelvic floor tests

Pelvic floor dysfunction is suggested by the inability to evacuate the rectum, a feeling of persistent rectal fullness, rectal pain, the need to extract stool from the rectum digitally, application of pressure on the posterior wall of the vagina, support of the perineum during straining, and excessive straining. These significant symptoms should be contrasted with the sense of incomplete rectal evacuation, which is common in IBS.

Formal psychological evaluation may identify eating disorders, "control issues," depression, or post-traumatic stress disorders that may respond to cognitive or other intervention and may be important in restoring quality of life to patients who might present with chronic constipation.

A simple clinical test in the office to document a nonrelaxing puborectalis muscle is to have the patient strain to expel the index finger during a digital rectal examination. Motion of the puborectalis posteriorly during straining indicates proper coordination of the pelvic floor muscles.

Measurement of perineal descent is relatively easy to gauge clinically by placing the patient in the left decubitus position and watching the perineum to detect inadequate descent (<1.5 cm, a sign of pelvic floor dysfunction) or perineal ballooning during straining relative to bony landmarks (>4 cm, suggesting excessive perineal descent).

A useful overall test of evacuation is the balloon expulsion test. A balloon-tipped urinary catheter is placed and inflated with 50 mL of water. Normally, a patient can expel it while seated on a toilet or in the left lateral decubitus position. In the lateral position, the weight needed to facilitate expulsion of the balloon is determined; normally, expulsion occurs with <200 g added.

Anorectal manometry, when used in the evaluation of patients with severe constipation, may find an excessively high resting (>80 mmHg) or squeeze anal sphincter tone, suggesting anismus (anal sphincter spasm). This test also identifies rare syndromes, such as adult Hirschsprung's disease, by the absence of the rectoanal inhibitory reflex.

Defecography (a dynamic barium enema including lateral views obtained during barium expulsion) reveals "soft abnormalities" in many patients; the most relevant findings are the measured changes in rectoanal angle, anatomic defects of the rectum such as internal mucosal prolapse, and enteroceles or rectoceles. Surgically remediable conditions are identified in only a few patients. These include severe, whole-thickness intussusception with complete outlet obstruction due to funnel-shaped plugging at the anal canal or an extremely large rectocele that fills preferentially during attempts at defecation instead of expulsion of the barium through the anus. In summary, defecography requires an interested and experienced radiologist, and abnormalities are not pathognomonic for pelvic floor dysfunction. The most common cause of outlet obstruction is failure of the puborectalis muscle to relax; this is not identified by defecography but requires a dynamic study such as proctography. MRI is being developed as an alternative and provides more information about the structure and function of the pelvic floor, distal colorectum, and anal sphincters.

Dynamic imaging studies such as proctography during defecation or scintigraphic expulsion of artificial stool help measure perineal descent and the rectoanal angle during rest, squeezing, and straining, and scintigraphic expulsion quantitates the amount of "artificial stool" emptied. Lack of straightening of the rectoanal angle by at least 15° during defecation confirms pelvic floor dysfunction.

Neurologic testing (electromyography) is more helpful in the evaluation of patients with incontinence than of those with symptoms suggesting obstructed defecation. The absence of neurologic signs in the lower extremities suggests that any documented denervation of the puborectalis results from pelvic (e.g., obstetric) injury or from stretching of the pudendal nerve by chronic, long-standing straining. Constipation is common among patients with spinal cord injuries, neurologic diseases such as Parkinson's disease, multiple sclerosis, and diabetic neuropathy.

Spinal-evoked responses during electrical rectal stimulation or stimulation of external anal sphincter contraction by applying magnetic stimulation over the lumbosacral cord identify patients with limited sacral neuropathies with sufficient residual nerve conduction to attempt biofeedback training.

In summary, a balloon expulsion test is an important screening test for anorectal dysfunction. If positive, an anatomic evaluation of the rectum or anal sphincters and an assessment of pelvic floor relaxation are the tools for evaluating patients in whom obstructed defecation is suspected.

TREATMENT Constipation

After the cause of constipation is characterized, a treatment decision can be made. Slow-transit constipation requires aggressive medical or surgical treatment; anismus or pelvic floor dysfunction usually responds to biofeedback management (Fig. 6-4). However, only ~60% of patients with severe constipation are found to have such a physiologic disorder (half with colonic transit delay and half with evacuation disorder). Patients with spinal cord injuries or other neurologic disorders require a dedicated bowel regimen that often includes rectal stimulation, enema therapy, and carefully timed laxative therapy.

Patients with slow-transit constipation are treated with bulk, osmotic, prokinetic, secretory, and stimulant laxatives including fiber, psyllium, milk of magnesia, lactulose, polyethylene glycol (colonic lavage solution), lubiprostone, and bisacodyl. Newer treatment aimed

at enhancing motility and secretion may have application in circumstances such as constipation-predominant IBS in females or severe constipation. If a 3- to 6-month trial of medical therapy fails and patients continue to have documented slow-transit constipation unassociated with obstructed defecation, the patients should be considered for laparoscopic colectomy with ileorectostomy; however, this should not be undertaken if there is continued evidence of an evacuation disorder or a generalized GI dysmotility. Referral to a specialized center for further tests of colonic motor function is warranted. The decision to resort to surgery is facilitated in the presence of megacolon and megarectum. The complications after surgery include small-bowel obstruction (11%) and fecal soiling, particularly at night during the first postoperative year. Frequency of defecation is 3–8 per day during the first year, dropping to 1–3 per day from the second year after surgery.

Patients who have a combined (evacuation and transit/motility) disorder should pursue pelvic floor retraining (biofeedback and muscle relaxation), psychological counseling, and dietetic advice first, followed by colectomy and ileorectostomy if colonic transit studies do not normalize and symptoms are intractable despite biofeedback and optimized medical therapy. In patients with pelvic floor dysfunction alone, biofeedback training has a 70–80% success rate, measured by the acquisition of comfortable stool habits. Attempts to manage pelvic floor dysfunction with operations (internal anal sphincter or puborectalis muscle division) have achieved only mediocre success and have been largely abandoned.

CHAPTER 7

GASTROINTESTINAL BLEEDING

Loren Laine

Bleeding from the gastrointestinal (GI) tract may present in five ways. *Hematemesis* is vomitus of red blood or "coffee-grounds" material. *Melena* is black, tarry, foul-smelling stool. *Hematochezia* is the passage of bright red or maroon blood from the rectum. *Occult GI bleeding* (GIB) may be identified in the absence of overt bleeding by a fecal occult blood test or the presence of iron deficiency. Finally, patients may present only with *symptoms of blood loss or anemia* such as lightheadedness, syncope, angina, or dyspnea.

SOURCES OF GASTROINTESTINAL BLEEDING

Upper gastrointestinal sources of bleeding

(Table 7-1) The annual incidence of hospital admissions for upper GIB (UGIB) in the United States and Europe is ~0.1%, with a mortality rate of ~5–10%. Patients rarely die from exsanguination; rather, they die

TABLE 7-1

SOURCES OF BLEEDING IN PATIENTS HOSPITALIZED FOR UPPER GI BLEEDING	
SOURCES OF BLEEDING	PROPORTION OF PATIENTS, %
Ulcers	31–67
Varices	6–39
Mallory-Weiss tears	2–8
Gastroduodenal erosions	2–18
Erosive esophagitis	1–13
Neoplasm	2–8
Vascular ectasias	0–6
No source identified	5–14

Source: Data on hospitalizations from year 2000 onward from Am J Gastroenterol 98:1494, 2003; Gastrointest Endosc 57:AB147, 2003; 60:875, 2004; Eur J Gastroenterol Hepatol 16:177, 2004; 17:641, 2005; J Clin Gastroenterol 42:128, 2008; World J Gastroenterol 14:5046, 2008; Dig Dis Sci 54:333, 2009.

due to decompensation from other underlying illnesses. The mortality rate for patients <60 years in the absence of major concurrent illness is <1%. Independent predictors of rebleeding and death in patients hospitalized with UGIB include increasing age, comorbidities, and hemodynamic compromise (tachycardia or hypotension).

Peptic ulcers are the most common cause of UGIB, accounting for up to ~50% of cases; an increasing proportion is due to nonsteroidal anti-inflammatory drugs (NSAIDs), with the prevalence of *Helicobacter pylori* decreasing. Mallory-Weiss tears account for ~5–10% of cases. The proportion of patients bleeding from varices varies widely from ~5 to 40%, depending on the population. Hemorrhagic or erosive gastropathy (e.g., due to NSAIDs or alcohol) and erosive esophagitis often cause mild UGIB, but major bleeding is rare.

▄▄▄ Peptic ulcers

In addition to clinical features, characteristics of an ulcer at endoscopy provide important prognostic information. One-third of patients with active bleeding or a nonbleeding visible vessel have further bleeding that requires urgent surgery if they are treated conservatively. These patients clearly benefit from endoscopic therapy with bipolar electrocoagulation; heater probe; injection therapy (e.g., absolute alcohol, 1:10,000 epinephrine); and/or clips with reductions in bleeding, hospital stay, mortality rate, and costs. In contrast, patients with clean-based ulcers have rates of recurrent bleeding approaching zero. If there is no other reason for hospitalization, such patients may be discharged on the first hospital day, following stabilization. Patients without clean-based ulcers should usually remain in the hospital for 3 days because most episodes of recurrent bleeding occur within 3 days.

Randomized controlled trials document that a high-dose, constant-infusion IV proton pump inhibitor (PPI) (e.g., omeprazole 80-mg bolus and 8-mg/h infusion), designed to sustain intragastric pH >6 and enhance clot stability, decreases further bleeding and mortality in patients with high-risk ulcers (active bleeding, non-bleeding visible vessel, adherent clot) when given after endoscopic therapy. Institution of PPI therapy at presentation in all patients with UGIB decreases high-risk ulcer characteristics (e.g., active bleeding) but does not significantly improve outcomes such as further bleeding, transfusions, or mortality as compared to initiating therapy only when high-risk ulcers are identified at the time of endoscopy.

Approximately one-third of patients with bleeding ulcers will rebleed within the next 1–2 years if no preventive strategies are employed. Prevention of recurrent bleeding focuses on the three main factors in ulcer pathogenesis, *H. pylori*, NSAIDs, and acid. Eradication of *H. pylori* in patients with bleeding ulcers decreases rates of rebleeding to <5%. If a bleeding ulcer develops in a patient taking NSAIDs, the NSAIDs should be discontinued, if possible. If NSAIDs must be continued or reinstituted, a cyclooxygenase 2 (COX-2) selective inhibitor (coxib) plus a PPI should be used. PPI co-therapy alone or a coxib alone is associated with an annual rebleeding rate of ~10% in patients with a recent bleeding ulcer, while combination of a coxib and PPI provides a further significant decrease in recurrent ulcer bleeding. Patients with cardiovascular disease who develop bleeding ulcers while taking low-dose aspirin should restart aspirin as soon as possible after their bleeding episode (e.g., ≤7 days). A randomized trial showed that failure to restart aspirin was associated with a nonsignificant difference in rebleeding (5% vs. 10% at 30 days), but a significant increase in mortality at 30 days (9% vs. 1%) and 8 weeks (13% vs. 1%) as compared to immediate reinstitution of aspirin. Patients with bleeding ulcers unrelated to *H. pylori* or NSAIDs should remain on full-dose antisecretory therapy indefinitely. Peptic ulcers are discussed in Chap. 14.

Mallory-Weiss tears

The classic history is vomiting, retching, or coughing preceding hematemesis, especially in an alcoholic patient. Bleeding from these tears, which are usually on the gastric side of the gastroesophageal junction, stops spontaneously in 80–90% of patients and recurs in only 0–7%. Endoscopic therapy is indicated for actively bleeding Mallory-Weiss tears. Angiographic therapy with embolization and operative therapy with oversewing of the tear are rarely required. Mallory-Weiss tears are discussed in Chap. 13.

Esophageal varices

Patients with variceal hemorrhage have poorer outcomes than patients with other sources of UGIB. Endoscopic therapy for acute bleeding and repeated sessions of endoscopic therapy to eradicate esophageal varices significantly reduce rebleeding and mortality. Ligation is the endoscopic therapy of choice for esophageal varices because it has less rebleeding, a lower mortality rate, fewer local complications, and it requires fewer treatment sessions to achieve variceal eradication than sclerotherapy.

Octreotide (50-μg bolus and 50-μg/h IV infusion for 2–5 days) further helps in the control of acute bleeding when used in combination with endoscopic therapy. Other vasoactive agents such as somatostatin and terlipressin, available outside the United States, are also effective. Antibiotic therapy (e.g., ceftriaxone) is also recommended for patients with cirrhosis presenting with UGIB because antibiotics decrease bacterial infections and mortality in this population. Over the long term, treatment with nonselective beta blockers decreases recurrent bleeding from esophageal varices. Chronic therapy with beta blockers plus endoscopic ligation is recommended for prevention of recurrent esophageal variceal bleeding.

In patients who have persistent or recurrent bleeding despite endoscopic and medical therapy, more invasive therapy with transjugular intrahepatic portosystemic shunt (TIPS) is recommended. Older studies indicate that most patients with TIPS developed shunt stenosis within 1–2 years and required reintervention to maintain shunt patency. The use of coated stents appears to decrease shunt dysfunction by ~50% in the first 2 years. A randomized comparison of TIPS (with uncoated stents) and distal splenorenal shunt in Child-Pugh class A or B cirrhotic patients with refractory variceal bleeding revealed no significant difference in rebleeding, encephalopathy, or survival, but had a much higher rate of reintervention with TIPS (82% vs. 11%). Therefore, decompressive surgery may be an option in patients with milder, well-compensated cirrhosis.

Portal hypertension is also responsible for bleeding from gastric varices, varices in the small and large intestine, and portal hypertensive gastropathy and enterocolopathy.

Hemorrhagic and erosive gastropathy ("gastritis")

Hemorrhagic and erosive gastropathy, often labeled gastritis, refers to endoscopically visualized subepithelial hemorrhages and erosions. These are mucosal lesions and, thus, do not cause major bleeding. They develop in various clinical settings, the most important of which are NSAID use, alcohol intake, and stress. Half of patients who chronically ingest NSAIDs have erosions (15–30% have ulcers), while up to 20% of actively drinking alcoholic patients with symptoms of UGIB have evidence of subepithelial hemorrhages or erosions.

Stress-related gastric mucosal injury occurs only in extremely sick patients: those who have experienced serious trauma, major surgery, burns covering more than one-third of the body surface area, major intracranial disease, or severe medical illness (i.e., ventilator dependence, coagulopathy). Significant bleeding probably does not develop unless ulceration occurs. The mortality rate in these patients is quite high because of their serious underlying illnesses.

The incidence of bleeding from stress-related gastric mucosal injury or ulceration has decreased dramatically in recent years, most likely due to better care of critically ill patients. Pharmacologic prophylaxis for bleeding may be considered in the high-risk patients mentioned earlier. Multiple trials document the efficacy of intravenous H_2-receptor antagonist therapy, which is more effective than sucralfate but not superior to a PPI immediate-release suspension given via nasogastric tube. Prophylactic therapy decreases bleeding but does not lower the mortality rate.

Other causes

Other less frequent causes of UGIB include erosive duodenitis, neoplasms, aortoenteric fistulas, vascular lesions [including hereditary hemorrhagic telangiectasias (Osler-Weber-Rendu) and gastric antral vascular ectasia ("watermelon stomach")], Dieulafoy's lesion (in which an aberrant vessel in the mucosa bleeds from a pinpoint mucosal defect), prolapse gastropathy (prolapse of proximal stomach into esophagus with retching, especially in alcoholics), and hemobilia or hemosuccus pancreaticus (bleeding from the bile duct or pancreatic duct).

Small-intestinal sources of bleeding

Small-intestinal sources of bleeding (bleeding from sites beyond the reach of the standard upper endoscope) are difficult to diagnose and are responsible for the majority of cases of obscure GIB. Fortunately, small-intestinal bleeding is uncommon. The most common causes in adults are vascular ectasias, tumors (e.g., adenocarcinoma, leiomyoma, lymphoma, benign polyps, carcinoid, metastases, and lipoma), and NSAID-induced erosions and ulcers. Other less common causes in adults include Crohn's disease, infection, ischemia, vasculitis, small-bowel varices, diverticula, Meckel's diverticulum, duplication cysts, and intussusception.

Meckel's diverticulum is the most common cause of significant lower GIB (LGIB) in children, decreasing in frequency as a cause of bleeding with age. In adults <40–50 years, small-bowel tumors often account for obscure GIB; in patients >50–60 years, vascular ectasias and NSAID-induced lesions are more commonly responsible.

Vascular ectasias should be treated with endoscopic therapy if possible. Surgical therapy can be used for vascular ectasias isolated to a segment of the small intestine when endoscopic therapy is unsuccessful. Although estrogen/progesterone compounds have been used for vascular ectasias, a double-blind trial found no benefit in prevention of recurrent bleeding. Isolated lesions, such as tumors, diverticula, or duplications, are generally treated with surgical resection.

Colonic sources of bleeding

The incidence of hospitalizations for LGIB is ≥20% that for UGIB. Hemorrhoids are probably the most common cause of LGIB; anal fissures also cause minor bleeding and pain. If these local anal processes, which rarely require hospitalization, are excluded, the most common causes of LGIB in adults are diverticula, vascular ectasias (especially in the proximal colon of patients >70 years), neoplasms (primarily adenocarcinoma), and colitis—most commonly infectious or idiopathic inflammatory bowel disease, but occasionally ischemic or radiation-induced. Uncommon causes include post-polypectomy bleeding, solitary rectal ulcer syndrome, NSAID-induced ulcers or colitis, trauma, varices (most commonly rectal), lymphoid nodular hyperplasia, vasculitis, and aortocolic fistulas. In children and adolescents, the most common colonic causes of significant GIB are inflammatory bowel disease and juvenile polyps.

Diverticular bleeding is abrupt in onset, usually painless, sometimes massive, and often from the right colon; minor and occult bleeding is not characteristic. Clinical reports suggest that bleeding colonic diverticula stop bleeding spontaneously in ~80% of patients and rebleed in about 20–25% of patients. Intraarterial vasopressin or embolization by superselective technique should stop bleeding in a majority of patients. If bleeding persists or recurs, segmental surgical resection is indicated.

Bleeding from right colonic vascular ectasias in the elderly may be overt or occult; it tends to be chronic and only occasionally is hemodynamically significant. Endoscopic hemostatic therapy may be useful in the treatment of vascular ectasias, as well as discrete bleeding ulcers and post-polypectomy bleeding, while endoscopic polypectomy, if possible, is used for bleeding colonic polyps. Surgical therapy is generally required for major, persistent, or recurrent bleeding from the wide variety of colonic sources of GIB that cannot be treated medically, angiographically, or endoscopically.

APPROACH TO THE PATIENT **Gastrointestinal Bleeding**

Measurement of the heart rate and blood pressure is the best way to initially assess a patient with GIB. Clinically significant bleeding leads to postural changes in heart rate or blood pressure, tachycardia, and, finally, recumbent hypotension. In contrast, the hemoglobin does not fall immediately with acute GIB, due to proportionate reductions in plasma and red cell volumes (i.e., "people bleed whole blood"). Thus, hemoglobin may be normal or only minimally decreased at the initial presentation of a severe bleeding episode. As extravascular fluid enters the vascular space to restore volume, the hemoglobin falls, but this process may take up to 72 h. Patients with slow, chronic GIB may have very low hemoglobin values despite normal blood pressure and heart rate. With the development of iron-deficiency anemia, the mean corpuscular volume will be low and red blood cell distribution width will increase.

DIFFERENTIATION OF UPPER FROM LOWER

GIB Hematemesis indicates an upper GI source of bleeding (above the ligament of Treitz). Melena indicates that blood has been present in the GI tract for at least 14 h (and as long as 3–5 days). The more proximal the bleeding site, the more likely melena will occur. Hematochezia usually represents a lower GI source of bleeding, although an upper GI lesion may bleed so briskly that blood does not remain in the bowel long enough for melena to develop. When hematochezia is the presenting symptom of UGIB, it is associated with hemodynamic instability and dropping hemoglobin. Bleeding lesions of the small bowel may present as melena or hematochezia. Other clues to UGIB include hyperactive bowel sounds and an elevated blood urea nitrogen level (due to volume depletion and blood proteins absorbed in the small intestine).

A nonbloody nasogastric aspirate may be seen in up to 18% of patients with UGIB—usually from a duodenal source. Even a bile-stained appearance does not exclude a bleeding postpyloric lesion because reports of bile in the aspirate are incorrect in ~50% of cases. Testing of aspirates that are not grossly bloody for occult blood is not useful.

DIAGNOSTIC EVALUATION OF THE PATIENT WITH GIB

Upper GIB (Fig. 7-1) History and physical examination are not usually diagnostic of the source of GIB. Upper endoscopy is the test of choice in patients with UGIB and should be performed urgently in patients who present with hemodynamic instability (hypotension, tachycardia, or postural changes in heart rate or blood pressure). Early endoscopy is also beneficial in cases of milder bleeding for management decisions. Patients with major bleeding and high-risk endoscopic findings (e.g., varices, ulcers with active bleeding or a visible vessel) benefit from endoscopic hemostatic therapy, while patients with low-risk lesions (e.g., clean-based ulcers, nonbleeding Mallory-Weiss tears, erosive or hemorrhagic gastropathy) who have stable vital signs and hemoglobin, and no other medical problems, can be discharged home.

Lower GIB (Fig. 7-2) Patients with hematochezia and hemodynamic instability should have upper endoscopy to rule out an upper GI source before evaluation of the lower GI tract. Patients with presumed LGIB may undergo early sigmoidoscopy for the detection of obvious, low-lying lesions. However, the procedure is difficult with brisk bleeding, and it is usually not possible

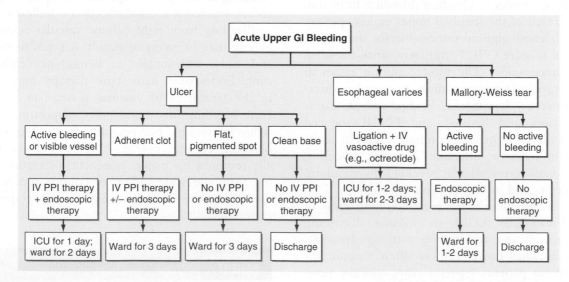

FIGURE 7-1

Suggested algorithm for patients with acute upper gastrointestinal bleeding. Recommendations on level of care and time of discharge assume patient is stabilized without further bleeding or other concomitant medical problems. ICU, intensive care unit; PPI, proton pump inhibitor.

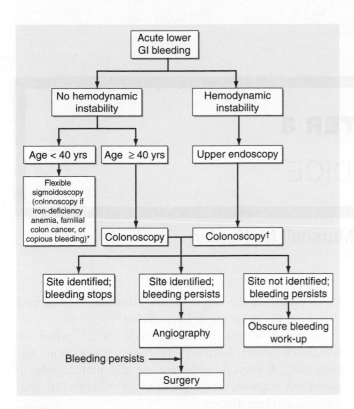

FIGURE 7-2
Suggested algorithm for patients with acute lower gastrointestinal bleeding. *Some suggest colonoscopy for any degree of rectal bleeding in patients <40 years as well. †If massive bleeding does not allow time for colonic lavage, proceed to angiography.

to identify the area of bleeding. Sigmoidoscopy is useful primarily in patients <40 years with minor bleeding.

Colonoscopy after an oral lavage solution is the procedure of choice in patients admitted with LGIB unless bleeding is too massive or unless sigmoidoscopy has disclosed an obvious actively bleeding lesion. ^{99m}Tc-labeled red cell scan allows repeated imaging for up to 24 h and may identify the general location of bleeding. However, radionuclide scans should be interpreted with caution because results, especially from later images, are highly variable. In active LGIB, angiography can detect the site of bleeding (extravasation of contrast into the gut) and permits treatment with embolization or intraarterial infusion of vasopressin. Even after bleeding has stopped, angiography may identify lesions with abnormal vasculature, such as vascular ectasias or tumors.

GIB of Obscure Origin Obscure GIB is defined as persistent or recurrent bleeding for which no source

has been identified by routine endoscopic and contrast x-ray studies; it may be overt (melena, hematochezia) or occult (iron-deficiency anemia). Current guidelines suggest angiography as the initial test for massive obscure bleeding, and video capsule endoscopy, which allows examination of the entire small intestine, for all others. Push enteroscopy, with a specially designed enteroscope or a pediatric colonoscope to inspect the entire duodenum and part of the jejunum, also may be considered as an initial evaluation. A systematic review of 14 trials comparing push enteroscopy to capsule revealed "clinically significant findings" in 26% and 56% of patients, respectively. However, in contrast to enteroscopy, lack of control of the capsule prevents its manipulation and full visualization of the intestine; in addition, tissue cannot be sampled and therapy cannot be applied.

If capsule endoscopy is positive, management (e.g., enteroscopy, laparoscopy) is dictated by the finding. If capsule is negative, current recommendations suggest patients may be either observed, or if their clinical course mandates (e.g., recurrent bleeding, need for transfusions or hospitalization), undergo further testing. Newer endoscopic techniques (e.g., double-balloon, single-balloon, and spiral enteroscopy) allow the endoscopist to examine, obtain specimens from, and provide therapy to much or all of the small intestine. Newer imaging techniques (CT and MR enterography) are now frequently being used in place of older specialized small-bowel radiographic exams (e.g., enteroclysis). Other tests include ^{99m}Tc-labeled red blood cell scintigraphy; angiography, which may be useful even if bleeding has subsided because it may disclose vascular anomalies or tumor vessels; and ^{99m}Tc-pertechnetate scintigraphy for diagnosis of Meckel's diverticulum (especially in young patients). When all tests are unrevealing, intraoperative endoscopy is indicated in patients with severe recurrent or persistent bleeding requiring repeated transfusions.

Positive Fecal Occult Blood Test Fecal occult blood testing is recommended only for colorectal cancer screening and may be used in average-risk adults (beginning at age 50) and in adults with a first-degree relative with colorectal neoplasm at ≥60 years or two second-degree relatives with colorectal cancer (beginning at age 40). A positive test necessitates colonoscopy. If evaluation of the colon is negative, further workup is not recommended unless iron-deficiency anemia or GI symptoms are present.

CHAPTER 8

JAUNDICE

Daniel S. Pratt ■ Marshall M. Kaplan

Jaundice, or icterus, is a yellowish discoloration of tissue resulting from the deposition of bilirubin. Tissue deposition of bilirubin occurs only in the presence of serum hyperbilirubinemia and is a sign of either liver disease or, less often, a hemolytic disorder. The degree of serum bilirubin elevation can be estimated by physical examination. Slight increases in serum bilirubin are best detected by examining the sclerae, which have a particular affinity for bilirubin due to their high elastin content. The presence of scleral icterus indicates a serum bilirubin of at least 51 μmol/L (3 mg/dL). The ability to detect scleral icterus is made more difficult if the examining room has fluorescent lighting. If the examiner suspects scleral icterus, a second place to examine is underneath the tongue. As serum bilirubin levels rise, the skin will eventually become yellow in light-skinned patients and even green if the process is long-standing; the green color is produced by oxidation of bilirubin to biliverdin.

The differential diagnosis for yellowing of the skin is limited. In addition to jaundice, it includes carotenoderma, the use of the drug quinacrine, and excessive exposure to phenols. Carotenoderma is the yellow color imparted to the skin by the presence of carotene; it occurs in healthy individuals who ingest excessive amounts of vegetables and fruits that contain carotene, such as carrots, leafy vegetables, squash, peaches, and oranges. Unlike jaundice, where the yellow coloration of the skin is uniformly distributed over the body, in carotenoderma, the pigment is concentrated on the palms, soles, forehead, and nasolabial folds. Carotenoderma can be distinguished from jaundice by the sparing of the sclerae. Quinacrine causes a yellow discoloration of the skin in 4–37% of patients treated with it. Unlike carotene, quinacrine can cause discoloration of the sclerae.

Another sensitive indicator of increased serum bilirubin is darkening of the urine, which is due to the renal excretion of conjugated bilirubin. Patients often describe their urine as tea- or cola-colored. Bilirubinuria indicates an elevation of the direct serum bilirubin fraction and, therefore, the presence of liver disease.

Increased serum bilirubin levels occur when an imbalance exists between bilirubin production and clearance. A logical evaluation of the patient who is jaundiced requires an understanding of bilirubin production and metabolism.

PRODUCTION AND METABOLISM OF BILIRUBIN

(See also Chap. 37) Bilirubin, a tetrapyrrole pigment, is a breakdown product of heme (ferroprotoporphyrin IX). About 70–80% of the 250–300 mg of bilirubin produced each day is derived from the breakdown of hemoglobin in senescent red blood cells. The remainder comes from prematurely destroyed erythroid cells in bone marrow and from the turnover of hemoproteins such as myoglobin and cytochromes found in tissues throughout the body.

The formation of bilirubin occurs in reticuloendothelial cells, primarily in the spleen and liver. The first reaction, catalyzed by the microsomal enzyme heme oxygenase, oxidatively cleaves the α bridge of the porphyrin group and opens the heme ring. The end products of this reaction are biliverdin, carbon monoxide, and iron. The second reaction, catalyzed by the cytosolic enzyme biliverdin reductase, reduces the central methylene bridge of biliverdin and converts it to bilirubin. Bilirubin formed in the reticuloendothelial cells is virtually insoluble in water. This is due to tight internal hydrogen bonding between the water-soluble moieties of bilirubin, proprionic acid carboxyl groups of one dipyrrolic half of the molecule with the imino and lactam groups of the opposite half. This configuration blocks solvent access to the polar residues of bilirubin and places the hydrophobic residues on the outside. To be transported in blood, bilirubin must be solubilized. This is accomplished by its reversible, non-covalent binding to albumin. Unconjugated bilirubin bound to albumin is transported to the liver, where it, but not the albumin, is taken up by hepatocytes via a process that at least partly involves carrier-mediated membrane transport. No specific bilirubin transporter has yet been identified (Chap. 37, Fig. 37-1).

After entering the hepatocyte, unconjugated bilirubin is bound in the cytosol to a number of proteins including proteins in the glutathione-S-transferase superfamily. These proteins serve both to reduce efflux of bilirubin back into the serum and to present the bilirubin for conjugation. In the endoplasmic reticulum, bilirubin is solubilized by conjugation to glucuronic acid, a process that disrupts the internal hydrogen bonds and yields bilirubin monoglucuronide and diglucuronide. The conjugation of glucuronic acid to bilirubin is catalyzed by bilirubin uridine diphosphate-glucuronosyl transferase (UDPGT). The now hydrophilic bilirubin conjugates diffuse from the endoplasmic reticulum to the canalicular membrane, where bilirubin monoglucuronide and diglucuronide are actively transported into canalicular bile by an energy-dependent mechanism involving the multiple drug resistance protein 2.

The conjugated bilirubin excreted into bile drains into the duodenum and passes unchanged through the proximal small bowel. Conjugated bilirubin is not taken up by the intestinal mucosa. When the conjugated bilirubin reaches the distal ileum and colon, it is hydrolyzed to unconjugated bilirubin by bacterial β-glucuronidases. The unconjugated bilirubin is reduced by normal gut bacteria to form a group of colorless tetrapyrroles called urobilinogens. About 80–90% of these products are excreted in feces, either unchanged or oxidized to orange derivatives called urobilins. The remaining 10–20% of the urobilinogens are passively absorbed, enter the portal venous blood, and are reexcreted by the liver. A small fraction (usually <3 mg/dL) escapes hepatic uptake, filters across the renal glomerulus, and is excreted in urine.

MEASUREMENT OF SERUM BILIRUBIN

The terms direct and indirect bilirubin, conjugated and unconjugated bilirubin, respectively, are based on the original van den Bergh reaction. This assay, or a variation of it, is still used in most clinical chemistry laboratories to determine the serum bilirubin level. In this assay, bilirubin is exposed to diazotized sulfanilic acid, splitting into two relatively stable dipyrrylmethene azopigments that absorb maximally at 540 nm, allowing for photometric analysis. The direct fraction is that which reacts with diazotized sulfanilic acid in the absence of an accelerator substance such as alcohol. The direct fraction provides an approximate determination of the conjugated bilirubin in serum. The total serum bilirubin is the amount that reacts after the addition of alcohol. The indirect fraction is the difference between the total and the direct bilirubin and provides an estimate of the unconjugated bilirubin in serum.

With the van den Bergh method, the normal serum bilirubin concentration usually is 17 μmol/L (<1 mg/dL). Up to 30%, or 5.1 μmol/L (0.3 mg/dL), of the total may be direct-reacting (conjugated) bilirubin. Total serum bilirubin concentrations are between 3.4 and 15.4 μmol/L (0.2 and 0.9 mg/dL) in 95% of a normal population.

Several new techniques, although less convenient to perform, have added considerably to our understanding of bilirubin metabolism. First, they demonstrate that in normal persons or those with Gilbert's syndrome, almost 100% of the serum bilirubin is unconjugated; <3% is monoconjugated bilirubin. Second, in jaundiced patients with hepatobiliary disease, the total serum bilirubin concentration measured by these new, more accurate methods is lower than the values found with diazo methods. This suggests that there are diazo-positive compounds distinct from bilirubin in the serum of patients with hepatobiliary disease. Third, these studies indicate that, in jaundiced patients with hepatobiliary disease, monoglucuronides of bilirubin predominate over the diglucuronides. Fourth, part of the direct-reacting bilirubin fraction includes conjugated bilirubin that is covalently linked to albumin. This albumin-linked bilirubin fraction (*delta fraction,* or *biliprotein*) represents an important fraction of total serum bilirubin in patients with cholestasis and hepatobiliary disorders. Albumin-bound conjugated bilirubin is formed in serum when hepatic excretion of bilirubin glucuronides is impaired and the glucuronides are present in serum in increasing amounts. By virtue of its tight binding to albumin, the clearance rate of albumin-bound bilirubin from serum approximates the half-life of albumin, 12–14 days, rather than the short half-life of bilirubin, about 4 h.

The prolonged half-life of albumin-bound conjugated bilirubin explains two previously unexplained enigmas in jaundiced patients with liver disease: (1) that some patients with conjugated hyperbilirubinemia do not exhibit bilirubinuria during the recovery phase of their disease because the bilirubin is covalently bound to albumin and therefore not filtered by the renal glomeruli, and (2) that the elevated serum bilirubin level declines more slowly than expected in some patients who otherwise appear to be recovering satisfactorily. Late in the recovery phase of hepatobiliary disorders, all the conjugated bilirubin may be in the albumin-linked form. Its value in serum falls slowly because of the long half-life of albumin.

MEASUREMENT OF URINE BILIRUBIN

Unconjugated bilirubin is always bound to albumin in the serum, is not filtered by the kidney, and is not found in the urine. Conjugated bilirubin is filtered at the glomerulus and the majority is reabsorbed by the proximal tubules; a small fraction is excreted in the urine. Any bilirubin found in the urine is conjugated bilirubin. The presence of bilirubinuria implies the presence of liver disease. A urine dipstick test (Ictotest) gives the same information as fractionation of the serum bilirubin. This test is very accurate. A false-negative test is possible in patients with prolonged cholestasis due to the predominance of conjugated bilirubin covalently bound to albumin.

APPROACH TO THE PATIENT | Bilirubin

The bilirubin present in serum represents a balance between input from production of bilirubin and hepatic/biliary removal of the pigment. Hyperbilirubinemia may result from (1) overproduction of bilirubin; (2) impaired uptake, conjugation, or excretion of bilirubin; or (3) regurgitation of unconjugated or conjugated bilirubin

from damaged hepatocytes or bile ducts. An increase in unconjugated bilirubin in serum results from either overproduction, impairment of uptake, or conjugation of bilirubin. An increase in conjugated bilirubin is due to decreased excretion into the bile ductules or backward leakage of the pigment. The initial steps in evaluating the patient with jaundice are to determine (1) whether the hyperbilirubinemia is predominantly conjugated or unconjugated in nature, and (2) whether other biochemical liver tests are abnormal. The thoughtful interpretation of limited data will allow for a rational evaluation of the patient (Fig. 8-1). This discussion will focus solely on the evaluation of the adult patient with jaundice.

ISOLATED ELEVATION OF SERUM BILIRUBIN

Unconjugated Hyperbilirubinemia The differential diagnosis of an isolated unconjugated hyperbilirubinemia is limited (Table 8-1). The critical determination

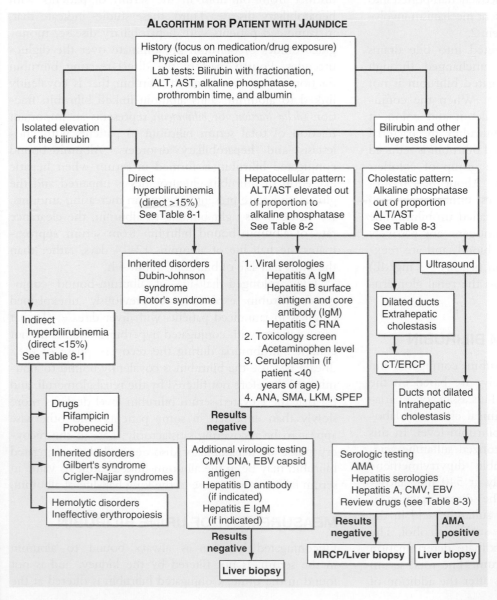

ALGORITHM FOR PATIENT WITH JAUNDICE

History (focus on medication/drug exposure)
Physical examination
Lab tests: Bilirubin with fractionation,
ALT, AST, alkaline phosphatase,
prothrombin time, and albumin

Isolated elevation of the bilirubin

Bilirubin and other liver tests elevated

Direct hyperbilirubinemia (direct >15%) See Table 8-1

Hepatocellular pattern: ALT/AST elevated out of proportion to alkaline phosphatase See Table 8-2

Cholestatic pattern: Alkaline phosphatase out of proportion ALT/AST See Table 8-3

Inherited disorders
Dubin-Johnson syndrome
Rotor's syndrome

1. Viral serologies
   Hepatitis A IgM
   Hepatitis B surface antigen and core antibody (IgM)
   Hepatitis C RNA
2. Toxicology screen
   Acetaminophen level
3. Ceruloplasmin (if patient <40 years of age)
4. ANA, SMA, LKM, SPEP

Ultrasound

Dilated ducts
Extrahepatic cholestasis

CT/ERCP

Ducts not dilated
Intrahepatic cholestasis

Indirect hyperbilirubinemia (direct <15%) See Table 8-1

Drugs
Rifampicin
Probenecid

Inherited disorders
Gilbert's syndrome
Crigler-Najjar syndromes

Hemolytic disorders
Ineffective erythropoiesis

Results negative

Additional virologic testing
CMV DNA, EBV capsid antigen
Hepatitis D antibody (if indicated)
Hepatitis E IgM (if indicated)

Serologic testing
AMA
Hepatitis serologies
Hepatitis A, CMV, EBV
Review drugs (see Table 8-3)

Results negative

Results negative

AMA positive

Results negative

Liver biopsy

MRCP/Liver biopsy

Liver biopsy

FIGURE 8-1

Evaluation of the patient with jaundice. ALT, alanine aminotransferase; AMA, antimitochondrial antibody; ANA, antinuclear antibody; AST, aspartate aminotransferase; CMV, cytomegalovirus; EBV, Epstein-Barr virus; LKM, liver-kidney microsomal antibody; MRCP, magnetic resonance cholangiopancreatography; SMA, smooth-muscle antibody; SPEP, serum protein electrophoresis.

TABLE 8-1

CAUSES OF ISOLATED HYPERBILIRUBINEMIA

I. Indirect hyperbilirubinemia
  A. Hemolytic disorders
    1. Inherited
      a. Spherocytosis, elliptocytosis
        Glucose-6-phosphate dehydrogenase and
        pyruvate kinase deficiencies
      b. Sickle cell anemia
    2. Acquired
      a. Microangiopathic hemolytic anemias
      b. Paroxysmal nocturnal hemoglobinuria
      c. Spur cell anemia
      d. Immune hemolysis
      e. Parasitic infections
        1. Malaria
        2. Babesiosis
  B. Ineffective erythropoiesis
    1. Cobalamin, folate, thalassemia, and severe iron
      deficiencies
  C. Drugs
    1. Rifampicin, probenecid, ribavirin
  D. Inherited conditions
    1. Crigler-Najjar types I and II
    2. Gilbert's syndrome
II. Direct hyperbilirubinemia
  A. Inherited conditions
    1. Dubin-Johnson syndrome
    2. Rotor's syndrome

is whether the patient is suffering from a hemolytic process resulting in an overproduction of bilirubin (hemolytic disorders and ineffective erythropoiesis) or from impaired hepatic uptake/conjugation of bilirubin (drug effect or genetic disorders).

Hemolytic disorders that cause excessive heme production may be either inherited or acquired. Inherited disorders include spherocytosis, sickle cell anemia, thalassemia, and deficiency of red cell enzymes such as pyruvate kinase and glucose-6-phosphate dehydrogenase. In these conditions, the serum bilirubin rarely exceeds 86 μmol/L (5 mg/dL). Higher levels may occur when there is coexistent renal or hepatocellular dysfunction or in acute hemolysis such as a sickle cell crisis. In evaluating jaundice in patients with chronic hemolysis, it is important to remember the high incidence of pigmented (calcium bilirubinate) gallstones found in these patients, which increases the likelihood of choledocholithiasis as an alternative explanation for hyperbilirubinemia.

Acquired hemolytic disorders include microangiopathic hemolytic anemia (e.g., hemolytic-uremic syndrome), paroxysmal nocturnal hemoglobinuria, spur cell anemia, and immune hemolysis and parasitic infections including malaria and babesiosis. Ineffective erythropoiesis occurs in cobalamin, folate, and iron deficiencies.

In the absence of hemolysis, the physician should consider a problem with the hepatic uptake or conjugation of bilirubin. Certain drugs, including rifampicin and probenecid, may cause unconjugated hyperbilirubinemia by diminishing hepatic uptake of bilirubin. Impaired bilirubin conjugation occurs in three genetic conditions: Crigler-Najjar syndrome, types I and II, and Gilbert's syndrome. *Crigler-Najjar type I* is an exceptionally rare condition found in neonates and characterized by severe jaundice [bilirubin >342 μmol/L (>20 mg/dL)] and neurologic impairment due to kernicterus, frequently leading to death in infancy or childhood. These patients have a complete absence of bilirubin UDPGT activity, usually due to mutations in the critical 3′ domain of the *UDPGT* gene, and are totally unable to conjugate, and hence cannot excrete, bilirubin. The only effective treatment is orthotopic liver transplantation. Use of gene therapy and allogeneic hepatocyte infusion are experimental approaches of future promise for this devastating disease.

Crigler-Najjar type II is somewhat more common than type I. Patients live into adulthood with serum bilirubin levels that range from 103–428 μmol/L (6–25 mg/dL). In these patients, mutations in the bilirubin *UDPGT* gene cause reduced but not completely absent activity of the enzyme. Bilirubin *UDPGT* activity can be induced by the administration of phenobarbital, which can reduce serum bilirubin levels in these patients. Despite marked jaundice, these patients usually survive into adulthood, although they may be susceptible to kernicterus under the stress of intercurrent illness or surgery.

Gilbert's syndrome is also marked by the impaired conjugation of bilirubin due to reduced bilirubin UDPGT activity to approximately one-third of normal. Gilbert's syndrome is very common, with a reported incidence of 3–12%. Patients with Gilbert's syndrome have a mild unconjugated hyperbilirubinemia with serum levels almost always <103 μmol/L (6 mg/dL). The serum levels may fluctuate, and jaundice is often identified only during periods of fasting. One molecular defect that has been identified in patients with Gilbert's syndrome is in the TATAA element in the 5′ promoter region of the bilirubin *UDPGT* gene upstream of exon 1. This defect alone is not necessarily sufficient for producing the clinical syndrome of Gilbert's as there are patients who are homozygous for this defect yet do not have the levels of hyperbilirubinemia typically seen in Gilbert's syndrome. An enhancer polymorphism that lowers transcriptional activity has been identified. The decrease in transcription caused by both mutations together may be critical for producing the syndrome. Unlike both Crigler-Najjar syndromes, Gilbert's syndrome is very common. The reported incidence is 3–7% of the population with males predominating over females by a ratio of 2–7:1.

Conjugated Hyperbilirubinemia Elevated conjugated hyperbilirubinemia is found in two rare inherited conditions: *Dubin-Johnson syndrome* and *Rotor's syndrome* (Table 8-1). Patients with both conditions present with asymptomatic jaundice, typically in the second generation of life. The defect in Dubin-Johnson syndrome is mutations in the gene for multiple drug resistance protein 2. These patients have altered excretion of bilirubin into the bile ducts. Rotor's syndrome seems to be a problem with the hepatic storage of bilirubin. Differentiating between these syndromes is possible, but clinically unnecessary, due to their benign nature.

ELEVATION OF SERUM BILIRUBIN WITH OTHER LIVER TEST ABNORMALITIES
The remainder of this chapter will focus on the evaluation of the patient with a conjugated hyperbilirubinemia in the setting of other liver test abnormalities. This group of patients can be divided into those with a primary hepatocellular process and those with intra- or extrahepatic cholestasis. Being able to make this differentiation will guide the physician's evaluation (Fig. 8-1). This differentiation is made on the basis of the history and physical examination as well as the pattern of liver test abnormalities.

History A complete medical history is perhaps the single most important part of the evaluation of the patient with unexplained jaundice. Important considerations include the use of or exposure to any chemical or medication, either physician-prescribed, over-the-counter, complementary or alternative medicines such as herbal and vitamin preparations, or other drugs such as anabolic steroids. The patient should be carefully questioned about possible parenteral exposures, including transfusions, intravenous and intranasal drug use, tattoos, and sexual activity. Other important questions include recent travel history; exposure to people with jaundice; exposure to possibly contaminated foods; occupational exposure to hepatotoxins; alcohol consumption; the duration of jaundice; and the presence of any accompanying symptoms such as arthralgias, myalgias, rash, anorexia, weight loss, abdominal pain, fever, pruritus, and changes in the urine and stool. While none of these latter symptoms are specific for any one condition, they can suggest a particular diagnosis. A history of arthralgias and myalgias predating jaundice suggests hepatitis, either viral or drug-related. Jaundice associated with the sudden onset of severe right upper quadrant pain and shaking chills suggests choledocholithiasis and ascending cholangitis.

Physical Examination The general assessment should include assessment of the patient's nutritional status. Temporal and proximal muscle wasting suggests long-standing diseases such as pancreatic cancer or cirrhosis. Stigmata of chronic liver disease, including spider nevi, palmar erythema, gynecomastia, caput medusae, Dupuytren's contractures, parotid gland enlargement, and testicular atrophy are commonly seen in advanced alcoholic (Laennec's) cirrhosis and occasionally in other types of cirrhosis. An enlarged left supraclavicular node (Virchow's node) or periumbilical nodule (Sister Mary Joseph's nodule) suggests an abdominal malignancy. Jugular venous distention, a sign of right-sided heart failure, suggests hepatic congestion. Right pleural effusion, in the absence of clinically apparent ascites, may be seen in advanced cirrhosis.

The abdominal examination should focus on the size and consistency of the liver, whether the spleen is palpable and hence enlarged, and whether there is ascites present. Patients with cirrhosis may have an enlarged left lobe of the liver, which is felt below the xiphoid, and an enlarged spleen. A grossly enlarged nodular liver or an obvious abdominal mass suggests malignancy. An enlarged tender liver could be viral or alcoholic hepatitis; an infiltrative process such as amyloid; or, less often, an acutely congested liver secondary to right-sided heart failure. Severe right upper quadrant tenderness with respiratory arrest on inspiration (Murphy's sign) suggests cholecystitis or, occasionally, ascending cholangitis. Ascites in the presence of jaundice suggests either cirrhosis or malignancy with peritoneal spread.

Laboratory Tests When the physician encounters a patient with unexplained jaundice, there is a battery of tests that are helpful in the initial evaluation. These include total and direct serum bilirubin with fractionation, aminotransferases, alkaline phosphatase, albumin, and prothrombin time tests. Enzyme tests [alanine aminotransferase (ALT), aspartate aminotransferase (AST), and alkaline phosphatase (ALP)] are helpful in differentiating between a hepatocellular process and a cholestatic process (Table 36-1; Fig. 8-1), a critical step in determining what additional workup is indicated. Patients with a hepatocellular process generally have a disproportionate rise in the aminotransferases compared to the ALP. Patients with a cholestatic process have a disproportionate rise in the ALP compared to the aminotransferases. The bilirubin can be prominently elevated in both hepatocellular and cholestatic conditions and, therefore, is not necessarily helpful in differentiating between the two.

In addition to the enzyme tests, all jaundiced patients should have additional blood tests, specifically an albumin level and a prothrombin time, to assess liver function. A low albumin level suggests a chronic process such as cirrhosis or cancer. A normal albumin level is suggestive of a more acute process such as viral hepatitis or choledocholithiasis. An elevated prothrombin time indicates either vitamin K deficiency due to prolonged jaundice and malabsorption of vitamin K or significant hepatocellular dysfunction. The failure of the prothrombin time to correct with parenteral administration of vitamin K indicates severe hepatocellular injury.

The results of the bilirubin, enzyme tests, albumin, and prothrombin time tests will usually indicate whether a jaundiced patient has a hepatocellular or a cholestatic disease, as well as some indication of the duration and severity of the disease. The causes and evaluation of hepatocellular and cholestatic diseases are quite different.

Hepatocellular Conditions Hepatocellular diseases that can cause jaundice include viral hepatitis, drug or environmental toxicity, alcohol, and end-stage cirrhosis from any cause (Table 8-2). Wilson's disease, once believed to occur primarily in young adults, should be considered in all adults if no other cause of jaundice is found. Autoimmune hepatitis is typically seen in young to middle-aged women but may affect men and women of any age. Alcoholic hepatitis can be differentiated from viral and toxin-related hepatitis by the pattern of the aminotransferases. Patients with alcoholic hepatitis typically have an AST:ALT ratio of at least 2:1. The AST rarely exceeds 300 U/L. Patients with acute viral hepatitis and toxin-related injury severe enough to produce jaundice typically have aminotransferases >500 U/L, with the ALT greater than or equal to the AST. The degree of aminotransferase elevation can occasionally help in differentiating between hepatocellular and cholestatic processes. While ALT and AST values less than 8 times normal may be seen in either hepatocellular or cholestatic liver disease, values 25 times normal or higher are seen primarily in acute hepatocellular diseases. Patients with jaundice

TABLE 8-2

HEPATOCELLULAR CONDITIONS THAT MAY PRODUCE JAUNDICE
Viral hepatitis
Hepatitis A, B, C, D, and E
Epstein-Barr virus
Cytomegalovirus
Herpes simplex
Alcohol
Drug toxicity
Predictable, dose-dependent (e.g., acetaminophen)
Unpredictable, idiosyncratic (e.g., isoniazid)
Environmental toxins
Vinyl chloride
Jamaica bush tea—pyrrolizidine alkaloids
Kava Kava
Wild mushrooms—*Amanita phalloides* or *A. verna*
Wilson's disease
Autoimmune hepatitis

from cirrhosis can have normal or only slight elevations of the aminotransferases.

When the physician determines that the patient has a hepatocellular disease, appropriate testing for acute viral hepatitis includes a hepatitis A IgM antibody, a hepatitis B surface antigen and core IgM antibody, and a hepatitis C viral RNA test. It can take many weeks for the hepatitis C antibody to become detectable, making it an unreliable test if acute hepatitis C is suspected. Depending on circumstances, studies for hepatitis D and E, Epstein-Barr virus (EBV), and cytomegalovirus (CMV) may be indicated. Ceruloplasmin is the initial screening test for Wilson's disease. Testing for autoimmune hepatitis usually includes an antinuclear antibody and measurement of specific immunoglobulins.

Drug-induced hepatocellular injury can be classified either as predictable or unpredictable. Predictable drug reactions are dose-dependent and affect all patients who ingest a toxic dose of the drug in question. The classic example is acetaminophen hepatotoxicity. Unpredictable or idiosyncratic drug reactions are not dose-dependent and occur in a minority of patients. A great number of drugs can cause idiosyncratic hepatic injury. Environmental toxins are also an important cause of hepatocellular injury. Examples include industrial chemicals such as vinyl chloride, herbal preparations containing pyrrolizidine alkaloids (Jamaica bush tea) and Kava Kava, and the mushrooms *Amanita phalloides* or *A. verna* that contain highly hepatotoxic amatoxins.

Cholestatic Conditions When the pattern of the liver tests suggests a cholestatic disorder, the next step is to determine whether it is intra- or extrahepatic cholestasis (Fig. 8-1). Distinguishing intrahepatic from extrahepatic cholestasis may be difficult. History, physical examination, and laboratory tests are often not helpful. The next appropriate test is an ultrasound. The ultrasound is inexpensive, does not expose the patient to ionizing radiation, and can detect dilation of the intra- and extrahepatic biliary tree with a high degree of sensitivity and specificity. The absence of biliary dilatation suggests intrahepatic cholestasis, while the presence of biliary dilatation indicates extrahepatic cholestasis. False-negative results occur in patients with partial obstruction of the common bile duct or in patients with cirrhosis or primary sclerosing cholangitis (PSC) where scarring prevents the intrahepatic ducts from dilating.

Although ultrasonography may indicate extrahepatic cholestasis, it rarely identifies the site or cause of obstruction. The distal common bile duct is a particularly difficult area to visualize by ultrasound because of overlying bowel gas. Appropriate next tests include CT, magnetic resonance cholangiography (MRCP), and endoscopic retrograde cholangiopancreatography (ERCP). CT scanning and MRCP are better than ultrasonography for assessing the head of the pancreas and for identifying choledocholithiasis in the distal common bile duct, particularly when the ducts are not dilated. ERCP is the "gold standard" for identifying choledocholithiasis. It is performed by introducing a side-viewing endoscope perorally into the duodenum. The ampulla of Vater is visualized, and a catheter is advanced through the ampulla. Injection of dye allows for the visualization of the common bile duct and the pancreatic duct. Beyond its diagnostic capabilities, ERCP allows for therapeutic interventions, including the removal of common bile duct stones and the placement of stents. In patients in whom ERCP is unsuccessful and there is a high likelihood of the need for a therapeutic intervention, transhepatic cholangiography can provide the same information and allow for intervention. MRCP has replaced ERCP as the initial diagnostic test in cases where the need for intervention is felt to be small.

In patients with apparent *intrahepatic cholestasis*, the diagnosis is often made by serologic testing in combination with percutaneous liver biopsy. The list of possible causes of intrahepatic cholestasis is long and varied (Table 8-3). A number of conditions that typically cause a hepatocellular pattern of injury can also present as a cholestatic variant. Both hepatitis B and C can cause a cholestatic hepatitis (fibrosing cholestatic hepatitis). This disease variant has been reported in patients who have undergone solid organ transplantation. Hepatitis A, alcoholic hepatitis, EBV, and CMV may also present as cholestatic liver disease.

Drugs may cause intrahepatic cholestasis, a variant of drug-induced hepatitis. Drug-induced cholestasis is usually reversible after eliminating the offending drug, although it may take many months for cholestasis to resolve. Drugs most commonly associated with cholestasis are the anabolic and contraceptive steroids. Cholestatic hepatitis has been reported with chlorpromazine, imipramine, tolbutamide, sulindac, cimetidine, and erythromycin estolate. It also occurs in patients taking trimethoprim; sulfamethoxazole; and penicillin-based antibiotics such as ampicillin, dicloxacillin, and clavulinic acid. Rarely, cholestasis may be chronic and associated with progressive fibrosis despite early discontinuation of the drug. Chronic cholestasis has been associated with chlorpromazine and prochlorperazine.

Primary biliary cirrhosis is an autoimmune disease predominantly of middle-aged women in which there is a progressive destruction of interlobular bile ducts. The diagnosis is made by the presence of the antimitochondrial antibody that is found in 95% of patients. *Primary sclerosing cholangitis* is characterized by the destruction and fibrosis of larger bile ducts. The disease may involve only the intrahepatic ducts and present as intrahepatic cholestasis. However, in 95% of patients with

TABLE 8-3

CHOLESTATIC CONDITIONS THAT MAY PRODUCE JAUNDICE

I. Intrahepatic
  A. Viral hepatitis
    1. Fibrosing cholestatic hepatitis—hepatitis B and C
    2. Hepatitis A, Epstein-Barr virus, cytomegalovirus
  B. Alcoholic hepatitis
  C. Drug toxicity
    1. Pure cholestasis—anabolic and contraceptive steroids
    2. Cholestatic hepatitis—chlorpromazine, erythromycin estolate
    3. Chronic cholestasis—chlorpromazine and prochlorperazine
  D. Primary biliary cirrhosis
  E. Primary sclerosing cholangitis
  F. Vanishing bile duct syndrome
    1. Chronic rejection of liver transplants
    2. Sarcoidosis
    3. Drugs
  G. Inherited
    1. Progressive familial intrahepatic cholestasis
    2. Benign recurrent cholestasis
  H. Cholestasis of pregnancy
  I. Total parenteral nutrition
  J. Nonhepatobiliary sepsis
  K. Benign postoperative cholestasis
  L. Paraneoplastic syndrome
  M. Venoocclusive disease
  N. Graft-versus-host disease
  O. Infiltrative disease
    1. TB
    2. Lymphoma
    3. Amyloid
  P. Infections
    1. Malaria
    2. Leptospirosis
II. Extrahepatic
  A. Malignant
    1. Cholangiocarcinoma
    2. Pancreatic cancer
    3. Gallbladder cancer
    4. Ampullary cancer
    5. Malignant involvement of the porta hepatis lymph nodes
  B. Benign
    1. Choledocholithiasis
    2. Postoperative biliary structures
    3. Primary sclerosing cholangitis
    4. Chronic pancreatitis
    5. AIDS cholangiopathy
    6. Mirizzi's syndrome
    7. Parasitic disease (ascariasis)

PSC, both intra- and extrahepatic ducts are involved. The diagnosis of PSC is made by imaging the biliary tree. The pathognomonic findings are multiple strictures of bile ducts with dilatations proximal to the strictures.

Approximately 75% of patients with PSC have inflammatory bowel disease.

The *vanishing bile duct syndrome* and *adult bile ductopenia* are rare conditions in which there are a decreased number of bile ducts seen in liver biopsy specimens. The histologic picture is similar to that found in primary biliary cirrhosis. This picture is seen in patients who develop chronic rejection after liver transplantation and in those who develop graft-versus-host disease after bone marrow transplantation. Vanishing bile duct syndrome also occurs in rare cases of sarcoidosis, in patients taking certain drugs including chlorpromazine, and idiopathically.

There are also familial forms of intrahepatic cholestasis. The familial intrahepatic cholestatic syndromes include *progressive familial intrahepatic cholestasis* (PFIC) *types 1–3*, and *benign recurrent cholestasis* (BRC). PFIC1 and BRC are autosomal recessive diseases that result from mutations in the *ATP8B1* gene that encodes a protein belonging to the subfamily of P-type ATPases; the exact function of this protein remains poorly defined. While PFIC1 is a progressive condition that manifests in childhood, BRC presents later than PFIC1 and is marked by recurrent episodes of jaundice and pruritus; the episodes are self-limited but can be debilitating. PFIC2 is caused by mutations in the *ABCB11* gene, which encodes the bile salt export pump, and PFIC3 is caused by mutations in the multidrug-resistant P-glycoprotein 3. *Cholestasis of pregnancy* occurs in the second and third trimesters and resolves after delivery. Its cause is unknown, but the condition is probably inherited and cholestasis can be triggered by estrogen administration.

Other causes of intrahepatic cholestasis include total parenteral nutrition (TPN); nonhepatobiliary sepsis; benign postoperative cholestasis; and a paraneoplastic syndrome associated with a number of different malignancies, including Hodgkin's disease, medullary thyroid cancer, renal cell cancer, renal sarcoma, T cell lymphoma, prostate cancer, and several gastrointestinal malignancies. The term *Stauffer's syndrome* has been used for intrahepatic cholestasis specifically associated with renal cell cancer. In patients developing cholestasis in the intensive care unit, the major considerations should be sepsis, shock liver, and TPN jaundice. Jaundice occurring after bone marrow transplantation is most likely due to venoocclusive disease or graft-versus-host disease.

Jaundice with associated liver dysfunction can be seen in severe cases of *Plasmodium falciparum*. The jaundice in these cases is a combination of indirect hyperbilirubinemia from hemolysis and both cholestatic and hepatocellular jaundice. Poor outcomes are seen in these cases when the jaundice is accompanied by encephalopathy and renal failure. Weil's disease, a severe presentation of leptospirosis, is marked by jaundice with renal failure, fever, headache, and muscle pain.

Causes of *extrahepatic cholestasis* can be split into malignant and benign (Table 8-3). Malignant causes include pancreatic, gallbladder, ampullary, and cholangiocarcinoma. The latter is most commonly associated with PSC and is exceptionally difficult to diagnose because its appearance is often identical to that of PSC. Pancreatic and gallbladder tumors, as well as cholangiocarcinoma, are rarely resectable and have poor prognoses. Ampullary carcinoma has the highest surgical cure rate of all the tumors that present as painless jaundice. Hilar lymphadenopathy due to metastases from other cancers may cause obstruction of the extrahepatic biliary tree.

Choledocholithiasis is the most common cause of extrahepatic cholestasis. The clinical presentation can range from mild right upper quadrant discomfort with only minimal elevations of the enzyme tests to ascending cholangitis with jaundice, sepsis, and circulatory collapse. PSC may occur with clinically important strictures limited to the extrahepatic biliary tree. In cases where there is a dominant stricture, patients can be effectively managed with serial endoscopic dilatations. Chronic pancreatitis rarely causes strictures of the distal common bile duct, where it passes through the head of the pancreas. AIDS cholangiopathy is a condition, usually due to infection of the bile duct epithelium with CMV or cryptosporidia, which has a cholangiographic appearance similar to that of PSC. These patients usually present with greatly elevated serum alkaline phosphatase levels (mean, 800 IU/L), but the bilirubin is often near normal. These patients do not typically present with jaundice.

SUMMARY

The goal of this chapter is not to provide an encyclopedic review of all of the conditions that can cause jaundice. Rather, it is intended to provide a framework that helps a physician to evaluate the patient with jaundice in a logical way (Fig. 8-1).

Simply stated, the initial step is to obtain appropriate blood tests to determine if the patient has an isolated elevation of serum bilirubin. If so, is the bilirubin elevation due to an increased unconjugated or conjugated fraction? If the hyperbilirubinemia is accompanied by other liver test abnormalities, is the disorder hepatocellular or cholestatic? If cholestatic, is it intra- or extrahepatic? All of these questions can be answered with a thoughtful history, physical examination, and interpretation of laboratory and radiologic tests and procedures.

CHAPTER 9

ABDOMINAL SWELLING AND ASCITES

Kathleen E. Corey ■ Lawrence S. Friedman

ABDOMINAL SWELLING

Abdominal swelling is a manifestation of numerous diseases. Patients may complain of bloating or abdominal fullness and may note increasing abdominal girth on the basis of increased clothing or belt size. Abdominal discomfort is often reported, but pain is less frequent. When abdominal pain does accompany swelling, it is frequently the result of an intraabdominal infection, peritonitis, or pancreatitis. Patients with abdominal distention from ascites (fluid in the abdomen) may report the new onset of an inguinal or umbilical hernia. Dyspnea may result from pressure against the diaphragm and the inability to expand the lungs fully.

The causes of abdominal swelling can be remembered conveniently by the *six Fs*: flatus, fat, fluid, fetus, feces, or a "fatal growth" (often a neoplasm).

FLATUS

Abdominal swelling may be the result of increased intestinal gas. The normal small intestine contains approximately 200 mL of gas made up of nitrogen, oxygen, carbon dioxide, hydrogen, and methane. Nitrogen and oxygen are consumed (swallowed), whereas carbon dioxide, hydrogen, and methane are produced intraluminally by bacterial fermentation. Increased intestinal gas can occur in a number of conditions. Aerophagia, the swallowing of air, can result in increased amounts of oxygen and nitrogen in the small intestine and lead to abdominal swelling. Aerophagia typically results from gulping food; chewing gum; smoking; or as a response to anxiety, which leads to repetitive belching. In some cases, increased intestinal gas is the result of bacterial metabolism of excess fermentable substances such as lactose and other oligosaccharides that can lead to production of hydrogen, carbon dioxide, or methane. In many cases, the precise cause of abdominal distention cannot be determined. In some persons, particularly those with irritable bowel syndrome

and bloating, the subjective sense of abdominal pressure is attributable to impaired intestinal transit of gas rather than increased gas volume. Abdominal distention, an objective increase in girth, is the result of a lack of coordination between diaphragmatic contraction and anterior abdominal wall relaxation in response to an increase in intraabdominal volume loads. Occasionally, increased lumbar lordosis accounts for apparent abdominal distention.

FAT

Weight gain with an increase in abdominal fat can result in an increase in abdominal girth and can be perceived as abdominal swelling. Abdominal fat may be the result of an imbalance between calorie intake and energy expenditure associated with a poor diet and sedentary lifestyle and also can be a manifestation of certain diseases such as Cushing's syndrome. Excess abdominal fat has been associated with an increased risk of insulin resistance and cardiovascular disease.

FLUID

Fluid within the abdominal cavity, or ascites, often results in abdominal distention and is discussed in detail later in the chapter

FETUS

Pregnancy results in increased abdominal girth. Typically, an increase in abdominal size is first noted at 12 to 14 weeks of gestation, when the uterus moves from the pelvis into the abdomen. Abdominal distention may be seen before this point as a result of fluid retention and relaxation of the abdominal muscles.

FECES

Increased stool in the colon, in the setting of severe constipation or intestinal obstruction, also leads to increased abdominal girth. These conditions often are accompanied by abdominal pain, nausea, and vomiting and can be diagnosed by imaging studies.

FATAL GROWTH

An abdominal mass can result in abdominal swelling. Enlargement of the intraabdominal organs, specifically the liver (hepatomegaly) or spleen (splenomegaly), or an abdominal aortic aneurysm can result in abdominal distention. Bladder distention also may result in abdominal swelling. In addition, malignancies, abscesses, or cysts can grow to sizes that lead to increased abdominal girth.

HISTORY AND PHYSICAL EXAMINATION

Determining the etiology of abdominal swelling begins with history-taking and a physical examination. Patients should be questioned regarding symptoms suggestive of malignancy, including weight loss, night sweats, and anorexia. Inability to pass stool or flatus together with nausea or vomiting suggest bowel obstruction, severe constipation, or an ileus (lack of peristalsis). Increased eructation and flatus may point toward aerophagia or increased intestinal production of gas. Patients should be questioned about risk factors for or symptoms of chronic liver disease, including excessive alcohol use and jaundice, which suggest ascites. Patients should also be asked about other symptoms of medical conditions, including heart failure and tuberculosis, which may cause ascites.

Physical examination should assess for signs of systemic disease. The presence of lymphadenopathy, especially supraclavicular lymphadenopathy (Virchow's node), suggests metastatic abdominal malignancy. Care also should be taken during the cardiac examination to evaluate for elevation of jugular venous pressure (JVP); Kussmaul's sign (elevation of the JVP during inspiration); or a pericardial knock, which may be seen in heart failure or constrictive pericarditis, as well as a murmur of tricuspid regurgitation. Spider angiomas, palmar erythema, dilated superficial veins around the umbilicus (caput medusae), and gynecomastia suggest chronic liver disease.

The abdominal examination should begin with inspection for the presence of uneven distention or an obvious mass. Auscultation should follow. The absence of bowel sounds or the presence of high-pitched localized bowel sounds point toward an ileus or intestinal obstruction. An umbilical venous hum may suggest the presence of portal hypertension, and a harsh bruit over the liver is heard rarely in patients with hepatocellular carcinoma or alcoholic hepatitis. Abdominal swelling caused by intestinal gas can be differentiated from

swelling caused by fluid or a solid mass by percussion; an abdomen filled with gas is tympanic, whereas an abdomen containing a mass or fluid is dull to percussion. The absence of abdominal dullness, however, does not exclude ascites, because a minimum of 1500 mL of ascites is required for detection on physical examination. Finally, the abdomen should be palpated to assess for tenderness, a mass, enlargement of the spleen or liver, or presence of a nodular liver suggesting cirrhosis or tumor. Light palpation of the liver may detect pulsations suggesting retrograde vascular flow from the heart in patients with right-sided heart failure, particularly tricuspid regurgitation.

IMAGING AND LABORATORY EVALUATION

Abdominal x-rays can be used to detect dilated loops of bowel, suggesting intestinal obstruction or ileus. An abdominal ultrasound can detect as little as 100 mL of ascites, hepatosplenomegaly, a nodular liver, or a mass. Ultrasound is often inadequate to detect retroperitoneal lymphadenopathy or a pancreatic lesion because of overlying bowel gas. If malignancy or pancreatic disease is suspected, CT can be performed. CT may also detect changes associated with advanced cirrhosis and portal hypertension (Fig. 9-1).

Laboratory evaluation should include liver biochemical testing, a serum albumin level, a prothrombin time

FIGURE 9-1

CT of a patient with a cirrhotic, nodular liver (white arrow), splenomegaly (yellow arrow), and ascites (arrowheads).

(international normalized ratio) to assess hepatic function, and a complete blood count to evaluate for the presence of cytopenias that may result from portal hypertension or leukocytosis, anemia, and thrombocytosis that may result from systemic infection. Serum amylase and lipase levels should be checked to evaluate the patient for acute pancreatitis. Urinary protein quantitation is indicated when nephrotic syndrome, which may cause ascites, is suspected.

In selected cases, measurement of the hepatic venous pressure gradient (pressure across the liver between the portal and hepatic veins) can be obtained via cannulation of the hepatic vein to confirm that ascites is caused by cirrhosis (see Chap. 42). In some cases, a liver biopsy may be necessary to confirm cirrhosis.

ASCITES

PATHOGENESIS IN CIRRHOSIS

Ascites in patients with cirrhosis is the result of portal hypertension and renal salt and water retention. Portal hypertension signifies elevation of the pressure within the portal vein. According to Ohm's law, pressure is the product of resistance and flow. Increased hepatic resistance occurs by several mechanisms. First, the development of hepatic fibrosis, which defines cirrhosis, disrupts the normal architecture of the hepatic sinusoids and impedes normal blood flow through the liver. Second, activation of hepatic stellate cells, which mediate fibrogenesis, leads to smooth muscle contraction and fibrosis. Finally, cirrhosis is associated with a decrease in endothelial nitric oxide synthetase (eNOS) production, which results in decreased nitric oxide production and increased intrahepatic vasoconstriction.

The development of cirrhosis is also associated with increased systemic circulating levels of nitric oxide (contrary to the decrease seen intrahepatically) as well as increased levels of vascular endothelial growth factor and tumor necrosis factor that result in splanchnic arterial vasodilatation. Vasodilatation of the splanchnic circulation results in pooling of blood and a decrease in the effective circulating volume, which is perceived by the kidneys as hypovolemia. Compensatory vasoconstriction via release of antidiuretic hormone ensues, thereby leading to free water retention and activation of the sympathetic nervous system and renin angiotensin aldosterone system, leading in turn to renal sodium and water retention.

PATHOGENESIS IN THE ABSENCE OF CIRRHOSIS

Ascites in the absence of cirrhosis generally results from peritoneal carcinomatosis, peritoneal infection, or

FIGURE 9-2
CT of a patient with peritoneal carcinomatosis (white arrow) and ascites (yellow arrow).

pancreatic disease. Peritoneal carcinomatosis can result from primary peritoneal malignancies such as mesothelioma or sarcoma, abdominal malignancies such as gastric or colonic adenocarcinoma, or metastatic disease from breast or lung carcinoma or melanoma **(Fig. 9-2)**. The tumor cells lining the peritoneum produce a protein-rich fluid that contributes to the development of ascites. Fluid from the extracellular space is drawn into the peritoneum, further contributing to the development of ascites. Tuberculous peritonitis causes ascites via a similar mechanism; tubercles deposited on the peritoneum exude a proteinaceous fluid. Pancreatic ascites results from leakage of pancreatic enzymes into the peritoneum.

CAUSES

Cirrhosis accounts for 84% of cases of ascites. Cardiac ascites, peritoneal carcinomatosis, and "mixed" ascites resulting from cirrhosis and a second disease account for 10 to 15% of cases. Less common causes of ascites include massive hepatic metastasis, infection (tuberculosis, Chlamydia), pancreatitis, and renal disease (nephrotic syndrome). Rare causes of ascites include hypothyroidism and familial Mediterranean fever.

EVALUATION

Once the presence of ascites has been confirmed, the etiology of the ascites is best determined by paracentesis. Paracentesis is a bedside procedure in which a needle or small catheter is passed transcutaneously to extract ascitic fluid from the peritoneum. The lower quadrants are the most frequent sites for paracentesis. Occasionally, an infraumbilical approach is used. The left lower quadrant is preferred because of the greater depth of ascites and thinner abdominal wall. Paracentesis is a safe procedure even in patients with coagulopathy; complications, including abdominal wall hematomas, hypotension, hepatorenal syndrome, and infection, are infrequent.

Once ascitic fluid has been extracted, its gross appearance should be examined. Turbid fluid can result from infection or tumor cells within the fluid. White, milky fluid indicates the presence of triglycerides in levels >200 mg/dL (and often >1000 mg/dL), which is the hallmark of *chylous ascites*. Chylous ascites results from lymphatic disruption that may occur with trauma, cirrhosis, tumor, tuberculosis, or certain congenital abnormalities. Dark brown fluid can reflect a high bilirubin concentration and indicates biliary tract perforation. Black fluid may indicate the presence of pancreatic necrosis or metastatic melanoma.

The ascitic fluid should be sent for measurement of the albumin and total protein levels, cell and differential counts, and, if infection is suspected, Gram's stain and culture, with inoculation of the fluid into blood culture bottles at the patient's bedside to maximize the yield. In addition, a serum albumin level should be sent simultaneously to permit calculation of the *serum-ascites albumin gradient (SAAG)*.

The SAAG is useful for distinguishing ascites caused by portal hypertension from nonportal hypertensive ascites (Fig. 9-3). The SAAG reflects the pressure within the hepatic sinusoids and correlates with the hepatic venous pressure gradient. The SAAG is calculated by subtracting the ascitic albumin from the serum albumin and does not change with diuresis. A SAAG ≥1.1 g/dL reflects the presence of portal hypertension and indicates that the ascites is from an increased pressure in the hepatic sinusoids. According to Starling's law, a high SAAG reflects the oncotic pressure that

counterbalances the portal pressure. Possible causes include cirrhosis, cardiac ascites, sinusoidal obstruction syndrome (venoocclusive disease), massive liver metastasis, or hepatic vein thrombosis (Budd-Chiari syndrome). A SAAG <1.1 g/dL indicates that the ascites is not related to portal hypertension as in tuberculous peritonitis, peritoneal carcinomatosis, or pancreatic ascites.

For high-SAAG (≥1.1) ascites, the ascitic protein level can provide further clues to the etiology (see Fig. 9-3). An ascitic protein level of ≥2.5 g/dL indicates that the hepatic sinusoids are normal and allows passage of protein into the ascites, as occurs in cardiac ascites, sinusoidal obstruction syndrome, or early Budd-Chiari syndrome. An ascitic protein level <2.5 g/dL indicates that the hepatic sinusoids have been damaged and scarred and no longer allow passage of protein, as occurs with cirrhosis, late Budd-Chiari syndrome, or massive liver metastases. Pro-brain-type natriuretic peptide (BNP) is a natriuretic hormone released by the heart as a result of increased volume and ventricular wall stretch. High levels of BNP in serum occur in heart failure and may be useful in identifying congestive heart failure as the cause of high-SAAG ascites.

Further tests are indicated only in specific clinical circumstances. When secondary peritonitis resulting from a perforated hollow viscus is suspected, ascitic glucose and lactate dehydrogenase (LDH) levels can be sent. In contrast to "spontaneous" bacterial peritonitis (SBP), which may complicate cirrhotic ascites, secondary peritonitis is suggested by an ascitic glucose level <50 mg/dL, an ascitic LDH greater than the serum LDH level, and multiple pathogens on ascitic fluid culture. When pancreatic ascites is suspected, an ascitic amylase should be measured and is typically >1000 mg/dL. Cytology can be useful in the diagnosis of peritoneal carcinomatosis. At least 50 mL of fluid should be obtained and sent for immediate processing. Tuberculous peritonitis can be difficult to diagnose by paracentesis. A smear for acid-fast bacilli has a sensitivity of only 0 to 3%, and a culture increases the sensitivity for diagnosis to 35 to

FIGURE 9-3
Algorithm for the diagnosis of ascites according to the serum-ascites albumin gradient (SAAG). IVC, inferior vena cava.

50%. In patients without cirrhosis, an elevated ascitic adenosine deaminase level has a sensitivity of more than 90% when a cut-off value of 30 to 45 U/L is used. When the cause of ascites remains uncertain, laparotomy or laparoscopy with peritoneal biopsies for histology and culture remains the gold standard.

TREATMENT Ascites

The initial treatment of cirrhotic ascites is restriction of sodium intake to 2 g/d. When sodium restriction alone is inadequate to control ascites, oral diuretics, typically the combination of spironolactone and furosemide, are used. Spironolactone is an aldosterone antagonist that inhibits Na^+ resorption in the distal convoluted tubule of the kidney. Use of spironolactone may be limited by hyponatremia, hyperkalemia, and painful gynecomastia. If the gynecomastia is distressing, amiloride, 5–40 mg/d, may be substituted for spironolactone. Furosemide is a loop diuretic that is generally combined with spironolactone in a ratio of 40:100; maximal daily doses of spironolactone and furosemide are generally 400 mg and 160 mg, respectively.

Refractory cirrhotic ascites is defined by the persistence of ascites despite sodium restriction and maximal (or maximally tolerated) diuretic use. Refractory ascites can be managed by serial large volume paracentesis (LVP) or a transjugular intrahepatic peritoneal shunt (TIPS), a radiologically placed portosystemic shunt to decompress the hepatic sinusoids. TIPS is superior to LVP in reducing the reaccumulation of ascites but is associated with an increased frequency of hepatic encephalopathy with no difference in mortality rates.

Malignant ascites does not respond to sodium restriction or diuretics. Patients must undergo serial LVPs, transcutaneous drainage catheter placement, or, rarely, creation of a peritovenous shunt (a shunt from the abdominal cavity to the vena cava).

Ascites caused by tuberculous peritonitis is treated with standard antituberculosis therapy. Noncirrhotic ascites of other causes is treated by correction of the precipitating condition.

COMPLICATIONS

Spontaneous bacterial peritonitis (SBP) is a common and potentially lethal complication of cirrhotic ascites. SBP also can occasionally complicate ascites caused by nephrotic syndrome, heart failure, acute hepatitis, and acute liver failure but is rare in malignant ascites. Patients with SBP generally note an increase in abdominal girth; however, abdominal tenderness is found in only 40% of patients, and rebound tenderness is rare. Patients may present with fever, nausea, vomiting, or the new onset of or exacerbation of preexisting hepatic encephalopathy.

SBP is defined by a polymorphonuclear neutrophil (PMN) count of $\geq250/mm^3$ in the ascitic fluid. Ascitic fluid cultures typically reveal one bacterial pathogen. The presence of multiple pathogens in the setting of an elevated ascitic PMN count suggests secondary peritonitis from a ruptured viscus or abscess. The presence of multiple pathogens without an elevated PMN count suggests bowel perforation from the paracentesis needle. SBP is generally the result of enteric bacteria that have translocated across an edematous bowel wall. The most common pathogens are Gram-negative rods, including *Escherichia coli* and *Klebsiella*, as well as streptococci and enterococci.

Treatment of SBP with an antibiotic such as intravenous cefotaxime is effective against gram-negative and Gram-positive aerobes. Five days of treatment are sufficient if the patient improves clinically.

Cirrhotic patients with a history of SBP, an ascitic fluid total protein concentration <1 g/dL, or active gastrointestinal bleeding should receive prophylactic antibiotics to prevent SBP; oral norfloxacin is commonly used. Diuresis increases the activity of ascitic fluid protein opsonins and may decrease the risk of SBP.

Hepatic hydrothorax occurs when ascites, often caused by cirrhosis, migrates via fenestrae in the diaphragm into the pleural space and can result in shortness of breath, hypoxia, and infection. Treatment is similar to that of cirrhotic ascites and includes sodium restriction, diuretics, and, if needed, thoracentesis or TIPS placement. Chest tube placement should be avoided.

CHAPTER 10

INVOLUNTARY WEIGHT LOSS

Russell G. Robertson ■ J. Larry Jameson

Involuntary weight loss (IWL) is frequently insidious and can have important implications, often serving as a harbinger of serious underlying disease. Clinically important weight loss is defined as the loss of 10 pounds (4.5 kg) or >5% of one's body weight over a period of 6–12 months. IWL is encountered in up to 8% of all adult outpatients and 27% of frail persons age 65 years and older. There is no identifiable cause in up to one-quarter of patients despite extensive investigation. Conversely, up to half of people who claim to have lost weight have no documented evidence of weight loss. People with no known cause of weight loss generally have a better prognosis than do those with known causes, particularly when the source is neoplastic. Weight loss in older persons is associated with a variety of deleterious effects, including hip fracture, pressure ulcers, impaired immune function, decreased functional status, and death. Not surprisingly, significant weight loss is associated with increased mortality, which can range from 9% to as high as 38% within 1 to 2.5 years in the absence of clinical awareness and attention.

PHYSIOLOGY OF WEIGHT REGULATION WITH AGING

(See also Chap. 57) Among healthy aging people, total body weight peaks in the sixth decade of life and generally remains stable until the ninth decade, after which it gradually falls. In contrast, lean body mass (fat-free mass) begins to decline at a rate of 0.3 kg per year in the third decade, and the rate of decline increases further beginning at age 60 in men and age 65 in women. These changes in lean body mass largely reflect the age-dependent decline in growth hormone secretion and, consequently, circulating levels of insulin-like growth factor type I (IGF-I) that occur with normal aging. In the healthy elderly, an increase in fat tissue balances the loss in lean body mass until very old age, when loss of both fat and skeletal muscle occurs. Age-dependent changes also occur at the cellular level. Telomeres shorten, and body cell mass—the fat-free portion of cells—declines steadily with aging.

Between ages 20 and 80, mean energy intake is reduced by up to 1200 kcal/d in men and 800 kcal/d in women. Decreased hunger is a reflection of reduced physical activity and loss of lean body mass, producing lower demand for calories and food intake. Several important age-associated physiologic changes also predispose elderly persons to weight loss, such as declining chemosensory function (smell and taste), reduced efficiency of chewing, slowed gastric emptying, and alterations in the neuroendocrine axis, including changes in levels of leptin, cholecystokinin, neuropeptide Y, and other hormones and peptides. These changes are associated with early satiety and a decline in both appetite and the hedonistic appreciation of food. Collectively, they contribute to the "anorexia of aging."

CAUSES OF INVOLUNTARY WEIGHT LOSS

Most causes of IWL belong to one of four categories: (1) malignant neoplasms, (2) chronic inflammatory or infectious diseases, (3) metabolic disorders (e.g., hyperthyroidism and diabetes), or (4) psychiatric disorders (Table 10-1). Not infrequently, more than one of these causes can be responsible for IWL. In most series, IWL is caused by malignant disease in a quarter of patients and by organic disease in one-third, with the remainder due to psychiatric disease, medications, or uncertain causes.

The most common malignant causes of IWL are gastrointestinal, hepatobiliary, hematologic, lung, breast, genitourinary, ovarian, and prostate. Half of all patients with cancer lose some body weight; one-third lose more than 5% of their original body weight, and up to 20% of all cancer deaths are caused directly by cachexia (through immobility and/or cardiac/respiratory failure).

TABLE 10-1

CAUSES OF INVOLUNTARY WEIGHT LOSS

Cancer
  Colon
  Hepatobiliary
  Hematologic
  Lung
  Breast
  Genitourinary
  Ovarian
  Prostate
Gastrointestinal disorders
  Malabsorption
  Peptic ulcer
  Inflammatory bowel
    disease
  Pancreatitis
  Obstruction/constipation
  Pernicious anemia
Endocrine and metabolic
  Hyperthyroidism
  Diabetes mellitus
  Pheochromocytoma
  Adrenal insufficiency
Cardiac disorders
  Chronic ischemia
  Chronic congestive
    heart
    failure
Respiratory disorders
  Emphysema
  Chronic obstructive
    pulmonary disease
Renal insufficiency
Rheumatologic disease
Infections
  HIV
  Tuberculosis
  Parasitic infection
  Subacute bacterial
    endocarditis

Medications
  Sedatives
  Antibiotics
  Nonsteroidal anti-
    inflammatory drugs
  Serotonin reuptake
    inhibitors
  Metformin
  Levodopa
  Angiotensin-converting
    enzyme inhibitors
  Other drugs
**Disorders of the mouth
  and teeth**
  Caries
  Dygeusia
Age-related factors
  Physiologic changes
  Visual impairment
  Decreased taste and smell
  Functional disabilities
Neurologic
  Stroke
  Parkinson's disease
  Neuromuscular disorders
  Dementia
Social
  Isolation
  Economic hardship
Psychiatric and behavioral
  Depression
  Anxiety
  Paranoia
  Bereavement
  Alcoholism
  Eating disorders
  Increased activity or
    exercise
Idiopathic

The greatest incidence of weight loss is seen among patients with solid tumors. Malignancy that reveals itself through significant weight loss usually has a very poor prognosis.

In addition to malignancies, gastrointestinal causes are among the most prominent causes of IWL. Peptic ulcer disease, inflammatory bowel disease, dysmotility syndromes, chronic pancreatitis, celiac disease, constipation, and atrophic gastritis are some of the more common entities. Oral and dental problems are easily overlooked and may manifest with halitosis, poor oral hygiene, xerostomia, inability to chew, reduced masticatory force, nonocclusion, temporomandibular joint syndrome, edentulousness, and pain due to caries or abscesses.

Tuberculosis, fungal diseases, parasites, subacute bacterial endocarditis, and HIV are well-documented causes of IWL. Cardiovascular and pulmonary diseases cause unintentional weight loss through increased metabolic demand and decreased appetite and caloric intake. Uremia produces nausea, anorexia, and vomiting. Connective tissue diseases may increase metabolic demand and disrupt nutritional balance. As the incidence of diabetes mellitus increases with aging, the associated glucosuria can contribute to weight loss. Hyperthyroidism in the elderly may have less prominent sympathomimetic features and may present as "apathetic hyperthyroidism" or T_3 toxicosis.

Neurologic injuries such as stroke, quadriplegia, and multiple sclerosis may lead to visceral and autonomic dysfunction that can impair caloric intake. Dysphagia from these neurologic insults is a common mechanism. Functional disability that compromises activities of daily living (ADLs) is a common cause of undernutrition in the elderly. Visual impairment from ophthalmic or central nervous system disorders such as a tremor can limit the ability of people to prepare and eat meals. IWL may be one of the earliest manifestations of Alzheimer's dementia.

Isolation and depression are significant causes of IWL that may manifest as an inability to care for oneself, including nutritional needs. A cytokine-mediated inflammatory metabolic cascade can be both a cause of and a manifestation of depression. Bereavement can be a cause of IWL and, when present, is more pronounced in men. More intense forms of mental illness such as paranoid disorders may lead to delusions about food and cause weight loss. Alcoholism can be a significant source of weight loss and malnutrition.

Elderly persons living in poverty may have to choose between purchasing food and purchasing medications. Institutionalization is an independent risk factor, as up to 30–50% of nursing home patients have inadequate food intake.

Medications can cause anorexia, nausea, vomiting, gastrointestinal distress, diarrhea, dry mouth, and changes in taste. This is particularly an issue in the elderly, many of whom take five or more medications.

ASSESSMENT

The four major manifestations of IWL are (1) anorexia (loss of appetite), (2) sarcopenia (loss of muscle mass), (3) cachexia (a syndrome that combines weight loss, loss of muscle and adipose tissue, anorexia, and weakness), and (4) dehydration. The current obesity epidemic adds complexity, as excess adipose tissue can mask the development of sarcopenia and delay awareness of the development of cachexia. If it is not possible to measure weight directly, a change in clothing size, corroboration of weight loss by a relative or friend, and a numeric estimate of weight loss provided by the patient are suggestive of true weight loss.

Initial assessment includes a comprehensive history and physical, a complete blood count, tests of liver enzyme levels, a C-reactive protein, erythrocyte sedimentation rate, renal function studies, thyroid function tests, chest radiography, and an abdominal ultrasound (Table 10-2). Age, sex, and risk factor–specific cancer screening tests, such as mammography and colonoscopy, should be performed. Patients at risk should have HIV testing. All elderly patients with weight loss should undergo screening for dementia and depression by using instruments such as the Mini-Mental State Examination and the Geriatric Depression Scale, respectively. The Mini-Nutritional Assessment (*www.mna-elderly.com*) and the Nutrition Screening Initiative (*www.aafp.org/afp/980301ap/edits.html*) are also available for the nutritional assessment of elderly patients. Almost all patients with a malignancy and >90% of those with other organic diseases have at least one laboratory abnormality. In patients presenting with substantial IWL, major organic and malignant diseases are unlikely when a baseline evaluation is completely normal. Careful follow-up rather than undirected testing is advised since the prognosis of weight loss of undetermined cause is generally favorable.

TABLE 10-2

ASSESSMENT AND TESTING FOR INVOLUNTARY WEIGHT LOSS	
Indications	**Laboratory**
5% weight loss in 30 d	Complete blood count
10% weight loss in 180 d	Comprehensive
Body mass index <21	electrolyte and meta-
25% of food left uneaten after 7 d	bolic panel, including liver and renal function
Change in fit of clothing	tests
Change in appetite, smell, or taste	Thyroid function tests
Abdominal pain, nausea, vomiting, diarrhea, constipation, dysphagia	Erythrocyte sedimentation rate
	C-reactive protein
Assessment	Ferritin
Complete physical exam, including dental evaluation	HIV testing, if indicated
Medication review	**Radiology**
Recommended cancer screening	Chest x-ray
Mini-Mental State Examination[a]	Abdominal ultrasound
Mini-Nutritional Assessment[a]	
Nutrition Screening Initiative[a]	
Simplified Nutritional Assessment Questionnaire[a]	
Observation of eating[a]	
Activities of daily living[a]	
Instrumental activities of daily living[a]	

[a]May be more specific to assess weight loss in the elderly.

TREATMENT　Unintentional Weight Loss

The first priority in managing weight loss is to identify and treat the underlying causes systematically. Treatment of underlying metabolic, psychiatric, infectious, or other systemic disorders may be sufficient to restore weight and functional status gradually. Medications that cause nausea or anorexia should be withdrawn or changed, if possible. For those with unexplained IWL, oral nutritional supplements such as high-energy drinks sometimes reverse weight loss. Advising patients to consume supplements between meals rather than with a meal may help minimize appetite suppression and facilitate increased overall intake. Orexigenic, anabolic, and anticytokine agents are under investigation. In selected patients, the antidepressant mirtazapine results in a significant increase in body weight, body fat mass, and leptin concentration. Patients with wasting conditions who can comply with an appropriate exercise program gain muscle protein mass, strength, and endurance and may be more capable of performing ADL.

SECTION II

EVALUATION OF THE PATIENT WITH ALIMENTARY TRACT SYNDROMES

CHAPTER 11
APPROACH TO THE PATIENT WITH GASTROINTESTINAL DISEASE

William L. Hasler ■ Chung Owyang

ANATOMIC CONSIDERATIONS

The gastrointestinal (GI) tract extends from the mouth to the anus and is composed of several organs with distinct functions. Specialized independently controlled thickened sphincters that assist in gut compartmentalization separate the organs. The gut wall is organized into well-defined layers that contribute to functional activities in each region. The mucosa is a barrier to luminal contents or as a site for transfer of fluids or nutrients. Gut smooth muscle mediates propulsion from one region to the next. Many GI organs possess a serosal layer that provides a supportive foundation but that also permits external input.

Interactions with other organ systems serve the needs both of the gut and the body. Pancreaticobiliary conduits deliver bile and enzymes into the duodenum. A rich vascular supply is modulated by GI tract activity. Lymphatic channels assist in gut immune activities. Intrinsic gut wall nerves provide the basic controls for propulsion and fluid regulation. Extrinsic neural input provides volitional or involuntary control to degrees that are specific for each gut region.

FUNCTIONS OF THE GASTROINTESTINAL TRACT

The GI tract serves two main functions—assimilating nutrients and eliminating waste. The gut anatomy is organized to serve these functions. In the mouth, food is processed, mixed with salivary amylase, and delivered to the gut lumen. The esophagus propels the bolus into the stomach; the lower esophageal sphincter prevents oral reflux of gastric contents. The esophageal mucosa has a protective squamous histology, which does not permit significant diffusion or absorption. Propulsive esophageal activities are exclusively aboral and coordinate with relaxation of the upper and lower esophageal sphincters on swallowing.

The stomach furthers food preparation by triturating and mixing the bolus with pepsin and acid. Gastric acid also sterilizes the upper gut. The proximal stomach serves a storage function by relaxing to accommodate the meal. The distal stomach exhibits phasic contractions that propel solid food residue against the pylorus, where it is repeatedly propelled proximally for further mixing before it is emptied into the duodenum. Finally, the stomach secretes intrinsic factor for vitamin B_{12} absorption.

The small intestine serves most of the nutrient absorptive function of the gut. The intestinal mucosa exhibits villus architecture to provide maximal surface area for absorption and is endowed with specialized enzymes and transporters. Triturated food from the stomach mixes with pancreatic juice and bile in the duodenum to facilitate digestion. Pancreatic juice contains the main enzymes for carbohydrate, protein, and fat digestion as well as bicarbonate to optimize the pH for activation of these enzymes. Bile secreted by the liver and stored in the gallbladder is essential for intestinal lipid digestion. The proximal intestine is optimized for rapid absorption of nutrient breakdown products and most minerals, while the ileum is better suited for absorption of vitamin B_{12} and bile acids. The small intestine also aids in waste elimination. Bile contains by-products of erythrocyte degradation, toxins, metabolized and unmetabolized medications, and cholesterol. Motor function of the small intestine delivers indigestible food residue and sloughed enterocytes into the colon for further processing. The small intestine terminates in the ileocecal junction, a sphincteric structure that prevents coloileal reflux and maintains small-intestinal sterility.

The colon prepares the waste material for controlled evacuation. The colonic mucosa dehydrates the stool, decreasing daily fecal volumes from 1000–1500 mL delivered from the ileum to 100–200 mL expelled from the rectum. The colonic lumen possesses a dense bacterial colonization that ferments undigested carbohydrates and short-chain fatty acids. Whereas transit times in the esophagus are on the order of seconds and times in the stomach and small intestine range from minutes to a few hours, propagation through the colon takes more than one day in most individuals. Colonic motor patterns exhibit a to-and-fro character that facilitates slow fecal desiccation. The proximal colon serves to mix and absorb fluid, while the distal colon exhibits peristaltic contractions and mass actions that function to expel the stool. The colon terminates in the anus, a structure with volitional and involuntary controls to permit retention of the fecal bolus until it can be released in a socially convenient setting.

EXTRINSIC MODULATION OF GUT FUNCTION

GI function is modified by influences outside of the gut. Unlike other organ systems, the gut is in continuity with the outside environment. Thus, protective mechanisms are vigilant against deleterious effects of foods, medications, toxins, and infectious organisms. Mucosal immune mechanisms include chronic lymphocyte and plasma cell populations in the epithelial layer and lamina propria backed up by lymph node chains to prevent noxious agents from entering the circulation. All substances absorbed into the bloodstream are filtered through the liver via the portal venous circulation. In the liver, many drugs and toxins are detoxified by a variety of mechanisms. Although intrinsic nerves control most basic gut activities, extrinsic neural input modulates many functions. Two activities under voluntary control are swallowing and defecation. Many normal GI reflexes involve extrinsic vagus or splanchnic nerve pathways. The brain gut axis further alters function in regions not under volitional regulation. As an example, stress has potent effects on gut motor, secretory, and sensory functions.

OVERVIEW OF GASTROINTESTINAL DISEASES

GI diseases develop as a result of abnormalities within or outside of the gut and range in severity from those that produce mild symptoms and no long-term morbidity to those with intractable symptoms or adverse outcomes. Diseases may be localized to one organ or exhibit diffuse involvement at many sites.

CLASSIFICATION OF GI DISEASES

GI diseases are manifestations of alterations in nutrient assimilation or waste evacuation or in the activities supporting these main functions.

Impaired digestion and absorption

Diseases of the stomach, intestine, biliary tree, and pancreas can disrupt digestion and absorption. The most common intestinal maldigestion syndrome, lactase deficiency, produces gas and diarrhea after dairy products and has no adverse outcomes. Other intestinal enzyme deficiencies produce similar symptoms after ingestion of other simple sugars. Conversely, celiac disease, bacterial overgrowth, infectious enteritis, Crohn's ileitis, and radiation damage, which affect digestion and/or absorption more diffusely, produce anemia, dehydration, electrolyte disorders, or malnutrition. Gastric hypersecretory conditions such as Zollinger-Ellison syndrome damage the intestinal mucosa, impair pancreatic enzyme activation, and accelerate transit due to excess gastric acid. Biliary obstruction from stricture or neoplasm impairs fat digestion. Impaired pancreatic enzyme release in chronic pancreatitis or pancreatic cancer decreases intraluminal digestion and can lead to malnutrition.

Altered secretion

Selected GI diseases result from dysregulation of gut secretion. Gastric acid hypersecretion occurs in Zollinger-Ellison syndrome, G cell hyperplasia, retained antrum syndrome, and some individuals with duodenal ulcers. Conversely, patients with atrophic gastritis or pernicious anemia release little or no gastric acid. Inflammatory and infectious small-intestinal and colonic diseases produce fluid loss through impaired absorption or enhanced secretion. Common intestinal and colonic hypersecretory conditions cause diarrhea and include acute bacterial or viral infection, chronic *Giardia* or cryptosporidia infections, small-intestinal bacterial overgrowth, bile salt diarrhea, microscopic colitis, diabetic diarrhea, and abuse of certain laxatives. Less common causes include large colonic villus adenomas and endocrine neoplasias with tumor overproduction of secretagogue transmitters like vasoactive intestinal polypeptide.

Altered gut transit

Impaired gut transit may be secondary to mechanical obstruction. Esophageal occlusion often results from acid-induced stricture or neoplasm. Gastric outlet obstruction develops from peptic ulcer disease or gastric cancer. Small-intestinal obstruction most commonly results from adhesions but may also occur with Crohn's disease, radiation- or drug-induced strictures, and less likely malignancy. The most common cause of colonic obstruction is colon cancer, although inflammatory strictures develop in patients with inflammatory bowel disease, after certain infections such as diverticulitis, or with some drugs.

Retardation of propulsion also develops from disordered motor function. Achalasia is characterized by impaired esophageal body peristalsis and incomplete lower esophageal sphincter relaxation. Gastroparesis is the symptomatic delay in gastric emptying of meals due to impaired gastric motility. Intestinal pseudoobstruction causes marked delays in small-bowel transit due to enteric nerve or intestinal smooth-muscle injury. Slow-transit constipation is produced by diffusely impaired colonic propulsion. Constipation also is produced by outlet abnormalities such as rectal prolapse, intussusception, or dyssynergia—a failure of anal or puborectalis relaxation upon attempted defecation.

Disorders of rapid propulsion are less common than those with delayed transit. Rapid gastric emptying occurs in postvagotomy dumping syndrome, with gastric hypersecretion, and in some cases of functional dyspepsia and cyclic vomiting syndrome. Exaggerated intestinal or colonic motor patterns may be responsible for diarrhea in irritable bowel syndrome. Accelerated transit with hyperdefecation is noted in hyperthyroidism.

Immune dysregulation

Many inflammatory GI conditions are consequences of altered gut immune function. The mucosal inflammation of celiac disease results from dietary ingestion of gluten-containing grains. Some patients with food allergy also exhibit altered immune populations. Eosinophilic esophagitis and eosinophilic gastroenteritis are inflammatory disorders with prominent mucosal eosinophils. Ulcerative colitis and Crohn's disease are disorders of uncertain etiology that produce mucosal injury primarily in the lower gut. The microscopic colitides, lymphocytic and collagenous colitis, exhibit colonic subepithelial infiltrates without visible mucosal damage. Bacterial, viral, and protozoal organisms may produce ileitis or colitis in selected patient populations.

Impaired gut blood flow

Different GI regions are at variable risk for ischemic damage from impaired blood flow. Rare cases of gastroparesis result from blockage of the celiac and superior mesenteric arteries. More commonly encountered are intestinal and colonic ischemia that are consequences of arterial embolus, arterial thrombosis, venous thrombosis, or hypoperfusion from dehydration, sepsis, hemorrhage, or reduced cardiac output. These may produce mucosal injury, hemorrhage, or even perforation. Some cases of radiation enterocolitis exhibit reduced mucosal blood flow.

Neoplastic degeneration

All GI regions are susceptible to malignant degeneration to varying degrees. In the United States, colorectal cancer is most common and usually presents after age 50 years. Worldwide, gastric cancer is prevalent especially in certain Asian regions. Esophageal cancer develops with chronic acid reflux or after an extensive alcohol or tobacco use history. Small-intestinal neoplasms are rare and occur with underlying inflammatory disease. Anal cancers arise after prior anal infection or inflammation. Pancreatic and biliary cancers elicit severe pain, weight loss, and jaundice and have poor prognoses. Hepatocellular carcinoma usually arises in the setting of chronic viral hepatitis or cirrhosis secondary to other causes. Most GI cancers exhibit carcinomatous histology; however, lymphomas and other cell types also are observed.

Disorders without obvious organic abnormalities

The most common GI disorders show no abnormalities on biochemical or structural testing and include irritable bowel syndrome, functional dyspepsia, functional chest pain, and functional heartburn. These disorders exhibit altered gut motor function; however, the pathogenic relevance of these abnormalities is uncertain. Exaggerated visceral sensory responses to noxious stimulation may cause discomfort in these disorders. Symptoms in other patients result from altered processing of visceral pain sensations in the central nervous system. Functional bowel patients with severe symptoms may exhibit significant emotional disturbances on psychometric testing. Subtle immunologic defects may contribute to functional symptoms as well.

Genetic influences

Although many GI diseases result from environmental factors, others exhibit hereditary components. Family members of inflammatory bowel disease patients show a genetic predisposition to disease development themselves. Colonic and esophageal malignancies arise in certain inherited disorders. Rare genetic dysmotility syndromes are described. Familial clustering is even observed in the functional bowel disorders, although this may be secondary learned familial illness behavior rather than a true hereditary factor.

SYMPTOMS OF GASTROINTESTINAL DISEASE

The most common GI symptoms are abdominal pain, heartburn, nausea and vomiting, altered bowel habits, GI bleeding, and jaundice (Table 11-1). Others are dysphagia, anorexia, weight loss, fatigue, and extraintestinal symptoms.

TABLE 11-1

COMMON CAUSES OF COMMON GI SYMPTOMS

ABDOMINAL PAIN	NAUSEA AND VOMITING	DIARRHEA	GI BLEEDING	OBSTRUCTIVE JAUNDICE
Appendicitis	Medications	Infection	Ulcer disease	Bile duct stones
Gallstone disease	GI obstruction	Poorly absorbed sugars	Esophagitis	Cholangiocarcinoma
Pancreatitis	Motor disorders	Inflammatory bowel disease	Varices	Cholangitis
Diverticulitis	Functional bowel disorder	Microscopic colitis	Vascular lesions	Sclerosing cholangitis
Ulcer disease	Enteric infection	Functional bowel disorder	Neoplasm	Ampullary stenosis
Esophagitis	Pregnancy	Celiac disease	Diverticula	Ampullary carcinoma
GI obstruction	Endocrine disease	Pancreatic insufficiency	Hemorrhoids	Pancreatitis
Inflammatory bowel disease	Motion sickness	Hyperthyroidism	Fissures	Pancreatic tumor
Functional bowel disorder	Central nervous system disease	Ischemia	Inflammatory bowel disease	
Vascular disease		Endocrine tumor	Infectious colitis	
Gynecologic causes				
Renal stone				

Abdominal pain

Abdominal pain results from GI disease and extraintestinal conditions involving the genitourinary tract, abdominal wall, thorax, or spine. Visceral pain generally is midline in location and vague in character, while parietal pain is localized and precisely described. Common inflammatory diseases with pain include peptic ulcer, appendicitis, diverticulitis, inflammatory bowel disease, and infectious enterocolitis. Other intraabdominal causes of pain include gallstone disease and pancreatitis. Noninflammatory visceral sources include mesenteric ischemia and neoplasia. The most common causes of abdominal pain are irritable bowel syndrome and functional dyspepsia.

Heartburn

Heartburn, a burning substernal sensation, is reported intermittently by at least 40% of the population. Classically, heartburn is felt to result from excess gastroesophageal reflux of acid. However, some cases exhibit normal esophageal acid exposure and may result from reflux of nonacidic material or heightened sensitivity of esophageal mucosal nerves.

Nausea and vomiting

Nausea and vomiting are caused by GI diseases, medications, toxins, acute and chronic infection, endocrine disorders, labyrinthine conditions, and central nervous system disease. The best-characterized GI etiologies relate to mechanical obstruction of the upper gut; however, disorders of propulsion including gastroparesis and intestinal pseudoobstruction also elicit prominent symptoms. Nausea and vomiting also are commonly reported by patients with irritable bowel syndrome and functional disorders of the upper gut (including chronic idiopathic nausea and functional vomiting).

Altered bowel habits

Altered bowel habits are common complaints of patients with GI disease. Constipation is reported as infrequent defecation, straining with defecation, passage of hard stools, or a sense of incomplete fecal evacuation. Causes of constipation include obstruction, motor disorders of the colon, medications, and endocrine diseases such as hypothyroidism and hyperparathyroidism. Diarrhea is reported as frequent defecation, passage of loose or watery stools, fecal urgency, or a similar sense of incomplete evacuation. The differential diagnosis of diarrhea is broad and includes infections, inflammatory causes, malabsorption, and medications. Irritable bowel syndrome produces constipation, diarrhea, or an alternating bowel pattern. Fecal mucus is common in irritable bowel syndrome, while pus characterizes inflammatory disease. Steatorrhea develops with malabsorption.

GI bleeding

Hemorrhage may develop from any gut organ. Most commonly, upper GI bleeding presents with melena or hematemesis, whereas lower GI bleeding produces passage of bright red or maroon stools. However, briskly bleeding upper sites can elicit voluminous red rectal bleeding, while slowly bleeding ascending colon sites may produce melena. Chronic slow GI bleeding may present with iron-deficiency anemia. The most common upper GI causes of bleeding are ulcer disease, gastroduodenitis, and esophagitis. Other etiologies include portal hypertensive causes, malignancy, tears across the gastroesophageal junction, and vascular lesions. The most prevalent lower GI sources of hemorrhage include hemorrhoids, anal fissures, diverticula, ischemic colitis, and arteriovenous malformations. Other causes include neoplasm, inflammatory bowel disease, infectious colitis, drug-induced colitis, and other vascular lesions.

Jaundice

Jaundice results from prehepatic, intrahepatic, or posthepatic disease. Posthepatic causes of jaundice include biliary diseases such as choledocholithiasis, acute cholangitis, primary sclerosing cholangitis, other strictures, and neoplasm and pancreatic disorders, such as acute and chronic pancreatitis, stricture, and malignancy.

Other symptoms

Other symptoms are manifestations of GI disease. Dysphagia, odynophagia, and unexplained chest pain suggest esophageal disease. A globus sensation is reported with esophagopharyngeal conditions, but also occurs with functional GI disorders. Weight loss, anorexia, and fatigue are nonspecific symptoms of neoplastic, inflammatory, gut motility, pancreatic, small-bowel mucosal, and psychiatric conditions. Fever is reported with inflammatory illness, but malignancies also evoke febrile responses. GI disorders also produce extraintestinal symptoms. Inflammatory bowel disease is associated with hepatobiliary dysfunction, skin and eye lesions, and arthritis. Celiac disease may present with dermatitis herpetiformis. Jaundice can produce pruritus. Conversely, systemic diseases can have GI consequences. Systemic lupus may cause gut ischemia, presenting with pain or bleeding. Overwhelming stress or severe burns may lead to gastric ulcer formation.

EVALUATION OF THE PATIENT WITH GASTROINTESTINAL DISEASE

Evaluation of the patient with GI disease begins with a careful history and examination. Subsequent investigation with a variety of tools designed to test gut structure or function are indicated in selected cases. Some patients exhibit normal findings on diagnostic testing. In these individuals, validated symptom profiles are employed to confidently diagnose a functional bowel disorder.

HISTORY

The history of the patient with suspected GI disease has several components. Symptom timing suggests specific etiologies. Symptoms of short duration commonly result from acute infection, toxin exposure, or abrupt inflammation or ischemia. Long-standing symptoms point to underlying chronic inflammatory or neoplastic conditions or functional bowel disorders. Symptoms from

mechanical obstruction, ischemia, inflammatory bowel disease, and functional bowel disorders are worsened by meals. Conversely, ulcer symptoms may be relieved by eating or antacids. Symptom patterns and duration may suggest underlying etiologies. Ulcer pain occurs at intermittent intervals lasting weeks to months, while biliary colic has a sudden onset and lasts up to several hours. Pain from acute inflammation as with acute pancreatitis is severe and persists for days to weeks. Meals elicit diarrhea in some cases of inflammatory bowel disease and irritable bowel syndrome. Defecation relieves discomfort in inflammatory bowel disease and irritable bowel syndrome. Functional bowel disorders are exacerbated by stress. Sudden awakening from sound sleep suggests organic rather than functional disease. Diarrhea from malabsorption usually improves with fasting, while secretory diarrhea persists without oral intake.

Symptom relation to other factors narrows the list of diagnostic possibilities. Obstructive symptoms with prior abdominal surgery raise concern for adhesions, whereas loose stools after gastrectomy or gallbladder excision suggest dumping syndrome or postcholecystectomy diarrhea. Symptom onset after travel prompts a search for enteric infection. Medications may produce pain, altered bowel habits, or GI bleeding. Lower GI bleeding likely results from neoplasms, diverticula, or vascular lesions in an older person and from anorectal abnormalities or inflammatory bowel disease in a younger individual. Celiac disease is prevalent in people of northern European descent, while inflammatory bowel disease is more common in certain Jewish populations. A sexual history may raise concern for sexually transmitted diseases or immunodeficiency.

For more than two decades, working groups have been convened to devise symptom criteria to improve the confident diagnosis of functional bowel disorders and to minimize the numbers of unnecessary diagnostic tests performed. The most widely accepted symptom-based criteria are the Rome criteria. When tested against findings of structural investigations, the Rome criteria exhibit diagnostic specificities exceeding 90% for many of the functional bowel disorders.

PHYSICAL EXAMINATION

The physical exam complements information from the history. Abnormal vital signs provide diagnostic clues and determine the need for acute intervention. Fever suggests inflammation or neoplasm. Orthostasis is found with significant blood loss, dehydration, sepsis, or autonomic neuropathy. Skin, eye, or joint findings may point to specific diagnoses. Neck exam with swallowing assessment evaluates dysphagia. Cardiopulmonary disease may present with abdominal pain or nausea; thus lung and cardiac exams are important. Pelvic examination tests for a gynecologic source of abdominal pain. Rectal exam may detect blood, indicating gut mucosal injury or neoplasm or a palpable inflammatory mass in appendicitis. Metabolic conditions and gut motor disorders have associated peripheral neuropathy.

Inspection of the abdomen may reveal distention from obstruction, tumor, or ascites or vascular abnormalities with liver disease. Ecchymoses develop with severe pancreatitis. Auscultation can detect bruits or friction rubs from vascular disease or hepatic tumors. Loss of bowel sounds signifies ileus, while high-pitched, hyperactive sounds characterize intestinal obstruction. Percussion assesses liver size and can detect shifting dullness from ascites. Palpation assesses for hepatosplenomegaly as well as neoplastic or inflammatory masses. Abdominal exam is helpful in evaluating unexplained pain. Intestinal ischemia elicits severe pain but little tenderness. Patients with visceral pain may exhibit generalized discomfort, while those with parietal pain or peritonitis have directed pain, often with involuntary guarding, rigidity, or rebound. Patients with musculoskeletal abdominal wall pain may note tenderness exacerbated by Valsalva or straight-leg lift maneuvers.

TOOLS FOR PATIENT EVALUATION

Laboratory, radiographic, and functional tests can assist in diagnosis of suspected GI disease. The GI tract also is amenable to internal evaluation with upper and lower endoscopy and to examination of luminal contents. Histopathologic exams of GI tissues complement these tests.

Laboratory

Selected laboratory tests facilitate the diagnosis of GI disease. Iron-deficiency anemia suggests mucosal blood loss, while vitamin B_{12} deficiency results from small-intestinal, gastric, or pancreatic disease. Either also can result from inadequate oral intake. Leukocytosis and increased sedimentation rates and C-reactive proteins are found in inflammatory conditions, while leukopenia is seen in viremic illness. Severe vomiting or diarrhea elicits electrolyte disturbances, acid-base abnormalities, and elevated blood urea nitrogen. Pancreaticobiliary or liver disease is suggested by elevated pancreatic or liver chemistries. Thyroid chemistries, cortisol, and calcium levels are obtained to exclude endocrinologic causes of GI symptoms. Pregnancy testing is considered for women with unexplained nausea. Serologic tests can screen for celiac disease, inflammatory bowel disease, rheumatologic diseases like lupus or scleroderma, and paraneoplastic dysmotility syndromes. Hormone levels are obtained for suspected endocrine neoplasia. Intra-abdominal malignancies produce other tumor markers including the carcinoembryonic antigen CA 19-9 and α-fetoprotein. Blood testing also monitors medication

therapy in some diseases, as with thiopurine metabolite levels in inflammatory bowel disease. Other body fluids are sampled under certain circumstances. Ascitic fluid is analyzed for infection, malignancy, or findings of portal hypertension. Cerebrospinal fluid is obtained for suspected central nervous system causes of vomiting. Urine samples screen for carcinoid, porphyria, and heavy metal intoxication.

Luminal contents

Luminal contents can be examined for diagnostic clues. Stool samples are cultured for bacterial pathogens, examined for leukocytes and parasites, or tested for *Giardia* antigen. Duodenal aspirates can be examined for parasites or cultured for bacterial overgrowth. Fecal fat is quantified in possible malabsorption. Stool electrolytes can be measured in diarrheal conditions. Laxative screens are done when laxative abuse is suspected. Gastric acid is quantified to rule out Zollinger-Ellison syndrome. Esophageal pH testing is done for refractory symptoms of acid reflux, whereas impedance techniques assess for nonacidic reflux. Pancreatic juice is analyzed for enzyme or bicarbonate content to exclude pancreatic exocrine insufficiency.

Endoscopy

The gut is accessible with endoscopy, which can provide the diagnosis of the causes of bleeding, pain, nausea and vomiting, weight loss, altered bowel function, and fever. **Table 11-2** lists the most common indications for the major endoscopic procedures. Upper endoscopy evaluates the esophagus, stomach, and duodenum, while colonoscopy assesses the colon and distal ileum. Upper endoscopy is advocated as the initial structural test performed in patients with suspected ulcer disease, esophagitis, neoplasm, malabsorption, and Barrett's metaplasia because of its ability to directly visualize as well as biopsy the abnormality. Colonoscopy is the procedure of choice for colon cancer screening and surveillance as well as diagnosis of colitis secondary to infection, ischemia, radiation, and inflammatory bowel disease. Sigmoidoscopy examines the colon up to the splenic flexure and is currently used to exclude distal colonic inflammation or obstruction in young patients not at significant risk for colon cancer. For elusive GI bleeding secondary to arteriovenous malformations or superficial ulcers, small-intestinal examination is performed with push enteroscopy, capsule endoscopy, or double-balloon enteroscopy. Capsule endoscopy also can visualize small-intestinal Crohn's disease in individuals with negative barium radiography. Endoscopic retrograde cholangiopancreaticography (ERCP) provides diagnoses of pancreatic and biliary disease. Endoscopic ultrasound is useful for evaluating extent of disease in

TABLE 11-2

COMMON INDICATIONS FOR ENDOSCOPY

UPPER ENDOSCOPY	COLONOSCOPY	ENDOSCOPIC RETROGRADE CHOLANGIOPANCREATOGRAPHY	ENDOSCOPIC ULTRASOUND	CAPSULE ENDOSCOPY	DOUBLE BALLOON ENDOSCOPY
Dyspepsia despite treatment	Cancer screening	Jaundice	Staging of malignancy	Obscure GI bleeding	Ablation of small-intestinal bleeding sources
Dyspepsia with signs of organic disease	Lower GI bleeding	Postbiliary surgery complaints	Characterize and biopsy submucosal mass	Suspected Crohn's disease of the small intestine	Biopsy of suspicious small-intestinal masses/ulcers
Refractory vomiting	Anemia	Cholangitis	Bile duct stones		
Dysphagia	Diarrhea	Gallstone pancreatitis	Chronic pancreatitis		
Upper GI bleeding	Polypectomy	Pancreatic/biliary/ampullary tumor	Drain pseudocyst		
Anemia	Obstruction	Unexplained pancreatitis	Large gastric folds		
Weight loss	Biopsy radiologic abnormality	Pancreatitis with unrelenting pain	Anal continuity		
Malabsorption	Cancer surveillance: family history prior polyp/cancer, colitis	Fistulas			
Biopsy radiologic abnormality		Biopsy radiologic abnormality			
Polypectomy		Pancreaticobiliary drainage			
Place gastrostomy	Palliate neoplasm	Sample bile			
Barrett's surveillance	Remove foreign body	Sphincter of Oddi manometry			
Palliate neoplasm	Place stent across stenosis				
Sample duodenal tissue/fluid					
Remove foreign body					
Endoscopic mucosal resection or ablation of dysplastic Barrett's mucosa					
Place stent across stenosis					

GI malignancy as well as exclusion of choledocholithiasis, evaluation of pancreatitis, drainage of pancreatic pseudocysts, and assessment of anal continuity.

Radiography/nuclear medicine

Radiographic tests evaluate diseases of the gut and extraluminal structures. Oral or rectal contrast agents like barium provide mucosal definition from the esophagus to the rectum. Contrast radiography also assesses gut transit and pelvic floor dysfunction. Barium swallow is the initial procedure for evaluation of dysphagia to exclude subtle rings or strictures and assess for achalasia, whereas small-bowel contrast radiology reliably diagnoses intestinal tumors and Crohn's ileitis. Contrast enemas are performed when colonoscopy is unsuccessful or contraindicated. Ultrasound and computed tomography (CT) evaluate regions not accessible by endoscopy or contrast studies, including the liver, pancreas, gallbladder, kidneys, and retroperitoneum. These tests are useful for diagnosis of mass lesions, fluid collections, organ enlargement, and in the case of ultrasound, gallstones. CT and magnetic resonance (MR) colonography are being evaluated as alternatives to colonoscopy for colon cancer screening. MR imaging assesses the pancreaticobiliary ducts to exclude neoplasm, stones, and sclerosing cholangitis, and the liver to characterize benign and malignant tumors. Specialized CT or MR enterography can assess intensity of inflammatory bowel disease. Angiography excludes mesenteric ischemia and determines spread of malignancy. Angiographic techniques also access the biliary tree in obstructive jaundice. CT and MR techniques can be used to screen for mesenteric occlusion, thereby limiting exposure to angiographic dyes. Positron emission tomography can facilitate distinguishing malignant from benign disease in several organ systems.

Scintigraphy both evaluates structural abnormalities and quantifies luminal transit. Radionuclide bleeding scans localize bleeding sites in patients with brisk hemorrhage so that therapy with endoscopy, angiography, or surgery may be directed. Radiolabeled leukocyte scans can search for intraabdominal abscesses not visualized on CT. Biliary scintigraphy is complementary to ultrasound in the assessment of cholecystitis. Scintigraphy to quantify esophageal and gastric emptying is well established, while techniques to measure small-intestinal or colonic transit are less widely used.

Histopathology

Gut mucosal biopsies obtained at endoscopy evaluate for inflammatory, infectious, and neoplastic disease. Deep rectal biopsies assist with diagnosis of Hirschsprung's disease or amyloid. Liver biopsy is indicated in cases with abnormal liver chemistries, unexplained jaundice, following liver transplant to exclude rejection, and to characterize the degree of inflammation in patients with chronic viral hepatitis prior to initiating antiviral therapy. Biopsies obtained during CT or ultrasound can evaluate for other intraabdominal conditions not accessible by endoscopy.

Functional testing

Tests of gut function provide important data when structural testing is nondiagnostic. In addition to gastric acid and pancreatic function testing, functional testing of motor activity is provided by manometric techniques. Esophageal manometry is useful for suspected achalasia, whereas small-intestinal manometry tests for pseudoobstruction. A wireless motility capsule is now available to measure transit and contractile activity in the stomach, small intestine, and colon in a single test. Anorectal manometry with balloon expulsion testing is employed for unexplained incontinence or constipation from outlet dysfunction. Anorectal manometry and electromyography also assess anal function in fecal incontinence. Biliary manometry tests for sphincter of Oddi dysfunction with unexplained biliary pain. Measurement of breath hydrogen while fasting and after oral mono- or oligosaccharide challenge can screen for carbohydrate intolerance and small-intestinal bacterial overgrowth.

TREATMENT   Gastrointestinal Disease

Management options for the patient with GI disease depend on the cause of symptoms. Available treatments include modifications in dietary intake, medications, interventional endoscopy or radiology techniques, surgery, and therapies directed to external influences.

NUTRITIONAL MANIPULATION Dietary modifications for GI disease include treatments that only reduce symptoms, therapies that correct pathologic defects, and measures that replace normal food intake with enteral or parenteral formulations. Changes that improve symptoms but do not reverse an organic abnormality include lactose restriction for lactase deficiency,

liquid meals in gastroparesis, carbohydrate restrictions with dumping syndrome, and high-fiber diets in irritable bowel syndrome. The gluten-free diet for celiac disease exemplifies a modification that serves as primary therapy to reduce mucosal inflammation. Enteral medium-chain triglycerides replace normal fats with short-gut syndrome or severe ileal disease. Perfusion of liquid meals through a gastrostomy is performed in those who cannot swallow safely. Enteral feeding through a jejunostomy is considered for gastric dysmotility syndromes that preclude feeding into the stomach. Intravenous hyperalimentation is employed for individuals with generalized gut malfunction who cannot tolerate or who cannot be sustained with enteral nutrition.

PHARMACOTHERAPY Several medications are available to treat GI diseases. Considerable health care resources are expended on over-the-counter remedies. Many prescription drug classes are offered as short-term or continuous therapy of GI illness. A plethora of alternative treatments have gained popularity in GI conditions for which traditional therapies provide incomplete relief.

Over-the-Counter Agents Over-the-counter agents are reserved for mild GI symptoms. Antacids and histamine H_2 antagonists decrease symptoms in gastroesophageal reflux and dyspepsia, whereas antiflatulents and adsorbents reduce gaseous symptoms. More potent acid inhibitors such as proton pump inhibitors are now available over the counter for treatment of chronic gastroesophageal reflux disease (GERD). Fiber supplements, stool softeners, enemas, and laxatives are used for constipation. Laxatives are categorized as stimulants, osmotic agents (including isotonic preparations containing polyethylene glycol), and poorly absorbed sugars. Nonprescription antidiarrheal agents include bismuth subsalicylate, kaolin-pectin combinations, and loperamide. Supplemental enzymes include lactase pills for lactose intolerance and bacterial α-galactosidase to treat excess gas. In general, use of a nonprescription preparation for more than a short time for chronic persistent symptoms should be supervised by a health care provider.

Prescription Drugs Prescription drugs for GI diseases are a major focus of attention from pharmaceutical companies. Potent acid suppressants including drugs that inhibit the proton pump are advocated for acid reflux when over-the-counter preparations are inadequate. Cytoprotective agents rarely are used for upper gut ulcers. Prokinetic drugs stimulate GI propulsion in gastroparesis and pseudoobstruction. Prosecretory drugs are prescribed for constipation refractory to other agents. Prescription antidiarrheals include opiate drugs, anticholinergic antispasmodics, tricyclics, bile acid binders, and serotonin antagonists. Antispasmodics and antidepressants also are useful for functional abdominal pain, whereas narcotics are used for pain control in organic conditions such as disseminated malignancy and chronic pancreatitis. Antiemetics in several classes reduce nausea and vomiting. Potent pancreatic enzymes decrease malabsorption and pain from pancreatic disease. Antisecretory drugs such as the somatostatin analogue octreotide treat hypersecretory states. Antibiotics treat ulcer disease secondary to *Helicobacter pylori*, infectious diarrhea, diverticulitis, intestinal bacterial overgrowth, and Crohn's disease. Some cases of irritable bowel syndrome (especially those with diarrhea) respond to nonabsorbable antibiotic therapy. Anti-inflammatory and immunosuppressive drugs are used in ulcerative colitis, Crohn's disease, microscopic colitis, refractory celiac disease, and gut vasculitis. Chemotherapy with or without radiotherapy is offered for GI malignancies. Most GI carcinomas respond poorly to such therapy, whereas lymphomas may be cured with such intervention.

Alternative Therapies Alternative treatments are marketed to treat selected GI symptoms. Ginger, acupressure, and acustimulation have been advocated for nausea, while pyridoxine has been investigated for nausea of first-trimester pregnancy. Probiotics containing active bacterial cultures are used as adjuncts in some cases of infectious diarrhea and irritable bowel syndrome. Probiotics that selectively nourish benign luminal bacteria may ultimately show benefit in functional disorders as well. Low-potency pancreatic enzyme preparations are sold as general digestive aids but have little evidence to support their efficacy.

ENTERIC THERAPIES/INTERVENTIONAL ENDOSCOPY AND RADIOLOGY Simple luminal interventions are commonly performed for GI diseases. Nasogastric tube suction decompresses the upper gut in ileus or mechanical obstruction. Nasogastric lavage of saline or water in the patient with upper GI hemorrhage determines the rate of bleeding and helps evacuate blood prior to endoscopy. Enteral feedings can be initiated through a nasogastric or nasoenteric tube. Enemas relieve fecal impaction or assist in gas evacuation in acute colonic pseudoobstruction. A rectal tube can be left in place to vent the distal colon in colonic pseudoobstruction and other colonic distention disorders.

In addition to its diagnostic role, endoscopy has therapeutic capabilities in certain settings. Cautery techniques can stop hemorrhage from ulcers, vascular malformations, and tumors. Injection with vasoconstrictor substances or sclerosants is used for bleeding ulcers, vascular malformations, varices, and hemorrhoids. Endoscopic encirclement of varices and hemorrhoids with constricting bands stops hemorrhage from these sites, while endoscopically placed clips can occlude arterial bleeding sites. Endoscopy can remove polyps or debulk lumen-narrowing malignancies. Endoscopic mucosal resection

and radio frequency techniques can remove or ablate some cases of Barrett's esophagus with dysplasia. Endoscopic sphincterotomy of the ampulla of Vater relieves symptoms of choledocholithiasis. Obstructions of the gut lumen and pancreaticobiliary tree are relieved by endoscopic dilatation or placement of plastic or expandable metal stents. In cases of acute colonic pseudoobstruction, colonoscopy is employed to withdraw luminal gas. Finally, endoscopy is commonly used to insert feeding tubes.

Radiologic measures also are useful in GI disease. Angiographic embolization or vasoconstriction decreases bleeding from sites not amenable to endoscopic intervention. Dilatation or stenting with fluoroscopic guidance relieves luminal strictures. Contrast enemas can reduce volvulus and evacuate air in acute colonic pseudoobstruction. CT and ultrasound help drain abdominal fluid collections, in many cases obviating the need for surgery. Percutaneous transhepatic cholangiography relieves biliary obstruction when ERCP is contraindicated. Lithotripsy can fragment gallstones in patients who are not candidates for surgery. In some instances, radiologic approaches offer advantages over endoscopy for gastroenterostomy placement. Finally, central venous catheters for parenteral nutrition may be placed using radiographic techniques.

SURGERY Surgery is performed to cure disease, control symptoms without cure, maintain nutrition, or palliate unresectable neoplasm. Medication-unresponsive ulcerative colitis, diverticulitis, cholecystitis, appendicitis, and intraabdominal abscess are curable with surgery, while only symptom control without cure is possible with Crohn's disease. Surgery is mandated for ulcer complications such as bleeding, obstruction, or perforation and intestinal obstructions that persist after conservative care. Fundoplication of the gastroesophageal junction is performed for severe ulcerative esophagitis and drug-refractory symptomatic acid reflux. Achalasia responds to operations to relieve lower esophageal sphincter pressure. Operations for motor disorders have been introduced including implanted electrical stimulators for gastroparesis and electrical devices and artificial sphincters for fecal incontinence. Surgery may be needed to place a jejunostomy for long-term enteral feedings. The threshold for performing surgery depends on the clinical setting. In all cases, the benefits of operation must be weighed against the potential for postoperative complications.

THERAPY DIRECTED TO EXTERNAL INFLUENCES In some conditions, GI symptoms respond to treatments directed outside the gut. Psychological therapies including psychotherapy, behavior modification, hypnosis, and biofeedback have shown efficacy in functional bowel disorders. Patients with significant psychological dysfunction and those with little response to treatments targeting the gut are likely to benefit from this form of therapy.

CHAPTER 12
GASTROINTESTINAL ENDOSCOPY

Louis Michel Wong Kee Song ■ Mark Topazian

Gastrointestinal endoscopy has been attempted for over 200 years, but the introduction of semirigid gastroscopes in the middle of the twentieth century marked the dawn of the modern endoscopic era. Since then, rapid advances in endoscopic technology have led to dramatic changes in the diagnosis and treatment of many digestive diseases. Innovative endoscopic devices and new endoscopic treatment modalities continue to expand the use of endoscopy in patient care.

Flexible endoscopes provide either an optical image (transmitted over fiberoptic bundles) or an electronic video image (generated by a charge-coupled device in the tip of the endoscope). Operator controls permit deflection of the endoscope tip; fiberoptic bundles bring light to the tip of the endoscope; and working channels allow washing, suctioning, and the passage of instruments. Progressive changes in the diameter and stiffness of endoscopes have improved the ease and patient tolerance of endoscopy.

ENDOSCOPIC PROCEDURES

UPPER ENDOSCOPY

Upper endoscopy, also referred to as esophagogastro-duodenoscopy (EGD), is performed by passing a flexible endoscope through the mouth into the esophagus, stomach, bulb, and second duodenum. The procedure is the best method of examining the upper gastrointestinal mucosa. While the upper gastrointestinal radiographic series has similar accuracy for diagnosis of duodenal ulcer (Fig. 12-1), EGD is superior for detection of gastric ulcers (Fig. 12-2) and flat mucosal lesions such as Barrett's esophagus (Fig. 12-3), and it permits directed biopsy and endoscopic therapy. Intravenous conscious sedation is given to most patients in

FIGURE 12-1
Duodenal ulcers. *A.* Ulcer with a clean base. ***B.*** Ulcer with a visible vessel (*arrow*) in a patient with recent hemorrhage.

the United States to ease the anxiety and discomfort of the procedure, although in many countries EGD is routinely performed with topical pharyngeal anesthesia only. Patient tolerance of unsedated EGD is improved by the use of an ultrathin, 5-mm diameter endoscope that can be passed transorally or transnasally.

FIGURE 12-2
Gastric ulcers. *A.* Benign gastric ulcer. ***B.*** Malignant gastric ulcer involving greater curvature of stomach.

FIGURE 12-3

Barrett's esophagus. A. Pink tongues of Barrett's mucosa extending proximally from the gastroesophageal junction. **B.** Barrett's esophagus with a suspicious nodule (*arrow*) identified during endoscopic surveillance. **C.** Histologic finding of intramucosal adenocarcinoma in the endoscopically resected nodule. Tumor extends into the esophageal submucosa (*arrow*). **D.** Barrett's esophagus with locally advanced adenocarcinoma.

COLONOSCOPY

Colonoscopy is performed by passing a flexible colonoscope through the anal canal into the rectum and colon. The cecum is reached in >95% of cases, and the terminal ileum can often be examined. Colonoscopy is the gold standard for diagnosis of colonic mucosal disease. Colonoscopy has greater sensitivity than barium enema for colitis (**Fig. 12-4**), polyps (**Fig. 12-5**), and cancer (**Fig. 12-6**). CT colonography is an emerging technology that rivals colonoscopy's accuracy for detection of polyps and cancer. Conscious sedation is usually given before colonoscopy in the United States, although a willing patient and a skilled examiner can complete the procedure without sedation in many cases.

FLEXIBLE SIGMOIDOSCOPY

Flexible sigmoidoscopy is similar to colonoscopy but visualizes only the rectum and a variable portion of the left colon, typically to 60 cm from the anal verge. This procedure causes abdominal cramping, but it is brief and is usually performed without sedation. Flexible sigmoidoscopy is primarily used for evaluation of diarrhea and rectal outlet bleeding.

FIGURE 12-4

Causes of colitis. A. Chronic ulcerative colitis with diffuse ulcerations and exudates. **B.** Severe Crohn's colitis with deep ulcers. **C.** Pseudomembranous colitis with yellow, adherent pseudomembranes. **D.** Ischemic colitis with patchy mucosal edema, subepithelial hemorrhage, and cyanosis.

FIGURE 12-5
**Colonic polyps. *A.* Pedunculated colon polyp on a thick stalk covered with normal mucosa (*arrow*). *B.* Sessile rectal polyp.

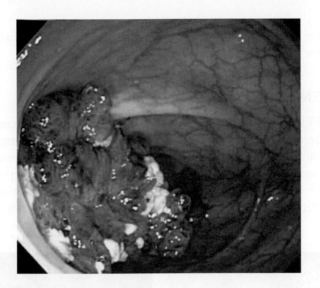

FIGURE 12-6
Colon adenocarcinoma growing into the lumen.

SMALL-BOWEL ENDOSCOPY

Three techniques are currently used to evaluate the small intestine, most often in patients presenting with presumed small-bowel bleeding. For *capsule endoscopy* the patient swallows a disposable capsule that contains a complementary metal oxide silicon (CMOS) chip camera. Color still images (Fig. 12-7) are transmitted wirelessly to an external receiver at several frames per second until the capsule's battery is exhausted or it is passed into the toilet. Although capsule endoscopy enables visualization of the jejunal and ileal mucosa beyond the reach of a conventional endoscope, it remains solely a diagnostic procedure at present.

Push enteroscopy is performed with a long endoscope similar in design to an upper endoscope. The enteroscope is pushed down the small bowel, sometimes with the help of a stiffening overtube that extends from the mouth to the small intestine. The proximal to mid-jejunum is usually reached, and the endoscope's instrument channel allows for biopsies or endoscopic therapy.

FIGURE 12-7
Capsule endoscopy image of jejunal vascular ectasia.

Deeper insertion into the small bowel can be accomplished by *single-* or *double-balloon enteroscopy* or *spiral enteroscopy* (Fig. 12-8). These instruments enable pleating of the small intestine onto an overtube. With balloon-assisted enteroscopy, the entire small bowel can be visualized in some patients when both the oral and anal routes of insertion are used. Biopsies and

FIGURE 12-8
Radiograph of a double-balloon enteroscope in the small intestine.

FIGURE 12-9

Nonsteroidal anti-inflammatory drug (NSAID)-induced proximal ileal stricture diagnosed by double-balloon endoscopy. *A.* Ileal stricture causing obstructive symptoms. *B.* Balloon dilatation of the ileal stricture. *C.* Appearance of stricture after dilatation.

endoscopic therapy can be performed throughout the visualized small bowel **(Fig. 12-9)**.

ENDOSCOPIC RETROGRADE CHOLANGIOPANCREATOGRAPHY (ERCP)

During ERCP, a side-viewing endoscope is passed through the mouth to the duodenum, the ampulla of Vater is identified and cannulated with a thin plastic catheter, and radiographic contrast material is injected into the bile duct and pancreatic duct under fluoroscopic guidance **(Fig. 12-10)**. When indicated, the sphincter of Oddi can be opened using the technique of endoscopic sphincterotomy **(Fig. 12-11)**. Stones can be retrieved from the ducts, biopsies can be performed, strictures can be dilated and/or stented **(Fig. 12-12)**, and ductal leaks can be stented **(Fig. 12-13)**. ERCP is often performed for therapy but remains important in diagnosis, especially for ductal strictures and bile duct stones.

ENDOSCOPIC ULTRASOUND (EUS)

EUS utilizes high-frequency ultrasound transducers incorporated into the tip of a flexible endoscope. Ultrasound images are obtained of the gut wall and adjacent organs, vessels, and lymph nodes. By sacrificing depth of ultrasound penetration and bringing the ultrasound transducer close to the area of interest via endoscopy,

FIGURE 12-10

Endoscopic retrograde cholangiopancreatography (ERCP) for bile duct stones with cholangitis. *A.* Faceted bile duct stones are demonstrated in the common bile duct. *B.* After endoscopic sphincterotomy, the stones are extracted with a Dormia basket. A small abscess communicates with the left hepatic duct.

FIGURE 12-11

Endoscopic sphincterotomy. *A.* A normal-appearing ampulla of Vater. *B.* Sphincterotomy is performed with electrocautery. *C.* Bile duct stones are extracted with a balloon catheter. *D.* Final appearance of the sphincterotomy.

FIGURE 12-12

Endoscopic diagnosis, staging, and palliation of hilar cholangiocarcinoma. A. Endoscopic retrograde cholangiopancreatography (ERCP) in a patient with obstructive jaundice demonstrates a malignant-appearing stricture of the biliary confluence extending into the left and right intrahepatic ducts. **B.** Intraductal ultrasound of the biliary stricture demonstrates marked bile duct wall thickening due to tumor (T) with partial encasement of the hepatic artery (*arrow*). **C.** Intraductal biopsy obtained during ERCP demonstrates malignant cells infiltrating the submucosa of the bile duct wall (*arrow*). **D.** Endoscopic placement of bilateral self-expanding metal stents (*arrow*) relieves the biliary obstruction. GB, gallbladder. (*Image C courtesy of Dr. Thomas Smyrk; with permission.*)

FIGURE 12-13

Bile leak (*arrow*) from a duct of Luschka after laparoscopic cholecystectomy. Contrast leaks from a small right intrahepatic duct into the gallbladder fossa, then flows into the pigtail of a percutaneous drainage catheter.

high-resolution images are obtained. EUS provides the most accurate preoperative local staging of esophageal, pancreatic, and rectal malignancies (**Fig. 12-14**), although it does not detect most distant metastases. EUS is also useful for diagnosis of bile duct stones, gallbladder disease, submucosal gastrointestinal lesions, and chronic pancreatitis. Fine-needle aspirates and core biopsies of masses and lymph nodes in the posterior mediastinum, abdomen, pancreas, retroperitoneum, and pelvis can be obtained under EUS guidance (**Fig. 12-15**).

NATURAL ORIFICE TRANSLUMINAL ENDOSCOPIC SURGERY (NOTES)

NOTES is an evolving collection of endoscopic methods that entail passage of an endoscope or its accessories through the wall of the gastrointestinal tract (e.g., stomach) to perform diagnostic or therapeutic interventions. Some NOTES procedures, such as percutaneous endoscopic gastrostomy (PEG) or endoscopic necrosectomy of pancreatic necrosis, are established clinical procedures; others, such as endoscopic appendectomy, cholecystectomy, and tubal ligation, are in development, and their ultimate clinical application is presently unclear. NOTES is currently an area of intense innovation and endoscopic research.

RISKS OF ENDOSCOPY

Medications used during conscious sedation may cause respiratory depression or allergic reactions. All endoscopic procedures carry some risk of bleeding and gastrointestinal perforation. These risks are quite low with diagnostic upper endoscopy and colonoscopy (<1:1000 procedures), although the risk is as high as 2:100 when therapeutic procedures such as polypectomy, control of hemorrhage, or stricture dilatation are performed. Bleeding and perforation are rare with flexible sigmoidoscopy. The risks for diagnostic EUS (without needle aspiration) are similar to the risks for diagnostic upper endoscopy.

Infectious complications are unusual with most endoscopic procedures. Some procedures carry a higher incidence of postprocedure bacteremia, and prophylactic antibiotics may be indicated (**Table 12-1**).

ERCP carries additional risks. Pancreatitis occurs in about 5% of patients undergoing ERCP and in up to 25% of patients with sphincter of Oddi dysfunction. Young anicteric patients with normal ducts are at increased risk. Post-ERCP pancreatitis is usually mild and self-limited but may rarely result in prolonged hospitalization, surgery, diabetes, or death. Bleeding occurs in 1% of endoscopic sphincterotomies. Ascending cholangitis, pseudocyst infection, retroperitoneal perforation, and abscess may occur as a result of ERCP.

FIGURE 12-14

Local staging of gastrointestinal cancers with endoscopic ultrasound. In each example the white arrowhead marks the primary tumor and the black arrow indicates the muscularis propria (mp) of the intestinal wall. *A.* T1 gastric cancer. The tumor does not invade the mp. *B.* T2 esophageal cancer. The tumor invades the mp. *C.* T3 esophageal cancer. The tumor extends through the mp into the surrounding tissue, and focally abuts the aorta. AO, aorta.

Clinical predictors of rebleeding help identify patients most likely to benefit from urgent endoscopy and endoscopic, angiographic, or surgical hemostasis.

Initial evaluation

The initial evaluation of the bleeding patient focuses on the magnitude of hemorrhage as reflected by the postural vital signs, the frequency of hematemesis or melena, and (in some cases) findings on nasogastric lavage. Decreases in hematocrit and hemoglobin lag behind the clinical course and are not reliable gauges of the magnitude of acute bleeding. This initial evaluation, completed well before the bleeding source is confidently identified, guides immediate supportive care of the patient and helps determine the timing of endoscopy. The severity of the initial hemorrhage is the most important indication for urgent endoscopy, since a large initial bleed increases the likelihood of ongoing or recurrent bleeding. Patients with resting hypotension, repeated hematemesis, bloody nasogastric aspirate that does not clear with large volume lavage, or orthostatic change in vital signs, or those requiring blood transfusions, should be considered for urgent endoscopy. In addition, patients with cirrhosis, coagulopathy, or respiratory or renal failure, and those over 70 years of age are more likely to have significant rebleeding.

Bedside evaluation also suggests an upper or lower gastrointestinal source of bleeding in most patients. Over 90% of patients with melena are bleeding proximal to the ligament of Treitz, and about 90% of patients with hematochezia are bleeding from the colon. Melena can result from bleeding in the small bowel or right colon, especially in older patients with slow colonic transit. Conversely, some patients with massive hematochezia may be bleeding from an upper gastrointestinal

FIGURE 12-15

Endoscopic ultrasound (EUS)-guided fine-needle aspiration (FNA). *A.* Ultrasound image of a 22-gauge needle passed through the duodenal wall and positioned in a hypoechoic pancreatic head mass. *B.* Micrograph of aspirated malignant cells. (*Image B courtesy of Dr. Michael R. Henry; with permission.*)

Percutaneous gastrostomy tube placement during EGD is associated with a 10–15% incidence of complications, most often wound infections. Fasciitis, pneumonia, bleeding, buried bumper syndrome, and colonic injury may result from gastrostomy tube placement.

URGENT ENDOSCOPY

ACUTE GASTROINTESTINAL HEMORRHAGE

Endoscopy is an important diagnostic and therapeutic technique for patients with acute gastrointestinal hemorrhage. Although gastrointestinal bleeding stops spontaneously in most cases, some patients will have persistent or recurrent hemorrhage that may be life-threatening.

TABLE 12-1

ANTIBIOTIC PROPHYLAXIS FOR ENDOSCOPIC PROCEDURES

PATIENT CONDITION	PROCEDURE CONTEMPLATED	GOAL OF PROPHYLAXIS	PERIPROCEDURAL ANTIBIOTIC PROPHYLAXIS
All cardiac conditions	Any endoscopic procedure	Prevention of infective endocarditis	Not indicated
Bile-duct obstruction in the absence of cholangitis	ERCP with complete drainage	Prevention of cholangitis	Not recommended
Bile-duct obstruction in absence of cholangitis	ERCP with anticipated incomplete drainage (e.g., PSC, hilar strictures)	Prevention of cholangitis	Recommended; continue antibiotics after the procedure
Sterile pancreatic fluid collection (e.g., pseudocyst, necrosis), which communicates with pancreatic duct	ERCP	Prevention of cyst infection	Recommended
Sterile pancreatic fluid collection	Transmural drainage	Prevention of cyst infection	Recommended
Solid lesion along upper GI tract	EUS-FNA	Prevention of local infection	Not recommended[a]
Solid lesion along lower GI tract	EUS-FNA	Prevention of local infection	Insufficient data to make firm recommendation[b]
Cystic lesions along GI tract (including mediastinum)	EUS-FNA	Prevention of cyst infection	Recommended
All patients	Percutaneous endoscopic feeding tube placement	Prevention of peristomal infection	Recommended
Cirrhosis with acute GI bleeding	Required for all patients, regardless of endoscopic procedures	Prevention of infectious complications and reduction of mortality	Upon admission[c]
Synthetic vascular graft and other nonvalvular cardiovascular devices	Any endoscopic procedure	Prevention of graft and device infection	Not recommended[d]
Prosthetic joints	Any endoscopic procedure	Prevention of septic arthritis	Not recommended[e]

[a]Low rates of bacteremia and local infection.
[b]Endoscopists may choose on a case-by-case basis.
[c]Risk for bacterial infection associated with cirrhosis and GI bleeding is well established.
[d]No reported cases of infection associated with endoscopy.
[e]Very low risk of infection.
Abbreviations: ERCP, endoscopic retrograde cholangiopancreatography; EUS-FNA, endoscopic ultrasound–fine-needle aspiration; PSC, primary sclerosing cholangitis.
Source: Adapted from S Banerjee et al: Gastrointest Endosc 67:719, 2008; with permission from Elsevier.

source, such as a gastric Dieulafoy's lesion or duodenal ulcer, with rapid intestinal transit. Early upper endoscopy should be considered in such patients.

Endoscopy should be performed after the patient has been resuscitated with intravenous fluids and transfusions as necessary. Marked coagulopathy or thrombocytopenia is usually treated before endoscopy, since correction of these abnormalities may lead to resolution of bleeding, and techniques for endoscopic hemostasis are limited in such patients. Metabolic derangements should also be addressed. Tracheal intubation for airway protection should be considered before upper endoscopy in patients with repeated recent hematemesis and suspected variceal hemorrhage.

Most patients with impressive hematochezia can undergo colonoscopy after a rapid colonic purge with a polyethylene glycol solution; the preparation fluid may be administered via a nasogastric tube. Colonoscopy has a higher diagnostic yield than radionuclide bleeding scans or angiography in lower gastrointestinal bleeding, and endoscopic therapy can be applied in some cases. In a minority of cases, endoscopic assessment is hindered by poor visualization due to persistent vigorous bleeding with recurrent hemodynamic instability, and other techniques (such as angiography or emergent subtotal colectomy) must be employed. In such patients, massive bleeding originating from an upper gastrointestinal source should also be considered and excluded by upper endoscopy. The anal and rectal mucosa should be visualized endoscopically early in the course of massive rectal bleeding, as bleeding lesions in or close to the anal canal may be identified that are amenable to endoscopic or surgical transanal hemostatic techniques.

Peptic ulcer

The endoscopic appearance of peptic ulcers provides useful prognostic information and guides the need for endoscopic therapy in patients with acute hemorrhage (Fig. 12-16). A clean-based ulcer is associated with a low, 3–5% risk of rebleeding; patients with melena and a clean-based ulcer are often discharged home from the emergency room or endoscopy suite if they are young, reliable, and otherwise healthy. Flat pigmented spots and adherent clots covering the ulcer base have a 10 and 20% risk of rebleeding, respectively. Endoscopic therapy is often considered for an ulcer with an adherent clot. When a platelet plug is seen protruding from a vessel wall in the base of an ulcer (so-called sentinel clot or visible vessel), the risk of rebleeding from the ulcer is 40%. This finding generally leads to endoscopic therapy to decrease the rebleeding rate. Occasionally, active spurting from an ulcer is seen with >90% risk of ongoing bleeding without therapy.

Endoscopic therapy of ulcers with high-risk stigmata typically lowers the rebleeding rate to 5–10%. Several hemostatic techniques are available, including injection of epinephrine or a sclerosant into and around the vessel, "coaptive coagulation" of the vessel in the base of the ulcer using a thermal probe that is pressed against the site of bleeding, placement of hemoclips, or a combination of these modalities. In conjunction with endoscopic therapy, the administration of a proton pump inhibitor decreases the risk of rebleeding and improves patient outcome.

Varices

Two complementary strategies guide therapy of bleeding varices: local treatment of the bleeding varices and treatment of the underlying portal hypertension. Local therapies, including endoscopic variceal sclerotherapy, endoscopic variceal band ligation, and balloon tamponade with a Sengstaken-Blakemore tube, effectively control acute hemorrhage in most patients, although therapies that decrease portal pressure (pharmacologic treatment, surgical shunts, or radiologically placed intrahepatic portosystemic shunts) also play an important role.

Endoscopic variceal ligation (EVL) is indicated for the prevention of a first bleed from large esophageal

FIGURE 12-16

Stigmata of hemorrhage in peptic ulcers. A. Gastric antral ulcer with a clean base. **B.** Duodenal ulcer with flat pigmented spots. **C.** Duodenal ulcer with a dense adherent clot. **D.** Gastric ulcer with a pigmented protuberance/visible vessel. **E.** Duodenal ulcer with active spurting (*arrow*).

FIGURE 12-17
Esophageal varices.

A   B

FIGURE 12-19
Dieulafoy's lesion. _A._ Actively spurting jejunal Dieulafoy's lesion. There is no underlying mucosal lesion. **_B._** Histology of a gastric Dieulafoy's lesion. A persistent caliber artery (_arrows_) is present in the gastric submucosa, immediately beneath the mucosa.

varices **(Fig. 12-17)**, particularly in patients in whom beta blockers are contraindicated or not tolerated (primary prophylaxis). EVL is also the preferred endoscopic therapy for control of active esophageal variceal bleeding and for subsequent eradication of esophageal varices (secondary prophylaxis). During EVL, a varix is suctioned into a cap fitted on the end of the endoscope, and a rubber band is released from the cap, ligating the varix. EVL controls acute hemorrhage in up to 90% of patients. Complications of EVL, such as postbanding ulcer bleeding and esophageal stenosis, are uncommon. Endoscopic variceal sclerotherapy (EVS) involves the injection of a sclerosing, thrombogenic solution into or next to the esophageal varices. EVS also controls acute hemorrhage in most patients but has a higher complication rate than EVL. These techniques are used when varices are actively bleeding during endoscopy or (more commonly) when varices are the only identifiable cause of acute hemorrhage. Bleeding from large gastric fundic varices **(Fig. 12-18)** is best treated with endoscopic cyanoacrylate ("glue") injection, since EVL or EVS of

these varices is associated with a high rebleeding rate. Complications of cyanoacrylate injection include infection and glue embolization to other organs, such as the lungs, brain, and spleen.

After treatment of the acute hemorrhage, an elective course of endoscopic therapy can be undertaken with the goal of eradicating esophageal varices and preventing rebleeding months to years later. However, this chronic therapy is less successful, preventing long-term rebleeding in ~50% of patients. Pharmacologic therapies that decrease portal pressure have similar efficacy, and the two modalities may be combined.

Dieulafoy's lesion

This lesion, also called _persistent caliber artery,_ is a large-caliber arteriole that runs immediately beneath the gastrointestinal mucosa and bleeds through a pinpoint mucosal erosion **(Fig. 12-19)**. Dieulafoy's lesion is seen most commonly on the lesser curvature of the proximal stomach, causes impressive arterial hemorrhage, and may be difficult to diagnose; it is often recognized only after repeated endoscopy for recurrent bleeding. Endoscopic therapy, such as thermal coagulation, is typically effective for control of bleeding and ablation of the underlying vessel once the lesion has been identified. Rescue therapies, such as angiographic embolization or surgical oversewing, are considered in situations where endoscopic therapy has failed.

Mallory-Weiss tear

A Mallory-Weiss tear is a linear mucosal rent near or across the gastroesophageal junction that is often associated with retching or vomiting **(Fig. 12-20)**. When the tear disrupts a submucosal arteriole, brisk hemorrhage may result. Endoscopy is the best method of diagnosis, and an actively bleeding tear can be treated

FIGURE 12-18
Gastric fundic varices.

FIGURE 12-20
Mallory-Weiss tear at the gastroesophageal junction.

endoscopically with epinephrine injection, coaptive coagulation, band ligation, or hemoclips. Unlike peptic ulcer, a Mallory-Weiss tear with a nonbleeding sentinel clot in its base rarely rebleeds and thus does not necessitate endoscopic therapy.

Vascular ectasias

Vascular ectasias are flat mucosal vascular anomalies that are best diagnosed by endoscopy. They usually cause slow intestinal blood loss and occur either in a sporadic fashion or in a well-defined pattern of distribution [e.g., gastric antral vascular ectasia (GAVE) or "watermelon stomach"] (Fig. 12–21). Cecal vascular ectasias (senile lesions), GAVE, and radiation-induced rectal ectasias are often responsive to local endoscopic ablative therapy, such as argon plasma coagulation. Patients with diffuse small-bowel vascular ectasias (associated with chronic renal failure and with hereditary hemorrhagic telangiectasia) may continue to bleed despite endoscopic treatment of easily accessible lesions by conventional endoscopy. These patients may benefit from deep enteroscopy with endoscopic therapy, pharmacologic treatment with octreotide or estrogen/progesterone therapy, or intraoperative enteroscopy.

Colonic diverticula

Diverticula form where nutrient arteries penetrate the muscular wall of the colon en route to the colonic mucosa (Fig. 12–22). The artery found in the base of a diverticulum may bleed, causing painless and impressive hematochezia. Colonoscopy is indicated in patients with hematochezia and suspected diverticular hemorrhage, since other causes of bleeding (such as vascular ectasias, colitis, and colon cancer) must be excluded. In addition, an actively bleeding diverticulum may be seen and treated during colonoscopy.

FIGURE 12-22
Colonic diverticula.

A   B   C

FIGURE 12-21
Gastrointestinal vascular ectasias. A. Gastric antral vascular ectasia ("watermelon stomach") characterized by stripes of prominent flat or raised vascular ectasias. **B.** Cecal vascular ectasias. **C.** Radiation-induced vascular ectasias of the rectum in a patient previously treated for prostate cancer.

GASTROINTESTINAL OBSTRUCTION AND PSEUDOOBSTRUCTION

Endoscopy is useful for evaluation and treatment of some forms of gastrointestinal obstruction. An important exception is small bowel obstruction due to surgical adhesions, which is generally not diagnosed or treated endoscopically. Esophageal, gastroduodenal, and colonic obstruction or pseudoobstruction can all be diagnosed and often managed endoscopically.

Acute esophageal obstruction

Esophageal obstruction by impacted food (Fig. 12-23) or an ingested foreign body is a potentially life-threatening event and represents an endoscopic emergency. Left untreated, the patient may develop esophageal ulceration, ischemia, and perforation. Patients with persistent esophageal obstruction often have hypersalivation and are usually unable to swallow water; endoscopy is generally the best initial test in such patients, since endoscopic removal of the obstructing material is usually possible, and the presence of an underlying esophageal pathology can often be determined. Radiographs of the chest and neck should be considered before endoscopy in patients with fever, obstruction for ≥24 h, or ingestion of a sharp object such as a fishbone. Radiographic contrast studies interfere with subsequent endoscopy and are not advisable in most patients with a clinical picture of esophageal obstruction. Occasionally, sublingual nifedipine or nitrates, or intravenous glucagon, may resolve an esophageal food impaction, but in most patients an underlying web, ring, or stricture is present and endoscopic removal of the obstructing food bolus is necessary.

Gastric outlet obstruction

Obstruction of the gastric outlet is commonly caused by gastric, duodenal, or pancreatic malignancy, or chronic

FIGURE 12-23
Esophageal food (meat) impaction.

FIGURE 12-24
Biliary and duodenal self-expanding metal stents (SEMS) for obstruction caused by pancreatic cancer. *A.* Endo- scopic retrograde cholangiopancreatography (ERCP) demonstrates a distal bile duct stricture (*arrow*). *B.* A biliary SEMS is placed. *C.* Contrast injection demonstrates a duodenal stricture (*arrow*). *D.* Biliary and duodenal SEMS in place.

peptic ulceration with stenosis of the pylorus. Patients vomit partially digested food many hours after eating. Gastric decompression with a nasogastric tube and subsequent lavage for removal of retained material is the first step in treatment. The diagnosis can then be confirmed with a saline load test, if desired. Endoscopy is useful for diagnosis and treatment. Patients with benign pyloric stenosis may be treated with endoscopic balloon dilatation of the pylorus, and a course of endoscopic dilatation results in long-term relief of symptoms in about 50% of patients. Malignant gastric outlet obstruction can be relieved with endoscopically placed expandable stents (Fig. 12-24) in patients with inoperable malignancy.

Colonic obstruction and pseudoobstruction

These both present with abdominal distention and discomfort; tympany; and a dilated, air-filled colon on plain abdominal radiography. The radiographic appearance can be characteristic of a particular condition, such as sigmoid volvulus (Fig. 12-25). Both structural obstruction and pseudoobstruction may lead to colonic perforation if untreated. Acute colonic pseudoobstruction is a form of colonic ileus that is usually attributable to electrolyte disorders, narcotic and anticholinergic

FIGURE 12-25
Sigmoid volvulus with the characteristic radiologic appearance of a "bent inner tube."

medications, immobility (as after surgery), and retroperitoneal hemorrhage or mass. Multiple causative factors are often present. Colonoscopy, water-soluble contrast enema, or CT may be used to look for an obstructing lesion and differentiate obstruction from pseudoobstruction. One of these diagnostic studies should be strongly considered if the patient does not have clear risk factors for pseudoobstruction, if radiographs do not show air in the rectum, or if the patient fails to improve when underlying causes of pseudoobstruction have been addressed. The risk of cecal perforation in pseudoobstruction rises when the cecal diameter exceeds 12 cm, and decompression of the colon may be achieved using intravenous neostigmine or via colonoscopic decompression **(Fig. 12-26)**. Most patients should receive a trial of conservative therapy (with correction of

electrolyte disorders, removal of offending medications, and increased mobilization) before undergoing an invasive decompressive procedure for colonic pseudoobstruction.

Colonic obstruction is an indication for urgent intervention. Emergent diverting colostomy may be performed with a subsequent second operation after bowel preparation to treat the underlying cause of obstruction. Colonoscopic placement of an expandable stent is an alternative that can relieve malignant obstruction without emergency surgery and permit bowel preparation for an elective one-stage operation **(Fig. 12-27)**.

ACUTE BILIARY OBSTRUCTION

The steady, severe pain that occurs when a gallstone acutely obstructs the common bile duct often brings patients to a hospital. The diagnosis of a ductal stone is suspected when the patient is jaundiced or when serum liver tests or pancreatic enzyme levels are elevated; it is confirmed by direct cholangiography (performed endoscopically, percutaneously, or during surgery). ERCP is currently the primary means of diagnosing and treating common bile duct stones in most hospitals in the United States (Figs. 12-10 and 12-11).

Bile duct imaging

While transabdominal ultrasound diagnoses only a minority of bile duct stones, magnetic resonance cholangiopancreatography (MRCP) and EUS are >90% accurate and have an important role in diagnosis. Examples of these modalities are shown in **Fig. 12-28**.

If the suspicion for a bile duct stone is high and urgent treatment is required (as in a patient with obstructive jaundice and biliary sepsis), ERCP is the procedure of choice, since it remains the gold standard for diagnosis and allows for immediate treatment. If a

FIGURE 12-26
Acute colonic pseudoobstruction. A. Acute colonic dilatation occurring in a patient soon after knee surgery. **B.** Colonoscopic placement of decompression tube with marked improvement in colonic dilatation.

FIGURE 12-27
Obstructing colonic carcinoma. A. Colonic adenocarcinoma causing marked luminal narrowing of the descending colon. **B.** Endoscopic placement of a self-expanding metal stent. **C.** Radiograph of expanded stent across the obstructing tumor with a residual waist (*arrow*). (*Image A courtesy of Dr. Glenn Alexander; with permission.*)

persistent bile duct stone is unlikely (as in a patient with gallstone pancreatitis), ERCP may be supplanted by less invasive imaging techniques, such as EUS or MRCP.

Ascending cholangitis

Charcot's triad of jaundice, abdominal pain, and fever is present in about 70% of patients with ascending cholangitis and biliary sepsis. These patients are managed initially with fluid resuscitation and intravenous antibiotics.

Abdominal ultrasound is often performed to assess for gallbladder stones and bile duct dilation. However, the bile duct may not be dilated early in the course of acute biliary obstruction. Medical management usually improves the patient's clinical status, providing a window of approximately 24 h during which biliary drainage should be established, typically by ERCP. Undue delay can result in recrudescence of overt sepsis and increased morbidity and mortality rates. In addition to Charcot's triad, the additional presence of shock and

FIGURE 12-28
Methods of bile duct imaging. Arrows mark bile duct stones. Arrowheads indicate the common bile duct, and the asterisk marks the portal vein. **A.** Endoscopic ultrasound (EUS). **B.** Magnetic resonance cholangiopancreatography (MRCP). **C.** Helical computed tomography (CT).

confusion (Reynolds's pentad) is associated with high mortality rate and should prompt an urgent intervention to restore biliary drainage.

Gallstone pancreatitis

Gallstones may cause acute pancreatitis as they pass through the ampulla of Vater. The occurrence of gallstone pancreatitis usually implies passage of a stone into the duodenum, and only about 20% of patients harbor a persistent stone in the ampulla or the common bile duct. Retained stones are more common in patients with jaundice, rising serum liver tests following hospitalization, severe pancreatitis, or superimposed ascending cholangitis.

Urgent ERCP decreases the morbidity rate of gallstone pancreatitis in a subset of patients with retained bile duct stones. It is unclear whether the benefit of ERCP is mainly attributable to treatment and prevention of ascending cholangitis or to relief of pancreatic duct obstruction. ERCP is warranted early in the course of gallstone pancreatitis if ascending cholangitis is suspected, especially in a jaundiced patient. Urgent ERCP also appears to benefit patients predicted to have severe pancreatitis using a clinical index of severity such as the Glasgow or Ranson score. Since the benefit of ERCP is limited to patients with a retained bile duct stone, a strategy of initial MRCP or EUS for diagnosis decreases the utilization of ERCP in gallstone pancreatitis and improves clinical outcomes by limiting the occurrence of ERCP-related complications.

ELECTIVE ENDOSCOPY

DYSPEPSIA

Dyspepsia is a chronic or recurrent burning discomfort or pain in the upper abdomen that may be caused by diverse processes such as gastroesophageal reflux, peptic ulcer disease, and "nonulcer dyspepsia," a heterogeneous category that includes disorders of motility, sensation, and somatization. Gastric and esophageal malignancies are less common causes of dyspepsia. Careful history-taking allows accurate differential diagnosis of dyspepsia in only about half of patients. In the remainder, endoscopy can be a useful diagnostic tool, especially in patients whose symptoms are not resolved by an empirical trial of symptomatic treatment. Endoscopy should be performed at the outset in patients with dyspepsia and alarm features, such as weight loss or iron-deficiency anemia.

GASTROESOPHAGEAL REFLUX DISEASE (GERD)

When classic symptoms of gastroesophageal reflux are present, such as water brash and substernal heartburn, presumptive diagnosis and empirical treatment are often sufficient. Endoscopy is a sensitive test for diagnosis of esophagitis (**Fig. 12-29**), but will miss nonerosive reflux disease (NERD) since some patients have

A

B

C

D

FIGURE 12-29

Causes of esophagitis. A. Severe reflux esophagitis with mucosal ulceration and friability. **B.** Cytomegalovirus esophagitis. **C.** Herpes simplex virus esophagitis with target-type shallow ulcerations. **D.** Candida esophagitis with white plaques adherent to the esophageal mucosa.

symptomatic reflux without esophagitis. The most sensitive test for diagnosis of GERD is 24-h ambulatory pH monitoring. Endoscopy is indicated in patients with reflux symptoms refractory to antisecretory therapy; in those with alarm symptoms such as dysphagia, weight loss, or gastrointestinal bleeding; and in those with recurrent dyspepsia after treatment that is not clearly due to reflux on clinical grounds alone. Endoscopy may be considered in patients with long-standing (≥10 years) GERD with frequent symptoms, as they have a sixfold increased risk of harboring Barrett's esophagus compared to a patient with <1 year of reflux symptoms. Patients with Barrett's esophagus (Fig. 12-3) generally undergo a surveillance program of periodic endoscopy with biopsies to detect dysplasia or early carcinoma.

Barrett's esophagus

Barrett's esophagus is specialized columnar metaplasia that replaces the normal squamous mucosa of the distal esophagus in some persons with GERD. Barrett's epithelium is a major risk factor for adenocarcinoma of the esophagus and is readily detected endoscopically, due to proximal displacement of the squamocolumnar junction (Fig. 12-3). A screening EGD for Barrett's esophagus may be considered in patients with a chronic history (>10 year) of GERD symptoms. Endoscopic biopsy is the gold standard for confirmation of Barrett's esophagus, and for dysplasia or cancer arising in Barrett's mucosa. Endoscopic therapies such as endoscopic mucosal resection (EMR), endoscopic submucosal dissection (ESD), photodynamic therapy (PDT), and radiofrequency ablation (RFA) are effective modalities for treatment of high-grade dysplasia and intramucosal cancer in Barrett's esophagus.

PEPTIC ULCER

Peptic ulcer classically causes epigastric gnawing or burning, often occurring nocturnally and promptly relieved by food or antacids. Although endoscopy is the most sensitive diagnostic test for peptic ulcer, it is not a cost-effective strategy in young patients with ulcer-like dyspeptic symptoms unless endoscopy is available at low cost. Patients with suspected peptic ulcer should be evaluated for *Helicobacter pylori* infection. Serology (past or present infection), urea breath testing (current infection), and stool tests are noninvasive and less costly than endoscopy with biopsy. Patients with alarm symptoms and those with persistent symptoms despite treatment should undergo endoscopy to exclude gastric malignancy and other etiologies.

FIGURE 12-30
Peptic esophageal stricture associated with ulceration and scarring of the distal esophagus.

NONULCER DYSPEPSIA

Nonulcer dyspepsia may be associated with bloating and, unlike peptic ulcer, tends not to remit and recur. Most patients describe marginal relief on acid-reducing, prokinetic, or anti-*Helicobacter* therapy, and are referred for endoscopy to exclude a refractory ulcer and assess for other causes. Although endoscopy is useful for excluding other diagnoses, its impact on the treatment of patients with nonulcer dyspepsia is limited.

DYSPHAGIA

About 50% of patients presenting with difficulty swallowing have a mechanical obstruction; the remainder has a motility disorder, such as achalasia or diffuse esophageal spasm. Careful history-taking often points to a presumptive diagnosis and leads to the appropriate use of diagnostic tests. Esophageal strictures (Fig. 12-30) typically cause progressive dysphagia, first for solids, then for liquids; motility disorders often cause intermittent dysphagia for both solids and liquids. Some underlying disorders have characteristic historic features: Schatzki's ring (Fig. 12-31) causes episodic dysphagia for solids, typically at the beginning of a meal; oropharyngeal motor disorders typically present with difficulty initiating deglutition (*transfer dysphagia*) and nasal reflux or coughing with swallowing; and achalasia may cause nocturnal regurgitation of undigested food.

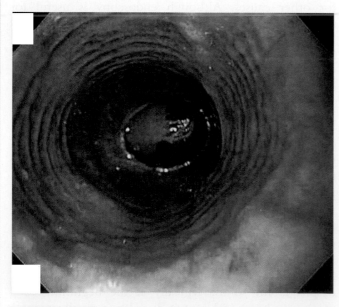

FIGURE 12-31
Schatzki's ring at the gastroesophageal junction.

When mechanical obstruction is suspected, endoscopy is a useful initial diagnostic test, since it permits immediate biopsy and/or dilatation of strictures, masses, or rings. The presence of linear furrows and multiple corrugated rings throughout a narrowed esophagus (*feline esophagus*) should raise suspicion for eosinophilic esophagitis, an increasingly recognized cause for recurrent dysphagia and food impaction **(Fig. 12-32)**. Blind or forceful passage of an endoscope may lead to

perforation in a patient with stenosis of the cervical esophagus or a Zenker's diverticulum, but gentle passage of an endoscope under direct visual guidance is reasonably safe. Endoscopy can miss a subtle stricture or ring in some patients.

When transfer dysphagia is evident or an esophageal motility disorder is suspected, esophageal radiography and/or a video-swallow study are the best initial diagnostic tests. The oropharyngeal swallowing mechanism, esophageal peristalsis, and the lower esophageal sphincter can all be assessed. In some disorders, subsequent esophageal manometry may also be important for diagnosis.

ANEMIA AND OCCULT BLOOD IN THE STOOL

Iron-deficiency anemia may be attributed to poor iron absorption (as in celiac sprue) or, more commonly, chronic blood loss. Intestinal bleeding should be strongly suspected in men and postmenopausal women with iron-deficiency anemia, and colonoscopy is indicated in such patients, even in the absence of detectable occult blood in the stool. Approximately 30% will have large colonic polyps, 10% will have colorectal cancer, and a few additional patients will have colonic vascular lesions. When a convincing source of blood loss is not found in the colon, upper gastrointestinal endoscopy should be considered; if no lesion is found, duodenal biopsies should be obtained to exclude sprue **(Fig. 12-33)**. Small bowel evaluation with capsule endoscopy or deep enteroscopy may be appropriate if both EGD and colonoscopy are unrevealing **(Fig. 12-34)**.

Tests for occult blood in the stool detect hemoglobin or the heme moiety and are most sensitive for

FIGURE 12-32
Eosinophilic esophagitis with multiple circular rings of the esophagus creating a corrugated appearance, and an impacted grape at the narrowed esophagogastric junction. The diagnosis requires biopsy with histologic finding of >15–20 eosinophils/high-power field.

FIGURE 12-33
Scalloped duodenal folds in a patient with celiac sprue.

FIGURE 12-34
Capsule endoscopy images of a mildly scalloped jejunal fold (left) and an ileal tumor (right) in a patient with celiac sprue. (*Images courtesy of Dr. Elizabeth Rajan; with permission.*)

colonic blood loss, although they will also detect larger amounts of upper gastrointestinal bleeding. Patients over age 50 with occult blood in normal-appearing stool should undergo colonoscopy to diagnose or exclude colorectal neoplasia. The diagnostic yield is lower than in iron-deficiency anemia. Whether upper endoscopy is also indicated depends on the patient's symptoms.

The small intestine may be the source of chronic intestinal bleeding, especially if colonoscopy and upper endoscopy are not diagnostic. The utility of small bowel evaluation varies with the clinical setting and is most important in patients in whom bleeding causes chronic or recurrent anemia. In contrast to the low diagnostic yield of small bowel radiography, positive findings on capsule endoscopy are seen in 50–70% of patients with suspected small-intestinal bleeding. The most common finding is mucosal vascular ectasias. Deep enteroscopy may follow capsule endoscopy for biopsy of lesions or to provide specific therapy, such as argon plasma coagulation of vascular ectasias (Fig. 12-35).

The majority of colon cancers develop from pre-existing colonic adenomas, and colorectal cancer can be largely prevented by the detection and removal of adenomatous polyps. The choice of screening strategy for an asymptomatic person depends on personal and family history. Individuals with inflammatory bowel disease, a history of colorectal polyps or cancer, family members with adenomatous polyps or cancer, or certain familial cancer syndromes (**Fig. 12-36**) are at increased risk for colorectal cancer. An individual without these factors is generally considered at average risk.

Screening strategies are summarized in **Table 12-2**. While stool tests for occult blood have been shown to decrease mortality rate from colorectal cancer, they do not detect some cancers and many polyps, and direct visualization of the colon is a more effective screening

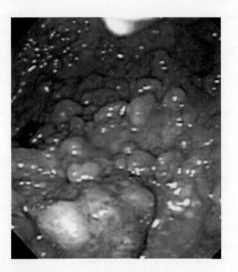

FIGURE 12-36
Innumerable colon polyps of various sizes in a patient with familial adenomatous polyposis syndrome.

A   *B*

FIGURE 12-35
A. Mid-jejunal vascular ectasia identified by double-balloon endoscopy. *B.* Ablation of vascular ectasia with argon plasma coagulation.

TABLE 12-2

COLORECTAL CANCER SCREENING STRATEGIES

	CHOICES/RECOMMENDATIONS	COMMENTS
Average-Risk Patients		
Asymptomatic individuals ≥50 years of age (≥45 years of age for African Americans)	Colonoscopy every 10 years[a]	Preferred cancer prevention strategy
	Annual fecal immunochemical test (FIT) for occult bleeding, fecal DNA testing every 3 years	Cancer detection strategy; fails to detect many polyps and some cancers
	CT colonography every 5 years	Evolving technology (see text)
	Flexible sigmoidoscopy every 5 years	Fails to detect proximal colon polyps and cancers
	Double-contrast barium enema every 5 years	Less sensitive than colonoscopy or CT colonography, misses some rectosigmoid polyps and cancers
Personal History of Polyps or Colorectal Cancer		
1 or 2 small (<1 cm) adenomas with low-grade dysplasia	Repeat colonoscopy in 5 years	Assuming complete polyp resection
3 to 9 adenomas, or any adenoma ≥1 cm or containing high-grade dysplasia or villus features	Repeat colonoscopy in 3 years; subsequent colonoscopy based on findings	Assuming complete polyp resection
≥10 adenomas	Colonoscopy in <3 years based on clinical judgment	Consider evaluation for FAP or HNPCC; see recommendations below
Piecemeal removal of a sessile polyp	Exam in 2 to 6 months to verify complete removal	
Small (<1 cm) hyperplastic polyps of sigmoid and rectum	Colonoscopy in 10 years	
>2 serrated polyps, or any serrated or hyperplastic polyp ≥1 cm	Repeat colonoscopy in 3 years	
Incompletely removed serrated polyp ≥1 cm	Exam in 2 to 6 months to verify complete removal	
Colon cancer	Evaluate entire colon around the time of resection, then repeat colonoscopy in 3 years	
Inflammatory Bowel Disease		
Long-standing (>8 years) ulcerative colitis or Crohn's colitis, or left-sided ulcerative colitis of >15 years' duration	Colonoscopy with biopsies every 1 to 3 years	
Family History of Polyps or Colorectal Cancer		
First-degree relatives with only small tubular adenomas	Same as average risk	
Single first-degree relative with CRC or advanced adenoma at age ≥60 years	Same as average risk	
Single first-degree relative with CRC or advanced adenoma at age <60 years, OR two first-degree relatives with CRC or advanced adenomas at any age	Colonoscopy every 5 years beginning at age 40 years or 10 years younger than age at diagnosis of the youngest affected relative	
FAP	Sigmoidoscopy or colonoscopy annually, beginning at age 10–12 years	Consider genetic counseling and testing
HNPCC	Colonoscopy every 2 years beginning at age 20–25 years until age 40, then annually thereafter	Consider histologic evaluation for microsatellite instability in tumor specimens of patients who meet Bethesda criteria; consider genetic counseling and testing

[a]Assumes good colonic preparation and complete exam to cecum.

Abbreviations: CRC, colorectal cancer; FAP, familial adenomatous polyposis; HNPCC, hereditary nonpolyposis colorectal cancer.

Source: Adapted from SJ Winawer et al: Gastroenterology 130:1872, 2006 and B Levin et al: CA Cancer J Clin 58:130, 2008.

strategy. Either sigmoidoscopy or colonoscopy may be used for cancer screening in asymptomatic average-risk individuals. The use of sigmoidoscopy was based on the historical finding that the majority of colorectal cancers occurred in the rectum and left colon, and that patients with right-sided colon cancers had left-sided polyps. Over the past several decades, however, the distribution of colon cancers has changed, with proportionally fewer rectal and left-sided cancers than in the past. Large studies of colonoscopy for screening of average-risk individuals show that cancers are roughly equally distributed between left and right colon and half of patients with right-sided lesions have no polyps in the left colon. Visualization of the entire colon thus appears to be the optimal strategy for colorectal cancer screening and prevention.

Virtual colonoscopy (VC) is a radiologic technique that images the colon with CT following rectal insufflation of the colonic lumen. Computer rendering of CT images generates an electronic display of a virtual "flight" along the colonic lumen, simulating colonoscopy (**Fig. 12-37**). Comparative studies of virtual and routine colonoscopy have shown conflicting results, but technical refinements have improved the performance characteristics of VC. The use of VC for colorectal cancer screening may become more widespread in the future, particularly at institutions with demonstrated skill with this technique. Findings detected during virtual colonoscopy often require subsequent conventional colonoscopy for confirmation and treatment.

DIARRHEA

Most cases of diarrhea are acute, self-limited, and due to infections or medication. Chronic diarrhea (lasting >6 weeks) is more often due to a primary inflammatory, malabsorptive, or motility disorder; is less likely to resolve spontaneously; and generally requires diagnostic evaluation. Patients with chronic diarrhea or severe, unexplained acute diarrhea often undergo endoscopy if stool tests for pathogens are unrevealing. The choice of endoscopic testing depends on the clinical setting.

Patients with colonic symptoms and findings such as bloody diarrhea, tenesmus, fever, or leukocytes in stool generally undergo sigmoidoscopy or colonoscopy to assess for colitis (Fig. 12-4). Sigmoidoscopy is an appropriate initial test in most patients. Conversely, patients with symptoms and findings suggesting small-bowel disease, such as large-volume watery stools, substantial weight loss, and malabsorption of iron, calcium, or fat may undergo upper endoscopy with duodenal aspirates for assessment of bacterial overgrowth and biopsies for assessment of mucosal diseases, such as celiac sprue.

Many patients with chronic diarrhea do not fit either of these patterns. In the setting of a long-standing history of alternating constipation and diarrhea dating to early adulthood, without findings such as blood in the stool or anemia, a diagnosis of irritable bowel syndrome may be made without direct visualization of the bowel. Steatorrhea and upper abdominal pain may prompt evaluation of the pancreas rather than the gut. Patients whose chronic diarrhea is not easily categorized often undergo initial colonoscopy to examine the entire colon and terminal ileum for inflammatory or neoplastic disease (**Fig. 12-38**).

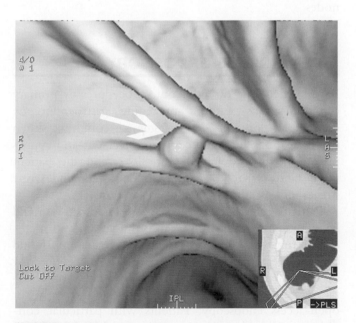

FIGURE 12-37
Virtual colonoscopy image of a colon polyp (*arrow*). (*Image courtesy of Dr. Jeff Fidler; with permission.*)

FIGURE 12-38
Ulcerated ileal carcinoid tumor.

FIGURE 12-39
Internal hemorrhoids with bleeding (*arrow*) as seen on a retroflexed view of the rectum.

MINOR HEMATOCHEZIA

Bright red blood passed with or on formed brown stool usually has a rectal, anal, or distal sigmoid source **(Fig. 12-39)**. Patients with even trivial amounts of hematochezia should be investigated with flexible sigmoidoscopy and anoscopy to exclude polyps or cancers in the distal colon. Patients reporting red blood on the toilet tissue only, without blood in the toilet or on the stool, are generally bleeding from a lesion in the anal canal. Careful external inspection, digital examination, and proctoscopy with anoscopy are sufficient for diagnosis in most cases.

PANCREATITIS

About 20% of patients with pancreatitis have no identified cause after routine clinical investigation (including a review of medication and alcohol use, measurement of serum triglyceride and calcium levels, abdominal ultrasonography, and CT). Endoscopic assessment leads to a specific diagnosis in the majority of such patients, often altering clinical management. Endoscopic investigation is particularly appropriate if the patient has had more than one episode of pancreatitis.

Microlithiasis, or the presence of microscopic crystals in bile, is a leading cause of previously unexplained acute pancreatitis and is sometimes seen during abdominal ultrasonography as layering sludge or flecks of floating, echogenic material in the gallbladder. Gallbladder bile can be obtained for microscopic analysis by administering a cholecystokinin analogue during endoscopy, causing contraction of the gallbladder. Bile is suctioned from the duodenum as it drains from the papilla, and the darkest fraction is examined for cholesterol crystals or bilirubinate granules. The combination of EUS of the gallbladder and bile microscopy is probably the most sensitive means of diagnosing microlithiasis.

Previously undetected chronic pancreatitis, pancreatic malignancy, or pancreas divisum may be diagnosed by either ERCP or EUS. Sphincter of Oddi dysfunction or stenosis is a potential cause for pancreatitis and can be diagnosed by manometric studies performed during ERCP. Autoimmune pancreatitis may require EUS-guided pancreatic biopsy for histologic diagnosis.

Severe pancreatitis often results in pancreatic fluid collections. Both pseudocysts and areas of organized pancreatic necrosis can be drained into the stomach or duodenum endoscopically, using transpapillary and transmural endoscopic techniques. Pancreatic necrosis can be treated by direct endoscopic necrosectomy.

CANCER STAGING

Local staging of esophageal, gastric, pancreatic, bile duct, and rectal cancers can be obtained with EUS (Fig. 12-14). EUS with fine-needle aspiration (Fig. 12-15) currently provides the most accurate preoperative assessment of local tumor and nodal staging, but it does not detect most distant metastases. Details of the local tumor stage can guide treatment decisions including resectability and need for neoadjuvant therapy. EUS with transesophageal needle biopsy may also be used to assess the presence of non–small cell lung cancer in mediastinal nodes.

OPEN-ACCESS ENDOSCOPY

Direct scheduling of endoscopic procedures by primary care physicians without preceding gastroenterology consultation, or *open-access endoscopy*, is common. When the indications for endoscopy are clear-cut and appropriate, the procedural risks are low, and the patient understands what to expect, open-access endoscopy streamlines patient care and decreases costs.

Patients referred for open-access endoscopy should have a recent history, physical examination, and medication review. A copy of such an evaluation should be available when the patient comes to the endoscopy suite. Patients with unstable cardiovascular or respiratory conditions should not be referred directly for open-access endoscopy. Patients with particular conditions and undergoing certain procedures should be prescribed prophylactic antibiotics prior to endoscopy (Table 12-1). In addition, patients taking anticoagulants and/or antiplatelet drugs may require adjustment of these agents before endoscopy based on the procedure risk for bleeding and condition risk for a thromboembolic event (**Figs. 12-40** and **12-41**). Common indications for open-access EGD include dyspepsia resistant to a trial of appropriate therapy; dysphagia; gastrointestinal bleeding; and persistent anorexia or early

satiety. Open-access colonoscopy is often requested in men or postmenopausal women with iron-deficiency anemia, in patients over age 50 with occult blood in the stool, in patients with a previous history of colorectal adenomatous polyps or cancer, and for colorectal cancer screening. Flexible sigmoidoscopy is commonly performed as an open-access procedure.

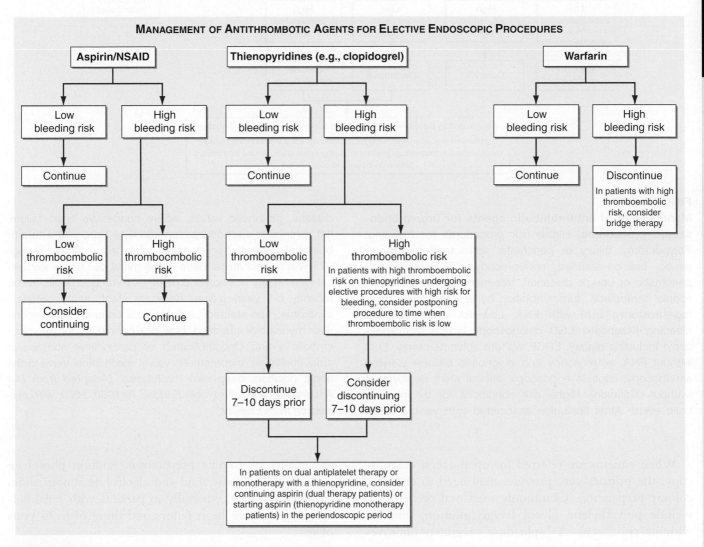

FIGURE 12-40

Management of antithrombotic agents for elective endoscopic procedures. Higher-risk procedures for bleeding: Polypectomy, biliary or pancreatic sphincterotomy, therapeutic balloon-assisted enteroscopy, PEG placement, pneumatic or bougie dilatation, treatment of varices, endoscopic hemostasis, tumor ablation by any technique, cystogastrostomy, EUS with FNA. Low-risk procedures for bleeding: Diagnostic (EGD, colonoscopy, flexible sigmoidoscopy) including biopsy, ERCP without sphincterotomy, EUS without FNA, enteroscopy and diagnostic balloon-assisted enteroscopy, capsule endoscopy, enteral stent deployment (without dilatation). Higher-risk conditions for thromboembolic event: Atrial fibrillation associated with valvular heart disease, prosthetic valves,

active congestive heart failure, left ventricular ejection fraction <35%, a history of a thromboembolic event, hypertension, diabetes mellitus, or age >75 years; mechanical valve in the mitral position; mechanical valve in any position and previous thromboembolic event; recently (<1 year) placed coronary stent; acute coronary syndrome; non-stented percutaneous coronary intervention after myocardial infarction. Low-risk conditions for thromboembolic event: Uncomplicated or paroxysmal nonvalvular atrial fibrillation; bioprosthetic valve; mechanical valve in the aortic position; deep vein thrombosis. (*Adapted from MA Anderson et al: Gastrointest Endosc 70:1060, 2009; with permission from Elsevier.*)

MANAGEMENT OF ANTITHROMBOTIC AGENTS FOR URGENT ENDOSCOPIC PROCEDURES

If unable to delay procedure for 7–10 days, hold as many as possible up to 7–10 days

In patients on dual antiplatelet therapy or monotherapy with a thienopyridine, consider continuing aspirin (dual therapy patients) or starting aspirin (thienopyridine monotherapy patients) in the periendoscopic period

FIGURE 12-41

Management of antithrombotic agents for urgent endoscopic procedures. Higher-risk procedures for bleeding: Polypectomy, biliary or pancreatic sphincterotomy, therapeutic balloon-assisted entero-scopy, PEG placement, pneumatic or bougie dilatation, treatment of varices, endoscopic hemostasis, tumor ablation by any technique, cystogastrostomy, EUS with FNA. Low-risk procedures for bleeding: Diagnostic (EGD, colonoscopy, flexible sigmoidoscopy) including biopsy, ERCP without sphincterotomy, EUS without FNA, enteroscopy and diagnostic balloon-assisted enteroscopy, capsule endoscopy, enteral stent deployment (without dilatation). Higher-risk conditions for thromboembolic event: Atrail fibrillation associated with valvular heart disease, prosthetic valves, active congestive heart failure, left ventricular ejection fraction <35%, a history of a thromboembolic event, hypertension, diabetes mellitus, or age >75 years; mechanical valve in the mitral position; mechanical valve in any position and previous thromboembolic event; recently (>1 year) placed coronary stent; acute coronary syndrome; non-stented percutaneous coronary intervention after myocardial infarction. Low-risk conditions for thromboembolic event: Uncomplicated or paroxysmal nonvalvular atrial fibrillation; bioprosthetic valve; mechanical valve in the aortic position, deep vein thrombosis. (*Adapted from MA Anderson et al: Gastrointest Endosc 70:1060, 2009; with permission from Elsevier.*)

When patients are referred for open–access colonoscopy, the primary care provider may need to choose a colonic preparation. Commonly used oral preparations include polyethylene glycol lavage solution, with or without citric acid. A "split-dose" regimen improves the quality of colonic preparation. Sodium phosphate purgatives may cause fluid and electrolyte abnormalities and renal toxicity, especially in patients with renal failure or congestive heart failure and those over 70 years of age.

SECTION III

DISORDERS OF THE ALIMENTARY TRACT

CHAPTER 13

DISEASES OF THE ESOPHAGUS

Peter J. Kahrilas ■ Ikuo Hirano

ESOPHAGEAL STRUCTURE AND FUNCTION

The esophagus is a hollow muscular tube coursing through the posterior mediastinum joining the hypopharynx to the stomach with a sphincter at each end. It functions to transport food and fluid between these ends, otherwise remaining empty. The physiology of swallowing, esophageal motility, and oral and pharyngeal dysphagia are described in Chap. 4. Esophageal diseases can be manifested by impaired function or pain. Key functional impairments are swallowing disorders and excessive gastroesophageal reflux. Pain, sometimes indistinguishable from cardiac chest pain, can result from inflammation, infection, dysmotility, or neoplasm.

SYMPTOMS OF ESOPHAGEAL DISEASE

The clinical history remains central to the evaluation of esophageal symptoms. A thoughtfully obtained history will often expedite management. Important details include weight gain or loss, gastrointestinal bleeding, dietary habits including the timing of meals, smoking, and alcohol consumption. The major esophageal symptoms are heartburn, regurgitation, chest pain, dysphagia, odynophagia, and globus sensation.

Heartburn (pyrosis), the most common esophageal symptom, is characterized by a discomfort or burning sensation behind the sternum that arises from the epigastrium and may radiate toward the neck. Heartburn is an intermittent symptom, most commonly experienced after eating, during exercise, and while lying recumbent. The discomfort is relieved with drinking water or antacid but can occur frequently and interfere with normal activities including sleep. The association between heartburn and gastroesophageal reflux disease (GERD) is so strong that empirical therapy for GERD has become accepted management. However, the term "heartburn" is often misused and/or referred to with other terms such as "indigestion" or "repeating," making it important to clarify the intended meaning.

Regurgitation is the effortless return of food or fluid into the pharynx without nausea or retching. Patients report a sour or burning fluid in the throat or mouth that may also contain undigested food particles. Bending, belching, or maneuvers that increase intraabdominal pressure can provoke regurgitation. A clinician needs to discriminate among regurgitation, vomiting, and rumination. *Vomiting* is preceded by nausea and accompanied by retching. *Rumination* is a behavior in which recently swallowed food is regurgitated and then reswallowed repetitively for up to an hour. Although there is some linkage between rumination and mental deficiency, the behavior is also exhibited by unimpaired individuals who sometimes even find it pleasurable.

Chest pain is a common esophageal symptom with characteristics similar to cardiac pain, sometimes making this distinction difficult. Esophageal pain is usually experienced as a pressure type sensation in the mid chest, radiating to the mid back, arms, or jaws. The similarity to cardiac pain is likely because the two organs share a nerve plexus and the nerve endings in the esophageal wall have poor discriminative ability among stimuli. Esophageal distention or even chemo-stimulation (e.g., with acid) will often be perceived as chest pain. Gastroesophageal reflux is the most common cause of esophageal chest pain.

Esophageal *dysphagia* (see also Chap. 4) is often described as a feeling of food "sticking" or even lodging in the chest. Important distinctions are between uniquely solid food dysphagia as opposed to liquid and solid, episodic versus constant dysphagia, and progressive versus static dysphagia. If the dysphagia is for liquids as well as solid food, it suggests a motility disorder such as achalasia. Conversely, uniquely solid food dysphagia is suggestive of a stricture, ring, or tumor. Of note, a patient's localization of food hang-up in the esophagus is notoriously imprecise. Approximately 30% of distal esophageal obstructions are perceived as cervical dysphagia. In such instances, the absence of concomitant symptoms generally associated with oropharyngeal dysphagia such as aspiration, nasopharyngeal regurgitation, cough, drooling, or obvious neuromuscular compromise should suggest an esophageal etiology.

Odynophagia is pain either caused by or exacerbated by swallowing. Odynophagia is more common with pill or infectious esophagitis than with reflux esophagitis and should prompt a search for these entities. When odynophagia does occur in GERD, it is likely related to an esophageal ulcer or deep erosion.

Globus sensation, alternatively labeled "globus hystericus," is the perception of a lump or fullness in the throat that is felt irrespective of swallowing. Although such patients are frequently referred for an evaluation of dysphagia, globus sensation is often relieved by the act of swallowing. As implied by its alternative name (globus hystericus), globus sensation often occurs in the setting of anxiety or obsessive-compulsive disorders. Clinical experience teaches that it is often attributable to GERD.

Water brash is excessive salivation resulting from a vagal reflex triggered by acidification of the esophageal mucosa. This is not a common symptom. Afflicted individuals will describe the unpleasant sensation of the mouth rapidly filling with salty thin fluid, often in the setting of concomitant heartburn.

DIAGNOSTIC STUDIES

ENDOSCOPY

Endoscopy, also known as esophagogastroduodenoscopy (EGD) is the best test for the evaluation of the proximal gastrointestinal tract. Modern instruments produce high-quality color images of the esophageal, gastric, and duodenal lumen. Endoscopes also have an instrumentation channel through which biopsy forceps, sclerotherapy catheters, balloon dilators, or cautery devices can be utilized. The key advantages of endoscopy over barium radiography are: (1) increased sensitivity for the detection of mucosal lesions, (2) vastly increased sensitivity for the detection of abnormalities mainly identifiable by an abnormal color such as Barrett's metaplasia, (3) the ability to obtain biopsy specimens for histologic examination of suspected abnormalities, and (4) the ability to dilate strictures during the examination. The main disadvantage of endoscopy is that it usually necessitates the use of conscious

sedation with medicines such as midazolam (Versed), meperidine (Demerol), or fentanyl.

RADIOGRAPHY

Contrast radiography of the esophagus, stomach, and duodenum can demonstrate barium reflux, hiatal hernia, mucosal granularity, erosions, ulcerations, and strictures. The sensitivity of radiography compared with endoscopy for detecting esophagitis reportedly ranges from 22 95%, with higher grades of esophagitis (i.e., ulceration or stricture) exhibiting greater detection rates. Conversely, the sensitivity of barium radiography for detecting esophageal strictures is greater than that of endoscopy, especially when the study is done in conjunction with barium-soaked bread or a 13-mm barium tablet. Barium studies also provide an assessment of esophageal function and morphology that may be undetected on endoscopy. Hypopharyngeal pathology and disorders of the cricopharyngeal muscle are better appreciated on radiographic examination, particularly with videofluoroscopic recording. The major shortcoming of barium radiography is that it rarely obviates the need for endoscopy. Either a positive or a negative study is usually followed by an endoscopic evaluation either to clarify findings in the case of a positive examination or to add a level of certainty in the case of a negative one.

ENDOSCOPIC ULTRASOUND

Endoscopic ultrasound (EUS) instruments combine an endoscope with an ultrasound transducer to create a transmural image of the tissue surrounding the endoscope tip. The key advantage of EUS over alternative radiologic imaging techniques is much greater resolution attributable to the proximity of the ultrasound transducer to the area being examined. Available devices can provide either radial imaging (360-degree, cross-sectional) or a curved linear image that can guide fine-needle aspiration of imaged structures such as lymph nodes or tumors. Major esophageal applications of EUS are to stage esophageal cancer, to evaluate dysplasia in Barrett's esophagus, and to assess submucosal tumors.

ESOPHAGEAL MANOMETRY

Esophageal manometry, or motility testing, entails positioning a pressure sensing catheter within the esophagus and then observing the contractility following test swallows. The upper and lower esophageal sphincters appear as zones of high pressure that relax on swallowing while the intersphincteric esophagus exhibits peristaltic contractions. Manometry is used to diagnose

Pressure Topography Plot

Conventional line tracings

FIGURE 13-1

High-resolution esophageal pressure topography (*right*) and conventional manometry (*left*) of a normal swallow.

LES, lower esophageal sphincter; E, esophageal body; UES, upper esophageal sphincter.

motility disorders (achalasia, diffuse esophageal spasm) and to assess peristaltic integrity prior to the surgery for reflux disease. Technological advances have rebranded esophageal manometry as high-resolution esophageal pressure topography **(Fig. 13-1)**. Manometry can also be combined with intraluminal impedance monitoring. Impedance recordings utilize a catheter with a series of paired electrodes. Esophageal luminal contents in contact with the electrodes decrease (liquid) or increase (air) the impedance signal allowing detection of anterograde or retrograde transit of esophageal bolus transit.

REFLUX TESTING

GERD is often diagnosed in the absence of endoscopic esophagitis, which would otherwise define the disease. This occurs in the settings of partially treated disease, an abnormally sensitive esophageal mucosa, or without obvious explanation. In such instances, reflux testing can demonstrate excessive esophageal exposure to refluxed gastric juice, the physiologic abnormality of GERD. This can be done by ambulatory 24- to 48-h esophageal pH recording using either a wireless pH-sensitive transmitter that is anchored to the esophageal mucosa or with a transnasally positioned wire electrode with the tip stationed in the distal esophagus. Either way, the outcome is expressed as the percentage of the day that the pH was less than 4 (indicative of recent acid reflux), with values exceeding 5% indicative of GERD. Reflux testing is useful with atypical symptoms or an inexplicably poor response to therapy. Intraluminal impedance monitoring can be added to pH monitoring to detect reflux events irrespective of whether or not they are acidic, potentially increasing the sensitivity of the study.

STRUCTURAL DISORDERS

HIATAL HERNIA

Hiatus hernia is a herniation of viscera, most commonly the stomach, into the mediastinum through the esophageal hiatus of the diaphragm. Four types of hiatus hernia are distinguished with type I, or sliding hiatal hernia comprising at least 95% of the overall total. A sliding hiatal hernia is one in which the gastroesophageal junction and gastric cardia slide upward as a result of weakening of the phrenoesophageal ligament attaching the gastroesophageal junction to the diaphragm at the hiatus. True to its name, sliding hernias enlarge with increased intraabdominal pressure, swallowing, and respiration. The incidence of sliding hernias increases with age and conceptually, results from wear and tear: increased intraabdominal pressure from abdominal obesity, pregnancy, etc., and hereditary factors predisposing to the condition. The main significance of sliding hernias is the propensity of affected individuals to have GERD.

Types II, III, and IV hiatal hernias are all subtypes of paraesophageal hernia in which the herniation into the mediastinum includes a visceral structure other than the gastric cardia. With type II and III paraesophageal hernias, the gastric fundus also herniates with the distinction being that in type II, the gastroesophageal junction remains fixed at the hiatus, while type III is a mixed sliding/paraesophageal hernia. With type IV hiatal hernias, viscera other than the stomach herniate into the mediastinum, most commonly the colon. With type II and III paraesophageal hernias, the stomach inverts as it herniates and large paraesophageal hernias can lead to an upside down stomach, gastric volvulus, and even strangulation of the stomach. Because of this risk, surgical repair is often advocated for large paraesophageal hernias.

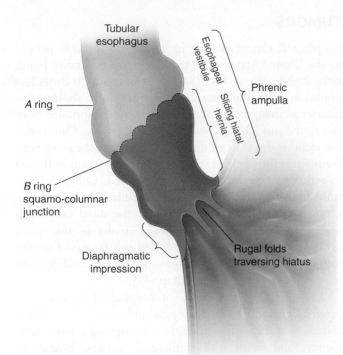

FIGURE 13-2
Radiographic anatomy of the gastroesophageal junction.

RINGS AND WEBS

A lower esophageal mucosal ring, also called a *B ring*, is a thin membranous narrowing at the squamocolumnar mucosal junction **(Fig. 13-2)**. Its origin is unknown, but B rings are demonstrable in about 15% of people and are usually asymptomatic. When the lumen diameter is less than 13 mm, distal rings are usually associated with episodic solid food dysphagia and are called *Schatzki's rings*. Patients typically present older than 40 years, consistent with an acquired rather than congenital origin. Schatzki's ring is one of the most common causes of intermittent food impaction, also known as "steakhouse syndrome" as meat is a typical instigator. Symptomatic rings are easily treated by dilatation.

Web-like constrictions higher in the esophagus can be of congenital or inflammatory origin. Asymptomatic cervical esophageal webs are demonstrated in about 10% of people and typically originate along the anterior aspect of the esophagus. When circumferential, they can cause intermittent dysphagia to solids similar to Schatzki's rings and are similarly treated with dilatation. The combination of symptomatic proximal esophageal webs and iron-deficiency anemia in middle-aged women constitutes Plummer-Vinson syndrome.

DIVERTICULA

Esophageal diverticula are categorized by location with the most common being epiphrenic, hypopharyngeal (Zenker's), and mid esophageal. Epiphrenic and Zenker's diverticula are false diverticula involving herniation of the mucosa and submucosa through the muscular layer of the esophagus. These lesions result from increased intraluminal pressure associated with distal obstruction. In the case of Zenker's, the obstruction is a stenotic cricopharyngeus muscle (upper esophageal sphincter) and the hypopharyngeal herniation most commonly occurs in an area of natural weakness known as *Killian's triangle* **(Fig. 13-3)**. Small Zenker's diverticula are usually asymptomatic, but when they enlarge sufficiently to retain food and saliva they can be associated with dysphagia, halitosis, and aspiration. Treatment is by surgical diverticulectomy and cricopharyngeal myotomy or a

FIGURE 13-3
Examples of small (*left*) and large (*middle, right*) Zenker's diverticulum arising from Killian's triangle in the distal hypopharynx. Smaller diverticula are evident only during the swallow, whereas larger ones retain food and fluid.

marsupialization procedure in which an endoscopic stapling device is used to divide the cricopharyngeus.

Epiphrenic diverticula are usually associated with achalasia or a distal esophageal stricture. Mid-esophageal diverticula may be caused by traction from adjacent inflammation (classically tuberculosis) in which case they are true diverticula involving all layers of the esophageal wall, or by pulsion associated with esophageal motor disorders. Mid-esophageal and epiphrenic diverticula are usually asymptomatic until they enlarge sufficiently to retain food and cause dysphagia and regurgitation. Symptoms attributable to the diverticula tend to correlate more with the underlying esophageal disorder than the size of the diverticula. Large diverticula can be removed surgically, usually in conjunction with a myotomy if the underlying cause is achalasia. Diffuse intramural esophageal diverticulosis is a rare entity that results from dilatation of the excretory ducts of submucosal esophageal glands **(Fig. 13-4)**. Esophageal candidiasis and proximal esophageal strictures are commonly found in association with this disorder.

FIGURE 13-4
Intramural esophageal pseudodiverticulosis associated with chronic obstruction. Invaginations of contrast into the esophageal wall outline deep esophageal glands.

TUMORS

Esophageal cancer occurs in about 4.5:100,000 people in the United States with the associated mortality being only slightly less at 4.4:100,000. It is about 10 times less common than colorectal cancer but kills about one-quarter as many patients. These statistics emphasize both the rarity and lethality of esophageal cancer. One notable trend is the shift of dominant esophageal cancer type from squamous cell to adenocarcinoma, strongly linked to reflux disease and Barrett's metaplasia. Other distinctions between cell types are the predilection for adenocarcinoma to affect white males in the distal esophagus and squamous cell to affect black males in the more proximal esophagus with the added risk factors of smoking, alcohol consumption, caustic injury, and human papilloma virus infection (Chap. 49).

The typical presentation of esophageal cancer is of progressive solid food dysphagia and weight loss. Associated symptoms may include odynophagia, iron deficiency, and, with mid-esophageal tumors, hoarseness from left recurrent laryngeal nerve injury. Generally, these are indications of locally invasive or even metastatic disease manifest by tracheoesophageal fistulas, and vocal cord paralysis. Even when detected as a small lesion, esophageal cancer has poor survival because of the abundant esophageal lymphatics leading to regional lymph node metastases.

Benign esophageal tumors are uncommon and usually discovered incidentally. In decreasing frequency of occurrence, cell types include leiomyomas, fibrovascular polyps, squamous papillomas, granular cell, lipomas, neurofibromas, and inflammatory fibroid polyps. These generally become symptomatic only when they are associated with dysphagia and merit removal only under the same circumstances.

CONGENITAL ANOMALIES

The most common congenital esophageal anomaly is esophageal atresia, occurring in about 1 in 5000 live births. Atresia can occur in several permutations, the common denominator being developmental failure of fusion between the proximal and distal esophagus associated with a tracheoesophageal fistula, most commonly with the distal segment excluded. Alternatively, there can be an H-type configuration in which esophageal fusion has occurred, but with a tracheoesophageal fistula. Esophageal atresia is usually recognized and corrected surgically within the first few days of life. Later life complications include dysphagia from anastomotic strictures or absent peristalsis and reflux, which can be severe. Less common developmental anomalies include congenital esophageal stenosis, webs, and duplications.

Dysphagia can also result from congenital abnormalities that cause extrinsic compression of the esophagus. In dysphagia lusoria, the esophagus is compressed by an aberrant right subclavian artery arising from the descending aorta and passing behind the esophagus. Alternatively vascular rings may surround and constrict the esophagus.

Heterotopic gastric mucosa, also known as an esophageal inlet patch, is a focus of gastric type epithelium in the proximal cervical esophagus; the estimated prevalence is 4.5%. The inlet patch is thought to result from incomplete replacement of embryonic columnar epithelium with squamous epithelium. The majority of patches are asymptomatic, but acid production can occur as most contain fundic type gastric epithelium with parietal cells.

ESOPHAGEAL MOTILITY DISORDERS

Esophageal motility disorders are diseases attributable to esophageal neuromuscular dysfunction commonly associated with dysphagia, chest pain, or heartburn. The major entities are achalasia, diffuse esophageal spasm (DES), and GERD. Motility disorders can also be secondary to broader disease processes as is the case with pseudoachalasia, Chagas' disease, and scleroderma. Not included in this discussion are diseases affecting the pharynx and proximal esophagus, impairment of which is almost always part of a more global neuromuscular disease process.

ACHALASIA

Achalasia is a rare disease caused by loss of ganglion cells within the esophageal myenteric plexus with a population incidence of about 1:100,000 and usually presenting between age 25 and 60. With long-standing disease, virtual aganglionosis is noted. Excitatory (cholinergic) ganglionic neurons are variably affected and inhibitory (nitric oxide) ganglionic neurons are necessarily involved. Functionally, inhibitory neurons mediate deglutitive lower esophageal sphincter (LES) relaxation and the sequential propagation of peristalsis. Their absence leads to impaired deglutitive LES relaxation and absent peristalsis. Increasing evidence suggests that the ultimate cause of ganglion cell degeneration in achalasia is an autoimmune process attributable to a latent infection with human herpes simplex virus 1 combined with genetic susceptibility.

Long-standing achalasia is characterized by progressive dilatation and sigmoid deformity of the esophagus with hypertrophy of the LES. Clinical manifestations may include dysphagia, regurgitation, chest pain, and weight loss. Most patients report solid and liquid food dysphagia. Regurgitation occurs when food, fluid, and secretions are retained in the dilated esophagus. Patients with advanced achalasia are at risk for bronchitis, pneumonia, or lung abscess from chronic regurgitation and aspiration. Chest pain is frequent early in the course of achalasia, thought to result from esophageal spasm. Patients describe a squeezing, pressure-like retrosternal pain, sometimes radiating to the neck, arms, jaw, and back. Paradoxically, some patients complain of heartburn that may be a chest pain equivalent. Treatment of achalasia is less effective in relieving chest pain than it is in relieving dysphagia or regurgitation.

The differential diagnosis of achalasia includes DES, Chagas' disease, and pseudoachalasia. Chagas' disease is endemic in areas of central Brazil, Venezuela, and northern Argentina, spread by the bite of the reduvid (kissing) bug that transmits the protozoan, *Trypanosoma cruzi*. The chronic phase of the disease develops years after infection and results from destruction of autonomic ganglion cells throughout the body, including the heart, gut, urinary tract, and respiratory tract. Tumor infiltration, most commonly seen with carcinoma in the gastric fundus or distal esophagus can mimic idiopathic achalasia. The resultant "pseudoachalasia" accounts for up to 5% of suspected cases and is more likely with advanced age, abrupt onset of symptoms (<1 year), and weight loss. Hence, endoscopy should be part of the evaluation of achalasia. When the clinical suspicion for pseudoachalasia is high and endoscopy nondiagnostic, CT scanning or endoscopic ultrasonography may be of value. Rarely, pseudoachalasia can result from a paraneoplastic syndrome with circulating antineuronal antibodies.

Achalasia is diagnosed by barium swallow x-ray and/or esophageal manometry; endoscopy has a relatively minor role other than to exclude pseudoachalasia. The barium swallow x-ray appearance is of a dilated esophagus with poor emptying, an air-fluid level, and tapering at the LES giving it a beak-like appearance (Fig. 13-5). Occasionally, an epiphrenic diverticulum is observed. In long-standing achalasia, the esophagus may assume a sigmoid configuration. The diagnostic criteria for achalasia with esophageal manometry are impaired LES relaxation and absent peristalsis. High-resolution manometry has somewhat advanced this diagnosis; three subtypes of achalasia are differentiated based on the pattern of pressurization in the nonperistaltic esophagus (Fig. 13-6). Because manometry identifies early disease before esophageal dilatation and food retention, it is the most sensitive diagnostic test.

There is no known way of preventing or reversing achalasia. Therapy is directed at reducing LES pressure so that gravity and esophageal pressurization promote esophageal emptying. Peristalsis rarely, if ever, returns. LES pressure can be reduced by pharmacological therapy, forceful dilatation, or surgical myotomy. No large, controlled trials of the therapeutic alternatives exist and the optimal approach is debated. Pharmacological

FIGURE 13-5

Achalasia with esophageal dilatation, tapering at the gastroesophageal junction and an air-fluid level within the esophagus. The example on the left shows sigmoid deformity with very advanced disease.

therapies are relatively ineffective but are often used as temporizing therapies. Nitrates or calcium channel blockers are administered before eating, advising caution because of their effects on blood pressure. Botulinum toxin, injected into the LES under endoscopic guidance, inhibits acetylcholine release from nerve endings and improves dysphagia in about 66% of cases for at least 6 months. Sildenafil, or alternative phosphodiesterase inhibitors, effectively decrease LES pressure, but practicalities limit their clinical use in achalasia.

The only durable therapies for achalasia are pneumatic dilatation and Heller myotomy. Pneumatic dilatation, with a reported efficacy ranging from 32–98%, is an endoscopic technique using a noncompliant, cylindrical balloon dilator positioned across the LES and inflated to a diameter of 3–4 cm. The major complication is perforation with a reported incidence of 1–5%. The most common surgical procedure for achalasia is laparoscopic Heller myotomy, usually performed in conjunction with an antireflux procedure (partial fundoplication); good to excellent results are reported in 62–100% of cases. Occasionally, patients with advanced disease fail to respond to pneumatic dilatation or Heller myotomy. In such refractory cases, esophageal resection with gastric pull-up or interposition of a segment of transverse colon may be the only option other than gastrostomy feeding.

In untreated or inadequately treated achalasia, esophageal dilatation predisposes to stasis esophagitis. Prolonged stasis esophagitis is the likely explanation for the association between achalasia and esophageal squamous cell cancer. Tumors develop after years of achalasia, usually in the setting of a greatly dilated esophagus with the overall squamous cell cancer risk increased 17-fold compared to controls.

FIGURE 13-6

Three subtypes of achalasia: classic (A), with esophageal compression (B), and spastic achalasia (C) imaged with pressure topography. All are characterized by impaired lower esophageal sphincter (LES) relaxation and absent peristalsis. However, classic achalasia has minimal pressurization of the esophageal body while substantial fluid pressurization is observed in achalasia with esophageal compression and spastic esophageal contractions are observed with spastic achalasia.

DIFFUSE ESOPHAGEAL SPASM (DES)

DES is manifested by episodes of dysphagia and chest pain attributable to abnormal esophageal contractions with normal deglutitive LES relaxation. Beyond that, there is little consensus. The pathophysiology and natural history of DES are ill defined. Radiographically,

FIGURE 13-7

Diffuse esophageal spasm. The characteristic "corkscrew" esophagus results from spastic contraction of the circular muscle in the esophageal wall; more precisely, this is actually a helical array of muscle. These findings are also seen with spastic achalasia.

DES has been characterized by tertiary contractions or a "corkscrew esophagus" (Fig. 13-7), but in many instances these abnormalities are actually indicative of achalasia. Manometrically, a variety of defining features have been proposed including uncoordinated ("spastic") activity in the distal esophagus, spontaneous and repetitive contractions, or high amplitude and prolonged contractions. Greatest consensus exists with the concept that simultaneous contractions define DES. All of these definitions lead to patients with a variety

of disorders being diagnosed as DES. In fact, high-resolution manometry suggests that DES, when defined in a restrictive fashion (Fig. 13-8), is actually much less common than achalasia and suspected cases are often incorrectly categorized achalasia.

Esophageal chest pain closely mimics angina pectoris. Features suggesting esophageal pain include pain that is nonexertional, prolonged, interrupts sleep, is meal-related, is relieved with antacids, and is accompanied by heartburn, dysphagia, or regurgitation. However, all of these features exhibit overlap with cardiac pain, which still must be the primary consideration. Furthermore, even within the spectrum of esophageal diseases, both chest pain and dysphagia are also characteristic of peptic or infectious esophagitis. Only after these more common entities have been excluded by evaluation and/or treatment should a diagnosis of DES be pursued.

Although the defining criteria are currently disputed, DES is diagnosed by manometry. Endoscopy is useful to identify alternative structural and inflammatory lesions that may cause chest pain. Radiographically, a "corkscrew esophagus," "rosary bead esophagus," pseudodiverticula, or curling can be indicative of DES, but these are also found with spastic achalasia. Given these vagaries of defining DES, and the resultant heterogeneity of patients identified for inclusion in therapeutic trials, it is not surprising that trial results have been disappointing. Only small, uncontrolled trials exist, reporting response to nitrates, calcium channel blockers, hydralazine, botulinum toxin, and anxiolytics. The only controlled trial showing efficacy was with an anxiolytic. Surgical therapy (long myotomy or even esophagectomy) should be considered only with severe weight loss or unbearable pain. These indications are extremely rare.

FIGURE 13-8

Esophageal pressure topography of the two major variants of esophageal spasm: spastic nutcracker (left) and diffuse esophageal spasm (right). Spastic nutcracker is defined by the extraordinarily vigorous and repetitive contractions with normal peristaltic onset. Diffuse esophageal spasm is similar but primarily defined by a rapid propagation at the onset of the contraction.

NONSPECIFIC MANOMETRIC FINDINGS

Manometric studies done to evaluate chest pain and/or dysphagia often report minor abnormalities (hypertensive or hypotensive peristalsis, hypertensive LES, etc.) that are insufficient to diagnose either achalasia or DES. These findings are of unclear significance. Reflux and psychiatric diagnoses, particularly anxiety and depression, are common among such individuals. A lower visceral pain threshold and symptoms of irritable bowel syndrome are noted in more than half of such patients. Consequently, therapy for these individuals should either target the most common esophageal disorder, GERD, or more global conditions such as depression or somatization neurosis that are found to be coexistent.

GASTROESOPHAGEAL REFLUX DISEASE (GERD)

The current conception of GERD is to encompass a family of conditions with the commonality that they are caused by the gastroesophageal reflux resulting in either troublesome symptoms or an array of potential esophageal and extraesophageal manifestations. It is estimated that 15% of adults in the United States are affected by GERD, although such estimates are based only on self-reported chronic heartburn. With respect to the esophagus, the spectrum of injury includes esophagitis, stricture, Barrett's esophagus, and adenocarcinoma (Fig. 13-9). Of particular concern is the rising incidence of esophageal adenocarcinoma, an epidemiologic trend that parallels the increasing incidence of GERD. There were about 8000 incident cases of esophageal adenocarcinoma in the United States in 2010 (half of all esophageal cancers); it is estimated that this disease burden has increased two- to sixfold in the last 20 years.

PATHOPHYSIOLOGY

The best-defined subset of GERD patients, albeit a minority overall, have esophagitis. Esophagitis occurs when refluxed gastric acid and pepsin cause necrosis of the esophageal mucosa causing erosions and ulcers. Note that some degree of gastroesophageal reflux is normal, physiologically intertwined with the

A Erosive esophagitis

B Esophageal stricture with chronic erosive esophagitis

C Barrett's esophagus

D Esophageal adenocarcinoma with Barrett's esophagus

FIGURE 13-9

Endoscopic appearance of (**A**) peptic esophagitis, (**B**) a peptic stricture, (**C**) Barrett's metaplasia, and (**D**) adenocarcinoma developing within an area of Barrett's esophagus.

mechanism of belching (transient LES relaxation), but esophagitis results from excessive reflux, often accompanied by impaired clearance of the refluxed gastric juice. Restricting reflux to that which is physiologically intended depends on the anatomic and physiologic integrity of the esophagogastric junction, a complex sphincter comprised of both the LES and the surrounding crural diaphragm. Three dominant mechanisms of esophagogastric junction incompetence are recognized: (1) transient LES relaxations (a vagovagal reflex in which LES relaxation is elicited by gastric distention), (2) LES hypotension, or (3) anatomic distortion of the esophagogastric junction inclusive of hiatus hernia. Of note, the third factor, esophagogastric junction anatomic disruption, is both significant unto itself and also because it interacts with the first two mechanisms. Transient LES relaxations account for at least 90% of reflux in normal subjects or GERD patients without hiatus hernia, but patients with hiatus hernia have a more heterogeneous mechanistic profile. Factors tending to exacerbate reflux regardless of mechanism are abdominal obesity, pregnancy, gastric hypersecretory states, delayed gastric emptying, disruption of esophageal peristalsis, and gluttony.

After acid reflux, peristalsis returns the refluxed fluid to the stomach and acid clearance is completed by titration of the residual acid by bicarbonate contained in swallowed saliva. Consequently, two causes of prolonged acid clearance are impaired peristalsis and reduced salivation. Impaired peristaltic emptying can be attributable to disrupted peristalsis or superimposed reflux associated with a hiatal hernia. With superimposed reflux, fluid retained within a sliding hiatal hernia refluxes back into the esophagus during swallow-related LES relaxation, a phenomenon that does not normally occur.

Inherent in the pathophysiologic model of GERD is that gastric juice is harmful to the esophageal epithelium. However, gastric acid hypersecretion is usually not a dominant factor in the development of esophagitis. An obvious exception is with Zollinger-Ellison syndrome, which is associated with severe esophagitis in about 50% of patients. Another caveat is with chronic *H. pylori* gastritis, which may have a protective effect by inducing atrophic gastritis with concomitant hypoacidity. Pepsin, bile, and pancreatic enzymes within gastric secretions can also injure the esophageal epithelium, but their noxious properties are either lessened in an acidic environment or dependent on acidity for activation. Bile warrants attention because it persists in refluxate despite acid-suppressing medications. Bile can transverse the cell membrane, imparting severe cellular injury in a weakly acidic environment, and has also been invoked as a cofactor in the pathogenesis of Barrett's metaplasia and adenocarcinoma. Hence, the causticity of gastric refluxate extends beyond hydrochloric acid.

SYMPTOMS

Heartburn and regurgitation are the typical symptoms of GERD. Somewhat less common are dysphagia and chest pain. In each case, multiple potential mechanisms for symptom genesis operate that extend beyond the basic concepts of mucosal erosion and activation of afferent sensory nerves. Specifically, hypersensitivity and functional pain are increasingly recognized as confounding factors. Nonetheless the dominant clinical strategy is of empirical treatment with acid inhibitors, reserving further evaluation for those who fail to respond. Important exceptions to this are patients with chest pain or persistent dysphagia, each of which may be indicative of more morbid conditions. With chest pain, cardiac disease must be carefully considered. In the case of persistent dysphagia, chronic reflux can lead to the development of a peptic stricture or adenocarcinoma, each of which benefits from early detection and/or specific therapy.

Extraesophageal syndromes with an established association to GERD include chronic cough, laryngitis, asthma, and dental erosions. A multitude of other conditions including pharyngitis, chronic bronchitis, pulmonary fibrosis, chronic sinusitis, cardiac arrhythmias, sleep apnea, and recurrent aspiration pneumonia have proposed associations with GERD. However, in both cases it is important to emphasize the word association as opposed to causation. In many instances the disorders likely coexist because of shared pathogenetic mechanisms rather than strict causality. Potential mechanisms for extraesophageal GERD manifestations are of either regurgitation with direct contact between the refluxate and supra-esophageal structures or via a vagovagal reflex wherein reflux activation of esophageal afferent nerves triggers efferent vagal reflexes such as bronchospasm, cough, or arrhythmias.

DIFFERENTIAL DIAGNOSIS

Although generally quite characteristic, symptoms from GERD need to be distinguished from symptoms related to infectious, pill, or eosinophilic esophagitis, peptic ulcer disease, dyspepsia, biliary colic, coronary artery disease, and esophageal motility disorders. It is especially important that coronary artery disease be given early consideration because of its potentially lethal implications. The remaining elements of the differential diagnosis can be addressed by endoscopy, upper gastrointestinal series, or biliary tract ultrasonography as appropriate. The distinction among etiologies of esophagitis is usually easily made by endoscopy with mucosal biopsies, which are necessary to evaluate for eosinophilic inflammation. In terms of endoscopic appearance, infectious esophagitis is diffuse and tends to involve the proximal esophagus far more frequently than does reflux esophagitis. The ulcerations seen in peptic esophagitis are usually solitary and distal, whereas infectious ulcerations are punctate and diffuse. Eosinophilic esophagitis characteristically exhibits multiple esophageal rings, linear furrows, or white punctate exudate. Esophageal ulcerations from pill esophagitis are usually singular and deep at points of luminal narrowing, especially near the carina, with sparing of the distal esophagus.

COMPLICATIONS

The complications of GERD are related to chronic esophagitis (bleeding and stricture) and the relationship between GERD and esophageal adenocarcinoma. However, both esophagitis and peptic strictures have become increasingly rare in the era of potent antisecretory medications. Conversely, the most severe histologic consequence of GERD is Barrett's metaplasia with the associated risk of esophageal adenocarcinoma, and the incidence of these lesions has increased, not decreased, in the era of potent acid suppression. Barrett's metaplasia, endoscopically recognized by tongues of reddish mucosa extending proximally from the gastroesophageal junction (Fig. 13-9) or histopathologically by the finding of specialized columnar metaplasia, is associated with at least a 20-fold increased risk for development of esophageal adenocarcinoma.

Barrett's metaplasia can progress to adenocarcinoma through the intermediate stages of low- and high-grade dysplasia (Fig. 13-10). Owing to this risk, areas of Barrett's and especially any included areas of mucosal irregularity should be extensively biopsied. The rate of cancer development is estimated at 0.5% per year, but vagaries in definition and of the extent of Barrett's metaplasia requisite to establish the diagnosis have contributed to variability and inconsistency in this risk assessment. The group at greatest risk is obese white males in their sixth decade of life. However, despite common practice, the utility of endoscopic screening and surveillance programs intended to control the adenocarcinoma risk has not been established. Also of note, no high-level evidence confirms that aggressive antisecretory therapy or antireflux surgery causes regression of Barrett's esophagus or prevents adenocarcinoma.

Although the management of Barrett's esophagus remains controversial, the finding of dysplasia in Barrett's, particularly high-grade dysplasia, mandates further intervention. In addition to the high rate of progression to adenocarcinoma, there is also a high prevalence of unrecognized coexisting cancer with high-grade dysplasia. Nonetheless, treatment remains controversial. Esophagectomy, intensive endoscopic surveillance, and mucosal ablation have all been advocated. Currently, most experts advocate esophagectomy as treatment for high-grade dysplasia in an otherwise healthy patient with minimal surgical risk. However, esophagectomy has a mortality ranging from 3–10%, along with substantial morbidity. That, along with increasing evidence of the effectiveness of endoscopic therapy with purpose-built radio frequency ablation devices, has led many to favor this therapy as a preferable alternative.

TREATMENT   Gastroesophageal Reflux Disease (GERD)

Lifestyle modifications are routinely advocated as GERD therapy. Broadly speaking, these fall into three categories: (1) avoidance of foods that reduce lower esophageal sphincter pressure, making them "refluxogenic" (these commonly include fatty foods, alcohol, spearmint, peppermint, tomato-based foods, possibly coffee and tea); (2) avoidance of acidic foods that are inherently irritating; and (3) adoption of behaviors to minimize reflux and/or heartburn. In general, minimal evidence supports the efficacy of these measures. However, clinical experience dictates that subsets of patients are benefitted by specific recommendations, based on their unique history and symptom profile. A patient

Barrett's metaplasia — Alcian blue stain

High-grade dysplasia — H&E stain

FIGURE 13-10
Histopathology of Barrett's metaplasia and Barrett's with high-grade dysplasia. H&E, hematoxylin and eosin.

with sleep disturbance from nighttime heartburn is likely to benefit from elevation of the head of the bed and avoidance of eating before retiring, but those recommendations are superfluous for a patient without nighttime symptoms. The most broadly applicable recommendation is for weight reduction. Even though the benefit with respect to reflux cannot be assured, the strong epidemiologic association between obesity and GERD and the secondary health gains of weight reduction are beyond dispute.

The dominant pharmacologic approach to GERD management is with inhibitors of gastric acid secretion and abundant data support the effectiveness of this approach. Pharmacologically reducing the acidity of gastric juice does not prevent reflux, but it ameliorates reflux symptoms and allows esophagitis to heal. The hierarchy of effectiveness among pharmaceuticals parallels their antisecretory potency. Proton pump inhibitors (PPIs), are more efficacious than histamine$_2$ receptor antagonists (H$_2$RAs), and both are superior to placebo. No major differences exist among PPIs, and only modest gain is achieved by increased dosage.

Paradoxically, the perceived frequency and severity of heartburn correlate poorly with the presence or severity of esophagitis. When GERD treatments are assessed in terms of resolving heartburn, both efficacy and differences among pharmaceuticals are less clearcut than with the objective of healing esophagitis. Although the same overall hierarchy of effectiveness exists, observed efficacy rates are lower and vary widely, likely reflective of patient heterogeneity.

Reflux symptoms tend to be chronic, irrespective of esophagitis. Thus, a common management strategy is indefinite treatment with PPIs or H$_2$RAs as necessary for symptom control. The side effects of PPI therapy are generally minimal. Vitamin B$_{12}$, calcium, and iron absorption may be compromised and susceptibility to enteric infections, particularly *Clostridium difficile* colitis, increased with treatment. Consequently, as with any medication, dosage should be minimized to that necessary.

Laparoscopic Nissen fundoplication, wherein the proximal stomach is wrapped around the distal esophagus to create an antireflux barrier, is a surgical alternative to the management of chronic GERD. Just as with PPI therapy, evidence on the utility of fundoplication is strongest for treating esophagitis and controlled trials suggest similar efficacy to PPI therapy. However, the benefits of fundoplication must be weighed against potential deleterious effects, including surgical morbidity and mortality, postoperative dysphagia, failure or breakdown requiring reoperation, an inability to belch, and increased bloating, flatulence, and bowel symptoms after surgery.

EOSINOPHILIC ESOPHAGITIS

Eosinophilic esophagitis (EoE) is increasingly recognized in adults and children around the world. Population-based studies suggest the prevalence to be in excess of 1:1000 with a predilection for white males. The increasing prevalence of EoE is attributable to a combination of an increasing incidence and a growing awareness of the condition. There is also an incompletely understood, but important, overlap between EoE and GERD that delays or confuses diagnosis of the disease in many cases.

EoE is diagnosed based on the combination of typical esophageal symptoms and esophageal mucosal biopsies demonstrating esophageal squamous epithelial infiltration with eosinophils. Secondary etiologies of esophageal eosinophilia including GERD, drug hypersensitivity, connective tissue disorders, hypereosinophilic syndrome and infection are excluded. Current evidence indicates that EoE is an allergic disorder induced by antigen sensitization in susceptible individuals. Studies have demonstrated an important role for dietary allergens in both the pathogenesis and treatment of EoE. Aeroallergens may also contribute but there is much less evidence in this regard. The natural history of the disorder is uncertain as are the consequences of not treating asymptomatic or minimally symptomatic patients.

EoE should be strongly considered in children and adults with dysphagia and food impactions, regardless of the presence or absence of heartburn. Other symptoms may include atypical chest pain and heartburn, particularly heartburn that is refractory to PPI therapy. An atopic history of food allergy, asthma, eczema, or allergic rhinitis is present in the majority of patients. Cytokines such as IL-5, eotaxin, and thymus and activation-related chemokine (TARC) may be elevated in the serum. The characteristic endoscopic findings include multiple esophageal rings, linear furrows, and punctate exudates (Fig. 13-11). Histologic confirmation is made with the demonstration of increased eosinophils in the esophageal mucosa (generally ≥15 eosinophils per high-power field) (Fig. 13-12). Fibrosis, narrow caliber esophagus, and stricture can occur with EoE, but the predictive variables for these are not known. Complications of disease include food impaction and esophageal perforation.

Treatments for EoE include dietary restrictions, PPIs, systemic or topical glucocorticoids, montelukast, immunomodulators, and endoscopic dilatation of strictures. Notably, allergy testing [radioallergosorbent test (RAST), skin prick testing] has demonstrated limited specificity in the identification of causative foods. Once esophageal eosinophilia is demonstrated, patients in whom GERD may be a confounding factor should undergo a trial of PPI therapy to determine if this results in clinical or histologic improvement. If symptoms and eosinophilia persist despite PPI therapy, other treatment options should

FIGURE 13-11

Endoscopic features of (A) eosinophilic esophagitis (EoE), (B) Candida esophagitis, (C) giant ulcer associated with HIV, and (D) a Schatzki's ring.

FIGURE 13-12

Histopathology of eosinophilic esophagitis (EoE) showing dense infiltration of the esophageal squamous epithelium with eosinophils. Eosinophilic inflammation can also be seen with gastroesophageal reflux disease (GERD); the optimal discriminatory threshold for EoE is greater than 15 eosinophils per high-power field.

be pursued. Topical glucocorticoids (fluticasone propionate or budesonide) are the most commonly used treatment in adults, but dietary restriction has proven effective primarily in pediatric studies. Systemic glucocorticoids are reserved for severely afflicted patients refractory to less morbid treatments. Esophageal dilation should be approached cautiously in patients with stricturing because of concerns for increased risk of esophageal mural disruption and perforation.

INFECTIOUS ESOPHAGITIS

With the increased use of immunosuppression for organ transplantation as well as chronic inflammatory diseases and chemotherapy along with the AIDS epidemic, infections with *Candida* species, herpesvirus, and cytomegalovirus (CMV) have become relatively common. Although rare, infectious esophagitis also occurs among the nonimmunocompromised, with herpes simplex and *Candida albicans* being the most common pathogens. Among AIDS patients, infectious esophagitis becomes more common as the CD4 count declines; cases are rare with the CD4 count >200 and common when <100. HIV itself may also be associated with a self-limited syndrome of acute esophageal ulceration with oral ulcers and a maculopapular skin rash at the time of seroconversion. Additionally, some patients with advanced disease have deep, persistent esophageal ulcers treated with oral glucocorticoids or thalidomide. However, with the widespread use of protease inhibitors, a reduction in these HIV complications has been noted.

Regardless of the infectious agent, odynophagia is a characteristic symptom of infectious esophagitis; dysphagia, chest pain, and hemorrhage are also common. Odynophagia is uncommon with reflux esophagitis, so its presence should always raise suspicion of an alternative etiology.

CANDIDA ESOPHAGITIS

Candida is normally found in the throat, but can become pathogenic and produce esophagitis in a compromised host; *C. albicans* is most common. *Candida* esophagitis also occurs with esophageal stasis secondary to esophageal motor disorders and diverticula. Patients complain of odynophagia and dysphagia. If oral thrush is present, empirical therapy is appropriate, but coinfection is common, and persistent symptoms should lead to prompt endoscopy with biopsy, which is the most useful diagnostic evaluation. *Candida* esophagitis has a characteristic appearance of white plaques with friability. Rarely, *Candida* esophagitis is complicated by bleeding, perforation, stricture, or systemic invasion. Oral fluconazole (200 mg on the first day, followed by 100 mg daily) for 7–14 days is the preferred treatment. Patients refractory to fluconazole may respond to itraconazole. Alternatively, poorly responsive patients or those who cannot swallow medications can be treated with an intravenous echinocandin (caspofungin 50 mg daily for 7–21 days). Amphotericin B (10–15 mg IV infusion for 6 h daily to a total dose of 300–500 mg) is used in severe cases.

HERPETIC ESOPHAGITIS

Herpes simplex virus type 1 or 2 may cause esophagitis. Vesicles on the nose and lips may coexist and are suggestive of a herpetic etiology. Varicella-zoster virus can also cause esophagitis in children with chickenpox or adults with zoster. The characteristic endoscopic findings are vesicles and small, punched-out ulcerations. Because herpes simplex infections are limited to squamous epithelium, biopsies from the ulcer margins are most likely to reveal the characteristic ground glass nuclei, eosinophilic Cowdry's type A inclusion bodies, and giant cells. Culture or polymerase chain reaction (PCR) assays are helpful to identify acyclovir-resistant strains. The infection is often self-limited after a 1–2 week period. Acyclovir (400 mg orally 5 times a day for 14–21 days) or valacyclovir (1 g orally tid for 7 days) reduces this morbidity. In patients with severe odynophagia, intravenous acyclovir (5 mg/kg every 8 h for 7–14 days), foscarnet (90 mg/kg intravenously bid for 2–4 weeks), or oral famciclovir is used.

CYTOMEGALOVIRUS

CMV esophagitis occurs only in immunocompromised patients, particularly transplant recipients. CMV is usually activated from a latent stage or may be acquired from transfusions. Endoscopically, CMV lesions appear as serpiginous ulcers in an otherwise normal mucosa, particularly in the distal esophagus. Biopsies of the ulcer bases have the highest diagnostic yield for finding the pathognomonic large nuclear or cytoplasmic inclusion bodies. Immunohistology with monoclonal antibodies to CMV and in situ hybridization tests are useful for early diagnosis. Ganciclovir, 5 mg/kg every 12 h intravenously, is the treatment of choice. Valganciclovir (900 mg bid), an oral formulation of ganciclovir, or foscarnet (90 mg/kg every 12 h intravenously) can also be used. Therapy is continued until healing, which may take 3–6 weeks.

MECHANICAL TRAUMA AND IATROGENIC INJURY

ESOPHAGEAL PERFORATION

Most cases of esophageal perforation are from instrumentation of the esophagus or trauma. Alternatively, forceful vomiting or retching can lead to spontaneous rupture at the gastroesophageal junction (Boerhaave's syndrome). More rarely, corrosive esophagitis or neoplasms lead to perforation. Instrumental perforation from endoscopy or nasogastric tube placement typically occurs in the hypopharynx or at the gastroesophageal junction. Perforation may also result at the site of stricture in the setting of endoscopic food disimpaction or esophageal dilation. Esophageal perforation causes pleuritic retrosternal pain that can be associated with pneumomediastinum and subcutaneous emphysema. Mediastinitis is a major complication of esophageal perforation, and prompt recognition is key to optimizing outcome. CT of the chest is most sensitive in detecting mediastinal air. Esophageal perforation is confirmed by a contrast swallow; usually Gastrografin followed by thin barium. Treatment includes nasogastric suction and parenteral broad-spectrum antibiotics with prompt surgical drainage and repair in noncontained leaks. Conservative therapy with NPO status and antibiotics without surgery may be appropriate in cases of minor instrumental perforation that are detected early. Endoscopic clipping or stent placement may be indicated in nonoperable cases such as perforated tumors.

MALLORY-WEISS TEAR

Vomiting, retching, or vigorous coughing can cause a nontransmural tear at the gastroesophageal junction that is a common cause of upper gastrointestinal bleeding. Most patients present with hematemesis. Antecedent vomiting is anticipated but not always evident. Bleeding usually abates spontaneously, but protracted bleeding may respond to local epinephrine or cauterization therapy, endoscopic clipping, or angiographic embolization. Surgery is rarely needed.

RADIATION ESOPHAGITIS

Radiation esophagitis can complicate treatment for thoracic cancers, especially breast and lung, with the risk proportional to radiation dosage. Radiosensitizing drugs such as doxorubicin, bleomycin, cyclophosphamide, and cisplatin also increase the risk. Dysphagia and odynophagia may last weeks to months after therapy. The esophageal mucosa becomes erythematous, edematous, and friable. Submucosal fibrosis and degenerative tissue changes and stricturing may occur years after the radiation exposure. Radiation exposure in excess of 5000 cGy has been associated with increased risk of esophageal stricture. Treatment for acute radiation esophagitis is supportive. Chronic strictures are managed with esophageal dilation.

CORROSIVE ESOPHAGITIS

Caustic esophageal injury from ingestion of alkali or, less commonly, acid can be accidental or from attempted suicide. Absence of oral injury does not exclude possible esophageal involvement. Thus, early endoscopic evaluation is recommended to assess and grade the injury to the esophageal mucosa. Severe corrosive injury may lead to esophageal perforation, bleeding, stricture, and death. Glucocorticoids have not been shown to improve the clinical outcome of acute corrosive esophagitis and are not recommended. Healing of more severe grades of caustic injury is commonly associated with severe stricture formation and often requires repeated dilatation.

PILL ESOPHAGITIS

Pill-induced esophagitis occurs when a swallowed pill fails to traverses the entire esophagus and lodges within the lumen. Generally, this is attributed to poor "pill taking habits": inadequate liquid with the pill, or lying down immediately after taking a pill. The most common location for the pill to lodge is in the mid-esophagus near the crossing of the aorta or carina. Extrinsic compression from these structures halts the movement of the pill or capsule. Since initially reported in 1970, more than 1000 cases of pill esophagitis have been reported, suggesting that this is not an unusual occurrence. A wide variety of medications are implicated with the most common being doxycycline, tetracycline, quinidine, phenytoin, potassium chloride, ferrous sulfate, nonsteroidal anti-inflammatory drugs (NSAIDs), and bisphosphonates. However, virtually any pill can result in pill esophagitis if taken carelessly.

Typical symptoms of pill esophagitis are the sudden onset of chest pain and odynophagia. Characteristically, the pain will develop over a period of hours or will awaken the individual from sleep. A classic history in the setting of ingestion of recognized pill offenders obviates the need for diagnostic testing in most patients. When endoscopy is performed, localized ulceration or inflammation is evident. Histologically, acute inflammation is typical. Chest CT imaging will sometimes reveal esophageal thickening consistent with transmural inflammation. Although the condition usually resolves within days to weeks, symptoms may persist for months and stricture can develop in severe cases. No specific therapy is known to hasten the healing process, but antisecretory medications are frequently prescribed to remove concomitant reflux as an aggravating factor. When healing results in stricture formation, dilatation is indicated.

FOREIGN BODIES AND FOOD IMPACTION

Food or foreign bodies may lodge in the esophagus causing complete obstruction, causing an inability to handle secretions (foaming at the mouth) and severe chest pain. Food impaction may occur due to stricture, carcinoma, Schatzki's ring, eosinophilic esophagitis, or simply inattentive eating. If it does not spontaneously resolve, impacted food is dislodged endoscopically. Use of meat tenderizer enzymes to facilitate passage of a meat bolus is discouraged because of potential esophageal injury. Glucagon (1 mg IV) is sometimes tried before endoscopic dislodgement. After emergent treatment patients should be evaluated for potential causes of the impaction with treatment rendered as indicated.

ESOPHAGEAL MANIFESTATIONS OF SYSTEMIC DISEASE

SCLERODERMA AND COLLAGEN VASCULAR DISEASES

Scleroderma esophagus (hypotensive LES and absent esophageal peristalsis) was initially described as a manifestation of scleroderma or other collagen vascular diseases and thought to be specific for these disorders. However, this nomenclature subsequently proved unfortunate and has been discarded because an estimated half of qualifying patients do not have an identifiable systemic disease, and reflux disease is often the only identifiable association. When scleroderma esophagus occurs as a manifestation of a collagen vascular disease, the histopathologic findings are of infiltration and destruction of the esophageal muscularis propria with collagen deposition and fibrosis. The pathogenesis of absent peristalsis and LES hypotension in the absence of a collagen vascular disease is unknown. Regardless of the underlying cause, the manometric abnormalities predispose patients to severe GERD due to inadequate LES barrier function combined with poor esophageal clearance of refluxed acid. Dysphagia may also be manifest but is generally mild and alleviated by eating in an upright position and using liquids to facilitate solid emptying.

DERMATOLOGIC DISEASES

A host of dermatologic disorders (pemphigus vulgaris, bullous pemphigoid, cicatricial pemphigoid, Behçet's syndrome, epidermolysis bullosa) can affect the oropharynx and esophagus, particularly the proximal esophagus, with blisters, bullae, webs, and strictures. Glucocorticoid treatment is usually effective. Erosive lichen planus, Stevens-Johnson syndrome, and graft-versus-host disease can also involve the esophagus. Esophageal dilatation may be necessary to treat strictures.

CHAPTER 14

PEPTIC ULCER DISEASE AND RELATED DISORDERS

John Del Valle

PEPTIC ULCER DISEASE

Burning epigastric pain exacerbated by fasting and improved with meals is a symptom complex associated with peptic ulcer disease (PUD). An *ulcer* is defined as disruption of the mucosal integrity of the stomach and/or duodenum leading to a local defect or excavation due to active inflammation. Ulcers occur within the stomach and/or duodenum and are often chronic in nature. Acid peptic disorders are very common in the United States, with 4 million individuals (new cases and recurrences) affected per year. Lifetime prevalence of PUD in the United States is ~12% in men and 10% in women. Moreover, an estimated 15,000 deaths per year occur as a consequence of complicated PUD. The financial impact of these common disorders has been substantial, with an estimated burden on direct and indirect health care costs of ~$10 billion per year in the United States.

GASTRIC PHYSIOLOGY

Despite the constant attack on the gastroduodenal mucosa by a host of noxious agents (acid, pepsin, bile acids, pancreatic enzymes, drugs, and bacteria), integrity is maintained by an intricate system that provides mucosal defense and repair.

Gastric anatomy

The gastric epithelial lining consists of rugae that contain microscopic gastric pits, each branching into four or five gastric glands made up of highly specialized epithelial cells. The makeup of gastric glands varies with their anatomic location. Glands within the gastric cardia comprise <5% of the gastric gland area and contain mucous and endocrine cells. The 75% of gastric glands

are found within the oxyntic mucosa and contain mucous neck, parietal, chief, endocrine, enterochromaffin, and enterochromaffin-like (ECL) cells **(Fig. 14-1)**. Pyloric glands contain mucous and endocrine cells (including gastrin cells) and are found in the antrum.

The parietal cell, also known as the oxyntic cell, is usually found in the neck, or isthmus, or in the oxyntic gland. The resting, or unstimulated, parietal cell has

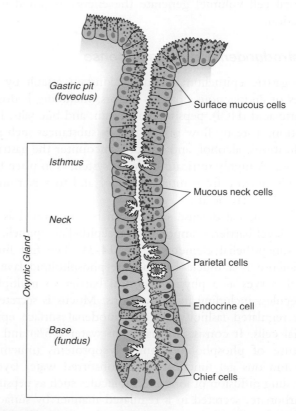

FIGURE 14-1

Diagrammatic representation of the oxyntic gastric gland. (*Adapted from S Ito, RJ Winchester: Cell Biol 16:541, 1963. © The Rockefeller University Press.*)

FIGURE 14-2

Gastric parietal cell undergoing transformation after secretagogue-mediated stimulation. cAMP, cyclic adenosine monophosphate. (*Adapted from SJ Hersey, G Sachs: Physiol Rev 75:155, 1995.*)

prominent cytoplasmic tubulovesicles and intracellular canaliculi containing short microvilli along its apical surface **(Fig. 14-2)**. H$^+$,K$^+$-adenosine triphosphatase (ATPase) is expressed in the tubulovesicle membrane; upon cell stimulation, this membrane, along with apical membranes, transforms into a dense network of apical intracellular canaliculi containing long microvilli. Acid secretion, a process requiring high energy, occurs at the apical canalicular surface. Numerous mitochondria (30–40% of total cell volume) generate the energy required for secretion.

Gastroduodenal mucosal defense

The gastric epithelium is under constant assault by a series of endogenous noxious factors, including hydrochloric acid (HCl), pepsinogen/pepsin, and bile salts. In addition, a steady flow of exogenous substances such as medications, alcohol, and bacteria encounter the gastric mucosa. A highly intricate biologic system is in place to provide defense from mucosal injury and to repair any injury that may occur.

The mucosal defense system can be envisioned as a three-level barrier, composed of preepithelial, epithelial, and subepithelial elements **(Fig. 14-3)**. The first line of defense is a mucus-bicarbonate-phospholipid layer, which serves as a physicochemical barrier to multiple molecules, including hydrogen ions. Mucus is secreted in a regulated fashion by gastroduodenal surface epithelial cells. It consists primarily of water (95%) and a mixture of phospholipids and glycoproteins (mucin). The mucous gel functions as a nonstirred water layer impeding diffusion of ions and molecules such as pepsin. Bicarbonate, secreted in a regulated manner by surface epithelial cells of the gastroduodenal mucosa into the mucous gel, forms a pH gradient ranging from 1 to 2 at the gastric luminal surface and reaching 6 to 7 along the epithelial cell surface.

Surface epithelial cells provide the next line of defense through several factors, including mucus production, epithelial cell ionic transporters that maintain intracellular pH and bicarbonate production, and intracellular tight junctions. Surface epithelial cells generate heat shock proteins that prevent protein denaturation and protect cells from certain factors such as increased temperature, cytotoxic agents, or oxidative stress. Epithelial cells also generate trefoil factor family peptides and cathelicidins, which also play a role in surface cell protection and regeneration. If the preepithelial barrier were breached, gastric epithelial cells bordering a site of injury can migrate to restore a damaged region (*restitution*). This process occurs independent of cell division and requires uninterrupted blood flow and an alkaline pH in the surrounding environment. Several growth factors, including epidermal growth factor (EGF), transforming growth factor (TGF) α, and basic fibroblast growth factor (FGF), modulate the process of restitution. Larger defects that are not effectively repaired by restitution require cell proliferation. Epithelial cell regeneration is regulated by prostaglandins and growth factors such as EGF and TGF-α. In tandem with epithelial cell renewal, formation of new vessels (*angiogenesis*) within the injured microvascular bed occurs. Both FGF and vascular endothelial growth factor (VEGF) are important in regulating angiogenesis in the gastric mucosa.

An elaborate microvascular system within the gastric submucosal layer is the key component of the subepithelial defense/repair system, providing HCO$_3^-$, which neutralizes the acid generated by the parietal cell. Moreover, this microcirculatory bed provides an adequate supply of micronutrients and oxygen while removing toxic metabolic by-products.

Prostaglandins play a central role in gastric epithelial defense/repair **(Fig. 14-4)**. The gastric mucosa contains abundant levels of prostaglandins that regulate the release of mucosal bicarbonate and mucus, inhibit parietal cell secretion, and are important in maintaining mucosal blood flow and epithelial cell restitution. Prostaglandins are derived from esterified arachidonic acid, which is formed from phospholipids (cell membrane) by the action of phospholipase A$_2$. A key enzyme that controls the rate-limiting step in prostaglandin synthesis is cyclooxygenase (COX), which is present in two isoforms (COX-1, COX-2), each having distinct characteristics regarding structure, tissue distribution, and expression. COX-1 is expressed in a host of tissues, including the stomach, platelets, kidneys, and endothelial cells. This isoform is expressed in a constitutive manner and plays an important role in maintaining the integrity of renal function, platelet aggregation, and gastrointestinal (GI) mucosal integrity. In contrast, the expression of COX-2 is inducible by inflammatory stimuli, and it is expressed in macrophages, leukocytes,

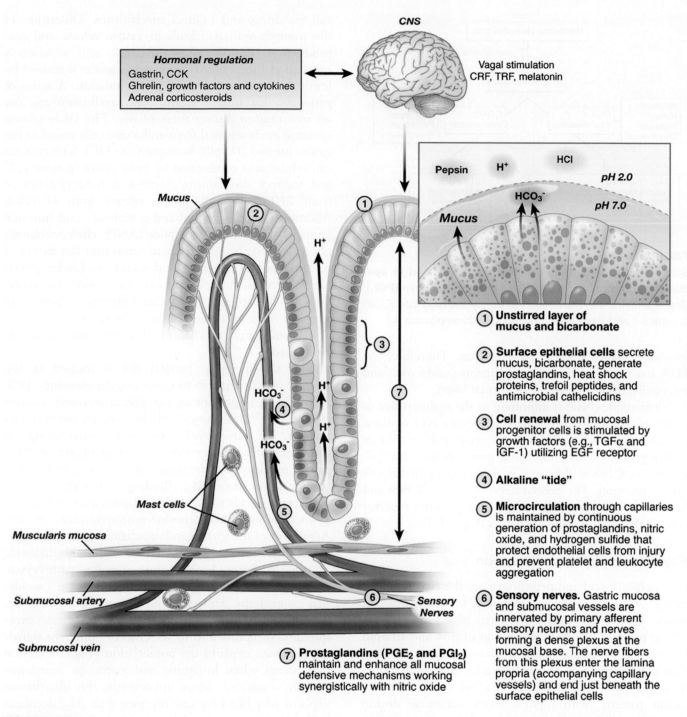

CNS

Vagal stimulation
CRF, TRF, melatonin

Hormonal regulation
Gastrin, CCK
Ghrelin, growth factors and cytokines
Adrenal corticosteroids

Pepsin   H⁺   HCl
                                 pH 2.0
                          HCO₃⁻
Mucus   **pH 7.0**

Mucus

H⁺

HCO₃⁻

H⁺

HCO₃⁻

H⁺

Mast cells

Muscularis mucosa

Submucosal artery

Submucosal vein

Sensory Nerves

① **Unstirred layer of mucus and bicarbonate**

② **Surface epithelial cells** secrete mucus, bicarbonate, generate prostaglandins, heat shock proteins, trefoil peptides, and antimicrobial cathelicidins

③ **Cell renewal** from mucosal progenitor cells is stimulated by growth factors (e.g., TGFα and IGF-1) utilizing EGF receptor

④ **Alkaline "tide"**

⑤ **Microcirculation** through capillaries is maintained by continuous generation of prostaglandins, nitric oxide, and hydrogen sulfide that protect endothelial cells from injury and prevent platelet and leukocyte aggregation

⑥ **Sensory nerves.** Gastric mucosa and submucosal vessels are innervated by primary afferent sensory neurons and nerves forming a dense plexus at the mucosal base. The nerve fibers from this plexus enter the lamina propria (accompanying capillary vessels) and end just beneath the surface epithelial cells

⑦ **Prostaglandins (PGE₂ and PGI₂)** maintain and enhance all mucosal defensive mechanisms working synergistically with nitric oxide

FIGURE 14-3

Components involved in providing gastroduodenal mucosal defense and repair. CCK, cholecystokinin; CRF, corticotropin-releasing factor; EGF, epidermal growth factor; HCl, hydrochloride; IGF, insulin-like growth factor; TGFα, transforming growth factor α; TRF, thyrotropin releasing factor. (*Modified and updated from Tarnawski A. Cellular and molecular mechanisms of mucosal defense and repair. In: Yoshikawa T, Arakawa T. Bioregulation and Its Disorders in the Gastrointestinal Tract. Tokyo, Japan: Blackwell Science, 1998:3–17.*)

fibroblasts, and synovial cells. The beneficial effects of nonsteroidal anti-inflammatory drugs (NSAIDs) on tissue inflammation are due to inhibition of COX-2; the toxicity of these drugs (e.g., GI mucosal ulceration and renal dysfunction) is related to inhibition of the

COX-1 isoform. The highly COX-2–selective NSAIDs have the potential to provide the beneficial effect of decreasing tissue inflammation while minimizing toxicity in the GI tract. Selective COX-2 inhibitors have had adverse effects on the cardiovascular system, leading to

FIGURE 14-4

Schematic representation of the steps involved in synthesis of prostaglandin E$_2$ (PGE$_2$) and prostacyclin (PGI$_2$). Characteristics and distribution of the cyclooxygenase (COX) enzymes 1 and 2 are also shown. TXA$_2$, thromboxane A$_2$.

increased risk of myocardial infarction. Therefore, the FDA has removed two of these agents (valdecoxib and rofecoxib) from the market (discussed later).

Nitric oxide (NO) is important in the maintenance of gastric mucosal integrity. The key enzyme NO synthase is constitutively expressed in the mucosa and contributes to cytoprotection by stimulating gastric mucus, increasing mucosal blood flow and maintaining epithelial cell barrier function. The central nervous system (CNS) and hormonal factors also play a role in regulating mucosal defense through multiple pathways (Fig. 14-3).

Physiology of gastric secretion

Hydrochloric acid and pepsinogen are the two principal gastric secretory products capable of inducing mucosal injury. Gastric acid and pepsinogen play a physiologic role in protein digestion, absorption of iron and vitamin B$_{12}$ as well as killing ingested bacteria. Acid secretion should be viewed as occurring under basal and stimulated conditions. Basal acid production occurs in a circadian pattern, with highest levels occurring during the night and lowest levels during the morning hours. Cholinergic input via the vagus nerve and histaminergic input from local gastric sources are the principal contributors to basal acid secretion. Stimulated gastric acid secretion occurs primarily in three phases based on the site where the signal originates (cephalic, gastric, and intestinal). Sight, smell, and taste of food are the components of the cephalic phase, which stimulates gastric secretion via the vagus nerve. The gastric phase is activated once food enters the stomach. This component of secretion is driven by nutrients (amino acids and amines) that directly stimulate the G cell to release gastrin, which in turn activates the parietal

cell via direct and indirect mechanisms. Distention of the stomach wall also leads to gastrin release and acid production. The last phase of gastric acid secretion is initiated as food enters the intestine and is mediated by luminal distention and nutrient assimilation. A series of pathways that inhibit gastric acid production are also set into motion during these phases. The GI hormone somatostatin is released from endocrine cells found in the gastric mucosa (D cells) in response to HCl. Somatostatin can inhibit acid production by both direct (parietal cell) and indirect mechanisms (decreased histamine release from ECL cells and gastrin release from G cells). Additional neural (central and peripheral) and humoral [amylin, atrial natriuretic peptide (ANP), cholecystokinin, ghrelin, obestatin, secretin, and serotonin] factors play a role in counterbalancing acid secretion. Under physiologic circumstances, these phases occur simultaneously. Ghrelin, the appetite-regulating hormone expressed in stomach, may stimulate gastric acid secretion through a vagal-mediated mechanism, but this remains to be confirmed.

The acid-secreting parietal cell is located in the oxyntic gland, adjacent to other cellular elements (ECL cell, D cell) important in the gastric secretory process (Fig. 14-5). This unique cell also secretes intrinsic factor (IF). The parietal cell expresses receptors for several stimulants of acid secretion, including histamine (H$_2$), gastrin (cholecystokinin B/gastrin receptor), and acetylcholine (muscarinic, M$_3$). Binding of histamine to the H$_2$ receptor leads to activation of adenylate cyclase and an increase in cyclic adenosine monophosphate (AMP). Activation of the gastrin and muscarinic receptors results in activation of the protein kinase C/phosphoinositide signaling pathway. Each of these signaling pathways in turn regulates a series of downstream kinase cascades that control the acid-secreting pump, H$^+$,K$^+$-ATPase. The discovery that different ligands and their corresponding receptors lead to activation of different signaling pathways explains the potentiation of acid secretion that occurs when histamine and gastrin or acetylcholine are combined. More importantly, this observation explains why blocking one receptor type (H$_2$) decreases acid secretion stimulated by agents that activate a different pathway (gastrin, acetylcholine). Parietal cells also express receptors for ligands that inhibit acid production (prostaglandins, somatostatin, and EGF). Histamine also stimulates gastric acid secretion indirectly by activating the histamine H$_3$ receptor on D cells, which inhibits somatostatin release.

The enzyme H$^+$,K$^+$-ATPase is responsible for generating the large concentration of H$^+$. It is a membrane-bound protein that consists of two subunits, α and β. The active catalytic site is found within the α subunit; the function of the β subunit is unclear. This enzyme uses the chemical energy of adenosine triphosphate

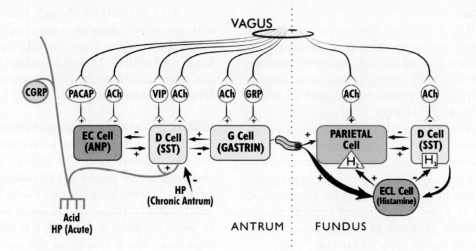

FIGURE 14-5

Regulation of gastric acid secretion at the cellular level. ACh, acetylcholine; ANP, atrial natriuretic peptide; CGRP, calcitonin gene-related peptide; EC, enterochromaffin; ECL, enterochromaffin-like; GRP, gastrin-releasing peptide; PACAP, pituitary adenylate-cyclase activating peptide; SST, somatostatin; VIP, vasoactive intestinal peptide.

(ATP) to transfer H^+ ions from parietal cell cytoplasm to the secretory canaliculi in exchange for K^+. The H^+,K^+-ATPase is located within the secretory canaliculus and in nonsecretory cytoplasmic tubulovesicles. The tubulovesicles are impermeable to K^+, which leads to an inactive pump in this location. The distribution of pumps between the nonsecretory vesicles and the secretory canaliculus varies according to parietal cell activity (Fig. 14-2). Proton pumps are recycled back to the inactive state in cytoplasmic vesicles once parietal cell activation ceases.

The chief cell, found primarily in the gastric fundus, synthesizes and secretes pepsinogen, the inactive precursor of the proteolytic enzyme pepsin. The acid environment within the stomach leads to cleavage of the inactive precursor to pepsin and provides the low pH (<2) required for pepsin activity. Pepsin activity is significantly diminished at a pH of 4 and irreversibly inactivated and denatured at a pH of ≥7. Many of the secretagogues that stimulate acid secretion also stimulate pepsinogen release. The precise role of pepsin in the pathogenesis of PUD remains to be established.

PATHOPHYSIOLOGIC BASIS OF PEPTIC ULCER DISEASE

PUD encompasses both gastric and duodenal ulcers. *Ulcers* are defined as breaks in the mucosal surface >5 mm in size, with depth to the submucosa. Duodenal ulcers (DUs) and gastric ulcers (GUs) share many common features in terms of pathogenesis, diagnosis, and treatment, but several factors distinguish them from one another.

Epidemiology

Duodenal ulcers

DUs are estimated to occur in 6–15% of the Western population. The incidence of DUs declined steadily from 1960 to 1980 and has remained stable since then. The death rates, need for surgery, and physician visits have decreased by >50% over the past 30 years. The reason for the reduction in the frequency of DUs is likely related to the decreasing frequency of *Helicobacter pylori*. Before the discovery of *H. pylori,* the natural history of DUs was typified by frequent recurrences after initial therapy. Eradication of *H. pylori* has greatly reduced these recurrence rates.

Gastric ulcers

GUs tend to occur later in life than duodenal lesions, with a peak incidence reported in the sixth decade. More than one-half of GUs occur in males and are less common than DUs, perhaps due to the higher likelihood of GUs being silent and presenting only after a complication develops. Autopsy studies suggest a similar incidence of DUs and GUs.

Pathology

Duodenal ulcers

DUs occur most often in the first portion of the duodenum (>95%), with ~90% located within 3 cm of the pylorus. They are usually ≤1 cm in diameter but can occasionally reach 3–6 cm (giant ulcer). Ulcers are sharply demarcated, with depth at times reaching the muscularis propria. The base of the ulcer often consists of a zone of eosinophilic necrosis with surrounding fibrosis. Malignant DUs are extremely rare.

Gastric ulcers

In contrast to DUs, GUs can represent a malignancy and should be biopsied upon discovery. Benign GUs are most often found distal to the junction between the antrum and the acid secretory mucosa. Benign GUs are quite rare in the gastric fundus and are histologically similar to DUs. Benign GUs associated with *H. pylori* are also associated with antral gastritis. In contrast, NSAID-related GUs are not accompanied by chronic active gastritis but may instead have evidence of a chemical gastropathy, typified by foveolar hyperplasia, edema of the lamina propria, and epithelial regeneration in the absence of *H. pylori*. Extension of smooth-muscle fibers into the upper portions of the mucosa, where they are not typically found, may also occur.

Pathophysiology

Duodenal ulcers

H. pylori and NSAID-induced injury account for the majority of DUs. Many acid secretory abnormalities have been described in DU patients. Of these, average basal and nocturnal gastric acid secretion appears to be increased in DU patients as compared to controls; however, the level of overlap between DU patients and control subjects is substantial. The reason for this altered secretory process is unclear, but *H. pylori* infection may contribute. Accelerated gastric emptying of liquids has been noted in some DU patients, but its role in DU formation, if any, is unclear. Bicarbonate secretion is significantly decreased in the duodenal bulb of patients with an active DU as compared to control subjects. *H. pylori* infection may also play a role in this process (discussed later).

Gastric ulcers

As in DUs, the majority of GUs can be attributed to either *H. pylori* or NSAID-induced mucosal damage. GUs that occur in the prepyloric area or those in the body associated with a DU or a duodenal scar are similar in pathogenesis to DUs. Gastric acid output (basal and stimulated) tends to be normal or decreased in GU patients. When GUs develop in the presence of minimal acid levels, impairment of mucosal defense factors may be present. Gastric ulcers have been classified based on their location: Type I occur in the gastric body and tend to be associated with low gastric acid production; type II occur in the antrum and gastric acid can vary from low to normal; type III occur within 3 cm of the pylorus and are commonly accompanied by duodenal ulcers and normal or high gastric acid production; and type IV are found in the cardia and are associated with low gastric acid production.

Abnormalities in resting and stimulated pyloric sphincter pressure with a concomitant increase in duodenal gastric reflux have been implicated in some GU patients. Although bile acids, lysolecithin, and pancreatic enzymes may injure gastric mucosa, a definite role for these in GU pathogenesis has not been established. Delayed gastric emptying of solids has been described in GU patients but has not been reported consistently

H. pylori and acid peptic disorders

Gastric infection with the bacterium *H. pylori* accounts for the majority of PUD (Chap. 26). This organism also plays a role in the development of gastric mucosa-associated lymphoid tissue (MALT) lymphoma and gastric adenocarcinoma. Although the entire genome of *H. pylori* has been sequenced, it is still not clear how this organism, which resides in the stomach, causes ulceration in the duodenum, or whether its eradication will lead to a decrease in gastric cancer.

The bacterium

The bacterium, initially named *Campylobacter pyloridis,* is a gram-negative microaerophilic rod found most commonly in the deeper portions of the mucous gel coating the gastric mucosa or between the mucous layer and the gastric epithelium. It may attach to gastric epithelium but under normal circumstances does not appear to invade cells. It is strategically designed to live within the aggressive environment of the stomach. It is S-shaped (~0.5–3 μm in size) and contains multiple sheathed flagella. Initially, *H. pylori* resides in the antrum but, over time, migrates toward the more proximal segments of the stomach. The organism is capable of transforming into a coccoid form, which represents a dormant state that may facilitate survival in adverse conditions. The genome of *H. pylori* (1.65 million base pairs) encodes ~1500 proteins. Among this multitude of proteins there are factors that are essential determinants of *H. pylori*–mediated pathogenesis and colonization such as the outer membrane protein (Hop proteins), urease, and the vacuolating cytotoxin (Vac A). Moreover, the majority of *H. pylori* strains contain a genomic fragment that encodes the cag pathogenicity island (cag-PAI). Several of the genes that make up cag-PAI encode components of a type IV secretion island that translocates Cag A into host cells. Once in the cell, Cag A activates a series of cellular events important in cell growth and cytokine production. *H. pylori* also has extensive genetic diversity that in turn enhances its ability to promote disease. The first step in infection by *H. pylori* is dependent on the bacteria's motility and its ability to produce urease. Urease produces ammonia from urea, an essential step in alkalinizing the surrounding pH. Additional bacterial factors include catalase, lipase, adhesins, platelet-activating factor, and pic B (induces cytokines). Multiple strains of *H. pylori* exist and are characterized by their ability to express several of these factors (Cag A, Vac A, etc.). It is possible that the different diseases related to *H. pylori* infection can be attributed to different strains of the organism with distinct pathogenic features.

Epidemiology

The prevalence of *H. pylori* varies throughout the world and depends largely on the overall standard of living in the region. In developing parts of the world, 80% of the population may be infected by the age of 20, whereas the prevalence is 20–50% in industrialized countries. In contrast, in the United States this organism is rare in childhood. The overall prevalence of *H. pylori* in the United States is ~30%, with individuals born before 1950 having a higher rate of infection than those born later. About 10% of Americans <30 years of age are colonized with the bacteria. The rate of infection with *H. pylori* in industrialized countries has decreased substantially in recent decades. The steady increase in the prevalence of *H. pylori* noted with increasing age is due primarily to a cohort effect, reflecting higher transmission during a period in which the earlier cohorts were children. It has been calculated through mathematical models that improved sanitation during the latter half of the nineteenth century dramatically decreased transmission of *H. pylori*. Moreover, with the present rate of intervention, the organism will be ultimately eliminated from the United States. Two factors that predispose to higher colonization rates include poor socioeconomic status and less education. These factors, not race, are responsible for the rate of *H. pylori* infection in blacks and Hispanic Americans being double the rate seen in whites of comparable age. Other risk factors for *H. pylori* infection are (1) birth or residence in a developing country, (2) domestic crowding, (3) unsanitary living conditions, (4) unclean food or water, and (5) exposure to gastric contents of an infected individual.

Transmission of *H. pylori* occurs from person to person, following an oral-oral or fecal-oral route. The risk of *H. pylori* infection is declining in developing countries. The rate of infection in the United States has fallen by >50% when compared to 30 years ago.

Pathophysiology

H. pylori infection is virtually always associated with a chronic active gastritis, but only 10–15% of infected individuals develop frank peptic ulceration. The basis for this difference is unknown, but is likely due to a combination of host and bacterial factors some of which are outlined here. Initial studies suggested that >90% of all DUs were associated with *H. pylori,* but *H. pylori* is present in only 30–60% of individuals with GUs and 50–70% of patients with DUs. The pathophysiology of ulcers not associated with *H. pylori* or NSAID ingestion [or the rare Zollinger-Ellison syndrome (ZES)] is becoming more relevant as the incidence of *H. pylori* is dropping, particularly in the Western world (discussed later).

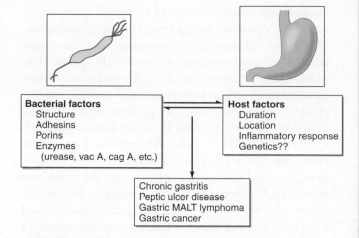

FIGURE 14-6
Outline of the bacterial and host factors important in determining *H. pylori*–induced gastrointestinal disease. MALT, mucosal-associated lymphoid tissue.

The particular end result of *H. pylori* infection (gastritis, PUD, gastric MALT lymphoma, gastric cancer) is determined by a complex interplay between bacterial and host factors (**Fig. 14-6**).

1. *Bacterial factors: H. pylori* is able to facilitate gastric residence, induce mucosal injury, and avoid host defense. Different strains of *H. pylori* produce different virulence factors. A specific region of the bacterial genome, the pathogenicity island (cag-PAI), encodes the virulence factors Cag A and pic B. Vac A also contributes to pathogenicity, although it is not encoded within the pathogenicity island. These virulence factors, in conjunction with additional bacterial constituents, can cause mucosal damage, in part through their ability to target the host immune cells. For example, Vac A targets human CD4 T cells, inhibiting their proliferation, and in addition can disrupt normal function of B cells, CD8 T cells, macrophages, and mast cells. Multiple studies have demonstrated that *H. pylori* strains that are cag-PAI positive are associated with a higher risk of peptic ulcer disease, premalignant gastric lesions, and gastric cancer than are strains that lack the cag-PAI. Urease, which allows the bacteria to reside in the acidic stomach, generates NH_3, which can damage epithelial cells. The bacteria produce surface factors that are chemotactic for neutrophils and monocytes, which in turn contribute to epithelial cell injury (discussed later). *H. pylori* makes proteases and phospholipases that break down the glycoprotein lipid complex of the mucous gel, thus reducing the efficacy of this first line of mucosal defense. *H. pylori* expresses adhesins (OMPs like BabA), which facilitate attachment of the bacteria to gastric epithelial cells. Although lipopolysaccharide (LPS) of gram-negative bacteria often plays an important role in the infection, *H. pylori* LPS has low

immunologic activity compared to that of other organisms. It may promote a smoldering chronic inflammation.

2. *Host factors:* Studies in twins suggest that there may be genetic predisposition to acquire *H. pylori*. The inflammatory response to *H. pylori* includes recruitment of neutrophils, lymphocytes (T and B), macrophages, and plasma cells. The pathogen leads to local injury by binding to class II major histocompatability complex (MHC) molecules expressed on gastric epithelial cells, leading to cell death (*apoptosis*). Moreover, bacterial strains that encode cag-PAI can introduce Cag A into the host cells, leading to further cell injury and activation of cellular pathways involved in cytokine production. Elevated concentrations of multiple cytokines are found in the gastric epithelium of *H. pylori*–infected individuals, including interleukin (IL) 1α/β, IL-2, IL-6, IL-8, tumor necrosis factor (TNF) α, and interferon (IFN-γ). *H. pylori* infection also leads to both a mucosal and a systemic humoral response, which does not lead to eradication of the bacteria but further compounds epithelial cell injury. Additional mechanisms by which *H. pylori* may cause epithelial cell injury include (1) activated neutrophil-mediated production of reactive oxygen or nitrogen species and enhanced epithelial cell turnover and (2) apoptosis related to interaction with T cells (T helper 1, or T$_H$1, cells) and IFN-γ.

The reason for *H. pylori*–mediated duodenal ulceration remains unclear. Studies suggest that *H. pylori* associated with duodenal ulceration may be more virulent. In addition, certain specific bacterial factors such as the duodenal ulcer-promoting gene A (*dupA*), may be associated with the development of duodenal ulcers. Another potential contributing factor is that gastric metaplasia in the duodenum of DU patients, which may be due to high acid exposure (discussed later), permits *H. pylori* to bind to it and produce local injury secondary to the host response. Another hypothesis is that *H. pylori* antral infection could lead to increased acid production, increased duodenal acid, and mucosal injury. Basal and stimulated [meal, gastrin-releasing peptide (GRP)] gastrin release are increased in *H. pylori*–infected individuals, and somatostatin-secreting D cells may be decreased. *H. pylori* infection might induce increased acid secretion through both direct and indirect actions of *H. pylori* and proinflammatory cytokines (IL-8, TNF, and IL-1) on G, D, and parietal cells (**Fig. 14–7**). Gastric ulcers, in contrast, are associated with *H. pylori* induced pangastritis and normal or low gastric acid secretion. *H. pylori* infection has also been associated with decreased duodenal mucosal bicarbonate production. Data supporting and contradicting each of these interesting theories have been demonstrated. Thus, the mechanism by which *H. pylori* infection of the stomach leads to duodenal ulceration remains to be established.

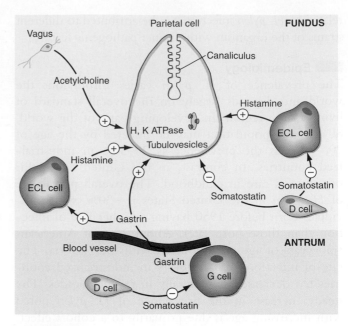

FIGURE 14-7
Summary of potential mechanisms by which *H. pylori* may lead to gastric secretory abnormalities. D, somatostatin cell; ECL, enterochromaffin-like cell; G, G cell. (*Adapted from J Calam et al: Gastroenterology 113:543, 1997.*)

In summary, the final effect of *H. pylori* on the GI tract is variable and determined by microbial and host factors. The type and distribution of gastritis correlate with the ultimate gastric and duodenal pathology observed. Specifically, the presence of antral-predominant gastritis is associated with DU formation; gastritis involving primarily the corpus predisposes to the development of GUs, gastric atrophy, and ultimately gastric carcinoma (**Fig. 14–8**).

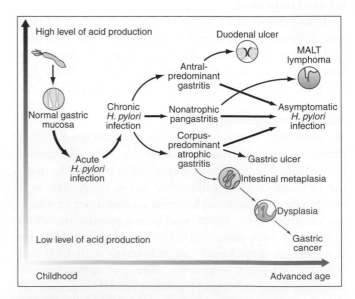

FIGURE 14-8
Natural history of *H. pylori* infection. (*Used with permission from S Suerbaum, P Michetti: N Engl J Med 347:1175, 2002.*)

NSAID-induced disease
Epidemiology

NSAIDs represent a group of the most commonly used medications in the United States. More than 30 billion over-the-counter tablets and over 100 million prescriptions are sold yearly in the United States alone. In fact, after the introduction of COX-2 inhibitors in the year 2000, the number of prescriptions written for NSAIDs was >111 million at a cost of $4.8 billion. Side effects and complications due to NSAIDs are considered the most common drug-related toxicities in the United States. The spectrum of NSAID-induced morbidity ranges from nausea and dyspepsia (prevalence reported as high as 50–60%) to a serious GI complication such as endoscopy-documented peptic ulceration (15–30% of individuals taking NSAIDs regularly) complicated by bleeding or perforation in as many as 1.5% of users per year. It is estimated that NSAID-induced GI bleeding accounts for 60,000 to 120,000 hospital admissions per year, and deaths related to NSAID-induced toxicity may be as high as 16,000 per year in the United States. Approximately 4–5% of patients develop symptomatic ulcers within 1 year. Unfortunately, dyspeptic symptoms do not correlate with NSAID-induced pathology. Over 80% of patients with serious NSAID-related complications did not have preceding dyspepsia. In view of the lack of warning signs, it is important to identify patients who are at increased risk for morbidity and mortality related to NSAID usage. Even 75 mg/d of aspirin may lead to serious GI ulceration; thus, no dose of NSAID is completely safe. Established risk factors include advanced age, history of ulcer, concomitant use of glucocorticoids, high-dose NSAIDs, multiple NSAIDs, concomitant use of anticoagulants, clopidogrel, and serious or multisystem disease. Possible risk factors include concomitant infection with *H. pylori,* cigarette smoking, and alcohol consumption.

Pathophysiology

Prostaglandins play a critical role in maintaining gastroduodenal mucosal integrity and repair. It therefore follows that interruption of prostaglandin synthesis can impair mucosal defense and repair, thus facilitating mucosal injury via a systemic mechanism. Animal studies have demonstrated that neutrophil adherence to the gastric microcirculation plays an essential role in the initiation of NSAID-induced mucosal injury. A summary of the pathogenetic pathways by which systemically administered NSAIDs may lead to mucosal injury is shown in **Fig. 14-9**.

Injury to the mucosa also occurs as a result of the topical encounter with NSAIDs. Aspirin and many NSAIDs are weak acids that remain in a nonionized lipophilic form when found within the acid environment of the stomach. Under these conditions, NSAIDs migrate across lipid membranes of epithelial cells,

FIGURE 14-9

Mechanisms by which NSAIDs may induce mucosal injury. *(Adapted from J Scheiman et al: J Clin Outcomes Management 3:23, 1996. Copyright 2003 Turner White Communications, Inc., www.turner-white.com. Used with permission.)*

leading to cell injury once trapped intracellularly in an ionized form. Topical NSAIDs can also alter the surface mucous layer, permitting back diffusion of H+ and pepsin, leading to further epithelial cell damage. Moreover, enteric-coated or buffered preparations are also associated with risk of peptic ulceration.

The interplay between *H. pylori* and NSAIDs in the pathogenesis of PUD is complex. Meta-analysis supports the conclusion that each of these aggressive factors is independent and synergistic risk factors for PUD and its complications such as GI bleeding. For example, eradication of *H. pylori* reduces the likelihood of GI complications in high-risk individuals to levels observed in individuals with average risk of NSAID-induced complications.

Pathogenetic factors unrelated to *H. pylori* and NSAID in acid peptic disease

Cigarette smoking has been implicated in the pathogenesis of PUD. Not only have smokers been found to have ulcers more frequently than do nonsmokers, but smoking appears to decrease healing rates, impair response to therapy, and increase ulcer-related complications such as perforation. The mechanism responsible for increased ulcer diathesis in smokers is unknown. Theories have included altered gastric emptying, decreased proximal duodenal bicarbonate production, increased risk for *H. pylori* infection, and cigarette-induced generation of noxious mucosal free radicals. Genetic predisposition may play a role in ulcer development. First-degree relatives of DU patients are three times as likely to develop an ulcer; however, the potential role of *H. pylori* infection in contacts is a major consideration. Increased frequency of blood group O and of the nonsecretor status have also been implicated as genetic risk factors for peptic diathesis. However, *H. pylori* preferentially binds to group O antigens. Psychological stress has been thought to contribute to PUD, but studies examining the role of psychological factors in its pathogenesis have generated conflicting results. Although PUD is associated with certain personality traits (neuroticism), these same traits are also present in individuals with nonulcer dyspepsia (NUD) and other functional and organic disorders.

Diet has also been thought to play a role in peptic diseases. Certain foods and beverages can cause dyspepsia, but no convincing studies indicate an association between ulcer formation and a specific diet. Specific chronic disorders have been shown to have a strong association with PUD: (1) systemic mastocytosis, (2) chronic pulmonary disease, (3) chronic renal failure,(4) cirrhosis, (5) nephrolithiasis, and (6) α_1-antitrypsin deficiency. Those with a possible association are (1) hyperparathyroidism, (2) coronary artery disease, (3) polycythemia vera, and (4) chronic pancreatitis.

Multiple factors play a role in the pathogenesis of PUD. The two predominant causes are *H. pylori* infection and NSAID ingestion. PUD not related to *H. pylori* or NSAIDs is increasing. Other less common causes of PUD are shown in Table 14-1. These etiologic agents should be considered as the incidence

TABLE 14-1

CAUSES OF ULCERS NOT CAUSED BY *HELICOBACTER PYLORI* AND NSAIDs

Pathogenesis of Non-Hp and Non-NSAID Ulcer Disease

Infection
Cytomegalovirus
Herpes simplex virus
H. heilmannii

Drug/Toxin
Bisphosphonates
Chemotherapy
Clopidogrel
Crack cocaine
Glucocorticoids (when combined with NSAIDs)
Mycophenolate mofetil
Potassium chloride

Miscellaneous
Basophilia in myeloproliferative disease
Duodenal obstruction (e.g., annular pancreas)
Infiltrating disease
Ischemia
Radiation therapy
Sarcoidosis
Crohn's disease
Idiopathic hypersecretory state

Abbreviations: Hp, *H. pylori*; NSAIDs, nonsteroidal anti-inflammatory drugs.

of *H. pylori* is decreasing. Independent of the inciting or injurious agent, peptic ulcers develop as a result of an imbalance between mucosal protection/repair and aggressive factors. Gastric acid plays an essential role in mucosal injury.

CLINICAL FEATURES

History

Abdominal pain is common to many GI disorders, including DU and GU, but has a poor predictive value for the presence of either DU or GU. Up to 10% of patients with NSAID-induced mucosal disease can present with a complication (bleeding, perforation, and obstruction) without antecedent symptoms. Despite this poor correlation, a careful history and physical examination are essential components of the approach to a patient suspected of having peptic ulcers.

Epigastric pain described as a burning or gnawing discomfort can be present in both DU and GU. The discomfort is also described as an ill-defined, aching sensation or as hunger pain. The typical pain pattern in DU occurs 90 min to 3 h after a meal and is frequently relieved by antacids or food. Pain that awakes the patient from sleep (between midnight and 3 A.M.) is the most discriminating symptom, with two-thirds of DU patients describing this complaint. Unfortunately, this symptom is also present in one-third of patients with NUD. The pain pattern in GU patients may be different from that in DU patients, where discomfort may actually be precipitated by food. Nausea and weight loss occur more commonly in GU patients. Endoscopy detects ulcers in <30% of patients who have dyspepsia.

The mechanism for development of abdominal pain in ulcer patients is unknown. Several possible explanations include acid-induced activation of chemical receptors in the duodenum, enhanced duodenal sensitivity to bile acids and pepsin, or altered gastroduodenal motility.

Variation in the intensity or distribution of the abdominal pain, as well as the onset of associated symptoms such as nausea and/or vomiting, may be indicative of an ulcer complication. Dyspepsia that becomes constant, is no longer relieved by food or antacids, or radiates to the back may indicate a penetrating ulcer (pancreas). Sudden onset of severe, generalized abdominal pain may indicate perforation. Pain worsening with meals, nausea, and vomiting of undigested food suggest gastric outlet obstruction. Tarry stools or coffee-ground emesis indicate bleeding.

Physical examination

Epigastric tenderness is the most frequent finding in patients with GU or DU. Pain may be found to the right of the midline in 20% of patients. Unfortunately, the predictive value of this finding is rather low. Physical examination is critically important for discovering evidence of ulcer complication. Tachycardia and orthostasis suggest dehydration secondary to vomiting or active GI blood loss. A severely tender, board-like abdomen suggests a perforation. Presence of a succussion splash indicates retained fluid in the stomach, suggesting gastric outlet obstruction.

PUD-related complications

Gastrointestinal bleeding

GI bleeding is the most common complication observed in PUD. It occurs in ~15% of patients and more often in individuals >60 years of age. The mortality rate is as high as 5–10%. The higher incidence in the elderly is likely due to the increased use of NSAIDs in this group. Up to 20% of patients with ulcer-related hemorrhage bleed without any preceding warning signs or symptoms.

Perforation

The second most common ulcer-related complication is perforation, being reported in as many as 6–7% of PUD patients. As in the case of bleeding, the incidence of perforation in the elderly appears to be increasing secondary to increased use of NSAIDs. *Penetration* is a form of perforation in which the ulcer bed tunnels into an adjacent organ. DUs tend to penetrate posteriorly into the pancreas, leading to pancreatitis, whereas GUs tend to penetrate into the left hepatic lobe. Gastrocolic fistulas associated with GUs have also been described.

Gastric outlet obstruction

Gastric outlet obstruction is the least common ulcer-related complication, occurring in 1–2% of patients. A patient may have relative obstruction secondary to ulcer-related inflammation and edema in the peripyloric region. This process often resolves with ulcer healing. A fixed, mechanical obstruction secondary to scar formation in the peripyloric areas is also possible. The latter requires endoscopic (balloon dilation) or surgical intervention. Signs and symptoms relative to mechanical obstruction may develop insidiously. New onset of early satiety, nausea, vomiting, increase of postprandial abdominal pain, and weight loss should make gastric outlet obstruction a possible diagnosis.

Differential diagnosis

The list of gastrointestinal and nongastrointestinal disorders that can mimic ulceration of the stomach or duodenum is quite extensive. The most commonly encountered diagnosis among patients seen for upper abdominal discomfort is NUD. NUD, also known as *functional dyspepsia* or *essential dyspepsia,* refers to a group of heterogeneous disorders typified by upper abdominal pain without the presence of an ulcer. Dyspepsia has been reported to occur in up to 30% of the U.S. population. Up to 60% of patients seeking medical care for dyspepsia have a negative diagnostic evaluation. The etiology of NUD is not established, and the potential role of *H. pylori* in NUD remains controversial.

Several additional disease processes that may present with "ulcer-like" symptoms include proximal GI tumors, gastroesophageal reflux, vascular disease, pancreaticobiliary disease (biliary colic, chronic pancreatitis), and gastroduodenal Crohn's disease.

Diagnostic evaluation

In view of the poor predictive value of abdominal pain for the presence of a gastroduodenal ulcer and the multiple disease processes that can mimic this disease, the clinician is often confronted with having to establish the presence of an ulcer. Documentation of an ulcer requires either a radiographic (barium study) or an endoscopic procedure. However, a large percentage of patients with symptoms suggestive of an ulcer have NUD; empirical therapy is appropriate for individuals who are otherwise healthy and <45 years of age, before embarking on a diagnostic evaluation (Chap. 5).

Barium studies of the proximal GI tract are still commonly used as a first test for documenting an ulcer. The sensitivity of older single-contrast barium meals for detecting a DU is as high as 80%, with a double-contrast study providing detection rates as high as 90%. Sensitivity for detection is decreased in small ulcers (<0.5 cm), presence of previous scarring, or in postoperative patients. A DU appears as a well-demarcated crater, most often seen in the bulb (**Fig. 14-10A**). A GU may represent benign or malignant disease. Typically, a benign GU also appears as a discrete crater with radiating mucosal folds originating from the ulcer margin (Fig. 14-10*B*). Ulcers >3 cm in size or those associated with a mass are more often malignant. Unfortunately, up to 8% of GUs that appear to be benign by radiographic appearance are malignant by endoscopy or surgery. Radiographic studies that show a GU must be followed by endoscopy and biopsy.

Endoscopy provides the most sensitive and specific approach for examining the upper GI tract (**Fig. 14-11**). In addition to permitting direct visualization of the mucosa, endoscopy facilitates photographic documentation of a mucosal defect and tissue biopsy to rule out malignancy (GU) or *H. pylori*. Endoscopic examination is particularly helpful in identifying lesions too small to detect by radiographic examination, for evaluation of atypical radiographic abnormalities, or to determine if an ulcer is a source of blood loss.

FIGURE 14-10
Barium study demonstrating: *A.* a benign duodenal ulcer; ***B.*** a benign gastric ulcer.

The methods for diagnosing *H. pylori* are briefly discussed here **(Table 14-2)**. Several biopsy urease tests have been developed (PyloriTek, CLOtest, Hpfast, Pronto Dry) that have a sensitivity and specificity of >90–95%. Several noninvasive methods for detecting this organism have been developed. Three types of studies routinely used include serologic testing, the ^{13}C- or ^{14}C-urea breath test, and the fecal *H. pylori* (Hp) antigen test. A urinary Hp antigen test, as well as a refined monoclonal antibody stool antigen test, appears promising.

Occasionally, specialized testing such as serum gastrin and gastric acid analysis or sham feeding may be needed

in individuals with complicated or refractory PUD [see "Zollinger-Ellison"]. Screening for aspirin or NSAIDs (blood or urine) may also be necessary in refractory *H. pylori*–negative PUD patients.

TREATMENT Peptic Ulcer Disease

Before the discovery of *H. pylori*, the therapy of PUD was centered on the old dictum by Schwartz of "no acid, no ulcer." Although acid secretion is still important in the pathogenesis of PUD, eradication of *H. pylori* and

FIGURE 14-11
Endoscopy demonstrating: *A.* a benign duodenal ulcer; ***B.*** a benign gastric ulcer.

TABLE 14-2

TESTS FOR DETECTION OF *H. PYLORI*

TEST	SENSITIVITY/ SPECIFICITY, %	COMMENTS
Invasive (Endoscopy/Biopsy Required)		
Rapid urease	80–95/95–100	Simple, false negative with recent use of PPIs, antibiotics, or bismuth compounds
Histology	80–90/>95	Requires pathology processing and staining; provides histologic information
Culture	—/—	Time-consuming, expensive, dependent on experience; allows determination of antibiotic susceptibility
Noninvasive		
Serology	>80/>90	Inexpensive, convenient; not useful for early follow-up
Urea breath test	>90/>90	Simple, rapid; useful for early follow-up; false negatives with recent therapy (see rapid urease test); exposure to low-dose radiation with ^{14}C test
Stool antigen	>90/>90	Inexpensive, convenient; not established for eradication but promising

Abbreviation: PPIs, proton pump inhibitors.

therapy/prevention of NSAID-induced disease is the mainstay of treatment. A summary of commonly used drugs for treatment of acid peptic disorders is shown in Table 14-3.

ACID NEUTRALIZING/INHIBITORY DRUGS

Antacids Before we understood the important role of histamine in stimulating parietal cell activity, neutralization of secreted acid with antacids constituted the main form of therapy for peptic ulcers. They are now rarely, if ever, used as the primary therapeutic agent but instead are often used by patients for symptomatic relief of dyspepsia. The most commonly used agents are mixtures of aluminum hydroxide and magnesium hydroxide. Aluminum hydroxide can produce constipation and phosphate depletion; magnesium hydroxide may cause loose stools. Many of the commonly used antacids (e.g., Maalox, Mylanta) have a combination of both aluminum and magnesium hydroxide in order to avoid these side effects. The magnesium-containing

TABLE 14-3

DRUGS USED IN THE TREATMENT OF PEPTIC ULCER DISEASE

DRUG TYPE/ MECHANISM	EXAMPLES	DOSE
Acid-suppressing drugs		
Antacids	Mylanta, Maalox, Tums, Gaviscon	100–140 meq/L 1 and 3 h after meals and hs
H$_2$ receptor antagonists	Cimetidine	400 mg bid
	Ranitidine	300 mg hs
	Famotidine	40 mg hs
	Nizatidine	300 mg hs
Proton pump inhibitors	Omeprazole	20 mg/d
	Lansoprazole	30 mg/d
	Rabeprazole	20 mg/d
	Pantoprazole	40 mg/d
	Esomeprazole	20 mg/d
Mucosal protective agents		
Sucralfate	Sucralfate	1 g qid
Prostaglandin analogue	Misoprostol	200 µg qid
Bismuth-containing compounds	Bismuth subsalicylate (BSS)	See anti-*H. pylori* regimens (Table 14-4)

Abbreviation: hs, at bedtime (*hora somni*).

preparation should not be used in chronic renal failure patients because of possible hypermagnesemia, and aluminum may cause chronic neurotoxicity in these patients.

Calcium carbonate and sodium bicarbonate are potent antacids with varying levels of potential problems. The long-term use of calcium carbonate (converts to calcium chloride in the stomach) can lead to milk-alkali syndrome (hypercalcemia, hyperphosphatemia with possible renal calcinosis and progression to renal insufficiency). Sodium bicarbonate may induce systemic alkalosis.

H$_2$ Receptor Antagonists Four of these agents are presently available (cimetidine, ranitidine, famotidine, and nizatidine), and their structures share homology with histamine. Although each has different potency, all will significantly inhibit basal and stimulated acid secretion to comparable levels when used at therapeutic doses. Moreover, similar ulcer-healing rates are achieved with each drug when used at the correct dosage. Presently, this class of drug is often used for treatment of active ulcers (4–6 weeks) in combination with antibiotics directed at eradicating *H. pylori* (discussed later).

Cimetidine was the first H$_2$ receptor antagonist used for the treatment of acid peptic disorders. The initial recommended dosing profile for cimetidine was

300 mg qid. Subsequent studies have documented the efficacy of using 800 mg at bedtime for treatment of active ulcer, with healing rates approaching 80% at 4 weeks. Cimetidine may have weak antiandrogenic side effects resulting in reversible gynecomastia and impotence, primarily in patients receiving high doses for prolonged periods of time (months to years, as in ZES). In view of cimetidine's ability to inhibit cytochrome P450, careful monitoring of drugs such as warfarin, phenytoin, and theophylline is indicated with long-term usage. Other rare reversible adverse effects reported with cimetidine include confusion and elevated levels of serum aminotransferases, creatinine, and serum prolactin. Ranitidine, famotidine, and nizatidine are more potent H_2 receptor antagonists than cimetidine. Each can be used once a day at bedtime for ulcer prevention, which was commonly done before the discovery of *H. pylori* and the development of proton pump inhibitors (PPIs). Patients may develop tolerance to H_2 blockers, a rare event with PPIs (discussed later). Comparable nighttime dosing regimens are ranitidine 300 mg, famotidine 40 mg, and nizatidine 300 mg.

Additional rare, reversible systemic toxicities reported with H_2 receptor antagonists include pancytopenia, neutropenia, anemia, and thrombocytopenia, with a prevalence rate varying from 0.01–0.2%. Cimetidine and ranitidine (to a lesser extent) can bind to hepatic cytochrome P450; famotidine and nizatidine do not.

Proton Pump (H^+,K^+-ATPase) Inhibitors

Omeprazole, esomeprazole, lansoprazole, rabeprazole, and pantoprazole are substituted benzimidazole derivatives that covalently bind and irreversibly inhibit H^+,K^+-ATPase. Esomeprazole, the newest member of this drug class, is the S-enantiomer of omeprazole, which is a racemic mixture of both S- and R-optical isomers. These are the most potent acid inhibitory agents available. Omeprazole and lansoprazole are the PPIs that have been used for the longest time. Both are acid-labile and are administered as enteric-coated granules in a sustained-release capsule that dissolves within the small intestine at a pH of 6. Lansoprazole is available in an orally disintegrating tablet that can be taken with or without water, an advantage for individuals who have significant dysphagia. Absorption kinetics are similar to the capsule. In addition, a lansoprazole-naproxen combination preparation that has been made available is targeted at decreasing NSAID-related GI injury (discussed later). Omeprazole is available as nonenteric-coated granules mixed with sodium bicarbonate in a powder form that can be administered orally or via gastric tube. The sodium bicarbonate has two purposes: to protect the omeprazole from acid degradation and to promote rapid gastric alkalinization and subsequent proton pump activation, which facilitates rapid action

of the PPI. Pantoprazole and rabeprazole are available as enteric-coated tablets. Pantoprazole is also available as a parenteral formulation for intravenous use. These agents are lipophilic compounds; upon entering the parietal cell, they are protonated and trapped within the acid environment of the tubulovesicular and canalicular system. These agents potently inhibit all phases of gastric acid secretion. Onset of action is rapid, with a maximum acid inhibitory effect between 2 and 6 hours after administration and duration of inhibition lasting up to 72–96 hours. With repeated daily dosing, progressive acid inhibitory effects are observed, with basal and secretagogue-stimulated acid production being inhibited by >95% after 1 week of therapy. The half-life of PPIs is ~18 hours; thus, it can take between 2 and 5 days for gastric acid secretion to return to normal levels once these drugs have been discontinued. Because the pumps need to be activated for these agents to be effective, their efficacy is maximized if they are administered before a meal (except for the immediate-release formulation of omeprazole) (e.g., in the morning before breakfast). Mild to moderate hypergastrinemia has been observed in patients taking these drugs. Carcinoid tumors developed in some animals given the drugs preclinically; however, extensive experience has failed to demonstrate gastric carcinoid tumor development in humans. Serum gastrin levels return to normal levels within 1–2 weeks after drug cessation. Rebound gastric acid hypersecretion has been described in *H. pylori*-negative individuals after discontinuation of PPIs. It occurs even after relatively short-term usage (2 months) and may last for up to 2 months after the PPI has been discontinued. The mechanism involves gastrin-induced hyperplasia and hypertrophy of histamine-secreting ECL cells. The clinical relevance of this observation is that individuals may have worsening symptoms of gastroesophageal reflux disease (GERD) or dyspepsia upon stopping the PPI. Gradual tapering of the PPI and switching to an H_2 receptor antagonist may prevent this from occurring. *H. pylori*–induced inflammation and concomitant decrease in acid production may explain why this does not occur in *H. pylori*–positive patients. IF production is also inhibited, but vitamin B_{12}-deficiency anemia is uncommon, probably because of the large stores of the vitamin. As with any agent that leads to significant hypochlorhydria, PPIs may interfere with absorption of drugs such as ketoconazole, ampicillin, iron, and digoxin. Hepatic cytochrome P450 can be inhibited by the earlier PPIs (omeprazole, lansoprazole). Rabeprazole, pantoprazole, and esomeprazole do not appear to interact significantly with drugs metabolized by the cytochrome P450 system. The overall clinical significance of this observation is not definitely established. Caution should be taken when using theophylline, warfarin, diazepam, atazanavir, and phenytoin concomitantly with PPIs. Long-term acid suppression, especially with PPIs, has been associated with a higher incidence of community-acquired pneumonia as well as community- and hospital-acquired *Clostridium difficile*–associated disease. These observations require confirmation but should alert the practitioner to take caution when recommending these agents for long-term use, especially in elderly patients at risk for developing pneumonia or *C. difficile* infection. A population-based study revealed that long-term use of PPIs was associated with the development of hip fractures in older women. The absolute risk of fracture remained low despite an observed increase associated with the dose and duration of acid suppression. The mechanism for this observation is not clear and this finding must be confirmed before making broad recommendations regarding the discontinuation of these agents in patients who benefit from them. PPIs may exert a negative effect on the anti-platelet effect of clopidogrel. Although the evidence is mixed and inconclusive, a small increase in mortality and readmission rate for coronary events is seen in patients receiving a PPI while on clopidogrel. The mechanism involves the competition of the PPI and clopidogrel with the same cytochrome P450 (CYP2C19). Whether this is a class effect of PPIs is unclear; there appears to be at least a theoretical advantage of pantoprazole over the other PPIs, but this has not been confirmed. This drug interaction is particularly relevant in light of the common use of aspirin and clopidogrel for prevention of coronary events and the efficacy of PPIs in preventing GI bleeding in these patients. The FDA has made several recommendations while awaiting further evidence to clarify the impact of PPI therapy on clopidogrel use. Health care providers should continue to prescribe clopidogrel to patients who require it and should reevaluate the need for starting or continuing treatment with a PPI. From a practical standpoint additional recommendations to consider include: Patients taking clopidogrel with aspirin, especially with other GI risk factors for bleeding, should receive GI protective therapy. Although high-dose H$_2$ blockers have been considered an option, these do not appear to be as effective as PPIs. If PPIs are to be given, there should be a 12-h separation between administration of the PPI and clopidogrel to minimize competition of the two agents with the involved cytochrome P450. One option is to give the PPI 30 min before breakfast and the clopidogrel at bedtime. Insufficient data are available to firmly recommend one PPI over another.

Two new formulations of acid inhibitory agents are being developed. Tenatoprazole is a PPI containing an imidazopyridine ring instead of a benzimidazole ring, which promotes irreversible proton pump inhibition. This agent has a longer half-life than the other PPIs and

may be beneficial for inhibiting nocturnal acid secretion, which has significant relevance in GERD. A second new class of agents is the potassium-competitive acid pump antagonists (P-CABs). These compounds inhibit gastric acid secretion via potassium competitive binding of the H$^+$,K$^+$-ATPase.

CYTOPROTECTIVE AGENTS

Sucralfate Sucralfate is a complex sucrose salt in which the hydroxyl groups have been substituted by aluminum hydroxide and sulfate. This compound is insoluble in water and becomes a viscous paste within the stomach and duodenum, binding primarily to sites of active ulceration. Sucralfate may act by several mechanisms: serving as a physicochemical barrier, promoting a trophic action by binding growth factors such as EGF, enhancing prostaglandin synthesis, stimulating mucus and bicarbonate secretion, and enhancing mucosal defense and repair. Toxicity from this drug is rare, with constipation being most common (2–3%). It should be avoided in patients with chronic renal insufficiency to prevent aluminum-induced neurotoxicity. Hypophosphatemia and gastric bezoar formation have also been reported rarely. Standard dosing of sucralfate is 1 g qid.

Bismuth-Containing Preparations Sir William Osler considered bismuth-containing compounds the drug of choice for treating PUD. The resurgence in the use of these agents is due to their effect against *H. pylori*. Colloidal bismuth subcitrate (CBS) and bismuth subsalicylate (BSS, Pepto-Bismol) are the most widely used preparations. The mechanism by which these agents induce ulcer healing is unclear. Adverse effects with short-term usage include black stools, constipation, and darkening of the tongue. Long-term usage with high doses, especially with the avidly absorbed CBS, may lead to neurotoxicity. These compounds are commonly used as one of the agents in an anti-*H. pylori* regimen (discussed later).

Prostaglandin Analogues In view of their central role in maintaining mucosal integrity and repair, stable prostaglandin analogues were developed for the treatment of PUD. The mechanism by which this rapidly absorbed drug provides its therapeutic effect is through enhancement of mucosal defense and repair. The most common toxicity noted with this drug is diarrhea (10–30% incidence). Other major toxicities include uterine bleeding and contractions; misoprostol is contraindicated in women who may be pregnant, and women of childbearing age must be made clearly aware of this potential drug toxicity. The standard therapeutic dose is 200 µg qid.

Miscellaneous Drugs A number of drugs including anticholinergic agents and tricyclic antidepressants were used for treating acid peptic disorders but in light of their toxicity and the development of potent antisecretory agents, these are rarely, if ever, used today.

THERAPY OF *H. PYLORI* Extensive effort has been made in determining who of the many individuals with *H. pylori* infection should be treated. The common conclusion arrived at by multiple consensus conferences around the world is that *H. pylori* should be eradicated in patients with documented PUD. This holds true independent of time of presentation (first episode or not), severity of symptoms, presence of confounding factors such as ingestion of NSAIDs, or whether the ulcer is in remission. Some have advocated treating patients with a history of documented PUD who are found to be *H. pylori*–positive by serology or breath testing. Over one-half of patients with gastric MALT lymphoma experience complete remission of the tumor in response to *H. pylori* eradication. Treating patients with NUD, to prevent gastric cancer or patients with GERD requiring long-term acid suppression, remains controversial. Guidelines from the American College of Gastroenterology suggest eradication of *H. pylori* in patients who have undergone resection of early gastric cancer. The role of *H. pylori* eradication as a means to prevent gastric cancer is still controversial although data suggest a benefit of early eradication of *H. pylori* for prevention of gastric cancer in patients with peptic ulcer disease.

Multiple drugs have been evaluated in the therapy of *H. pylori*. No single agent is effective in eradicating the organism. Combination therapy for 14 days provides the greatest efficacy. A shorter course administration (7–10 days), although attractive, has not proved as successful as the 14-day regimens. The agents used with the greatest frequency include amoxicillin, metronidazole, tetracycline, clarithromycin, and bismuth compounds.

The physician's goal in treating PUD is to provide relief of symptoms (pain or dyspepsia), promote ulcer healing, and ultimately prevent ulcer recurrence and complications. The greatest impact of understanding the role of *H. pylori* in peptic disease has been the ability to prevent recurrence. Documented eradication of *H. pylori* in patients with PUD is associated with a dramatic decrease in ulcer recurrence to <10–20% as compared to 59% in GU patients and 67% in DU patients when the organism is not eliminated. Eradication of the organism may lead to diminished recurrent ulcer bleeding. The impact of its eradication on ulcer perforation is unclear.

Suggested treatment regimens for *H. pylori* are outlined in **Table 14-4**. Choice of a particular regimen will be influenced by several factors, including efficacy, patient tolerance, existing antibiotic resistance, and cost

TABLE 14-4

REGIMENS RECOMMENDED FOR ERADICATION OF *H. PYLORI* INFECTION	
DRUG	**DOSE**
Triple Therapy	
1. Bismuth subsalicylate *plus*	2 tablets qid
Metronidazole *plus*	250 mg qid
Tetracycline[a]	500 mg qid
2. Ranitidine bismuth citrate *plus*	400 mg bid
Tetracycline *plus*	500 mg bid
Clarithromycin or metronidazole	500 mg bid
3. Omeprazole (lansoprazole) *plus*	20 mg bid (30 mg bid)
Clarithromycin *plus*	250 or 500 mg bid
Metronidazole[b] *or*	500 mg bid
Amoxicillin[c]	1 g bid
Quadruple Therapy	
Omeprazole (lansoprazole)	20 mg (30 mg) daily
Bismuth subsalicylate	2 tablets qid
Metronidazole	250 mg qid
Tetracycline	500 mg qid

[a]Alternative: use prepacked Helidac (see text).
[b]Alternative: use prepacked Prevpac (see text).
[c]Use either metronidazole or amoxicillin, not both.

of the drugs. The aim for initial eradication rates should be 85–90%. Dual therapy [PPI plus amoxicillin, PPI plus clarithromycin, ranitidine bismuth citrate (Tritec) plus clarithromycin] is not recommended in view of studies demonstrating eradication rates of <80–85%. The combination of bismuth, metronidazole, and tetracycline was the first triple regimen found effective against *H. pylori*. The combination of two antibiotics plus either a PPI, H$_2$ blocker, or bismuth compound has comparable success rates. Addition of acid suppression assists in providing early symptom relief and may enhance bacterial eradication.

Triple therapy, although effective, has several drawbacks, including the potential for poor patient compliance and drug-induced side effects. Compliance is being addressed by simplifying the regimens so that patients can take the medications twice a day. Simpler (dual therapy) and shorter regimens (7 and 10 days) are not as effective as triple therapy for 14 days. Two anti-*H. pylori* regimens are available in prepackaged formulation: Prevpac (lansoprazole, clarithromycin, and amoxicillin) and Helidac (BSS, tetracycline, and metronidazole). The contents of the Prevpac are to be taken twice per day for 14 days, whereas Helidac constituents are taken four times per day with an antisecretory agent (PPI or H$_2$ blocker), also for at least 14 days.

Side effects have been reported in up to 20–30% of patients on triple therapy. Bismuth may cause black stools, constipation, or darkening of the tongue. The most feared complication with amoxicillin is pseudomembranous colitis, but this occurs in <1–2% of patients. Amoxicillin can also lead to antibiotic-associated diarrhea, nausea, vomiting, skin rash, and allergic reaction. Tetracycline has been reported to cause rashes and, very rarely, hepatotoxicity and anaphylaxis.

One important concern with treating patients who may not need therapy is the potential for development of antibiotic-resistant strains. The incidence and type of antibiotic-resistant *H. pylori* strains vary worldwide. Strains resistant to metronidazole, clarithromycin, amoxicillin, and tetracycline have been described, with the latter two being uncommon. Antibiotic-resistant strains are the most common cause for treatment failure in compliant patients. Unfortunately, in vitro resistance does not predict outcome in patients. Culture and sensitivity testing of *H. pylori* is not performed routinely. Although resistance to metronidazole has been found in as many as 30% of isolates in North America and 80% in developing countries, triple therapy is effective in eradicating the organism in >50% of patients infected with a resistant strain. Clarithromycin resistance is seen in 13% of individuals in the United States, with resistance to amoxicillin being <1% and resistance to both metronidazole and clarithromycin in the 5% range.

Failure of *H. pylori* eradication with triple therapy in a compliant patient is usually due to infection with a resistant organism. Quadruple therapy (Table 14-4), where clarithromycin is substituted for metronidazole (or vice versa), should be the next step. The combination of pantoprazole, amoxicillin, and rifabutin for 10 days has also been used successfully (86% cure rate) in patients infected with resistant strains. Additional regimens considered for second-line therapy include levofloxacin-based triple therapy (levofloxacin, amoxicillin, PPI) for 10 days and furazolidone-based triple therapy (furazolidone, amoxicillin, PPI) for 14 days. Unfortunately, there is no universally accepted treatment regimen recommended for patients who have failed two courses of antibiotics. If eradication is still not achieved in a compliant patient, then culture and sensitivity of the organism should be considered. Additional factors that may lower eradication rates include the patient's country of origin (higher in Northeast Asia than other parts of Asia or Europe) and cigarette smoking. In addition, meta-analysis suggests that even the most effective regimens (quadruple therapy including PPI, bismuth, tetracycline, and metronidazole and triple therapy including PPI, clarithromycin, and amoxicillin) may have suboptimal eradication rates (<80%), thus demonstrating the need for the development of more efficacious treatments.

In view of the observation that 15–25% of patients treated with first-line therapy may still remain infected with the organism, new approaches to treatment have been explored. One promising approach is sequential therapy. This regimen consists of 5 days of amoxicillin and a PPI, followed by an additional 5 days of PPI plus tinidazole and clarithromycin. Initial studies have demonstrated eradication rates of >90% with good patient tolerance. Confirmation of these findings and applicability of this approach in the United States are needed.

Reinfection after successful eradication of *H. pylori* is rare in the United States (<1% per year). If recurrent infection occurs within the first 6 months after completing therapy, the most likely explanation is recrudescence as opposed to reinfection.

THERAPY OF NSAID-RELATED GASTRIC OR DUODENAL INJURY Medical intervention for NSAID-related mucosal injury includes treatment of an active ulcer and primary prevention of future injury. Recommendations for the treatment and primary prevention of NSAID-related mucosal injury are listed in Table 14-5. Ideally, the injurious agent should be stopped as the first step in the therapy of an active NSAID-induced ulcer. If that is possible, then treatment with one of the acid inhibitory agents (H_2 blockers, PPIs) is indicated. Cessation of NSAIDs is not always possible because of the patient's severe underlying disease. Only PPIs can heal GUs or DUs, independent of whether NSAIDs are discontinued.

The approach to primary prevention has included avoiding the agent, using NSAIDs that are theoretically less injurious, and/or the use of concomitant medical therapy to prevent NSAID-induced injury. Several nonselective NSAIDs that are associated with a lower likelihood of GI toxicity include diclofenac, aceclofenac, and

TABLE 14-5

RECOMMENDATIONS FOR TREATMENT OF NSAID-RELATED MUCOSAL INJURY

CLINICAL SETTING	RECOMMENDATION
Active ulcer	
NSAID discontinued	H_2 receptor antagonist or PPI
NSAID continued	PPI
Prophylactic therapy	Misoprostol
	PPI
	Selective COX-2 inhibitor
H. pylori infection	Eradication if active ulcer present or there is a past history of peptic ulcer disease

Abbreviations: COX-2, isoenzyme of cyclooxygenase; PPI, proton pump inhibitor.

ibuprofen, although the beneficial effect may be eliminated if higher dosages of the agents are used. Primary prevention of NSAID-induced ulceration can be accomplished by misoprostol (200 μg qid) or a PPI. High-dose H_2 blockers (famotidine, 40 mg bid) have also shown some promise in preventing endoscopically documented ulcers, although PPIs are superior. The highly selective COX-2 inhibitors, celecoxib and rofecoxib, are 100 times more selective inhibitors of COX-2 than standard NSAIDs, leading to gastric or duodenal mucosal injury that is comparable to placebo; their utilization led to an increase in cardiovascular events and withdrawal from the market. Additional caution was engendered when the CLASS study demonstrated that the advantage of celecoxib in preventing GI complications was offset when low-dose aspirin was used simultaneously. Therefore, gastric protection therapy is required in individuals taking COX-2 inhibitors and aspirin prophylaxis. Finally, much of the work demonstrating the benefit of COX-2 inhibitors and PPIs on GI injury has been performed in individuals of average risk; it is unclear if the same level of benefit will be achieved in high-risk patients. For example, concomitant use of warfarin and a COX-2 inhibitor was associated with rates of GI bleeding similar to those observed in patients taking nonselective NSAIDs. A combination of factors, including withdrawal of the majority of COX-2 inhibitors from the market, the observation that low-dose aspirin appears to diminish the beneficial effect of COX-2 selective inhibitors, and the growing use of aspirin for prophylaxis of cardiovascular events, have significantly altered the approach to gastric protective therapy during the use of NSAIDs. A set of guidelines for the approach to the use of NSAIDs was published by the American College of Gastroenterology and is shown in Table 14-6. Individuals who are not at risk for cardiovascular events, do not use aspirin, and are without risk for GI complications can receive nonselective NSAIDs without gastric protection. In those without cardiovascular risk factors but with a high potential risk (prior GI bleeding or multiple GI risk factors) for NSAID-induced GI toxicity, cautious use of a selective COX-2 inhibitor and co-therapy with misoprostol or high-dose PPI is recommended. Individuals at moderate GI risk without cardiac risk factors can be treated with a COX-2 inhibitor alone or with a nonselective NSAID with misoprostol or a PPI. Individuals with cardiovascular risk factors, who require low-dose aspirin and have low potential for NSAID-induced toxicity, should be considered for a non-NSAID agent or use of a traditional NSAID in combination with gastric protection, if warranted. Finally, individuals with cardiovascular and GI risks who require aspirin must be considered for non-NSAID therapy, but if that is not an option, then gastric protection with any type of NSAID

TABLE 14-6

GUIDE TO NSAID THERAPY

	NO/LOW NSAID GI RISK	NSAID GI RISK
No CV risk (no aspirin)	Traditional NSAID	Coxib *or* Traditional NSAID + PPI *or* misoprostol Consider non-NSAID therapy
CV risk (consider aspirin)	Traditional NSAID + PPI *or* misoprostol if GI risk warrants gastroprotection Consider non-NSAID therapy	A gastroprotective agent must be added if a traditional NSAID is prescribed Consider non-NSAID therapy

Abbreviations: CV, cardiovascular; GI, gastrointestinal; NSAID, nonsteroidal anti-inflammatory drug; PPI, proton pump inhibitor.
Source: Adapted from AM Fendrick: Am J Manag Care 10:740, 2004. Reproduced with permission of INTELLISPHERE, LLC via Copyright Clearance Center.

must be considered. Any patient, regardless of risk status, who is being considered for long-term traditional NSAID therapy, should also be considered for *H. pylori* testing and treatment if positive.

APPROACH AND THERAPY: SUMMARY
Controversy continues regarding the best approach to the patient who presents with dyspepsia (Chap. 5). The discovery of *H. pylori* and its role in pathogenesis of ulcers has added a new variable to the equation. Previously, if a patient <50 years of age presented with dyspepsia and without alarming signs or symptoms suggestive of an ulcer complication or malignancy, an empirical therapeutic trial with acid suppression was commonly recommended. Although this approach is practiced by some today, an approach presently gaining approval for the treatment of patients with dyspepsia is outlined in Fig. 14-12. The referral to a gastroenterologist is for the potential need of endoscopy and subsequent evaluation and treatment if the endoscopy is negative.

Once an ulcer (GU or DU) is documented, the main issue at stake is whether *H. pylori* or an NSAID is involved. With *H. pylori* present, independent of the NSAID status, triple therapy is recommended for 14 days, followed by continued acid-suppressing drugs (H_2 receptor antagonist or PPIs) for a total of 4–6 weeks. Selection of patients for documentation of *H. pylori* eradication (organisms gone at least 4 weeks after completing antibiotics) is an area of some debate. The test of choice for documenting eradication is the urea breath

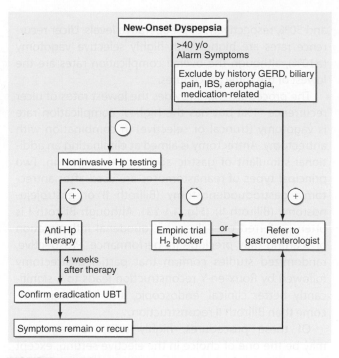

FIGURE 14-12

Overview of new-onset dyspepsia. Hp, *Helicobacter pylori*; UBT, urea breath test; IBS, irritable bowel syndrome. (*Adapted from BS Anand and DY Graham: Endoscopy 31:215, 1999.*)

test (UBT). The stool antigen assay may also hold promise for this purpose, but the data have not been as clear cut as in the case of using the stool antigen test for primary diagnosis, especially if one considers patients who live in areas of low *H. pylori* prevalence. Further studies are warranted, but if the UBT is not available, a stool antigen should be considered to document eradication. The patient must be off antisecretory agents when being tested for eradication of *H. pylori* with UBT or stool antigen. Serologic testing is not useful for the purpose of documenting eradication since antibody titers fall slowly and often do not become undetectable. Two approaches toward documentation of eradication exist: (1) Test for eradication only in individuals with a complicated course or in individuals who are frail or with multisystem disease who would do poorly with an ulcer recurrence, and (2) test all patients for successful eradication. Some recommend that patients with complicated ulcer disease, or who are frail, should be treated with long-term acid suppression, thus making documentation of *H. pylori* eradication a moot point. In view of this discrepancy in practice, it would be best to discuss with the patient the different options available.

Several issues differentiate the approach to a GU versus a DU. GUs, especially of the body and fundus, have the potential of being malignant. Multiple biopsies of a GU should be taken initially; even if these are negative for

neoplasm, repeat endoscopy to document healing at 8–12 weeks should be performed, with biopsy if the ulcer is still present. About 70% of GUs eventually found to be malignant undergo significant (usually incomplete) healing.

The majority (>90%) of GUs and DUs heal with the conventional therapy outlined earlier. A GU that fails to heal after 12 weeks and a DU that does not heal after 8 weeks of therapy should be considered refractory. Once poor compliance and persistent *H. pylori* infection have been excluded, NSAID use, either inadvertent or surreptitious, must be excluded. In addition, cigarette smoking must be eliminated. For a GU, malignancy must be meticulously excluded. Next, consideration should be given to a gastric acid hypersecretory state such as ZES (see "Zollinger-Ellison Syndrome,") or the idiopathic form, which can be excluded with gastric acid analysis. Although a subset of patients have gastric acid hypersecretion of unclear etiology as a contributing factor to refractory ulcers, ZES should be excluded with a fasting gastrin or secretin stimulation test (discussed later). More than 90% of refractory ulcers (either DUs or GUs) heal after 8 weeks of treatment with higher doses of PPI (omeprazole, 40 mg/d; lansoprazole 30–60 mg/d). This higher dose is also effective in maintaining remission. Surgical intervention may be a consideration at this point; however, other rare causes of refractory ulcers must be excluded before recommending surgery. Rare etiologies of refractory ulcers that may be diagnosed by gastric or duodenal biopsies include ischemia, Crohn's disease, amyloidosis, sarcoidosis, lymphoma, eosinophilic gastroenteritis, or infection [cytomegalovirus (CMV), tuberculosis, or syphilis].

SURGICAL THERAPY Surgical intervention in PUD can be viewed as being either elective, for treatment of medically refractory disease, or as urgent/emergent, for the treatment of an ulcer-related complication. The development of pharmacologic and endoscopic approaches for the treatment of peptic disease and its complications has led to a substantial decrease in the number of operations needed for this disorder. Refractory ulcers are an exceedingly rare occurrence. Surgery is more often required for treatment of an ulcer-related complication.

Hemorrhage is the most common ulcer-related complication, occurring in ~15–25% of patients. Bleeding may occur in any age group but is most often seen in older patients (sixth decade or beyond). The majority of patients stop bleeding spontaneously, but endoscopic therapy (Chap. 12) is necessary in some. Parenterally and orally administered PPIs also decrease ulcer rebleeding in patients who have undergone endoscopic therapy. Patients unresponsive or refractory to endoscopic intervention will require surgery (~5% of transfusion-requiring patients).

Free peritoneal perforation occurs in ~2–3% of DU patients. As in the case of bleeding, up to 10% of these patients will not have antecedent ulcer symptoms. Concomitant bleeding may occur in up to 10% of patients with perforation, with mortality being increased substantially. Peptic ulcer can also penetrate into adjacent organs, especially with a posterior DU, which can penetrate into the pancreas, colon, liver, or biliary tree.

Pyloric channel ulcers or DUs can lead to gastric outlet obstruction in ~2–3% of patients. This can result from chronic scarring or from impaired motility due to inflammation and/or edema with pylorospasm. Patients may present with early satiety, nausea, vomiting of undigested food, and weight loss. Conservative management with nasogastric suction, intravenous hydration/nutrition, and antisecretory agents is indicated for 7–10 days with the hope that a functional obstruction will reverse. If a mechanical obstruction persists, endoscopic intervention with balloon dilation may be effective. Surgery should be considered if all else fails.

SPECIFIC OPERATIONS FOR DUODENAL ULCERS Surgical treatment is designed to decrease gastric acid secretion. Operations most commonly performed include (1) vagotomy and drainage (by pyloroplasty, gastroduodenostomy, or gastrojejunostomy), (2) highly selective vagotomy (which does not require a drainage procedure), and (3) vagotomy with antrectomy. The specific procedure performed is dictated by the underlying circumstances: elective vs. emergency, the degree and extent of duodenal ulceration, and the expertise of the surgeon. Moreover, the trend has been toward minimally invasive and anatomy-preserving operations.

Vagotomy is a component of each of these procedures and is aimed at decreasing acid secretion through ablating cholinergic input to the stomach. Unfortunately, both truncal and selective vagotomy (preserves the celiac and hepatic branches) result in gastric atony despite successful reduction of both basal acid output (BAO, decreased by 85%) and maximal acid output (MAO, decreased by 50%). Drainage through pyloroplasty or gastroduodenostomy is required in an effort to compensate for the vagotomy-induced gastric motility disorder. This procedure has an intermediate complication rate and a 10% ulcer recurrence rate. To minimize gastric dysmotility, highly selective vagotomy (also known as parietal cell, super-selective, or proximal vagotomy) was developed. Only the vagal fibers innervating the portion of the stomach that contains parietal cells is transected, thus leaving fibers important for regulating gastric motility intact. Although this procedure leads to an immediate decrease in both BAO and stimulated acid output, acid secretion recovers over time. By the end of the first postoperative year, basal and stimulated acid output are ~30

and 50%, respectively, of preoperative levels. Ulcer recurrence rates are higher with highly selective vagotomy (≥10%), although the overall complication rates are the lowest of the three procedures.

The procedure that provides the lowest rates of ulcer recurrence (1%) but has the highest complication rate is vagotomy (truncal or selective) in combination with antrectomy. Antrectomy is aimed at eliminating an additional stimulant of gastric acid secretion, gastrin. Two principal types of reanastomoses are used after antrectomy: gastroduodenostomy (Billroth I) or gastrojejunostomy (Billroth II) (Fig. 14-13). Although Billroth I is often preferred over II, severe duodenal inflammation or scarring may preclude its performance. Prospective, randomized studies confirm that partial gastrectomy followed by Roux-en-Y reconstruction leads to a significantly better clinical, endoscopic, and histologic outcome than Billroth II reconstruction.

Of these procedures, highly selective vagotomy may be the one of choice in the elective setting, except in situations where ulcer recurrence rates are high (prepyloric ulcers and those refractory to medical therapy). Selection of vagotomy and antrectomy may be more appropriate in these circumstances.

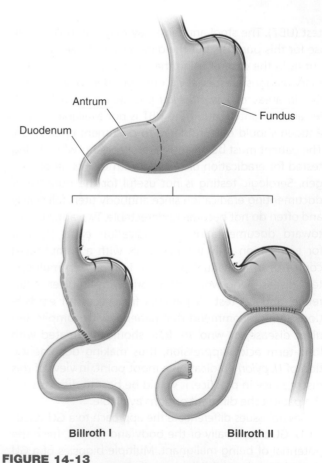

FIGURE 14-13
Schematic representation of Billroth I and II procedures.

These procedures have been traditionally performed by standard laparotomy. The advent of laparoscopic surgery has led several surgical teams to successfully perform highly selective vagotomy, truncal vagotomy/pyloroplasty, and truncal vagotomy/antrectomy through this approach. An increase in the number of laparoscopic procedures for treatment of PUD has occurred. Laparoscopic repair of perforated peptic ulcers is safe, feasible for the experienced surgeon and is associated with decreased postoperative pain, although it does take longer than an open approach. Moreover, no difference between the two approaches is noted in postoperative complications or length of hospital stay.

Specific Operations for Gastric Ulcers The location and the presence of a concomitant DU dictate the operative procedure performed for a GU. Antrectomy (including the ulcer) with a Billroth I anastomosis is the treatment of choice for an antral ulcer. Vagotomy is performed only if a DU is present. Although ulcer excision with vagotomy and drainage procedure has been proposed, the higher incidence of ulcer recurrence makes this a less desirable approach. Ulcers located near the esophagogastric junction may require a more radical approach, a subtotal gastrectomy with a Roux-en-Y esophagogastrojejunostomy (Csende's procedure). A less aggressive approach, including antrectomy, intraoperative ulcer biopsy, and vagotomy (Kelling-Madlener procedure), may be indicated in fragile patients with a high GU. Ulcer recurrence approaches 30% with this procedure.

Surgery-Related Complications Complications seen after surgery for PUD are related primarily to the extent of the anatomic modification performed. Minimal alteration (highly selective vagotomy) is associated with higher rates of ulcer recurrence and less GI disturbance. More aggressive surgical procedures have a lower rate of ulcer recurrence but a greater incidence of GI dysfunction. Overall, morbidity and mortality related to these procedures are quite low. Morbidity associated with vagotomy and antrectomy or pyloroplasty is ≤5%, with mortality ~1%. Highly selective vagotomy has lower morbidity and mortality rates of 1 and 0.3%, respectively.

In addition to the potential early consequences of any intraabdominal procedure (bleeding, infection, thromboembolism), gastroparesis, duodenal stump leak, and efferent loop obstruction can be observed.

Recurrent ulceration The risk of ulcer recurrence is directly related to the procedure performed. Ulcers that recur after partial gastric resection tend to develop at the anastomosis (stomal or marginal ulcer). Epigastric abdominal pain is the most frequent presenting complaint (>90%). Severity and duration of pain tend to be more progressive than observed with DUs before surgery.

Ulcers may recur for several reasons, including incomplete vagotomy, inadequate drainage, retained antrum, and, less likely, persistent or recurrent *H. pylori* infection. ZES should have been excluded preoperatively. Surreptitious use of NSAIDs is an important reason for recurrent ulcers after surgery, especially if the initial procedure was done for an NSAID-induced ulcer. Once *H. pylori* and NSAIDs have been excluded as etiologic factors, the question of incomplete vagotomy or retained gastric antrum should be explored. For the latter, fasting plasma gastrin levels should be determined. If elevated, retained antrum or ZES (discussed later) should be considered. Incomplete vagotomy can be ruled out by gastric acid analysis coupled with sham feeding. In this test, gastric acid output is measured while the patient sees, smells, and chews a meal (without swallowing). The cephalic phase of gastric secretion, which is mediated by the vagus, is being assessed with this study. An increase in gastric acid output in response to sham feeding is evidence that the vagus nerve is intact. A rise in serum pancreatic polypeptide >50% within 30 min of sham feeding is also suggestive of an intact vagus nerve.

Medical therapy with H_2 blockers will heal postoperative ulceration in 70–90% of patients. The efficacy of PPIs has not been fully assessed in this group, but one may anticipate greater rates of ulcer healing compared to those obtained with H_2 blockers. Repeat operation (complete vagotomy, partial gastrectomy) may be required in a small subgroup of patients who have not responded to aggressive medical management.

Afferent loop syndromes Two types of afferent loop syndrome can occur in patients who have undergone partial gastric resection with Billroth II anastomosis. The more common of the two is bacterial overgrowth in the afferent limb secondary to stasis. Patients may experience postprandial abdominal pain, bloating, and diarrhea with concomitant malabsorption of fats and vitamin B_{12}. Cases refractory to antibiotics may require surgical revision of the loop. The less common afferent loop syndrome can present with severe abdominal pain and bloating that occur 20–60 min after meals. Pain is often followed by nausea and vomiting of bile-containing material. The pain and bloating may improve after emesis. The cause of this clinical picture is theorized to be incomplete drainage of bile and pancreatic secretions from an afferent loop that is partially obstructed. Cases refractory to dietary measures may need surgical revision.

Dumping syndrome Dumping syndrome consists of a series of vasomotor and GI signs and symptoms and occurs in patients who have undergone vagotomy and drainage (especially Billroth procedures). Two phases of dumping, early and late, can occur. Early dumping takes place 15–30 min after meals and consists of crampy abdominal discomfort, nausea, diarrhea, belching, tachycardia, palpitations, diaphoresis, light-headedness, and, rarely, syncope. These signs and symptoms arise from the rapid emptying of hyperosmolar gastric contents into the small intestine, resulting in a fluid shift into the gut lumen with plasma volume contraction and acute intestinal distention. Release of vasoactive GI hormones (vasoactive intestinal polypeptide, neurotensin, motilin) is also theorized to play a role in early dumping.

The late phase of dumping typically occurs 90 min to 3 h after meals. Vasomotor symptoms (light-headedness, diaphoresis, palpitations, tachycardia, and syncope) predominate during this phase. This component of dumping is thought to be secondary to hypoglycemia from excessive insulin release.

Dumping syndrome is most noticeable after meals rich in simple carbohydrates (especially sucrose) and high osmolarity. Ingestion of large amounts of fluids may also contribute. Up to 50% of postvagotomy and drainage patients will experience dumping syndrome to some degree. Signs and symptoms often improve with time, but a severe protracted picture can occur in up to 1% of patients.

Dietary modification is the cornerstone of therapy for patients with dumping syndrome. Small, multiple (six) meals devoid of simple carbohydrates coupled with elimination of liquids during meals is important. Antidiarrheals and anticholinergic agents are complementary to diet. Guar and pectin, which increase the viscosity of intraluminal contents, may be beneficial in more symptomatic individuals. Acarbose, an α-glucosidase inhibitor that delays digestion of ingested carbohydrates, has also been shown to be beneficial in the treatment of the late phases of dumping. The somatostatin analogue octreotide has been successful in diet-refractory cases. This drug is administered subcutaneously (50 μg tid), titrated according to clinical response. A long-acting depot formulation of octreotide can be administered once every 28 days and provides symptom relief comparable to the short-acting agent. In addition, patient weight gain and quality of life appear to be superior with the long-acting form.

Postvagotomy diarrhea Up to 10% of patients may seek medical attention for the treatment of postvagotomy diarrhea. This complication is most commonly observed after truncal vagotomy. Patients may complain of intermittent diarrhea that occurs typically 1–2 h after meals. Occasionally the symptoms may be severe and relentless. This is due to a motility disorder from interruption of the vagal fibers supplying the luminal gut. Other contributing factors may include decreased absorption of nutrients (discussed later), increased

excretion of bile acids, and release of luminal factors that promote secretion. Diphenoxylate or loperamide is often useful in symptom control. The bile salt–binding agent cholestyramine may be helpful in severe cases. Surgical reversal of a 10-cm segment of jejunum may yield a substantial improvement in bowel frequency in a subset of patients.

Bile reflux gastropathy A subset of postpartial gastrectomy patients who present with abdominal pain, early satiety, nausea, and vomiting will have mucosal erythema of the gastric remnant as the only finding. Histologic examination of the gastric mucosa reveals minimal inflammation but the presence of epithelial cell injury. This clinical picture is categorized as bile or alkaline reflux gastropathy/gastritis. Although reflux of bile is implicated as the reason for this disorder, the mechanism is unknown. Prokinetic agents, cholestyramine, and sucralfate have been somewhat effective treatments. Severe refractory symptoms may require using either nuclear scanning with ^{99m}Tc-HIDA to document reflux or an alkaline challenge test, where 0.1 N NaOH is infused into the stomach in an effort to reproduce the patient's symptoms. Surgical diversion of pancreaticobiliary secretions away from the gastric remnant with a Roux-en-Y gastrojejunostomy consisting of a long (50–60 cm) Roux limb has been used in severe cases. Bilious vomiting improves, but early satiety and bloating may persist in up to 50% of patients.

Maldigestion and malabsorption Weight loss can be observed in up to 60% of patients after partial gastric resection. A significant component of this weight reduction is due to decreased oral intake. However, mild steatorrhea can also develop. Reasons for maldigestion/malabsorption include decreased gastric acid production, rapid gastric emptying, decreased food dispersion in the stomach, reduced luminal bile concentration, reduced pancreatic secretory response to feeding, and rapid intestinal transit.

Decreased serum vitamin B_{12} levels can be observed after partial gastrectomy. This is usually not due to deficiency of IF, since a minimal amount of parietal cells (source of IF) are removed during antrectomy. Reduced vitamin B_{12} may be due to competition for the vitamin by bacterial overgrowth or inability to split the vitamin from its protein-bound source due to hypochlorhydria.

Iron-deficiency anemia may be a consequence of impaired absorption of dietary iron in patients with a Billroth II gastrojejunostomy. Absorption of iron salts is normal in these individuals; thus, a favorable response to oral iron supplementation can be anticipated. Folate deficiency with concomitant anemia can also develop in these patients. This deficiency may be secondary to decreased absorption or diminished oral intake.

Malabsorption of vitamin D and calcium resulting in osteoporosis and osteomalacia is common after partial gastrectomy and gastrojejunostomy (Billroth II). Osteomalacia can occur as a late complication in up to 25% of postpartial gastrectomy patients. Bone fractures occur twice as commonly in men after gastric surgery as in a control population. It may take years before x-ray findings demonstrate diminished bone density. Elevated alkaline phosphatase, reduced serum calcium, bone pain, and pathologic fractures may be seen in patients with osteomalacia. The high incidence of these abnormalities in this subgroup of patients justifies treating them with vitamin D and calcium supplementation indefinitely. Therapy is especially important in females.

Gastric adenocarcinoma The incidence of adenocarcinoma in the gastric stump is increased 15 years after resection. Some have reported a four- to fivefold increase in gastric cancer 20–25 years after resection. The pathogenesis is unclear but may involve alkaline reflux, bacterial proliferation, or hypochlorhydria. The role of endoscopic screening is not clear, and most guidelines do not support its use.

RELATED CONDITIONS

ZOLLINGER–ELLISON SYNDROME

Severe peptic ulcer diathesis secondary to gastric acid hypersecretion due to unregulated gastrin release from a non-β cell endocrine tumor (gastrinoma) defines the components of ZES. Initially, ZES was typified by aggressive and refractory ulceration in which total gastrectomy provided the only chance for enhancing survival. Today it can be cured by surgical resection in up to 30% of patients.

Epidemiology

The incidence of ZES varies from 0.1–1% of individuals presenting with PUD. Males are more commonly affected than females, and the majority of patients are diagnosed between ages 30 and 50. Gastrinomas are classified into sporadic tumors (more common) and those associated with multiple endocrine neoplasia (MEN) type I (discussed later). The widespread availability and use of PPIs has led to a decreased patient referral for gastrinoma evaluation, delay in diagnosis, and an increase in false-positive diagnoses of ZES.

Pathophysiology

Hypergastrinemia originating from an autonomous neoplasm is the driving force responsible for the clinical manifestations in ZES. Gastrin stimulates acid secretion through gastrin receptors on parietal cells and by inducing histamine release from ECL cells. Gastrin also has a trophic action on gastric epithelial cells. Long-standing hypergastrinemia leads to markedly increased gastric acid secretion through both parietal cell stimulation and increased parietal cell mass. The increased gastric acid output leads to peptic ulcer diathesis, erosive esophagitis, and diarrhea.

Tumor distribution

Although early studies suggested that the vast majority of gastrinomas occurred within the pancreas, a significant number of these lesions are extrapancreatic. Over 80% of these tumors are found within the hypothetical gastrinoma triangle (confluence of the cystic and common bile ducts superiorly, junction of the second and third portions of the duodenum inferiorly, and junction of the neck and body of the pancreas medially). Duodenal tumors constitute the most common nonpancreatic lesion; between 50 and 75% of gastrinomas are found here. Duodenal tumors are smaller, slower growing, and less likely to metastasize than pancreatic lesions. Less-common extrapancreatic sites include stomach, bones, ovaries, heart, liver, and lymph nodes. More than 60% of tumors are considered malignant, with up to 30–50% of patients having multiple lesions or metastatic disease at presentation. Histologically, gastrin-producing cells appear well-differentiated, expressing markers typically found in endocrine neoplasms (chromogranin, neuron-specific enolase).

Clinical manifestations

Gastric acid hypersecretion is responsible for the signs and symptoms observed in patients with ZES. Peptic ulcer is the most common clinical manifestation, occurring in >90% of gastrinoma patients. Initial presentation and ulcer location (duodenal bulb) may be indistinguishable from common PUD. Clinical situations that should create suspicion of gastrinoma are ulcers in unusual locations (second part of the duodenum and beyond), ulcers refractory to standard medical therapy, ulcer recurrence after acid-reducing surgery, ulcers presenting with frank complications (bleeding, obstruction, and perforation), or ulcers in the absence of H. pylori or NSAID ingestion. Symptoms of esophageal origin are present in up to two-thirds of patients with ZES, with a spectrum ranging from mild esophagitis to frank ulceration with stricture and Barrett's mucosa.

Diarrhea, the next most common clinical manifestation, is found in up to 50% of patients. Although diarrhea often occurs concomitantly with acid peptic disease, it may also occur independent of an ulcer. Etiology of the diarrhea is multifactorial, resulting from marked volume overload to the small bowel, pancreatic enzyme inactivation by acid, and damage of the intestinal epithelial surface by acid. The epithelial damage can lead to a mild degree of maldigestion and malabsorption of nutrients. The diarrhea may also have a secretory component due to the direct stimulatory effect of gastrin on enterocytes or the co-secretion of additional hormones from the tumor such as vasoactive intestinal peptide.

Gastrinomas can develop in the presence of MEN I syndrome (Chap. 52) in ~25% of patients. This autosomal dominant disorder involves primarily three organ sites: the parathyroid glands (80–90%), pancreas (40–80%), and pituitary gland (30–60%). The genetic defect in MEN I is in the long arm of chromosome 11 (11q11-q13). In view of the stimulatory effect of calcium on gastric secretion, the hyperparathyroidism and hypercalcemia seen in MEN I patients may have a direct effect on ulcer disease. Resolution of hypercalcemia by parathyroidectomy reduces gastrin and gastric acid output in gastrinoma patients. An additional distinguishing feature in ZES patients with MEN I is the higher incidence of gastric carcinoid tumor development (as compared to patients with sporadic gastrinomas). Gastrinomas tend to be smaller, multiple, and located in the duodenal wall more often than is seen in patients with sporadic ZES. Establishing the diagnosis of MEN I is critical not only from the standpoint of providing genetic counseling to the patient and his or her family but also to the surgical approach recommended.

Diagnosis

The first step in the evaluation of a patient suspected of having ZES is to obtain a fasting gastrin level. A list of clinical scenarios that should arouse suspicion regarding this diagnosis is shown in Table 14-7. Fasting gastrin levels are usually <150 pg/mL. Virtually all gastrinoma patients will have a gastrin level >150–200 pg/mL. Measurement of fasting gastrin should be repeated to confirm the clinical suspicion.

Multiple processes can lead to an elevated fasting gastrin level: gastric hypochlorhydria or achlorhydria (the most frequent), with or without pernicious anemia; retained gastric antrum; G cell hyperplasia; gastric outlet obstruction; renal insufficiency; massive small-bowel obstruction; and conditions such as rheumatoid arthritis, vitiligo, diabetes mellitus, and pheochromocytoma. Gastric acid induces feedback inhibition of gastrin release. A decrease in acid production will subsequently lead to failure of the feedback inhibitory pathway, resulting in net hypergastrinemia. Gastrin levels will thus be high in patients using antisecretory agents for the treatment of acid peptic disorders and dyspepsia. *H. pylori* infection can also cause hypergastrinemia. Although a fasting gastrin >10 times normal is highly suggestive of ZES, two-thirds of patients will

TABLE 14-7

WHEN TO OBTAIN A FASTING SERUM GASTRIN LEVEL

Multiple ulcers
Ulcers in unusual locations; associated with severe esophagitis; resistant to therapy with frequent recurrences; in the absence of NSAID ingestion or *H. pylori* infection
Ulcer patients awaiting surgery
Extensive family history for peptic ulcer disease
Postoperative ulcer recurrence
Basal hyperchlorhydria
Unexplained diarrhea or steatorrhea
Hypercalcemia
Family history of pancreatic islet, pituitary, or parathyroid tumor
Prominent gastric or duodenal folds

have fasting gastrin levels that overlap with levels found in the more common disorders outlined earlier.

The next step in establishing a biochemical diagnosis of gastrinoma is to assess acid secretion. Nothing further needs to be done if decreased acid output is observed. In contrast, normal or elevated gastric acid output suggests a need for additional tests. Up to 12% of patients with common PUD may have comparable levels of acid secretion. A BAO/MAO ratio >0.6 is highly suggestive of ZES, but a ratio <0.6 does not exclude the diagnosis. Pentagastrin is no longer available in the United States, making measurement of MAO virtually impossible. An endoscopic method for measuring gastric acid output has been developed but requires further validation. If the technology for measuring gastric acid secretion is not available, a basal gastric pH ≥3 virtually excludes a gastrinoma.

Gastrin provocative tests have been developed in an effort to differentiate between the causes of hypergastrinemia and are especially helpful in patients with indeterminate acid secretory studies. The tests are the secretin stimulation test and the calcium infusion study. The most sensitive and specific gastrin provocative test for the diagnosis of gastrinoma is the secretin study. An increase in gastrin of ≥120 pg within 15 min of secretin injection has a sensitivity and specificity of >90% for ZES. PPI–induced hypochlorhydria or achlorhydria may lead to a false-positive secretin test, thus this agent must be stopped for 1 week before testing.

The calcium infusion study is less sensitive and specific than the secretin test, which coupled with it being a more cumbersome study with greater potential for adverse effects, relegates it to rare utilization in the cases where the patient's clinical characteristics are highly suggestive of ZES, but the secretin stimulation is inconclusive.

Tumor localization

Once the biochemical diagnosis of gastrinoma has been confirmed, the tumor must be located. Multiple imaging studies have been utilized in an effort to enhance tumor localization (Table 14-8). The broad range of sensitivity is due to the variable success rates achieved by the different investigative groups. Endoscopic ultrasound (EUS) permits imaging of the pancreas with a high degree of resolution (<5 mm). This modality is particularly helpful in excluding small neoplasms within the pancreas and in assessing the presence of surrounding lymph nodes and vascular involvement, but it is not very sensitive for finding duodenal lesions. Several types of endocrine tumors express cell-surface receptors for somatostatin. This permits the localization of gastrinomas by measuring the uptake of the stable somatostatin analogue ^{111}In-pentreotide (OctreoScan) with sensitivity and specificity rates of >85%.

Up to 50% of patients have metastatic disease at diagnosis. Success in controlling gastric acid hypersecretion has shifted the emphasis of therapy toward providing a surgical cure. Detecting the primary tumor and excluding metastatic disease are critical in view of this paradigm shift. Once a biochemical diagnosis has been confirmed, the patient should first undergo an abdominal CT scan, MRI, or OctreoScan (depending on availability) to exclude metastatic disease. Once metastatic disease has been excluded, an experienced endocrine surgeon may opt for exploratory laparotomy with intraoperative ultrasound or transillumination. In other centers, careful examination of the peripancreatic area with EUS, accompanied by endoscopic exploration of the duodenum for primary tumors, will be performed before surgery. Selective arterial secretin injection may

be a useful adjuvant for localizing tumors in a subset of patients.

TREATMENT Zollinger-Ellison Syndrome

Treatment of functional endocrine tumors is directed at ameliorating the signs and symptoms related to hormone overproduction, curative resection of the neoplasm, and attempts to control tumor growth in metastatic disease.

PPIs are the treatment of choice and have decreased the need for total gastrectomy. Initial PPI doses tend to be higher than those used for treatment of GERD or PUD. The initial dose of omeprazole, lansoprazole, rabeprazole or esomeprazole should be in the range of 60 mg in divided doses in a 24-h period. Dosing can be adjusted to achieve a BAO <10 meq/h (at the drug trough) in surgery-naive patients and to <5 meq/h in individuals who have previously undergone an acid-reducing operation. Although the somatostatin analogue has inhibitory effects on gastrin release from receptor-bearing tumors and inhibits gastric acid secretion to some extent, PPIs have the advantage of reducing parietal cell activity to a greater degree. Despite this, octreotide may be considered as adjunctive therapy to the PPI in patients with tumors that express somatostatin receptors and have peptic symptoms that are difficult to control with high-dose PPI.

The ultimate goal of surgery would be to provide a definitive cure. Improved understanding of tumor distribution has led to immediate cure rates as high as 60% with 10-year disease-free intervals as high as 34% in sporadic gastrinoma patients undergoing surgery. A positive outcome is highly dependent on the experience of the surgical team treating these rare tumors. Surgical therapy of gastrinoma patients with MEN I remains controversial because of the difficulty in rendering these patients disease-free with surgery. In contrast to the encouraging postoperative results observed in patients with sporadic disease, only 6% of MEN I patients are disease free 5 years after an operation. Some groups suggest surgery only if a clearly identifiable, nonmetastatic lesion is documented by structural studies. Others advocate a more aggressive approach, where all patients free of hepatic metastasis are explored and all detected tumors in the duodenum are resected; this is followed by enucleation of lesions in the pancreatic head, with a distal pancreatectomy to follow. The outcome of the two approaches has not been clearly defined. Laparoscopic surgical interventions may provide attractive approaches in the future.

Therapy of metastatic endocrine tumors in general remains suboptimal; gastrinomas are no exception.

TABLE 14-8

SENSITIVITY OF IMAGING STUDIES IN ZOLLINGER-ELLISON SYNDROME

	SENSITIVITY, %	
STUDY	PRIMARY GASTRINOMA	METASTATIC GASTRINOMA
Ultrasound	21–28	14
CT scan	55–70	>85
Selective angiography	35–68	33–86
Portal venous sampling	70–90	N/A
SASI	55–78	41
MRI	55–70	>85
OctreoScan	67–86	80–100
EUS	80–100	N/A

Abbreviations: CT, computed tomography; EUS, endoscopic ultrasonography; MRI, magnetic resonance imaging; OctreoScan, imaging with ^{111}In-pentreotide; SASI, selective arterial secretin injection.

In light of the observation that in many instances tumor growth is indolent and that many individuals with metastatic disease remain relatively stable for significant periods of time, many advocate not instituting systemic tumor targeted therapy until evidence of tumor progression or refractory symptoms not controlled with PPIs are noted. Medical approaches including biological therapy (IFN-α, long-acting somatostatin analogues, peptide receptor radionuclides), systemic chemotherapy (streptozotocin, 5-fluorouracil, and doxorubicin), and hepatic artery embolization may lead to significant toxicity without a substantial improvement in overall survival. ^{111}In-pentetreotide has been used in the therapy of metastatic neuroendocrine tumors; further studies are needed. Several novel therapies are being explored, including radiofrequency or cryoablation of liver lesions and use of agents that block the vascular endothelial growth receptor pathway (bevacizumab, sunitinib) or the mammalian target of rapamycin (Chap. 52).

Surgical approaches including debulking surgery and liver transplantation for hepatic metastasis have also produced limited benefit.

The overall 5- and 10-year survival rates for gastrinoma patients are 62–75% and 47–53%, respectively. Individuals with the entire tumor resected or those with a negative laparotomy have 5- and 10-year survival rates >90%. Patients with incompletely resected tumors have 5- and 10-year survival rates of 43% and 25%, respectively. Patients with hepatic metastasis have <20% survival at 5 years. Favorable prognostic indicators include primary duodenal wall tumors, isolated lymph node tumor, and undetectable tumor upon surgical exploration. Poor outcome is seen in patients with shorter disease duration; higher gastrin levels (>10,000 pg/mL); large pancreatic primary tumors (>3 cm); metastatic disease to lymph nodes, liver, and bone; and Cushing's syndrome. Rapid growth of hepatic metastases is also predictive of poor outcome.

STRESS-RELATED MUCOSAL INJURY

Patients suffering from shock, sepsis, massive burns, severe trauma, or head injury can develop acute erosive gastric mucosal changes or frank ulceration with bleeding. Classified as stress-induced gastritis or ulcers, injury is most commonly observed in the acid-producing (fundus and body) portions of the stomach. The most common presentation is GI bleeding, which is usually minimal but can occasionally be life threatening. Respiratory failure requiring mechanical ventilation and underlying coagulopathy are risk factors for bleeding, which tends to occur 48–72 h after the acute injury or insult.

Histologically, stress injury does not contain inflammation or *H. pylori*; thus, "gastritis" is a misnomer.

Although elevated gastric acid secretion may be noted in patients with stress ulceration after head trauma (Cushing's ulcer) and severe burns (Curling's ulcer), mucosal ischemia and breakdown of the normal protective barriers of the stomach also play an important role in the pathogenesis. Acid must contribute to injury in view of the significant drop in bleeding noted when acid inhibitors are used as prophylaxis for stress gastritis.

Improvement in the general management of intensive care unit patients has led to a significant decrease in the incidence of GI bleeding due to stress ulceration. The estimated decrease in bleeding is from 20–30% to <5%. This improvement has led to some debate regarding the need for prophylactic therapy. The limited benefit of medical (endoscopic, angiographic) and surgical therapy in a patient with hemodynamically compromising bleeding associated with stress ulcer/gastritis supports the use of preventive measures in high-risk patients (mechanically ventilated, coagulopathy, multiorgan failure, or severe burns). Maintenance of gastric pH >3.5 with continuous infusion of H_2 blockers or liquid antacids administered every 2–3 h are viable options. Tolerance to the H_2 blocker is likely to develop; thus, careful monitoring of the gastric pH and dose adjustment is important if H_2 blockers are used. Sucralfate slurry (1 g every 4–6 h) has also been somewhat successful but requires a gastric tube and may lead to constipation and aluminum toxicity. Sucralfate use in endotracheal intubated patients has also been associated with aspiration pneumonia. PPIs are the treatment of choice for stress prophylaxis. Oral PPI is the best option if the patient can tolerate enteral administration. Pantoprazole is available as an intravenous formulation for individuals in whom enteral administration is not possible. If bleeding occurs despite these measures, endoscopy, intraarterial vasopressin, or embolization are options. If all else fails, then surgery should be considered. Although vagotomy and antrectomy may be used, the better approach would be a total gastrectomy, which has an exceedingly high mortality rate in this setting.

GASTRITIS

The term *gastritis* should be reserved for histologically documented inflammation of the gastric mucosa. Gastritis is not the mucosal erythema seen during endoscopy and is not interchangeable with "dyspepsia." The etiologic factors leading to gastritis are broad and heterogeneous. Gastritis has been classified based on time course (acute versus chronic), histologic features, and anatomic distribution or proposed pathogenic mechanism (Table 14-9).

The correlation between the histologic findings of gastritis, the clinical picture of abdominal pain or dyspepsia, and endoscopic findings noted on gross

TABLE 14-9

CLASSIFICATION OF GASTRITIS

I. Acute gastritis	II. Chronic atrophic gastritis
A. Acute *H. pylori* infection	A. Type A: Autoimmune, body-predominant
B. Other acute infectious gastritides	B. Type B: *H. pylori*–related, antral-predominant
1. Bacterial (other than *H. pylori*)	C. Indeterminant
2. *H. heilmannii*	III. Uncommon forms of gastritis
3. Phlegmonous	A. Lymphocytic
4. Mycobacterial	B. Eosinophilic
5. Syphilitic	C. Crohn's disease
6. Viral	D. Sarcoidosis
7. Parasitic	E. Isolated granulomatous gastritis
8. Fungal	

inspection of the gastric mucosa is poor. Therefore, there is no typical clinical manifestation of gastritis.

Acute gastritis

The most common causes of acute gastritis are infectious. Acute infection with *H. pylori* induces gastritis. However, *H. pylori* acute gastritis has not been extensively studied. It is reported as presenting with sudden onset of epigastric pain, nausea, and vomiting, and limited mucosal histologic studies demonstrate a marked infiltrate of neutrophils with edema and hyperemia. If not treated, this picture will evolve into one of chronic gastritis. Hypochlorhydria lasting for up to 1 year may follow acute *H. pylori* infection.

Bacterial infection of the stomach or phlegmonous gastritis is a rare, potentially life-threatening disorder characterized by marked and diffuse acute inflammatory infiltrates of the entire gastric wall, at times accompanied by necrosis. Elderly individuals, alcoholics, and AIDS patients may be affected. Potential iatrogenic causes include polypectomy and mucosal injection with India ink. Organisms associated with this entity include streptococci, staphylococci, *Escherichia coli*, *Proteus*, and *Haemophilus* species. Failure of supportive measures and antibiotics may result in gastrectomy.

Other types of infectious gastritis may occur in immunocompromised individuals such as AIDS patients. Examples include herpetic (herpes simplex) or CMV gastritis. The histologic finding of intranuclear inclusions would be observed in the latter.

Chronic gastritis

Chronic gastritis is identified histologically by an inflammatory cell infiltrate consisting primarily of lymphocytes and plasma cells, with very scant neutrophil involvement. Distribution of the inflammation may be patchy, initially involving superficial and glandular portions of the gastric mucosa. This picture may progress to more severe glandular destruction, with atrophy and metaplasia. Chronic gastritis has been classified according to histologic characteristics. These include superficial atrophic changes and gastric atrophy.

The early phase of chronic gastritis is *superficial gastritis*. The inflammatory changes are limited to the lamina propria of the surface mucosa, with edema and cellular infiltrates separating intact gastric glands. The next stage is *atrophic gastritis*. The inflammatory infiltrate extends deeper into the mucosa, with progressive distortion and destruction of the glands. The final stage of chronic gastritis is *gastric atrophy*. Glandular structures are lost, and there is a paucity of inflammatory infiltrates. Endoscopically, the mucosa may be substantially thin, permitting clear visualization of the underlying blood vessels.

Gastric glands may undergo morphologic transformation in chronic gastritis. Intestinal metaplasia denotes the conversion of gastric glands to a small intestinal phenotype with small-bowel mucosal glands containing goblet cells. The metaplastic changes may vary in distribution from patchy to fairly extensive gastric involvement. Intestinal metaplasia is an important predisposing factor for gastric cancer (Chap. 49).

Chronic gastritis is also classified according to the predominant site of involvement. Type A refers to the body-predominant form (autoimmune) and type B is the antral-predominant form (*H. pylori*–related). This classification is artificial in view of the difficulty in distinguishing between these two entities. The term *AB gastritis* has been used to refer to a mixed antral/body picture.

■ Type A gastritis

The less common of the two forms involves primarily the fundus and body, with antral sparing. Traditionally, this form of gastritis has been associated with pernicious anemia in the presence of circulating antibodies against parietal cells and IF; thus, it is also called *autoimmune gastritis*. *H. pylori* infection can lead to a similar distribution of gastritis. The characteristics of an autoimmune picture are not always present.

Antibodies to parietal cells have been detected in >90% of patients with pernicious anemia and in up to 50% of patients with type A gastritis. The parietal cell antibody is directed against H^+,K^+-ATPase. T cells are also implicated in the injury pattern of this form of gastritis. A subset of patients infected with *H. pylori* develop antibodies against H^+,K^+-ATPase, potentially leading to the atrophic gastritis pattern seen in some patients infected with this organism. The mechanism is thought to involve molecular mimicry between *H. pylori* LPS and H^+,K^+-ATPase.

Parietal cell antibodies and atrophic gastritis are observed in family members of patients with pernicious anemia. These antibodies are observed in up to 20% of individuals over age 60 and in ~20% of patients with vitiligo and Addison's disease. About one-half of patients with pernicious anemia have antibodies to thyroid antigens, and about 30% of patients with thyroid disease have circulating antiparietal cell antibodies. Anti-IF antibodies are more specific than parietal cell antibodies for type A gastritis, being present in ~40% of patients with pernicious anemia. Another parameter consistent with this form of gastritis being autoimmune in origin is the higher incidence of specific familial histocompatibility haplotypes such as HLA-B8 and HLA-DR3.

The parietal cell–containing gastric gland is preferentially targeted in this form of gastritis, and achlorhydria results. Parietal cells are the source of IF, the lack of which will lead to vitamin B_{12} deficiency and its sequelae (megaloblastic anemia, neurologic dysfunction).

Gastric acid plays an important role in feedback inhibition of gastrin release from G cells. Achlorhydria, coupled with relative sparing of the antral mucosa (site of G cells), leads to hypergastrinemia. Gastrin levels can be markedly elevated (>500 pg/mL) in patients with pernicious anemia. ECL cell hyperplasia with frank development of gastric carcinoid tumors may result from gastrin trophic effects. Hypergastrinemia and achlorhydria may also be seen in nonpernicious anemia–associated type A gastritis.

Type B gastritis

Type B, or antral-predominant, gastritis is the more common form of chronic gastritis. H. pylori infection is the cause of this entity. Although described as "antral-predominant," this is likely a misnomer in view of studies documenting the progression of the inflammatory process toward the body and fundus of infected individuals. The conversion to a pangastritis is time-dependent, estimated to require 15–20 years. This form of gastritis increases with age, being present in up to 100% of persons over age 70. Histology improves after H. pylori eradication. The number of H. pylori organisms decreases dramatically with progression to gastric atrophy, and the degree of inflammation correlates with the level of these organisms. Early on, with antral-predominant findings, the quantity of H. pylori is highest and a dense chronic inflammatory infiltrate of the lamina propria is noted, accompanied by epithelial cell infiltration with polymorphonuclear leukocytes (**Fig. 14-14**).

Multifocal atrophic gastritis, gastric atrophy with subsequent metaplasia, has been observed in chronic H. pylori–induced gastritis. This may ultimately lead to development of gastric adenocarcinoma (Fig. 14-8; Chap. 49). H. pylori infection is now considered an independent risk factor for gastric cancer. Worldwide epidemiologic studies have documented a higher incidence of H. pylori infection in patients with adenocarcinoma of the stomach as compared to control subjects.

FIGURE 14-14

Chronic gastritis and _H. pylori_ organisms. Steiner silver stain of superficial gastric mucosa, showing abundant darkly stained microorganisms layered over the apical portion of the surface epithelium. Note that there is no tissue invasion.

Seropositivity for H. pylori is associated with a three- to sixfold increased risk of gastric cancer. This risk may be as high as ninefold after adjusting for the inaccuracy of serologic testing in the elderly. The mechanism by which H. pylori infection leads to cancer is unknown, but it appears to be related to the chronic inflammation induced by the organism. Eradication of H. pylori as a general preventative measure for gastric cancer is being evaluated but is not yet recommended.

Infection with H. pylori is also associated with development of a low-grade B cell lymphoma, gastric MALT lymphoma. The chronic T cell stimulation caused by the infection leads to production of cytokines that promote the B cell tumor. The tumor should be initially staged with a CT scan of the abdomen and EUS. Tumor growth remains dependent on the presence of H. pylori, and its eradication is often associated with complete regression of the tumor. The tumor may take more than a year to regress after treating the infection. Such patients should be followed by EUS every 2–3 months. If the tumor is stable or decreasing in size, no other therapy is necessary. If the tumor grows, it may have become a high-grade B cell lymphoma. When the tumor becomes a high-grade aggressive lymphoma histologically, it loses responsiveness to H. pylori eradication.

TREATMENT Chronic Gastritis

Treatment in chronic gastritis is aimed at the sequelae and not the underlying inflammation. Patients with pernicious anemia will require parenteral vitamin B_{12} supplementation on a long-term basis. Eradication of H. pylori is not routinely recommended unless PUD or a low-grade MALT lymphoma is present.

Miscellaneous forms of gastritis

Lymphocytic gastritis is characterized histologically by intense infiltration of the surface epithelium with lymphocytes. The infiltrative process is primarily in the body of the stomach and consists of mature T cells and plasmacytes. The etiology of this form of chronic gastritis is unknown. It has been described in patients with celiac sprue, but whether there is a common factor associating these two entities is unknown. No specific symptoms suggest lymphocytic gastritis. A subgroup of patients have thickened folds noted on endoscopy. These folds are often capped by small nodules that contain a central depression or erosion; this form of the disease is called *varioliform gastritis*. *H. pylori* probably plays no significant role in lymphocytic gastritis. Therapy with glucocorticoids or sodium cromoglycate has obtained unclear results.

Marked eosinophilic infiltration involving any layer of the stomach (mucosa, muscularis propria, and serosa) is characteristic of *eosinophilic gastritis*. Affected individuals will often have circulating eosinophilia with clinical manifestation of systemic allergy. Involvement may range from isolated gastric disease to diffuse eosinophilic gastroenteritis. Antral involvement predominates, with prominent edematous folds being observed on endoscopy. These prominent antral folds can lead to outlet obstruction. Patients can present with epigastric discomfort, nausea, and vomiting. Treatment with glucocorticoids has been successful.

Several systemic disorders may be associated with *granulomatous gastritis*. Gastric involvement has been observed in Crohn's disease. Involvement may range from granulomatous infiltrates noted only on gastric biopsies to frank ulceration and stricture formation. Gastric Crohn's disease usually occurs in the presence of small-intestinal disease. Several rare infectious processes can lead to granulomatous gastritis, including histoplasmosis, candidiasis, syphilis, and tuberculosis. Other unusual causes of this form of gastritis include sarcoidosis, idiopathic granulomatous gastritis, and eosinophilic granulomas involving the stomach. Establishing the specific etiologic agent in this form of gastritis can be difficult, at times requiring repeat endoscopy with biopsy and cytology. Occasionally, a surgically obtained full-thickness biopsy of the stomach may be required to exclude malignancy.

MÉNÉTRIER'S DISEASE

Ménétrier's disease is a rare entity characterized by large, tortuous gastric mucosal folds. The differential diagnosis of large gastric folds includes ZES, malignancy, infectious etiologies (CMV, histoplasmosis, syphilis), and infiltrative disorders such as sarcoidosis. The mucosal folds in Ménétrier's disease are often most prominent in the body and fundus. Histologically, massive foveolar hyperplasia (hyperplasia of surface and glandular mucous cells) is noted, which replaces most of the chief and parietal cells. This hyperplasia produces the prominent folds observed. The pits of the gastric glands elongate and may become extremely tortuous. Although the lamina propria may contain a mild chronic inflammatory infiltrate, Ménétrier's disease is not considered a form of gastritis. The etiology of this unusual clinical picture is unknown. Overexpression of growth factors such as TGF-α may be involved in the process.

Epigastric pain, at times accompanied by nausea, vomiting, anorexia, and weight loss, are signs and symptoms in patients with Ménétrier's disease. Occult GI bleeding may occur, but overt bleeding is unusual and, when present, is due to superficial mucosal erosions. Twenty to 100% of patients (depending on time of presentation) develop a protein-losing gastropathy accompanied by hypoalbuminemia and edema. Gastric acid secretion is usually reduced or absent because of the replacement of parietal cells. Large gastric folds are readily detectable by either radiographic (barium meal) or endoscopic methods. Endoscopy with deep mucosal biopsy (and cytology) is required to establish the diagnosis and exclude other entities that may present similarly. A nondiagnostic biopsy may lead to a surgically obtained full-thickness biopsy to exclude malignancy.

TREATMENT   Ménétrier's Disease

Medical therapy with anticholinergic agents, prostaglandins, PPIs, prednisone, and H_2 receptor antagonists yields varying results. Anticholinergics decrease protein loss. A high-protein diet should be recommended to replace protein loss in patients with hypoalbuminemia. Ulcers should be treated with a standard approach. Severe disease with persistent and substantial protein loss may require total gastrectomy. Subtotal gastrectomy is performed by some; it may be associated with higher morbidity and mortality secondary to the difficulty in obtaining a patent and long-lasting anastomosis between normal and hyperplastic tissues.

ACKNOWLEDGMENTS

The author acknowledges the contribution of material to this chapter by Dr. Lawrence Friedman and Dr. Walter Peterson from their chapter on this subject in the 14th edition of Harrison's Principles of Internal Medicine.

CHAPTER 15

DISORDERS OF ABSORPTION

Henry J. Binder

Disorders of absorption constitute a broad spectrum of conditions with multiple etiologies and varied clinical manifestations. Almost all of these clinical problems are associated with *diminished* intestinal absorption of one or more dietary nutrients and are often referred to as the *malabsorption syndrome.* This term is not ideal as it represents a pathophysiologic state, does *not* provide an etiologic explanation for the underlying problem, and should not be considered an adequate final diagnosis. The only clinical situations in which absorption is *increased* are hemochromatosis and Wilson's disease, in which absorption of iron and copper, respectively, are increased.

Most, but not all, malabsorption syndromes are associated with *steatorrhea,* an increase in stool fat excretion of >6% of dietary fat intake. Some malabsorption disorders are not associated with steatorrhea: primary lactase deficiency, a congenital absence of the small intestinal brush border disaccharidase enzyme lactase, is associated with lactose "malabsorption," and pernicious anemia is associated with a marked decrease in intestinal absorption of cobalamin (vitamin B_{12}) due to an absence of gastric parietal cell intrinsic factor required for cobalamin absorption.

Disorders of absorption must be included in the differential diagnosis of diarrhea (Chap. 6). First, diarrhea is frequently associated with and/or is a consequence of the diminished absorption of one or more dietary nutrients. The diarrhea may be secondary either to the intestinal process that is responsible for the steatorrhea or to steatorrhea per se. Thus, celiac disease (discussed later) is associated with both extensive morphologic changes in the small intestinal mucosa and reduced absorption of several dietary nutrients; in contrast, the diarrhea of steatorrhea is the result of the effect of nonabsorbed dietary fatty acids on intestinal, usually colonic, ion transport. For example, oleic acid and ricinoleic acid (a bacterially hydroxylated fatty acid that is also the active ingredient in castor oil, a widely used laxative) induce active colonic Cl ion secretion, most likely secondary

to increasing intracellular Ca. In addition, diarrhea per se may result in mild steatorrhea (<11 g fat excretion while on a 100-g fat diet). Second, most patients will indicate that they have diarrhea, not that they have fat malabsorption. Third, many intestinal disorders that have diarrhea as a prominent symptom (e.g., ulcerative colitis, traveler's diarrhea secondary to an enterotoxin produced by *Escherichia coli*) do not necessarily have diminished absorption of any dietary nutrient.

Diarrhea as a *symptom* (i.e., when used by patients to describe their bowel movement pattern) may be a decrease in stool consistency, an increase in stool volume, an increase in number of bowel movements, or any combination of these three changes. In contrast, diarrhea as a *sign* is a quantitative increase in stool water or weight of >200–225 mL or gram per 24 h, when a Western-type diet is consumed. Individuals consuming a diet with higher fiber content may normally have a stool weight of up to 400 g/24 h. Thus, the clinician must clarify what an individual patient means by diarrhea. Some 10% of patients referred to gastroenterologists for further evaluation of unexplained diarrhea do not have an increase in stool water when it is determined quantitatively. Such patients may have small, frequent, somewhat loose bowel movements with stool urgency that is indicative of proctitis but do not have an increase in stool weight or volume.

It is also critical to establish whether a patient's diarrhea is secondary to diminished absorption of one or more dietary nutrients, in contrast to diarrhea that is due to small- and/or large-intestinal fluid and electrolyte secretion. The former has often been termed *osmotic diarrhea,* while the latter has been referred to as *secretory diarrhea.* Unfortunately, both secretory and osmotic elements can be present simultaneously in the same disorder; thus, this separation is not always precise. Nonetheless, two studies—determination of stool electrolytes and observation of the effect of a fast on stool output—can help make this distinction.

The demonstration of the effect of prolonged (>24 h) fasting on stool output can be very effective in suggesting that a *dietary nutrient* is responsible for the individual's diarrhea. A secretory diarrhea associated with enterotoxin-induced traveler's diarrhea would not be affected by prolonged fasting, as enterotoxin-induced stimulation of intestinal fluid and electrolyte secretion is not altered by eating. In contrast, diarrhea secondary to lactose malabsorption in primary lactase deficiency would undoubtedly cease during a prolonged fast. Thus, a substantial decrease in stool output while fasting during a quantitative stool collection of at least 24 h is presumptive evidence that the diarrhea is related to malabsorption of a dietary nutrient. The persistence of stool output while fasting indicates that the diarrhea is likely secretory and that the cause of diarrhea is *not* a dietary nutrient. Either a luminal (e.g., *E. coli* enterotoxin) or circulating (e.g., vasoactive intestinal peptide) secretagogue could be responsible for the patient's diarrhea persisting unaltered during a prolonged fast. The observed effects of fasting can be compared and correlated with stool electrolyte and osmolality determinations.

Measurement of stool electrolytes and osmolality requires the comparison of stool Na^+ and K^+ concentrations determined in liquid stool to the stool osmolality to determine the presence or absence of a so-called stool osmotic gap. The following formula is used:

$$2 \times (stool\ [Na^+] + stool\ [K^+]) \leq stool\ osmolality$$

The cation concentrations are doubled to estimate stool anion concentrations. The presence of a significant osmotic gap suggests the presence in stool water of a substance (or substances) other than Na/K anions that is presumably responsible for the patient's diarrhea. Originally, stool osmolality was measured, but it is almost invariably greater than the required 290–300 mosmol/kg H_2O, reflecting bacterial degradation of nonabsorbed carbohydrate either immediately before defecation or in the stool jar while awaiting chemical analysis, even when the stool is refrigerated. As a result, the stool osmolality should be assumed to be 300 mosmol/kg H_2O. A low stool osmolality (<290 mosmol/kg H_2O) reflects the addition of either dilute urine or water indicating either collection of urine and stool together or so-called factitious diarrhea, a form of Münchausen's syndrome. When the calculated difference is >50, an osmotic gap is present, suggesting that the diarrhea is due to a nonabsorbed dietary nutrient, e.g., a fatty acid and/or carbohydrate. When this difference is <25, it is presumed that a dietary nutrient is not responsible for the diarrhea. Since elements of both osmotic (i.e., malabsorption of a dietary nutrient) and secretory diarrhea may be present, this separation at times is less clear-cut at the bedside than when used as a teaching example. Ideally, the presence of an osmotic gap will be associated with a marked decrease in stool output during a prolonged fast, while the absence of an osmotic gap will likely be present in an individual whose stool output had not been reduced substantially during a period of fasting.

NUTRIENT DIGESTION AND ABSORPTION

The lengths of the small intestine and colon are ~300 cm and ~80 cm, respectively. However, the effective functional surface area is approximately 600-fold greater than that of a hollow tube as a result of the presence of folds, villi (in the small intestine), and microvilli. The functional surface area of the small intestine is somewhat greater than that of a doubles tennis court. In addition to nutrient digestion and absorption, the intestinal epithelia have several other functions:

1. *Barrier and immune defense.* The intestine is exposed to a large number of potential antigens and enteric and invasive microorganisms, and it is extremely effective preventing the entry of almost all these agents. The intestinal mucosa also synthesizes and secretes secretory IgA.
2. *Fluid and electrolyte absorption and secretion.* The intestine absorbs ~7–8 L of fluid daily, comprising dietary fluid intake (1–2 L/d) and salivary, gastric, pancreatic, biliary, and intestinal fluid (6–7 L/d). Several stimuli, especially bacteria and bacterial enterotoxins, induce fluid and electrolyte secretion that may lead to diarrhea (Chap. 23).
3. *Synthesis and secretion of several proteins.* The intestinal mucosa is a major site for the production of proteins, including apolipoproteins.
4. *Production of several bioactive amines and peptides.* The intestine is one of the largest endocrine organs in the body and produces several amines (e.g., 5-hydroxytryptophan) and peptides that serve as paracrine and hormonal mediators of intestinal function.

The small and large intestines are distinct anatomically (villi are present in the small intestine but are absent in the colon) and functionally (nutrient digestion and absorption take place in the small intestine but not in the colon). No precise anatomic characteristics separate duodenum, jejunum, and ileum, although certain nutrients are absorbed exclusively in specific areas of the small intestine. However, villous cells in the small intestine (and surface epithelial cells in the colon) and crypt cells have distinct anatomic and functional characteristics. Intestinal epithelial cells are continuously renewed, with new proliferating epithelial cells at the base of the crypt migrating over 48–72 h to the tip of the villus (or surface of the colon), where they are well-developed epithelial cells with digestive and absorptive function. This high rate of cell turnover explains the relatively rapid resolution of diarrhea and other digestive tract side effects during chemotherapy as new cells not exposed to these toxic agents are produced. Equally important is the paradigm of separation of villous/surface cell and crypt cell function: Digestive hydrolytic enzymes are present primarily in the brush border of villous epithelial cells. Absorptive and secretory functions are also separated, with villous/surface cells primarily, but not exclusively, being the site for absorptive function, while secretory function is present in crypts of both the small and large intestine.

Nutrients, minerals, and vitamins are absorbed by one or more active transport mechanisms. Active transport mechanisms are energy-dependent and mediated by membrane transport proteins. These processes will result in the *net* movement of a substance against or in the absence of an electrochemical concentration gradient. Intestinal absorption of amino acids and monosaccharides, e.g., glucose, is also a specialized form of active transport—*secondary active transport*. The movement of these actively transported nutrients against a concentration gradient is Na^+-dependent and is due to a Na^+ gradient across the apical membrane. The Na^+ gradient is maintained by Na^+, K^+-adenosine triphosphatase (ATPase), the so-called Na^+ pump located on the basolateral membrane, which extrudes Na^+ and maintains low intracellular [Na] as well as the Na^+ gradient across the apical membrane. As a result, active glucose absorption and glucose-stimulated Na^+ absorption require both the apical membrane transport protein, SGLT1, and the basolateral Na^+, K^+-ATPase. In addition to glucose absorption being Na^+-dependent, glucose also stimulates Na^+ and fluid absorption, which is the physiologic basis of oral rehydration therapy for the treatment of diarrhea (Chap. 6).

The mechanisms of intestinal fluid and electrolyte absorption and secretion are discussed in Chap. 6.

Although the intestinal epithelial cells are crucial mediators of absorption and ion and water flow, the several cell types in the lamina propria (e.g., mast cells, macrophages, myofibroblasts) and the enteric nervous system interact with the epithelium to regulate mucosal cell function. The function of the intestine is the result of the integrated responses of and interactions between both intestinal epithelial cells and intestinal muscle.

ENTEROHEPATIC CIRCULATION OF BILE ACIDS

Bile acids are not present in the diet but are synthesized in the liver by a series of enzymatic steps that also include cholesterol catabolism. Indeed, interruption of the enterohepatic circulation of bile acids can reduce

serum cholesterol levels by 10% before a new steady state is established. Bile acids are either primary or secondary: Primary bile acids are synthesized in the liver from cholesterol, and secondary bile acids are synthesized from primary bile acids in the intestine by colonic bacterial enzymes. The two primary bile acids in humans are cholic acid and chenodeoxycholic acid; the two most abundant secondary bile acids are deoxycholic acid and lithocholic acid. Approximately 500 mg of bile acids are synthesized in the liver daily, conjugated to either taurine or glycine to form tauroconjugated or glycoconjugated bile acids, respectively, and secreted into the duodenum in bile. The primary functions of bile acids are (1) to promote bile flow, (2) to solubilize cholesterol and phospholipid in the gallbladder by mixed micelle formation, and (3) to enhance dietary lipid digestion and absorption by forming mixed micelles in the proximal small intestine.

Bile acids are primarily absorbed by an active, Na^+-dependent process that is located exclusively in the ileum, though bile acids can also be absorbed to a lesser extent by non-carrier-mediated transport processes in the jejunum, ileum, and colon. Conjugated bile acids that enter the colon are deconjugated by colonic bacterial enzymes to unconjugated bile acids and are rapidly absorbed by nonionic diffusion. Colonic bacterial enzymes also dehydroxylate bile acids to secondary bile acids.

Bile acids absorbed from the intestine return to the liver via the portal vein where they are re-secreted (Fig. 15-1). Bile acid synthesis is largely autoregulated by 7α-hydroxylase, the initial enzyme in cholesterol degradation. A decrease in the amount of bile acids returning to the liver from the intestine is associated with an increase in bile acid synthesis/cholesterol catabolism, which helps keep the bile acid pool size relatively constant. However, the capacity to increase bile acid synthesis is limited to about two to two and a half-fold (discussed later). The bile acid pool size is approximately 4 g and is circulated via the enterohepatic circulation about twice during each meal, or six to eight times during a 24-h period. A relatively small quantity of bile acids is not absorbed and is excreted in stool daily; this fecal loss is matched by hepatic bile acid synthesis.

Defects in any of the steps of the enterohepatic circulation of bile acids can result in a decrease in duodenal concentration of conjugated bile acids and, as a result, steatorrhea. Thus, steatorrhea can be caused by abnormalities in bile acid synthesis and excretion, their physical state in the intestinal lumen, and reabsorption (Table 15-1).

Synthesis

Decreased bile acid synthesis and steatorrhea have been demonstrated in chronic liver disease, but steatorrhea is often not a major component of the illness of these patients.

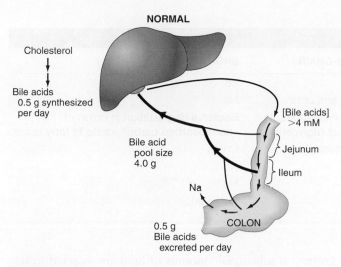

NORMAL

Cholesterol

Bile acids
0.5 g synthesized
per day

Bile acid
pool size
4.0 g

[Bile acids]
>4 mM

Jejunum

Ileum

Na

COLON

0.5 g
Bile acids
excreted per day

FIGURE 15-1

Schematic representation of the enterohepatic circulation of bile acids. Bile acid synthesis is cholesterol catabolism and occurs in the liver. Bile acids are secreted in bile and are stored in the gallbladder between meals and at night. Food in the duodenum induces the release of cholecystokinin, a potent stimulus for gallbladder contraction resulting in bile acid entry into the duodenum. Bile acids are primarily absorbed via a Na-dependent transport process that is located only in the ileum. A relatively small quantity of bile acids (~500 mg) is not absorbed in a 24-h period and is lost in stool. Fecal bile acid losses are matched by bile acid synthesis. The bile acid pool (the total amount of bile acids in the body) is ~4 g and is circulated twice during each meal or six to eight times in a 24-h period.

Secretion

Although bile acid secretion may be reduced or absent in biliary obstruction, steatorrhea is rarely a significant medical problem in these patients. In contrast, primary biliary cirrhosis represents a defect in canalicular excretion of organic anions, including bile acids, and not infrequently is associated with steatorrhea and

TABLE 15-1

DEFECTS IN ENTEROHEPATIC CIRCULATION OF BILE ACIDS

PROCESS	PATHOPHYSIOLOGIC DEFECT	DISEASE EXAMPLE
Synthesis	Decreased hepatic function	Cirrhosis
Biliary secretion	Altered canalicular function	Primary biliary cirrhosis
Maintenance of conjugated bile acids	Bacterial overgrowth	Jejunal diverticulosis
Reabsorption	Abnormal ileal function	Crohn's disease

its consequences, e.g., chronic bone disease. Thus, the osteopenia/osteomalacia and other chronic bone abnormalities often present in patients with primary biliary cirrhosis and other cholestatic syndromes are secondary to steatorrhea that then leads to calcium and vitamin D malabsorption as well as to the effects of cholestasis (e.g., bile acids and inflammatory cytokines).

Maintenance of conjugated bile acids

In bacterial overgrowth syndromes associated with diarrhea, steatorrhea, and macrocytic anemia, a colonic type of bacterial flora is increased in the small intestine. The steatorrhea is primarily a result of the decrease in conjugated bile acids secondary to their deconjugation by colonic-type bacteria. Two complementary explanations account for the resulting impairment of micelle formation: (1) unconjugated bile acids are rapidly absorbed in the jejunum by nonionic diffusion, resulting in a reduced concentration of duodenal bile acids; and (2) the critical micellar concentration (CMC) of unconjugated bile acids is higher than that of conjugated bile acids, and therefore unconjugated bile acids are less effective than conjugated bile acids in micelle formation.

Reabsorption

Ileal dysfunction caused by either Crohn's disease or surgical resection results in a decrease in bile acid reabsorption in the ileum and an *increase* in the delivery of bile acids to the large intestine. The resulting clinical consequences—diarrhea with or without steatorrhea—are determined by the *degree* of ileal dysfunction and the *response* of the enterohepatic circulation to bile acid losses **(Table 15-2)**. Patients with limited ileal disease

TABLE 15-2

COMPARISON OF BILE ACID AND FATTY ACID DIARRHEA

	BILE ACID DIARRHEA	FATTY ACID DIARRHEA
Extent of ileal disease	Limited	Extensive
Ileal bile acid absorption	Reduced	Reduced
Fecal bile acid excretion	Increased	Increased
Fecal bile acid loss compensated by hepatic synthesis	Yes	No
Bile acid pool size	Normal	Reduced
Intraduodenal [bile acid]	Normal	Reduced
Steatorrhea	None or mild	>20 g
Response to cholestyramine	Yes	No
Response to low-fat diet	No	Yes

TABLE 15-3

COMPARISON OF DIFFERENT TYPES OF FATTY ACIDS			
	LONG-CHAIN	**MEDIUM-CHAIN**	**SHORT-CHAIN**
Carbon chain length	>12	8–12	<8
Present in diet	In large amounts	In small amounts	No
Origin	In diet as triglycerides	Only in small amounts in diet as triglycerides	Bacterial degradation in colon of nonabsorbed carbohydrate to fatty acids
Primary site of absorption	Small intestine	Small intestine	Colon
Requires pancreatic lipolysis	Yes	No	No
Requires micelle formation	Yes	No	No
Presence in stool	Minimal	No	Substantial

or resection will often have diarrhea but not steatorrhea. The diarrhea, a result of bile acids in the colon stimulating active Cl secretion, has been called *bile acid diarrhea,* or choleretic enteropathy, and responds promptly to cholestyramine, an anion-binding resin. Such patients do not develop steatorrhea because hepatic synthesis of bile acids increases to compensate for the rate of fecal bile acid losses, resulting in maintenance of both the bile acid pool size and the intraduodenal concentrations of bile acids. In contrast, patients with greater degrees of ileal disease and/or resection will often have diarrhea and steatorrhea that do not respond to cholestyramine. In this situation, ileal disease is also associated with increased amounts of bile acids entering the colon; however, hepatic synthesis can no longer increase sufficiently to maintain the bile acid pool size. As a consequence, the intraduodenal concentration of bile acids is also reduced to less than the CMC, resulting in impaired micelle formation and steatorrhea. This second situation is often called *fatty acid diarrhea.* Cholestyramine may not be effective (and may even increase the diarrhea by further depleting the intraduodenal bile acid concentration); however, a low-fat diet to reduce fatty acids entering the colon can be effective. Two clinical features, the length of ileum removed and the degree of steatorrhea, can predict whether an individual patient will respond to cholestyramine. Unfortunately, these predictors are imperfect, and a therapeutic trial of cholestyramine is often necessary to establish whether an individual patient will benefit from cholestyramine. Table 15-2 contrasts the characteristics of bile acid diarrhea (small ileal dysfunction) and fatty acid diarrhea (large ileal dysfunction).

LIPIDS

Steatorrhea is caused by one or more defects in the digestion and absorption of dietary fat. Average intake of dietary fat in the United States is approximately 120–150 g/d, and fat absorption is linear to dietary fat intake. The total load of fat presented to the small intestine is considerably greater, as substantial amounts of lipid are secreted in bile each day. (Enterohepatic circulation of bile acids is discussed earlier.) Three types of fatty acids compose fats: long-chain fatty acids (LCFAs), medium-chain fatty acids (MCFAs), and short-chain fatty acids (SCFAs) **(Table 15-3)**. Dietary fat is exclusively composed of long-chain triglycerides (LCTs), i.e., glycerol that is bound via ester-linkages to three LCFAs. While the majority of dietary LCFAs have carbon chain lengths of 16 or 18, fatty acids of carbon chain length >12 are metabolized in the same manner; saturated and unsaturated fatty acids are handled identically.

Assimilation of dietary lipid requires three integrated processes: (1) an intraluminal, or digestive, phase; (2) a mucosal, or absorptive, phase; and (3) a delivery, or postabsorptive, phase. An abnormality at any site of this process can cause steatorrhea **(Table 15-4)**. Therefore,

TABLE 15-4

DEFECTS IN LIPID DIGESTION AND ABSORPTION IN STEATORRHEA		
PHASE: PROCESS	**PATHOPHYSIOLOGIC DEFECT**	**DISEASE EXAMPLE**
Digestive		
Lipolysis formation	Decreased lipase secretion	Chronic pancreatitis
Micelle formation	Decreased intraduodenal bile acids	See Table 15-1
Absorptive		
Mucosal uptake and reesterification	Mucosal dysfunction	Celiac disease
Postabsorptive		
Chylomicron formation	Absent betalipoproteins	Abetalipoproteinemia
Delivery from intestine	Abnormal lymphatics	Intestinal lymphangiectasia

Pancreas	Liver	Jejunal Mucosa	Lymphatics
Lipolysis	Micellar Solubilization with Bile Acid	Absorption	Delivery

FIGURE 15-2

Schematic representation of lipid digestion and absorption. Dietary lipid is in the form of long-chain triglycerides (LCTs). The overall process can be divided into (1) a digestive phase that includes both lipolysis and micelle formation requiring pancreatic lipase and conjugated bile acids, respectively, in the duodenum; (2) an absorptive phase for mucosal uptake and reesterification; and (3) a postabsorptive phase that includes chylomicron formation and exit from the intestinal epithelial cell via lymphatics. (*Courtesy of John M. Dietschy, MD; with permission.*)

it is essential that any patient with steatorrhea be evaluated to identify the specific physiologic defect in overall lipid digestion–absorption, as therapy will be determined by the specific cause of the steatorrhea.

The digestive phase has two components, *lipolysis* and *micellar formation*. Although dietary lipid is in the form of LCTs, the intestinal mucosa does not absorb triglycerides; they must first be hydrolyzed **(Fig. 15-2)**. The initial step in lipid digestion is the formation of emulsions of finely dispersed lipid, which is accomplished by mastication and gastric contractions. Lipolysis, the hydrolysis of triglycerides to free fatty acids, monoglycerides, and glycerol by lipase, is initiated in the stomach by lingual and gastric lipases that have a pH optimum of 4.5–6.0. About 20–30% of total lipolysis occurs in the stomach. Lipolysis is completed in the duodenum and jejunum by pancreatic lipase, which is inactivated by a pH <7.0. Pancreatic lipolysis is greatly enhanced by the presence of a second pancreatic enzyme, colipase, which facilitates the movement of lipase to the triglyceride.

Impaired lipolysis can lead to steatorrhea and can occur in the presence of pancreatic insufficiency due to chronic pancreatitis in adults or cystic fibrosis in children and adolescents. Normal lipolysis can be maintained by approximately 5% of maximal pancreatic lipase secretion; thus, steatorrhea is a late manifestation of these disorders. A reduction in intraduodenal pH can also result in altered lipolysis as pancreatic lipase is inactivated at pH <7. Thus, ~15% of patients with gastrinoma (Chap. 14) with substantial increases in gastric acid secretion from ectopic production of gastrin (usually from an islet cell adenoma) have diarrhea, and some will have steatorrhea believed secondary to acid-inactivation of pancreatic lipase. Similarly, patients with chronic pancreatitis (who have reduced lipase secretion) often have a decrease in pancreatic bicarbonate secretion, which will also result in a decrease in intraduodenal pH and inactivation of endogenous pancreatic lipase or of therapeutically administered lipase.

Overlying the microvillus membrane of the small intestine is the so-called unstirred water layer, a relatively stagnant aqueous phase that must be traversed by the products of lipolysis that are primarily water–insoluble. Water-soluble mixed micelles provide a mechanism for the water-insoluble products of lipolysis to reach the luminal plasma membrane of villous epithelial cells, the site for lipid absorption. Mixed micelles are molecular aggregates composed of fatty acids, monoglycerides, phospholipids, cholesterol, and conjugated bile acids. Mixed micelles are formed when the concentration of conjugated bile acids is greater than its CMC, which differs among the several bile acids present in the small intestinal lumen. Conjugated bile acids, synthesized in the liver and excreted into the duodenum in bile, are regulated by the enterohepatic circulation (see above). Steatorrhea can result from impaired movement of fatty acids across the unstirred aqueous fluid layer in two situations: (1) an increase in the relative thickness of the unstirred water layer that occurs in bacterial overgrowth syndromes (discussed later) secondary to functional stasis (e.g., scleroderma); and (2) a decrease in the *duodenal* concentration of conjugated bile acids below its CMC, resulting in impaired micelle formation. Thus, steatorrhea can be caused by one or more defects in the enterohepatic circulation of bile acids.

Uptake and reesterification constitute the *absorptive phase* of lipid digestion-absorption. Although passive diffusion has been thought responsible, a carrier-mediated process may mediate fatty acid and monoglyceride uptake. Regardless of the uptake process, fatty acids and monoglycerides are reesterified by a series of enzymatic steps in the endoplasmic reticulum to form triglycerides, the form in which lipid exits from the intestinal epithelial cell. Impaired lipid absorption as a result of either mucosal inflammation (e.g., celiac disease) and/or intestinal resection can also lead to steatorrhea.

The reesterified triglycerides require the formation of *chylomicrons* to permit their exit from the small-intestinal epithelial cell and their delivery to the liver via the *lymphatics*. Chylomicrons are composed of β-lipoprotein and contain triglycerides, cholesterol, cholesterol esters, and phospholipids and enter the lymphatics, not the portal vein. Defects in the *postabsorptive phase* of lipid digestion-absorption can also result in steatorrhea, but these disorders are uncommon. Abetalipoproteinemia, or acanthocytosis, is a rare disorder of impaired synthesis of β-lipoprotein associated with abnormal erythrocytes (acanthocytes), neurologic problems, and steatorrhea. Lipolysis, micelle formation, and lipid uptake are all normal in patients with abetalipoproteinemia, but the reesterified triglyceride cannot exit from the epithelial cell because of the failure to produce chylomicrons. Small-intestinal biopsies of these rare patients in the postprandial state reveal lipid-laden small-intestinal epithelial cells that become perfectly normal in appearance following a 72–96 h fast. Similarly, abnormalities of intestinal lymphatics (e.g., intestinal lymphangiectasia) may also be associated with steatorrhea as well as protein loss (discussed later). Steatorrhea can result from defects at any of the several steps in lipid digestion-absorption.

The mechanism of lipid digestion-absorption outlined earlier is limited to *dietary* lipid that is almost exclusively in the form of LCTs (Table 15-3). Medium-chain triglycerides (MCTs), composed of fatty acids with carbon chain lengths of 8–12, are present in large amounts in coconut oil and are used as a nutritional supplement. MCTs can be digested and absorbed by a different pathway from LCTs and at one time held promise as an important treatment of steatorrhea of almost all etiologies. Unfortunately, their therapeutic effects have been less than expected because their use is often not associated with an increase in body weight for reasons that are not completely understood.

MCTs, in contrast to LCTs, do not require pancreatic lipolysis as the triglyceride can be absorbed intact by the intestinal epithelial cell. Further, micelle formation is not necessary for the absorption of MCTs or medium-chain fatty acids, if hydrolyzed by pancreatic lipase. MCTs are absorbed more efficiently than LCTs for the following reasons: (1) The rate of MCT absorption is greater than that of long-chain fatty acids; (2) medium-chain fatty acids following absorption are not reesterified; (3) following absorption, MCTs are hydrolyzed to medium-chain fatty acids; (4) MCTs do not require chylomicron formation for their exit from the intestinal epithelial cells; and (5) their route of exit is via the portal vein and not via lymphatics. Thus, the absorption of MCTs is greater than that of LCTs in pancreatic insufficiency, conditions with reduced intraduodenal bile acid concentrations, small-intestinal mucosal disease, abetalipoproteinemia, and intestinal lymphangiectasia.

SCFAs are not dietary lipids but are synthesized by colonic bacterial enzymes from nonabsorbed carbohydrate and are the anions in highest concentration in stool (between 80 and 130 m*M*). The SCFAs present in stool are primarily acetate, propionate, and butyrate, whose carbon chain lengths are 2, 3, and 4, respectively. Butyrate is the primary nutrient for colonic epithelial cells, and its deficiency may be associated with one or more colitides. SCFAs conserve calories and carbohydrate, because carbohydrates not completely absorbed in the small intestine will not be absorbed in the large intestine due to the absence of both disaccharidases and SGLT1, the transport protein that mediates monosaccharide absorption. In contrast, SCFAs are rapidly absorbed and stimulate colonic Na-Cl and fluid absorption. Most non–*Clostridium difficile* antibiotic-associated diarrhea is due to antibiotic suppression of colonic microbiota, with a resulting decrease in SCFA production. As *C. difficile* accounts for about 15–20% of all antibiotic-associated diarrhea, a relative decrease in colonic production of SCFA is likely the cause of most antibiotic-associated diarrhea.

The clinical manifestations of steatorrhea are a consequence of both the underlying disorder responsible for the development of steatorrhea and steatorrhea per se. Depending on the degree of steatorrhea and the level of dietary intake, significant fat malabsorption may lead to weight loss. Steatorrhea per se can be responsible for diarrhea; if the primary cause of the steatorrhea has not been identified, a low-fat diet can often ameliorate the diarrhea by decreasing fecal fat excretion. Steatorrhea is often associated with fat-soluble vitamin deficiency, which will require replacement with water-soluble preparations of these vitamins.

Disorders of absorption may also be associated with malabsorption of other dietary nutrients, most often carbohydrates, with or without a decrease in dietary lipid digestion and absorption. Therefore, knowledge of the mechanism of the digestion and absorption of carbohydrates, proteins, and other minerals and vitamins is useful in the evaluation of patients with altered intestinal nutrient absorption.

CARBOHYDRATES

Carbohydrates in the diet are present in the form of starch, disaccharides (sucrose and lactose), and glucose. Carbohydrates are absorbed only in the small intestine and only in the form of monosaccharides. Therefore, before their absorption, starch and disaccharides must first be digested by pancreatic amylase and intestinal brush border disaccharidases to monosaccharides. Monosaccharide absorption occurs by a Na-dependent process mediated by the brush border transport protein SGLT1.

Lactose malabsorption is the only clinically important disorder of carbohydrate absorption. Lactose, the disaccharide present in milk, requires digestion by brush border lactase to its two constituent monosaccharides, glucose and galactose. Lactase is present in almost all species in the postnatal period but then disappears throughout the animal kingdom, except in humans. Lactase activity persists in many individuals throughout life. Two different types of lactase deficiency exist—primary and secondary. In *primary lactase deficiency,* a genetically determined decrease or absence of lactase is noted, while all other aspects of both intestinal absorption and brush border enzymes are normal. In a number of non-white groups, primary lactase deficiency is common in adulthood. Table 15-5 presents the incidence of primary lactase deficiency in several ethnic groups. Northern European and North American whites are the only groups to maintain small-intestinal lactase activity throughout adult life. The persistence of lactase is the abnormality due to a defect in the regulation of its maturation. In contrast, *secondary lactase deficiency* occurs in association with small-intestinal mucosal disease with abnormalities in both structure and function of other brush border enzymes and transport processes. Secondary lactase deficiency is often seen in celiac disease.

As lactose digestion is rate-limiting compared to glucose/galactose absorption, lactase deficiency is associated with significant lactose malabsorption. Some individuals with lactose malabsorption develop symptoms such as diarrhea, abdominal pain, cramps, and/or flatus. Most individuals with primary lactase deficiency do not have symptoms. Since lactose intolerance may be associated with symptoms suggestive of irritable bowel syndrome, persistence of such symptoms in an individual with lactose intolerance while on a strict lactose-free diet would suggest that the individual's symptoms were related to irritable bowel syndrome.

Development of symptoms of lactose intolerance is related to several factors:

1. *Amount of lactose in the diet.*
2. *Rate of gastric emptying.* Symptoms are more likely when gastric emptying is rapid than when gastric emptying is slower. Therefore, it is more likely that skim milk will be associated with symptoms of lactose intolerance than will whole milk, as the rate of gastric emptying following skim milk intake is more rapid. Similarly, the diarrhea observed following subtotal gastrectomy is often a result of lactose intolerance, as gastric emptying is accelerated in patients with a gastrojejunostomy.
3. *Small-intestinal transit time.* Although the small and large intestine contribute to the development of symptoms, many of the symptoms of lactase deficiency are related to the interaction of colonic bacteria and nonabsorbed lactose. More rapid small-intestinal transit makes symptoms more likely.
4. *Colonic compensation by production of SCFAs from nonabsorbed lactose.* Reduced levels of colonic microflora, which can occur following antibiotic use, will also be associated with increased symptoms following lactose ingestion, especially in a lactase-deficient individual.

Glucose-galactose or monosaccharide malabsorption may also be associated with diarrhea and is due to a congenital absence of SGLT1. Diarrhea is present when individuals with this disorder ingest carbohydrates that contain actively transported monosaccharides (e.g., glucose, galactose) but not monosaccharides that are not actively transported (e.g., fructose). Fructose is absorbed by the brush border transport protein GLUT 5, a facilitated diffusion process that is not Na-dependent and is distinct from SGLT1. In contrast, some individuals develop diarrhea as a result of consuming large quantities of sorbitol, a sugar used in diabetic candy; sorbitol is only minimally absorbed due to the absence of an intestinal absorptive transport mechanism for sorbitol.

PROTEINS

Protein is present in food almost exclusively as polypeptides and requires extensive hydrolysis to di- and tripeptides and amino acids before absorption. Proteolysis occurs in both the stomach and small intestine; it is mediated by pepsin secreted as pepsinogen by gastric chief cells and trypsinogen and other peptidases from pancreatic acinar cells. These proenzymes, pepsinogen and trypsinogen, must be activated to pepsin (by pepsin in the presence of a pH <5) and to trypsin (by the intestinal brush border enzyme enterokinase

TABLE 15-5

PRIMARY LACTASE DEFICIENCY IN DIFFERENT ADULT ETHNIC GROUPS	
ETHNIC GROUP	**PREVALENCE OF LACTASE DEFICIENCY, %**
Northern European	5–15
Mediterranean	60–85
African black	85–100
American black	45–80
American white	10–25
Native American	50–95
Mexican American	40–75
Asian	90–100

Source: From FJ Simons: Am J Dig Dis 23:963, 1978.

and subsequently by trypsin), respectively. Proteins are absorbed by separate transport systems for di- and tripeptides and for different types of amino acids, e.g., neutral and dibasic. Alterations in either protein or amino acid digestion and absorption are rarely observed clinically, even in the presence of extensive small-intestinal mucosal inflammation. However, three rare genetic disorders involve protein digestion–absorption: (1) *Enterokinase deficiency* is due to an absence of the brush border enzyme that converts the proenzyme trypsinogen to trypsin and is associated with diarrhea, growth retardation, and hypoproteinemia. (2) *Hartnup syndrome*, a defect in neutral amino acid transport, is characterized by a pellagra-like rash and neuropsychiatric symptoms. (3) *Cystinuria*, a defect in dibasic amino acid transport, is associated with renal calculi and chronic pancreatitis.

APPROACH TO THE PATIENT   Malabsorption

The clues provided by the history, symptoms, and initial preliminary observations will serve to limit extensive, ill-focused, and expensive laboratory and imaging studies. For example, a clinician evaluating a patient with symptoms suggestive of malabsorption, who recently had extensive small-intestinal resection for mesenteric ischemia, should direct the initial assessment almost exclusively to define whether a short bowel syndrome might explain the entire clinical picture. Similarly, the development of a pattern of bowel movements suggestive of steatorrhea in a patient with long-standing alcohol abuse and chronic pancreatitis should lead toward assessing pancreatic exocrine function.

The classic picture of malabsorption is rarely seen today in most parts of the United States. As a consequence, diseases with malabsorption must be suspected in individuals with less severe symptoms and signs and with subtle evidence of the altered absorption of only a *single* nutrient rather than obvious evidence of the malabsorption of multiple nutrients.

Although diarrhea can be caused by changes in fluid and electrolyte movement in either the small or the large intestine, dietary nutrients are absorbed almost exclusively in the small intestine. Therefore, the demonstration of diminished absorption of a dietary nutrient provides unequivocal evidence of small-intestinal disease, although colonic dysfunction may also be present (e.g., Crohn's disease may involve both small and large intestine). Dietary nutrient absorption may be segmental or diffuse along the small intestine and is site-specific. Thus, for example, calcium, iron, and folic acid are exclusively absorbed by active transport processes in the proximal small intestine, especially the duodenum;

in contrast, the active transport mechanisms for both cobalamin and bile acids are present only in the ileum. Therefore, in an individual who years previously had had an intestinal resection, the details of which are not presently available, a presentation with evidence of calcium, folic acid, and/or iron malabsorption but without cobalamin deficiency would make it likely that the duodenum and proximal jejunum, but not ileum, had been resected.

Some nutrients, e.g., glucose, amino acids, and lipids, are absorbed throughout the small intestine, though their rate of absorption is greater in the proximal than in the distal segments. However, following segmental resection of the small intestine, the remaining segments undergo both morphologic and functional "adaptation" to enhance absorption. Such adaptation is secondary to the presence of luminal nutrients and hormonal stimuli and may not be complete in humans for several months following the resection. Adaptation is critical for survival in individuals who have undergone massive resection of the small intestine and/or colon.

Establishing the presence of steatorrhea and identifying its specific cause are often quite difficult. The "gold standard" still remains a timed, quantitative stool fat determination. On a practical basis, stool collections are invariably difficult and often incomplete, as nobody wants to handle stool. A qualitative test—Sudan III stain—has long been available to establish the presence of an increase in stool fat. This test is rapid and inexpensive but, as a qualitative test, does not establish the degree of fat malabsorption and is best used as a preliminary screening study. Many of the blood, breath, and isotopic tests that have been developed (1) do not directly measure fat absorption; (2) have excellent sensitivity when steatorrhea is obvious and severe but have poor sensitivity when steatorrhea is mild (e.g., stool chymotrypsin, elastase, that can potentially distinguish pancreatic from nonpancreatic etiologies of steatorrhea); or (3) have not survived the transition from the research laboratory to commercial application.

Despite this situation, the use of routine laboratory studies (i.e., complete blood count, prothrombin time, serum protein determination, alkaline phosphatase) may suggest the presence of dietary nutrient depletion, especially iron, folate, cobalamin, and vitamins D and K. Additional studies include measurement of serum carotene, cholesterol, albumin, iron, folate, and cobalamin levels. The serum carotene level can also be reduced if the patient has poor dietary intake of leafy vegetables.

If steatorrhea and/or altered absorption of other nutrients are suspected, the history, clinical observations, and laboratory testing can help detect deficiency of a nutrient, especially the fat-soluble vitamins A, D, E, or K. Thus, evidence of metabolic bone disease with elevated alkaline phosphatase and/or reduced serum calcium levels would suggest vitamin D malabsorption. A deficiency of vitamin K would be suggested by an elevated prothrombin time in an individual without liver disease who was not taking anticoagulants. Macrocytic anemia would lead to evaluation of whether cobalamin or folic acid malabsorption was present. The presence of iron-deficiency anemia in the absence of occult bleeding from the gastrointestinal tract in either a male or a non-menstruating female would require evaluation of iron malabsorption and the exclusion of celiac disease, as iron is absorbed exclusively in the proximal small intestine.

At times, however, a timed (72 h) quantitative stool collection, preferably on a defined diet, must be obtained to determine stool fat content and establish the presence of steatorrhea. The presence of steatorrhea then requires further assessment to establish the pathophysiologic process(es) responsible for the defect in dietary lipid digestion-absorption (Table 15-4). Some of the other studies include the Schilling test, D-xylose test, duodenal mucosal biopsy, small-intestinal radiologic examination, and tests of pancreatic exocrine function.

THE SCHILLING TEST This test is performed to determine the cause of cobalamin malabsorption. Unfortunately, the Schilling test has not been available commercially in the United States for the past few years. Since understanding the physiology and pathophysiology of cobalamin absorption is very valuable to enhance one's understanding of aspects of gastric, pancreatic, and ileal function, discussion of the Schilling test is provided in Chap. 16.

URINARY D-XYLOSE TEST The urinary D-xylose test for carbohydrate absorption provides an assessment of proximal small-intestinal mucosal function. D-Xylose, a pentose, is absorbed almost exclusively in the proximal small intestine. The D-xylose test is usually performed by giving 25 g D-xylose and collecting urine for 5 h. An abnormal test (<4.5 g excretion) primarily reflects the presence of duodenal/jejunal mucosal disease. The D-xylose test can also be abnormal in patients with blind loop syndrome (as a consequence primarily of abnormal intestinal mucosa) and, as a false-positive study, in patients with large collections of fluid in a third space (i.e., ascites, pleural fluid). The ease of obtaining a mucosal biopsy of the small intestine by endoscopy and the false-negative rate of the D-xylose test have led to its diminished use. When small-intestinal mucosal disease is suspected, a small-intestinal mucosal biopsy should be performed.

RADIOLOGIC EXAMINATION Radiologic examination of the small intestine using barium contrast (small-bowel series or study) can provide important information in the evaluation of the patient with presumed or suspected malabsorption. These studies are most often performed in conjunction with the examination of the esophagus, stomach, and duodenal bulb, and insufficient barium is given to the patient to permit an adequate examination of the small-intestinal mucosa, especially the ileum. As a result, many gastrointestinal radiologists alter the procedure of a barium contrast examination of the small intestine by performing either a small-bowel series in which a large amount of barium is given by mouth without concurrent examination of the esophagus and stomach or an enteroclysis study in which a large amount of barium is introduced into the duodenum via a fluoroscopically placed tube. In addition, many of the diagnostic features initially described by radiologists to denote the presence of small-intestinal disease (e.g., flocculation, segmentation) are rarely seen with current barium suspensions. Nonetheless, in skilled hands barium contrast examination of the small intestine can yield important information. For example, with extensive mucosal disease, dilation of intestine can be seen, as dilution of barium from increased intestinal fluid secretion (Fig. 15-3). A normal barium contrast study does *not* exclude the possibility of small-intestinal disease. However, a small-bowel series remains a useful examination to look for anatomic abnormalities, such as strictures and fistulas (as in Crohn's disease) or blind loop syndrome (e.g., multiple jejunal diverticula), and to define the extent of a previous surgical resection. Other imaging studies to assess the integrity of small intestinal morphology are CT enteroclysis and magnetic resonance (MR) enteroclysis, while capsule endoscopy and double-barrel enteroscopy are other useful aids in the diagnostic assessment of small-intestinal pathology.

BIOPSY OF SMALL-INTESTINAL MUCOSA A small-intestinal mucosal biopsy is essential in the evaluation of a patient with documented steatorrhea or chronic diarrhea (lasting >3 weeks) (Chap. 6). The ready availability of endoscopic equipment to examine the stomach and duodenum has led to its almost uniform use as the preferred method to obtain histologic material of proximal small-intestinal mucosa. The primary indications for a small-intestinal biopsy are (1) evaluation of a patient either with documented or suspected steatorrhea or with chronic diarrhea, and (2) diffuse or focal abnormalities of the small intestine defined on a small-intestinal series. Lesions seen on small-bowel biopsy can be classified into three different categories (Table 15-6):

1. *Diffuse, specific lesions.* Relatively few diseases associated with altered nutrient absorption have specific histopathologic abnormalities on small-intestinal mucosal biopsy, and they are uncommon. Whipple's disease is characterized by the presence of periodic

FIGURE 15-3
Barium contrast small-intestinal radiologic examinations. *A.* Normal individual. ***B.*** Celiac sprue. ***C.*** Jejunal diverticulosis. ***D.*** Crohn's disease. (*Courtesy of Morton Burrell, MD, Yale University; with permission.*)

acid–Schiff (PAS)–positive macrophages in the lamina propria, while the bacilli that are also present may require electron-microscopic examination for identification (Fig. 15-4). *Abetalipoproteinemia* is characterized by a normal mucosal appearance except for the presence of mucosal absorptive cells that contain lipid postprandially and disappear following a prolonged period of either fat-free intake or fasting. *Immune globulin deficiency* is associated with a variety of histopathologic findings on small-intestinal mucosal biopsy. The characteristic feature is the absence of or substantial reduction in the number of plasma cells in the lamina propria; the mucosal architecture may be either perfectly normal or flat (i.e., villous atrophy). As patients with immune globulin deficiency are often infected with *Giardia lamblia*, *Giardia* trophozoites may also be seen in the biopsy.

2. *Patchy, specific lesions.* Several diseases show abnormal small-intestinal mucosa with a patchy distribution.

As a result, biopsies obtained randomly or in the absence of abnormalities visualized endoscopically may not reveal the diagnostic features. Intestinal *lymphoma* can at times be diagnosed on mucosal biopsy by the identification of malignant lymphoma cells in the lamina propria and submucosa. The presence of dilated lymphatics in the submucosa and sometimes in the lamina propria indicates the presence of *lymphangiectasia* associated with hypoproteinemia secondary to protein loss into the intestine. *Eosinophilic gastroenteritis* comprises a heterogeneous group of disorders with a spectrum of presentations and symptoms with an eosinophilic infiltrate of the lamina propria, with or without peripheral eosinophilia. The patchy nature of the infiltrate as well as its presence in the submucosa often leads to an absence of histopathologic findings on mucosal biopsy. As the involvement of the duodenum in *Crohn's disease* is also submucosal and not necessarily continuous,

TABLE 15-6

DISEASE THAT CAN BE DIAGNOSED BY SMALL-INTESTINAL MUCOSAL BIOPSIES

LESIONS	PATHOLOGIC FINDINGS
Diffuse, Specific	
Whipple's disease	Lamina propria contains macrophages containing PAS+ material
Agammaglobulinemia	No plasma cells; either normal or absent villi ("flat mucosa")
Abetalipoproteinemia	Normal villi; epithelial cells vacuolated with fat postprandially
Patchy, Specific	
Intestinal lymphoma	Malignant cells in lamina propria and submucosa
Intestinal lymphangiectasia	Dilated lymphatics; clubbed villi
Eosinophilic gastroenteritis	Eosinophil infiltration of lamina propria and mucosa
Amyloidosis	Amyloid deposits
Crohn's disease	Noncaseating granulomas
Infection by one or more microorganisms (see text)	Specific organisms
Mastocytosis	Mast cell infiltration of lamina propria
Diffuse, Nonspecific	
Celiac disease	Short or absent villi; mononuclear infiltrate; epithelial cell damage; hypertrophy of crypts
Tropical sprue	Similar to celiac disease
Bacterial overgrowth	Patchy damage to villi; lymphocyte infiltration
Folate deficiency	Short villi; decreased mitosis in crypts; megalocytosis
Vitamin B$_{12}$ deficiency	Similar to folate deficiency
Radiation enteritis	Similar to folate deficiency
Zollinger-Ellison syndrome	Mucosal ulceration and erosion from acid
Protein-calorie malnutrition	Villous atrophy; secondary bacterial overgrowth
Drug-induced enteritis	Variable histology

Abbreviation: PAS+, periodic acid–Schiff positive.

mucosal biopsies are not the most direct approach to the diagnosis of duodenal Crohn's disease (Chap. 17). Amyloid deposition can be identified by Congo Red stain in some patients with *amyloidosis* involving the duodenum.

3. Several microorganisms can be identified on small-intestinal biopsies, establishing a correct diagnosis. At times the small biopsy is performed to establish the diagnosis of the infection, e.g., Whipple's disease or giardiasis. In most other instances the infection is picked up incidentally during the workup of diarrhea or other abdominal symptoms. Many of these infections occur in immunocompromised patients with diarrhea and include *Cryptosporidium, Isospora belli, Microsporidia, Cyclospora, Toxoplasma,* cytomegalovirus, adenovirus, *Mycobacterium avium-intracellulare,* and *G. lamblia.* In immunocompromised patients, when *Candida, Aspergillus, Cryptococcus,* or *Histoplasma* organisms are seen on duodenal biopsy, their presence generally reflects systemic infection. Apart from Whipple's disease and infections in the immunocompromised host, the small bowel biopsy is seldom used as the primary mode to diagnose infection. Even giardiasis is more easily diagnosed with duodenal aspirates and/or stool antigen studies than by duodenal biopsy.

4. *Diffuse, nonspecific lesions. Celiac disease* presents with a characteristic mucosal appearance on duodenal/proximal jejunal mucosal biopsy that is *not* diagnostic of the disease. The diagnosis of celiac disease is established by clinical, histologic, and immunologic response to a gluten-free diet. *Tropical sprue* is associated with histologic findings similar to those of celiac disease after a tropical or subtropical exposure but does not respond to gluten restriction; most often symptoms improve with antibiotics and folate administration.

Patients with steatorrhea require assessment of *pancreatic exocrine function,* which is often abnormal in chronic pancreatitis. The secretin test that collects pancreatic secretions by duodenal intubation following intravenous administration of secretin is the only test that directly measures pancreatic exocrine function but is available only at few specialized centers. Endoscopic approaches provide excellent assessment of pancreatic duct anatomy but do *not* assess exocrine function (Chap. 47).

Table 15-7 summarizes the results of the D-xylose test, Schilling test, and small-intestinal mucosal biopsy in patients with five different causes of steatorrhea.

SPECIFIC DISEASE ENTITIES

CELIAC DISEASE

Celiac disease is a common cause of malabsorption of one or more nutrients. Though originally considered largely a disease in whites, especially those of European descent, recent observations have established that celiac disease is a common disease with protean manifestations, a worldwide distribution, and an estimated incidence in the United States that is as high as 1:113 people. Its incidence has increased over the past 50 years. Celiac disease has had several other names, including nontropical sprue, celiac sprue, adult celiac disease, and gluten-sensitive enteropathy. The etiology of celiac disease

FIGURE 15-4
Small-intestinal mucosal biopsies. *A.* Normal individual. ***B.*** Untreated celiac sprue. ***C.*** Treated celiac sprue. ***D.*** Intestinal lymphangiectasia. ***E.*** Whipple's disease. ***F.*** Lymphoma. ***G.*** Giardiasis. (*Courtesy of Marie Robert, MD, Yale University; with permission.*)

is not known, but environmental, immunologic, and genetic factors are important. Celiac disease is considered an "iceberg" disease with a small number of individuals with classical symptoms and manifestations related to nutrient malabsorption, and a varied natural history, with the onset of symptoms occurring at ages ranging from the first year of life through the eighth decade. A much larger number of individuals have manifestations that are not obviously related to intestinal malabsorption, e.g., anemia, osteopenia, infertility, neurologic symptoms ("atypical celiac disease"); while an even larger group is essentially asymptomatic although with abnormal small-intestinal histopathology and serologies (discussed later) and as is referred to as having "silent" celiac disease.

The hallmark of celiac disease is the presence of an abnormal small-intestinal biopsy (Fig. 15-4) and the response of the condition—symptoms and the histologic changes on the small-intestinal biopsy—to the elimination of gluten from the diet. The histologic changes have a proximal-to-distal intestinal distribution of severity, which probably reflects the exposure of the intestinal mucosa to varied amounts of dietary gluten; the symptoms do not necessarily correlate with histologic changes especially as many newly diagnosed patients with celiac disease may be asymptomatic.

The symptoms of celiac disease may appear with the introduction of cereals in an infant's diet, although spontaneous remissions often occur during the second

TABLE 15-7

RESULTS OF DIAGNOSTIC STUDIES IN DIFFERENT CAUSES OF STEATORRHEA

	D-XYLOSE TEST	SCHILLING TEST	DUODENAL MUCOSAL BIOPSY
Chronic pancreatitis	Normal	50% abnormal; if abnormal, normal with pancreatic enzymes	Normal
Bacterial overgrowth syndrome	Normal or only modestly abnormal	Often abnormal; if abnormal, normal after antibiotics	Usually normal
Ileal disease	Normal	Abnormal	Normal
Celiac disease	Decreased	Normal	Abnormal: probably "flat"
Intestinal lymphangiectasia	Normal	Normal	Abnormal: "dilated lymphatics"

decade of life that may be either permanent or followed by the reappearance of symptoms over several years. Alternatively, the symptoms of celiac disease may first become evident at almost any age throughout adulthood. In many patients, frequent spontaneous remissions and exacerbations occur. The symptoms range from significant malabsorption of multiple nutrients, with diarrhea, steatorrhea, weight loss, and the consequences of nutrient depletion (i.e., anemia and metabolic bone disease), to the absence of any gastrointestinal symptoms but with evidence of the depletion of a single nutrient (e.g., iron or folate deficiency, osteomalacia, edema from protein loss). Asymptomatic relatives of patients with celiac disease have been identified as having this disease either by small-intestinal biopsy or by serologic studies [e.g., antiendomysial antibodies, tissue transglutaminase (tTG)]. The availability of these "celiac serologies" has led to a substantial increase in the diagnosis of celiac disease, and the diagnosis is now being made primarily in patients without "classic" symptoms but with atypical and subclinical presentations.

Etiology

The etiology of celiac disease is not known, but environmental, immunologic, and genetic factors all appear to contribute to the disease. One *environmental* factor is the clear association of the disease with gliadin, a component of gluten that is present in wheat, barley, and rye. In addition to the role of gluten restriction in treatment, the instillation of gluten into both normal-appearing rectum and distal ileum of patients with celiac disease results in morphologic changes within hours.

An *immunologic* component in the pathogenesis of celiac disease is critical and involves both adaptive and innate immune responses. Serum antibodies—IgA antigliadin, IgA antiendomysial, and IgA anti-tTG antibodies—are present, but it is not known whether such antibodies are primary or secondary to the tissue damage. The antiendomysial antibody has 90–95% sensitivity and 90–95% specificity; the antigen recognized by the antiendomysial antibody is tTG, which deaminates gliadin, which is presented to HLA-DQ2 or HLA-DQ8 (discussed later). Antibody studies are frequently used to identify patients with celiac disease; patients with these antibodies should undergo duodenal biopsy. This autoantibody has not been linked to a pathogenetic mechanism (or mechanisms) responsible for celiac disease. Nonetheless, this antibody is useful in establishing the true prevalence of celiac disease in the general population. A 4-week treatment with prednisolone of a patient with celiac disease who continues to eat gluten will induce a remission and convert the "flat" abnormal duodenal biopsy to a more normal-appearing one. In addition, gliadin peptides interact with gliadin-specific T cells that mediate tissue injury and induce the release of one or more cytokines (e.g., IFN-γ) that cause tissue injury.

Genetic factor(s) are also involved in celiac disease. The incidence of symptomatic celiac disease varies widely in different population groups (high in whites, low in blacks and Asians) and is 10% in first-degree relatives of celiac disease patients; however, serologic studies provide clear evidence that celiac disease is present worldwide. Furthermore, all patients with celiac disease express the HLA-DQ2 or HLA-DQ8 allele, though only a minority of people expressing DQ2/DQ8 have celiac disease. Absence of DQ2/DQ8 excludes the diagnosis of celiac disease.

Diagnosis

A small-intestinal biopsy is required to establish a diagnosis of celiac disease (Fig. 15-4). A biopsy should be performed in patients with symptoms and laboratory findings suggestive of nutrient malabsorption and/or deficiency and with a positive endomysial antibody test. Since the presentation of celiac disease is often subtle, without overt evidence of malabsorption or nutrient deficiency, a relatively low threshold to perform a biopsy is important. It is more prudent to perform a biopsy than to obtain another test of intestinal absorption, which can never completely exclude or establish this diagnosis.

The diagnosis of celiac disease requires the presence of characteristic histologic changes on small-intestinal biopsy together with a prompt clinical and histologic response following the institution of a gluten-free diet. If serologic studies have detected the presence of IgA antiendomysial or tTG antibodies, they too should disappear after a gluten-free diet is started. With the increase in number of patients diagnosed with celiac disease that have been largely identified by serologic studies, the spectrum of histologic changes seen on duodenal biopsy has increased and includes findings that are not as severe as the classic changes shown in Fig. 15-4. The classical changes seen on duodenal/jejunal biopsy are restricted to the mucosa and include (1) an increase in the number of intraepithelial lymphocytes; (2) absence or reduced height of villi, resulting in a flat appearance with increased crypt cell proliferation, resulting in crypt hyperplasia and loss of villous structure, with consequent villous, but not mucosal, atrophy; (3) cuboidal appearance and nuclei that are no longer oriented basally in surface epithelial cells; and (4) increased lymphocytes and plasma cells in the lamina propria (Fig. 15-4B). Although these features are characteristic of celiac disease, they are *not* diagnostic because a similar appearance can be seen in tropical sprue, eosinophilic enteritis, and milk-protein intolerance in children and occasionally in lymphoma, bacterial overgrowth, Crohn's disease, and gastrinoma with acid hypersecretion. However, the presence of a characteristic histologic appearance that reverts toward normal following the initiation of a gluten-free diet establishes the diagnosis of celiac disease (Fig. 15-4C). Readministration of gluten with or without an additional small-intestinal biopsy is not necessary.

Failure to respond to gluten restriction

The most common cause of persistent symptoms in a patient who fulfills all the criteria for the diagnosis of celiac disease is continued intake of gluten. Gluten is ubiquitous, and significant effort must be made to exclude all gluten from the diet. Use of rice in place of wheat flour is very helpful, and several support groups provide important aid to patients with celiac disease and to their families. More than 90% of patients who have the characteristic findings of celiac disease will respond to complete dietary gluten restriction. The remainder constitute a heterogeneous group (whose condition is often called *refractory celiac disease or refractory sprue*) that includes some patients who (1) respond to restriction of other dietary protein, e.g., soy; (2) respond to glucocorticoids; (3) are "temporary" (i.e., the clinical and morphologic findings disappear after several months or years); or (4) fail to respond to all measures and have a fatal outcome, with or without documented

complications of celiac disease, such as development of intestinal T cell lymphoma.

Mechanism of diarrhea

The diarrhea in celiac disease has several pathogenetic mechanisms. Diarrhea may be secondary to (1) steatorrhea, which is primarily a result of the changes in jejunal mucosal function; (2) secondary lactase deficiency, a consequence of changes in jejunal brush border enzymatic function; (3) bile acid malabsorption resulting in bile acid–induced fluid secretion in the colon, in cases with more extensive disease involving the ileum; and (4) endogenous fluid secretion resulting from crypt hyperplasia. Patients with more severe involvement with celiac disease may obtain temporary improvement with *dietary lactose and fat restriction* while awaiting the full effects of total gluten restriction, which is primary therapy.

Associated diseases

Celiac disease is associated with dermatitis herpetiformis (DH), though the association has not been explained. Patients with DH have characteristic papulovesicular lesions that respond to dapsone. Almost all patients with DH have histologic changes in the small intestine consistent with celiac disease, although usually much milder and less diffuse in distribution. Most patients with DH have mild or no gastrointestinal symptoms. In contrast, relatively few patients with celiac disease have DH.

Celiac disease is also associated with diabetes mellitus type 1; IgA deficiency; Down syndrome; and Turner's syndrome. The clinical importance of the association with diabetes is that although severe watery diarrhea without evidence of malabsorption is most often diagnosed as diarrhea," assay of antiendomysial antibodies and/or a small-intestinal biopsy must be considered to exclude celiac disease.

Complications

The most important complication of celiac disease is the development of cancer. An increased incidence of both gastrointestinal and nongastrointestinal neoplasms as well as intestinal lymphoma exists in patients with celiac disease. For unexplained reasons the occurrence of lymphoma in patients with celiac disease is higher in Ireland and the United Kingdom than in the United States. The possibility of lymphoma must be considered whenever a patient with celiac disease previously doing well on a gluten-free diet is no longer responsive to gluten restriction or a patient who presents with clinical and histologic features consistent with celiac disease does not respond to a gluten-free diet. Other complications of celiac disease include the development of intestinal ulceration independent of lymphoma and so-called refractory sprue (discussed earlier) and collagenous sprue. In *collagenous sprue,* a layer of collagen-like material is present beneath the basement membrane; patients with collagenous sprue generally do not respond to a gluten-free diet and often have a poor prognosis.

TROPICAL SPRUE

Tropical sprue is a poorly understood syndrome that affects both expatriates and natives in certain but not all tropical areas and is manifested by chronic diarrhea, steatorrhea, weight loss, and nutritional deficiencies, including those of both folate and cobalamin. This disease affects 5–10% of the population in some tropical areas.

Chronic diarrhea in a tropical environment is most often caused by infectious agents including *G. lamblia, Yersinia enterocolitica, C. difficile, Cryptosporidium parvum,* and *Cyclospora cayetanensis,* among other organisms. Tropical sprue should not be entertained as a possible diagnosis until the presence of cysts and trophozoites has been excluded in three stool samples.

Chronic infections of the gastrointestinal tract and diarrhea in patients with and without AIDS are discussed in Chap. 23.

The small-intestinal mucosa in individuals living in tropical areas is not identical to that of individuals who reside in temperate climates. Biopsies reveal a mild alteration of villous architecture with a modest increase in mononuclear cells in the lamina propria, which on occasion can be as severe as that seen in celiac disease. These changes are observed both in native residents and in expatriates living in tropical regions and are usually associated with mild decreases in absorptive function, but they revert to "normal" when an individual moves or returns to a temperate area. Some have suggested that the changes seen in tropical enteropathy and in tropical sprue represent different ends of the spectrum of a single entity, but convincing evidence to support this concept is lacking.

Etiology

Because tropical sprue responds to antibiotics, the consensus is that it may be caused by one or more infectious agents. Nonetheless, the etiology and pathogenesis of tropical sprue are uncertain. First, its occurrence is not evenly distributed in all tropical areas; rather, it is found in specific locations, including southern India, the Philippines, and several Caribbean islands (e.g., Puerto Rico, Haiti), but is rarely observed in Africa, Jamaica, or Southeast Asia. Second, an occasional individual will not develop symptoms of tropical sprue until long after having left an endemic area. This is the reason why the original term for celiac disease (often referred to as celiac sprue) was *nontropical sprue* to distinguish it from tropical sprue. Third, multiple microorganisms have been identified on jejunal aspirate with relatively little consistency among studies. *Klebsiella pneumoniae, Enterobacter cloacae,* or *E. coli* have been implicated in some studies of tropical sprue, while other studies have favored a role for a toxin produced by one or more of these bacteria. Fourth, the incidence of tropical sprue appears to have decreased substantially during the past two or three decades, perhaps related to improved sanitation in many tropical countries during this time. One speculation for the reduced occurrence is the wider use of antibiotics in acute diarrhea, especially in travelers to tropical areas from temperate countries. Fifth, the role of folic acid deficiency in the pathogenesis of tropical sprue requires clarification. Folic acid is absorbed exclusively in the duodenum and proximal jejunum, and most patients with tropical sprue have evidence of folate malabsorption and depletion. Although folate deficiency can cause changes in small-intestinal mucosa that are corrected by folate replacement, several earlier studies reporting that tropical sprue could be cured by folic acid did not provide an explanation for the "insult" that was initially responsible for folate malabsorption.

The clinical pattern of tropical sprue varies in different areas of the world (e.g., India vs. Puerto Rico). Not infrequently, individuals in South India initially will report the occurrence of an acute enteritis before the development of steatorrhea and malabsorption. In contrast, in Puerto Rico a most insidious onset of symptoms and a more dramatic response to antibiotics is seen when compared to some other locations. Tropical sprue in different areas of the world may not be the same disease, and similar clinical entities may have different etiologies.

Diagnosis

The diagnosis of tropical sprue is best made by the presence of an abnormal small-intestinal mucosal biopsy in an individual with chronic diarrhea and evidence of malabsorption who is either residing or has recently lived in a tropical country. The small-intestinal biopsy in tropical sprue does not have pathognomonic features but resembles, and can often be indistinguishable from, that seen in celiac disease (Fig. 15-4). The biopsy in tropical sprue will have less villous architectural alteration and more mononuclear cell infiltrate in the lamina propria. In contrast to celiac disease, the histologic features of tropical sprue are present with a similar degree of severity throughout the small intestine, and a gluten-free diet does not result in either clinical or histologic improvement in tropical sprue.

172

TREATMENT Tropical Sprue

Broad-spectrum antibiotics and folic acid are most often curative, especially if the patient leaves the tropical area and does not return. Tetracycline should be used for up to 6 months and may be associated with improvement within 1–2 weeks. Folic acid alone will induce a hematologic remission as well as improvement in appetite, weight gain, and some morphologic changes in small-intestinal biopsy. Because of the presence of marked folate deficiency, folic acid is most often given together with antibiotics.

SHORT BOWEL SYNDROME

This is a descriptive term for the myriad clinical problems that occur following resection of varying lengths of small intestine; or on rare occasions, it may be congenital, e.g., microvillous inclusion disease. The factors that determine both the type and degree of symptoms include (1) the specific segment (jejunum vs. ileum) resected, (2) the length of the resected segment, (3) the integrity of the ileocecal valve, (4) whether any large intestine has also been removed, (5) residual disease in the remaining small and/or large intestine (e.g., Crohn's disease, mesenteric artery disease), and (6) the degree of adaptation in the remaining intestine. Short bowel syndrome can occur at any age from neonates through the elderly. *Intestinal failure* is the inability to maintain nutrition without parenteral support.

Three different situations in adults demand intestinal resections: (1) mesenteric vascular disease, including atherosclerosis, thrombotic phenomena, and vasculitides; (2) primary mucosal and submucosal disease, e.g., Crohn's disease; and (3) operations without preexisting small intestinal disease, such as trauma.

Following resection of the small intestine, the residual intestine undergoes adaptation of both structure and function that may last for up to 6–12 months. Continued intake of dietary nutrients and calories is required to stimulate adaptation via direct contact with intestinal mucosa, the release of one or more intestinal hormones, and pancreatic and biliary secretions. Thus, enteral nutrition with calorie administration must be maintained, especially in the early postoperative period, even if an extensive intestinal resection requiring parenteral nutrition (PN) had been performed. The subsequent ability of such patients to absorb nutrients will not be known for several months, until adaptation is completed.

Multiple factors besides the absence of intestinal mucosa (required for lipid, fluid, and electrolyte absorption) contribute to the diarrhea and steatorrhea in these patients. Removal of the ileum and especially the ileocecal valve is often associated with more severe diarrhea than jejunal resection. Without part or all of the ileum,

diarrhea can be caused by an increase in bile acids entering the colon, leading to their stimulation of colonic fluid and electrolyte secretion. Absence of the ileocecal valve is also associated with a decrease in intestinal transit time and bacterial overgrowth from the colon. The presence of the colon (or a major portion) is associated with substantially less diarrhea and lower likelihood of intestinal failure as a result of fermentation of nonabsorbed carbohydrates to SCFAs. The latter are absorbed in the colon and stimulate Na and water absorption, improving overall fluid balance. Lactose intolerance as a result of the removal of lactase-containing mucosa as well as gastric hypersecretion may also contribute to the diarrhea.

In addition to diarrhea and/or steatorrhea, a range of nonintestinal symptoms is also observed in some patients. A significant increase in renal calcium oxalate calculi is observed in patients with a small-intestinal resection with an intact colon and is due to an increase in oxalate absorption by the large intestine, with subsequent hyperoxaluria (called *enteric hyperoxaluria*). Two possible mechanisms for the increase in oxalate absorption in the colon have been suggested: (1) bile acids and fatty acids that increase colonic mucosal permeability, resulting in increased oxalate absorption; and (2) increased fatty acids that bind calcium, resulting in increased soluble oxalate that is then absorbed. Since oxalate is high in relatively few foods (e.g., spinach, rhubarb, tea), dietary restrictions alone are not adequate treatment. Cholestyramine, an anion-binding resin, and calcium have proved useful in reducing the hyperoxaluria. Similarly, an increase in cholesterol gallstones is related to a decrease in the bile acid pool size, which results in the generation of cholesterol supersaturation in gallbladder bile. Gastric hypersecretion of acid occurs in many patients following large resections of the small intestine. The etiology is unclear but may be related to either reduced hormonal inhibition of acid secretion or increased gastrin levels due to reduced small-intestinal catabolism of circulating gastrin. The resulting gastric acid secretion may be an important factor contributing to the diarrhea and steatorrhea. A reduced pH in the duodenum can inactivate pancreatic lipase and/or precipitate duodenal bile acids, thereby increasing steatorrhea, and an increase in gastric secretion can create a volume overload relative to the reduced small-intestinal absorptive capacity. Inhibition of gastric acid secretion with proton pump inhibitors can help in reducing the diarrhea and steatorrhea but only for the first 6 months.

TREATMENT Short Bowel Syndrome

Treatment of short bowel syndrome depends on the severity of symptoms and whether the individual is able to maintain caloric and electrolyte balance with oral intake alone. Initial treatment includes judicious use of opiates (including codeine) to reduce stool output and to establish an effective diet. An initial diet should be low-fat and high-carbohydrate, if the colon is in situ, to minimize the diarrhea from fatty acid stimulation of colonic fluid secretion. MCTs (discussed earlier), a low-lactose diet, and various soluble fiber-containing diets should also be tried. In the absence of an ileocecal valve, the possibility of bacterial overgrowth must be considered and treated. If gastric acid hypersecretion is contributing to the diarrhea and steatorrhea, a proton pump inhibitor may be helpful. Usually none of these therapeutic approaches will provide an instant solution, but they can reduce disabling diarrhea.

The patient's vitamin and mineral status must also be monitored; replacement therapy should be initiated if indicated. Fat-soluble vitamins, folate, cobalamin, calcium, iron, magnesium, and zinc are the most critical factors to monitor on a regular basis. If these approaches are not successful, home PN is an established therapy that can be maintained for many years. Small intestinal transplantation is becoming established as a possible approach for individuals with extensive intestinal resection who cannot be maintained without PN, i.e., "intestinal failure." Considerable attention has been directed to the potential effectiveness of trophic hormones, e.g., glucagon-like peptide 2 (GLP-2), to improve absorptive function.

BACTERIAL OVERGROWTH SYNDROME

Bacterial overgrowth syndrome comprises a group of disorders with diarrhea, steatorrhea, and macrocytic anemia whose common feature is the proliferation of colonic-type bacteria within the small intestine. This bacterial proliferation is due to stasis caused by impaired peristalsis (*functional stasis*), changes in intestinal anatomy (*anatomic stasis*), or direct communication between the small and large intestine. These conditions have also been referred to as *stagnant bowel syndrome* or *blind loop syndrome*.

Pathogenesis

The manifestations of bacterial overgrowth syndromes are a direct consequence of the presence of increased amounts of a colonic-type bacterial flora, such as *E. coli* or *Bacteroides*, in the small intestine. *Macrocytic anemia* is due to cobalamin, not folate, deficiency. Most bacteria require cobalamin for growth, and increasing concentrations of bacteria use up the relatively small amounts of dietary cobalamin. *Steatorrhea* is due to impaired micelle formation as a consequence of a reduced intraduodenal concentration of conjugated bile acids and the

presence of unconjugated bile acids. Certain bacteria, e.g., *Bacteroides*, deconjugate conjugated bile acids to unconjugated bile acids. Unconjugated bile acids will be absorbed more rapidly than conjugated bile acids, and, as a result, the intraduodenal concentration of bile acids will be reduced. In addition, the CMC of unconjugated bile acids is higher than that of conjugated bile acids, resulting in a decrease in micelle formation. *Diarrhea* is due, at least in part, to the steatorrhea, when it is present. However, some patients manifest diarrhea *without* steatorrhea, and it is assumed that the colonic-type bacteria in these patients are producing one or more bacterial enterotoxins that are responsible for fluid secretion and diarrhea.

Etiology

The etiology of these different disorders is bacterial proliferation in the small intestinal lumen secondary to either anatomic or functional stasis or to a communication between the relatively sterile small intestine and the colon with its high levels of aerobic and anaerobic bacteria. Several examples of *anatomic* stasis have been identified: (1) one or more diverticula (both duodenal and jejunal) (Fig. 15-3C); (2) fistulas and strictures related to Crohn's disease (Fig. 15-3D); (3) a proximal duodenal afferent loop following a subtotal gastrectomy and gastrojejunostomy; (4) a bypass of the intestine, e.g., jejunoileal bypass for obesity; and (5) dilation at the site of a previous intestinal anastomosis. These anatomic derangements are often associated with the presence of a segment (or segments) of intestine out of continuity of propagated peristalsis, resulting in stasis and bacterial proliferation. Bacterial overgrowth syndromes can also occur in the *absence* of an anatomic blind loop when *functional* stasis is present. Impaired peristalsis and bacterial overgrowth in the absence of a blind loop occur in scleroderma, where motility abnormalities exist in both the esophagus and small intestine. Functional stasis and bacterial overgrowth can also occur in association with diabetes mellitus and in the small intestine when a direct connection exists between the small and large intestine, including an ileocolonic resection, or occasionally following an enterocolic anastomosis that permits entry of bacteria into the small intestine as a result of bypassing the ileocecal valve.

Diagnosis

The diagnosis may be suspected from the combination of a low serum cobalamin level and an elevated serum folate level, as enteric bacteria frequently produce folate compounds that will be absorbed in the duodenum. Ideally, the diagnosis of the bacterial overgrowth syndrome is the demonstration of increased levels of aerobic and/or anaerobic colonic-type bacteria in a jejunal aspirate obtained by intubation. This specialized test is rarely available. Breath hydrogen testing with lactulose (a nondigestible disaccharide) administration has also been used to detect bacterial overgrowth. The Schilling test can also diagnose bacterial overgrowth (see Chap. 16) but is also not available routinely. Often the diagnosis is suspected clinically and confirmed by response to treatment.

TREATMENT   Bacterial Overgrowth Syndrome

Primary treatment should be directed, if at all possible, to the surgical correction of an anatomic blind loop. In the absence of functional stasis, it is important to define the anatomic relationships responsible for stasis and bacterial overgrowth. For example, bacterial overgrowth secondary to strictures, one or more diverticula, or a proximal afferent loop can potentially be cured by surgical correction of the anatomic state. In contrast, the functional stasis of scleroderma or certain anatomic stasis states (e.g., multiple jejunal diverticula) cannot be corrected surgically, and these conditions should be treated with broad-spectrum antibiotics. Tetracycline used to be the initial treatment of choice; due to increasing resistance, however, other antibiotics such as metronidazole, amoxicillin/clavulanic acid, and cephalosporins have been employed. The antibiotic should be given for approximately 3 weeks or until symptoms remit. Although the natural history of these conditions is chronic, antibiotics should not be given continuously. Symptoms usually remit within 2–3 weeks of initial antibiotic therapy. Therapy need not be repeated until symptoms recur. In the presence of frequent recurrences, several treatment strategies exist, but the use of antibiotics for 1 week per month, whether or not symptoms are present, is often most effective.

Unfortunately, therapy for bacterial overgrowth syndrome is largely empirical, with an absence of clinical trials on which to base rational decisions regarding the antibiotic choice, the duration of treatment, and/or the best approach for treating recurrences. Bacterial overgrowth may also occur as a component of another chronic disease, e.g., Crohn's disease, radiation enteritis, or short bowel syndrome. Treatment of the bacterial overgrowth in these settings will not cure the underlying problem but may be very important in ameliorating a subset of clinical problems that are related to bacterial overgrowth.

WHIPPLE'S DISEASE

Whipple's disease is a chronic multisystem disease associated with diarrhea, steatorrhea, weight loss, arthralgia, and central nervous system (CNS) and cardiac problems; it is caused by the bacteria *Tropheryma whipplei*. Until the identification of *T. whipplei* by polymerase chain reaction, the hallmark of Whipple's disease had been the presence of PAS-positive macrophages in the small intestine (Fig. 15-4E) and other organs with evidence of disease.

Etiology

Whipple's disease is caused by a small gram-positive bacillus, *T. whipplei*. The bacillus, an Actinobacteria, has low virulence but high infectivity, and relatively minimal symptoms are observed compared to the extent of the bacilli in multiple tissues.

Clinical presentation

The onset of Whipple's disease is insidious and is characterized by diarrhea, steatorrhea, abdominal pain, weight loss, migratory large-joint arthropathy, and fever as well as ophthalmologic and CNS symptoms. The development of dementia is a relatively late symptom and an extremely poor prognostic sign, especially in patients who relapse following the induction of a remission with antibiotics. For unexplained reasons, the disease occurs primarily in middle-aged white men. The steatorrhea in these patients is generally believed secondary to both small-intestinal mucosal injury and lymphatic obstruction secondary to the increased number of PAS-positive macrophages in the lamina propria of the small intestine.

Diagnosis

The diagnosis of Whipple's disease is suggested by a multisystem disease in a patient with diarrhea and steatorrhea. Obtaining tissue biopsies from the small intestine and/or other organs that may be involved (e.g., liver, lymph nodes, heart, eyes, CNS, or synovial membranes), based on the patient's symptoms, is the primary approach to establish the diagnosis of Whipple's disease. The presence of PAS-positive macrophages containing the characteristic small (0.25—1–2 mm) bacilli is suggestive of this diagnosis. However, Whipple's disease can be confused with the PAS-positive macrophages containing *M. avium* complex, which may be a cause of diarrhea in AIDS. The presence of the *T. whipplei* bacillus outside of macrophages is a more important indicator of active disease than is their presence within the macrophages. *T. whipplei* has now been successfully grown in culture.

TREATMENT   Whipple's Disease

The treatment for Whipple's disease is prolonged use of antibiotics. The current drug of choice is double-strength trimethoprim/sulfamethoxazole for approximately 1 year. PAS-positive macrophages can persist following successful treatment, and the presence of bacilli outside of macrophages is indicative of persistent infection or an early sign of recurrence. Recurrence of disease activity, especially with dementia, is an extremely poor prognostic sign and requires an antibiotic that crosses the blood-brain barrier. If trimethoprim/sulfamethoxazole is not tolerated, chloramphenicol is an appropriate second choice.

PROTEIN-LOSING ENTEROPATHY

Protein-losing enteropathy is not a specific disease but rather a group of gastrointestinal and nongastrointestinal disorders with hypoproteinemia and edema in the absence of either proteinuria or defects in protein synthesis, e.g., chronic liver disease. These diseases are characterized by excess protein loss into the gastrointestinal tract. Normally, about 10% of total protein catabolism occurs via the gastrointestinal tract. Evidence of increased protein loss into the gastrointestinal tract occurs in more than 65 different diseases, which can be classified into three groups: (1) mucosal ulceration, such that the protein loss primarily represents exudation across damaged mucosa, e.g., ulcerative colitis, gastrointestinal carcinomas, and peptic ulcer; (2) nonulcerated mucosa, but with evidence of mucosal damage so that the protein loss represents loss across epithelia with altered permeability, e.g., celiac disease and Ménétrier's disease in the small intestine and stomach, respectively; and (3) lymphatic dysfunction, representing either primary lymphatic disease or secondary to partial lymphatic obstruction that may occur as a result of enlarged lymph nodes or cardiac disease.

Diagnosis

The diagnosis of protein-losing enteropathy is suggested by the presence of peripheral edema and low serum albumin and globulin levels in the absence of renal and hepatic disease. An individual with protein-losing enteropathy only rarely has selective loss of *only* albumin or *only* globulins. Therefore, marked reduction of serum albumin with normal serum globulins should not initiate an evaluation for protein-losing enteropathy but should suggest the presence of renal and/or hepatic disease. Likewise, reduced serum globulins with normal serum albumin levels are more likely a result of reduced globulin synthesis rather than enhanced globulin loss into the intestine. Documentation of an increase in protein loss into the gastrointestinal tract has been established by the administration of one of several radiolabeled proteins and its quantitation in stool during a 24- or 48-h period. Unfortunately, none of these radiolabeled proteins is available for routine clinical use. α_1-Antitrypsin, a protein that accounts for ~4% of total serum proteins and is resistant to proteolysis, can be used to document enhanced rates of serum protein loss into the intestinal tract but cannot be used to assess gastric protein loss due to its degradation in an acid milieu. α_1-Antitrypsin clearance is measured by determining

stool volume and both stool and plasma α_1-antitrypsin concentrations. In addition to the loss of protein via abnormal and distended lymphatics, peripheral lymphocytes may also be lost via lymphatics, resulting in a relative lymphopenia. Thus, the presence of lymphopenia in a patient with hypoproteinemia supports the presence of increased loss of protein into the gastrointestinal tract.

Patients with increased protein loss into the gastrointestinal tract from lymphatic obstruction often have steatorrhea and diarrhea. The steatorrhea is a result of altered lymphatic flow as lipid-containing chylomicrons exit from intestinal epithelial cells via intestinal lymphatics (Table 15-4; Fig. 15-4). In the absence of mechanical or anatomic lymphatic obstruction, intrinsic intestinal lymphatic dysfunction, with or without lymphatic dysfunction in the peripheral extremities, has been named *intestinal lymphangiectasia*. Similarly, about 50% of individuals with intrinsic peripheral lymphatic disease (Milroy's disease) will also have intestinal lymphangiectasia and hypoproteinemia. Other than steatorrhea and enhanced protein loss into the gastrointestinal tract, all other aspects of intestinal absorptive function are normal in intestinal lymphangiectasia.

Other causes

Patients who appear to have idiopathic protein-losing enteropathy without any evidence of gastrointestinal disease should be examined for cardiac disease—especially right-sided valvular disease and chronic pericarditis. On occasion, hypoproteinemia can be the only presentation for these two types of heart disease. Ménétrier's disease (also called *hypertrophic gastropathy*) is an uncommon entity that involves the body and fundus of the stomach and is characterized by large gastric folds, reduced gastric acid secretion, and, at times, enhanced protein loss into the stomach.

TREATMENT Protein-Losing Enteropathy

As excess protein loss into the gastrointestinal tract is most often secondary to a specific disease, treatment should be directed primarily to the underlying disease process and not to the hypoproteinemia. For example, if significant hypoproteinemia with resulting peripheral edema is secondary to either celiac disease or ulcerative colitis, a gluten-free diet or mesalamine, respectively, would be the initial therapy. When enhanced protein loss is secondary to lymphatic obstruction, it is critical to establish the nature of this obstruction. Identification of mesenteric nodes or lymphoma may be possible by imaging studies. Similarly, it is important to exclude cardiac disease as a cause of protein-losing enteropathy either by echosonography or, on occasion, by a right-heart catheterization.

TABLE 15-8

CLASSIFICATION OF MALABSORPTION SYNDROMES

Inadequate digestion
  Postgastrectomy[a]
  Deficiency or inactivation of pancreatic lipase
    Exocrine pancreatic insufficiency
      Chronic pancreatitis
      Pancreatic carcinoma
      Cystic fibrosis
      Pancreatic insufficiency—congenital or acquired
    Gastrinoma—acid inactivation of lipase[a]
    Drugs—orlistat

Reduced intraduodenal bile acid concentration/impaired
  micelle formation
  Liver disease
    Parenchymal liver disease
    Cholestatic liver disease
  Bacterial overgrowth in small intestine:
    Anatomic stasis   Functional stasis
      Afferent loop   Diabetes[a]
      Stasis/blind   Scleroderma[a]
        loop/strictures/   Intestinal
        fistulae   pseudoobstruction
  Interrupted enterohepatic circulation of bile salts
    Ileal resection
    Crohn's disease[a]
  Drugs (bind or precipitate bile salts)—neomycin,
    cholestyramine, calcium carbonate

Impaired mucosal absorption/mucosal loss or defect
  Intestinal resection or bypass[a]
  Inflammation, infiltration, or infection:
    Crohn's disease[a]   Celiac disease
    Amyloidosis   Collagenous sprue
    Scleroderma[a]   Whipple's disease[a]
    Lymphoma[a]   Radiation enteritis[a]
    Eosinophilic enteritis   Folate and vitamin B$_{12}$ deficiency
    Mastocytosis   Infections—giardiasis
    Tropical sprue   Graft-versus-host disease
  Genetic disorders
    Disaccharidase deficiency
    Agammaglobulinemia
    Abetalipoproteinemia
    Hartnup's disease
    Cystinuria

Impaired nutrient delivery to and/or from intestine:
  Lymphatic obstruction   Circulatory disorders
    Lymphoma[a]   Congestive heart failure
    Lymphangiectasia   Constrictive pericarditis
                           Mesenteric artery atherosclerosis
                           Vasculitis

Endocrine and metabolic disorders
  Diabetes[a]
  Hypoparathyroidism
  Adrenal insufficiency
  Hyperthyroidism
  Carcinoid syndrome

[a]Malabsorption caused by more than one mechanism.

TABLE 15-9

PATHOPHYSIOLOGY OF CLINICAL MANIFESTATIONS OF MALABSORPTION DISORDERS

SYMPTOM OR SIGN	MECHANISM
Weight loss/malnutrition	Anorexia, malabsorption of nutrients
Diarrhea	Impaired absorption or secretion of water and electrolytes; colonic fluid secretion secondary to unabsorbed dihydroxy bile acids and fatty acids
Flatus	Bacterial fermentation of unabsorbed carbohydrate
Glossitis, cheilosis, stomatitis	Deficiency of iron, vitamin B$_{12}$, folate, and vitamin A
Abdominal pain	Bowel distention or inflammation, pancreatitis
Bone pain	Calcium, vitamin D malabsorption, protein deficiency, osteoporosis
Tetany, paresthesia	Calcium and magnesium malabsorption
Weakness	Anemia, electrolyte depletion (particularly K$^+$)
Azotemia, hypotension	Fluid and electrolyte depletion
Amenorrhea, decreased libido	Protein depletion, decreased calories, secondary hypopituitarism
Anemia	Impaired absorption of iron, folate, vitamin B$_{12}$
Bleeding	Vitamin K malabsorption, hypoprothrombinemia
Night blindness/xerophthalmia	Vitamin A malabsorption
Peripheral neuropathy	Vitamin B$_{12}$ and thiamine deficiency
Dermatitis	Deficiency of vitamin A, zinc, and essential fatty acids

The increased protein loss that occurs in intestinal lymphangiectasia is a result of distended lymphatics associated with lipid malabsorption. Treatment of the hypoproteinemia is accomplished by a low-fat diet and the administration of MCTs (Table 15-3), which do not exit from the intestinal epithelial cells via lymphatics but are delivered to the body via the portal vein.

SUMMARY

A pathophysiologic classification of the many conditions that can produce malabsorption is given in **Table 15-8**. A summary of the pathophysiology of the various clinical manifestations of malabsorption is given in **Table 15-9**.

SECTION III Disorders of the Alimentary Tract

CHAPTER 16

THE SCHILLING TEST

Henry J. Binder

The Schilling test is performed to determine the cause for cobalamin malabsorption. Unfortunately, this test has not been available commercially in the United States for the last few years. Since understanding the physiology and pathophysiology of cobalamin absorption is very valuable for enhancing one's understanding of aspects of gastric, pancreatic, and ileal function, discussion of the Schilling test is provided as supplemental information to Chap. 15. Since cobalamin absorption requires multiple steps, including gastric, pancreatic, and ileal processes, the Schilling test also can be used to assess the integrity of those other organs. Cobalamin is present primarily in meat. Except in strict vegans, *dietary* cobalamin deficiency is exceedingly uncommon. Dietary cobalamin is bound in the stomach to a glycoprotein called *R-binder protein*, which is synthesized in both the stomach and the salivary glands. This cobalamin–R binder complex is formed in the acid milieu of the stomach. Cobalamin absorption has an absolute requirement for intrinsic factor, another glycoprotein synthesized and released by gastric parietal cells, to promote its uptake by specific cobalamin receptors on the brush border of ileal enterocytes. Pancreatic protease enzymes split the cobalamin–R binder complex to release cobalamin in the proximal small intestine, where cobalamin then is bound by intrinsic factor.

As a consequence, cobalamin absorption may be abnormal in the following:

1. *Pernicious anemia*, a disease in which immunologically mediated atrophy of gastric parietal cells leads to an absence of both gastric acid and intrinsic factor secretion.
2. *Chronic pancreatitis* as a result of deficiency of pancreatic proteases to split the cobalamin–R binder complex. Although 50% of patients with chronic pancreatitis have been reported to have an abnormal Schilling test that was corrected by pancreatic enzyme replacement, the presence of a cobalamin-responsive

macrocytic anemia in chronic pancreatitis is extremely rare. Although this probably reflects a difference in the digestion/absorption of cobalamin in food versus that in a crystalline form, the Schilling test still can be used to assess pancreatic exocrine function.

3. *Achlorhydria*, or absence of another factor secreted with acid that is responsible for splitting cobalamin away from the proteins in food to which it is bound. Up to one-third of individuals >60 years of age have marginal vitamin B_{12} absorption because of the inability to release cobalamin from food; these people have no defects in absorbing crystalline vitamin B_{12}.
4. *Bacterial overgrowth syndromes*, which are most often secondary to stasis in the small intestine, leading to bacterial utilization of cobalamin (often referred to as *stagnant bowel syndrome*; see later).
5. *Ileal dysfunction* (as a result of either inflammation or prior intestinal resection) due to impaired function of the mechanism of cobalamin–intrinsic factor uptake by ileal intestinal epithelial cells.

The Schilling test is performed by administering ^{58}Co-labeled cobalamin orally and collecting urine for 24 h, and it is dependent on normal renal and bladder function. Urinary excretion of cobalamin will reflect cobalamin absorption provided that intrahepatic binding sites for cobalamin are fully occupied. To ensure saturation of hepatic cobalamin binding sites so that all absorbed radiolabeled cobalamin will be excreted in urine, 1 mg of cobalamin is administered intramuscularly 1 h after ingestion of the radiolabeled cobalamin. The Schilling test may be abnormal (usually defined as <10% excretion in 24 h) in pernicious anemia, chronic pancreatitis, blind loop syndrome, and ileal disease (Table 16-1). Therefore, whenever an abnormal Schilling test is found, ^{58}Co-labeled cobalamin should be administered on another occasion bound to intrinsic factor, with pancreatic enzymes, or after a 5-day course

TABLE 16-1

DIFFERENTIAL RESULTS OF SCHILLING TEST IN SEVERAL DISEASES ASSOCIATED WITH COBALAMIN (CBL) MALABSORPTION				
	^{58}CO-CBL	WITH INTRINSIC FACTOR	WITH PANCREATIC ENZYMES	AFTER 5 DAYS OF ANTIBIOTICS
Pernicious anemia	Reduced	Normal	Reduced	Reduced
Chronic pancreatitis	Reduced	Reduced	Normal	Reduced
Bacterial overgrowth	Reduced	Reduced	Reduced	Normal
Ileal disease	Reduced	Reduced	Reduced	Reduced

of antibiotics (often tetracycline). A variation of the Schilling test can detect failure to split cobalamin from food proteins. The labeled cobalamin is cooked together with a scrambled egg and administered orally. People with achlorydria will excrete <10% of the labeled cobalamin in the urine. In addition to establishing the etiology for cobalamin deficiency, the Schilling test can be used to help delineate the pathologic process responsible for steatorrhea by assessing ileal, pancreatic, and small-intestinal luminal function. Unfortunately, the Schilling test is performed infrequently because of the unavailability of human intrinsic factor.

CHAPTER 17
INFLAMMATORY BOWEL DISEASE

Sonia Friedman ■ Richard S. Blumberg

Inflammatory bowel disease (IBD) is an immune-mediated chronic intestinal condition. Ulcerative colitis (UC) and Crohn's disease (CD) are the two major types of IBD.

EPIDEMIOLOGY

The incidence of IBD varies within different geographic areas. CD and UC both occur at the highest incidence in Europe, the United Kingdom, and North America. In North America, incidence rates range from 2.2–14.3 cases per 100,000 person years for UC and from 3.1–14.6 cases per 100,000 person-years for CD (Table 17-1). Prevalence ranges from 37–246 cases per 100,000 person-years for UC and from

TABLE 17-1

EPIDEMIOLOGY OF IBD		
	ULCERATIVE COLITIS	**CROHN'S DISEASE**
Incidence (North America) per person-years	2.2–14.3:100,000	3.1–14.6:100,000
Age of onset	15–30 & 60–80	15–30 & 60–80
Ethnicity	Jewish > non-Jewish white > African American > Hispanic > Asian	
Male/female ratio	1:1	1.1–1.8:1
Smoking	May prevent disease	May cause disease
Oral contraceptives	No increased risk	Odds ratio 1.4
Appendectomy	Protective	Not protective
Monozygotic twins	6% concordance	58% concordance
Dizygotic twins	0% concordance	4% concordance

26–199 cases per 100,000 person-years for CD. In Europe, incidence ranges from 1.5–20.3 cases per 100,000 person-years for UC and from 0.7–9.8 cases for CD; prevalence ranges from 21.4–243 cases for UC and from 8.3–214 cases per 100,000 person-years for CD. IBD has been rare in other areas except Israel, Australia, and South Africa. The incidence of IBD, especially UC, is rising in Japan, South Korea, Singapore, northern India, and Latin America, areas previously thought to have low incidence. The incidence of UC has increased sixfold in the past two decades in Hong Kong. Reports from the United States, Poland, Denmark, and South Korea indicate that the incidence of pediatric IBD is increasing rapidly as well. The highest mortality is during the first years of disease and in long-duration disease due to the risk of colon cancer. In a Danish population study, the standardized mortality ratios for CD and UC were 1.31 and 1.1, respectively.

The peak age of onset of UC and CD is between 15 and 30 years. A second peak occurs between the ages of 60 and 80. The male to female ratio for UC is 1:1 and for CD is 1.1–1.8:1. UC and CD have two- to four-fold increased frequency in Jewish populations in the United States, Europe, and South Africa. Furthermore, disease frequency differs within the Jewish populations. The prevalence of IBD in Ashkenazi Jews is about twice that of Israeli-born, Sephardic, or Asian Jews. The prevalence decreases progressively in non-Jewish white, African-American, Hispanic, and Asian populations. Urban areas have a higher prevalence of IBD than rural areas, and high socioeconomic classes have a higher prevalence than lower socioeconomic classes.

The effects of cigarette smoking are different in UC and CD. The risk of UC in smokers is 40% that of nonsmokers. Additionally, former smokers have a 1.7-fold increased risk for UC than people who have never smoked. In contrast, smoking is associated with a twofold increased risk of CD. Oral contraceptives are also linked to CD; the odds ratio of CD for oral

179

contraceptive users is about 1.4. Appendectomy is protective against UC but is associated with an increased risk of CD. This elevated risk in CD is observed early after an appendectomy, which is diminished thereafter, making it likely that it reflects diagnostic problems in patients with incipient CD.

IBD is a familial disease in 5–10% of patients. Some of these patients may exhibit early onset disease during the first decade of life and, in CD, a concordance of anatomic site and clinical type within families. In the remainder of patients, IBD is observed in the absence of a family history (i.e., sporadic disease). If a patient has IBD, the lifetime risk that a first-degree relative will be affected is ~10%. If two parents have IBD, each child has a 36% chance of being affected. In twin studies, 58% of monozygotic twins are concordant for CD and 6% are concordant for UC, whereas 4% of dizygotic twins are concordant for CD and none are concordant for UC. In a recent twin study from Germany, the relative risk of a monozygotic twin developing Crohn's disease if his or her twin was affected was 738. The risks of developing IBD are higher in first-degree relatives of Jewish versus non-Jewish patients: 7.8% versus 5.2% for CD and 4.5% versus 1.6% for UC.

Additional evidence for genetic predisposition to IBD comes from its association with certain genetic syndromes. UC and CD are both associated with Turner's syndrome, and Hermansky-Pudlak syndrome is associated with granulomatous colitis. Glycogen storage disease type 1b can present with Crohn's-like lesions of the large and small bowel. Severe immunodeficiency disorders such as Wiskott-Aldrich syndrome and chronic granulomatous disease are associated with IBD. Immune dysregulation, polyendocrinopathy, enteropathy, X-linked (IPEX) syndrome is associated with a severe enteropathy and autoimmunity (Table 17-2). Other immunodeficiency disorders such as hypogammaglobulinemia, selective IgA deficiency, and hereditary angioedema, also exhibit an increased association with IBD.

ETIOLOGY AND PATHOGENESIS

A consensus hypothesis is that in genetically predisposed individuals, both exogenous factors (e.g., composition of normal intestinal microbiota) and endogenous host factors (e.g., intestinal epithelial cell barrier function, innate and adaptive immune function) interact to cause a chronic state of dysregulated mucosal immune function that is further modified by specific environmental factors (e.g., smoking, enteropathogens). Although chronic activation of the mucosal immune system may represent an appropriate response to an unidentified infectious agent, a search for such an agent has thus far been unrewarding in IBD. As such, IBD is currently considered an inappropriate immune response to the endogenous commensal microbiota within the intestines, with or without some component of autoimmunity. Importantly, the normal intestines contain a large number of immune cells in a chronic state of so-called physiologic inflammation, in which the gut is restrained from full immunologic responses to the commensal microbiota and dietary antigens by very powerful regulatory pathways that function within the immune system (e.g., FoxP3⁺ T regulatory cells). During the course of infections in the normal host, full activation of the gut-associated lymphoid tissues occurs but is rapidly superseded by dampening of the immune response and tissue repair. In IBD this process may not be regulated normally.

TABLE 17-2

PRIMARY GENETIC DISORDERS ASSOCIATED WITH IBD		
NAME	GENETIC ASSOCIATION	PHENOTYPE
Turner's syndrome	Loss of part or all of X chromosome	Associated with UC and colonic CD
Hermansky-Pudlak syndrome	Autosomal recessive chromosome 10q23	Granulomatous colitis, oculocutaneous albinism, platelet dysfunction, pulmonary fibrosis
Wiskott-Aldrich syndrome (WAS)	X-linked recessive disorder, loss of WAS protein function	Colitis, immunodeficiency, severely dysfunctional platelets, and thrombocytopenia
Glycogen storage disease	Deficiency of the glucose-6-phosphate transport protein type B1	Granulomatous colitis, presents in infancy with hypoglycemia, growth failure, hepatomegaly, and neutropenia
Immune dysregulation polyendocrinopathy, enteropathy X-linked (IPEX)	Loss of FoxP3 transcription factor and T regulatory cell function	UC-like autoimmune enteropathy, with endocrinopathy (neonatal type 1 diabetes or thyroiditis), dermatitis
Early-onset IBD	Deficient IL-10 receptor function	Severe, refractory IBD in early life

Abbreviations: CD, Crohn's disease; IBD, inflammatory bowel disease; IL, interleukin; UC, ulcerative colitis; WASP, Wiskott-Aldrich syndrome protein.

GENETIC CONSIDERATIONS

IBD is a polygenic disorder that gives rise to multiple clinical subgroups within UC and CD. A variety of genetic approaches including candidate gene studies, linkage analysis and genome-wide association studies that focus on the identification of disease-associated, single-nucleotide polymorphisms (SNP) within the human genome have identified Approximately 100 disease-associated loci on many different chromosomes (Table 17-3). About one-third of these genetic risk factors are shared between CD and UC accounting for the overlapping immunopathogenesis and consequently epidemiologic observations of both diseases in the same families and similarities in response to therapies. Because the specific causal variants for each gene or locus are largely unknown, it is not clear whether the similarities in the genetic risk factors associated with CD and UC that are observed are shared at structural or functional levels. Similarly, many of the genetic risk factors identified are also observed to be associated with risk for other immune-mediated diseases suggesting that related immunogenetic pathways are involved in the pathogenesis of multiple different disorders accounting for the common responsiveness to similar types of biologic therapies (e.g., anti-tumor necrosis factor therapies) and possibly the simultaneous occurrence of these disorders. The diseases and the genetic risk factors that are shared with IBD include rheumatoid arthritis (*TNFAIP3*), psoriasis (*IL23R, IL12B*), ankylosing spondylitis (*IL23R*), type 1 diabetes mellitus (*IL10, PTPN2*), asthma (*ORMDL3*), and systemic lupus erythematosus (*TNFAIP3, IL10*).

The genetic factors defined to date that are recognized to mediate risk for IBD have highlighted the importance of several common mechanisms of disease (Table 17-3). These include the following: Those genes that are associated with innate immunity

TABLE 17-3

GENETIC LOCI ASSOCIATED WITH CD AND/OR UC

Chr	PUTATIVE GENE	GENE NAME	PROTEIN FUNCTION	CD	UC
Innate Immunity and Autophagy					
1q23	*ITLN1*	Intelectin 1	Bacterial binding	+	
2q37	*ATG16L1*	ATG16 autophagy related 16-like 1	Autophagy	+	
5q33	*IRGM*	Immunity-related GTPase family, M	Autophagy	+	
9p24	*JAK2*	Janus kinase 2	IL-6R & IL-23R signaling	+	+
12q12	*LRRK2*	Leucine-rich repeat kinase 2	Autophagy ?	+	
16q12	*NOD2*	Nucleotide-binding oligomerization domain containing 2	Bacterial sensing	+	
17q21	*STAT3*	Signal transducer and activator of transcription 3	IL-6R, IL-23R & IL-10R signaling	+	+
ER Stress and Metabolism					
5q31	*SLC22A5*	Solute carrier family 22, member 5	β carnitine transporter	+	
7p21	*AGR2*	Anterior gradient 2	ER stress	+	+
17q21	*ORMDL3*	Orosomucoid related member 1-like 3	ER stress	+	+
22q12	*XBP1*	X-box binding protein 1	ER stress	+	+
Adaptive Immunity					
1p31	*IL23R*	Interleukin 23 receptor	Th17 cell stimulation	+	+
1q32	*IL10*	Interleukin-10	Treg associated cytokine		+
5q33	*IL12B*	Interleukin 12B	IL-12 p40 chain of IL-12/IL-23	+	+
18p11	*PTPN2*	Protein tyrosine phosphatase, nonreceptor type 2	T cell regulation	+	
Inflammation					
3p21	*MST1*	Macrophage stimulating 1	Macrophage activation	+	+
5p13	*PTGER4*	Prostaglandin E receptor 4	PGE2 receptor	+	+
6q23	*TNFAIP3*	Tumor necrosis factor, alpha-induced protein 3 (A20)	Toll-like receptor regulation	+	
6q27	*CCR6*	Chemokine (C-C motif) receptor 6	Dendritic cell migration	+	

Abbreviations: CD, Crohn's disease; ER, endoplasmic reticulum; GTPase, guanosine triphosphatase; IL, interleukin; UC, ulcerative colitis.
Source: Adapted from A Kaser et al: Ann Rev Immunol 28:573, 2010.

CHAPTER 17 Inflammatory Bowel Disease

and autophagy (e.g., *NOD2, ATG16L1, IRGM, JAK2, STAT3*) that function in innate immune cells (both parenchymal and hematopoietic) to respond to and clear bacteria, mycobacteria, and viruses; those that are associated with endoplasmic reticulum (ER) and metabolic stress (e.g., *XBP1, ORMDL3, OCTN*), which serve to regulate the secretory activity of cells involved in responses to the commensal microbiota such as Paneth and goblet cells and the manner in which intestinal cells respond to the metabolic products of bacteria; those that are associated with the regulation of adaptive immunity (e.g., *IL23R, IL12B, IL10, PTPN2*), which regulate the balance between inflammatory and regulatory cytokines; and, finally, those that are involved in the development and resolution of inflammation (e.g., *MST1, CCR6, TNFAIP3, PTGER4*) and ultimately leukocyte recruitment and inflammatory mediator production. Some of these loci are associated with specific subtypes of disease such as the association between *NOD2* polymorphisms and fibrostenosing CD, especially within the ileum. However, the clinical utility of these genetic risk factors for the diagnosis or determination of prognosis and therapeutic responses remains to be defined.

DEFECTIVE IMMUNE REGULATION IN IBD

The mucosal immune system is normally unreactive to luminal contents due to oral (mucosal) tolerance. When soluble antigens are administered orally rather than subcutaneously or intramuscularly, antigen-specific nonresponsiveness is induced. Multiple mechanisms are involved in the induction of oral tolerance and include deletion or anergy of antigen-reactive T cells or induction of CD4$^+$ T cells that suppress gut inflammation (e.g., T regulatory cells expressing the FoxP3 transcription factor) that secrete anti-inflammatory cytokines such as interleukin (IL) 10 and transforming growth factor β (TGF-β). Oral tolerance may be responsible for the lack of immune responsiveness to dietary antigens and the commensal microbiota in the intestinal lumen. In IBD this suppression of inflammation is altered, leading to uncontrolled inflammation. The mechanisms of this regulated immune suppression are incompletely known.

Gene knockout ($^{-/-}$) or transgenic (Tg) mouse models of IBD have revealed that deleting specific cytokines (e.g., IL-2, IL-10, TGF-β) or their receptors, deleting molecules associated with T cell antigen recognition (e.g., T cell antigen receptors), or interfering with intestinal epithelial cell barrier function and the regulation of responses to commensal bacteria (e.g., XBP1, N-cadherin, mucus glycoprotein, or NFκB) leads to spontaneous colitis or enteritis. In the majority of

circumstances, intestinal inflammation in these animal models requires the presence of the commensal microbiota. Thus, a variety of specific alterations can lead to immune activation by commensal microbiota and inflammation directed at the intestines in mice. How these relate to human IBD remains to be defined but are consistent with inappropriate responses of the genetically susceptible host to the commensal bacteria.

In both UC and CD, an inflammatory pathway thus likely emerges from the genetic predisposition that is associated with inappropriate innate immune sensing and reactivity to commensal bacteria together with inadequate regulatory pathways that lead to activated CD4$^+$ T cells in the lamina propria that secrete excessive quantities of inflammatory cytokines relative to anti-inflammatory cytokines. Some cytokines activate other inflammatory cells (macrophages and B cells) and others act indirectly to recruit other lymphocytes, inflammatory leukocytes, and mononuclear cells from the bloodstream into the gut through interactions between homing receptors on leukocytes (e.g., α^{4}β$_7$ integrin) and addressins on vascular endothelium (e.g., MadCAM1). CD4$^+$ T helper (T$_H$) cells that promote inflammation are of three major types, all of which may be associated with colitis in animal models and perhaps humans: T$_H$1 cells (secrete interferon [IFN] γ), T$_H$2 cells (secrete IL-4, IL-5, IL-13), and T$_H$17 cells (secrete IL-17, IL-21). T$_H$1 cells induce transmural granulomatous inflammation that resembles CD, T$_H$2 cells, and related natural killer T cells that secrete IL-13 induce superficial mucosal inflammation resembling UC, and T$_H$17 cells may be responsible for neutrophilic recruitment. Each of these T cell subsets cross-regulate each other. The T$_H$1 cytokine pathway is initiated by IL-12, a key cytokine in the pathogenesis of experimental models of mucosal inflammation. IL-4 and IL-23, together with IL-6 and TGF-β, induce T$_H$2 and T$_H$17 cells, respectively. Activated macrophages secrete tumor necrosis factor (TNF and IL-6). Thus, use of antibodies to block proinflammatory cytokines (e.g., anti-TNF, anti-IL-12, anti-IL-23, anti-IL-6, anti-IFN-γ) or molecules associated with leukocyte recruitment (e.g., anti-α^{4}β$_7$) or use of cytokines that inhibit inflammation and promote regulatory T cells (e.g., IL-10) or promote intestinal barrier function may be beneficial to humans with intestinal inflammation.

THE INFLAMMATORY CASCADE IN IBD

Once initiated in IBD by abnormal innate immune sensing of bacteria by parenchymal cells (e.g., intestinal epithelial cells) and hematopoietic cells (e.g., dendritic cells), the immune inflammatory response is perpetuated by T cell activation. A sequential cascade of inflammatory mediators extends the response; each step is a potential target for therapy. Inflammatory cytokines such as IL-1, IL-6, and TNF, have diverse effects on tissues. They promote fibrogenesis, collagen production, activation of tissue metalloproteinases, and the production of other inflammatory mediators; they also activate the coagulation cascade in local blood vessels (e.g., increased production of von Willebrand's factor). These cytokines are normally produced in response to infection but are usually turned off or inhibited at the appropriate time to limit tissue damage. In IBD their activity is not regulated, resulting in an imbalance between the proinflammatory and anti-inflammatory mediators. Therapies such as the 5-aminosalicylic acid (5-ASA) compounds are potent inhibitors of these inflammatory mediators through inhibition of transcription factors such as NFκB that regulate their expression.

EXOGENOUS FACTORS

IBD may have an as yet undefined infectious etiology. Observational studies suggest that multiple pathogens (e.g., *Salmonella*, *Shigella*, *Campylobacter*, *Clostridium difficile* spp.) may initiate IBD by triggering an inflammatory response that the mucosal immune system may fail to control. However, in an IBD patient, the normal microbiota is likely perceived inappropriately as if it were a pathogen. Alterations in the composition of the commensal microbiota are observed in both CD and UC. However, whether these changes are primary or secondary to inflammation is unknown. Anaerobic organisms, particularly *Bacteroides* and *Clostridia* species, and some aerobic species such as *Escherichia* may be responsible for the induction of inflammation. This notion is supported by the immune response in patients with CD to a number of bacterial antigens. In addition, agents that alter the intestinal flora such as metronidazole, ciprofloxacin, and elemental diets, may improve CD. CD also responds to fecal diversion, demonstrating the ability of luminal contents to exacerbate disease. Conversely, other organisms, so-called probiotics (e.g., *Faecalibacterium prausnitzii*, *Lactobacillus*, *Bifidobacterium*, *Taenia suis,* and *Saccharomyces boulardii* spp.), may inhibit inflammation in animal models and humans.

Psychosocial factors can contribute to worsening of symptoms. Major life events such as illness or death in the family, divorce or separation, interpersonal conflict, or other major loss are associated with an increase in IBD symptoms such as pain, bowel dysfunction, and bleeding. Acute daily stress can worsen bowel symptoms even after controlling for major life events. When measured with validated psychological scales, patients with active IBD have lower psychological well-being and mastery as well as higher distress than non-IBD controls.

PATHOLOGY

ULCERATIVE COLITIS: MACROSCOPIC FEATURES

UC is a mucosal disease that usually involves the rectum and extends proximally to involve all or part of the colon. About 40–50% of patients have disease limited to the rectum and rectosigmoid, 30–40% have disease extending beyond the sigmoid but not involving the whole colon, and 20% have a total colitis. Proximal spread occurs in continuity without areas of uninvolved mucosa. When the whole colon is involved, the inflammation extends 2–3 cm into the terminal ileum in 10–20% of patients. The endoscopic changes of *backwash ileitis* are superficial and mild and are of little clinical significance. Although variations in macroscopic activity may suggest skip areas, biopsies from normal-appearing mucosa are usually abnormal. Thus, it is important to obtain multiple biopsies from apparently uninvolved mucosa, whether proximal or distal, during endoscopy. One caveat is that effective medical therapy can change the appearance of the mucosa such that either skip areas or the entire colon can be microscopically normal.

With mild inflammation, the mucosa is erythematous and has a fine granular surface that resembles sandpaper. In more severe disease, the mucosa is hemorrhagic, edematous, and ulcerated (**Fig. 17-1**). In long-standing disease, inflammatory polyps (pseudopolyps) may be present as a result of epithelial regeneration. The mucosa

FIGURE 17-1

Ulcerative colitis. Diffuse (nonsegmental) mucosal disease, with broad areas of ulceration. The bowel wall is not thickened, and there is no cobblestoning. (*Courtesy of Dr. R Odze, Division of Gastrointestinal Pathology, Department of Pathology, Brigham and Women's Hospital, Boston, Massachusetts; with permission.*)

CHAPTER 17 Inflammatory Bowel Disease

may appear normal in remission, but in patients with many years of disease it appears atrophic and featureless, and the entire colon becomes narrowed and shortened. Patients with fulminant disease can develop a toxic colitis or megacolon where the bowel wall thins and the mucosa is severely ulcerated; this may lead to perforation.

ULCERATIVE COLITIS: MICROSCOPIC FEATURES

Histologic findings correlate well with the endoscopic appearance and clinical course of UC. The process is limited to the mucosa and superficial submucosa, with deeper layers unaffected except in fulminant disease. In UC, two major histologic features suggest chronicity and help distinguish it from infectious or acute self-limited colitis. First, the crypt architecture of the colon is distorted; crypts may be bifid and reduced in number, often with a gap between the crypt bases and the muscularis mucosae. Second, some patients have basal plasma cells and multiple basal lymphoid aggregates. Mucosal vascular congestion, with edema and focal hemorrhage, and an inflammatory cell infiltrate of neutrophils, lymphocytes, plasma cells, and macrophages may be present. The neutrophils invade the epithelium, usually in the crypts, giving rise to cryptitis and, ultimately, to crypt abscesses (Fig. 17-2). Ileal changes in patients with backwash ileitis include villous atrophy and crypt regeneration with increased inflammation, increased neutrophil and mononuclear inflammation

in the lamina propria, and patchy cryptitis and crypt abscesses.

CROHN'S DISEASE: MACROSCOPIC FEATURES

CD can affect any part of the gastrointestinal (GI) tract from the mouth to the anus. Some 30–40% of patients have small bowel disease alone, 40–55% have disease involving both the small and large intestines, and 15–25% have colitis alone. In the 75% of patients with small intestinal disease, the terminal ileum is involved in 90%. Unlike UC, which almost always involves the rectum, the rectum is often spared in CD. CD is segmental with skip areas in the midst of diseased intestine (Fig. 17-3). Perirectal fistulas, fissures, abscesses, and anal stenosis are present in one-third of patients with CD, particularly those with colonic involvement. Rarely, CD may also involve the liver and the pancreas.

Unlike UC, CD is a transmural process. Endoscopically, aphthous or small superficial ulcerations characterize mild disease; in more active disease, stellate ulcerations fuse longitudinally and transversely to demarcate islands of mucosa that frequently are histologically normal. This "cobblestone" appearance is characteristic of CD, both endoscopically and by barium radiography. As in UC, pseudopolyps can form in CD.

Active CD is characterized by focal inflammation and formation of fistula tracts, which resolve by fibrosis and stricturing of the bowel. The bowel wall thickens and becomes narrowed and fibrotic, leading to chronic,

FIGURE 17-2
Medium power view of colonic mucosa in ulcerative colitis showing diffuse mixed inflammation, basal lymphoplasmacytosis, crypt atrophy and irregularity, and superficial erosion. These features are typical of chronic active ulcerative colitis. (*Courtesy of Dr. R Odze, Division of Gastrointestinal Pathology, Department of Pathology, Brigham and Women's Hospital, Boston, Massachusetts; with permission.*)

FIGURE 17-3
Crohn's disease of the colon showing thickening of the wall, with stenosis, linear serpiginous ulcers, and cobblestoning of the mucosa. (*Courtesy of Dr. R Odze, Division of Gastrointestinal Pathology, Department of Pathology, Brigham and Women's Hospital, Boston, Massachusetts; with permission.*)

FIGURE 17-4

Medium power view of Crohn's colitis showing mixed acute and chronic inflammation, crypt atrophy, and multiple small epithelioid granulomas in the mucosa. (*Courtesy of Dr. R Odze, Division of Gastrointestinal Pathology, Department of Pathology, Brigham and Women's Hospital, Boston, Massachusetts; with permission.*)

recurrent bowel obstructions. Projections of thickened mesentery encase the bowel ("creeping fat"), and serosal and mesenteric inflammation promotes adhesions and fistula formation.

CROHN'S DISEASE: MICROSCOPIC FEATURES

The earliest lesions are aphthoid ulcerations and focal crypt abscesses with loose aggregations of macrophages, which form noncaseating granulomas in all layers of the bowel wall (Fig. 17-4). Granulomas can be seen in lymph nodes, mesentery, peritoneum, liver, and pancreas. Although granulomas are a pathognomonic feature of CD, they are rarely found on mucosal biopsies. Surgical resection reveals granulomas in about one-half of cases. Other histologic features of CD include submucosal or subserosal lymphoid aggregates, particularly away from areas of ulceration, gross and microscopic skip areas, and transmural inflammation that is accompanied by fissures that penetrate deeply into the bowel wall and sometimes form fistulous tracts or local abscesses.

CLINICAL PRESENTATION

ULCERATIVE COLITIS

Signs and symptoms

The major symptoms of UC are diarrhea, rectal bleeding, tenesmus, passage of mucus, and crampy abdominal pain. The severity of symptoms correlates with the extent of disease. Although UC can present acutely, symptoms usually have been present for weeks to months. Occasionally, diarrhea and bleeding are so intermittent and mild that the patient does not seek medical attention.

Patients with proctitis usually pass fresh blood or blood-stained mucus, either mixed with stool or streaked onto the surface of a normal or hard stool. They also have tenesmus, or urgency with a feeling of incomplete evacuation, but rarely have abdominal pain. With proctitis or proctosigmoiditis, proximal transit slows, which may account for the constipation commonly seen in patients with distal disease.

When the disease extends beyond the rectum, blood is usually mixed with stool or grossly bloody diarrhea may be noted. Colonic motility is altered by inflammation with rapid transit through the inflamed intestine. When the disease is severe, patients pass a liquid stool containing blood, pus, and fecal matter. Diarrhea is often nocturnal and/or postprandial. Although severe pain is not a prominent symptom, some patients with active disease may experience vague lower abdominal discomfort or mild central abdominal cramping. Severe cramping and abdominal pain can occur with severe attacks of the disease. Other symptoms in moderate to severe disease include anorexia, nausea, vomiting, fever, and weight loss.

Physical signs of proctitis include a tender anal canal and blood on rectal examination. With more extensive disease, patients have tenderness to palpation directly over the colon. Patients with a toxic colitis have severe pain and bleeding, and those with megacolon have hepatic tympany. Both may have signs of peritonitis if a perforation has occurred. The classification of disease activity is shown in Table 17–4.

Laboratory, endoscopic, and radiographic features

Active disease can be associated with a rise in acute-phase reactants (C-reactive protein [CRP]), platelet count, and erythrocyte sedimentation rate (ESR), and a decrease in hemoglobin. Fecal lactoferrin is a highly sensitive and specific marker for detecting intestinal inflammation. Fecal calprotectin levels correlate well with histologic inflammation, predict relapses, and detect pouchitis. In severely ill patients, the serum albumin level will fall rather quickly. Leukocytosis may be present but is not a specific indicator of disease activity. Proctitis or proctosigmoiditis rarely causes a rise in CRP. Diagnosis relies upon the patient's history; clinical symptoms; negative stool examination for bacteria, *C. difficile* toxin, and ova and parasites; sigmoidoscopic appearance (see Fig. 12-4*A*); and histology of rectal or colonic biopsy specimens.

TABLE 17-4

ULCERATIVE COLITIS: DISEASE PRESENTATION			
	MILD	**MODERATE**	**SEVERE**
Bowel movements	<4 per day	4–6 per day	>6 per day
Blood in stool	Small	Moderate	Severe
Fever	None	<37.5°C mean (<99.5°F)	>37.5°C mean (>99.5°F)
Tachycardia	None	<90 mean pulse	>90 mean pulse
Anemia	Mild	>75%	≤75%
Sedimentation rate	<30 mm		>30 mm
Endoscopic appearance	Erythema, decreased vascular pattern, fine granularity	Marked erythema, coarse granularity, absent vascular markings, contact bleeding, no ulcerations	Spontaneous bleeding, ulcerations

Sigmoidoscopy is used to assess disease activity and is usually performed before treatment. If the patient is not having an acute flare, colonoscopy is used to assess disease extent and activity (Fig. 17-5). Endoscopically mild disease is characterized by erythema, decreased vascular pattern, and mild friability. Moderate disease is characterized by marked erythema, absent vascular pattern, friability and erosions, and severe disease by spontaneous bleeding and ulcerations. Histologic features change more slowly than clinical features but can also be used to grade disease activity.

The earliest radiologic change of UC seen on single-contrast barium enema is a fine mucosal granularity. With increasing severity, the mucosa becomes thickened, and superficial ulcers are seen. Deep ulcerations can appear as "collar-button" ulcers, which indicate that the ulceration has penetrated the mucosa. Haustral folds may be normal in mild disease, but as activity progresses they become edematous and thickened. Loss of haustration can occur, especially in patients with long-standing disease. In addition, the colon becomes shortened and narrowed. Polyps in the colon may be postinflammatory polyps or pseudopolyps, adenomatous polyps, or carcinoma.

CT scanning is not as helpful as endoscopy and barium enema in making the diagnosis of UC, but typical findings include mild mural thickening (<1.5 cm), inhomogeneous wall density, absence of small-bowel thickening, increased perirectal and presacral fat, target appearance of the rectum, and adenopathy.

Complications

Only 15% of patients with UC present initially with catastrophic illness. Massive hemorrhage occurs with severe attacks of disease in 1% of patients, and treatment for the disease usually stops the bleeding. However, if a patient requires 6–8 units of blood within 24–48 h, colectomy is indicated. *Toxic megacolon* is defined as a transverse or right colon with a diameter of >6 cm, with loss of haustration in patients with severe attacks of UC. It occurs in about 5% of attacks and can be triggered by electrolyte abnormalities and narcotics. About 50% of acute dilations will resolve with medical therapy alone, but urgent colectomy is required for those that do not improve. Perforation is the most dangerous of the local complications, and the physical signs of peritonitis may not be obvious, especially if the patient is receiving glucocorticoids. Although perforation is rare, the mortality rate for perforation complicating a toxic megacolon is about 15%. In addition, patients can develop a toxic colitis and such severe ulcerations that the bowel may perforate without first dilating.

Strictures occur in 5–10% of patients and are always a concern in UC because of the possibility of underlying neoplasia. Although benign strictures can form from

FIGURE 17-5
Colonoscopy with acute ulcerative colitis: Severe colon inflammation with erythema, friability, and exudates. (*Courtesy of Dr. M. Hamilton, Gastroenterology Division, Department of Medicine, Brigham and Women's Hospital, Boston, Massachusetts; with permission.*)

the inflammation and fibrosis of UC, strictures that are impassable with the colonoscope should be presumed malignant until proven otherwise. A stricture that prevents passage of the colonoscope is an indication for surgery. UC patients occasionally develop anal fissures, perianal abscesses, or hemorrhoids, but the occurrence of extensive perianal lesions should suggest CD.

CROHN'S DISEASE

Signs and symptoms

Although CD usually presents as acute or chronic bowel inflammation, the inflammatory process evolves toward one of two patterns of disease: a fibrostenotic obstructing pattern or a penetrating fistulous pattern, each with different treatments and prognoses. The site of disease influences the clinical manifestations.

Ileocolitis

Because the most common site of inflammation is the terminal ileum, the usual presentation of ileocolitis is a chronic history of recurrent episodes of right lower quadrant pain and diarrhea. Sometimes the initial presentation mimics acute appendicitis with pronounced right lower quadrant pain, a palpable mass, fever, and leukocytosis. Pain is usually colicky; it precedes and is relieved by defecation. A low-grade fever is usually noted. High-spiking fever suggests intraabdominal abscess formation. Weight loss is common—typically 10–20% of body weight—and develops as a consequence of diarrhea, anorexia, and fear of eating.

An inflammatory mass may be palpated in the right lower quadrant of the abdomen. The mass is composed of inflamed bowel, adherent and indurated mesentery, and enlarged abdominal lymph nodes. Extension of the mass can cause obstruction of the right ureter or bladder inflammation, manifested by dysuria and fever. Edema, bowel wall thickening, and fibrosis of the bowel wall within the mass account for the radiographic "string sign" of a narrowed intestinal lumen.

Bowel obstruction may take several forms. In the early stages of disease, bowel wall edema and spasm produce intermittent obstructive manifestations and increasing symptoms of postprandial pain. Over several years, persistent inflammation gradually progresses to fibrostenotic narrowing and stricture. Diarrhea will decrease and be replaced by chronic bowel obstruction. Acute episodes of obstruction occur as well, precipitated by bowel inflammation and spasm or sometimes by impaction of undigested food or medication. These episodes usually resolve with intravenous fluids and gastric decompression.

Severe inflammation of the ileocecal region may lead to localized wall thinning, with microperforation and fistula formation to the adjacent bowel, the skin, or the

urinary bladder, or to an abscess cavity in the mesentery. Enterovesical fistulas typically present as dysuria or recurrent bladder infections or, less commonly, as pneumaturia or fecaluria. Enterocutaneous fistulas follow tissue planes of least resistance, usually draining through abdominal surgical scars. Enterovaginal fistulas are rare and present as dyspareunia or as a feculent or foul-smelling, often painful vaginal discharge. They are unlikely to develop without a prior hysterectomy.

Jejunoileitis

Extensive inflammatory disease is associated with a loss of digestive and absorptive surface, resulting in malabsorption and steatorrhea. Nutritional deficiencies can also result from poor intake and enteric losses of protein and other nutrients. Intestinal malabsorption can cause anemia, hypoalbuminemia, hypocalcemia, hypomagnesemia, coagulopathy, and hyperoxaluria with nephrolithiasis in patients with an intact colon. Many patients need to take oral and often intravenous iron. Vertebral fractures are caused by a combination of vitamin D deficiency, hypocalcemia, and prolonged glucocorticoid use. Pellagra from niacin deficiency can occur in extensive small-bowel disease, and malabsorption of vitamin B_{12} can lead to megaloblastic anemia and neurologic symptoms. Other important nutrients to measure and replete if low are folate and vitamins A, E, and K. Levels of minerals such as zinc, selenium, copper, and magnesium are often low in patients with extensive small-bowel inflammation or resections and these should be repleted as well. Most patients should take a daily multivitamin, calcium, and vitamin D supplements.

Diarrhea is characteristic of active disease; its causes include (1) bacterial overgrowth in obstructive stasis or fistulization, (2) bile-acid malabsorption due to a diseased or resected terminal ileum, and (3) intestinal inflammation with decreased water absorption and increased secretion of electrolytes.

Colitis and perianal disease

Patients with colitis present with low-grade fevers, malaise, diarrhea, crampy abdominal pain, and sometimes hematochezia. Gross bleeding is not as common as in UC and appears in about one-half of patients with exclusively colonic disease. Only 1–2% bleed massively. Pain is caused by passage of fecal material through narrowed and inflamed segments of the large bowel. Decreased rectal compliance is another cause for diarrhea in Crohn's colitis patients. Toxic megacolon is rare but may be seen with severe inflammation and short duration disease.

Stricturing can occur in the colon in 4–16% of patients and produce symptoms of bowel obstruction. If the endoscopist is unable to traverse a stricture in Crohn's colitis, surgical resection should be considered, especially if the patient has symptoms of chronic obstruction. Colonic disease may fistulize into the stomach or duodenum, causing feculent vomiting, or to the proximal or mid-small bowel, causing malabsorption by "short circuiting" and bacterial overgrowth. Ten percent of women with Crohn's colitis will develop a rectovaginal fistula.

Perianal disease affects about one-third of patients with Crohn's colitis and is manifested by incontinence, large hemorrhoidal tags, anal strictures, anorectal fistulae, and perirectal abscesses. Not all patients with perianal fistula will have endoscopic evidence of colonic inflammation.

Gastroduodenal disease

Symptoms and signs of upper GI tract disease include nausea, vomiting, and epigastric pain. Patients usually have an *Helicobacter pylori*–negative gastritis. The second portion of the duodenum is more commonly involved than the bulb. Fistulas involving the stomach or duodenum arise from the small or large bowel and do not necessarily signify the presence of upper GI tract involvement. Patients with advanced gastroduodenal CD may develop a chronic gastric outlet obstruction.

Laboratory, endoscopic, and radiographic features

Laboratory abnormalities include elevated ESR and CRP. In more severe disease, findings include hypoalbuminemia, anemia, and leukocytosis.

Endoscopic features of CD include rectal sparing, aphthous ulcerations, fistulas, and skip lesions. Colonoscopy allows examination and biopsy of mass lesions or strictures and biopsy of the terminal ileum. Upper endoscopy is useful in diagnosing gastroduodenal involvement in patients with upper tract symptoms. Ileal or colonic strictures may be dilated with balloons introduced through the colonoscope. Strictures ≤4 cm and those at a anastomotic sites respond better to endoscopic dilation. The perforation rate is as high as 10%. Most endoscopists dilate only fibrotic strictures and not those associated with active inflammation. Wireless capsule endoscopy (WCE) allows direct visualization of the entire small-bowel mucosa (Fig. 17-6). The diagnostic yield of detecting lesions suggestive of active CD is higher with WCE than CT enterography or small-bowel series. WCE cannot be used in the setting of a small-bowel stricture. Capsule retention occurs in <1% of patients with suspected CD, but retention rates of 4–6% are seen in patients with established CD.

In CD, early radiographic findings in the small bowel include thickened folds and aphthous ulcerations. "Cobblestoning" from longitudinal and transverse ulcerations most frequently involves the small bowel. In more advanced disease, strictures, fistulas, inflammatory masses, and abscesses may be detected. The earliest macroscopic findings of colonic CD are aphthous

FIGURE 17-6

Wireless capsule endoscopy image in a patient with Crohn's disease of the ileum shows ulcerations and narrowing of the intestinal lumen. (*Courtesy of Dr. S Reddy, Gastroenterology Division, Department of Medicine, Brigham and Women's Hospital, Boston, Massachusetts; with permission.*)

ulcers. These small ulcers are often multiple and separated by normal intervening mucosa. As the disease progresses, aphthous ulcers become enlarged, deeper, and occasionally connected to one another, forming longitudinal stellate, serpiginous, and linear ulcers (see Fig. 12-4B).

The transmural inflammation of CD leads to decreased luminal diameter and limited distensibility. As ulcers progress deeper, they can lead to fistula formation. The radiographic "string sign" represents long areas of circumferential inflammation and fibrosis, resulting in long segments of luminal narrowing. The segmental nature of CD results in wide gaps of normal or dilated bowel between involved segments.

CT enterography combines the improved spatial and temporal resolution of multidetector-row CT with large volumes of ingested neutral enteric contrast material to permit visualization of the entire small bowel and lumen. Unlike routine CT, which is used to detect the extraenteric complications of CD such as fistula and abscess, CT enterography clearly depicts the small-bowel inflammation associated with CD by displaying mural hyperenhancement, stratification, and thickening; engorged vasa recta; and perienteric inflammatory changes (Figs. 17-7 and 17-8). CT enterography is the first-line test for the evaluation of suspected CD and its complications. As an initial test in children or in adults with multiple radiation exposures, MR

FIGURE 17-7

Coronal contrast-enhanced multidetector computed tomography (MDCT) image obtained after oral administration of 1350 cc of neutral oral contrast material shows dilation of small-bowel loops, segmental mucosal hyperenhancement, and interloop sinus tracts (*white arrow*) and mesenteric fat stranding. (*Courtesy of Dr. K Mortele, Gastrointestinal Radiology, Department of Radiology, Brigham and Women's Hospital, Boston, Massachusetts; with permission.*)

enterography is comparable to CT in diagnostic accuracy. Pelvic MRI is superior to CT for demonstrating pelvic lesions such as ischiorectal abscesses and perianal fistulae (Fig. 17-9).

Complications

Because CD is a transmural process, serosal adhesions develop that provide direct pathways for fistula formation and reduce the incidence of free perforation. Perforation occurs in 1–2% of patients, usually in the ileum but occasionally in the jejunum or as a complication of toxic megacolon. The peritonitis of free perforation, especially colonic, may be fatal. Intraabdominal and pelvic abscesses occur in 10–30% of patients with Crohn's disease at some time in the course of their illness. CT-guided percutaneous drainage of the abscess is standard therapy. Despite adequate drainage, most patients need resection of the offending bowel segment. Percutaneous drainage has an especially high failure rate in abdominal

FIGURE 17-8

Coronal contrast-enhanced multidetector computed tomography (MDCT) image obtained after oral administration of 1350 cc of neutral oral contrast material shows mucosal hyperenhancement of the terminal ileum with narrowing and mild prestenotic dilatation. (*Courtesy of Dr. K Mortele, Gastrointestinal Radiology, Department of Radiology, Brigham and Women's Hospital, Boston, Massachusetts; with permission.*)

wall abscesses. Systemic glucocorticoid therapy increases the risk of intraabdominal and pelvic abscesses in CD patients who have never had an operation. Other complications include intestinal obstruction in 40%, massive hemorrhage, malabsorption, and severe perianal disease.

Serologic markers

Patients with Crohn's disease show a wide variation in the way they present and progress over time. Some patients present with mild disease activity and do well with generally safe and mild medications, but many others exhibit more severe disease and can develop serious complications that will require surgery. Current and developing biologic therapies can help halt progression of disease and give patients with moderate to severe Crohn's disease a better quality of life. There are potential risks of biologic therapies such as infection and malignancy, and it would be optimal to determine at the time of diagnosis which patients will require more aggressive medical therapy. This same argument holds true for UC patients as well.

FIGURE 17-9

Axial T2-weighted MR image obtained in a 37-year-old man with Crohn's disease shows a linear fluid-filled perianal fistula (*arrow*) in the right ischioanal fossa. (*Courtesy of Dr. K Mortele, Gastrointestinal Radiology, Department of Radiology, Brigham and Women's Hospital, Boston, Massachusetts; with permission.*)

Subsets of patients with differing immune responses to microbial antigens have been described. These include antibodies to *Escherichia coli* (*E. coli*) outer membrane porin protein C (OmpC), which is found in 55% of CD patients, an antibody to I_2, a homologue of the bacterial transcription-factor families from a *Pseudomonas fluorescens*–associated sequence that is found in 50–54% of CD patients, as well as anti–*Saccharomyces cerevisiae* (ASCA) and autoantigens (perinuclear antineutrophil antibody [pANCA]). A novel immune response, antiflagellin (anti-CBir1) has been identified in approximately 50% of Crohn's patients and has been suggested to represent a unique subgroup of CD patients.

Unfortunately, these serologic markers are only marginally useful in helping to make the diagnosis of UC or CD and in predicting the course of disease. For success in diagnosing IBD and in differentiating between CD and UC, the efficacy of these serologic tests depends upon the prevalence of IBD in a specific population. pANCA positivity is found in about 60–70% of UC patients and 5–10% of CD patients; 5–15% of first-degree relatives of UC patients are pANCA positive, whereas only 2–3% of the general population is pANCA positive.

Sixty to seventy percent of CD patients, 10–15% of UC patients, and up to 5% of non-IBD controls are ASCA-positive. In a patient population with a combined prevalence of UC and CD of 62%, pANCA/

ASCA serology showed a sensitivity of 64% and a specificity of 94%. Positive and negative predictive values (PPVs and NPVs) for pANCA/ASCA also vary based on the prevalence of IBD in a given population. For the patient population with a prevalence of IBD of 62%, the PPV is 94%, and the NPV is 63%.

Combining these diagnostic assays may improve the ability to diagnose CD. In a referral population of CD patients, 85% had an antibody to at least one antigen (pANCA, ASCA, OmpC, and I_2); only 4% responded to all four. Some evidence suggests that antibody positivity may help predict disease phenotype. ASCA positivity is associated with an increased rate of early CD complications; OmpC-positive patients are more likely to have internal perforating disease; and I_2-positive patients are more likely to have fibrostenosing disease. Patients positive for I_2, OmpC, and ASCA are the most likely to have undergone small-bowel surgery.

Anti-Cbir1 expression is associated with small-bowel disease, fibrostenosing, and internal penetrating disease. Children with CD positive for all four immune responses (ASCA+, OmpC+, I_2+, and anti-Cbir1+) may have more aggressive disease and a shorter time to progression to internal perforating and/or stricturing disease. However, larger prospective studies in both children and adults have not yet been performed and compared to CRP or other markers.

Clinical factors described at diagnosis are more helpful than serologies at predicting the natural history of Crohn's disease. The initial requirement for glucocorticoid use, an age at diagnosis below 40 years and the presence of perianal disease at diagnosis, have been shown to be independently associated with subsequent disabling CD after 5 years. Except in special circumstances (such as before consideration of an ileoanal pouch anastomosis [IPAA] in a patient with indeterminate colitis), serologic markers have only minimal clinical utility.

DIFFERENTIAL DIAGNOSIS OF UC AND CD

UC and CD have similar features to many other diseases. In the absence of a key diagnostic test, a combination of features is used (**Table 17-5**). Once a diagnosis of IBD is made, distinguishing between UC and CD is impossible initially in up to 15% of cases. These are termed *indeterminate colitis*. Fortunately, in most cases, the true nature of the underlying colitis becomes evident later in the course of the patient's disease. Approximately 5% (range 1–20%) of colon resection specimens are difficult to classify as either UC or CD because they exhibit overlapping histologic features.

TABLE 17-5

DIFFERENT CLINICAL, ENDOSCOPIC, AND RADIOGRAPHIC FEATURES

	ULCERATIVE COLITIS	CROHN'S DISEASE
Clinical		
Gross blood in stool	Yes	Occasionally
Mucus	Yes	Occasionally
Systemic symptoms	Occasionally	Frequently
Pain	Occasionally	Frequently
Abdominal mass	Rarely	Yes
Significant perineal disease	No	Frequently
Fistulas	No	Yes
Small intestinal obstruction	No	Frequently
Colonic obstruction	Rarely	Frequently
Response to antibiotics	No	Yes
Recurrence after surgery	No	Yes
ANCA-positive	Frequently	Rarely
ASCA-positive	Rarely	Frequently
Endoscopic		
Rectal sparing	Rarely	Frequently
Continuous disease	Yes	Occasionally
"Cobblestoning"	No	Yes
Granuloma on biopsy	No	Occasionally
Radiographic		
Small bowel significantly abnormal	No	Yes
Abnormal terminal ileum	No	Yes
Segmental colitis	No	Yes
Asymmetric colitis	No	Yes
Stricture	Occasionally	Frequently

Abbreviations: ANCA, antineutrophil cytoplasm antibody; ASCA, anti-*Saccharomyces cerevisiae* antibody.

TABLE 17-6

DISEASES THAT MIMIC IBD

Infectious Etiologies

Bacterial	**Mycobacterial**	**Viral**
Salmonella	Tuberculosis	Cytomegalovirus
Shigella	*Mycobacterium avium*	Herpes simplex
Toxigenic		HIV
Escherichia coli	**Parasitic**	**Fungal**
Campylobacter	Amebiasis	Histoplasmosis
Yersinia	*Isospora*	*Candida*
Clostridium difficile	*Trichuris trichiura*	*Aspergillus*
Gonorrhea	Hookworm	
Chlamydia trachomatis	*Strongyloides*	

Noninfectious Etiologies

Inflammatory	**Neoplastic**	**Drugs and Chemicals**
Appendicitis	Lymphoma	NSAIDs
Diverticulitis	Metastatic carcinoma	Phosphosoda
Diversion colitis		Cathartic colon
Collagenous/lymphocytic colitis	Carcinoma of the ileum	Gold
Ischemic colitis	Carcinoid	Oral contraceptives
Radiation colitis/enteritis	Familial polyposis	Cocaine
Solitary rectal ulcer syndrome		Chemotherapy
Eosinophilic gastroenteritis		
Neutropenic colitis		
Behçet's syndrome		
Graft-versus-host disease		

Abbreviation: NSAIDs, nonsteroidal anti-inflammatory drugs.

INFECTIOUS DISEASE

Infections of the small intestines and colon can mimic CD or UC. They may be bacterial, fungal, viral, or protozoal in origin (Table 17-6). *Campylobacter* colitis can mimic the endoscopic appearance of severe UC and can cause a relapse of established UC. *Salmonella* can cause watery or bloody diarrhea, nausea, and vomiting. Shigellosis causes watery diarrhea, abdominal pain, and fever followed by rectal tenesmus and by the passage of blood and mucus per rectum. All three are usually self-limited, but 1% of patients infected with *Salmonella* become asymptomatic carriers. *Yersinia enterocolitica* infection occurs mainly in the terminal ileum and causes mucosal ulceration, neutrophil invasion, and thickening of the ileal wall. Other bacterial infections that may mimic IBD include *C. difficile,* which presents with watery diarrhea, tenesmus, nausea, and vomiting; and

E. coli, three categories of which can cause colitis. These are enterohemorrhagic, enteroinvasive, and enteroadherent *E. coli,* all of which can cause bloody diarrhea and abdominal tenderness. Diagnosis of bacterial colitis is made by sending stool specimens for bacterial culture and *C. difficile* toxin analysis. Gonorrhea, *Chlamydia,* and syphilis can also cause proctitis.

GI involvement with mycobacterial infection occurs primarily in the immunosuppressed patient but may occur in patients with normal immunity. Distal ileal and cecal involvement predominates, and patients present with symptoms of small-bowel obstruction and a tender abdominal mass. The diagnosis is made most directly by colonoscopy with biopsy and culture. *Mycobacterium avium-intracellulare* complex infection occurs in advanced stages of HIV infection and in other immunocompromised states; it usually manifests as a systemic infection with diarrhea, abdominal pain, weight loss, fever, and malabsorption. Diagnosis is established by acid-fast smear and culture of mucosal biopsies.

Although most of the patients with viral colitis are immunosuppressed, cytomegalovirus (CMV) and herpes simplex proctitis may occur in immunocompetent individuals. CMV occurs most commonly in the esophagus, colon, and rectum but may also involve the small intestine. Symptoms include abdominal pain, bloody diarrhea, fever, and weight loss. With severe disease, necrosis and perforation can occur. Diagnosis is made by identification of characteristic intranuclear inclusions in mucosal cells on biopsy. Herpes simplex infection of the GI tract is limited to the oropharynx, anorectum, and perianal areas. Symptoms include anorectal pain, tenesmus, constipation, inguinal adenopathy, difficulty with urinary voiding, and sacral paresthesias. Diagnosis is made by rectal biopsy with identification of characteristic cellular inclusions and viral culture. HIV itself can cause diarrhea, nausea, vomiting, and anorexia. Small intestinal biopsies show partial villous atrophy; small-bowel bacterial overgrowth and fat malabsorption may also be noted.

Protozoan parasites include *Isospora belli,* which can cause a self-limited infection in healthy hosts but causes a chronic profuse, watery diarrhea, and weight loss in AIDS patients. *Entamoeba histolytica* or related species infect about 10% of the world's population; symptoms include abdominal pain, tenesmus, frequent loose stools containing blood and mucus, and abdominal tenderness. Colonoscopy reveals focal punctate ulcers with normal intervening mucosa; diagnosis is made by biopsy or serum amebic antibodies. Fulminant amebic colitis is rare but has a mortality rate of >50%.

Other parasitic infections that may mimic IBD include hookworm (*Necator americanus*), whipworm (*T. trichiura*), and *Strongyloides stercoralis*. In severely immunocompromised patients, *Candida* or *Aspergillus* can be identified in the submucosa. Disseminated histoplasmosis can involve the ileocecal area.

NONINFECTIOUS DISEASE

Diverticulitis can be confused with CD clinically and radiographically. Both diseases cause fever, abdominal pain, tender abdominal mass, leukocytosis, elevated ESR, partial obstruction, and fistulas. Perianal disease or ileitis on small-bowel series favors the diagnosis of CD. Significant endoscopic mucosal abnormalities are more likely in CD than in diverticulitis. Endoscopic or clinical recurrence following segmental resection favors CD. Diverticular-associated colitis is similar to CD, but mucosal abnormalities are limited to the sigmoid and descending colon.

Ischemic colitis is commonly confused with IBD. The ischemic process can be chronic and diffuse, as in UC, or segmental, as in CD. Colonic inflammation due to ischemia may resolve quickly or may persist and result in transmural scarring and stricture formation. Ischemic bowel disease should be considered in the elderly following abdominal aortic aneurysm repair or when a patient has a hypercoagulable state or a severe cardiac or peripheral vascular disorder. Patients usually present with sudden onset of left lower quadrant pain, urgency to defecate, and the passage of bright red blood per rectum. Endoscopic examination often demonstrates a normal-appearing rectum and a sharp transition to an area of inflammation in the descending colon and splenic flexure.

The effects of radiotherapy on the GI tract can be difficult to distinguish from IBD. Acute symptoms can occur within 1–2 weeks of starting radiotherapy. When the rectum and sigmoid are irradiated, patients develop bloody, mucoid diarrhea and tenesmus, as in distal UC. With small-bowel involvement, diarrhea is common. Late symptoms include malabsorption and weight loss. Stricturing with obstruction and bacterial overgrowth may occur. Fistulas can penetrate the bladder, vagina, or abdominal wall. Flexible sigmoidoscopy reveals mucosal granularity, friability, numerous telangiectasias, and occasionally discrete ulcerations. Biopsy can be diagnostic.

Solitary rectal ulcer syndrome is uncommon and can be confused with IBD. It occurs in persons of all ages and may be caused by impaired evacuation and failure of relaxation of the puborectalis muscle. Single or multiple ulcerations may arise from anal sphincter overactivity, higher intrarectal pressures during defecation, and digital removal of stool. Patients complain of constipation with straining and pass blood and mucus per rectum. Other symptoms include abdominal pain, diarrhea, tenesmus, and perineal pain. Ulceration as large as 5 cm in diameter is usually seen anteriorly or anteriorlaterally 3–15 cm from the anal verge. Biopsies can be diagnostic.

Several types of colitis are associated with nonsteroidal anti-inflammatory drugs (NSAIDs), including de novo colitis, reactivation of IBD, and proctitis caused by use of suppositories. Most patients with NSAID-related colitis present with diarrhea and abdominal pain, and complications include stricture, bleeding, obstruction, perforation, and fistulization. Withdrawal of these agents is crucial, and in cases of reactivated IBD, standard therapies are indicated.

THE ATYPICAL COLITIDES

Two atypical colitides—collagenous colitis and lymphocytic colitis—have completely normal endoscopic appearances. Collagenous colitis has two main histologic components: increased subepithelial collagen deposition and colitis with increased intraepithelial lymphocytes. The female to male ratio is 9:1, and most patients present in the sixth or seventh decades of life. The main symptom is chronic watery diarrhea. Treatments range from sulfasalazine or mesalamine and Lomotil to bismuth to budesonide to prednisone for refractory disease.

Lymphocytic colitis has features similar to collagenous colitis, including age at onset and clinical presentation, but it has almost equal incidence in men and women and no subepithelial collagen deposition on pathologic section. However, intraepithelial lymphocytes are increased. The frequency of celiac disease is increased in lymphocytic colitis and ranges from 9 to 27%. Celiac disease should be excluded in all patients with lymphocytic colitis, particularly if diarrhea does not respond to conventional therapy. Treatment is similar to that of collagenous colitis with the exception of a gluten-free diet for those who have celiac disease.

Diversion colitis is an inflammatory process that arises in segments of the large intestine that are excluded from the fecal stream. It usually occurs in patients with ileostomy or colostomy when a mucus fistula or a Hartmann's pouch has been created. Clinically, patients have mucus or bloody discharge from the rectum. Erythema, granularity, friability, and, in more severe cases, ulceration can be seen on endoscopy. Histopathology shows areas of active inflammation with foci of cryptitis and crypt abscesses. Crypt architecture is normal, which differentiates it from UC. It may be impossible to distinguish from CD. Short-chain fatty acid enemas may help in diversion colitis, but the definitive therapy is surgical reanastomosis.

EXTRAINTESTINAL MANIFESTATIONS

Up to one-third of IBD patients have at least one extraintestinal disease manifestation.

DERMATOLOGIC

Erythema nodosum (EN) occurs in up to 15% of CD patients and 10% of UC patients. Attacks usually correlate with bowel activity; skin lesions develop after the onset of bowel symptoms, and patients frequently have concomitant active peripheral arthritis. The lesions of EN are hot, red, tender nodules measuring 1–5 cm in diameter and are found on the anterior surface of the lower legs, ankles, calves, thighs, and arms. Therapy is directed toward the underlying bowel disease.

Pyoderma gangrenosum (PG) is seen in 1–12% of UC patients and less commonly in Crohn's colitis. Although it usually presents after the diagnosis of IBD, PG may occur years before the onset of bowel symptoms, run a course independent of the bowel disease, respond poorly to colectomy, and even develop years after proctocolectomy. It is usually associated with severe disease. Lesions are commonly found on the dorsal surface of the feet and legs but may occur on the arms, chest, stoma, and even the face. PG usually begins as a pustule and then spreads concentrically to rapidly undermine healthy skin. Lesions then ulcerate, with violaceous edges surrounded by a margin of erythema. Centrally, they contain necrotic tissue with blood and exudates. Lesions may be single or multiple and grow as large as 30 cm. They are sometimes very difficult to treat and often require intravenous (IV) antibiotics, intravenous, glucocorticoids, dapsone, azathioprine, thalidomide, IV cyclosporine, or infliximab.

Other dermatologic manifestations include pyoderma vegetans, which occurs in intertriginous areas; pyostomatitis vegetans, which involves the mucous membranes; Sweet's syndrome, a neutrophilic dermatosis; and metastatic CD, a rare disorder defined by cutaneous granuloma formation. Psoriasis affects 5–10% of patients with IBD and is unrelated to bowel activity consistent with the potential shared immunogenetic basis of these diseases. Perianal skin tags are found in 75–80% of patients with CD, especially those with colon involvement. Oral mucosal lesions, seen often in CD and rarely in UC, include aphthous stomatitis and "cobblestone" lesions of the buccal mucosa.

RHEUMATOLOGIC

Peripheral arthritis develops in 15–20% of IBD patients, is more common in CD, and worsens with exacerbations of bowel activity. It is asymmetric, polyarticular, and migratory and most often affects large joints of the upper and lower extremities. Treatment is directed at reducing bowel inflammation. In severe UC, colectomy frequently cures the arthritis.

Ankylosing spondylitis (AS) occurs in about 10% of IBD patients and is more common in CD than UC. About two-thirds of IBD patients with AS express the HLA-B27 antigen. The AS activity is not related to bowel activity and does not remit with glucocorticoids or colectomy. It most often affects the spine and pelvis, producing symptoms of diffuse low-back pain, buttock pain, and morning stiffness. The course is continuous and progressive, leading to permanent skeletal damage and deformity. Infliximab reduces spinal inflammation and improves functional status and quality of life.

Sacroiliitis is symmetric, occurs equally in UC and CD, is often asymptomatic, does not correlate with bowel activity, and does not always progress to AS. Other rheumatic manifestations include hypertrophic osteoarthropathy, pelvic/femoral osteomyelitis, and relapsing polychondritis.

OCULAR

The incidence of ocular complications in IBD patients is 1–10%. The most common are conjunctivitis, anterior uveitis/iritis, and episcleritis. Uveitis is associated with both UC and Crohn's colitis, may be found during periods of remission, and may develop in patients following bowel resection. Symptoms include ocular pain, photophobia, blurred vision, and headache. Prompt intervention, sometimes with systemic glucocorticoids, is required to prevent scarring and visual impairment. Episcleritis is a benign disorder that presents with symptoms of mild ocular burning. It occurs in 3–4% of IBD patients, more commonly in Crohn's colitis, and is treated with topical glucocorticoids.

HEPATOBILIARY

Hepatic steatosis is detectable in about one-half of the abnormal liver biopsies from patients with CD and UC; patients usually present with hepatomegaly. Fatty liver usually results from a combination of chronic debilitating illness, malnutrition, and glucocorticoid therapy. Cholelithiasis occurs in 10–35% of CD patients with ileitis or ileal resection. Gallstone formation is caused by malabsorption of bile acids, resulting in depletion of the bile salt pool and the secretion of lithogenic bile.

Primary sclerosing cholangitis (PSC) is a disorder characterized by both intrahepatic and extrahepatic bile duct inflammation and fibrosis, frequently leading to biliary cirrhosis and hepatic failure; approximately 5% of patients with UC have PSC, but 50–75% of patients with PSC have IBD. PSC occurs less often in patients with CD. Although it can be recognized after the diagnosis of IBD, PSC can be detected earlier or even years after proctocolectomy. Consistent with this, the immunogenetic basis for PSC appears to be overlapping but distinct from UC based upon genome-wide association studies (GWAS) although both IBD and PSC are commonly pANCA positive. Most patients have no symptoms at the time of diagnosis; when symptoms are present, they consist of fatigue, jaundice, abdominal pain, fever, anorexia, and malaise. The traditional gold-standard diagnostic test is endoscopic retrograde cholangiopancreatography (ERCP), but magnetic resonance cholangiopancreatography (MRCP) is also sensitive and specific. MRCP is reasonable as an initial diagnostic test in children and can visualize irregularities, multifocal strictures, and dilatations of all levels of the biliary tree. In patients with PSC, both ERCP and MRCP demonstrate multiple bile duct strictures alternating with relatively normal segments.

The bile acid ursodeoxycholic acid (ursodiol) may reduce alkaline phosphatase and serum aminotransferase levels, but histologic improvement has been marginal. High doses (25–30 mg/kg per day) may decrease the risk of colorectal dysplasia and cancer in patients with UC and PSC. Endoscopic stenting may be palliative for cholestasis secondary to bile duct obstruction. Patients with symptomatic disease develop cirrhosis and liver failure over 5–10 years and eventually require liver transplantation. PSC patients have a 10–15% lifetime risk of developing cholangiocarcinoma and then cannot be transplanted. Patients with IBD and PSC are at increased risk of colon cancer and should be surveyed yearly by colonoscopy and biopsy.

In addition, cholangiography is normal in a small percentage of patients who have a variant of PSC known as *small duct primary sclerosing cholangitis*. This variant (sometimes referred to as "pericholangitis") is probably a form of PSC involving small caliber bile ducts. It has similar biochemical and histologic features to classic PSC. It appears to have a significantly better prognosis than classic PSC, although it may evolve into classic PSC. Granulomatous hepatitis and hepatic amyloidosis are much rarer extraintestinal manifestations of IBD.

UROLOGIC

The most frequent genitourinary complications are calculi, ureteral obstruction, and ileal bladder fistulas. The highest frequency of nephrolithiasis (10–20%) occurs in patients with CD following small-bowel resection. Calcium oxalate stones develop secondary to hyperoxaluria, which results from increased absorption of dietary oxalate. Normally, dietary calcium combines with luminal oxalate to form insoluble calcium oxalate, which is eliminated in the stool. In patients with ileal dysfunction, however, nonabsorbed fatty acids bind calcium and leave oxalate unbound. The unbound oxalate is then delivered to the colon, where it is readily absorbed, especially in the presence of inflammation.

METABOLIC BONE DISORDERS

Low bone mass occurs in 3–30% of IBD patients. The risk is increased by glucocorticoids, cyclosporine, methotrexate, and total parenteral nutrition (TPN). Malabsorption and inflammation mediated by IL-1, IL-6, TNF, and other inflammatory mediators also contribute to low bone density. An increased incidence of hip, spine, wrist, and rib fractures has been noted: 36% in CD and 45% in UC. The absolute risk of an osteoporotic fracture is about 1% per person per year. Fracture rates, particularly in the spine and hip, were highest among the elderly (age >60). One study noted an odds ratio of vertebral fracture to be 1.72 and hip fracture 1.59. The disease severity predicted the risk of a fracture. Only 13% of IBD patients who had a fracture were on any kind of antifracture treatment. Up to 20% of bone mass can be lost per year with chronic glucocorticoid use. The effect is dosage-dependent. Budesonide may also suppress the pituitary-adrenal axis and thus carries a risk of causing osteoporosis.

Osteonecrosis is characterized by death of osteo-cytes and adipocytes and eventual bone collapse. The pain is aggravated by motion and swelling of the joints. It affects the hips more often than knees and shoulders, and in one series 4.3% of patients developed osteo-necrosis within 6 months of starting glucocorticoids. Diagnosis is made by bone scan or MRI, and treatment consists of pain control, cord decompression, osteot-omy, and joint replacement.

THROMBOEMBOLIC DISORDERS

Patients with IBD have an increased risk of both venous and arterial thrombosis even if the disease is not active. Factors responsible for the hypercoagulable state have included abnormalities of the platelet-endothelial inter-action, hyperhomocysteinemia, alterations in the coag-ulation cascade, impaired fibrinolysis, involvement of tissue factor-bearing microvesicles, disruption of the normal coagulation system by autoantibodies, as well as a genetic predisposition. A spectrum of vasculitides involving small, medium, and large vessels has also been observed.

OTHER DISORDERS

More common cardiopulmonary manifestations include endocarditis, myocarditis, pleuropericarditis, and inter-stitial lung disease. A secondary or reactive amyloidosis can occur in patients with long-standing IBD, especially in patients with CD. Amyloid material is deposited systemically and can cause diarrhea, constipation, and renal failure. The renal disease can be successfully treated with colchicine. Pancreatitis is a rare extra-intestinal manifestation of IBD and results from duo-denal fistulas; ampullary CD; gallstones; PSC; drugs such as 6-mercaptopurine, azathioprine, or, very rarely, 5-ASA agents; autoimmune pancreatitis; and primary CD of the pancreas.

| TREATMENT | Inflammatory Bowel Disease |

5-ASA AGENTS The mainstay of therapy for mild to moderate UC is sulfasalazine and the other 5-ASA agents. These agents are effective at inducing and main-taining remission in UC. They may have a limited role in inducing remission in CD but no clear role in mainte-nance of CD. The most convincing evidence for the use of sulfasalazine is treatment of active Crohn's disease involving the colon. Sulfasalazine was originally devel-oped to deliver both antibacterial (sulfapyridine) and anti-inflammatory (5-ASA) therapy into the connective tissues of joints and the colonic mucosa. The molecular

structure provides a convenient delivery system to the colon by allowing the intact molecule to pass through the small intestine after only partial absorption, and to be broken down in the colon by bacterial azo reduc-tases that cleave the azo bond linking the sulfa and 5-ASA moieties. Sulfasalazine is effective treatment for mild to moderate UC, but its high rate of side effects limits its use. Although sulfasalazine is more effective at higher doses, at 6 or 8 g/d up to 30% of patients expe-rience allergic reactions or intolerable side effects such as headache, anorexia, nausea, and vomiting that are attributable to the sulfapyridine moiety. Hypersensi-tivity reactions, independent of sulfapyridine levels, include rash, fever, hepatitis, agranulocytosis, hypersen-sitivity pneumonitis, pancreatitis, worsening of colitis, and reversible sperm abnormalities. Sulfasalazine can also impair folate absorption, and patients should be given folic acid supplements.

Newer sulfa-free aminosalicylate preparations deliver increased amounts of the pharmacologically active ingredient of sulfasalazine (5-ASA, mesalamine) to the site of active bowel disease while limiting systemic tox-icity. Peroxisome proliferator activated receptor γ (PPAR-γ) may mediate 5-ASA therapeutic action by decreasing nuclear localization of NFκB. Sulfa-free aminosalicylate formulations include alternative azo-bonded carriers, 5-ASA dimers, pH-dependent tablets, and delayed-release and controlled-release preparations. Each has the same efficacy as sulfasalazine when equimolar con-centrations are used. Olsalazine is composed of two 5-ASA radicals linked by an azo bond, which is split in the colon by bacterial reduction, and two 5-ASA molecules are released. Olsalazine is similar in effec-tiveness to sulfasalazine in treating UC, but up to 17% of patients experience nonbloody diarrhea caused by increased secretion of fluid in the small bowel. Balsalazide contains an azo bond binding mesalamine to the carrier molecule 4-aminobenzoyl-β-alanine; it is effective in the colon.

Asacol is an enteric-coated form of mesalamine with the 5-ASA being released at pH >7. The disintegration of Asacol is variable, with complete breakup of the tab-let occurring in many different parts of the gut ranging from the small intestine to the splenic flexure; it has increased gastric residence when taken with a meal. Pentasa is another mesalamine formulation that uses an ethylcellulose coating to allow water absorption into small beads containing the mesalamine. Water dissolves the 5-ASA, which then diffuses out of the bead into the lumen. Disintegration of the capsule occurs in the stomach. The microspheres then disperse throughout the entire tract from the small intestine through the distal colon in both fasted and fed conditions. Additional formulations of mesalamine continue to be developed. A once-a-day formulation of mesalamine (Multi-Matrix System [MMX], marketed in the United States as Lialda) is designed to release mesalamine in the colon. The MMX technology incorporates mesalamine into a lipophilic matrix within a hydrophilic matrix encapsulated in a polymer resistant to degradation at a low pH (<7) to delay release throughout the colon. The safety profile appears to be comparable to other 5-ASA formulations. A formulation containing encapsulated mesalamine granules (Apriso) was approved for use in the United States. Apriso delivers mesalamine to the terminal ileum and colon via a proprietary extended-release mechanism (Intellicor). The outer coating (Eudragit L) dissolves at a pH >6. In addition, there is a polymer matrix core that aids in sustained release throughout the colon. Since Lialda and Apriso are given once daily, an anticipated benefit is improved compliance compared with two to four daily doses required for other mesalamine preparations. Unencapsulated versions of mesalamine (Salofalk® Granu-Stix) have been in use in Europe for induction and maintenance of remission for several years.

Appropriate doses of Asacol and other 5-ASA compounds are shown in Table 17-7. Some 50–75% of patients with mild to moderate UC improve when treated with 5-ASA doses equivalent to 2 g/d of mesalamine; the dose response continues up to at least 4.8 g/d. As a general rule, 5-ASA agents act within 2–4 weeks. 5-ASA doses equivalent to 1.5–4 g/d of mesalamine maintain remission in 50–75% of patients with UC.

Topical mesalamine enemas are effective in mild-to-moderate distal UC. Clinical response occurs in up to 80% of UC patients with colitis distal to the splenic flexure. Combination therapy with mesalamine in both oral and enema form is more effective than either treatment alone for both distal and extensive UC. Mesalamine suppositories are effective in treating proctitis.

GLUCOCORTICOIDS The majority of patients with moderate-to-severe UC benefit from oral or parenteral glucocorticoids. Prednisone is usually started at doses of 40–60 mg/d for active UC that is unresponsive to 5-ASA therapy. Parenteral glucocorticoids may be administered as hydrocortisone, 300 mg/d, or methylprednisolone, 40–60 mg/d. Topically applied glucocorticoids are also beneficial for distal colitis and may serve as an adjunct in those who have rectal involvement plus more proximal disease. Hydrocortisone enemas or foam may control active disease, although they have no proven role as maintenance therapy. These glucocorticoids are significantly absorbed from the rectum and can lead to adrenal suppression with prolonged administration. Topical 5-ASA therapy is more effective than topical steroid therapy in the treatment of distal UC.

Glucocorticoids are also effective for treatment of moderate-to-severe CD and induce a 60–70% remission rate compared to a 30% placebo response. The systemic effects of standard glucocorticoid formulations have led to the development of more potent formulations that are less well-absorbed and have increased first-pass metabolism. Controlled ileal-release budesonide has been nearly equal to prednisone for ileocolonic CD with fewer glucocorticoid side effects. Budesonide is used for 2–3 months at a dose of 9 mg/d, then tapered.

TABLE 17-7

ORAL 5-ASA PREPARATIONS			
PREPARATION	FORMULATION	DELIVERY	DOSING PER DAY
Azo-Bond			
Sulfasalazine (500 mg) (Azulfidine)	Sulfapyridine-5-ASA	Colon	3–6 g (acute) 2–4 g (maintenance)
Olsalazine (250 mg) (Dipentum)	5-ASA-5-ASA	Colon	1–3 g
Balsalazide (750 mg) (Colazal)	Aminobenzoyl-alanine-5-ASA	Colon	6.75–9 g
Delayed-Release			
Mesalamine (400, 800 mg) (Asacol)	Eudragit S (pH 7)	Distal ileum-colon	2.4–4.8 g (acute) 1.6–4.8 g (maintenance)
Mesalamine (1.2 g) (Lialda)	MMX mesalamine (SPD476)	Ileum-colon	2.4–4.8 g
Controlled-Release			
Mesalamine (250, 500, 1000 mg) (Pentasa)	Ethylcellulose microgranules	Stomach-colon	2–4 g (acute) 1.5–4 g (maintenance)
Delayed and Extended-Release			
Mesalamine (0.375 g) (Apriso)	Intellicor extended-release mechanism	Ileum-colon	1.5 g (maintenance)

Budesonide 6 mg/d is effective in reducing relapse rates at 3–6 months but not at 12 months in CD patients with a medically induced remission.

Glucocorticoids play no role in maintenance therapy in either UC or CD. Once clinical remission has been induced, they should be tapered according to the clinical activity, normally at a rate of no more than 5 mg/week. They can usually be tapered to 20 mg/d within 4–5 weeks but often take several months to be discontinued altogether. The side effects are numerous, including fluid retention, abdominal striae, fat redistribution, hyperglycemia, subcapsular cataracts, osteonecrosis, osteoporosis, myopathy, emotional disturbances, and withdrawal symptoms. Most of these side effects, aside from osteonecrosis, are related to the dose and duration of therapy.

ANTIBIOTICS Antibiotics have no role in the treatment of active or quiescent UC. However, pouchitis, which occurs in about a third of UC patients after colectomy and IPAA, usually responds to treatment with metronidazole and/or ciprofloxacin.

Metronidazole is effective in active inflammatory, fistulous, and perianal CD and may prevent recurrence after ileal resection. The most effective dose is 15–20 mg/kg per day in three divided doses; it is usually continued for several months. Common side effects include nausea, metallic taste, and disulfiram-like reaction. Peripheral neuropathy can occur with prolonged administration (several months) and on rare occasions is permanent despite discontinuation. Ciprofloxacin (500 mg bid) is also beneficial for inflammatory, perianal, and fistulous CD but has recently been associated with Achilles tendinitis and rupture. Both ciprofloxacin and metronidazole antibiotics can be used as first-line drugs for short periods of time in active inflammatory, fistulizing and perianal CD.

AZATHIOPRINE AND 6-MERCAPTOPURINE
Azathioprine and 6-mercaptopurine (6-MP) are purine analogues commonly employed in the management of glucocorticoid-dependent IBD. Azathioprine is rapidly absorbed and converted to 6-MP, which is then metabolized to the active end product, thioinosinic acid, an inhibitor of purine ribonucleotide synthesis and cell proliferation. These agents also inhibit the immune response. Efficacy can be seen as early as 3–4 weeks but can take up to 4–6 months. Adherence can be monitored by measuring the levels of 6-thioguanine and 6-methyl-mercaptopurine, end products of 6-MP metabolism. Azathioprine (2–3 mg/kg per day) and 6-MP (1–1.5 mg/kg per day) have been employed successfully as glucocorticoid-sparing agents in up to two-thirds of UC and CD patients previously unable to be weaned from glucocorticoids. The role of these immunomodulators as maintenance therapy in UC and CD and for treating active perianal disease and fistulas in CD appears promising. In addition, 6-MP or azathioprine is effective for postoperative prophylaxis of CD.

Although azathioprine and 6-MP are usually well tolerated, pancreatitis occurs in 3–4% of patients, typically presents within the first few weeks of therapy, and is completely reversible when the drug is stopped. Other side effects include nausea, fever, rash, and hepatitis. Bone marrow suppression (particularly leukopenia) is dose-related and often delayed, necessitating regular monitoring of the complete blood cell count (CBC). Additionally, 1 in 300 individuals lacks thiopurine methyltransferase, the enzyme responsible for drug metabolism; an additional 11% of the population are heterozygotes with intermediate enzyme activity. Both are at increased risk of toxicity because of increased accumulation of thioguanine metabolites. Although 6-thioguanine and 6-methylmercaptopurine levels can be followed to determine correct drug dosing and reduce toxicity, weight-based dosing is an acceptable alternative. CBCs and liver function tests should be monitored frequently regardless of dosing strategy. IBD patients treated with azathioprine/6-MP are at a fourfold increased risk of developing a lymphoma. This increased risk could be a result of the medications, the underlying disease, or both.

METHOTREXATE Methotrexate (MTX) inhibits dihydrofolate reductase, resulting in impaired DNA synthesis. Additional anti-inflammatory properties may be related to decreased IL-1 production. Intramuscular (IM) or subcutaneous (SC) MTX (25 mg/week) is effective in inducing remission and reducing glucocorticoid dosage; 15 mg/week is effective in maintaining remission in active CD. Potential toxicities include leukopenia and hepatic fibrosis, necessitating periodic evaluation of CBCs and liver enzymes. The role of liver biopsy in patients on long-term MTX is uncertain but is probably limited to those with increased liver enzymes. Hypersensitivity pneumonitis is a rare but serious complication of therapy.

CYCLOSPORINE Cyclosporine (CSA) is a lipophilic peptide with inhibitory effects on both the cellular and humoral immune systems. CSA blocks the production of IL-2 by T-helper lymphocytes. CSA binds to cyclophilin, and this complex inhibits calcineurin, a cytoplasmic phosphatase enzyme involved in the activation of T cells. CSA also indirectly inhibits B cell function by blocking helper T cells. CSA has a more rapid onset of action than 6-MP and azathioprine.

CSA is most effective when given at 2–4 mg/kg per day IV in severe UC that is refractory to IV glucocorticoids, with 82% of patients responding. CSA can be an alternative to colectomy. The long-term success of oral CSA is not as dramatic, but if patients are started on 6-MP or azathioprine at the time of hospital discharge, remission can be maintained. For the 2 mg/kg dose, levels as measured by monoclonal radioimmunoassay or by the high performance liquid chromatography assay should be maintained between 150 and 350 ng/mL.

CSA may cause significant toxicity; renal function should be monitored frequently. Hypertension, gingival hyperplasia, hypertrichosis, paresthesias, tremors, headaches, and electrolyte abnormalities are common side effects. Creatinine elevation calls for dose reduction or discontinuation. Seizures may also complicate therapy, especially if the patient is hypomagnesemic or if serum cholesterol levels are <3.1 mmol/L (<120 mg/dL). Opportunistic infections, most notably *Pneumocystis carinii* pneumonia, may occur with combination immunosuppressive treatment; prophylaxis should be given. Major adverse events occurred in 15% of patients in one large study including nephrotoxicity not responding to dose adjustment, serious infections, seizures, anaphylaxis, and death of two patients. This high incidence suggests that vigorous monitoring by experienced clinicians at tertiary care centers may be required.

TACROLIMUS Tacrolimus is a macrolide antibiotic with immunomodulatory properties similar to CSA. It is 100 times as potent as CSA and is not dependent on bile or mucosal integrity for absorption. These pharmacologic properties enable tacrolimus to have good oral absorption despite proximal small-bowel Crohn's involvement. It has shown efficacy in children with refractory IBD and in adults with extensive involvement of the small bowel. It is also effective in adults with steroid-dependent or refractory UC and CD as well as refractory fistulizing CD.

BIOLOGIC THERAPIES Biologic therapy is often reserved for moderately to severely ill patients with Crohn's disease, who have failed other therapies. Patients who respond to biologic therapies enjoy an improvement in clinical symptoms, a better quality of life, less disability, fatigue, and depression, and fewer surgeries and hospitalizations.

Anti-TNF Therapy The first biologic therapy approved for Crohn's disease was infliximab, a chimeric IgG1 antibody against TNF-alpha, which is now also approved for treatment of moderately to severely active ulcerative colitis. Of active CD patients refractory to glucocorticoids, 6-MP, or 5-ASA, 65% will respond to IV infliximab (5 mg/kg); one-third will enter complete remission. The ACCENT I (A Crohn's Disease Clinical Trial Evaluating Infliximab in a New Long Term Treatment Regimen) study showed that of the patients who experience an initial response, 40% of these will maintain

remission for at least 1 year with repeated infusions of infliximab every 8 weeks.

Infliximab is also effective in CD patients with refractory perianal and enterocutaneous fistulas, with the ACCENT II trial showing a 68% response rate (50% reduction in fistula drainage) and a 50% complete remission rate. Reinfusion, typically every 8 weeks, is necessary to continue therapeutic benefits in many patients.

The development of antibodies to infliximab (ATI) is associated with an increased risk of infusion reactions and a decreased response to treatment. Current practice does not include giving on-demand or episodic infusions rather than periodic (every 8 weeks) infusions because patients are more likely to develop ATI. ATI are generally present when the quality of response or the response duration to infliximab infusion decreases. Decreasing the dosing intervals or increasing the dosage to 10 mg/kg may restore the efficacy of the drug.

The SONIC (Study of Biologic and Immunomodulator-Naïve Patients with Crohn's Disease) Trial compared infliximab plus azathioprine, infliximab alone, and azathioprine alone in immunomodulator and biologic naïve patients with moderate-to-severe Crohn's disease. At 1 year, of 508 randomized patients, the infliximab plus azathioprine group exhibited a steroid-free remission rate of 46% compared with 35% (infliximab alone) and 24% (azathioprine alone). There was also increased complete mucosal healing at week 26 with the combined approach relative to either infliximab or azathioprine alone (44% vs. 30% vs. 17%). The adverse events were equal between groups.

The annual risk of lymphoma (e.g., Hodgkin's and non-Hodgkin's lymphoma) with infliximab has been estimated to be anywhere from 5:10,000 to 20:10,000. The annual risk of lymphoma in the general population is 2:10,000. Forty-eight cases of malignancy were identified by the FDA in children and adolescents with the use of TNF blockers. Etanercept and infliximab were the only TNF blockers included in the analysis. Of the 48 cases, about 50% were lymphomas. Other malignancies such as leukemia, melanoma, and solid organ tumors were reported; malignancies rarely seen in children (e.g., leiomyosarcoma, hepatic malignancies, and renal cell carcinoma) were also observed. Of note, most of these cases (88%) were receiving other immunosuppressive medications (e.g., azathioprine and methotrexate).

Hepatosplenic T cell lymphoma is a nearly universally fatal lymphoma in patients with Crohn's disease. At least 12 cases involved immunomodulators alone, and 19 cases received combination therapy. There have been three reports in patients taking adalimumab alone without an immunomodulator. Patients tend to be young and almost all male.

The FDA also reviewed 147 postmarketing reports of leukemia (including acute myeloid leukemia, chronic lymphocytic leukemia, and chronic myeloid leukemia) and 69 cases of new-onset psoriasis (including pustular, palmoplantar) occurring in patients using TNF blockers. The FDA concluded that there is a possible association with both leukemia and new-onset psoriasis with the use of TNF blockers.

Other morbidities of infliximab include acute infusion reactions and severe serum sickness. All of the anti-TNF drugs are associated with an increased risk of infections, particularly reactivation of latent tuberculosis and opportunistic fungal infections including disseminated histoplasmosis and coccidioidomycosis. Rarely, infliximab and the other anti-TNF drugs have been associated with optic neuritis, seizures, new-onset or exacerbation of clinical symptoms, and radiographic evidence of central nervous system demyelinating disorders, including multiple sclerosis. They may exacerbate symptoms in patients with New York Heart Association functional class III/IV heart failure.

Infliximab has also shown efficacy in UC. In two large randomized, placebo-controlled trials, 37–49% of patients responded to infliximab and 22% and 20% of patients were able to maintain remission after 30 and 54 weeks, respectively. Patients received infliximab at 0, 2, and 6 weeks and then every 8 weeks until the end of the study.

Some patients losing response or not tolerating infliximab can be switched to adalimumab or certolizumab pegol. The GAIN (Gauging Infliximab Efficacy in Infliximab Non-Responders) trial evaluated patients who were previously treated with infliximab and became intolerant or who initially responded and lost response. Three-hundred and twenty-five patients were randomized to adalimumab or placebo. At 4 weeks, 21% of the adalimumab group and 7% of the placebo group were in remission. In clinical practice, this remission rate in the adalimumab group increases over time with a dose increase to 40 mg weekly instead of every other week.

Adalimumab is a recombinant human monoclonal IgG1 antibody containing only human peptide sequences and is injected subcutaneously. Adalimumab binds TNF and neutralizes its function by blocking the interaction between TNF and its cell-surface receptor. Therefore, it seems to have a similar mechanism of action to infliximab but with less immunogenicity. Adalimumab has been approved for treatment of moderate to severe CD. CHARM (Crohn's Trial of the Fully Human Adalimumab for Remission Maintenance) is an adalimumab maintenance study in patients who responded to adalimumab induction therapy. About 50% of the patients in this trial were previously treated with infliximab. Remission rates ranged from 42–48% of infliximab naïve patients at 1 year compared with remission rates of 31–34% in the patients who had previously received infliximab. Certolizumab pegol is a PEGylated form of an anti-TNF antibody administered SC once monthly. SC certolizumab pegol was effective for induction of clinical response in patients with active inflammatory CD. In the PRECISE II (The PEGylated Antibody Fragment Evaluation in Crohn's Disease) trial of maintenance therapy with certolizumab in patients who responded to certolizumab induction, the results were similar to the CHARM trial. At week 26, the subgroup of patients who were infliximab naïve had a response of 69% as compared to 44% in patients who had previously received infliximab.

At least one-third of patients do not respond to infliximab, but no published controlled trial has examined infliximab nonresponders for a response to other anti-TNF agents. If a patient does not have an initial response to any anti-TNF therapy, currently it must be considered futile to try another. Before the approval of natalizumab, the only option for this group of patients was surgery.

Natalizumab Integrins are expressed on the surface of leukocytes and serve as mediators of leukocyte adhesion to vascular endothelium. Alpha4 (α4) integrin along with its beta1 (β1) or beta7 (β7) subunit interact with endothelial ligands, termed adhesion molecules or vascular addressins. Interaction between α4β7 and mucosal addressin cellular adhesion molecule (MAdCAM-1) is important in lymphocyte tracking to gut mucosa. Natalizumab is a recombinant humanized immunoglobulin G4 antibody against α4 integrin that is effective in the induction and maintenance of remission in CD patients. It was approved February 2008 for the treatment of patients with CD refractory or intolerant to anti-TNF therapy. In the ENACT-2 (Evaluation of Natalizumab in Active Crohn's Disease Therapy) study, 354 patients who had a response to natalizumab in ENACT-1 were enrolled into maintenance therapy with an infusion of natalizumab or placebo every 4 weeks through week 56. Natalizumab patients were more likely to have a response (61% vs. 28% placebo) and remission (44% vs. 26% placebo). However, 3 cases of progressive multifocal leukoencephalopathy (PML) associated with the JC polyoma virus in the clinical trials and 102 cases in the postmarketing setting have been reported to date. One case occurred in a patient with Crohn's disease and 104 in patients with multiple sclerosis. The annual risk of PML associated with natalizumab is approximately 1:1000. Patients and caregivers must now adhere to the TOUCH Treatment Program, which details strict criteria including no concomitant 6-MP, azathioprine, or MTX, no glucocorticoids for longer than 6 months, the signing of consent forms, and a monthly check by nurses for symptoms of PML.

THERAPIES IN DEVELOPMENT Other therapies currently in development include monoclonal antibodies against IL-12 and IL-23. IL-12, derived from intestinal antigen presenting cells, initiates T_H1 mediated inflammation. IL-23 is a cytokine composed of a unique p19 subunit together with the p40 subunit of IL-12, which is also upregulated in CD mucosa and promotes T_H17 cells and inhibits T regulatory cells. Therefore, both IL-12 and IL-23 biologic activity can be inhibited by neutralizing IL-12 p40 with specific antibodies. The discovery of IL-23R as an IBD susceptibility gene strengthens the case for the use of IL-23 directed immunotherapy in IBD. Clinical trials are under way. Other promising therapies included those directed at IL-6 and the class of selective adhesion molecule inhibitors (e.g., anti-α4β7 and anti-MadCAM1 antibodies).

NUTRITIONAL THERAPIES Dietary antigens may stimulate the mucosal immune response. Patients with active CD respond to bowel rest, along with TPN. Bowel rest and TPN are as effective as glucocorticoids at inducing remission of active CD but are not effective as maintenance therapy. Enteral nutrition in the form of elemental or peptide-based preparations is also as effective as glucocorticoids or TPN, but these diets are not palatable. Enteral diets may provide the small intestine with nutrients vital to cell growth and do not have the complications of TPN. In contrast to CD, dietary intervention does not reduce inflammation in UC. Standard medical management of UC and CD is shown in Fig. 17-10.

SURGICAL THERAPY

Ulcerative Colitis Nearly one-half of patients with extensive chronic UC undergo surgery within the first 10 years of their illness. The indications for surgery are listed in Table 17-8. Morbidity is about 20% in elective, 30% for urgent, and 40% for emergency proctocolectomy. The risks are primarily hemorrhage, contamination and

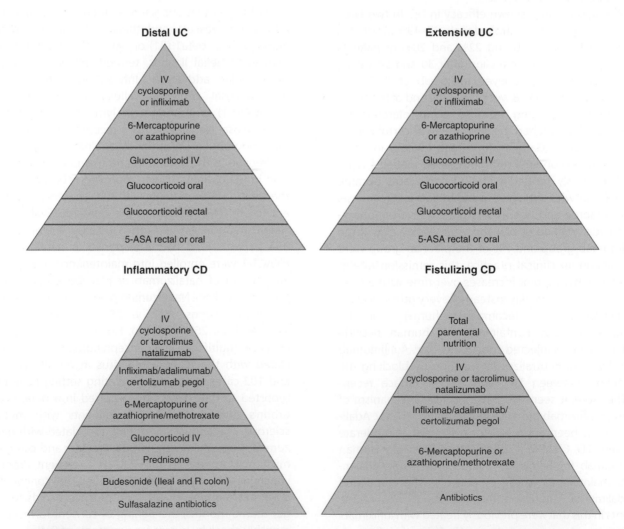

FIGURE 17-10
Medical management of IBD. 5-ASA, 5-aminosalicylic acid; CD, Crohn's disease; UC, ulcerative colitis.

TABLE 17-8

INDICATIONS FOR SURGERY	
ULCERATIVE COLITIS	**CROHN'S DISEASE**
Intractable disease	Small Intestine
Fulminant disease	Stricture and obstruction
Toxic megacolon	unresponsive to medical
Colonic perforation	therapy
Massive colonic	Massive hemorrhage
hemorrhage	Refractory fistula
Extracolonic disease	Abscess
Colonic obstruction	Colon and rectum
Colon cancer prophylaxis	Intractable disease
Colon dysplasia or cancer	Fulminant disease
	Perianal disease
	unresponsive to medical
	therapy
	Refractory fistula
	Colonic obstruction
	Cancer prophylaxis
	Colon dysplasia or cancer

sepsis, and neural injury. The operation of choice is an IPAA.

Because UC is a mucosal disease, the rectal mucosa can be dissected and removed down to the dentate line of the anus or about 2 cm proximal to this landmark. The ileum is fashioned into a pouch that serves as a neorectum. This ileal pouch is then sutured circumferentially to the anus in an end-to-end fashion. If performed carefully, this operation preserves the anal sphincter and maintains continence. The overall operative morbidity is 10%, with the major complication being bowel obstruction. Pouch failure necessitating conversion to permanent ileostomy occurs in 5–10% of patients. Some inflamed rectal mucosa is usually left behind, and thus endoscopic surveillance is necessary. Primary dysplasia of the ileal mucosa of the pouch has occurred rarely.

Patients with IPAA usually have about 6–10 bowel movements a day. On validated quality-of-life indices, they report better performance in sports and sexual activities than ileostomy patients. The most frequent complication of IPAA is pouchitis in about 30–50% of patients with UC. This syndrome consists of increased stool frequency, watery stools, cramping, urgency, nocturnal leakage of stool, arthralgias, malaise, and fever. Pouch biopsies may distinguish true pouchitis from underlying CD. Although pouchitis usually responds to antibiotics, 3–5% of patients remain refractory and may require steroids, immunomodulators, anti-TNF therapy or even pouch removal. A highly concentrated probiotic preparation with four strains of *Lactobacillus,* three strains of *Bifidobacterium,* and one strain of *Streptococcus salivarius* can prevent the recurrence of pouchitis when taken daily.

Crohn's Disease Most patients with CD require at least one operation in their lifetime. The need for surgery is related to duration of disease and the site of involvement. Patients with small-bowel disease have an 80% chance of requiring surgery. Those with colitis alone have a 50% chance. Surgery is an option only when medical treatment has failed or complications dictate its necessity. The indications for surgery are shown in Table 17-8.

Small intestinal disease Because CD is chronic and recurrent, with no clear surgical cure, as little intestine as possible is resected. Current surgical alternatives for treatment of obstructing CD include resection of the diseased segment and strictureplasty. Surgical resection of the diseased segment is the most frequently performed operation, and in most cases primary anastomosis can be done to restore continuity. If much of the small bowel has already been resected and the strictures are short, with intervening areas of normal mucosa, strictureplasties should be done to avoid a functionally insufficient length of bowel. The strictured area of intestine is incised longitudinally and the incision sutured transversely, thus widening the narrowed area. Complications of strictureplasty include prolonged ileus, hemorrhage, fistula, abscess, leak, and restricture.

There is evidence that mesalamine, nitro-imidazole antibiotics, 6-MP/azathioprine, and infliximab are all superior to placebo for the prevention of postoperative recurrence of Crohn's disease. Mesalamine is the least effective and the side effects of the nitro-imidazole antibiotics limit their use. Risk factors for early recurrence of disease include cigarette smoking, penetrating disease (internal fistulas, abscesses or other evidence of penetration through the wall of the bowel), early recurrence since a previous surgery, multiple surgeries, or a young age at the time of the first surgery. Aggressive postoperative treatment with 6-MP/azathioprine or infliximab should be considered for this group of patients. It is also recommended to evaluate for endoscopic recurrence of Crohn's disease via a colonoscopy, if possible, 6 months after surgery.

Colorectal disease A greater percentage of patients with Crohn's colitis require surgery for intractability, fulminant disease, and anorectal disease. Several alternatives are available, ranging from the use of a temporary loop ileostomy to resection of segments of diseased colon or even the entire colon and rectum. For patients with segmental involvement, segmental colon resection with primary anastomosis can be performed. In 20–25% of patients with extensive colitis, the rectum is spared sufficiently to consider rectal preservation. Most surgeons believe that an IPAA is contraindicated in CD due to the high incidence of pouch failure.

A diverting colostomy may help heal severe perianal disease or rectovaginal fistulas, but disease almost always recurs with reanastomosis. These patients often require a total proctocolectomy and ileostomy.

INFLAMMATORY BOWEL DISEASE AND PREGNANCY

Patients with quiescent UC and CD have normal fertility rates; the fallopian tubes can be scarred by the inflammatory process of CD, especially on the right side because of the proximity of the terminal ileum. In addition, perirectal, perineal, and rectovaginal abscesses and fistulae can result in dyspareunia. Infertility in men can be caused by sulfasalazine but reverses when treatment is stopped. In women who have had pouch surgery, most studies show that the fertility rate is reduced to about one-third of normal. This is due to scarring or occlusion of the fallopian tubes secondary to pelvic inflammation.

In mild or quiescent UC and CD, fetal outcome is nearly normal. Spontaneous abortions, stillbirths, and developmental defects are increased with increased disease activity, not medications. The courses of CD and UC during pregnancy mostly correlate with disease activity at the time of conception. Patients should be in remission for 6 months before conceiving. Most CD patients can deliver vaginally, but cesarean section may be the preferred route of delivery for patients with anorectal and perirectal abscesses and fistulas to reduce the likelihood of fistulas developing or extending into the episiotomy scar.

Sulfasalazine, mesalamine, and balsalazide are safe for use in pregnancy and nursing, but additional folate supplementation must be given with sulfasalazine. Topical 5-ASA agents are also safe during pregnancy and nursing. Glucocorticoids are generally safe for use during pregnancy and are indicated for patients with moderate to severe disease activity. The amount of glucocorticoids received by the nursing infant is minimal. The safest antibiotics to use for CD in pregnancy for short periods of time (weeks, not months) are ampicillin and cephalosporin. Metronidazole can be used in the second or third trimester. Ciprofloxacin causes cartilage lesions in immature animals and should be avoided because of the absence of data on its effects on growth and development in humans.

6-MP and azathioprine pose minimal or no risk during pregnancy, but experience is limited. If the patient cannot be weaned from the drug or has an exacerbation that requires 6-MP/azathioprine during pregnancy, she should continue the drug with informed consent. Breast milk contained negligible levels of 6-MP/azathioprine when measured in a limited number of patients.

Little data exist on CSA in pregnancy. In a small number of patients with severe IBD treated with IV CSA during pregnancy, 80% of pregnancies were successfully completed without development of renal toxicity, congenital malformations, or developmental defects. However, because of the lack of data, CSA should probably be avoided unless the patient would otherwise require surgery. Methotrexate is contraindicated in pregnancy and nursing. No increased risk of stillbirths, miscarriages, or spontaneous abortions has been seen with infliximab, adalimumab, or certolizumab, all class B drugs. The anti-TNF drugs are relatively safe in nursing as well because they do not pass into breast milk. Natalizumab is a class C drug, and there is limited data on pregnancy.

Surgery in UC should be performed only for emergency indications, including severe hemorrhage, perforation, and megacolon refractory to medical therapy. Total colectomy and ileostomy carry a 50–60% risk of postoperative spontaneous abortion. Fetal mortality is also high in CD requiring surgery. Patients with IPAAs have increased nighttime stool frequency during pregnancy that resolves postpartum. Transient small-bowel obstruction or ileus has been noted in up to 8% of patients with ileostomies.

CANCER IN INFLAMMATORY BOWEL DISEASE

ULCERATIVE COLITIS

Patients with long-standing UC are at increased risk for developing colonic epithelial dysplasia and carcinoma (**Fig. 17-11**).

FIGURE 17-11

Medium power view of low-grade dysplasia in a patient with chronic ulcerative colitis. Low-grade dysplastic crypts are interspersed among regenerating crypts. (*Courtesy of Dr. R Odze, Division of Gastrointestinal Pathology, Department of Pathology, Brigham and Women's Hospital, Boston, Massachusetts; with permission.*)

The risk of neoplasia in chronic UC increases with duration and extent of disease. The risk of cancer, as measured in tertiary referral centers, rises 0.5–1% per year after 8–10 years of disease in patients with pancolitis. The only prospective surveillance study reported a lower rate of cancer; 2.5% at 20 years of disease, 7.6% at 30 years of disease, and 10.8% at 40 years. The rates of colon cancer are higher than in the general population, and colonoscopic surveillance is the standard of care.

Annual or biennial colonoscopy with multiple biopsies is recommended for patients with >8–10 years of pancolitis or 12–15 years of left-sided colitis and has been widely employed to screen and survey for subsequent dysplasia and carcinoma. Risk factors for cancer in UC include long-duration disease, extensive disease, family history of colon cancer, PSC, a colon stricture, and the presence of postinflammatory pseudopolyps on colonoscopy.

CROHN'S DISEASE

Risk factors for developing cancer in Crohn's colitis are long-duration and extensive disease, bypassed colon segments, colon strictures, PSC, and family history of colon cancer. The cancer risks in CD and UC are probably equivalent for similar extent and duration of disease. In patients with extensive Crohn's colitis, the cumulative risk of detecting an initial finding of any definite dysplasia or cancer after a negative screening colonoscopy is 25% by the tenth surveillance examination. The cumulative risk of detecting an initial finding of flat high-grade dysplasia (HGD) or cancer after a negative screening colonoscopy is 7% by the ninth surveillance examination. Thus, the same endoscopic surveillance strategy used for UC is recommended for patients with chronic Crohn's colitis. A pediatric colonoscope can be used to pass narrow strictures in CD patients, but surgery should be considered in symptomatic patients with impassable strictures.

MANAGEMENT OF DYSPLASIA AND CANCER

Dysplasia can be flat or polypoid. If flat HGD is encountered on colonoscopic surveillance, the usual treatment for UC is colectomy and for CD is either colectomy or segmental resection. If flat low-grade dysplasia (LGD) is found (Fig. 17-11), most investigators recommend immediate colectomy. Adenomas may occur coincidently in UC and CD patients with chronic colitis and can be removed endoscopically provided that biopsies of the surrounding mucosa are free of dysplasia. New techniques such as high definition and magnification colonoscopes and dye sprays have increased the rate of dysplasia detection. In the future, endoscopists may be able to do targeted rather than segmental biopsies in patients with chronic Crohn's or ulcerative colitis.

IBD patients are also at greater risk for other malignancies. Patients with CD may have an increased risk of non-Hodgkin's lymphoma, leukemia, and myelodysplastic syndromes. Severe chronic, complicated perianal disease in CD patients may be associated with an increased risk of cancer in the lower rectum and anal canal (squamous cell cancers). Although the absolute risk of small-bowel adenocarcinoma in CD is low (2.2% at 25 years in one study), patients with long-standing, extensive, small-bowel disease should consider screening.

CHAPTER 18

IRRITABLE BOWEL SYNDROME

Chung Owyang

Irritable bowel syndrome (IBS) is a functional bowel disorder characterized by abdominal pain or discomfort and altered bowel habits in the absence of detectable structural abnormalities. No clear diagnostic markers exist for IBS, thus the diagnosis of the disorder is based on clinical presentation. In 2006, the Rome II criteria for the diagnosis of IBS were revised (Table 18-1). Throughout the world, about 10–20% of adults and adolescents have symptoms consistent with IBS, and most studies show a female predominance. IBS symptoms tend to come and go over time and often overlap with other functional disorders such as fibromyalgia, headache, backache, and genitourinary symptoms. Severity of symptoms varies and can significantly impair quality of life, resulting in high health care costs. Advances in basic, mechanistic, and clinical investigations have improved our understanding of this disorder and its physiologic and psychosocial determinants. Altered gastrointestinal (GI) motility, visceral hyperalgesia, disturbance of brain-gut interaction, abnormal central processing, autonomic and hormonal events, genetic and environmental factors, and psychosocial disturbances are variably involved, depending on the individual. This progress may result in improved methods of treatment.

CLINICAL FEATURES

IBS is a disorder that affects all ages, although most patients have their first symptoms before age 45. Older individuals have a lower reporting frequency. Women are diagnosed with IBS two to three times as often as men and make up 80% of the population with severe IBS. As indicated in Table 18-1, pain or abdominal discomfort is a key symptom for the diagnosis of IBS. These symptoms should be improved with defecation and/or have their onset associated with a change in frequency or form of stool. Painless diarrhea or constipation does not fulfill the diagnostic criteria to be classified as IBS. Supportive symptoms that are not part of the diagnostic criteria include defecation straining, urgency or a feeling of incomplete bowel movement, passing mucus, and bloating.

Abdominal pain

According to the current IBS diagnostic criteria, abdominal pain or discomfort is a prerequisite clinical feature of IBS. Abdominal pain in IBS is highly variable in intensity and location. It is frequently episodic and crampy, but it may be superimposed on a background of constant ache. Pain may be mild enough to be ignored or it may interfere with daily activities. Despite this, malnutrition due to inadequate caloric intake is exceedingly rare with IBS. Sleep deprivation is also unusual because abdominal pain is almost uniformly present only during waking hours. However, patients with severe IBS frequently wake repeatedly during the night; thus, nocturnal pain is a poor discriminating factor between organic and functional bowel disease. Pain is often exacerbated by eating or emotional stress and

TABLE 18-1

DIAGNOSTIC CRITERIA FOR IRRITABLE BOWEL SYNDROME[a]
Recurrent abdominal pain or discomfort[b] at least 3 days per month in the last 3 months associated with *two or more* of the following: 1. Improvement with defecation 2. Onset associated with a change in frequency of stool 3. Onset associated with a change in form (appearance) of stool

[a]Criteria fulfilled for the last 3 months with symptom onset at least 6 months prior to diagnosis.
[b]Discomfort means an uncomfortable sensation not described as pain. In pathophysiology research and clinical trials, a pain/discomfort frequency of at least 2 days a week during screening evaluation is required for subject eligibility.
Source: Adapted from GF Longstreth et al: Gastroenterology 130: 1480, 2006.

improved by passage of flatus or stools. In addition, female patients with IBS commonly report worsening symptoms during the premenstrual and menstrual phases.

Altered bowel habits

Alteration in bowel habits is the most consistent clinical feature in IBS. The most common pattern is constipation alternating with diarrhea, usually with one of these symptoms predominating. At first, constipation may be episodic, but eventually it becomes continuous and increasingly intractable to treatment with laxatives. Stools are usually hard with narrowed caliber, possibly reflecting excessive dehydration caused by prolonged colonic retention and spasm. Most patients also experience a sense of incomplete evacuation, thus leading to repeated attempts at defecation in a short time span. Patients whose predominant symptom is constipation may have weeks or months of constipation interrupted with brief periods of diarrhea. In other patients, diarrhea may be the predominant symptom. Diarrhea resulting from IBS usually consists of small volumes of loose stools. Most patients have stool volumes of <200 mL. Nocturnal diarrhea does not occur in IBS. Diarrhea may be aggravated by emotional stress or eating. Stool may be accompanied by passage of large amounts of mucus. Bleeding is not a feature of IBS unless hemorrhoids are present, and malabsorption or weight loss does not occur.

Bowel pattern subtypes are highly unstable. In a patient population with ~33% prevalence rates of IBS–diarrhea predominant (IBS-D), IBS–constipation predominant (IBS-C), and IBS–mixed (IBS-M) forms, 75% of patients change subtypes and 29% switch between IBS-C and IBS-D over 1 year. The heterogeneity and variable natural history of bowel habits in IBS increase the difficulty of conducting pathophysiology studies and clinical trials.

Gas and flatulence

Patients with IBS frequently complain of abdominal distention and increased belching or flatulence, all of which they attribute to increased gas. Although some patients with these symptoms actually may have a larger amount of gas, quantitative measurements reveal that most patients who complain of increased gas generate no more than a normal amount of intestinal gas. Most IBS patients have impaired transit and tolerance of intestinal gas loads. In addition, patients with IBS tend to reflux gas from the distal to the more proximal intestine, which may explain the belching.

Some patients with bloating may also experience visible distention with increase in abdominal girth. Both symptoms are more common among female patients and in those with higher overall Somatic Symptom Checklist scores. IBS patients who experienced bloating alone have been shown to have lower thresholds for pain and desire to defecate compared to those with concomitant distention irrespective of bowel habit. When patients were grouped according to sensory threshold, hyposensitive individuals had distention significantly more than those with hypersensitivity and this was observed more in the constipation subgroup. This suggests that the pathogenesis of bloating and distention may not be the same.

Upper gastrointestinal symptoms

Between 25 and 50% of patients with IBS complain of dyspepsia, heartburn, nausea, and vomiting. This suggests that other areas of the gut apart from the colon may be involved. Prolonged ambulant recordings of small-bowel motility in patients with IBS show a high incidence of abnormalities in the small bowel during the diurnal (waking) period; nocturnal motor patterns are not different from those of healthy controls. The overlap between dyspepsia and IBS is great. The prevalence of IBS is higher among patients with dyspepsia (31.7%) than among those who reported no symptoms of dyspepsia (7.9%). Conversely, among patients with IBS, 55.6% reported symptoms of dyspepsia. In addition, the functional abdominal symptoms can change over time. Those with predominant dyspepsia or IBS can flux between the two. Although the prevalence of functional gastrointestinal disorders is stable over time, the turnover in symptom status is high. Many episodes of symptom disappearance are due to subjects changing symptoms rather than total symptom resolution. Thus it is conceivable that functional dyspepsia and IBS are two manifestations of a single, more extensive digestive system disorder. Furthermore, IBS symptoms are prevalent in noncardiac chest pain patients, suggesting overlap with other functional gut disorders.

PATHOPHYSIOLOGY

The pathogenesis of IBS is poorly understood, although roles of abnormal gut motor and sensory activity, central neural dysfunction, psychological disturbances, mucosal inflammation, stress, and luminal factors have been proposed.

Gastrointestinal motor abnormalities

Studies of colonic myoelectrical and motor activity under unstimulated conditions have not shown consistent abnormalities in IBS. In contrast, colonic motor abnormalities are more prominent under stimulated conditions in IBS. IBS patients may exhibit increased rectosigmoid motor activity for up to 3 h after eating.

Similarly, inflation of rectal balloons both in IBS-D and IBS-C patients leads to marked and prolonged distention-evoked contractile activity. Recordings from the transverse, descending, and sigmoid colon showed that the motility index and peak amplitude of high-amplitude propagating contractions (HAPCs) in diarrhea-prone IBS patients were greatly increased compared to those in healthy subjects and were associated with rapid colonic transit and accompanied by abdominal pain.

Visceral hypersensitivity

As with studies of motor activity, IBS patients frequently exhibit exaggerated sensory responses to visceral stimulation. Postprandial pain has been temporally related to entry of the food bolus into the cecum in 74% of patients. Rectal balloon inflation produces nonpainful and painful sensations at lower volumes in IBS patients than in healthy controls without altering rectal tension, suggestive of visceral afferent dysfunction in IBS. Similar studies show gastric and esophageal hypersensitivity in patients with nonulcer dyspepsia and noncardiac chest pain, raising the possibility that these conditions have a similar pathophysiologic basis. Lipids lower the thresholds for the first sensation of gas, discomfort, and pain in IBS patients. Hence, postprandial symptoms in IBS patients may be explained in part by a nutrient-dependent exaggerated sensory component of the gastrocolonic response. In contrast to enhanced gut sensitivity, IBS patients do not exhibit heightened sensitivity elsewhere in the body. Thus, the afferent pathway disturbances in IBS appear to be selective for visceral innervation with sparing of somatic pathways. The mechanisms responsible for visceral hypersensitivity are still under investigation. It has been proposed that these exaggerated responses may be due to (1) increased end-organ sensitivity with recruitment of "silent" nociceptors; (2) spinal hyperexcitability with activation of nitric oxide and possibly other neurotransmitters; (3) endogenous (cortical and brainstem) modulation of caudad nociceptive transmission; and (4) over time, the possible development of long-term hyperalgesia due to development of neuroplasticity, resulting in permanent or semipermanent changes in neural responses to chronic or recurrent visceral stimulation (Table 18-2).

TABLE 18-2

PROPOSED MECHANISMS FOR VISCERAL HYPERSENSITIVITY	
End-organ sensitivity	Long-term hyperalgesia
"Silent" nociceptors	Tonic cortical regulation
CNS modulation	Neuroplasticity
Cortex	
Brainstem	

Abbreviation: CNS, central nervous system.

Central neural dysregulation

The role of central nervous system (CNS) factors in the pathogenesis of IBS is strongly suggested by the clinical association of emotional disorders and stress with symptom exacerbation and the therapeutic response to therapies that act on cerebral cortical sites. Functional brain imaging studies such as MRI have shown that in response to distal colonic stimulation, the mid-cingulate cortex—a brain region concerned with attention processes and response selection—shows greater activation in IBS patients. Modulation of this region is associated with changes in the subjective unpleasantness of pain. In addition, IBS patients also show preferential activation of the prefrontal lobe, which contains a vigilance network within the brain that increases alertness. These may represent a form of cerebral dysfunction leading to the increased perception of visceral pain.

Abnormal psychological features

Abnormal psychiatric features are recorded in up to 80% of IBS patients, especially in referral centers; however, no single psychiatric diagnosis predominates. Most of these patients demonstrated exaggerated symptoms in response to visceral distention, and this abnormality persists even after exclusion of psychological factors.

Psychological factors influence pain thresholds in IBS patients, as stress alters sensory thresholds. An association between prior sexual or physical abuse and development of IBS has been reported. Abuse is associated with greater pain reporting, psychological distress, and poor health outcome. Brain functional MRI studies show greater activation of the posterior and middle dorsal cingulate cortex, which is implicated in affect processing in IBS patients with a past history of sexual abuse.

Thus, patients with IBS frequently demonstrate increased motor reactivity of the colon and small bowel to a variety of stimuli and altered visceral sensation associated with lowered sensation thresholds. These may result from CNS—enteric nervous system dysregulation (Fig. 18-1).

Post-infectious IBS

IBS may be induced by GI infection. In an investigation of 544 patients with confirmed bacterial gastroenteritis, one-quarter developed IBS subsequently. Conversely, about a third of IBS patients experienced an acute "gastroenteritis-like" illness at the onset of their chronic IBS symptomatology. This group of "postinfective" IBS occurs more commonly in females and affects younger rather than older patients. Risk factors for developing post-infectious IBS include, in order of importance, prolonged duration of initial illness, toxicity of infecting bacterial strain, smoking, mucosal markers

FIGURE 18-1

Therapeutic targets for irritable bowel syndrome. Patients with mild to moderate symptoms usually have intermittent symptoms that correlate with altered gut physiology. Treatments include gut-acting pharmacologic agents such as antispasmodics, antidiarrheals, fiber supplements, and gut serotonin modulators. Patients who have severe symptoms usually have constant pain and psychosocial difficulties. This group of patients is best managed with antidepressants and other psychosocial treatments. CNS, central nervous system; ENS, enteric nervous system.

of inflammation, female gender, depression, hypochondriasis, and adverse life events in the preceding 3 months. Age older than 60 years might protect against post-infectious IBS, whereas treatment with antibiotics has been associated with increased risk. The microbes involved in the initial infection are *Campylobacter*, *Salmonella*, and *Shigella*. Those patients with *Campylobacter* infection who are toxin-positive are more likely to develop postinfective IBS. Increased rectal mucosal enteroendocrine cells, T lymphocytes, and increased gut permeability are acute changes following *Campylobacter* enteritis that could persist for more than a year and may contribute to postinfective IBS.

Immune activation and mucosal inflammation

Some patients with IBS display persistent signs of low-grade mucosal inflammation with activated lymphocytes, mast cells, and enhanced expression of proinflammatory cytokines. These abnormalities may contribute to abnormal epithelial secretion and visceral hypersensitivity. Interestingly, clinical studies have shown increased intestinal permeability in patients with IBS-D. Psychological stress and anxiety can increase the release of proinflammatory cytokine and this in turn may alter intestinal permeability. This provides a functional link between psychological stress, immune activation, and symptom generation in patients with IBS.

Altered gut flora

A high prevalence of small intestinal bacterial overgrowth in IBS patients has been noted based on positive lactulose hydrogen breath test. This finding, however, has been challenged by a number of other studies that found no increased incidence of bacterial overgrowth based on jejunal aspirate culture. Abnormal H_2 breath test can occur because of small bowel rapid transit and may lead to erroneous interpretation. Hence, the role of testing for small intestinal bacterial overgrowth in IBS patients remains unclear.

A number of studies found significant differences between the molecular profile of the fecal microbiota of IBS patients compared with that of healthy subjects. Several bacterial genera with *Lactobacillus* sequence appear to be absent from IBS, and *Collinsella* sequences were greatly reduced in this group of patients. Currently it is unclear whether such changes are causal, consequential, or merely the result of constipation and diarrhea. In addition, the stability of the changes in the microbiota needs to be determined.

Abnormal serotonin pathways

The serotonin (5HT)-containing enterochromaffin cells in the colon are increased in a subset of IBS-D patients compared to healthy individuals or patients with ulcerative colitis. Furthermore, postprandial plasma 5HT levels were significantly higher in this group of patients compared to healthy controls. Since serotonin plays an important role in the regulation of GI motility and visceral perception, the increased release of serotonin may contribute to the postprandial symptoms of these patients and provides a rationale for the use of serotonin antagonists in the treatment of this disorder.

APPROACH TO THE PATIENT   **Irritable Bowel Syndrome**

Because IBS is a disorder for which no pathognomonic abnormalities have been identified, its diagnosis relies on recognition of positive clinical features and elimination of other organic diseases. A careful history and physical examination are frequently helpful in establishing the diagnosis. Clinical features suggestive of IBS include the following: recurrence of lower abdominal pain with altered bowel habits over a period of time without progressive deterioration, onset of symptoms during periods of stress or emotional upset, absence of other systemic symptoms such as fever and weight loss, and small-volume stool without any evidence of blood.

On the other hand, the appearance of the disorder for the first time in old age, progressive course from time of onset, persistent diarrhea after a 48-h fast, and presence of nocturnal diarrhea or steatorrheal stools argue against the diagnosis of IBS.

Because the major symptoms of IBS—abdominal pain, abdominal bloating, and alteration in bowel habits—are common complaints of many GI organic disorders, the list of differential diagnoses is a long one. The quality, location, and timing of pain may be helpful to suggest specific disorders. Pain due to IBS that occurs in the epigastric or periumbilical area must be differentiated from biliary tract disease, peptic ulcer disorders, intestinal ischemia, and carcinoma of the stomach and pancreas. If pain occurs mainly in the lower abdomen, the possibility of diverticular disease of the colon, inflammatory bowel disease (including ulcerative colitis and Crohn's disease), and carcinoma of the colon must be considered. Postprandial pain accompanied by bloating, nausea, and vomiting suggests gastroparesis or partial intestinal obstruction. Intestinal infestation with *Giardia lamblia* or other parasites may cause similar symptoms. When diarrhea is the major complaint, the possibility of lactase deficiency, laxative abuse, malabsorption, celiac sprue, hyperthyroidism, inflammatory bowel disease, and infectious diarrhea must be ruled out. On the other hand, constipation may be a side effect of many different drugs, such as anticholinergic, antihypertensive, and antidepressant medications. Endocrinopathies such as hypothyroidism and hypoparathyroidism must also be considered in the differential diagnosis of constipation, particularly if other systemic signs or symptoms of these endocrinopathies are present. In addition, acute intermittent porphyria and lead poisoning may present in a fashion similar to IBS, with painful constipation as the major complaint. These possibilities are suspected on the basis of their clinical presentations and are confirmed by appropriate serum and urine tests.

Few tests are required for patients who have typical IBS symptoms and no alarm features. Unnecessary investigations may be costly and even harmful. The American Gastroenterological Association has delineated factors to be considered when determining the aggressiveness of the diagnostic evaluation. These include the duration of symptoms, the change in symptoms over time, the age and sex of the patient, the referral status of the patient, prior diagnostic studies, a family history of colorectal malignancy, and the degree of psychosocial dysfunction. Thus, a younger individual with mild symptoms requires a minimal diagnostic evaluation, while an older person or an individual with rapidly progressive symptoms should undergo a more thorough exclusion of organic disease. Most patients should have a complete blood count and sigmoidoscopic examination; in addition, stool specimens should be examined for ova and parasites in those who have diarrhea. In patients with persistent diarrhea not responding to simple anti-diarrhea agents, a sigmoid colon biopsy should be performed to rule out microscopic colitis. In those aged >40 years, an air-contrast barium enema or colonoscopy should also be performed. If the main symptoms are diarrhea and increased gas, the possibility of lactase deficiency should be ruled out with a hydrogen breath test or with evaluation after a 3-week lactose-free diet. Some patients with IBS-D may have undiagnosed celiac sprue. Because the symptoms of celiac sprue respond to a gluten-free diet, testing for celiac sprue in IBS may prevent years of morbidity and attendant expense. Decision-analysis studies show that serology testing for celiac sprue in patients with IBS-D has an acceptable cost when the prevalence of celiac sprue is >1% and is the dominant strategy when the prevalence is >8%. In patients with concurrent symptoms of dyspepsia, upper GI radiographs or esophagogastroduodenoscopy may be advisable. In patients with postprandial right upper quadrant pain, an ultrasonogram of the gallbladder should be obtained. Laboratory features that argue against IBS include evidence of anemia, elevated sedimentation rate, presence of leukocytes or blood in stool, and stool volume >200–300 mL/d. These findings would necessitate other diagnostic considerations.

TREATMENT   Irritable Bowel Syndrome

PATIENT COUNSELING AND DIETARY ALTERATIONS Reassurance and careful explanation of the functional nature of the disorder and of how to avoid obvious food precipitants are important first steps in patient counseling and dietary change. Occasionally, a meticulous dietary history may reveal substances (such as coffee, disaccharides, legumes, and cabbage) that aggravate symptoms. Excessive fructose and artificial sweeteners, such as sorbitol or mannitol, may cause diarrhea, bloating, cramping, or flatulence. As a therapeutic trial, patients should be encouraged to eliminate any foodstuffs that appear to produce symptoms. However patients should avoid nutritionally depleted diets. Patients with IBS-D anecdotally report symptom improvement after initiating a low-carbohydrate diet. A prospective study has shown marked symptomatic improvement in stool frequency, consistency, pain scores, and quality of life following 4 weeks of a very-low-carbohydrate (CHO) diet (20 g CHO/day). This diet may be tried in IBS patients who report intolerance to certain carbohydrates.

Stool-Bulking Agents High-fiber diets and bulking agents, such as bran or hydrophilic colloid, are frequently used in treating IBS. The water-holding action of fibers may contribute to increased stool bulk because of the ability of fiber to increase fecal output of bacteria.

Fiber also speeds up colonic transit in most persons. In diarrhea-prone patients, whole-colonic transit is faster than average; however, dietary fiber can delay transit. Furthermore, because of their hydrophilic properties, stool-bulking agents bind water and thus prevent both excessive hydration and dehydration of stool. The latter observation may explain the clinical experience that a high-fiber diet relieves diarrhea in some IBS patients. Fiber supplementation with psyllium has been shown to reduce perception of rectal distention, indicating that fiber may have a positive effect on visceral afferent function.

The beneficial effects of dietary fiber on colonic physiology suggest that dietary fiber should be an effective treatment for IBS patients, but controlled trials of dietary fiber have produced variable results. This is not surprising since IBS is a heterogeneous disorder, with some patients being constipated and other having predominant diarrhea. Most investigations report increases in stool weight, decreases in colonic transit times, and improvement in constipation. Others have noted benefits in patients with alternating diarrhea and constipation, pain, and bloating. However, most studies observe no responses in patients with diarrhea- or pain-predominant IBS. It is possible that different fiber preparations may have dissimilar effects on selected symptoms in IBS. A cross-over comparison of different fiber preparations found that psyllium produced greater improvements in stool pattern and abdominal pain than bran. Furthermore, psyllium preparations tend to produce less bloating and distention. Despite the equivocal data regarding efficacy, most gastroenterologists consider stool-bulking agents worth trying in patients with IBS-C.

Antispasmodics Clinicians have observed that anticholinergic drugs may provide temporary relief for symptoms such as painful cramps related to intestinal spasm. Although controlled clinical trials have produced mixed results, evidence generally supports beneficial effects of anticholinergic drugs for pain. A meta-analysis of 26 double-blind clinical trials of antispasmodic agents in IBS reported better global improvement (62%) and abdominal pain reductions (64%) compared to placebo (35% and 45%, respectively), suggesting efficacy in some patients. The drugs are most effective when prescribed in anticipation of predictable pain. Physiologic studies demonstrate that anticholinergic drugs inhibit the gastrocolic reflex; hence, postprandial pain is best managed by giving antispasmodics 30 min before meals so that effective blood levels are achieved shortly before the anticipated onset of pain. Most anticholinergics contain natural belladonna alkaloids, which may cause xerostomia, urinary hesitancy and retention, blurred vision, and drowsiness. They should be used in the elderly with caution. Some physicians prefer to use synthetic anticholinergics such as dicyclomine that have less effect on mucous membrane secretions and produce fewer undesirable side effects.

Antidiarrheal Agents Peripherally acting opiate-based agents are the initial therapy of choice for IBS-D. Physiologic studies demonstrate increases in segmenting colonic contractions, delays in fecal transit, increases in anal pressures, and reductions in rectal perception with these drugs. When diarrhea is severe, especially in the painless diarrhea variant of IBS, small doses of loperamide, 2–4 mg every 4–6 h up to a maximum of 12 g/d, can be prescribed. These agents are less addictive than paregoric, codeine, or tincture of opium. In general, the intestines do not become tolerant of the antidiarrheal effect of opiates, and increasing doses are not required to maintain antidiarrheal potency. These agents are most useful if taken before anticipated stressful events that are known to cause diarrhea. However, not infrequently, a high dose of loperamide may cause cramping because of increases in segmenting colonic contractions. Another anti-diarrhea agent that may be used in IBS patients is the bile acid binder cholestyramine resin.

Antidepressant Drugs In addition to their mood-elevating effects, antidepressant medications have several physiologic effects that suggest they may be beneficial in IBS. In IBS-D patients, the tricyclic antidepressant imipramine slows jejunal migrating motor complex transit propagation and delays orocecal and whole-gut transit, indicative of a motor inhibitory effect. Some studies also suggest that tricyclic agents may alter visceral afferent neural function.

A number of studies indicate that tricyclic antidepressants may be effective in some IBS patients. In a 2-month study of desipramine, abdominal pain improved in 86% of patients compared to 59% given placebo. Another study of desipramine in 28 IBS patients showed improvement in stool frequency, diarrhea, pain, and depression. When stratified according to the predominant symptoms, improvements were observed in IBS-D patients, with no improvement being noted in IBS-C patients. The beneficial effects of the tricyclic compounds in the treatment of IBS appear to be independent of their effects on depression. The therapeutic benefits for the bowel symptoms occur faster and at a lower dosage. The efficacy of antidepressant agents in other chemical classes in the management of IBS is less well evaluated. In contrast to tricyclic agents, the selective serotonin reuptake inhibitor (SSRI) paroxetine accelerates orocecal transit, raising the possibility that this drug class may be useful in IBS-C patients. The SSRI citalopram blunts perception of rectal distention and reduces the magnitude of the gastrocolonic response in healthy volunteers. A small placebo-controlled study of citalopram in IBS patients reported reductions in pain. However, these findings could not be confirmed in another randomized controlled trial which showed that citalopram at 20 mg/d for 4 weeks was not superior to placebo in treating non-depressed IBS patients. Hence, the efficacy of SSRIs in the treatment of IBS needs further confirmation.

Antiflatulence Therapy The management of excessive gas is seldom satisfactory, except when there is obvious aerophagia or disaccharidase deficiency. Patients should be advised to eat slowly and not chew gum or drink carbonated beverages. Bloating may decrease if an associated gut syndrome such as IBS or constipation is improved. If bloating is accompanied by diarrhea and worsens after ingesting dairy products, fresh fruits, vegetables, or juices, further investigation or a dietary exclusion trial may be worthwhile. Avoiding flatogenic foods, exercising, losing excess weight, and taking activated charcoal are safe but unproven remedies. Data regarding the use of surfactants such as simethicone are conflicting. Antibiotics may help in a subgroup of IBS patients with predominant symptoms of bloating. Beano, an over-the-counter oral β-glycosidase solution, may reduce rectal passage of gas without decreasing bloating and pain. Pancreatic enzymes reduce bloating, gas, and fullness during and after high-calorie, high-fat meal ingestion.

Modulation of Gut Flora Antibiotic treatment benefits a subset of IBS patients. In a double-blind randomized placebo controlled study, neomycin dosed at 500 mg twice daily for 10 days was more effective than placebo at improving symptom scores among IBS patients. The non-absorbed oral antibiotic rifaximin is the most thoroughly studied antibiotic for the treatment of IBS. Patients receiving rifaximin at a dose of 400 mg three times daily experienced substantial improvement of global IBS symptoms over placebo. Rifaximin is the only antibiotic with demonstrated sustained benefit beyond therapy cessation in IBS patients. The drug has a favorable safety and tolerability profile compared with systemic antibiotics. However, currently there is still insufficient data to recommend routine use of this antibiotic in the treatment of IBS.

Since altered colonic flora may contribute to the pathogenesis of IBS, this has led to great interest in using probiotics to naturally alter the flora. *Bifidobacterium infantis* 35624 showed significant improvement in the composite score for abdominal pain, bloating/distention, and/or bowel movement compared with placebo in two placebo-controlled trials. Currently, there are inadequate data to comment on the efficacy of other probiotics.

Serotonin Receptor Agonists and Antagonists
Serotonin receptor antagonists have been evaluated as therapies for IBS-D. Serotonin acting on 5-HT3 receptors enhances the sensitivity of afferent neurons projecting from the gut. In humans, a 5-HT3 receptor antagonist such as alosetron reduces perception of painful visceral stimulation in IBS. It also induces rectal relaxation, increases rectal compliance, and delays colonic transit. Meta-analysis of 14 randomized controlled trials of alosetron or cilansetron showed that these antagonists are more effective than placebo in achieving global improvement in IBS symptoms and relief of abdominal pain and discomfort. These agents are more likely to cause constipation in IBS patients with diarrhea alternating with constipation. In addition, 0.2% of patients using 5HT3 antagonist developed ischemic colitis versus none in the control group. In postrelease surveillance, 84 cases of ischemic colitis were observed, including 44 cases that required surgery and 4 deaths. As a consequence, the medication was voluntarily withdrawn by the manufacturer in 2000. Alosetron has been reintroduced under a new risk-management program where patients have to sign a patient-physician agreement. This has significantly limited its usage.

Novel 5-HT4 receptor agonists such as tegaserod exhibit prokinetic activity by stimulating peristalsis. In IBS patients with constipation, tegaserod accelerated intestinal and ascending colon transit. Clinical trials involving >4000 IBS-C patients reported reductions in discomfort and improvements in constipation and bloating, compared to placebo. Diarrhea is the major side effect. However, tegaserod has been withdrawn from the market; a meta-analysis revealed an increase in serious cardiovascular events.

Chloride Channel Activators Lubiprostone is a bicyclic fatty acid that stimulates chloride channels in the apical membrane of intestinal epithelial cells. Chloride secretion induces passive movement of sodium and water into the bowel lumen and improves bowel function. Oral lubiprostone was effective in the treatment of patients with constipation-predominant IBS in large phase II and phase III randomized double-blinded placebo-controlled multicenter trials. Responses were significantly greater in patients receiving lubiprostone 8 μg twice daily for 3 months than in those receiving placebo. In general, the drug was quite well tolerated. The major side effects are nausea and diarrhea. Lubiprostone is a new class of compounds for treatment of chronic constipation with or without IBS.

SUMMARY The treatment strategy of IBS depends on the severity of the disorder (Table 18-3). Most of the IBS patients have mild symptoms. They are usually

TABLE 18-3

SPECTRUM OF SEVERITY IN IBS

	MILD	MODERATE	SEVERE
Clinical Features			
Prevalence	70%	25%	5%
Correlations with gut physiology	+++	++	+
Symptoms constant	0	+	+++
Psychosocial difficulties	0	+	+++
Health care issues	+	++	+++
Practice type	Primary	Specialty	Referral

TABLE 18-4

POSSIBLE DRUGS FOR A DOMINANT SYMPTOM IN IBS

SYMPTOM	DRUG	DOSE
Diarrhea	Loperamide	2–4 mg when necessary/maximum 12 g/d
	Cholestyramine resin	4 g with meals
	Alosetron[a]	0.5–1 mg bid (for severe IBS, women)
Constipation	Psyllium husk	3–4 g bid with meals, then adjust
	Methylcellulose	2 g bid with meals, then adjust
	Calcium polycarbophil	1 g qd to qid
	Lactulose syrup	10–20 g bid
	70% sorbitol	15 mL bid
	Polyethylene glycol 3350	17 g in 250 mL water qd
	Lubiprostone (Amitiza)	24 mg bid
	Magnesium hydroxide	30–60 mL qd
Abdominal pain	Smooth-muscle relaxant	qd to qid ac
	Tricyclic antidepressants	Start 25–50 mg hs, then adjust
	Selective serotonin reuptake inhibitors	Begin small dose, increase as needed

[a]Available only in the United States.
Source: Adapted from GF Longstreth et al: Gastroenterology 130:1480, 2006.

cared for in primary care practices, have little or no psychosocial difficulties, and do not seek health care often. Treatment usually involves education, reassurance, and dietary/lifestyle changes. A smaller portion have moderate symptoms that are usually intermittent and correlate with altered gut physiology, e.g., worsened with eating or stress and relieved by defecation. Treatments include gut-acting pharmacologic agents such as antispasmodics, antidiarrheals, fiber supplements, and the newer gut serotonin modulators (Table 18-4). A small proportion of IBS patients have severe and refractory symptoms, are usually seen in referral centers, and frequently have constant pain and psychosocial difficulties (Fig. 18-1). This group of patients is best managed with antidepressants and other psychological treatments (Table 18-4).

CHAPTER 19

DIVERTICULAR DISEASE AND COMMON ANORECTAL DISORDERS

Susan L. Gearhart

DIVERTICULAR DISEASE

Incidence and epidemiology

Among Western populations, diverticulosis of the colon affects nearly one-half of individuals older than age 60 years. Fortunately, only 20% of patients with diverticulosis develop symptomatic disease. However, in the United States, diverticular disease results in >200,000 hospitalizations annually, making it the fifth most costly gastrointestinal disorder. The incidence of the disease is on the rise, mainly among young patients. The mean age at presentation of the disease is 59 years. Although the prevalence among females and males is similar, males tend to present at a younger age. Diverticulosis is rare in underdeveloped countries, where diets include more fiber and roughage. However, shortly following migration to the United States, immigrants will develop diverticular disease at the same rate as U.S. natives.

Anatomy and pathophysiology

Two types of diverticula occur in the intestine: true and false (or pseudodiverticula). A true diverticulum is a saclike herniation of the entire bowel wall, whereas a pseudodiverticulum involves only a protrusion of the mucosa through the muscularis propria of the colon (Fig. 19-1). The type of diverticulum affecting the colon is the pseudodiverticulum. The protrusion occurs at the point where the nutrient artery, or *vasa recti*, penetrates through the muscularis propria, resulting in a break in the integrity of the colonic wall. Diverticula commonly affect the sigmoid colon; only 5% of persons exhibit pancolonic diverticula. This anatomic restriction may be a result of the relative high-pressure zone within the muscular sigmoid colon. Thus, higher-amplitude

FIGURE 19-1

Gross and microscopic view of sigmoid diverticular disease. Arrows mark an inflamed diverticulum with the diverticular wall made up only of mucosa.

contractions combined with constipated, high-fat-content stool within the sigmoid lumen results in the creation of these diverticula. *Diverticulitis* is inflammation of a diverticulum. The cause is not well understood and is probably multifactorial. The predominant theory is the retention of particulate material within the diverticular sac and the formation of a fecalith. Consequently, the vasa recti is either compressed or eroded, leading to either perforation or bleeding.

Presentation, evaluation, and management of diverticular bleeding

Hemorrhage from a colonic diverticulum is the most common cause of hematochezia in patients >60 years, yet only 20% of patients with diverticulosis will have gastrointestinal bleeding. Patients at increased risk for bleeding tend to be hypertensive, have atherosclerosis, and regularly use nonsteroidal anti-inflammatory agents. Most bleeds are self-limited and stop spontaneously with bowel rest. The lifetime risk of rebleeding is 25%.

Localization of diverticular bleeding should include colonoscopy, which may be both diagnostic and therapeutic in the management of mild to moderate diverticular bleeding. If the patient is stable, massive bleeding is best managed by angiography. Mesenteric angiography can localize the bleeding site and occlude the bleeding vessel successfully with a coil in 80% of cases. The patient can then be followed closely with repetitive colonoscopy, if necessary, looking for evidence of colonic ischemia. Alternatively, a segmental resection of the colon can be undertaken to eliminate the risk of further bleeding. This may be advantageous in patients on chronic blood thinners. However, with newer techniques of highly selective coil embolization, the rate of colonic ischemia is <10% and the risk of acute rebleeding is <25%. Long-term results (40 months) indicate that more than 50% of patients with acute diverticular bleeds have had definitive treatment with highly selective angiography.

As another alternative, a selective infusion of vasopressin can be given to stop the hemorrhage, although this has been associated with significant complications, including myocardial infarction and intestinal ischemia. Furthermore, bleeding recurs in 50% of patients once the infusion is stopped. Localization studies indicate that bleeding as a result of colonic diverticulosis is more often seen from the right colon. For this reason, patients with presumed bleeding from diverticular disease requiring emergent surgery without localization should undergo a total abdominal colectomy. If the patient is unstable or has had a 6-unit bleed within 24 h, current recommendations are that surgery should be performed. In patients without severe comorbidities, surgical resection can be performed with a primary anastomosis.

TABLE 19-1

PRESENTATION OF DIVERTICULAR DISEASE

Uncomplicated Diverticular Disease—75%

Abdominal pain
Fever
Leukocytosis
Anorexia/obstipation

Complicated Diverticular Disease—25%

Abscess 16%
Perforation 10%
Stricture 5%
Fistula 2%

A higher anastomotic leak rate has been reported in patients who received >10 units of blood.

Presentation, evaluation, and staging of diverticulitis

Acute uncomplicated diverticulitis characteristically presents with fever, anorexia, left lower quadrant abdominal pain, and obstipation (Table 19-1). In <25% of cases, patients may present with generalized peritonitis indicating the presence of a diverticular perforation. If a pericolonic abscess has formed, the patient may have abdominal distention and signs of localized peritonitis. Laboratory investigations will demonstrate a leukocytosis. Rarely, a patient may present with an air-fluid level in the left lower quadrant on plain abdominal film. This is a giant diverticulum of the sigmoid colon and is managed with resection to avoid impending perforation.

The diagnosis of diverticulitis is best made on CT with the following findings: sigmoid diverticula, thickened colonic wall >4 mm, and inflammation within the pericolic fat ± the collection of contrast material or fluid. In 16% of patients, an abdominal abscess may be present. Symptoms of irritable bowel syndrome (IBS) may mimic those of diverticulitis. Therefore, suspected diverticulitis that does not meet CT criteria or is not associated with a leukocytosis or fever is not diverticular disease. Other conditions that can mimic diverticular disease include an ovarian cyst, endometriosis, acute appendicitis, and pelvic inflammatory disease.

Barium enema or colonoscopy should not be performed in the acute setting because of the higher risk of colonic perforation associated with insufflation or insertion of barium-based contrast material under pressure. A sigmoid malignancy can masquerade as diverticular disease. Therefore, a colonoscopy should be performed ~6 weeks after an attack of diverticular disease.

Complicated diverticular disease is defined as diverticular disease associated with an abscess or perforation and

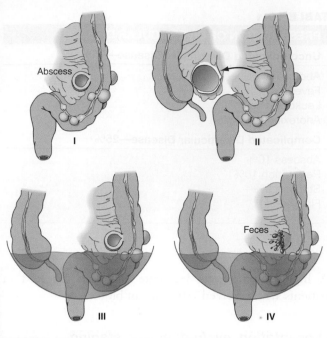

FIGURE 19-2

Hinchey classification of diverticulitis. Stage I: Perforated diverticulitis with a confined paracolic abscess. Stage II: Perforated diverticulitis that has closed spontaneously with distant abscess formation. Stage III: Noncommunicating perforated diverticulitis with fecal peritonitis (the diverticular neck is closed off and therefore contrast will not freely expel on radiographic images). Stage IV: Perforation and free communication with the peritoneum, resulting in fecal peritonitis.

less commonly with a fistula (Table 19-1). Perforated diverticular disease is staged using the Hinchey classification system **(Fig. 19-2)**. This staging system was developed to predict outcomes following the surgical management of complicated diverticular disease. In complicated diverticular disease with fistula formation, common locations include cutaneous, vaginal, or vesicle fistulas. These conditions present with either passage of stool through the skin or vagina or the presence of air in the urinary stream (pneumaturia). Colovaginal fistulas are more common in women who have undergone a hysterectomy.

TREATMENT ▸ Diverticular Disease

MEDICAL MANAGEMENT Asymptomatic diverticular disease discovered on imaging studies or at the time of colonoscopy is best managed by diet alterations. Patients should be instructed to eat a fiber-enriched diet that includes 30 g of fiber each day. Supplementary fiber products such as Metamucil, Fibercon, or Citrucel are useful. The incidence of complicated diverticular disease appears to be increased in patients who smoke. Therefore, patients should be encouraged to refrain from smoking. The historical recommendation to avoid eating nuts is not based on more than anecdotal data.

Symptomatic uncomplicated diverticular disease with confirmation of inflammation and infection within the colon should be treated initially with antibiotics and bowel rest. Nearly 75% of patients hospitalized for acute diverticulitis will respond to nonoperative treatment with a suitable antimicrobial regimen. The current recommended antimicrobial coverage is trimethoprim/sulfamethoxazole or ciprofloxacin and metronidazole targeting aerobic gram-negative rods and anaerobic bacteria. Unfortunately, these agents do not cover enterococci, and the addition of ampicillin to this regimen for nonresponders is recommended. Alternatively, single-agent therapy with a third-generation penicillin such as IV piperacillin or oral penicillin/clavulanic acid may be effective. The usual course of antibiotics is 7–10 days. Patients should remain on a limited diet until their pain resolves.

For long-term medical management of uncomplicated diverticular disease, rifaximin (a poorly absorbed broad-spectrum antibiotic), when compared to fiber alone, is associated with 30% less frequent recurrent symptoms from uncomplicated diverticular disease. Furthermore, the use of probiotics has been shown to decrease the incidence of recurrent attacks. Culture data from patients on probiotics noted a decrease in the presence of *Clostridium* species and an increase in *Lactobacillus* and *Bifidobacterium* strains.

SURGICAL MANAGEMENT Preoperative risk factors influencing postoperative mortality rates include higher American Society of Anesthesiologists (ASA) physical status class (Table 19-2) and preexisting organ failure. In patients who are low risk (ASA P1 and P2), surgical therapy can be offered to those who do not rapidly improve on medical therapy. For uncomplicated diverticular disease, studies indicate that medical therapy can be continued beyond two attacks without an increased

TABLE 19-2

AMERICAN SOCIETY OF ANESTHESIOLOGISTS PHYSICAL STATUS CLASSIFICATION SYSTEM	
P1	A normal healthy patient
P2	A patient with mild systemic disease
P3	A patient with severe systemic disease
P4	A patient with severe systemic disease that is a constant threat to life
P5	A moribund patient who is not expected to survive without the operation
P6	A declared brain-dead patient whose organs are being removed for donor purposes

risk of perforation requiring a colostomy. However, patients on immunosuppressive therapy, in chronic renal failure, or with a collagen-vascular disease have a fivefold greater risk of perforation during recurrent attacks. Surgical therapy is indicated in all low-surgical-risk patients with complicated diverticular disease.

The goals of surgical management of diverticular disease include controlling sepsis, eliminating complications such as fistula or obstruction, removing the diseased colonic segment, and restoring intestinal continuity. These goals must be obtained while minimizing morbidity rate, length of hospitalization, and cost in addition to maximizing survival and quality of life. Table 19-3 lists the operations most commonly indicated based upon Hinchey classification and the predicted morbidity and mortality rates. Surgical objectives include removal of the diseased sigmoid down to the rectosigmoid junction. Failure to do this may result in recurrent disease. The current options for uncomplicated diverticular disease include an open sigmoid resection or a laparoscopic sigmoid resection. The benefits of laparoscopic resection over open surgical techniques include early discharge (by at least 1 day), less narcotic use, less postoperative complications, and an earlier return to work.

FIGURE 19-3
Methods of surgical management of complicated diverticular disease. *(1)* Drainage, omental pedicle graft, and proximal diversion. *(2)* Hartmann's procedure. *(3)* Sigmoid resection with coloproctostomy. *(4)* Sigmoid resection with coloproctostomy and proximal diversion.

TABLE 19-3

OUTCOME FOLLOWING SURGICAL THERAPY FOR COMPLICATED DIVERTICULAR DISEASE			
HINCHEY STAGE	OPERATIVE PROCEDURE	ANASTOMOTIC LEAK RATE, %	OVERALL MORBIDITY RATE, %
I	Resection with primary anastomosis without diverting stoma	3.8	22
II	Resection with primary anastomosis +/− diversion	3.8	30
III	Hartmann's procedure vs. diverting colostomy and omental pedal graft	—	0 vs. 6 mortality
IV	Hartmann's procedure vs. diverting colostomy and omental pedicle graft	—	6 vs. 2 mortality

The options for the surgical management of complicated diverticular disease (Fig. 19-3) include the following: (1) proximal diversion of the fecal stream with an ileostomy or colostomy and sutured omental patch with drainage, (2) resection with colostomy and mucous fistula or closure of distal bowel with formation of a Hartmann's pouch, (3) resection with anastomosis (coloproctostomy), or (4) resection with anastomosis and diversion (coloproctostomy with loop ileostomy or colostomy). Laparoscopic techniques have been employed for complicated diverticular disease; however, higher conversion rates to open techniques have been reported.

Patients with Hinchey stages I and II disease are managed with percutaneous drainage followed by resection with anastomosis about 6 weeks later. Percutaneous drainage is recommended for abscesses ≥5 cm with a well-defined wall that is accessible. Paracolic abscesses <5 cm in size may resolve with antibiotics alone. Contraindications to percutaneous drainage are no percutaneous access route, pneumoperitoneum, and fecal peritonitis. Urgent operative intervention is undertaken if patients develop generalized peritonitis, and most will need to be managed with a Hartmann's procedure. In selected cases, nonoperative therapy may be considered. In one nonrandomized study, nonoperative management of isolated paracolic abscesses (Hinchey stage I) was associated with only a 20% recurrence rate at 2 years. More than 80% of patients with distant abscesses (Hinchey stage II) required surgical resection for recurrent symptoms.

Hinchey stage III disease is managed with a Hartmann's procedure or with primary anastomosis and proximal diversion. If the patient has significant comorbidities, making operative intervention risky, a limited procedure including intraoperative peritoneal lavage (irrigation), omental patch to the oversewn perforation, and proximal diversion of the fecal stream with either an ileostomy or transverse colostomy can be performed. No anastomosis of any type should be attempted in Hinchey stage IV disease. A limited approach to these patients is associated with a decreased mortality rate.

Recurrent symptoms

Recurrent abdominal symptoms following surgical resection for diverticular disease occur in 10% of patients. Recurrent diverticular disease develops in patients following inadequate surgical resection. A retained segment of diseased rectosigmoid colon is associated with twice the incidence of recurrence. IBS may also cause recurrence of initial symptoms. Patients undergoing surgical resection for presumed diverticulitis and symptoms of abdominal cramping and irregular loose bowel movements consistent with IBS have functionally poorer outcomes.

COMMON DISEASES OF THE ANORECTUM

RECTAL PROLAPSE (PROCIDENTIA)

Incidence and epidemiology

Rectal prolapse is six times more common in women than in men. The incidence of rectal prolapse peaks in women >60 years. Women with rectal prolapse have a higher incidence of associated pelvic floor disorders including urinary incontinence, rectocele, cystocele, and enterocele. About 20% of children with rectal prolapse will have cystic fibrosis. All children presenting with prolapse should undergo a sweat chloride test. Less common associations include Ehlers-Danlos syndrome, solitary rectal ulcer syndrome, congenital hypothyroidism, and Hirschsprung's disease.

Anatomy and pathophysiology

Rectal prolapse (procidentia) is a circumferential, full-thickness protrusion of the rectal wall through the anal orifice. It is often associated with a redundant sigmoid colon, pelvic laxity, and a deep rectovaginal septum (pouch of Douglas). Initially, rectal prolapse was felt to be the result of early internal rectal intussusception, which occurs in the upper to mid rectum. This was considered to be the first step in an inevitable progression to full-thickness external prolapse. However, only 1 of 38 patients with internal prolapse followed for >5 years developed full-thickness prolapse. Others have suggested that full-thickness prolapse is the result of damage to the nerve supply to the pelvic floor muscles or pudendal nerves from repeated stretching with straining to defecate. Damage to the pudendal nerves would weaken the pelvic floor muscles, including the external anal sphincter muscles. Bilateral pudendal nerve injury is more significantly associated with prolapse and incontinence than unilateral injury.

Presentation and evaluation

In external prolapse, the majority of patient complaints include anal mass, bleeding per rectum, and poor perianal hygiene. Prolapse of the rectum usually occurs following defecation and will spontaneously reduce or require the patient to manually reduce the prolapse. Constipation occurs in ~30–67% of patients with rectal prolapse. Differing degrees of fecal incontinence occur in 50–70% of patients. Patients with internal rectal prolapse will present with symptoms of both constipation and incontinence. Other associated findings include outlet obstruction (anismus) in 30%, colonic inertia in 10%, and solitary rectal ulcer syndrome in 12%.

Office evaluation is best performed after the patient has been given an enema, which enables the prolapse to protrude. An important distinction should be made between full-thickness rectal prolapse and isolated mucosal prolapse associated with hemorrhoidal disease (Fig. 19-4). Mucosal prolapse is known for radial grooves rather than circumferential folds around the anus and is due to increased laxity of the connective tissue between the submucosa and underlying muscle of the anal canal. The evaluation of prolapse should also include cystoproctography and colonoscopy. These examinations evaluate for associated pelvic floor disorders and rule out a malignancy or a polyp as the lead point for prolapse. If rectal prolapse is associated with chronic constipation, the patient should undergo a defecating proctogram and a sitzmark study. This will evaluate for the presence of anismus or colonic inertia. Anismus is the result of attempting to defecate against a closed pelvic floor and is also known as *nonrelaxing puborectalis*. This can be seen when straightening of the rectum fails to occur on fluoroscopy while the patient is attempting to defecate. In colonic inertia, a sitzmark study will demonstrate retention of >20% of markers on abdominal x-ray 5 days after swallowing. For patients

FIGURE 19-4

Degree of rectal prolapse. Mucosal prolapse only (***A, B,*** sagittal view). Full-thickness prolapse associated with redundant rectosigmoid and deep pouch of Douglas (***C, D,*** sagittal view).

with fecal incontinence, endoanal ultrasound and manometric evaluation, including pudendal nerve testing of their anal sphincter muscles, may be performed before surgery for prolapse (see "Fecal Incontinence").

| TREATMENT | Rectal Prolapse |

The medical approach to the management of rectal prolapse is limited and includes stool-bulking agents or fiber supplementation to ease the process of evacuation. Surgical correction of rectal prolapse is the mainstay of therapy. Two approaches are commonly considered, transabdominal and transperineal. Transabdominal approaches have been associated with lower recurrence rates, but some patients with significant comorbidities are better served by a transperineal approach.

Common transperineal approaches include a transanal proctectomy (Altmeier procedure), mucosal proctectomy (Delorme procedure), or placement of a Tirsch wire encircling the anus. The goal of the transperineal approach is to remove the redundant rectosigmoid colon. Common transabdominal approaches include presacral suture or mesh rectopexy (Ripstein)

with (Frykman-Goldberg) or without resection of the redundant sigmoid. Transabdominal procedures can be performed effectively with laparoscopic techniques without increased incidence of recurrence. The goal of the transabdominal approach is to restore normal anatomy by removing redundant bowel and reattaching the supportive tissue of the rectum to the presacral fascia. The final alternative is abdominal proctectomy with end-sigmoid colostomy. Colon resection, in general, is reserved for patients with constipation and outlet obstruction. If total colonic inertia is present, as defined by a history of constipation and a positive sitzmark study, a subtotal colectomy with an ileosigmoid or rectal anastomosis may be required at the time of rectopexy.

Previously, the presence of internal rectal prolapse identified on imaging studies has been considered a nonsurgical disorder and biofeedback was recommended. However, only one-third of patients will have successful resolution of symptoms from biofeedback. Two surgical procedures have been shown to be more effective than biofeedback. The STARR (stapled transanal rectal resection) procedure (Fig. 19-5) is performed through the anus in patients with internal prolapse. A circular stapling device is inserted through the anus; the internal prolapse is identified and ligated with the stapling device. The laparoscopic ventral rectopexy (LVR) (Fig. 19-6) is performed by creating an opening in the peritoneum on the left side of the rectosigmoid and carrying this opening down anterior on the rectum into the pouch of Douglas. No rectal mobilization is performed, thus avoiding any autonomic nerve injury.

FIGURE 19-5

Stapled transanal rectal resection. Schematic of placement of the circular stapling device.

FIGURE 19-6
Laparoscopic ventral rectopexy (LVR). To reduce the internal prolapse and close any rectovaginal septal defect, the pouch of Douglas is opened and mesh is secured to the anterolateral rectum, vaginal fornix, and sacrum. (*From D'Hoore et al: Br J Surg 91:1500, 2004.*)

Mesh is secured to the anterior and lateral portion of the rectum, the vaginal fornix, and the sacral promontory, allowing for closure of the rectovaginal septum and correction of the internal prolapse. In both procedures, recurrence at 1 year was low (<10%) and symptoms improved in more than three-fourths of patients.

FECAL INCONTINENCE

Incidence and epidemiology

Fecal incontinence is the involuntary passage of fecal material >10 mL for at least 1 month. The prevalence of fecal incontinence in the United States is 0.5–11%. The majority of patients are women. A higher incidence of incontinence is seen among parous women. One-half of patients with fecal incontinence also suffer from urinary incontinence. The majority of incontinence is a result of obstetric injury to the pelvic floor, either while carrying a fetus or during the delivery. An anatomic sphincter defect may occur in up to 32% of women following childbirth regardless of visible damage to the perineum. Risk factors at the time of delivery include prolonged labor, the use of forceps, and the

TABLE 19-4

MEDICAL CONDITIONS THAT CONTRIBUTE TO SYMPTOMS OF FECAL INCONTINENCE
Neurologic Disorders
• Dementia
• Brain tumor
• Stroke
• Multiple sclerosis
• Tabes dorsalis
• Cauda equina lesions
Skeletal Muscle Disorders
• Myasthenia gravis
• Myopathies, muscular dystrophy
Miscellaneous
• Hypothyroidism
• Irritable bowel syndrome
• Sedation
• Severe diarrhea

need for an episiotomy. Medical conditions known to contribute to the development of fecal incontinence are listed in **Table 19-4**.

Anatomy and pathophysiology

The anal sphincter complex is made up of the internal and external anal sphincter. The internal sphincter is smooth muscle and a continuation of the circular fibers of the rectal wall. It is innervated by the intestinal myenteric plexus and is therefore not under voluntary control. The external anal sphincter is formed in continuation with the levator ani muscles and is under voluntary control. The pudendal nerve supplies motor innervation to the external anal sphincter. Obstetric injury may result in tearing of the muscle fibers anteriorly at the time of the delivery. This results in an obvious anterior defect on endoanal ultrasound. Injury may also be the result of stretching of the pudendal nerves. The majority of patients who suffer from fecal incontinence following obstetric injury do so several years following the birth of their last child.

Presentation and evaluation

Patients may suffer with varying degrees of fecal incontinence. Minor incontinence includes incontinence to flatus and occasional seepage of liquid stool. Major incontinence is frequent inability to control solid waste. As a result of fecal incontinence, patients suffer from poor perianal hygiene. Beyond the immediate problems associated with fecal incontinence, these patients are often withdrawn and suffer from depression. For this reason, quality-of-life measures have become an important component in the evaluation of patients with fecal incontinence.

The evaluation of fecal incontinence should include a thorough history and physical examination, anal manometry, pudendal nerve terminal motor latency (PNTML), and endoanal ultrasound. Unfortunately, all of these investigations are user-dependent. Centers that care for patients with fecal incontinence will have an anorectal physiology laboratory that uses standardized methods of evaluating anorectal physiology. Anal manometry measures resting and squeeze pressures within the anal canal using an intraluminal water-perfused catheter. Pudendal nerve studies evaluate the function of the nerves innervating the anal canal using a finger electrode placed in the anal canal. Stretch injuries to these nerves will result in a delayed response of the sphincter muscle to a stimulus, indicating a prolonged latency. Finally, ultrasound will evaluate the extent of the injury to the sphincter muscles before surgical repair. Only PNTML has been shown to consistently predict outcome following surgical intervention.

Rarely does a pelvic floor disorder exist alone. The majority of patients with fecal incontinence will have a degree of urinary incontinence. Similarly, fecal incontinence is a part of the spectrum of pelvic organ prolapse. For this reason, patients may present with symptoms of obstructed defecation as well as fecal incontinence. Careful evaluation including cinedefecography should be performed to search for other associated defects. Surgical repair of incontinence without attention to other associated defects may decrease the success of the repair.

TREATMENT   Fecal Incontinence

The "gold standard" for the treatment of fecal incontinence with an isolated sphincter defect is overlapping sphincteroplasty. The external anal sphincter muscle and scar tissue as well as any identifiable internal sphincter muscle are dissected free from the surrounding adipose and connective tissue and then an overlapping repair is performed in an attempt to rebuild the muscular ring and restore its function. Other newer approaches include radio frequency therapy to the anal canal to aid in the development of collagen fibers and provide tensile strength to the sphincter muscles. Sacral nerve stimulation and the artificial bowel sphincter are both adaptations of procedures developed for the management of urinary incontinence. Sacral nerve stimulation is ideally suited for patients with intact but weak anal sphincters. A temporary nerve stimulator is placed on the third sacral nerve. If there is at least a 50% improvement in symptoms, a permanent nerve stimulator is placed under the skin. The artificial bowel sphincter is a cuff and reservoir apparatus that allows for manual inflation of a cuff placed around the anus, increasing anal tone. This allows the patient to manually close off the anal canal until defecation is necessary.

Long-term results following overlapping sphincteroplasty show about a 50% failure rate over 5 years. Poorer outcome has been seen in patients with prolonged PNTML. Long-term results for sacral stimulation have been promising; however, the indications for this procedure are presently limited in the United States. Unfortunately, the artificial bowel sphincter has been associated with a 30% infection rate.

HEMORRHOIDAL DISEASE
Incidence and epidemiology

Symptomatic hemorrhoids affect >1 million individuals in the Western world per year. The prevalence of hemorrhoidal disease is not selective for age or sex. However, age is known to have a deleterious effect on the anal canal. The prevalence of hemorrhoidal disease is less in underdeveloped countries. The typical low-fiber, high-fat Western diet is associated with constipation and straining and the development of symptomatic hemorrhoids.

Anatomy and pathophysiology

Hemorrhoidal cushions are a normal part of the anal canal. The vascular structures contained within this tissue aid in continence by preventing damage to the sphincter muscle. Three main hemorrhoidal complexes traverse the anal canal—the left lateral, the right anterior, and the right posterior. Engorgement and straining leads to prolapse of this tissue into the anal canal. Over time, the anatomic support system of the hemorrhoidal complex weakens, exposing this tissue to the outside of the anal canal where it is susceptible to injury. Hemorrhoids are commonly classified as internal or external. Although small external cushions do exist, the standard classification of hemorrhoidal disease is based on the progression of the disease from their normal internal location to the prolapsing external position (Table 19-5).

Presentation and evaluation

Patients commonly present to a physician for two reasons: bleeding and protrusion. Pain is less common than with fissures and, if present, is described as a dull ache from engorgement of the hemorrhoidal tissue. Severe pain may indicate a thrombosed hemorrhoid. Hemorrhoidal bleeding is described as bright red blood seen either in the toilet or upon wiping. Occasional patients can present with significant bleeding, which may be a cause of

TABLE 19-5

THE STAGING AND TREATMENT OF HEMORRHOIDS

STAGE	DESCRIPTION OF CLASSIFICATION	TREATMENT
I	Enlargement with bleeding	Fiber supplementation Cortisone suppository Sclerotherapy
II	Protrusion with spontaneous reduction	Fiber supplementation Cortisone suppository
III	Protrusion requiring manual reduction	Fiber supplementation Cortisone suppository Banding Operative hemorrhoidectomy (stapled or traditional)
IV	Irreducible protrusion	Fiber supplementation Cortisone suppository Operative hemorrhoidectomy

anemia; however, the presence of a colonic neoplasm must be ruled out. Patients who present with a protruding mass complain about inability to maintain perianal hygiene and are often concerned about the presence of a malignancy.

The diagnosis of hemorrhoidal disease is made on physical examination. Inspection of the perianal region for evidence of thrombosis or excoriation is performed, followed by a careful digital examination. Anoscopy is performed paying particular attention to the known position of hemorrhoidal disease. The patient is asked to strain. If this is difficult for the patient, the maneuver can be performed while sitting on a toilet. The physician is notified when the tissue prolapses. It is important to differentiate the circumferential appearance of a full-thickness rectal prolapse from the radial nature of prolapsing hemorrhoids (see "Rectal Prolapse"). The stage and location of the hemorrhoidal complexes are defined.

TREATMENT   Hemorrhoidal Disease

The treatment for bleeding hemorrhoids is based upon the stage of the disease (Table 19-5). In all patients with bleeding, the possibility of other causes must be considered. In young patients without a family history of colorectal cancer, the hemorrhoidal disease may be treated first and a colonoscopic examination performed if the bleeding continues. Older patients who have not had colorectal cancer screening should undergo colonoscopy or flexible sigmoidoscopy.

With rare exceptions, the acutely thrombosed hemorrhoid can be excised within the first 72 h by performing an elliptical excision. Sitz baths, fiber, and stool softeners are prescribed. Additional therapy for bleeding hemorrhoids includes banding, sclerotherapy, excisional hemorrhoidectomy, and stapled hemorrhoidectomy. Sensation begins at the dentate line; therefore, banding or sclerotherapy can be performed without discomfort in the office. Bands are placed around the engorged tissue, causing ischemia and fibrosis. This aids in fixing the tissue proximally in the anal canal. Patients may complain of a dull ache for 24 h following band application. During sclerotherapy, 1–2 mL of a sclerosant (usually sodium tetradecyl sulfate) is injected using a 25-gauge needle into the submucosa of the hemorrhoidal complex. Care must be taken not to inject the anal canal circumferentially, or stenosis may occur. The sutured and stapled hemorrhoidectomies are equally effective in the treatment of symptomatic third- and fourth-degree hemorrhoids. However, because the sutured hemorrhoidectomy involves the removal of redundant tissue down to the anal verge, unpleasant anal skin tags are removed as well. The stapled hemorrhoidectomy is associated with less discomfort; however, this procedure does not remove anal skin tags. No procedures on hemorrhoids should be done in patients who are immunocompromised or who have active proctitis. Furthermore, emergent hemorrhoidectomy for bleeding hemorrhoids is associated with a higher complication rate.

Acute complications associated with the treatment of hemorrhoids include pain, infection, recurrent bleeding, and urinary retention. Care should be taken to place bands properly and to avoid overhydration in patients undergoing operative hemorrhoidectomy. Late complications include fecal incontinence as a result of injury to the sphincter during the dissection. Anal stenosis may develop from overzealous excision, with loss of mucosal skin bridges for reepithelialization. Finally, an *ectropion* (prolapse of rectal mucosa from the anal canal) may develop. Patients with an ectropion complain of a "wet" anus as a result of inability to prevent soiling once the rectal mucosa is exposed below the dentate line.

ANORECTAL ABSCESS

Incidence and epidemiology

The development of a perianal abscess is more common in men than women by a ratio of 3:1. The peak incidence is in the third to fifth decade of life. Perianal pain associated with the presence of an abscess accounts for 15% of office visits to a colorectal surgeon. The disease is more prevalent in immunocompromised patients such as those with diabetes, hematologic disorders, or inflammatory bowel disease (IBD) and persons who are

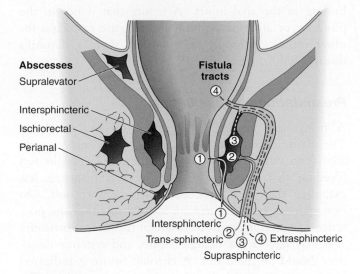

Abscesses
Supralevator
Intersphincteric
Ischiorectal
Perianal

Fistula tracts
④
③
①②

① Intersphincteric
② Trans-sphincteric ③ ④ Extrasphincteric
Suprasphincteric

FIGURE 19-7
Common locations of anorectal abscess *(left)* and fistula in ano *(right)*.

HIV positive. These disorders should be considered in patients with recurrent perianal infections.

Anatomy and pathophysiology

An anorectal abscess is an abnormal fluid-containing cavity in the anorectal region. Anorectal abscess results from an infection involving the glands surrounding the anal canal. Normally, these glands release mucus into the anal canal, which aids in defecation. When stool accidentally enters the anal glands, the glands become infected and an abscess develops. Anorectal abscesses are perianal in 40–50% of patients, ischiorectal in 20–25%, intersphincteric in 2–5%, and supralevator in 2.5% **(Fig. 19-7)**.

Presentation and evaluation

Perianal pain and fever are the hallmarks of an abscess. Patients may have difficulty voiding and have blood in the stool. A prostatic abscess may present with similar complaints, including dysuria. Patients with a prostatic abscess will often have a history of recurrent sexually transmitted diseases. On physical examination, a large fluctuant area is usually readily visible. Routine laboratory evaluation shows an elevated white blood cell count. Diagnostic procedures are rarely necessary unless evaluating a recurrent abscess. A CT scan or MRI has an accuracy of 80% in determining incomplete drainage. If there is a concern about the presence of IBD, a rigid or flexible sigmoidoscopic examination may be done at the time of drainage to evaluate for inflammation within the rectosigmoid region. A more complete evaluation for Crohn's disease would include a full colonoscopy and small-bowel series.

Office drainage of an uncomplicated anorectal abscess may suffice. A small incision close to the anal verge is made and a Mallenkot drain is advanced into the abscess cavity. For patients who have a complicated abscess or who are diabetic or immunocompromised, drainage should be performed in an operating room under anesthesia. These patients are at greater risk for developing necrotizing fasciitis. The course of antibiotics is controversial but should be at least 2 weeks in patients who are immunocompromised or have prosthetic heart valves, artificial joints, diabetes, or IBD.

FISTULA IN ANO

Incidence and epidemiology

The incidence and prevalence of fistulating perianal disease parallels the incidence of anorectal abscess. Some 30–40% of abscesses will give rise to fistula in ano. While the majority of the fistulas are cryptoglandular in origin, 10% are associated with IBD, tuberculosis, malignancy, and radiation.

Anatomy and pathophysiology

A fistula in ano is defined as a communication of an abscess cavity with an identifiable internal opening within the anal canal. This identifiable opening is most commonly located at the dentate line where the anal glands enter the anal canal. Patients experiencing continuous drainage following the treatment of a perianal abscess likely have a fistula in ano. These fistulas are classified by their relationship to the anal sphincter muscles, with 70% being intersphincteric, 23% transsphincteric, 5% suprasphincteric, and 2% extrasphincteric (Fig. 19-7).

Presentation and evaluation

A patient with a fistula in ano will complain of constant drainage from the perianal region. The drainage may increase with defecation. Perianal hygiene is difficult to maintain. Examination under anesthesia is the best way to evaluate a fistula. At the time of the examination, anoscopy is performed to look for an internal opening. Diluted hydrogen peroxide will aid in identifying such an opening. In lieu of anesthesia, MRI with an endoanal coil will also identify tracts in 80% of the cases. After drainage of an abscess with insertion of a Mallenkot catheter, a fistulagram through the catheter can be obtained in search of an occult fistula tract. Goodsall's rule states that a posterior external fistula will enter the anal canal in the posterior midline, whereas an anterior fistula will enter at the nearest crypt. A fistula exiting

>3 cm from the anal verge may have a complicated upward extension and may not obey Goodsall's rule.

TREATMENT Fistula In Ano

A newly diagnosed draining fistula is best managed with placement of a seton, a vessel loop or silk tie placed through the fistula tract, which maintains the tract open and quiets down the surrounding inflammation that occurs from repeated blockage of the tract. Once the inflammation is less, the exact relationship of the fistula tract to the anal sphincters can be ascertained. A simple fistulotomy can be performed for intersphincteric and low (less than one-third of the muscle) transsphincteric fistulas without compromising continence. For a higher transsphincteric fistula, an anorectal advancement flap in combination with a drainage catheter or fibrin glue may be used. Very long (>2 cm) and narrow tracts respond better to fibrin glue than shorter tracts. Simple ligation of the internal fistula tract (LIFT procedure) has also been used in the management of simple fistula with good success.

Patients should be maintained on stool-bulking agents, nonnarcotic pain medication, and sitz baths following surgery for a fistula. Early complications from these procedures include urinary retention and bleeding. Later complications are rare (<10%) and include temporary and permanent incontinence. Recurrence following fistulotomy is 0–18% and following anorectal advancement flap and the LIFT procedure is 20–30%.

ANAL FISSURE

Incidence and epidemiology

Anal fissures occur at all ages but are more common in the third through the fifth decades. A fissure is the most common cause of rectal bleeding in infancy. The prevalence is equal in males and females. It is associated with constipation, diarrhea, infectious etiologies, perianal trauma, and Crohn's disease.

Anatomy and pathophysiology

Trauma to the anal canal occurs following defecation. This injury occurs in the anterior or, more commonly, the posterior anal canal. Irritation caused by the trauma to the anal canal results in an increased resting pressure of the internal sphincter. The blood supply to the sphincter and anal mucosa enters laterally. Therefore, increased anal sphincter tone results in a relative ischemia in the region of the fissure and leads to poor

healing of the anal injury. A fissure that is not in the posterior or anterior position should raise suspicion for other causes, including tuberculosis, syphilis, Crohn's disease, and malignancy.

Presentation and evaluation

A fissure can be easily diagnosed on history alone. The classic complaint is pain, which is strongly associated with defecation and is relentless. The bright red bleeding that can be associated with a fissure is less extensive than that associated with hemorrhoids. On examination, most fissures are located in either the posterior or anterior position. A lateral fissure is worrisome as it may have a less benign nature, and systemic disorders should be ruled out. A chronic fissure is indicated by the presence of a hypertrophied anal papilla at the proximal end of the fissure and a sentinel pile or skin tag at the distal end. Often the circular fibers of the hypertrophied internal sphincter are visible within the base of the fissure. If anal manometry is performed, elevation in anal resting pressure and a sawtooth deformity with paradoxical contractions of the sphincter muscles are pathognomonic.

TREATMENT Anal Fissure

The management of the acute fissure is conservative. Stool softeners for those with constipation, increased dietary fiber, topical anesthetics, glucocorticoids, and sitz baths are prescribed and will heal 60–90% of fissures. Chronic fissures are those present for >6 weeks. These can be treated with modalities aimed at decreasing the anal canal resting pressure including nifedipine or nitroglycerin ointment applied three times a day, and botulinum toxin type A, up to 20 units, injected into the internal sphincter on each side of the fissure. Surgical management includes anal dilatation and lateral internal sphincterotomy. Usually, one-third of the internal sphincter muscle is divided; it is easily identified because it is hypertrophied. Recurrence rates from medical therapy are higher, but this is offset by a risk of incontinence following sphincterotomy. Lateral internal sphincterotomy may lead to incontinence more commonly in women.

ACKNOWLEDGMENT

We would like to thank Cory Sandore for providing some illustrations for this chapter. Gregory Bulkley, MD, contributed to this chapter in the 16th edition of Harrison's Principles of Internal Medicine.

CHAPTER 20
MESENTERIC VASCULAR INSUFFICIENCY

Susan L. Gearhart

INTESTINAL ISCHEMIA

INCIDENCE AND EPIDEMIOLOGY

Intestinal ischemia is an uncommon vascular disease associated with a high mortality. It is categorized according to etiology: (1) arteriooclusive mesenteric ischemia (AOMI), (2) nonocclusive mesenteric ischemia (NOMI), and (3) mesenteric venous thrombosis (MVT). Acute intestinal ischemia is more common than its counterpart, chronic arterial ischemia. Risk factors for acute arterial ischemia include atrial fibrillation, recent myocardial infarction, valvular heart disease, and recent cardiac or vascular catheterization. The increased incidence of intestinal ischemia seen in Western countries parallels the incidence of atherosclerosis and the aging population. With the exception of strangulated small-bowel obstruction, ischemic colitis is the most common form of acute ischemia and the most prevalent gastrointestinal disease complicating cardiovascular surgery. The incidence of ischemic colitis following elective aortic repair is 5–9%, and the incidence triples in patients following emergent repair. Other less common forms of intestinal ischemia include chronic mesenteric angina associated with atherosclerotic disease and MVT. The latter is associated with the presence of a hypercoagulable state including protein C or S deficiency, antithrombin III deficiency, polycythemia vera, and carcinoma.

ANATOMY AND PATHOPHYSIOLOGY

Intestinal ischemia occurs when insufficient perfusion to intestinal tissue produces ischemic tissue injury. The blood supply to the intestines is depicted in **Fig. 20-1**. To prevent ischemic injury, extensive collateralization occurs between major mesenteric trunks and branches of the mesenteric arcades **(Table 20-1)**. Collateral vessels within the small bowel are numerous and meet within the duodenum and the bed of the pancreas. Collateral vessels within the colon meet at the splenic flexure and descending/sigmoid colon. These areas, which are inherently at risk for decreased blood flow, are known as *Griffiths' point* and *Sudeck's*

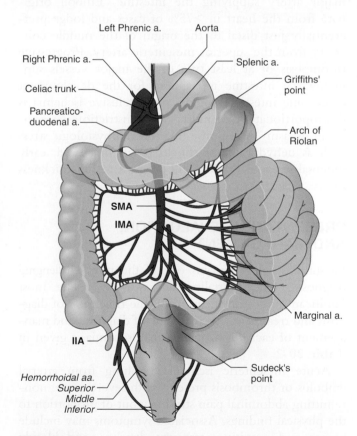

FIGURE 20-1
Blood supply to the intestines includes the celiac artery, superior mesenteric artery (SMA), inferior mesenteric artery (IMA), and branches of the internal iliac artery (IIA). Griffiths' and Sudeck's points, indicated by shaded areas, are watershed areas within the colonic blood supply and common locations for ischemia.

223

TABLE 20-1

COLLATERAL ARTERIAL INTESTINAL BLOOD FLOW			
INVOLVED CIRCULATION	MESENTERIC ARTERY	ADJOINING ARTERY	COLLATERAL ARTERY
Systemic	Celiac	Descending aorta	Phrenic
Systemic	IMA	Hypogastric	Middle hemorrhoidal
Mesenteric	Celiac	SMA	Superior/inferior pancreaticoduodenal
Mesenteric	SMA	IMA	Arch of Riolan
Mesenteric	SMA	Celiac/IMA	Intramesenteric
Mesenteric	SMA	IMA	Marginal

Abbreviations: IMA, inferior mesenteric artery; SMA, superior mesenteric artery.

point, respectively, and are the most common locations for colonic ischemia (Fig. 20-1, shaded areas). The splanchnic circulation can receive up to 30% of the cardiac output. Protective responses to prevent intestinal ischemia include abundant collateralization, autoregulation of blood flow, and the ability to increase oxygen extraction from the blood.

Occlusive ischemia is a result of disruption of blood flow by an embolus or progressive thrombosis in a major artery supplying the intestine. Emboli originate from the heart in >75% of cases and lodge preferentially just distal to the origin of the middle colic artery from the superior mesenteric artery. Progressive thrombosis of at least two of the major vessels supplying the intestine is required for the development of chronic intestinal angina. Nonocclusive ischemia is disproportionate mesenteric vasoconstriction (arteriolar vasospasm) in response to a severe physiologic stress such as dehydration or shock. If left untreated, early mucosal stress ulceration will progress to full-thickness injury.

PRESENTATION, EVALUATION, AND MANAGEMENT

Intestinal ischemia remains one of the most challenging diagnoses. The mortality rate is >50%. The most significant indicator of survival is the timeliness of diagnosis and treatment. An overview of diagnosis and management of each form of intestinal ischemia is given in **Table 20-2**.

Acute mesenteric ischemia resulting from arterial embolus or thrombosis presents with severe acute, nonremitting abdominal pain strikingly out of proportion to the physical findings. Associated symptoms may include nausea and vomiting, transient diarrhea, and bloody stools. With the exception of minimal abdominal distention and hypoactive bowel sounds, early abdominal examination is unimpressive. Later findings will demonstrate peritonitis and cardiovascular collapse. In the evaluation of acute intestinal ischemia, routine laboratory tests should be obtained, including complete blood count, serum chemistry, coagulation profile, arterial blood gas, amylase, lipase, lactic acid, blood type and cross match, and cardiac enzymes. Regardless of the need for urgent surgery, emergent admission to a monitored bed or intensive care unit is recommended for resuscitation and further evaluation. If the diagnosis of intestinal ischemia is being considered, consultation with a surgical service is necessary.

Other diagnostic modalities that may be useful in diagnosis but should not delay surgical therapy include electrocardiogram (ECG), abdominal radiographs, CT, and mesenteric angiography. More recently, mesentery duplex scanning and visible light spectroscopy during colonoscopy have been demonstrated to be beneficial. The ECG may demonstrate an arrhythmia, indicating the possible source of the emboli. A plain abdominal film may show evidence of free intraperitoneal air, indicating a perforated viscus and the need for emergent exploration. Earlier features of intestinal ischemia seen on abdominal radiographs include bowel-wall edema, known as "thumbprinting." If the ischemia progresses, air can be seen within the bowel wall (*pneumatosis intestinalis*) and within the portal venous system. Other features include calcifications of the aorta and its tributaries, indicating atherosclerotic disease. With the administration of oral and IV contrast, dynamic CT with three-dimensional reconstruction is a highly sensitive test for intestinal ischemia. In acute embolic disease, mesenteric angiography is best performed intraoperatively. A mesenteric duplex scan demonstrating a high peak velocity of flow in the superior mesenteric artery (SMA) is associated with an ~80% positive predictive value of mesenteric ischemia. More significantly, a negative duplex scan virtually precludes the diagnosis of mesenteric ischemia. Duplex imaging serves as a screening test; further investigations with angiography are needed. Endoscopic techniques using visible light spectroscopy can be used in the diagnosis of chronic ischemia.

The "gold standard" for the diagnosis and management of acute arterial occlusive disease is laparotomy. Surgical exploration should not be delayed if suspicion of acute occlusive mesenteric ischemia is high or

TABLE 20-2

OVERVIEW OF THE MANAGEMENT OF ACUTE INTESTINAL ISCHEMIA

CONDITION	KEY TO EARLY DIAGNOSIS	TREATMENT OF UNDERLYING CAUSE	TREATMENT OF SPECIFIC LESION	TREATMENT OF SYSTEMIC CONSEQUENCES
Arterial embolus	Early laparotomy	Anticoagulation Cardioversion Proximal thrombectomy Aneurysmectomy	Laparotomy Embolectomy Vascular bypass Assess viability and resect dead bowel	Ensure hydration Give antibiotics Reverse acidosis Optimize oxygen delivery Support cardiac output Treat other embolic sites Avoid vasoconstrictors
Arterial thrombosis	Duplex ultrasound Angiography	Anticoagulation Hydration	Endovascular stent Endarterectomy/ thrombectomy or vascular bypass Assess viability and resect dead bowel	Give antibiotics Reverse acidosis Optimize oxygen delivery Support cardiac output Avoid vasoconstrictors
Venous thrombosis	Spiral CT	Anticoagulation Massive hydration	Anticoagulation ± laparotomy/ thrombectomy/ portasystemic shunt Assess viability and resect dead bowel	Give antibiotics Reverse acidosis Optimize oxygen delivery Support cardiac output Avoid vasoconstrictors
Nonocclusive mesenteric ischemia	Vasospasm: Angiography Hypoperfusion: Spiral CT or colonoscopy	Ensure hydration Support cardiac output Avoid vasoconstrictors Ablate renin-angiotensin axis	Vasospasm: Intraarterial vasodilators Hypoperfusion: Delayed laparotomy Assess viability and resect dead bowel	Ensure hydration Give antibiotics Reverse acidosis Optimize oxygen delivery Support cardiac output Avoid vasoconstrictors

Source: Modified from GB Bulkley, in JL Cameron (ed): *Current Surgical Therapy*, 2nd ed. Toronto, BC Decker, 1986.

evidence of clinical deterioration or frank peritonitis is present. The goal of operative exploration is to resect compromised bowel and restore blood supply. Intraoperative or preoperative arteriography and systemic heparinization may assist the vascular surgeon in restoring blood supply to the compromised bowel. The entire length of the small and large bowel beginning at the ligament of Treitz should be evaluated. The pattern of intestinal ischemia may indicate the level of arterial occlusion. In the case of SMA occlusion where the embolus usually lies just proximal to the origin of the middle colic artery, the proximal jejunum is often spared while the remainder of the small bowel to the transverse colon will be ischemic. The surgical management of acute mesenteric ischemia of the small bowel is attempted embolectomy via intraoperative angiography or arteriotomy. Although more commonly applied to chronic disease, acute thrombosis may be managed with angioplasty, with or without endovascular stent placement. If this is unsuccessful, a bypass from the aorta to the superior mesenteric artery is performed.

Nonocclusive or vasospastic mesenteric ischemia presents with generalized abdominal pain, anorexia, bloody stools, and abdominal distention. Often these patients are obtunded, and physical findings may not assist in the diagnosis. The presence of a leukocytosis, metabolic acidosis, elevated amylase or creatinine phosphokinase levels, and/or lactic acidosis are useful in support of the diagnosis of advanced intestinal ischemia; however, these markers may not be indicative of either reversible ischemia or frank necrosis. Investigational markers for intestinal ischemia include D-dimer, glutathione S-transferase, platelet activating factor (PAF), and mucosal pH monitoring. Regardless of the need for urgent surgery, emergent admission to a monitored bed or intensive care unit is recommended for resuscitation and further evaluation. Early manifestations of intestinal ischemia include fluid sequestration within the bowel wall leading to a loss of interstitial volume. Aggressive fluid resuscitation may be necessary. To optimize oxygen delivery, nasal O_2 and blood transfusions may be given. Broad-spectrum antibiotics should be given to provide sufficient coverage for enteric pathogens, including gram-negative and anaerobic organisms. Frequent monitoring of the patient's vital signs, urine output, blood gases, and lactate levels is paramount, as is frequent abdominal examination. All vasoconstricting agents should be avoided; fluid resuscitation is the intervention of choice to maintain hemodynamics.

If ischemic colitis is a concern, colonoscopy should be performed to assess the integrity of the colon mucosa. Visualization of the rectosigmoid region may demonstrate decreased mucosal integrity, associated more commonly with nonocclusive mesenteric ischemia, or, on occasion, occlusive disease as a result of acute loss of inferior mesenteric arterial flow following aortic surgery. Ischemia of the colonic mucosa is graded as *mild* with minimal mucosal erythema or as *moderate* with pale mucosal ulcerations and evidence of extension to the muscular layer of the bowel wall. *Severe* ischemic colitis presents with severe ulcerations resulting in black or green discoloration of the mucosa, consistent with full-thickness bowel-wall necrosis. The degree of reversibility can be predicted from the mucosal findings: Mild erythema is nearly 100% reversible, moderate ~50%, and frank necrosis is simply dead bowel. Followup colonoscopy can be performed to rule out progression of ischemic colitis.

Laparotomy for nonocclusive mesenteric ischemia is warranted for signs of peritonitis or worsening endoscopic findings and if the patient's condition does not improve with aggressive resuscitation. Ischemic colitis is optimally treated with resection of the ischemic bowel and formation of a proximal stoma. Primary anastomosis should not be performed in patients with acute intestinal ischemia.

Patients with MVT may present with a gradual or sudden onset. Symptoms include vague abdominal pain, nausea, and vomiting. Examination findings include abdominal distention with mild to moderate tenderness and signs of dehydration. The diagnosis of mesenteric thrombosis is frequently made on abdominal spiral CT with oral and IV contrast. Findings on CT include bowel-wall thickening and ascites. Intravenous contrast will demonstrate a delayed arterial phase and clot within the superior mesenteric vein. The goal of management is to optimize hemodynamics and correct electrolyte abnormalities with massive fluid resuscitation. Intravenous antibiotics as well as anticoagulation should be initiated. If laparotomy is performed and MVT is suspected, heparin anticoagulation is immediately initiated and compromised bowel is resected. Of all acute intestinal disorders, mesenteric venous insufficiency is associated with the best prognosis.

Chronic intestinal ischemia presents with intestinal angina or abdominal pain associated with need for increased blood flow to the intestine. Patients report abdominal cramping and pain following ingestion of a meal. Weight loss and chronic diarrhea may also be noted. Abdominal pain without weight loss is not chronic mesenteric angina. Physical examination will often reveal the presence of an abdominal bruit as well as other manifestations of atherosclerosis. Duplex ultrasound evaluation of the mesenteric vessels has gained in popularity. In the absence of obesity and an increased bowel gas pattern, the radiologist may be able to identify flow disturbances within the vessels or the lack of a vasodilation response to feeding. This tool is frequently used as a screening test for patients with symptoms suggestive of chronic mesenteric ischemia. The gold standard for confirmation of mesenteric arterial occlusion is mesenteric angiography. Evaluation with mesenteric angiography allows for identification and possible intervention for the treatment of thrombus within the vessel lumen and will also evaluate the patency of remaining mesenteric vessels. The use of mesenteric angiography may be limited in the presence of renal failure or contrast allergy. Magnetic resonance angiography is an alternative if the administration of contrast dye is contraindicated.

The management of chronic intestinal ischemia includes medical management of atherosclerotic disease by lipid-lowering medications, exercise, and cessation of smoking. A full cardiac evaluation should be performed before intervention. Newer endovascular procedures may avoid an operative intervention in selected patient populations. Angioplasty with endovascular stenting in the treatment of chronic mesenteric ischemia is associated with an 80% long-term success rate. In patients requiring surgical exploration, the approach used is determined by the mesenteric angiogram. The entire length of the small and large bowel should be evaluated, beginning at the ligament of Treitz. Restoration of blood flow at the time of laparotomy is accomplished with mesenteric bypass.

Determination of intestinal viability intraoperatively in patients with suspected intestinal ischemia can be challenging. After revascularization, the bowel wall should be observed for return of a pink color and peristalsis. Palpation of major arterial vessels can be performed as well as applying a doppler flowmeter to the antimesenteric border of the bowel wall, but neither is a definitive indicator of viability. In equivocal cases, 1 g of IV sodium fluorescein is administered and the pattern of bowel reperfusion is observed under ultraviolet illumination with a standard (3600 A) Wood's lamp. An area of nonfluorescence >5 mm in diameter suggests nonviability. If doubt persists, reexploration performed 24–48 h following surgery will allow demarcation of nonviable bowel. Primary intestinal anastomosis in patients with ischemic bowel is always worrisome, and reanastomosis should be deferred to the time of second-look laparotomy.

Acknowledgments

We thank Cory Sandore for providing some illustrations for this chapter. Gregory Bulkley contributed to this chapter in the 16th edition of Harrison's Principles of Internal Medicine.

CHAPTER 21

ACUTE INTESTINAL OBSTRUCTION

William Silen

ETIOLOGY AND CLASSIFICATION

In 75% of patients, acute intestinal obstruction results from adhesive bands or internal hernias secondary to previous abdominal surgery or from external hernias. The incidence of acute intestinal obstruction requiring hospital admission within the first few postoperative weeks is 5–25%, and 10–50% of these patients will require surgical intervention. The incidence of postoperative intestinal obstruction may be lower following laparoscopic surgery than open procedures. However, the laparoscopic gastric bypass procedure may be associated with an unexpected high rate of intestinal obstruction, with a higher reoperative rate. Other causes of intestinal obstruction not related to previous abdominal surgery include lesions *intrinsic* to the wall of the intestine, e.g., diverticulitis, carcinoma, and regional enteritis; and luminal obstruction, e.g., gallstone obstruction and intussusception.

Two other conditions that must be differentiated from acute intestinal obstruction include *adynamic ileus* and *primary intestinal pseudo-obstruction*. Adynamic ileus is mediated via the hormonal component of the sympathoadrenal system and may occur after any peritoneal insult; its severity and duration will be dependent to some degree on the type of peritoneal injury. Hydrochloric acid, colonic contents, and pancreatic enzymes are among the most irritating to the peritoneum, whereas blood and urine are less so. Adynamic ileus occurs to some degree after any abdominal operation. Retroperitoneal hematoma, particularly associated with vertebral fracture, may cause severe adynamic ileus, and the latter may occur with other retroperitoneal conditions, such as ureteral calculus or severe pyelonephritis. Thoracic diseases, including lower-lobe pneumonia, fractured ribs, and myocardial infarction, frequently produce adynamic ileus, as do electrolyte disturbances, particularly potassium depletion. Finally, intestinal ischemia, whether from vascular occlusion or intestinal distention itself, may perpetuate an adynamic ileus.

Intestinal pseudo-obstruction is a chronic motility disorder that frequently mimics mechanical obstruction. This condition is often exacerbated by narcotic use.

PATHOPHYSIOLOGY

Distention of the intestine is caused by the accumulation of gas and fluid proximal to and within the obstructed segment. Between 70 and 80% of intestinal gas consists of swallowed air, and because this is composed mainly of nitrogen, which is poorly absorbed from the intestinal lumen, removal of air by continuous gastric suction is a useful adjunct in the treatment of intestinal distention. The accumulation of fluid proximal to the obstructing mechanism results not only from ingested fluid, swallowed saliva, gastric juice, and biliary and pancreatic secretions but also from interference with normal sodium and water transport. During the first 12–24 h of obstruction, a marked depression of flux from lumen to blood of sodium and water occurs in the distended proximal intestine. After 24 h, sodium and water move into the lumen, contributing further to the distention and fluid losses. Intraluminal pressure rises from a normal of 2–4 cmH$_2$O to 8–10 cmH$_2$O. The loss of fluids and electrolytes may be extreme, and unless replacement is prompt, hypovolemia, renal insufficiency, and shock may result. Vomiting, accumulation of fluids within the lumen, and the sequestration of fluid into the edematous intestinal wall and peritoneal cavity as a result of impairment of venous return from the intestine all contribute to massive loss of fluid and electrolytes.

A "closed loop" is the most feared complication of acute intestinal obstruction. Closed-loop obstruction results when the lumen is occluded at two points by a single mechanism such as a fascial hernia or adhesive band, thus producing a closed loop, the blood supply of which is also often occluded by the hernia or band. During peristalsis, when a "closed loop" is present, pressures reach 30–60 cmH$_2$O. Strangulation of the closed loop is common in association with marked distention proximal to the involved loop. A form of closed-loop obstruction is encountered when complete obstruction of the colon exists in the presence of a competent ileocecal valve (85% of individuals). Although the blood supply of the colon is not entrapped within the obstructing mechanism, distention of the cecum is extreme because of its greater diameter (Laplace's law), and impairment of the intramural blood supply is considerable, with consequent gangrene of the cecal wall. Once impairment of blood supply to the gastrointestinal tract occurs, bacterial invasion supervenes, and peritonitis develops. The systemic effects of extreme distention include elevation of the diaphragm with restricted ventilation and subsequent atelectasis. Venous return via the inferior vena cava may also be impaired.

SYMPTOMS

Mechanical intestinal obstruction is characterized by cramping midabdominal pain, which tends to be more severe the higher the obstruction. The pain occurs in paroxysms, and the patient is relatively comfortable in the intervals between the pains. Audible borborygmi are often noted by the patient simultaneously with the paroxysms of pain. The pain may become less severe as distention progresses, probably because motility is impaired in the edematous intestine. When strangulation is present, the pain is usually more localized and may be steady and severe without a colicky component, a fact that often causes delay in diagnosis of obstruction. Vomiting is almost invariable, and it is earlier and more profuse the higher the obstruction. The vomitus initially contains bile and mucus and remains as such if the obstruction is high in the intestine. With low ileal obstruction, the vomitus becomes feculent, i.e., orange-brown in color with a foul odor, which results from the overgrowth of bacteria proximal to the obstruction. Hiccups (singultus) are common. Obstipation and failure to pass gas by rectum are invariably present when the obstruction is complete, although some stool and gas may be passed spontaneously or after an enema shortly after onset of the complete obstruction. Diarrhea is occasionally observed in partial obstruction. Blood in the stool is rare but does occur in cases of intussusception.

In *adynamic ileus* as well as *colonic pseudo-obstruction*, colicky pain is absent and only discomfort from distention is evident. Vomiting may be frequent but is rarely profuse. Complete obstipation may or may not occur. Singultus (hiccups) is common.

PHYSICAL FINDINGS

Abdominal distention is the hallmark of all forms of intestinal obstruction. It is least marked in cases of obstruction high in the small intestine and most marked in colonic obstruction. In early obstruction of the small and large intestine, tenderness and rigidity are usually minimal; the temperature is rarely >37.8°C (100°F). The appearance of shock, tenderness, rigidity, and fever indicates that contamination of the peritoneum with infected intestinal content has occurred. Hernial orifices should always be carefully examined for the presence of a mass. Auscultation may reveal loud, high-pitched borborygmi coincident with colicky pain, but this finding is often absent late in strangulating or nonstrangulating obstruction. A quiet abdomen does not eliminate the possibility of obstruction, nor does it necessarily establish the diagnosis of adynamic ileus. The presence of a palpable abdominal mass usually signifies a closed-loop strangulating small-bowel obstruction; the tense fluid-filled loop is the palpable lesion.

LABORATORY AND X-RAY FINDINGS

Laboratory and radiographic studies are used to help differentiate the two important clinical aspects of this disorder: strangulation vs. nonstrangulation and partial vs. complete obstruction. Leukocytosis, with shift to the left, usually occurs when strangulation is present, but a normal white blood cell count does not exclude strangulation. Elevation of the serum amylase level is encountered occasionally in all forms of intestinal obstruction. Radiographic images demonstrating distention of fluid- and gas-filled loops of small intestine usually arranged in a "stepladder" pattern with air-fluid levels and an absence or paucity of colonic gas are pathognomonic for small-bowel obstruction. Complete obstruction is suggested when passage of gas or stool per rectum has ceased and when gas is absent in the distal intestine by x-ray. A general haze due to peritoneal fluid and sometimes a "coffee bean"–shaped mass are seen in strangulating closed loop obstruction. A thin barium upper gastrointestinal series may help to differentiate partial from complete obstruction. However, thick barium given by mouth should be avoided when the obstruction is considered to be high grade or complete since retained barium sulfate may become inspissated and either make an incomplete obstruction complete or be aspirated into the tracheobronchial tree. CT is the most commonly used modality to evaluate patients for intestinal obstruction but differentiating adynamic ileus, partial obstruction, and complete obstruction may be difficult (**Fig. 21-1**). The sensitivity and specificity of CT for strangulating obstruction are low (50 and 80%, respectively).

Common causes of colonic obstruction can be seen on abdominal radiographic series. These films may demonstrate a "bird's beak" sign when a sigmoid volvulus has occurred or an enlarged cecum when a cecal

FIGURE 21-1
CT with oral and intravenous contrast demonstrating **(A)** evidence of small-bowel dilatation with air-fluid levels consistent with a small-bowel obstruction; **(B)** a partial small-bowel obstruction from an incarcerated ventral hernia (*arrow*); and **(C)** decompressed bowel seen distal to the hernia (*arrow*).

torsion or bascule is present. Colonic obstruction with a competent ileocecal valve is easily recognized because distention with gas is mainly confined to the colon. Gastrografin enema may help in demonstrating a complete colonic obstruction. Furthermore, *barium should*

never be given by mouth to a patient with a possible colonic obstruction until that possibility has been excluded.

229

TREATMENT	Acute Intestinal Obstruction

SMALL-INTESTINAL OBSTRUCTION The overall mortality rate for obstruction of the small intestine is about 10%. While the mortality rate for nonstrangulating obstruction is 5–8%, the mortality rate for a strangulating obstruction ranges from 20 to 75%. Since strangulating small-bowel obstruction is always complete, surgical interventions should always be undertaken in such patients after suitable preparation. Before operating, fluid and electrolyte balance should be restored and decompression instituted by means of a nasogastric tube. Replacement of potassium is especially important because intake is nil and losses in vomitus are large. A long intestinal tube is not indicated. Operative intervention may be undertaken successfully by laparoscopic techniques with a decreased incidence of wound complications. However, laparoscopic lysis of adhesions is associated with a longer operative time and higher conversion to open rate when compared to other laparoscopic procedures. Alternatively, lysis of adhesions can be achieved through an open abdominal incision. In general, >50% of adhesions that occur are found at the previous incision site. Purely nonoperative therapy is safe only in the presence of incomplete obstruction and is best used in patients without increasing abdominal pain or leukocytosis. The overall recurrence of small-bowel obstruction is 16%. Population-based studies show that although the surgical management of small-bowel obstruction is associated with longer hospital stays, the rate of readmission for obstruction is lower. However, regardless of treatment type, following the index admission, only 20% of patients required readmission within a 5-year follow-up period.

COLONIC OBSTRUCTION The mortality rate for colonic obstruction is about 20%. As in small-bowel obstruction, nonoperative treatment is contraindicated unless the obstruction is incomplete. Incomplete obstruction can be treated with colonoscopic decompression and placement of a metallic stent if a malignant lesion is present. The success rate approaches 90% depending on the location of the obstruction, with left-sided lesions being more successfully stented than right-sided lesions. In general, the colonic stent is considered to be a temporary solution or a "bridge to surgery," which allows for colonic preparation before surgical intervention. When obstruction is complete, early operation is mandatory, especially when the ileocecal valve is competent, because of the concern for cecal perforation. Cecal perforation is more likely if the cecal diameter is >10 cm on plain abdominal film.

Decisions regarding the operative management of colonic obstruction are based on the cause of the obstruction and the patient's overall well-being. For obstruction on the left side of the colon, operative management strategies include either decompression by cecostomy or transverse colostomy or resection with end-colostomy formation (Hartmann's procedure). Primary resection of obstructing left-sided lesions with on-table washout of the colon has also been accomplished safely. For a lesion of the right or transverse colon, primary resection and anastomosis can be performed safely because distention of the ileum with consequent discrepancy in size and hazard in suture are usually not present. Furthermore, the bacterial and stool content is less on the right side of the colon, decreasing the chance of infection.

ADYNAMIC ILEUS This type of ileus usually responds to nonoperative decompression and treatment of the primary disease. The prognosis is usually good. Correction of electrolyte abnormalities should be instituted (i.e., potassium, magnesium). Successful decompression of a colonic ileus has been accomplished by repetitive colonoscopy. Neostigmine is also effective in cases of colonic ileus that have not responded to other conservative treatment. Rarely, adynamic colonic distention may become so great that cecostomy is required if cecal gangrene is feared.

CHAPTER 22

ACUTE APPENDICITIS AND PERITONITIS

William Silen

ACUTE APPENDICITIS

INCIDENCE AND EPIDEMIOLOGY

With more than 250,000 appendectomies performed annually, appendicitis is the most common abdominal surgical emergency in the United States. The peak incidence of acute appendicitis is in the second and third decades of life; it is relatively rare at the extremes of age. However, perforation is more common in infancy and in the elderly, during which periods mortality rates are highest. Males and females are equally affected, except between puberty and age 25, when males predominate in a 3:2 ratio. The incidence of appendicitis has remained stable in the United States over the last 30 years, while the incidence of appendicitis is much lower in underdeveloped countries, especially parts of Africa, and in lower socioeconomic groups. The mortality rate in the United States decreased eightfold between 1941 and 1970 but has remained at <1 per 100,000 since then.

PATHOGENESIS

Appendicitis is believed to occur as a result of appendiceal luminal obstruction. Obstruction is most commonly caused by a fecalith, which results from accumulation and inspissation of fecal matter around vegetable fibers. Enlarged lymphoid follicles associated with viral infections (e.g., measles), inspissated barium, worms (e.g., pinworms, *Ascaris*, and *Taenia*), and tumors (e.g., carcinoid or carcinoma) may also obstruct the lumen. Other common pathologic findings include appendiceal ulceration. The cause of the ulceration is unknown, although a viral etiology has been postulated. Infection with *Yersinia* organisms may cause the disease, since high complement fixation antibody titers have been found in up to 30% of cases of proven appendicitis. Luminal bacteria multiply and invade the appendiceal wall as venous engorgement and subsequent arterial compromise result

from the high intraluminal pressures. Finally, gangrene and perforation occur. If the process evolves slowly, adjacent organs such as the terminal ileum, cecum, and omentum may wall off the appendiceal area so that a localized abscess will develop, whereas rapid progression of vascular impairment may cause perforation with free access to the peritoneal cavity. Subsequent rupture of primary appendiceal abscesses may produce fistulas between the appendix and bladder, small intestine, sigmoid, or cecum. Occasionally, acute appendicitis may be the first manifestation of Crohn's disease.

While chronic infection of the appendix with tuberculosis, amebiasis, and actinomycosis may occur, a useful clinical aphorism states that *chronic appendiceal inflammation is not usually the cause of prolonged abdominal pain of weeks' or months' duration*. In contrast, recurrent acute appendicitis does occur, often with complete resolution of inflammation and symptoms between attacks. Recurrent acute appendicitis may also occur if a long appendiceal stump is left after initial appendectomy.

CLINICAL MANIFESTATIONS

The sequence of abdominal discomfort and anorexia associated with acute appendicitis is pathognomonic. The pain is described as being located in the periumbilical region initially and then migrating to the right lower quadrant. This classic sequence of symptoms occurs in only 66% of patients. The differential diagnoses for periumbilical and right lower quadrant pain is listed in Table 22-1. The periumbilical abdominal pain is of the visceral type, resulting from distention of the appendiceal lumen. This pain is carried on slow-conducting C fibers and is usually poorly localized in the periumbilical or epigastric region. In general, this visceral pain is mild, often cramping and usually lasting 4–6 h, but it may not be noted by stoic individuals. As inflammation spreads to the parietal peritoneal surfaces, the pain

TABLE 22-1

THE ANATOMIC ORIGIN OF PERIUMBILICAL AND RIGHT LOWER QUADRANT PAIN IN THE DIFFERENTIAL DIAGNOSIS OF APPENDICITIS

Periumbilical

Appendicitis
Small-bowel obstruction
Gastroenteritis
Mesenteric ischemia

Right Lower Quadrant

Gastrointestinal causes	Gynecologic causes
Appendicitis	Ovarian tumor/torsion
Inflammatory bowel disease	Pelvic inflammatory disease
Right-sided diverticulitis	Renal causes
Gastroenteritis	Pyelonephritis
Inguinal hernia	Perinephritic abscess
	Nephrolithiasis

becomes somatic, steady, and more severe and aggravated by motion or cough. Parietal afferent nerves are A delta fibers, which are fast-conducting and unilateral. These fibers localize the pain to the *right lower quadrant*. *Anorexia* is very common; a hungry patient almost invariably does not have acute appendicitis. *Nausea* and *vomiting* occur in 50–60% of cases, but vomiting is usually self-limited. Change in bowel habit is of little diagnostic value, since any or no alteration may be observed, although the presence of diarrhea caused by an inflamed appendix in juxtaposition to the sigmoid may cause diagnostic difficulties. Urinary frequency and dysuria occur if the appendix lies adjacent to the bladder.

Physical findings vary with time after onset of the illness and according to the location of the appendix, which may be situated deep in the pelvic cul-de-sac; in the right lower quadrant in any relation to the peritoneum, cecum, and small intestine; in the right upper quadrant (especially during pregnancy); or even in the left lower quadrant. *The diagnosis cannot be established unless tenderness can be elicited.* While tenderness is sometimes absent in the early visceral stage of the disease, it ultimately always develops and is found in any location corresponding to the position of the appendix. Typically, tenderness to palpation will often occur at McBurney's point, anatomically located on a line one-third of the way between the anterior iliac spine and the umbilicus. Abdominal tenderness may be completely absent if a retrocecal or pelvic appendix is present, in which case the sole physical finding may be tenderness in the flank or on rectal or pelvic examination. Referred rebound tenderness is often present and is most likely to be absent early in the illness. Flexion of the right hip and guarded movement by the patient are due to parietal peritoneal involvement. Hyperesthesia of the skin of the right lower quadrant and a positive psoas or obturator sign are often late findings and are rarely of diagnostic value.

The temperature is usually normal or slightly elevated (37.2°–38°C [99°–100.5°F]), but a temperature >38.3°C (101°F) should suggest perforation. Tachycardia is commensurate with the elevation of the temperature. Rigidity and tenderness become more marked as the disease progresses to perforation and localized or diffuse peritonitis. Distention is rare unless severe diffuse peritonitis has developed. A mass may develop if localized perforation has occurred but will not usually be detectable before 3 days after onset. Earlier presence of a mass suggests carcinoma of the cecum or Crohn's disease. Perforation is rare before 24 h after onset of symptoms, but the rate may be as high as 80% after 48 h.

Although moderate leukocytosis of 10,000–18,000 cells/µL is frequent (with a concomitant left shift), the absence of leukocytosis does not rule out acute appendicitis. Leukocytosis of >20,000 cells/µL suggests probable perforation. Anemia and blood in the stool suggest a primary diagnosis of carcinoma of the cecum, especially in elderly individuals. The urine may contain a few white or red blood cells without bacteria if the appendix lies close to the right ureter or bladder. Urinalysis is most useful in excluding genitourinary conditions that may mimic acute appendicitis.

Radiographs are rarely of value except when an opaque fecalith (5% of patients) is observed in the right lower quadrant (especially in children). Consequently, abdominal films are not routinely obtained unless other conditions such as intestinal obstruction or ureteral calculus may be present. The diagnosis may also be established by the ultrasonic demonstration of an enlarged and thick-walled appendix. Ultrasound is most useful to exclude ovarian cysts, ectopic pregnancy, or tuboovarian abscess. Several studies have recently demonstrated the benefit of contrast-enhanced or nonenhanced CT over ultrasound and plain radiographs in the diagnosis of acute appendicitis. The findings on CT will include a thickened appendix with periappendiceal stranding and often the presence of a fecalith (**Figs. 22-1** and **22-2**). The reported positive predictive value of CT is 95–97% and the overall accuracy is 90–98%. Furthermore, nonvisualization of the appendix on CT is associated with the findings of a normal appendix 98% of the time. Free peritoneal air is uncommon, even in perforated appendicitis.

While the typical historic sequence and physical findings are present in 50–60% of cases, a wide variety of atypical patterns of disease are encountered, especially at the age extremes and during pregnancy. Infants under 2 years of age have a 70–80% incidence of

FIGURE 22-1
CT with oral and intravenous contrast of acute appendicitis.
There is thickening of the wall of the appendix and periappendiceal stranding (*arrow*).

perforation and generalized peritonitis. This is thought to be the result of a delay in diagnosis. Any infant or child with diarrhea, vomiting, and abdominal pain is highly suspect. Fever is much more common in this age group, and abdominal distention is often the only physical finding. In the elderly, pain and tenderness are often blunted, and thus the diagnosis is also frequently delayed and leads to a 30% incidence of perforation in patients older than age 70 years. Elderly patients often present initially with a slightly painful mass (a primary

FIGURE 22-2
Appendiceal fecolith (*arrow*).

appendiceal abscess) or with adhesive intestinal obstruction 5 or 6 days after a previously undetected perforated appendix.

Appendicitis occurs about once in every 500–2000 pregnancies and is the most common extrauterine condition requiring abdominal operation. The diagnosis may be missed or delayed because of the frequent occurrence of mild abdominal discomfort and nausea and vomiting during pregnancy, and because of the gradual shift of the appendix from the right lower quadrant to the right upper quadrant during the second and third trimester of pregnancy. Appendicitis tends to be most common during the second trimester. The diagnosis is best made with ultrasound, which is 80% accurate; however, if perforation has already occurred, the accuracy of ultrasound decreases to 30%. Early intervention is warranted because the incidence of fetal loss with a normal appendix is 1.5%. With perforation, the incidence of fetal loss is 20–35%.

DIFFERENTIAL DIAGNOSIS

Acute appendicitis has been labeled the *masquerader*, and the diagnosis is often more difficult to make in young females. Obtaining a good history, including sexual activity and the presence of a vaginal discharge, will help differentiate acute appendicitis from pelvic inflammatory disease (PID). The presence of a malodorous vaginal discharge and gram-negative intracellular diplococci are pathognomonic for PID. Pain on movement of the cervix is also more specific for PID but may occur in appendicitis if perforation has occurred or if the appendix lies adjacent to the uterus or adnexa. *Rupture of a graafian follicle* (mittelschmerz) occurs at midcycle and will produce pain and tenderness more diffuse and usually of a less severe degree than in appendicitis. *Rupture of a corpus luteum cyst* is identical clinically to rupture of a graafian follicle but develops about the time of menstruation. The presence of an adnexal mass, evidence of blood loss, and a positive pregnancy test help differentiate *ruptured tubal pregnancy*. *Twisted ovarian cyst* and *endometriosis* are occasionally difficult to distinguish from appendicitis. In all these female conditions, ultrasonography and laparoscopy may be of great value.

Acute mesenteric lymphadenitis and *acute gastroenteritis* are the diagnoses usually given when enlarged, slightly reddened lymph nodes at the root of the mesentery and a normal appendix are encountered at operation in a patient who usually has right lower quadrant tenderness. Retrospectively, these patients may have had a higher temperature, diarrhea, more diffuse pain and abdominal tenderness, and a lymphocytosis. Between cramps, the abdomen is completely relaxed. Children seem to be affected more frequently than adults. Some of these patients have infection with *Y. pseudotuberculosis* or *Y. enterocolitica*, in which case the diagnosis can be established by culture of the mesenteric nodes or by serologic titers. In *Salmonella* gastroenteritis, the abdominal findings are similar, although the pain may be more severe and more localized, and fever and chills are common. The occurrence of similar symptoms among other members of the family may be helpful. *Regional enteritis* (Crohn's disease) is usually associated with a more prolonged history, often with previous exacerbations regarded as episodes of gastroenteritis unless the diagnosis has been established previously. Often an inflammatory mass is palpable. In addition, acute cholecystitis, perforated ulcer, acute pancreatitis, acute diverticulitis, strangulating intestinal obstruction, ureteral calculus, and pyelonephritis may present diagnostic difficulties.

TREATMENT   Acute Appendicitis

If the diagnosis is in question, 4–6 h of observation with serial abdominal exams is always more beneficial than harmful. Antibiotics should not be administered when the diagnosis is in question, since they will only mask the perforation. The treatment of presumed acute appendicitis is early operation and appendectomy as soon as the patient can be prepared. Appendectomy is frequently accomplished laparoscopically and is associated with less postoperative narcotic use and earlier discharge. It is acceptable to have a 15–20% incidence of a normal appendix at the time of appendectomy to avoid perforation. The use of early laparoscopy instead of close clinical observation has not shown a clinical benefit in the management of patients with nonspecific abdominal pain.

A different approach is indicated if a palpable mass is found 3–5 days after the onset of symptoms. This finding usually represents the presence of a phlegmon or abscess, and complications from attempted surgical excision are frequent. Such patients treated with broad-spectrum antibiotics, drainage of abscesses >3 cm, parenteral fluids, and bowel rest usually show resolution of symptoms within 1 week. *Interval appendectomy* can be performed safely 6–12 weeks later. A randomized clinical trial has demonstrated that antibiotics alone can effectively treat acute, nonperforated appendicitis in 86% of male patients. However, antibiotics alone were associated with a higher recurrence rate than when followed by surgical intervention. If the mass enlarges or the patient becomes more toxic, the abscess should be drained. Free perforation is associated with generalized peritonitis and its complications, including subphrenic, pelvic, or other abscesses, and can be avoided by early diagnosis. The mortality rate for nonperforated appendicitis is 0.1%, little more than the risk of general anesthesia; for perforated appendicitis, mortality is 3% (and can reach 15% in the elderly).

ACUTE PERITONITIS

Peritonitis is an inflammation of the peritoneum; it may be localized or diffuse in location, acute or chronic in natural history, and infectious or aseptic in pathogenesis. Acute peritonitis is most often infectious and is usually related to a perforated viscus (and called *secondary peritonitis*). When no intraabdominal source is identified, infectious peritonitis is called *primary* or *spontaneous*. Acute peritonitis is associated with decreased intestinal motor activity, resulting in distention of the intestinal lumen with gas and fluid (adynamic ileus). The accumulation of fluid in the bowel together with the lack of oral intake leads to rapid intravascular volume depletion with effects on cardiac, renal, and other systems.

ETIOLOGY

Infectious agents gain access to the peritoneal cavity through a perforated viscus, a penetrating wound of the abdominal wall, or external introduction of a foreign object that is or becomes infected (e.g., a chronic peritoneal dialysis catheter). In the absence of immune compromise, host defenses are capable of eradicating small contaminations. The conditions that most commonly result in the introduction of bacteria into the peritoneum are ruptured appendix, ruptured diverticulum, perforated peptic ulcer, incarcerated hernia, gangrenous gallbladder, volvulus, bowel infarction, cancer, inflammatory bowel disease, or intestinal obstruction. However, a wide range of mechanisms may play a role **(Table 22-2)**. Bacterial peritonitis can also occur in the apparent absence of an intraperitoneal source of bacteria (primary or spontaneous bacterial peritonitis). This condition occurs in the setting of ascites and liver cirrhosis in 90% of the cases, usually in patients with ascites with low protein concentration (<1 g/L) (Chap. 42). Bacterial peritonitis is discussed in detail in Chap. 25.

Aseptic peritonitis may be due to peritoneal irritation by abnormal presence of physiologic fluids (e.g., gastric juice, bile, pancreatic enzymes, blood, or urine) or sterile foreign bodies (e.g., surgical sponges or instruments, starch from surgical gloves) in the peritoneal cavity or as a complication of rare systemic diseases such as lupus erythematosus, porphyria, or familial Mediterranean fever. Chemical irritation of the peritoneum is greatest for acidic gastric juice and pancreatic enzymes. Secondary bacterial infection is common in chemical peritonitis.

CLINICAL FEATURES

The cardinal manifestations of peritonitis are acute abdominal pain and tenderness, usually with fever.

TABLE 22-2

CONDITIONS LEADING TO SECONDARY BACTERIAL PERITONITIS

Perforations of bowel	Perforations or leaking of other organs
Trauma, blunt or penetrating	Pancreas—pancreatitis
Inflammation	Gallbladder—cholecystitis
Appendicitis	Urinary bladder—trauma, rupture
Diverticulitis	Liver—bile leak after biopsy
Peptic ulcer disease	Fallopian tubes—salpingitis
Inflammatory bowel disease	Bleeding into the peritoneal cavity
Iatrogenic	**Disruption of integrity of peritoneal cavity**
Endoscopic perforation	Trauma
Anastomotic leaks	Continuous ambulatory peritoneal dialysis (indwelling catheter)
Catheter perforation	
Vascular	Intraperitoneal chemotherapy
Embolus	Perinephric abscess
Ischemia	Iatrogenic—postoperative, foreign body
Obstructions	
Adhesions	
Strangulated hernias	
Volvulus	
Intussusception	
Neoplasms	
Ingested foreign body, toothpick, fish bone	

The location of the pain depends on the underlying cause and whether the inflammation is localized or generalized. Localized peritonitis is most common in uncomplicated appendicitis and diverticulitis, and physical findings are limited to the area of inflammation. Generalized peritonitis is associated with widespread inflammation and diffuse abdominal tenderness and rebound. Rigidity of the abdominal wall is common in both localized and generalized peritonitis. Bowel sounds are usually but not always absent. Tachycardia, hypotension, and signs of dehydration are common. Leukocytosis and marked acidosis are common laboratory findings. Plain abdominal films may show dilation of large and small bowel with edema of the bowel wall. Free air under the diaphragm is associated with a perforated viscus. CT and/or ultrasonography can identify the presence of free fluid or an abscess. When ascites is present, diagnostic paracentesis with cell count (>250 neutrophils/μL is usual in peritonitis), protein and lactate dehydrogenase levels, and culture is essential. In elderly and immunosuppressed patients, signs of peritoneal irritation may be more difficult to detect.

THERAPY AND PROGNOSIS

Treatment relies on rehydration, correction of electrolyte abnormalities, antibiotics, and surgical correction of the underlying defect. Mortality rates are <10% for uncomplicated peritonitis associated with a perforated ulcer or ruptured appendix or diverticulum in an otherwise healthy person. Mortality rates of ≥40% have been reported for elderly people, those with underlying illnesses, and when peritonitis has been present for >48 h.

SECTION IV

INFECTIONS OF THE ALIMENTARY TRACT

CHAPTER 23

ACUTE INFECTIOUS DIARRHEAL DISEASES AND BACTERIAL FOOD POISONING

Regina C. LaRocque ■ Edward T. Ryan ■ Stephen B. Calderwood

Ranging from a mild annoyance to a devastating dehydrating illness, acute diarrheal disease is a leading cause of illness globally, with an estimated 4.6 billion episodes worldwide per year. Diarrheal disease ranks second only to lower respiratory infection as the most common infectious cause of death worldwide. Among children <5 years old, diarrheal disease is a particularly important cause of death. Every year nearly 2 million children in this age group die of diarrheal disease; the majority of these young children are impoverished and live in resource-poor areas. By contributing to malnutrition and thereby reducing resistance to other infectious agents, diarrheal disease is also an indirect factor in a far greater burden of disease.

The wide range of clinical manifestations of acute gastrointestinal illnesses is matched by the wide variety of infectious agents involved, including viruses, bacteria, and parasitic pathogens (Table 23-1). This chapter discusses factors that enable gastrointestinal pathogens to cause disease, reviews host defense mechanisms, and delineates an approach to the evaluation and treatment of patients presenting with acute diarrhea. Individual organisms causing acute gastrointestinal illnesses are discussed in detail in subsequent chapters.

PATHOGENIC MECHANISMS

Enteric pathogens have developed a variety of tactics to overcome host defenses. Understanding the virulence factors employed by these organisms is important in the diagnosis and treatment of clinical disease.

Inoculum size

The number of microorganisms that must be ingested to cause disease varies considerably from species to species. For *Shigella*, enterohemorrhagic *Escherichia coli*, *Giardia lamblia*, or *Entamoeba*, as few as 10–100 bacteria or cysts can produce infection, while 10^5–10^8 *Vibrio cholerae* organisms must be ingested orally to cause disease. The infective dose of *Salmonella* varies widely, depending on the species, host, and food vehicle. The ability of organisms to overcome host defenses has important implications for transmission; *Shigella*, enterohemorrhagic *E. coli*, *Entamoeba*, and *Giardia* can spread by person-to-person contact, whereas under some circumstances *Salmonella* may have to grow in food for several hours before reaching an effective infectious dose.

Adherence

Many organisms must adhere to the gastrointestinal mucosa as an initial step in the pathogenic process; thus, organisms that can compete with the normal bowel flora and colonize the mucosa have an important advantage in causing disease. Specific cell-surface proteins involved in attachment of bacteria to intestinal cells are important virulence determinants. *V. cholerae*, for example, adheres to the brush border of small-intestinal enterocytes via specific surface adhesins, including the toxin-coregulated pilus and other accessory colonization factors. Enterotoxigenic *E. coli*, which causes watery diarrhea, produces an adherence protein called *colonization factor antigen* that is necessary for colonization of the upper small intestine by the organism prior to the production of enterotoxin. Enteropathogenic *E. coli*, an agent of diarrhea in young children, and enterohemorrhagic *E. coli*, which causes hemorrhagic colitis and the hemolytic-uremic syndrome, produce virulence determinants that allow these organisms to attach to and efface the brush border of the intestinal epithelium.

TABLE 23-1

GASTROINTESTINAL PATHOGENS CAUSING ACUTE DIARRHEA

MECHANISM	LOCATION	ILLNESS	STOOL FINDINGS	EXAMPLES OF PATHOGENS INVOLVED
Noninflammatory (enterotoxin)	Proximal small bowel	Watery diarrhea	No fecal leukocytes; mild or no increase in fecal lactoferrin	*Vibrio cholerae*, enterotoxigenic *Escherichia coli* (LT and/or ST), enteroaggregative *E. coli*, *Clostridium perfringens*, *Bacillus cereus*, *Staphylococcus aureus*, *Aeromonas hydrophila*, *Plesiomonas shigelloides*, rotavirus, norovirus, enteric adenoviruses, *Giardia lamblia*, *Cryptosporidium* spp., *Cyclospora* spp., microsporidia
Inflammatory (invasion or cytotoxin)	Colon or distal small bowel	Dysentery or inflammatory diarrhea	Fecal polymorpho-nuclear leukocytes; substantial increase in fecal lactoferrin	*Shigella* spp., *Salmonella* spp., *Campylobacter jejuni*, enterohemorrhagic *E. coli*, enteroinvasive *E. coli*, *Yersinia enterocolitica*, *Listeria monocytogenes*, *Vibrio parahaemolyticus*, *Clostridium difficile*, *A. hydrophila*, *P. shigelloides*, *Entamoeba histolytica*, *Klebsiella oxytoca*
Penetrating	Distal small bowel	Enteric fever	Fecal mononuclear leukocytes	*Salmonella typhi*, *Y. enterocolitica*

Abbreviations: LT, heat-labile enterotoxin; ST, heat-stable enterotoxin.
Source: After TS Steiner, RL Guerrant: Principles and syndromes of enteric infection, in Mandell, Douglas, and Bennett's Principles and Practice of Infectious Diseases, 7th ed, GL Mandell et al (eds). Philadelphia, Churchill Livingstone, 2010, pp 1335–1351.

Toxin production

The production of one or more exotoxins is important in the pathogenesis of numerous enteric organisms. Such toxins include *enterotoxins*, which cause watery diarrhea by acting directly on secretory mechanisms in the intestinal mucosa; *cytotoxins*, which cause destruction of mucosal cells and associated inflammatory diarrhea; and *neurotoxins*, which act directly on the central or peripheral nervous system.

The prototypical enterotoxin is cholera toxin, a heterodimeric protein composed of one A and five B subunits. The A subunit contains the enzymatic activity of the toxin, while the B subunit pentamer binds holotoxin to the enterocyte surface receptor, the ganglioside G_{M1}. After the binding of holotoxin, a fragment of the A subunit is translocated across the eukaryotic cell membrane into the cytoplasm, where it catalyzes the ADP-ribosylation of a GTP-binding protein and causes persistent activation of adenylate cyclase. The end result is an increase of cyclic AMP in the intestinal mucosa, which increases Cl^- secretion and decreases Na^+ absorption, leading to a loss of fluid and the production of diarrhea.

Enterotoxigenic strains of *E. coli* may produce a protein called *heat-labile enterotoxin* (LT) that is similar to cholera toxin and causes secretory diarrhea by the same mechanism. Alternatively, enterotoxigenic strains of *E. coli* may produce *heat-stable enterotoxin* (ST), one form of which causes diarrhea by activation of guanylate cyclase and elevation of intracellular cyclic GMP.

Some enterotoxigenic strains of *E. coli* produce both LT and ST.

Bacterial cytotoxins, in contrast, destroy intestinal mucosal cells and produce the syndrome of dysentery, with bloody stools containing inflammatory cells. Enteric pathogens that produce such cytotoxins include *Shigella dysenteriae* type 1, *Vibrio parahaemolyticus*, and *Clostridium difficile*. *S. dysenteriae* type 1 and Shiga toxin–producing strains of *E. coli* produce potent cytotoxins and have been associated with outbreaks of hemorrhagic colitis and hemolytic–uremic syndrome.

Neurotoxins are usually produced by bacteria outside the host and therefore cause symptoms soon after ingestion. Included are the staphylococcal and *Bacillus cereus* toxins, which act on the central nervous system to produce vomiting.

Invasion

Dysentery may result not only from the production of cytotoxins but also from bacterial invasion and destruction of intestinal mucosal cells. Infections due to *Shigella* and enteroinvasive *E. coli* are characterized by the organisms' invasion of mucosal epithelial cells, intraepithelial multiplication, and subsequent spread to adjacent cells. *Salmonella* causes inflammatory diarrhea by invasion of the bowel mucosa but generally is not associated with the destruction of enterocytes or the full clinical syndrome of dysentery. *Salmonella typhi* and *Yersinia enterocolitica* can penetrate intact intestinal mucosa, multiply intracellularly in Peyer's patches and intestinal lymph nodes, and then disseminate through the bloodstream to cause enteric fever, a syndrome characterized by fever, headache, relative bradycardia, abdominal pain, splenomegaly, and leukopenia.

HOST DEFENSES

Given the enormous number of microorganisms ingested with every meal, the normal host must combat a constant influx of potential enteric pathogens. Studies of infections in patients with alterations in defense mechanisms have led to a greater understanding of the variety of ways in which the normal host can protect itself against disease.

Normal flora

The large numbers of bacteria that normally inhabit the intestine act as an important host defense by preventing colonization by potential enteric pathogens. Persons with fewer intestinal bacteria, such as infants who have not yet developed normal enteric colonization or patients receiving antibiotics, are at significantly greater risk of developing infections with enteric pathogens. The composition of the intestinal flora is as important as the number of organisms present. More than 99% of the normal colonic flora is made up of anaerobic bacteria, and the acidic pH and volatile fatty acids produced by these organisms appear to be critical elements in resistance to colonization.

Gastric acid

The acidic pH of the stomach is an important barrier to enteric pathogens, and an increased frequency of infections due to *Salmonella*, *G. lamblia*, and a variety of helminths has been reported among patients who have undergone gastric surgery or are achlorhydric for some other reason. Neutralization of gastric acid with antacids, proton pump inhibitors, or H_2 blockers—a common practice in the management of hospitalized patients—similarly increases the risk of enteric colonization. In addition, some microorganisms can survive the extreme acidity of the gastric environment; rotavirus, for example, is highly stable to acidity.

Intestinal motility

Normal peristalsis is the major mechanism for clearance of bacteria from the proximal small intestine. When intestinal motility is impaired (e.g., by treatment with opiates or other antimotility drugs, anatomic abnormalities, or hypomotility states), the frequency of bacterial overgrowth and infection of the small bowel with enteric pathogens is increased. Some patients whose

treatment for *Shigella* infection consists of diphenoxylate hydrochloride with atropine (Lomotil) experience prolonged fever and shedding of organisms, while patients treated with opiates for mild *Salmonella* gastroenteritis have a higher frequency of bacteremia than those not treated with opiates.

Immunity

Both cellular immune responses and antibody production play important roles in protection from enteric infections. Humoral immunity to enteric pathogens consists of systemic IgG and IgM as well as secretory IgA. The mucosal immune system may be the first line of defense against many gastrointestinal pathogens. The binding of bacterial antigens to the luminal surface of M cells in the distal small bowel and the subsequent presentation of antigens to subepithelial lymphoid tissue lead to the proliferation of sensitized lymphocytes. These lymphocytes circulate and populate all of the mucosal tissues of the body as IgA-secreting plasma cells.

Genetic determinants

Host genetic variation influences susceptibility to diarrheal diseases. People with blood group O show increased susceptibility to disease due to *V. cholerae*, *Shigella*, *E. coli* O157, and norovirus. Polymorphisms in genes encoding inflammatory mediators have been associated with the outcome of infection with enteroaggregative *E. coli*, enterotoxin-producing *E. coli*, *Salmonella*, *C. difficile*, and *V. cholerae*.

APPROACH TO THE PATIENT | **Infectious Diarrhea or Bacterial Food Poisoning**

The approach to the patient with possible infectious diarrhea or bacterial food poisoning is shown in **Fig. 23-1**.

HISTORY The answers to questions with high discriminating value can quickly narrow the range of potential causes of diarrhea and help determine whether treatment is needed. Important elements of the narrative history are detailed in Fig. 23-1.

PHYSICAL EXAMINATION The examination of patients for signs of dehydration provides essential information about the severity of the diarrheal illness and the need for rapid therapy. Mild dehydration is indicated by thirst, dry mouth, decreased axillary sweat, decreased urine output, and slight weight loss. Signs of moderate dehydration include an orthostatic fall in blood pressure, skin tenting, and sunken eyes (or, in infants, a sunken fontanelle). Signs of severe dehydration include lethargy, obtundation, feeble pulse, hypotension, and frank shock.

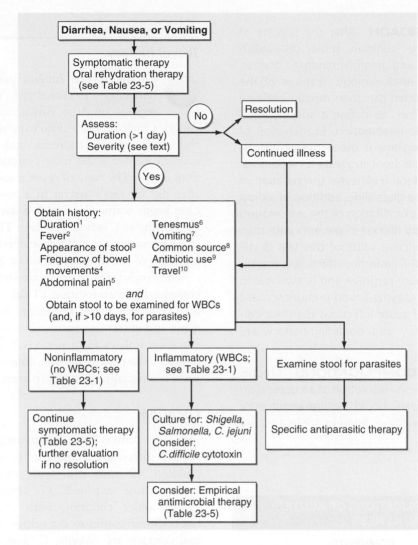

FIGURE 23-1

Clinical algorithm for the approach to patients with community-acquired infectious diarrhea or bacterial food poisoning. Key to superscripts: **1.** Diarrhea lasting >2 weeks is generally defined as chronic; in such cases, many of the causes of acute diarrhea are much less likely, and a new spectrum of causes needs to be considered. **2.** Fever often implies invasive disease, although fever and diarrhea may also result from infection outside the gastrointestinal tract, as in malaria. **3.** Stools that contain blood or mucus indicate ulceration of the large bowel. Bloody stools without fecal leukocytes should alert the laboratory to the possibility of infection with Shiga toxin–producing enterohemorrhagic *Escherichia coli*. Bulky white stools suggest a small-intestinal process that is causing malabsorption. Profuse "rice-water" stools suggest cholera or a similar toxigenic process. **4.** Frequent stools over a given period can provide the first warning of impending dehydration. **5.** Abdominal pain may be most severe in inflammatory processes like those due to *Shigella*, *Campylobacter*, and necrotizing toxins. Painful abdominal muscle cramps, caused by electrolyte loss, can develop in severe cases of cholera. Bloating is common in giardiasis. An appendicitis-like syndrome should prompt a culture for *Yersinia enterocolitica* with cold enrichment. **6.** Tenesmus (painful rectal spasms with a strong urge to defecate but little passage of stool) may be a feature of cases with proctitis, as in shigellosis or amebiasis. **7.** Vomiting implies an acute infection (e.g., a toxin-mediated illness or food poisoning) but can also be prominent in a variety of systemic illnesses (e.g., malaria) and in intestinal obstruction. **8.** Asking patients whether anyone else they know is sick is a more efficient means of identifying a common source than is constructing a list of recently eaten foods. If a common source seems likely, specific foods can be investigated. See text for a discussion of bacterial food poisoning. **9.** Current antibiotic therapy or a recent history of treatment suggests *Clostridium difficile* diarrhea (Chap. 24). Stop antibiotic treatment if possible and consider tests for *C. difficile* toxins. Antibiotic use may increase the risk of other infections, such as salmonellosis. **10.** See text for a discussion of traveler's diarrhea. (*After TS Steiner, RL Guerrant: Principles and syndromes of enteric infection, in Mandell, Douglas, and Bennett's Principles and Practice of Infectious Diseases, 7th ed, GL Mandell et al [eds]. Philadelphia, Churchill Livingstone, 2010, pp 1335–1351; RL Guerrant, DA Bobak: N Engl J Med 325:327, 1991; with permission.*)

DIAGNOSTIC APPROACH After the severity of illness is assessed, the clinician must distinguish between *inflammatory* and *noninflammatory* disease. Using the history and epidemiologic features of the case as guides, the clinician can then rapidly evaluate the need for further efforts to define a specific etiology and for therapeutic intervention. Examination of a stool sample may supplement the narrative history. Grossly bloody or mucoid stool suggests an inflammatory process. A test for fecal leukocytes (preparation of a thin smear of stool on a glass slide, addition of a drop of methylene blue, and examination of the wet mount) can suggest inflammatory disease in patients with diarrhea, although the predictive value of this test is still debated. A test for fecal lactoferrin, which is a marker of fecal leukocytes, is more sensitive and is available in latex agglutination and enzyme-linked immunosorbent assay formats. Causes of acute infectious diarrhea, categorized as inflammatory and noninflammatory, are listed in Table 23-1.

POST-DIARRHEA COMPLICATIONS Chronic complications may follow the resolution of an acute diarrheal episode. The clinician should inquire about prior diarrheal illness if the conditions listed in Table 23-2 are observed.

TABLE 23-2

POST-DIARRHEA COMPLICATIONS OF ACUTE INFECTIOUS DIARRHEAL ILLNESS

COMPLICATION	COMMENTS
Chronic diarrhea • Lactase deficiency • Small-bowel bacterial overgrowth • Malabsorption syndromes (tropical and celiac sprue)	Occurs in ~1% of travelers with acute diarrhea • Protozoa account for ~1/3 of cases
Initial presentation or exacerbation of inflammatory bowel disease	May be precipitated by traveler's diarrhea
Irritable bowel syndrome	Occurs in ~10% of travelers with traveler's diarrhea
Reactive arthritis (formerly known as Reiter's syndrome)	Particularly likely after infection with invasive organisms (*Shigella, Salmonella, Campylobacter, Yersinia*)
Hemolytic-uremic syndrome (hemolytic anemia, thrombocytopenia, and renal failure)	Follows infection with Shiga toxin–producing bacteria (*Shigella dysenteriae* type 1 and enterohemorrhagic *Escherichia coli*)
Guillain-Barré syndrome	Particularly likely after *Campylobacter* infection

EPIDEMIOLOGY

Travel history

Of the several million people who travel from temperate industrialized countries to tropical regions of Asia, Africa, and Central and South America each year, 20–50% experience a sudden onset of abdominal cramps, anorexia, and watery diarrhea; thus *traveler's diarrhea* is the most common travel-related infectious illness. The time of onset is usually 3 days to 2 weeks after the traveler's arrival in a resource-poor area; most cases begin within the first 3–5 days. The illness is generally self-limited, lasting 1–5 days. The high rate of diarrhea among travelers to underdeveloped areas is related to the ingestion of contaminated food or water.

The organisms that cause traveler's diarrhea vary considerably with location (Table 23-3), as does the pattern of antimicrobial resistance. In all areas, enterotoxigenic and enteroaggregative strains of *E. coli* are the most common isolates from persons with the classic secretory traveler's diarrhea syndrome. Infection with *Campylobacter jejuni* is especially common in areas of Asia.

Location

Day-care centers have particularly high attack rates of enteric infections. Rotavirus is most common among children <2 years old, with attack rates of 75–100% among those exposed. *G. lamblia* is more common among older children, with somewhat lower attack rates. Other common organisms, often spread by fecal-oral contact, are *Shigella, C. jejuni,* and *Cryptosporidium*. A characteristic feature of infection among children attending day-care centers is the high rate of secondary cases among family members.

Similarly, hospitals are sites in which enteric infections are concentrated. Diarrhea is one of the most common manifestations of nosocomial infections. *C. difficile* is the predominant cause of nosocomial diarrhea among adults in the United States. *Klebsiella oxytoca* has been identified as a cause of antibiotic-associated hemorrhagic colitis. Viral pathogens, especially rotavirus, can spread rapidly in pediatric wards. Enteropathogenic *E. coli* has been associated with outbreaks of diarrhea in nurseries for newborns. One-third of elderly patients in chronic-care institutions develop a significant diarrheal illness each year; more than one-half of these cases are caused by cytotoxin-producing *C. difficile*. Antimicrobial therapy can predispose to pseudomembranous colitis by altering the normal colonic flora and allowing the multiplication of *C. difficile* (Chap. 24).

Age

Globally, most morbidity and mortality from enteric pathogens involves children <5 years of age. Breast-fed

TABLE 23-3

CAUSES OF TRAVELER'S DIARRHEA

ETIOLOGIC AGENT	APPROXIMATE PERCENTAGE OF CASES	COMMENTS
BACTERIA	**50–75**	
Enterotoxigenic *Escherichia coli*	10–45	Single most important agent
Enteroaggregative *E. coli*	5–35	Emerging enteric pathogen with worldwide distribution
Campylobacter jejuni	5–25	More common in Asia
Shigella	0–15	Major cause of dysentery
Salmonella	0–15	
Others	0–5	Including *Aeromonas*, *Plesiomonas*, and *Vibrio cholerae*
VIRUSES	**0–20**	
Norovirus	0–10	Associated with cruise ships
Rotavirus	0–5	Particularly common among children
PARASITES	**0–10**	
Giardia lamblia	0–5	Affects hikers and campers who drink from freshwater streams; contaminates water supplies in Russia
Cryptosporidium	0–5	Resistant to chlorine treatment
Entamoeba histolytica	<1	
Cyclospora	<1	
OTHER	**0–10**	
Acute food poisoning[a]	0–5	
No pathogen identified	10–50	

[a]For etiologic agents, see Table 23-4.
Source: After DR Hill et al: Clin Infect Dis 43:1499, 2006.

infants are protected from contaminated food and water and derive some protection from maternal antibodies, but their risk of infection rises dramatically when they begin to eat solid foods. Exposure to rotavirus is universal, with most children experiencing their first infection in the first or second year of life. Older children and adults are more commonly infected with norovirus. Other organisms with higher attack rates among children than among adults include enterotoxigenic, enteropathogenic,

and enterohemorrhagic *E. coli*; *Shigella*; *C. jejuni*; and *G. lamblia*.

Host immune status

Immunocompromised hosts are at elevated risk of acute and chronic infectious diarrhea. Individuals with defects in cell-mediated immunity (including those with AIDS) are at particularly high risk of invasive enteropathies, including salmonellosis, listeriosis, and cryptosporidiosis. Individuals with hypogammaglobulinemia are at particular risk of *C. difficile* colitis and giardiasis. Patients with cancer are more likely to develop *C. difficile* infection as a result of chemotherapy and frequent hospitalizations. Infectious diarrhea can be life-threatening in immunocompromised hosts, with complications including bacteremia and metastatic seeding of infection. Furthermore, dehydration may compromise renal function and increase the toxicity of immunosuppressive drugs.

Bacterial food poisoning

If the history and the stool examination indicate a noninflammatory etiology of diarrhea and there is evidence of a common-source outbreak, questions concerning the ingestion of specific foods and the time of onset of the diarrhea after a meal can provide clues to the bacterial cause of the illness. Potential causes of bacterial food poisoning are shown in **Table 23-4**.

Bacterial disease caused by an enterotoxin elaborated outside the host, such as that due to *Staphylococcus aureus* or *B. cereus*, has the shortest incubation period (1–6 h) and generally lasts <12 h. Most cases of staphylococcal food poisoning are caused by contamination from infected human carriers. Staphylococci can multiply at a wide range of temperatures; thus, if food is left to cool slowly and remains at room temperature after cooking, the organisms will have the opportunity to form enterotoxin. Outbreaks following picnics where potato salad, mayonnaise, and cream pastries have been served offer classic examples of staphylococcal food poisoning. Diarrhea, nausea, vomiting, and abdominal cramping are common, while fever is less so.

B. cereus can produce either a syndrome with a short incubation period—the *emetic* form, mediated by a staphylococcal type of enterotoxin—or one with a longer incubation period (8–16 h)—the *diarrheal* form, caused by an enterotoxin resembling *E. coli* LT, in which diarrhea and abdominal cramps are characteristic but vomiting is uncommon. The emetic form of *B. cereus* food poisoning is associated with contaminated fried rice; the organism is common in uncooked rice, and its heat-resistant spores survive boiling. If cooked rice is not refrigerated, the

TABLE 23-4

BACTERIAL FOOD POISONING

INCUBATION PERIOD, ORGANISM	SYMPTOMS	COMMON FOOD SOURCES
1–6 h		
Staphylococcus aureus	Nausea, vomiting, diarrhea	Ham, poultry, potato or egg salad, mayonnaise, cream pastries
Bacillus cereus	Nausea, vomiting, diarrhea	Fried rice
8–16 h		
Clostridium perfringens	Abdominal cramps, diarrhea (vomiting rare)	Beef, poultry, legumes, gravies
B. cereus	Abdominal cramps, diarrhea (vomiting rare)	Meats, vegetables, dried beans, cereals
>16 h		
Vibrio cholerae	Watery diarrhea	Shellfish, water
Enterotoxigenic *Escherichia coli*	Watery diarrhea	Salads, cheese, meats, water
Enterohemorrhagic *E. coli*	Bloody diarrhea	Ground beef, roast beef, salami, raw milk, raw vegetables, apple juice
Salmonella spp.	Inflammatory diarrhea	Beef, poultry, eggs, dairy products
Campylobacter jejuni	Inflammatory diarrhea	Poultry, raw milk
Shigella spp.	Dysentery	Potato or egg salad, lettuce, raw vegetables
Vibrio parahaemolyticus	Dysentery	Mollusks, crustaceans

spores can germinate and produce toxin. Frying before serving may not destroy the preformed, heat-stable toxin.

Food poisoning due to *Clostridium perfringens* also has a slightly longer incubation period (8–14 h) and results from the survival of heat-resistant spores in inadequately cooked meat, poultry, or legumes. After ingestion, toxin is produced in the intestinal tract, causing moderately severe abdominal cramps and diarrhea; vomiting is rare, as is fever. The illness is self-limited, rarely lasting >24 h.

Not all food poisoning has a bacterial cause. Nonbacterial agents of short-incubation food poisoning include capsaicin, which is found in hot peppers, and a variety of toxins found in fish and shellfish.

LABORATORY EVALUATION

Many cases of noninflammatory diarrhea are self-limited or can be treated empirically, and in these instances the clinician may not need to determine a specific etiology. Potentially pathogenic *E. coli* cannot be distinguished from normal fecal flora by routine culture, and tests to detect enterotoxins are not available in most clinical laboratories. In situations in which cholera is a concern, stool should be cultured on selective media such as thiosulfate–citrate–bile salts–sucrose (TCBS) or tellurite-taurocholate-gelatin (TTG) agar. A latex agglutination test has made the rapid detection of rotavirus in stool practical for many laboratories, while reverse-transcriptase polymerase chain reaction and specific antigen enzyme immunoassays have been developed for the identification of norovirus. Stool specimens should be examined by immunofluorescence-based rapid assays or (less sensitive) standard microscopy for *Giardia* cysts or *Cryptosporidium* if the level of clinical suspicion regarding the involvement of these organisms is high.

All patients with fever and evidence of inflammatory disease acquired outside the hospital should have stool cultured for *Salmonella*, *Shigella*, and *Campylobacter*. *Salmonella* and *Shigella* can be selected on MacConkey agar as non-lactose-fermenting (colorless) colonies or can be grown on *Salmonella-Shigella* agar or in selenite enrichment broth, both of which inhibit most organisms except these pathogens. Evaluation of nosocomial diarrhea should initially focus on *C. difficile*; stool culture for other pathogens in this setting has an extremely low yield and is not cost-effective. Toxins A and B produced by pathogenic strains of *C. difficile* can be detected by rapid enzyme immunoassays and latex agglutination tests (Chap. 24). Isolation of *C. jejuni* requires inoculation of fresh stool onto selective growth medium and incubation at 42°C in a microaerophilic atmosphere. In many laboratories in the United States, *E. coli* O157:H7 is among the most common pathogens isolated from visibly bloody stools. Strains of this enterohemorrhagic serotype can be identified in specialized laboratories by serotyping but also can be identified presumptively in hospital laboratories as lactose-fermenting, indole-positive colonies of sorbitol nonfermenters (white colonies) on sorbitol MacConkey plates. If the clinical presentation suggests the possibility of intestinal amebiasis, stool should be examined by a rapid antigen detection assay or by (less sensitive) microscopy.

TREATMENT Infectious Diarrhea or Bacterial Food Poisoning

In many cases, a specific diagnosis is not necessary or not available to guide treatment. The clinician can proceed with the information obtained from the history, stool examination, and evaluation of dehydration severity. Empirical regimens for the treatment of traveler's diarrhea are listed in Table 23-5. The mainstay of treatment is adequate rehydration. The treatment of cholera and other dehydrating diarrheal diseases was revolutionized by the promotion of oral rehydration solution (ORS), the efficacy of which depends on the fact that glucose-facilitated

absorption of sodium and water in the small intestine remains intact in the presence of cholera toxin. The use of ORS has reduced mortality rates for cholera from >50% (in untreated cases) to <1%. A number of ORS formulas have been used. Initial preparations were based on the treatment of patients with cholera and included a solution containing 3.5 g of sodium chloride, 2.5 g of sodium bicarbonate, 1.5 g of potassium chloride, and 20 g of glucose (or 40 g of sucrose) per liter of water. Such a preparation can still be used for the treatment of severe cholera. Many causes of secretory diarrhea, however, are associated with less electrolyte loss than occurs in cholera; beginning in 2002, the World Health Organization recommended a "reduced-osmolarity/reduced-salt" ORS that is better tolerated and more effective than classic ORS. This preparation contains 2.6 g of sodium chloride, 2.9 g of trisodium citrate, 1.5 g of potassium chloride,

TABLE 23-5

TREATMENT OF TRAVELER'S DIARRHEA ON THE BASIS OF CLINICAL FEATURES[a]

CLINICAL SYNDROME	SUGGESTED THERAPY
Watery diarrhea (no blood in stool, no fever), 1 or 2 unformed stools per day without distressing enteric symptoms	Oral fluids (oral rehydration solution, Pedialyte, Lytren, or flavored mineral water) and saltine crackers
Watery diarrhea (no blood in stool, no fever), 1 or 2 unformed stools per day with distressing enteric symptoms	Bismuth subsalicylate (for adults): 30 mL or 2 tablets (262 mg/tablet) every 30 min for 8 doses; or loperamide[b]: 4 mg initially followed by 2 mg after passage of each unformed stool, not to exceed 8 tablets (16 mg) per day (prescription dose) or 4 caplets (8 mg) per day (over-the-counter dose); drugs can be taken for 2 days
Watery diarrhea (no blood in stool, no distressing abdominal pain, no fever), >2 unformed stools per day	Antibacterial drug[c] plus (for adults) loperamide[b] (see dose above)
Dysentery (passage of bloody stools) or fever (>37.8°C)	Antibacterial drug[c]
Vomiting, minimal diarrhea	Bismuth subsalicylate (for adults; see dose above)
Diarrhea in infants (<2 years old)	Fluids and electrolytes (oral rehydration solution, Pedialyte, Lytren); continue feeding, especially with breast milk; seek medical attention for moderate dehydration, fever lasting >24 h, bloody stools, or diarrhea lasting more than several days

[a]All patients should take oral fluids (Pedialyte, Lytren, or flavored mineral water) plus saltine crackers. If diarrhea becomes moderate or severe, if fever persists, or if bloody stools or dehydration develops, the patient should seek medical attention.

[b]Loperamide should not be used by patients with fever or dysentery; its use may prolong diarrhea in patients with infection due to *Shigella* or other invasive organisms.

[c]The recommended antibacterial drugs are as follows:

Travel to high-risk country other than Thailand:
Adults: (1) A fluoroquinolone such as ciprofloxacin, 750 mg as a single dose or 500 mg bid for 3 days; levofloxacin, 500 mg as a single dose or 500 mg qd for 3 days; or norfloxacin, 800 mg as a single dose or 400 mg bid for 3 days. (2) Azithromycin, 1000 mg as a single dose or 500 mg qd for 3 days. (3) Rifaximin, 200 mg tid or 400 mg bid for 3 days (not recommended for use in dysentery).
Children: Azithromycin, 10 mg/kg on day 1, 5 mg/kg on days 2 and 3 if diarrhea persists. Alternative agent: furazolidone, 7.5 mg/kg per day in four divided doses for 5 days.

Travel to Thailand (with risk of fluoroquinolone-resistant *Campylobacter*):
Adults: Azithromycin (at above dose for adults). Alternative agent: a fluoroquinolone (at above doses for adults).
Children: Same as for children traveling to other areas (see above).
Source: After DR Hill et al: Clin Infect Dis 43:1499, 2006.

and 13.5 g of glucose (or 27 g of sucrose) per liter of water. ORS formulations containing rice or cereal as the carbohydrate source may be even more effective than glucose-based solutions. Patients who are severely dehydrated or in whom vomiting precludes the use of oral therapy should receive IV solutions such as Ringer's lactate.

Although most secretory forms of traveler's diarrhea (usually due to enterotoxigenic or enteroaggregative *E. coli* or to *Campylobacter*) can be treated effectively with rehydration, bismuth subsalicylate, or antiperistaltic agents, antimicrobial agents can shorten the duration of illness from 3–4 days to 24–36 h. Changes in diet have not been shown to have an impact on the duration of illness, while the efficacy of probiotics continues to be debated. Most individuals who present with dysentery (bloody diarrhea and fever) should be treated empirically with an antimicrobial agent (e.g., a fluoroquinolone or a macrolide) pending microbiologic analysis of stool. Individuals with shigellosis should be treated with a 3- to 7-day course. Individuals with *Campylobacter* infection often benefit from antimicrobial treatment as well. Because of increasing resistance of *Campylobacter* to fluoroquinolones, especially in parts of Asia, a macrolide antibiotic such as erythromycin or azithromycin may be preferred for this infection.

Treatment of salmonellosis must be tailored to the individual patient. Since administration of antimicrobial agents often prolongs intestinal colonization with *Salmonella*, these drugs are usually reserved for individuals at high risk of complications from disseminated salmonellosis, such as young children, patients with prosthetic devices, elderly patients, and immunocompromised persons. Antimicrobial agents should not be administered to individuals (especially children) in whom enterohemorrhagic *E. coli* infection is suspected. Laboratory studies of enterohemorrhagic *E. coli* strains have demonstrated that a number of antibiotics induce replication of Shiga toxin–producing lambdoid bacteriophages, thereby significantly increasing toxin production by these strains. Clinical studies have supported these laboratory results, and antibiotics may increase by twentyfold the risk of hemolytic-uremic syndrome and renal failure during enterohemorrhagic *E. coli* infection. A clinical clue in the diagnosis of the latter infection is bloody diarrhea with low fever or none at all.

PROPHYLAXIS

Improvements in hygiene to limit fecal-oral spread of enteric pathogens will be necessary if the prevalence of diarrheal diseases is to be significantly reduced in developing countries. Travelers can reduce their risk of diarrhea by eating only hot, freshly cooked food; by avoiding raw vegetables, salads, and unpeeled fruit; and by drinking only boiled or treated water and avoiding ice. Historically, few travelers to tourist destinations adhere to these dietary restrictions. Bismuth subsalicylate is an inexpensive agent for the prophylaxis of traveler's diarrhea; it is taken at a dosage of two tablets (525 mg) four times a day. Treatment appears to be effective and safe for up to 3 weeks, but adverse events such as temporary darkening of the tongue and tinnitus can occur. A meta-analysis suggests that probiotics may lessen the likelihood of traveler's diarrhea by ~15%. Prophylactic antimicrobial agents, although effective, are not generally recommended for the prevention of traveler's diarrhea except when travelers are immunosuppressed or have other underlying illnesses that place them at high risk for morbidity from gastrointestinal infection. The risk of side effects and the possibility of developing an infection with a drug-resistant organism or with more harmful, invasive bacteria make it more reasonable to institute an empirical short course of treatment if symptoms develop. If prophylaxis is indicated, the nonabsorbed antibiotic rifaximin can be considered for use in regions such as Latin America and Africa, where noninvasive *E. coli* predominates as the cause of traveler's diarrhea. Rifaximin is not effective against invasive enteropathogens.

The possibility of exerting a major impact on the worldwide morbidity and mortality associated with diarrheal diseases has led to intense efforts to develop effective vaccines against the common bacterial and viral enteric pathogens. An effective rotavirus vaccine is currently available. Vaccines against *S. typhi* and *V. cholerae* are also available, although the protection they offer is incomplete and/or short lived. At present, there is no effective commercially available vaccine against *Shigella*, enterotoxigenic *E. coli*, *Campylobacter*, nontyphoidal *Salmonella*, norovirus, or intestinal parasites.

ACKNOWLEDGMENTS

The substantial contributions of Joan R. Butterton, MD, an author of this chapter in previous editions of Harrison's Principles of Internal Medicine, are gratefully acknowledged.

CHAPTER 24

CLOSTRIDIUM DIFFICILE INFECTION, INCLUDING PSEUDOMEMBRANOUS COLITIS

Dale N. Gerding ■ Stuart Johnson

DEFINITION

Clostridium difficile infection (CDI) is a unique colonic disease that is acquired almost exclusively in association with antimicrobial use and the consequent disruption of the normal colonic flora. The most commonly diagnosed diarrheal illness acquired in the hospital, CDI results from the ingestion of spores of *C. difficile* that vegetate, multiply, and secrete toxins, causing diarrhea and pseudomembranous colitis (PMC).

ETIOLOGY AND EPIDEMIOLOGY

C. difficile is an obligately anaerobic, gram-positive, spore-forming bacillus whose spores are found widely in nature, particularly in the environment of hospitals and chronic-care facilities. CDI occurs most frequently in hospitals and nursing homes where the level of antimicrobial use is high and the environment is contaminated by *C. difficile* spores.

Clindamycin, ampicillin, and cephalosporins were the first antibiotics associated with CDI. The second- and third-generation cephalosporins, particularly cefotaxime, ceftriaxone, cefuroxime, and ceftazidime, are agents frequently responsible for this condition, and the fluoroquinolones (ciprofloxacin, levofloxacin, and moxifloxacin) are the most recent drug class to be implicated in hospital outbreaks. Penicillin/β-lactamase-inhibitor combinations such as ticarcillin/clavulanate and piperacillin/tazobactam pose significantly less risk. However, all antibiotics, including vancomycin and metronidazole (the agents most commonly used to treat CDI), have been found to carry a risk of subsequent CDI. Rare cases are reported in patients without prior antibiotic exposure.

C. difficile is acquired exogenously, most frequently in the hospital or nursing home, and is carried in the stool of symptomatic and asymptomatic patients. The rate of fecal colonization is often ≥20% among adult patients hospitalized for >1 week; in contrast, the rate is 1–3% among community residents. Community-onset CDI without recent hospitalization probably accounts for ≤10% of all cases. The risk of *C. difficile* acquisition increases in proportion to length of hospital stay. Asymptomatic fecal carriage of *C. difficile* in healthy neonates is very common, with rates often exceeding 50% during the first 6 months of life, but associated disease in this population is rare. Spores of *C. difficile* are found on environmental surfaces (where the organism can persist for months) and on the hands of hospital personnel who fail to practice good hand hygiene. Hospital epidemics of CDI have been attributed to a single *C. difficile* strain and to multiple strains present simultaneously. Other identified risk factors for CDI include older age, greater severity of underlying illness, gastrointestinal surgery, use of electronic rectal thermometers, enteral tube feeding, and antacid treatment. Use of proton pump inhibitors may be a risk factor, but this risk is probably modest, and no firm data have implicated these agents in patients who are not already receiving antibiotics.

PATHOLOGY AND PATHOGENESIS

Spores of toxigenic *C. difficile* are ingested, survive gastric acidity, germinate in the small bowel, and colonize the lower intestinal tract, where they elaborate two large toxins: toxin A (an enterotoxin) and toxin B (a cytotoxin). These toxins initiate processes resulting in the disruption of epithelial-cell barrier function, diarrhea, and pseudomembrane formation. Toxin A is a potent neutrophil chemoattractant, and both toxins glucosylate the GTP-binding proteins of the Rho subfamily that regulate the actin cell cytoskeleton. Data from studies using molecular disruption of toxin genes in isogenic mutants suggest that toxin B is the essential virulence

247

factor; this possibility, if confirmed, might account for the occurrence of clinical disease caused by toxin A–negative strains. Disruption of the cytoskeleton results in loss of cell shape, adherence, and tight junctions, with consequent fluid leakage. A third toxin, binary toxin CDT, was previously found in only ~6% of strains but is present in all isolates of the newly recognized epidemic strain (see "Global Considerations"); this toxin is related to *C. perfringens* iota toxin. Its role in the pathogenesis of CDI has not yet been defined.

The pseudomembranes of PMC are confined to the colonic mucosa and initially appear as 1- to 2-mm whitish-yellow plaques. The intervening mucosa appears unremarkable, but, as the disease progresses, the pseudomembranes coalesce to form larger plaques and become confluent over the entire colon wall (Fig. 24-1). The whole colon is usually involved, but 10% of patients have rectal sparing. Viewed microscopically, the pseudomembranes have a mucosal attachment point and contain necrotic leukocytes, fibrin, mucus, and cellular debris. The epithelium is eroded and necrotic in focal areas, with neutrophil infiltration of the mucosa.

Patients colonized with *C. difficile* were initially thought to be at high risk for CDI. However, four prospective studies have shown that colonized patients actually have a decreased risk of subsequent CDI. At least three events are proposed as essential for the

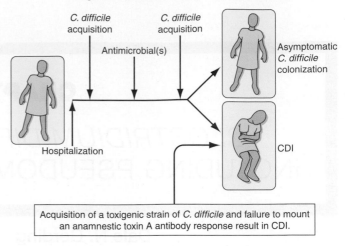

Pathogenesis model for *C. difficile* enteric disease

Acquisition of a toxigenic strain of *C. difficile* and failure to mount an anamnestic toxin A antibody response result in CDI.

FIGURE 24-2

Pathogenesis model for hospital-acquired *Clostridium difficile* infection (CDI). At least three events are integral to *C. difficile* pathogenesis. Exposure to antibiotics establishes susceptibility to infection. Once susceptible, the patient may acquire nontoxigenic (nonpathogenic) or toxigenic strains of *C. difficile* as a second event. Acquisition of toxigenic *C. difficile* may be followed by asymptomatic colonization or CDI, depending on one or more additional events, including an inadequate host anamnestic IgG response to *C. difficile* toxin A.

FIGURE 24-1

Autopsy specimen showing confluent pseudomembranes covering the cecum of a patient with pseudomembranous colitis. Note the sparing of the terminal ileum (*arrow*).

development of CDI (Fig. 24-2). Exposure to antimicrobial agents is the first event and establishes susceptibility to *C. difficile* infection. The second event is exposure to toxigenic *C. difficile*. Given that the majority of patients do not develop CDI after the first two events, a third event is clearly essential for its occurrence. Candidate third events include exposure to a *C. difficile* strain of particular virulence, exposure to antimicrobial agents especially likely to cause CDI, and an inadequate host immune response. The host anamnestic serum IgG antibody response to toxin A of *C. difficile* is the most likely third event that determines which patients develop diarrhea and which patients remain asymptomatic. The majority of humans first develop antibody to *C. difficile* toxins when colonized asymptomatically during the first year of life. Infants are thought not to develop symptomatic CDI because they lack suitable mucosal toxin receptors that develop later in life. In adulthood, serum levels of IgG antibody to toxin A increase more in response to infection in individuals who become asymptomatic carriers than in those who develop CDI. For persons who develop CDI, increasing levels of antitoxin A during treatment correlate with a lower risk of recurrence of CDI. A clinical trial using monoclonal antibodies to both toxin A and toxin B in addition to standard therapy showed rates of recurrence lower than those obtained with placebo plus standard therapy.

GLOBAL CONSIDERATIONS

 Rates and severity of CDI in the United States, Canada, and Europe have increased markedly since the year 2000. Rates in U.S. hospitals tripled between 2000 and 2005. Hospitals in Montreal, Quebec, have reported rates four times higher than the 1997 baseline, with directly attributable mortality of 6.9% (increased from 1.5%). An epidemic strain, variously known as toxinotype III, REA type BI, PCR ribotype 027, and pulsed-field type NAP1, is thought to account for much of the increase in incidence and has been found in North America, Europe, and Asia. The epidemic organism is characterized by (1) an ability to produce 16–23 times as much toxin A and toxin B as control strains in vitro; (2) the presence of a third toxin (binary toxin CDT); and (3) high-level resistance to all fluoroquinolones. New strains have been and will probably continue to be implicated in outbreaks; their emergence may be explained in part by patterns of antibiotic use, particularly in hospitals.

CLINICAL MANIFESTATIONS

Diarrhea is the most common manifestation caused by *C. difficile*. Stools are almost never grossly bloody and range from soft and unformed to watery or mucoid in consistency, with a characteristic odor. Patients may have as many as 20 bowel movements per day. Clinical and laboratory findings include fever in 28% of cases, abdominal pain in 22%, and leukocytosis in 50%. When adynamic ileus (which is seen on x-ray in ~20% of cases) results in cessation of stool passage, the diagnosis of CDI is frequently overlooked. A clue to the presence of unsuspected CDI in these patients is unexplained leukocytosis, with ≥15,000 white blood cells (WBCs)/μL. Such patients are at high risk for complications of *C. difficile* infection, particularly toxic megacolon and sepsis.

C. difficile diarrhea recurs after treatment in ~15–30% of cases, and this figure may be increasing. Recurrences may represent either relapses due to the same strain or reinfections with a new strain. Susceptibility to recurrence of clinical CDI is likely a result of continued disruption of the normal fecal flora caused by the antibiotic used to treat CDI.

DIAGNOSIS

The diagnosis of CDI is based on a combination of clinical criteria: (1) diarrhea (≥3 unformed stools per 24 h for ≥2 days) with no other recognized cause plus (2) toxin A or B detected in the stool, toxin-producing *C. difficile* detected in the stool by polymerase chain reaction (PCR) or culture, or pseudomembranes seen in the colon. PMC is a more advanced form of CDI and is visualized at endoscopy in only ~50% of patients with diarrhea who have a positive stool culture and toxin assay for *C. difficile* (Table 24-1). Endoscopy is a rapid

TABLE 24-1

RELATIVE SENSITIVITY AND SPECIFICITY OF DIAGNOSTIC TESTS FOR *CLOSTRIDIUM DIFFICILE* INFECTION (CDI)

TYPE OF TEST	RELATIVE SENSITIVITY[a]	RELATIVE SPECIFICITY[a]	COMMENT
Stool culture for *C. difficile*	++++	+++	Most sensitive test; specificity of ++++ if the *C. difficile* isolate tests positive for toxin; with clinical data, is diagnostic of CDI; turnaround time too slow for practical use
Cell culture cytotoxin test on stool	+++	++++	With clinical data, is diagnostic of CDI; highly specific but not as sensitive as stool culture; slow turnaround time
Enzyme immunoassay for toxin A or toxins A and B in stool	++ to +++	+++	With clinical data, is diagnostic of CDI; rapid results, but not as sensitive as stool culture or cell culture cytotoxin test
Enzyme immunoassay for *C. difficile* common antigen in stool	+++ to ++++	+++	Detects glutamate dehydrogenase found in toxigenic and nontoxigenic strains of *C. difficile* and other stool organisms; more sensitive and less specific than enzyme immunoassay for toxins; rapid results
PCR for *C. difficile* toxin B gene in stool	++++	++++	Detects toxigenic *C. difficile* in stool; newly approved for clinical testing, but appears to be more sensitive than enzyme immunoassay toxin testing and at least as specific
Colonoscopy or sigmoidoscopy	+	++++	Highly specific if pseudomembranes are seen; insensitive compared with other tests

[a]According to both clinical and test-based criteria.
Note: ++++, >90%; +++, 71–90%; ++, 51–70%; +, ~50%.

diagnostic tool in seriously ill patients with suspected PMC and an acute abdomen, but a negative result in this examination does not rule out CDI.

Despite the array of tests available for *C. difficile* and its toxins (Table 24-1), no single test has high sensitivity, high specificity, and rapid turnaround. Most laboratory tests for toxins, including enzyme immunoassays (EIAs), lack sensitivity. However, testing of multiple additional stool specimens is not recommended. PCR assays have now been approved for diagnostic testing and appear to be both rapid and sensitive while retaining high specificity. Empirical treatment is appropriate if CDI is strongly suspected on clinical grounds. Testing of asymptomatic patients is not recommended except for epidemiologic study purposes. In particular, so-called tests of cure following treatment are not recommended because many patients continue to harbor the organism and toxin after diarrhea has ceased and test results do not always predict recurrence of CDI. Thus these results should not be used to restrict placement of patients in long-term-care or nursing home facilities.

TREATMENT ▷ *Clostridium difficile* Infection

PRIMARY CDI When possible, discontinuation of any ongoing antimicrobial administration is recommended as the first step in treatment of CDI. Earlier studies indicated that 15–23% of patients respond to this simple measure. However, with the advent of the current epidemic strain and the associated rapid clinical deterioration of some patients, prompt initiation of specific CDI treatment has become the standard. General treatment guidelines include hydration and the avoidance of antiperistaltic agents and opiates, which may mask symptoms and possibly worsen disease. Nevertheless, antiperistaltic agents have been used safely with vancomycin or metronidazole for mild to moderate CDI.

All drugs, particularly vancomycin, should be given orally if possible. When IV metronidazole is administered, fecal bactericidal drug concentrations are achieved during acute diarrhea, and CDI treatment has been successful; however, in the presence of adynamic ileus, IV metronidazole treatment of PMC has failed. In previous randomized trials, diarrhea response rates to oral therapy with vancomycin or metronidazole were ≥94%, but four recent observational studies found that response rates for metronidazole had declined to 62–78%. Although the mean time to resolution of diarrhea is 2–4 days, the response to metronidazole may be much slower. Treatment should not be deemed a failure until a drug has been given for at least 6 days. On the basis of data for shorter courses of vancomycin, it is recommended that metronidazole and vancomycin be given for at least 10 days, although no controlled comparisons are available. Metronidazole is not approved for this indication by the U.S. Food and Drug Administration (FDA), but most patients with mild to moderate illness respond to 500 mg given by mouth three times a day for 10 days; extension of the treatment period may be needed for slow responders. In addition to the reports of increases in metronidazole failures, a prospective, randomized, double-blind, placebo-controlled study has demonstrated the superiority of vancomycin over metronidazole for treatment of severe CDI. The severity assessment score in that study included age as well as laboratory parameters (elevated temperature, low albumin level, or elevated WBC count), documentation of PMC by endoscopy, or treatment of CDI in the intensive care unit. Although a validated severity score is not yet available, it is important to initiate treatment with oral vancomycin for patients who appear seriously ill, particularly if they have a high WBC count (>15,000/µL) or a creatinine level that is ≥1.5 times higher than the premorbid value (Table 24-2). Small randomized trials of nitazoxanide, bacitracin, rifaximin, and fusidic acid for treatment of CDI have been conducted. While these drugs have not yet been extensively studied, shown to be superior, or approved by the FDA for this indication, they provide potential alternatives to vancomycin and metronidazole.

RECURRENT CDI Overall, ~15–30% of patients experience recurrences of CDI, either as relapses caused by the original organism or as reinfections following treatment. Recurrence rates are higher among patients ≥65 years old, those who continue to take antibiotics while being treated for CDI, and those who remain in the hospital after the initial episode of CDI. Patients who have a first recurrence of CDI have a high rate of second recurrence (33–65%). In the first recurrence, re-treatment with metronidazole is comparable to treatment with vancomycin (Table 24-2). Recurrent disease, once thought to be relatively mild, has now been documented to pose a significant (11%) risk of serious complications (shock, megacolon, perforation, colectomy, or death within 30 days). There is no standard treatment for multiple recurrences, but long or repeated metronidazole courses should be avoided because of potential neurotoxicity. Approaches include the administration of vancomycin followed by the yeast *Saccharomyces boulardii*; the administration of vancomycin followed by a synthetic fecal bacterial enema; and the intentional colonization of the patient with a nontoxigenic strain of *C. difficile*. None of these biotherapeutic approaches has been approved by the FDA for use in the United States. Other strategies include (1) the use of vancomycin in tapering doses or with pulse dosing every other day for 2–8 weeks and (2) sequential treatment with vancomycin (125 mg four times daily for

TABLE 24-2

RECOMMENDATIONS FOR THE TREATMENT OF *CLOSTRIDIUM DIFFICILE* INFECTION (CDI)

CLINICAL SETTING	TREATMENT(S)	COMMENTS
Initial episode, mild to moderate	Oral metronidazole (500 mg tid × 10–14 d)	
Initial episode, severe	Oral vancomycin (125 mg qid × 10–14 d)	Indicators of severe disease may include leukocytosis (≥15,000 white blood cells/μL) and a creatinine level ≥1.5 times the premorbid value.
Initial episode, severe complicated or fulminant	Vancomycin (500 mg PO or via nasogastric tube) plus metronidazole (500 mg IV q8h) *plus consider* Rectal instillation of vancomycin (500 mg in 100 mL of normal saline as a retention enema q6–8h)	Severe complicated or fulminant CDI is defined as severe CDI with the addition of hypotension, shock, ileus, or toxic megacolon. The duration of treatment may need to be >2 weeks and is dictated by response. Consider using IV tigecycline (50 mg q12h after a 100-mg loading dose) in place of metronidazole.
First recurrence	Same as for initial episode	
Second recurrence	Vancomycin in tapered/pulsed regimen	Typical taper/pulse regimen: 125 mg qid ×10–14 d, then bid × 1 week, then daily × 1 week, then q2–3d for 2–8 weeks
Multiple recurrences	Consider the following options: • Repeat vancomycin taper/pulse • Vancomycin (500 mg qid × 10 d) plus *Saccharomyces boulardii* (500 mg bid × 28 d) • Vancomycin (125 mg qid × 10–14 d); then stop vancomycin and start rifaximin (400 mg bid × 2 weeks) • Nitazoxanide (500 mg bid × 10 d) • Fecal transplantation • IV immunoglobulin (400 mg/kg)	The only controlled study of treatment for recurrent CDI used *S. boulardii* and showed borderline significance compared with placebo.

10–14 days) followed by rifaximin (400 mg twice daily for 14 days). IV immunoglobulin, which has also been used with some success, presumably provides antibodies to *C. difficile* toxins.

SEVERE COMPLICATED OR FULMINANT CDI Fulminant (rapidly progressive and severe) CDI presents the most difficult treatment challenge. Patients with fulminant disease often do not have diarrhea, and their illness mimics an acute surgical abdomen. Sepsis (hypotension, fever, tachycardia, leukocytosis) may result from severe CDI. An acute abdomen (with or without toxic megacolon) may include signs of obstruction, ileus, colon-wall thickening, and ascites on abdominal CT, often with peripheral-blood leukocytosis (≥20,000 WBCs/μL). With or without diarrhea, the differential diagnosis of an acute abdomen, sepsis, or toxic megacolon should include CDI if the patient has received antibiotics in the past 2 months. Cautious sigmoidoscopy or colonoscopy to visualize PMC and an abdominal CT examination are the best diagnostic tests in patients without diarrhea.

Medical management of fulminant CDI is suboptimal because of the difficulty of delivering metronidazole or vancomycin to the colon by the oral route in the presence of ileus (Table 24-2). The combination of vancomycin (given via nasogastric tube and by retention enema) plus IV metronidazole has been used with some success in uncontrolled studies, as has IV tigecycline in small-scale uncontrolled studies. Surgical colectomy may be life-saving if there is no response to medical management. If possible, colectomy should be performed before the serum lactate level reaches 5 mmol/L. The incidence of fulminant CDI requiring colectomy appears to be increasing in the evolving epidemic.

PROGNOSIS

The mortality rate attributed to CDI, previously found to be 0.6–3.5%, has reached 6.9% in recent outbreaks and is progressively higher with increasing age. Most patients recover, but recurrences are common.

PREVENTION AND CONTROL

Strategies for the prevention of CDI are of two types: those aimed at preventing transmission of the organism to the patient and those aimed at reducing the risk of CDI if the organism is transmitted. Transmission of *C. difficile* in clinical practice has been prevented by gloving of personnel, elimination of the use of contaminated electronic thermometers, and use of hypochlorite (bleach) solution for environmental decontamination of patients' rooms. Hand hygiene is critical; hand washing is recommended in CDI outbreaks because alcohol hand gels are not sporicidal. CDI outbreaks have been best controlled by restricting the use of specific antibiotics, such as clindamycin and second- and third-generation cephalosporins. Outbreaks of CDI due to clindamycin-resistant strains have resolved promptly when clindamycin use is restricted.

CHAPTER 25

INTRAABDOMINAL INFECTIONS
AND ABSCESSES

Miriam J. Baron ■ Dennis L. Kasper

Intraperitoneal infections generally arise because a normal anatomic barrier is disrupted. This disruption may occur when the appendix, a diverticulum, or an ulcer ruptures; when the bowel wall is weakened by ischemia, tumor, or inflammation (e.g., in inflammatory bowel disease); or with adjacent inflammatory processes, such as pancreatitis or pelvic inflammatory disease, in which enzymes (in the former case) or organisms (in the latter) may leak into the peritoneal cavity. Whatever the inciting event, once inflammation develops and organisms usually contained within the bowel or another organ enter the normally sterile peritoneal space, a predictable series of events takes place. Intraabdominal infections occur in two stages: peritonitis and—if the patient survives this stage and goes untreated—abscess formation. The types of microorganisms predominating in each stage of infection are responsible for the pathogenesis of disease.

PERITONITIS

Peritonitis is a life-threatening event that is often accompanied by bacteremia and sepsis syndrome. The peritoneal cavity is large but is divided into compartments. The upper and lower peritoneal cavities are divided by the transverse mesocolon; the greater omentum extends from the transverse mesocolon and from the lower pole of the stomach to line the lower peritoneal cavity. The pancreas, duodenum, and ascending and descending colon are located in the anterior retroperitoneal space; the kidneys, ureters, and adrenals are found in the posterior retroperitoneal space. The other organs, including liver, stomach, gallbladder, spleen, jejunum, ileum, transverse and sigmoid colon, cecum, and appendix, are within the peritoneal cavity. The cavity is lined with a serous membrane that can serve as

a conduit for fluids—a property exploited in peritoneal dialysis (Fig. 25-1). A small amount of serous fluid is normally present in the peritoneal space, with a protein content (consisting mainly of albumin) of <30 g/L and <300 white blood cells (WBCs, generally mononuclear cells) per microliter. In bacterial infections, leukocyte recruitment into the infected peritoneal cavity consists of an early influx of polymorphonuclear leukocytes (PMNs) and a prolonged subsequent phase of mononuclear cell migration. The phenotype of the infiltrating leukocytes during the course of inflammation is regulated primarily by resident-cell chemokine synthesis.

PRIMARY (SPONTANEOUS) BACTERIAL PERITONITIS

Peritonitis is either primary (without an apparent source of contamination) or secondary. The types of organisms found and the clinical presentations of these two processes are different. In adults, primary bacterial peritonitis (PBP) occurs most commonly in conjunction with cirrhosis of the liver (frequently the result of alcoholism). However, the disease has been reported in adults with metastatic malignant disease, postnecrotic cirrhosis, chronic active hepatitis, acute viral hepatitis, congestive heart failure, systemic lupus erythematosus, and lymphedema as well as in patients with no underlying disease. Although PBP virtually always develops in patients with preexisting ascites, it is, in general, an uncommon event, occurring in ≤10% of cirrhotic patients. The cause of PBP has not been established definitively but is believed to involve hematogenous spread of organisms in a patient in whom a diseased liver and altered portal circulation result in a defect in the usual filtration function. Organisms multiply in ascites, a good medium for growth. The proteins of the complement cascade have been found in peritoneal fluid, with lower

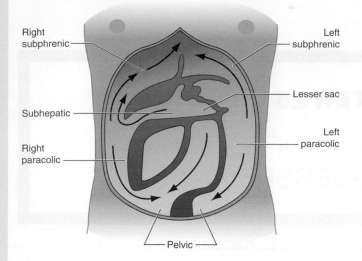

FIGURE 25-1

Diagram of the intraperitoneal spaces, showing the circulation of fluid and potential areas for abscess formation. Some compartments collect fluid or pus more often than others. These compartments include the pelvis (the lowest portion), the subphrenic spaces on the right and left sides, and Morrison's pouch, which is a posterosuperior extension of the subhepatic spaces and is the lowest part of the paravertebral groove when a patient is recumbent. The falciform ligament separating the right and left subphrenic spaces appears to act as a barrier to the spread of infection; consequently, it is unusual to find bilateral subphrenic collections. (*Reprinted with permission from B Lorber [ed]: Atlas of Infectious Diseases, vol VII: Intra-abdominal Infections, Hepatitis, and Gastroenteritis. Philadelphia, Current Medicine, 1996, p 1.13.*)

levels in cirrhotic patients than in patients with ascites of other etiologies. The opsonic and phagocytic properties of PMNs are diminished in patients with advanced liver disease.

The presentation of PBP differs from that of secondary peritonitis. The most common manifestation is fever, which is reported in up to 80% of patients. Ascites is found but virtually always predates infection. Abdominal pain, an acute onset of symptoms, and peritoneal irritation during physical examination can be helpful diagnostically, but the absence of any of these findings does not exclude this often-subtle diagnosis. Nonlocalizing symptoms (such as malaise, fatigue, or encephalopathy) without another clear etiology should also prompt consideration of PBP in a susceptible patient. It is vital to sample the peritoneal fluid of any cirrhotic patient with ascites and fever. The finding of >250 PMNs/μL is diagnostic for PBP, according to Conn (*http://jac.oxfordjournals.org/cgi/content/full/47/3/369*). This criterion does not apply to secondary peritonitis (see later in the chapter). The microbiology of PBP is also distinctive.

While enteric gram-negative bacilli such as *Escherichia coli* are most commonly encountered, gram-positive organisms such as streptococci, enterococci, or even pneumococci are sometimes found. In PBP, a single organism is typically isolated; anaerobes are found less frequently in PBP than in secondary peritonitis, in which a mixed flora including anaerobes is the rule. In fact, if PBP is suspected and multiple organisms including anaerobes are recovered from the peritoneal fluid, the diagnosis must be reconsidered and a source of secondary peritonitis sought.

The diagnosis of PBP is not easy. It depends on the exclusion of a primary intraabdominal source of infection. Contrast-enhanced CT is useful in identifying an intraabdominal source for infection. It may be difficult to recover organisms from cultures of peritoneal fluid, presumably because the burden of organisms is low. However, the yield can be improved if 10 mL of peritoneal fluid is placed directly into a blood culture bottle. Since bacteremia frequently accompanies PBP, blood should be cultured simultaneously. No specific radiographic studies are helpful in the diagnosis of PBP. A plain film of the abdomen would be expected to show ascites. Chest and abdominal radiography should be performed in patients with abdominal pain to exclude free air, which signals a perforation **(Fig. 25-2)**.

FIGURE 25-2

Pneumoperitoneum. Free air under the diaphragm on an upright chest film suggests the presence of a bowel perforation and associated peritonitis. (*Image courtesy of Dr. John Braver; with permission.*)

TREATMENT   Primary Bacterial Peritonitis

Treatment for PBP is directed at the isolate from blood or peritoneal fluid. Gram's staining of peritoneal fluid often gives negative results in PBP. Therefore, until culture results become available, therapy should cover gram-negative aerobic bacilli and gram-positive cocci. Third-generation cephalosporins such as cefotaxime (2 g q8h, administered IV) provide reasonable initial coverage in moderately ill patients. Broad-spectrum antibiotics, such as penicillin/β-lactamase inhibitor combinations (e.g., piperacillin/tazobactam, 3.375 g q6h IV for adults with normal renal function) or ceftriaxone (2 g q24h IV), are also options. Empirical coverage for anaerobes is not necessary. After the infecting organism is identified, therapy should be narrowed to target the specific pathogen. Patients with PBP usually respond within 72 h to appropriate antibiotic therapy. Antimicrobial treatment can be administered for as little as 5 days if rapid improvement occurs and blood cultures are negative, but a course of up to 2 weeks may be required for patients with bacteremia and for those whose improvement is slow. Persistence of WBCs in the ascitic fluid after therapy should prompt a search for additional diagnoses.

Prevention

Primary prevention

One observational study raises the concern that proton pump inhibitor (PPI) therapy may increase the risk of PBP. No prospective studies have yet addressed whether avoidance of PPI therapy may prevent PBP.

Secondary prevention

PBP has a high rate of recurrence. Up to 70% of patients experience a recurrence within 1 year. Antibiotic prophylaxis reduces this rate to <20% and improves short-term survival rates. Prophylactic regimens for adults with normal renal function include fluoroquinolones (ciprofloxacin, 750 mg weekly; norfloxacin, 400 mg/d) or trimethoprim-sulfamethoxazole (one double-strength tablet daily). However, long-term administration of broad-spectrum antibiotics in this setting has been shown to increase the risk of severe staphylococcal infections.

SECONDARY PERITONITIS

Secondary peritonitis develops when bacteria contaminate the peritoneum as a result of spillage from an intraabdominal viscus. The organisms found almost always constitute a mixed flora in which facultative gram-negative bacilli and anaerobes predominate, especially when the contaminating source is colonic. Early in the course of infection, when the host response is directed toward containment of the infection, exudate containing fibrin and PMNs is found. Early death in this setting is attributable to gram-negative bacillary sepsis and to potent endotoxins circulating in the bloodstream. Gram-negative bacilli, particularly *E. coli*, are common bloodstream isolates, but *Bacteroides fragilis* bacteremia also occurs. The severity of abdominal pain and the clinical course depend on the inciting process. The organisms isolated from the peritoneum also vary with the source of the initial process and the normal flora at that site. Secondary peritonitis can result primarily from chemical irritation and/or bacterial contamination. For example, as long as the patient is not achlorhydric, a ruptured gastric ulcer will release low-pH gastric contents that will serve as a chemical irritant. The normal flora of the stomach comprises the same organisms found in the oropharynx but in lower numbers. Thus, the bacterial burden in a ruptured ulcer is negligible compared with that in a ruptured appendix. The normal flora of the colon below the ligament of Treitz contains ~10^{11} anaerobic organisms/g of feces but only 10^8 aerobes/g; therefore, anaerobic species account for 99.9% of the bacteria. Leakage of colonic contents (pH 7–8) does not cause significant chemical peritonitis, but infection is intense because of the heavy bacterial load.

Depending on the inciting event, local symptoms may occur in secondary peritonitis—for example, epigastric pain from a ruptured gastric ulcer. In appendicitis (Chap. 22), the initial presenting symptoms are often vague, with periumbilical discomfort and nausea followed in a number of hours by pain more localized to the right lower quadrant. Unusual locations of the appendix (including a retrocecal position) can complicate this presentation further. Once infection has spread to the peritoneal cavity, pain increases, particularly with infection involving the parietal peritoneum, which is innervated extensively. Patients usually lie motionless, often with knees drawn up to avoid stretching the nerve fibers of the peritoneal cavity. Coughing and sneezing, which increase pressure within the peritoneal cavity, are associated with sharp pain. There may or may not be pain localized to the infected or diseased organ from which secondary peritonitis has arisen. Patients with secondary peritonitis generally have abnormal findings on abdominal examination, with marked voluntary and involuntary guarding of the anterior abdominal musculature. Later findings include tenderness, especially rebound tenderness. In addition, there may be localized findings in the area of the inciting event. In general, patients are febrile, with marked leukocytosis and a left shift of the WBCs to band forms.

While recovery of organisms from peritoneal fluid is easier in secondary than in primary peritonitis, a tap of the abdomen is rarely the procedure of choice in secondary peritonitis. An exception is in cases involving trauma, where the possibility of a hemoperitoneum may need to be excluded early. Emergent studies (such as abdominal CT) to find the source of peritoneal contamination should be undertaken if the patient is hemodynamically stable; unstable patients may require surgical intervention without prior imaging.

TREATMENT   Secondary Peritonitis

Treatment for secondary peritonitis includes early administration of antibiotics aimed particularly at aerobic gram-negative bacilli and anaerobes (discussed later). Mild to moderate disease can be treated with many drugs covering these organisms, including broad-spectrum penicillin/β-lactamase inhibitor combinations (e.g., ticarcillin/clavulanate, 3.1 g q4–6h IV), cefoxitin (2 g q4–6h IV), or a combination of a fluoroquinolone (e.g., levofloxacin, 750 mg q24h IV) or a third-generation cephalosporin (e.g., ceftriaxone, 2 g q24h IV) plus metronidazole (500 mg q8h IV). Patients in intensive care units should receive imipenem (500 mg q6h IV), meropenem (1 g q8h IV), or combinations of drugs, such as ampicillin plus metronidazole plus ciprofloxacin. The role of enterococci and *Candida* spp. in mixed infections is controversial. Secondary peritonitis usually requires both surgical intervention to address the inciting process and antibiotics to treat early bacteremia, to decrease the incidence of abscess formation and wound infection, and to prevent distant spread of infection. While surgery is rarely indicated in PBP in adults, it may be life-saving in secondary peritonitis. Recombinant human activated protein C has been shown to reduce mortality rates among patients with severe sepsis and may benefit some patients with secondary peritonitis.

Peritonitis may develop as a complication of abdominal surgeries. These infections may be accompanied by localizing pain and/or nonlocalizing symptoms such as fever, malaise, anorexia, and toxicity. As a nosocomial infection, postoperative peritonitis may be associated with organisms such as staphylococci, components of the gram-negative hospital microflora, and the microbes that cause PBP and secondary peritonitis, as described earlier.

PERITONITIS IN PATIENTS UNDERGOING CAPD

A third type of peritonitis arises in patients who are undergoing continuous ambulatory peritoneal dialysis (CAPD). Unlike PBP and secondary peritonitis, which are caused by endogenous bacteria, CAPD-associated peritonitis usually involves skin organisms. The pathogenesis of infection is similar to that of intravascular device–related infection, in which skin organisms migrate along the catheter, which both serves as an entry point and exerts the effects of a foreign body. Exit-site or tunnel infection may or may not accompany CAPD-associated peritonitis. Like PBP, CAPD-associated peritonitis is usually caused by a single organism. Peritonitis is, in fact, the most common reason for discontinuation of CAPD. Improvements in equipment design, especially the Y-set connector, have resulted in a decrease from one case of peritonitis per 9 months of CAPD to one case per 24 months.

The clinical presentation of CAPD peritonitis resembles that of secondary peritonitis in that diffuse pain and peritoneal signs are common. The dialysate is usually cloudy and contains >100 WBCs/μL, >50% of which are neutrophils. The most common organisms are *Staphylococcus* spp., which accounted for ~45% of cases in one series. Historically, coagulase-negative staphylococcal species were identified most commonly in these infections, but more recently these isolates have been decreasing in frequency. *Staphylococcus aureus* is more often involved among patients who are nasal carriers of the organism than among those who are not, and this organism is the most common pathogen in overt exit-site infections. Gram-negative bacilli and fungi such as *Candida* spp. are also found. Vancomycin-resistant enterococci and vancomycin-intermediate *S. aureus* have been reported to produce peritonitis in CAPD patients. The finding of more than one organism in dialysate culture should prompt evaluation for secondary peritonitis. As with PBP, culture of dialysate fluid in blood culture bottles improves the yield. To facilitate diagnosis, several hundred milliliters of removed dialysis fluid should be concentrated by centrifugation before culture.

TREATMENT   CAPD Peritonitis

Empirical therapy for CAPD peritonitis should be directed at *S. aureus*, coagulase-negative *Staphylococcus*, and gram-negative bacilli until the results of cultures are available. Guidelines issued in 2005 suggest that agents should be chosen on the basis of local experience with resistant organisms. In some centers, a first-generation cephalosporin such as cefazolin (for gram-positive bacteria) and a fluoroquinolone or a third-generation cephalosporin such as ceftazidime (for gram-negative bacteria) may be reasonable; in areas with high rates of infection with methicillin-resistant *S. aureus*, vancomycin should be used instead of cefazolin, and gram-negative coverage may need to be broadened. Broad coverage including vancomycin should be particularly considered for toxic patients and for those with exit-site infections. Loading doses are administered intraperitoneally; doses depend on the dialysis method and the patient's renal function. Antibiotics are given either continuously (i.e., with each exchange) or intermittently (i.e., once daily, with the dose allowed to remain in the peritoneal cavity for at least 6 h). If the patient is severely ill, IV antibiotics should be added at doses appropriate for the patient's degree of renal failure. The clinical response to an empirical treatment regimen should be rapid; if the patient has not responded after 48–96 h of treatment, catheter removal should be considered.

TUBERCULOUS PERITONITIS

Tuberculous peritonitis follows either the direct spread of the organism from ruptured lymph nodes and intraabdominal organs or hematogenous seeding. The coexistence of cirrhosis complicates the diagnosis. In tuberculous peritonitis, paracentesis reveals an exudate with high protein content and lymphocytic leukocytosis. Smear and culture are generally low yield but peritoneal biopsy often establishes the diagnosis with typical caseating granulomas and positive acid-fast stain.

INTRAABDOMINAL ABSCESSES

INTRAPERITONEAL ABSCESSES

Abscess formation is common in untreated peritonitis if overt gram-negative sepsis either does not develop or develops but is not fatal. In experimental models of abscess formation, mixed aerobic and anaerobic organisms have been implanted intraperitoneally. Without therapy directed at anaerobes, animals develop intraabdominal abscesses. As in humans, these experimental abscesses may stud the peritoneal cavity, lie within the omentum or mesentery, or even develop on the surface of or within viscera such as the liver.

Pathogenesis and immunity

There is often disagreement about whether an abscess represents a disease state or a host response. In a sense, it represents both: while an abscess is an infection in which viable infecting organisms and PMNs are contained in a fibrous capsule, it is also a process by which the host confines microbes to a limited space, thereby preventing further spread of infection. In any event, abscesses do cause significant symptoms, and patients with abscesses can be quite ill. Experimental work has helped to define both the host cells and the bacterial virulence factors responsible—most notably in the case of *B. fragilis*. This organism, although accounting for only 0.5% of the normal colonic flora, is the anaerobe most frequently isolated from intraabdominal infections, is especially prominent in abscesses, and is the most common anaerobic bloodstream isolate. On clinical grounds, therefore, *B. fragilis* appears to be uniquely

virulent. Moreover, *B. fragilis* acts alone to cause abscesses in animal models of intraabdominal infection, whereas most other *Bacteroides* species must act synergistically with a facultative organism to induce abscess formation.

Of the several virulence factors identified in *B. fragilis*, one is critical: the capsular polysaccharide complex (CPC) found on the bacterial surface. The CPC comprises at least eight distinct surface polysaccharides. Structural analysis of these polysaccharides has shown an unusual motif of oppositely charged sugars. Polysaccharides having these *zwitterionic* characteristics, such as polysaccharide A (PSA), evoke a host response in the peritoneal cavity that localizes bacteria into abscesses. *B. fragilis* and PSA have been found to adhere to primary mesothelial cells in vitro; this adherence, in turn, stimulates the production of tumor necrosis factor α (TNF-α) and intercellular adhesion molecule 1 (ICAM-1) by peritoneal macrophages. Although abscesses characteristically contain PMNs, the process of abscess induction depends on the stimulation of T lymphocytes by these unique zwitterionic polysaccharides. The stimulated CD4+ T lymphocytes secrete leukoattractant cytokines and chemokines. The alternative pathway of complement and fibrinogen also participate in abscess formation.

While antibodies to the CPC enhance bloodstream clearance of *B. fragilis*, CD4+ T cells are critical in immunity to abscesses. When administered subcutaneously, *B. fragilis* PSA has immunomodulatory characteristics and stimulates CD4+ T regulatory cells via an interleukin (IL) 2–dependent mechanism to produce IL-10. IL-10 downregulates the inflammatory response, thereby preventing abscess formation.

Clinical presentation

Of all intraabdominal abscesses, 74% are intraperitoneal or retroperitoneal and are not visceral. Most intraperitoneal abscesses result from fecal spillage from a colonic source, such as an inflamed appendix. Abscesses can also arise from other processes. They usually form within weeks of the development of peritonitis and may be found in a variety of locations—from omentum to mesentery, pelvis to psoas muscles, and subphrenic space to a visceral organ such as the liver, where they may develop either on the surface of the organ or within it. Periappendiceal and diverticular abscesses occur commonly. Diverticular abscesses are least likely to rupture. Infections of the female genital tract and pancreatitis are also among the more common causative events. When abscesses occur in the female genital tract—either as a primary infection (e.g., tuboovarian abscess) or as an infection extending into the pelvic cavity or peritoneum—*B. fragilis* figures prominently among the organisms isolated. *B. fragilis* is not found in large numbers in the normal vaginal flora. For example, it is encountered less commonly in pelvic

258

inflammatory disease and endometritis without an associated abscess. In pancreatitis with leakage of damaging pancreatic enzymes, inflammation is prominent. Therefore, clinical findings such as fever, leukocytosis, and even abdominal pain do not distinguish pancreatitis itself from complications such as pancreatic pseudocyst, pancreatic abscess (Chap. 48), or intraabdominal collections of pus. Especially in cases of necrotizing pancreatitis, in which the incidence of local pancreatic infection may be as high as 30%, needle aspiration under CT guidance is performed to sample fluid for culture. Many centers prescribe preemptive antibiotics for patients with necrotizing pancreatitis. Imipenem is frequently used for this purpose since it reaches high tissue levels in the pancreas (although it is not unique in this regard). If needle aspiration yields infected fluid in the setting of acute necrotizing pancreatitis, most experts agree that surgery is superior to percutaneous drainage. Infected pseudocysts that occur remotely from acute pancreatitis are unlikely to be associated with significant amounts of necrotic tissue and may be treated with either surgical or percutaneous catheter drainage in conjunction with appropriate antibiotic therapy.

Diagnosis

Scanning procedures have considerably facilitated the diagnosis of intraabdominal abscesses. Abdominal CT probably has the highest yield, although ultrasonography is particularly useful for the right upper quadrant, kidneys, and pelvis. Both indium-labeled WBCs and gallium tend to localize in abscesses and may be useful in finding a collection. Since gallium is taken up in the bowel, indium-labeled WBCs may have a slightly greater yield for abscesses near the bowel. Neither indium-labeled WBC nor gallium scans serve as a basis for a definitive diagnosis, however; both need to be followed by other, more specific studies, such as CT, if an area of possible abnormality is identified. Abscesses contiguous with or contained within diverticula are particularly difficult to diagnose with scanning procedures. Occasionally, a barium enema may detect a diverticular abscess not diagnosed by other procedures, although barium should not be injected if a perforation is suspected. If one study is negative, a second study sometimes reveals a collection. Although exploratory laparotomy has been less commonly used since the advent of CT, this procedure still must be undertaken on occasion if an abscess is strongly suspected on clinical grounds.

> **TREATMENT** Intraperitoneal Abscesses

An algorithm for the management of patients with intraabdominal (including intraperitoneal) abscesses is presented in **Fig. 25-3**. The treatment of intraabdominal

FIGURE 25-3
Algorithm for the management of patients with intraabdominal abscesses using percutaneous drainage. Antimicrobial therapy should be administered concomitantly. (*Reprinted with permission from B Lorber [ed]: Atlas of Infectious Diseases, vol VII: Intra-abdominal Infections, Hepatitis, and Gastroenteritis. Philadelphia, Current Medicine, 1996, p 1.30, as adapted from OD Rotstein, RL Simmons, in SL Gorbach et al [eds]: Infectious Diseases. Philadelphia, Saunders, 1992, p 668.*)

infections involves the determination of the initial focus of infection, the administration of broad-spectrum antibiotics targeting the organisms involved, and the performance of a drainage procedure if one or more definitive abscesses have formed. Antimicrobial therapy, in general, is adjunctive to drainage and/or surgical correction of an underlying lesion or process in intraabdominal abscesses. Unlike the intraabdominal abscesses resulting from most causes, for which drainage of some kind is generally required, abscesses associated with diverticulitis usually wall off locally after rupture of a diverticulum, so that surgical intervention is not routinely required.

A number of agents exhibit excellent activity against aerobic gram-negative bacilli. Since death in intraabdominal sepsis is linked to gram-negative bacteremia, empirical therapy for intraabdominal infection always needs to include adequate coverage of gram-negative aerobic, facultative, and anaerobic organisms. Even if anaerobes are not cultured from clinical specimens, they still must be covered by the therapeutic regimen. Empirical antibiotic therapy should be the same as that discussed earlier for secondary peritonitis.

VISCERAL ABSCESSES
Liver abscesses

The liver is the organ most subject to the development of abscesses. In one study of 540 intraabdominal

SECTION IV Infections of the Alimentary Tract

abscesses, 26% were visceral. Liver abscesses made up 13% of the total number, or 48% of all visceral abscesses. Liver abscesses may be solitary or multiple; they may arise from hematogenous spread of bacteria or from local spread from contiguous sites of infection within the peritoneal cavity. In the past, appendicitis with rupture and subsequent spread of infection was the most common source for a liver abscess. Currently, associated disease of the biliary tract is most common. Pylephlebitis (suppurative thrombosis of the portal vein), usually arising from infection in the pelvis but sometimes from infection elsewhere in the peritoneal cavity, is another common source for bacterial seeding of the liver.

Fever is the most common presenting sign of liver abscess. Some patients, particularly those with associated disease of the biliary tract, have symptoms and signs localized to the right upper quadrant, including pain, guarding, punch tenderness, and even rebound tenderness. Nonspecific symptoms, such as chills, anorexia, weight loss, nausea, and vomiting, may also develop. Only 50% of patients with liver abscesses, however, have hepatomegaly, right-upper-quadrant tenderness, or jaundice; thus, one-half of patients have no symptoms or signs to direct attention to the liver. Fever of unknown origin (FUO) may be the only manifestation of liver abscess, especially in the elderly. Diagnostic studies of the abdomen, especially the right upper quadrant, should be a part of any FUO workup. The single most reliable laboratory finding is an elevated serum concentration of alkaline phosphatase, which is documented in 70% of patients with liver abscesses. Other tests of liver function may yield normal results, but 50% of patients have elevated serum levels of bilirubin, and 48% have elevated concentrations of aspartate aminotransferase. Other laboratory findings include leukocytosis in 77% of patients, anemia (usually normochromic, normocytic) in 50%, and hypoalbuminemia in 33%. Concomitant bacteremia is found in one-third to one-half of patients. A liver abscess is sometimes suggested by chest radiography, especially if a new elevation of the right hemidiaphragm is seen; other suggestive findings include a right basilar infiltrate and a right pleural effusion.

Imaging studies are the most reliable methods for diagnosing liver abscesses. These studies include ultrasonography, CT **(Fig. 25-4)**, indium-labeled WBC or gallium scan, and MRI. More than one such study may be required. Organisms recovered from liver abscesses vary with the source. In liver infection arising from the biliary tree, enteric gram-negative aerobic bacilli and enterococci are common isolates. Unless previous surgery has been performed, anaerobes are not generally involved in liver abscesses arising from biliary infections. In contrast, in liver abscesses arising from pelvic and other intraperitoneal sources, a mixed flora including both aerobic and anaerobic species is common;

FIGURE 25-4
Multilocular liver abscess on CT scan. Multiple or multilocular abscesses are more common than solitary abscesses. (*Reprinted with permission from B Lorber [ed]: Atlas of Infectious Diseases, Vol VII: Intra-abdominal Infections, Hepatitis, and Gastroenteritis. Philadelphia, Current Medicine, 1996, Fig. 1.22.*)

B. fragilis is the species most frequently isolated. With hematogenous spread of infection, usually only a single organism is encountered; this species may be *S. aureus* or a streptococcal species such as *S. milleri*. Results of cultures obtained from drain sites are not reliable for defining the etiology of infections. Liver abscesses may also be caused by *Candida* spp.; such abscesses usually follow fungemia in patients receiving chemotherapy for cancer and often present when PMNs return after a period of neutropenia. Amebic liver abscesses are not an uncommon problem (Chap. 32). Amebic serologic testing gives positive results in >95% of cases; thus, a negative result helps to exclude this diagnosis.

TREATMENT Liver Abscesses

(Fig. 25-3) While drainage—either percutaneous (with a pigtail catheter kept in place) or surgical—is the mainstay of therapy for intraabdominal abscesses (including liver abscesses), there is growing interest in medical management alone for pyogenic liver abscesses. The drugs used for empirical therapy include the same ones used in intraabdominal sepsis and secondary bacterial peritonitis. Usually, blood cultures and a diagnostic aspirate of abscess contents should be obtained before the initiation of empirical therapy, with antibiotic choices adjusted when the results of Gram's staining and culture become available. Cases treated without definitive drainage generally require longer courses of antibiotic therapy. When percutaneous drainage was compared with open surgical drainage, the average length of hospital stay for the former was almost twice that for the latter, although both the time required for fever to resolve and the mortality rate were the same for the two procedures. The mortality rate was appreciable despite treatment, averaging 15%. Several factors predict the failure of percutaneous drainage and therefore may favor primary surgical intervention. These factors include the presence of multiple, sizable abscesses; viscous abscess contents that tend to plug the catheter; associated disease (e.g., disease of the biliary tract) requiring surgery; or the lack of a clinical response to percutaneous drainage in 4–7 days.

Treatment of candidal liver abscesses often entails initial administration of amphotericin B or liposomal amphotericin, with subsequent fluconazole therapy. In some cases, therapy with fluconazole alone (6 mg/kg daily) may be used—e.g., in clinically stable patients whose infecting isolate is susceptible to this drug.

Splenic abscesses

Splenic abscesses are much less common than liver abscesses. The incidence of splenic abscesses has ranged from 0.14% to 0.7% in various autopsy series. The clinical setting and the organisms isolated usually differ from those for liver abscesses. The degree of clinical suspicion for splenic abscess needs to be high, as this condition is frequently fatal if left untreated. Even in the most recently published series, diagnosis was made only at autopsy in 37% of cases. While splenic abscesses may arise occasionally from contiguous spread of infection or from direct trauma to the spleen, hematogenous spread of infection is more common. Bacterial endocarditis is the most common associated infection. Splenic abscesses can develop in patients who have received extensive immunosuppressive therapy (particularly those with malignancy involving the spleen) and in patients with hemoglobinopathies or other hematologic disorders (especially sickle cell anemia).

While ~50% of patients with splenic abscesses have abdominal pain, the pain is localized to the left upper quadrant in only one-half of these cases. Splenomegaly is found in ~50% of cases. Fever and leukocytosis are generally present; the development of fever preceded diagnosis by an average of 20 days in one series. Left-sided chest findings may include abnormalities to auscultation, and chest radiographic findings may include an infiltrate or a left-sided pleural effusion. CT scan of the abdomen has been the most sensitive diagnostic tool. Ultrasonography can yield the diagnosis but is less sensitive. Liver-spleen scan or gallium scan may also be useful. Streptococcal species are the most common bacterial isolates from splenic abscesses, followed by S. aureus—presumably reflecting the associated endocarditis. An increase in the prevalence of gram-negative aerobic isolates from

splenic abscesses has been reported; these organisms often derive from a urinary tract focus, with associated bacteremia, or from another intraabdominal source. Salmonella species are seen fairly commonly, especially in patients with sickle cell hemoglobinopathy. Anaerobic species accounted for only 5% of isolates in the largest collected series, but the reporting of a number of "sterile abscesses" may indicate that optimal techniques for the isolation of anaerobes were not employed.

TREATMENT Splenic Abscesses

Because of the high mortality figures reported for splenic abscesses, splenectomy with adjunctive antibiotics has traditionally been considered standard treatment and remains the best approach for complex, multilocular abscesses or multiple abscesses. However, percutaneous drainage has worked well for single, small (<3-cm) abscesses in some studies and may also be useful for patients with high surgical risk. Patients undergoing splenectomy should be vaccinated against encapsulated organisms (Streptococcus pneumoniae, Haemophilus influenzae, Neisseria meningitidis). The most important factor in successful treatment of splenic abscesses is early diagnosis.

Perinephric and renal abscesses

Perinephric and renal abscesses are not common: The former accounted for only ~0.02% of hospital admissions and the latter for ~0.2% in Altemeier's series of 540 intraabdominal abscesses. Before antibiotics became available, most renal and perinephric abscesses were hematogenous in origin, usually complicating prolonged bacteremia, with S. aureus most commonly recovered. Now, in contrast, >75% of perinephric and renal abscesses arise from a urinary tract infection. Infection ascends from the bladder to the kidney, with pyelonephritis occurring prior to abscess development. Bacteria may directly invade the renal parenchyma from medulla to cortex. Local vascular channels within the kidney may also facilitate the transport of organisms. Areas of abscess developing within the parenchyma may rupture into the perinephric space. The kidneys and adrenal glands are surrounded by a layer of perirenal fat that, in turn, is surrounded by Gerota's fascia, which extends superiorly to the diaphragm and inferiorly to the pelvic fat. Abscesses extending into the perinephric space may track through Gerota's fascia into the psoas or transversalis muscles, into the anterior peritoneal cavity, superiorly to the subdiaphragmatic space, or inferiorly to the pelvis. Of the risk factors that have been associated with the development of perinephric abscesses, the most important is concomitant nephrolithiasis obstructing urinary flow. Of patients with perinephric abscess, 20–60% have renal stones. Other structural abnormalities of the urinary tract, prior urologic surgery, trauma, and diabetes mellitus have also been identified as risk factors.

The organisms most frequently encountered in perinephric and renal abscesses are *E. coli*, *Proteus* spp., and *Klebsiella* spp. *E. coli*, the aerobic species most commonly found in the colonic flora, seems to have unique virulence properties in the urinary tract, including factors promoting adherence to uroepithelial cells. The urease of *Proteus* spp. splits urea, thereby creating a more alkaline and more hospitable environment for bacterial proliferation. *Proteus* spp. are frequently found in association with large struvite stones caused by the precipitation of magnesium ammonium sulfate in an alkaline environment. These stones serve as a nidus for recurrent urinary tract infection. While a single bacterial species is usually recovered from a perinephric or renal abscess, multiple species may also be found. If a urine culture is not contaminated with periurethral flora and is found to contain more than one organism, a perinephric abscess or renal abscess should be considered in the differential diagnosis. Urine cultures may also be polymicrobial in cases of bladder diverticulum.

Candida spp. can cause renal abscesses. This fungus may spread to the kidney hematogenously or by ascension from the bladder. The hallmark of the latter route of infection is ureteral obstruction with large fungal balls.

The presentation of perinephric and renal abscesses is quite nonspecific. Flank pain and abdominal pain are common. At least 50% of patients are febrile. Pain may be referred to the groin or leg, particularly with extension of infection. The diagnosis of perinephric abscess, like that of splenic abscess, is frequently delayed, and the mortality rate in some series is appreciable, although lower than in the past. Perinephric or renal abscess should be most seriously considered when a patient presents with symptoms and signs of pyelonephritis and remains febrile after 4 or 5 days of treatment. Moreover, when a urine culture yields a polymicrobial flora, when a patient is known to have renal stones, or when fever and pyuria coexist with a sterile urine culture, these diagnoses should be entertained.

Renal ultrasonography and abdominal CT are the most useful diagnostic modalities. If a renal or perinephric abscess is diagnosed, nephrolithiasis should be excluded, especially when a high urinary pH suggests the presence of a urea-splitting organism.

TREATMENT   Perinephric and Renal Abscesses

Treatment for perinephric and renal abscesses, like that for other intraabdominal abscesses, includes drainage of pus and antibiotic therapy directed at the organism(s) recovered. For perinephric abscesses, percutaneous drainage is usually successful.

Psoas abscesses

The psoas muscle is another location in which abscesses are encountered. Psoas abscesses may arise from a hematogenous source, by contiguous spread from an intraabdominal or pelvic process, or by contiguous spread from nearby bony structures (e.g., vertebral bodies). Associated osteomyelitis due to spread from bone to muscle or from muscle to bone is common in psoas abscesses. When Pott's disease was common, *Mycobacterium tuberculosis* was a frequent cause of psoas abscess. Currently, either *S. aureus* or a mixture of enteric organisms including aerobic and anaerobic gram-negative bacilli is usually isolated from psoas abscesses in the United States. *S. aureus* is most likely to be isolated when a psoas abscess arises from hematogenous spread or a contiguous focus of osteomyelitis; a mixed enteric flora is the most likely etiology when the abscess has an intraabdominal or pelvic source. Patients with psoas abscesses frequently present with fever, lower abdominal or back pain, or pain referred to the hip or knee. CT is the most useful diagnostic technique.

TREATMENT   Psoas Abscesses

Treatment includes surgical drainage and the administration of an antibiotic regimen directed at the inciting organism(s).

Pancreatic abscesses

See Chap. 48.

ACKNOWLEDGMENT

The substantial contributions of Dori F. Zaleznik, MD, to this chapter in previous editions of Harrison's Principles of Internal Medicine are gratefully acknowledged.

CHAPTER 26

HELICOBACTER PYLORI INFECTIONS

John C. Atherton ■ Martin J. Blaser

DEFINITION

Helicobacter pylori colonizes the stomachs of ~50% of the world's human population throughout their lifetimes. Colonization with this organism is the main risk factor for peptic ulceration (Chap. 14) as well as for gastric adenocarcinoma and gastric MALT (mucosa-associated lymphoid tissue) lymphoma (Chap. 49). Treatment for *H. pylori* has revolutionized the management of peptic ulcer disease, providing a permanent cure in most cases. Such treatment also represents first-line therapy for patients with low-grade gastric MALT lymphoma. Treatment of *H. pylori* is of no benefit in the treatment of gastric adenocarcinoma, but prevention of *H. pylori* colonization could potentially prevent gastric malignancy and peptic ulceration. In contrast, increasing evidence indicates that lifelong *H. pylori* colonization may offer some protection against complications of gastroesophageal reflux disease (GERD), including esophageal adenocarcinoma. Recent research has focused on whether *H. pylori* colonization is a risk factor for some extragastric diseases and whether it is protective against some recently emergent medical problems, such as asthma and obesity.

ETIOLOGIC AGENT

H. pylori is a gram-negative bacillus that has naturally colonized humans for at least 50,000 years—and probably throughout human evolution. It lives in gastric mucus, with a small proportion of the bacteria adherent to the mucosa and possibly a very small number of the organisms entering cells or penetrating the mucosa; its distribution is never systemic. Its spiral shape and flagella render *H. pylori* motile in the mucus environment. The organism has several acid-resistance mechanisms, most notably a highly expressed urease that catalyzes urea hydrolysis to produce buffering ammonia. *H. pylori* is microaerophilic (requiring low levels of oxygen), is slow-growing, and requires complex growth media in vitro. Publication of several complete genomic sequences of *H. pylori* since 1997 has led to significant advances in the understanding of the organism's biology.

A very small proportion of gastric *Helicobacter* infections are due to species other than *H. pylori*, possibly acquired as zoonoses. Whether these non-*pylori* gastric helicobacters cause disease remains controversial. In immunocompromised hosts, several nongastric (intestinal) *Helicobacter* species can cause disease with clinical features resembling those of *Campylobacter* infections; these species are covered in Chap. 29.

EPIDEMIOLOGY

The prevalence of *H. pylori* among adults is ~30% in the United States and other developed countries as opposed to >80% in most developing countries. In the United States, prevalence varies with age: ~50% of 60-year-old persons, ~20% of 30-year-old persons, and <10% of children are colonized. *H. pylori* is usually acquired in childhood. The age association is due mostly to a birth-cohort effect whereby current 60-year-olds were more commonly colonized as children than are current children. Spontaneous acquisition or loss of *H. pylori* in adulthood is uncommon. Other strong risk factors for *H. pylori* colonization are markers of crowding and maternal colonization. The low incidence among children in developed countries at present is due, at least in part, to decreased maternal colonization and increased use of antibiotics.

Humans are the only important reservoir of *H. pylori*. Children may acquire the organism from their parents (more often from the mother) or from other children. Whether transmission takes place more often by the fecal-oral or the oral-oral route is unknown, but *H. pylori* is easily cultured from vomitus and gastroesophageal refluxate and is less easily cultured from stool.

PATHOLOGY AND PATHOGENESIS

H. pylori colonization induces a tissue response in the stomach, *chronic superficial gastritis*, which includes infiltration of the mucosa by both mononuclear and polymorphonuclear cells. (The term *gastritis* should be used specifically to describe histologic features; it has also been used to describe endoscopic appearances and even symptoms, which do not correlate with microscopic findings or even with the presence of *H. pylori*.) Although *H. pylori* is capable of numerous adaptations that prevent excessive stimulation of the immune system, colonization is accompanied by a considerable persistent immune response, including the production of both local and systemic antibodies as well as cell-mediated responses. However, these responses are ineffective in clearing the bacterium. This inefficient clearing appears to be due in part to *H. pylori*'s downregulation of the immune system, which fosters its own persistence.

Most *H. pylori*–colonized persons do not develop clinical sequelae. That some persons develop overt disease whereas others do not is related to a combination of factors: bacterial strain differences, host susceptibility to disease, and environmental factors.

Several *H. pylori* virulence factors are more common among strains that are associated with disease than among those that are not. The *cag* island is a group of genes that encodes a bacterial secretion system through which a specific protein, CagA, is translocated into epithelial cells. CagA affects host cell signal transduction, inducing proliferative, cytoskeletal, and inflammatory changes; a proportion of transgenic mice expressing CagA in the stomach develop gastric adenocarcinoma. The secretion system also translocates soluble components of the peptidoglycan cell wall into the gastric epithelial cell; these components are recognized by the intracellular emergency bacterial receptor Nod1, which stimulates a proinflammatory cytokine response resulting in enhanced gastric inflammation. Patients with peptic ulcer disease or gastric adenocarcinoma are more likely than persons without these conditions to be colonized by *cag*-positive strains. The secreted *H. pylori* protein VacA occurs in several forms. Strains with the more active forms are more commonly isolated from patients with peptic ulcer disease or gastric carcinoma than from persons without these conditions. Other bacterial factors that are associated with increased disease risk include adhesins, such as BabA and SabA, and incompletely characterized genes, such as *dupA*.

The best-characterized host determinants of disease are genetic polymorphisms leading to enhanced activation of the innate immune response, such as polymorphisms in cytokine genes or genes encoding bacterial recognition proteins such as Toll-like receptors (TLRs). For example, colonized people with polymorphisms in the interleukin (IL) 1 gene that cause the production of large quantities of this cytokine in response to *H. pylori* infection are at increased risk of gastric adenocarcinoma. In addition, environmental cofactors are important in pathogenesis. Smoking increases the risks of ulcers and cancer in *H. pylori*–positive individuals. Diets high in salt and preserved foods increase cancer risk, whereas diets high in antioxidants and vitamin C are protective.

The pattern of gastric inflammation is associated with disease risk: antral-predominant gastritis is most closely linked with duodenal ulceration, whereas pangastritis is linked with gastric ulceration and adenocarcinoma. This difference probably explains why patients with duodenal ulceration are not at high risk of developing gastric adenocarcinoma later in life, despite being colonized by *H. pylori*.

How gastric colonization causes duodenal ulceration is now becoming clearer. *H. pylori*–induced inflammation diminishes the number of somatostatin-producing D cells. Since somatostatin inhibits gastrin release, gastrin levels are higher than in *H. pylori*–negative persons, and these higher levels lead to increased meal-stimulated acid secretion in the gastric corpus, which is only mildly inflamed in antral-predominant gastritis. How this increases duodenal ulcer risk remains controversial, but the increased acid secretion may contribute to the formation of the potentially protective gastric metaplasia found in the duodenum of duodenal ulcer patients. Gastric metaplasia in the duodenum may become colonized by *H. pylori* and subsequently inflamed and ulcerated.

The pathogenesis of gastric ulceration and that of gastric adenocarcinoma are less well understood, although both conditions arise in association with pan- or corpus-predominant gastritis. The hormonal changes described earlier still occur, but the inflammation in the gastric corpus means that it produces less acid (hypochlorhydria) despite hypergastrinemia. Gastric ulcers usually occur at the junction of antral and corpus-type mucosa, and this region is particularly inflamed. Gastric cancer probably stems from progressive DNA damage and the survival of abnormal epithelial cell clones. The DNA damage is thought to be due principally to reactive oxygen and nitrogen species arising from inflammatory cells and perhaps in relation to other bacteria that survive in a hypochlorhydric stomach. Longitudinal analyses of gastric biopsy specimens taken years apart from the same patient show that the common *intestinal* type of gastric adenocarcinoma follows stepwise changes from simple gastritis to gastric atrophy, intestinal metaplasia, and dysplasia. A second, *diffuse* type of gastric adenocarcinoma may arise directly from chronic gastritis alone.

CLINICAL MANIFESTATIONS

Essentially all *H. pylori*–colonized persons have gastric tissue responses, but fewer than 15% develop associated illnesses such as peptic ulceration, gastric adenocarcinoma, or gastric lymphoma **(Fig. 26-1)**.

264

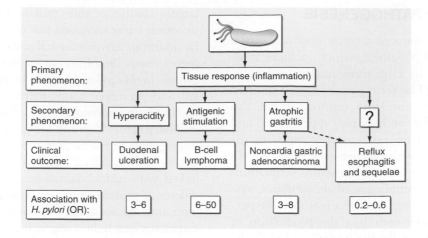

FIGURE 26-1

Schematic of the relationships between colonization with *Helicobacter pylori* and diseases of the upper gastrointestinal tract among persons in developed countries. Essentially all persons colonized with *H. pylori* develop a host response, which is generally termed chronic gastritis. The nature of the interaction of the host with the particular bacterial population determines the clinical outcome. *H. pylori* colonization increases the lifetime risk of peptic ulcer disease, noncardia gastric cancer, and B cell non-Hodgkin's gastric lymphoma [odds ratios (ORs) for all, >3]. In contrast, a growing body of evidence indicates that *H. pylori* colonization (especially with *cagA*⁺ strains) protects against adenocarcinoma of the esophagus (and the sometimes related gastric cardia) and premalignant lesions such as Barrett's esophagus (OR, <1). While the incidences of peptic ulcer disease (cases not due to nonsteroidal anti-inflammatory drugs) and noncardia gastric cancer are declining in developed countries, the incidence of adenocarcinoma of the esophagus is rapidly increasing. (*Adapted from MJ Blaser: Hypothesis: The changing relationships of Helicobacter pylori and humans: Implications for health and disease. J Infect Dis 179:1523, 1999, with permission.*)

Worldwide, >80% of duodenal ulcers and >60% of gastric ulcers are related to *H. pylori* colonization (Chap. 14, although the proportion of ulcers due to aspirin and nonsteroidal anti-inflammatory drugs (NSAIDs) is increasing, especially in developed countries. The main lines of evidence for an ulcer-promoting role for *H. pylori* are that (1) the presence of the organism is a risk factor for the development of ulcers, (2) non-NSAID-induced ulcers rarely develop in the absence of *H. pylori*, (3) eradication of *H. pylori* markedly reduces rates of ulcer relapse, and (4) experimental *H. pylori* infection of gerbils causes gastric ulceration.

Prospective nested case-control studies have shown that *H. pylori* colonization is a risk factor for adenocarcinomas of the distal (noncardia) stomach (Chap. 49). Long-term experimental infection of gerbils also may result in gastric adenocarcinoma. Moreover, the presence of *H. pylori* is strongly associated with primary gastric lymphoma, although this condition is much less common. Many low-grade gastric B cell lymphomas arising from MALT are driven by T cell proliferation, which in turn is driven by *H. pylori* antigen stimulation; *H. pylori* antigen–driven tumors may regress either fully or partially after *H. pylori* eradication but require careful long-term monitoring.

Many patients have upper gastrointestinal symptoms but have normal results in upper gastrointestinal endoscopy (so-called functional or nonulcer dyspepsia;

Chap. 14). Because *H. pylori* is common, some of these patients will be colonized with the organism. *H. pylori* eradication leads to symptom resolution a little (7%) more commonly than does placebo treatment. Whether such patients have peptic ulcers in remission at the time of endoscopy or whether a small subgroup of patients with true functional dyspepsia respond to *H. pylori* treatment is unclear.

Much interest has focused on a possible protective role for *H. pylori* against GERD (Chap. 13), Barrett's esophagus (Chap. 13), and adenocarcinoma of the esophagus and gastric cardia (Chap. 49). The main lines of evidence for this role are (1) that there is a temporal relationship between a falling prevalence of gastric *H. pylori* colonization and a rising incidence of these conditions and (2) that, in most studies, the prevalence of *H. pylori* colonization (especially with proinflammatory *cagA*⁺ strains) is significantly lower among patients with these esophageal diseases than among control subjects. The mechanism underlying this protective effect appears to include *H. pylori*–induced hypochlorhydria. Since, at the individual level, GERD symptoms may decrease, worsen, or remain unchanged after treatment targeting *H. pylori*, concerns about GERD should not affect decisions about *H. pylori* treatment when an indication exists.

H. pylori has an increasingly recognized role in other gastric pathologies. It may be one initial precipitant of

SECTION IV Infections of the Alimentary Tract

autoimmune gastritis and pernicious anemia and also may predispose some patients to iron deficiency through occult blood loss and/or hypochlorhydria and reduced iron absorption. In addition, several extragastrointestinal pathologies have been linked with *H. pylori* colonization, although evidence of causality is less strong. Several small studies of *H. pylori* treatment in idiopathic thrombocytopenic purpura have described improvement in or even normalization of platelet counts. Potentially important but even more controversial associations are with ischemic heart disease and cerebrovascular disease. However, the strength of these latter associations is reduced if confounding factors are taken into account, and most authorities consider the associations to be noncausal. Recent studies have shown an inverse association of *cagA*⁺ *H. pylori* with childhood-onset asthma, hay fever, and atopic disorders. Whether *H. pylori* status is merely a marker or is causally associated with protection against these diseases remains to be determined.

DIAGNOSIS

Tests for the presence of *H. pylori* can be divided into two groups: invasive tests, which require upper gastrointestinal endoscopy and are based on the analysis of gastric biopsy specimens, and noninvasive tests (Table 26-1). Endoscopy often is not performed in the initial management of young dyspeptic patients without "alarm" symptoms but is commonly used to exclude malignancy in older patients. If endoscopy is performed, the most convenient biopsy-based test is the biopsy urease test, in which one large or two small antral biopsy specimens are placed into a gel containing urea and an indicator. The presence of *H. pylori* urease leads to a pH alteration and therefore to a color change, which often occurs within minutes but can require up to 24 h. Histologic examination of biopsy specimens for *H. pylori* also is accurate, provided that a special stain (e.g., a modified Giemsa or silver stain) permitting optimal visualization of the organism is used. If biopsy specimens are obtained from both antrum and corpus, histologic study yields additional information, including the degree and pattern of inflammation, atrophy, metaplasia, and dysplasia. Microbiologic culture is most specific but may be insensitive because of difficulty with *H. pylori* isolation. Once the organism is cultured, its identity as *H. pylori* can be confirmed by its typical appearance on Gram's stain and its positive reactions in oxidase, catalase, and urease tests. Moreover, the organism's susceptibility to antibiotics can be determined, and this information can be clinically useful in difficult cases. The occasional biopsy specimens containing the less common non-*pylori* gastric helicobacters give only weakly positive results in the biopsy urease test. Positive identification of these bacteria requires visualization of the characteristic long, tight spirals in histologic sections.

Noninvasive *H. pylori* testing is the norm if gastric cancer does not need to be excluded by endoscopy. The most consistently accurate test is the urea breath test. In this simple test, the patient drinks a solution of urea labeled with the nonradioactive isotope ¹³C and then blows into a tube. If *H. pylori* urease is present, the urea

TABLE 26-1

TESTS COMMONLY USED TO DETECT *HELICOBACTER PYLORI*

TEST	ADVANTAGES	DISADVANTAGES
Invasive (Based on Endoscopic Biopsy)		
Biopsy urease test	Quick, simple	Some commercial tests not fully sensitive before 24 h
Histology	May give additional histologic information	Sensitivity dependent on experience and use of special stains
Culture	Permits determination of antibiotic susceptibility	Sensitivity dependent on experience
Noninvasive		
Serology	Inexpensive and convenient; not affected by recent antibiotics or proton pump inhibitors to the same extent as breath and stool tests	Cannot be used for early follow-up after treatment; some commercial kits inaccurate, and all less accurate than breath test
¹³C urea breath test	Inexpensive and simpler than endoscopy; useful for follow-up after treatment	Requires fasting; not as convenient as blood or stool tests
Stool antigen test	Inexpensive and convenient; useful for follow-up after treatment; may be useful in children	May be disliked by people from some cultures; may be slightly less accurate than urea breath test, particularly when used to assess treatment success

is hydrolyzed and labeled carbon dioxide is detected in breath samples. The stool antigen test, another simple assay, is more convenient and potentially less expensive than the urea breath test but has been slightly less accurate in some comparative studies. The simplest tests for ascertaining *H. pylori* status are serologic assays measuring specific IgG levels in serum by enzyme-linked immunosorbent assay or immunoblot. The best of these tests are as accurate as other diagnostic methods, but many commercial tests—especially rapid office tests—do not perform well.

The urea breath test, the stool antigen test, and biopsy-based tests can all be used to assess the success of treatment **(Fig. 26-2)**. However, because these tests are dependent on *H. pylori* load, their use <4 weeks after treatment may yield false-negative results. Furthermore, these tests are unreliable if performed within 4 weeks of intercurrent treatment with antibiotics or bismuth compounds or within 2 weeks of the discontinuation of proton pump inhibitor (PPI) treatment. In the assessment of treatment success, noninvasive tests are normally preferred; however, after gastric ulceration, endoscopy should be repeated to ensure healing and to exclude gastric carcinoma by further histologic sampling.

Serologic tests are not used to monitor treatment success, as the gradual drop in titer of *H. pylori*–specific antibodies is too slow to be of practical use.

TREATMENT   *H. pylori* Infections

The most clear-cut indications for treatment are *H. pylori*–related duodenal or gastric ulceration or low-grade gastric B cell lymphoma. *H. pylori* should be eradicated in patients with documented ulcer disease, whether or not the ulcers are currently active, to reduce the likelihood of relapse (Fig. 26-2). Many guidelines now recommend *H. pylori* eradication in uninvestigated simple dyspepsia following noninvasive diagnosis; others also recommend treatment in functional dyspepsia, in case the patient is one of the perhaps 7% (beyond placebo effects) to benefit from such treatment. Individuals with a strong family history of gastric cancer should be treated to eradicate *H. pylori* in the hope that their cancer risk will be reduced. Currently, widespread community screening for and treatment of *H. pylori* as primary prophylaxis for gastric cancer and peptic ulcers are not recommended, mainly because it is unclear whether treatment for *H. pylori* reduces the risk of cancer to that in persons who have never acquired the organism. The largest randomized controlled study to date (performed in China) showed no cancer risk reduction during the 7 years of follow-up, although a post hoc subgroup analysis documented improvement in the group of participants who did not already have gastric atrophy

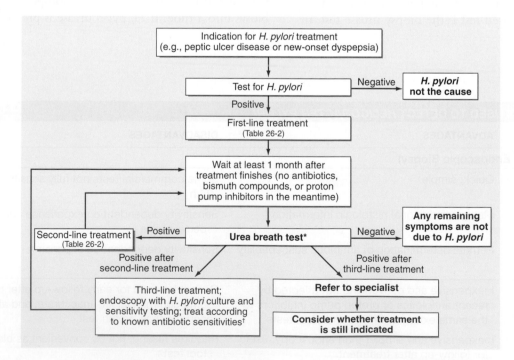

FIGURE 26-2
Algorithm for the management of *Helicobacter pylori* infection. *Occasionally, an endoscopy and a biopsy-based test are used instead of a urea breath test in follow-up after treatment. The main indication for these invasive tests is gastric ulceration;

in this condition, as opposed to duodenal ulceration, it is important to check healing and to exclude underlying gastric adenocarcinoma. †Some authorities now use empirical third-line regimens, several of which have been described.

or intestinal metaplasia. Other studies have found a reduced cancer risk after treatment, but the size of this effect in different populations remains unclear, and the results of further large-scale prospective interventional studies must be awaited. Other reasons for not treating *H. pylori* in asymptomatic populations at present include (1) the adverse side effects of the multiple-antibiotic regimens used (which are common and can be severe in rare cases); (2) antibiotic resistance, which may arise in *H. pylori* or other incidentally carried bacteria; (3) the anxiety that may arise in otherwise healthy people, especially if treatment is unsuccessful; and (4) the apparent existence of a subset of people who will develop GERD symptoms after treatment, although on average *H. pylori* treatment does not affect GERD symptoms or severity.

Although *H. pylori* is susceptible to a wide range of antibiotics in vitro, monotherapy is not usually successful, probably because of inadequate antibiotic delivery to the colonization niche. Failure of monotherapy has prompted the development of multidrug regimens, the most successful of which are triple and quadruple combinations. Initially these regimens produced *H. pylori* eradication rates of >90% in many trials; in recent years, however, resistance to key antibiotics has become more common, a trend leading to *H. pylori* eradication rates of only 75–80% for the most commonly used regimens.

Current regimens consist of a PPI or ranitidine bismuth citrate and two or three antimicrobial agents given for 7–14 days (Table 26-2). Research on optimizing drug combinations to increase efficacy continues, and it is likely that guidelines will change as the field develops and as countries increasingly individualize treatment to suit local antibiotic resistance patterns and economic needs. The two most important factors in successful *H. pylori* treatment are the patient's close compliance with the regimen and the use of drugs to which the patient's strain of *H. pylori* has not acquired resistance. Treatment failure following minor lapses in compliance is common and often leads to acquired resistance to metronidazole or clarithromycin. To stress the importance of compliance, written instructions should be given to the patient, and minor side effects of the regimen should be explained. Resistance to clarithromycin and, to a lesser extent, to metronidazole are of growing concern. Clarithromycin resistance is less prevalent but, if present, usually results in treatment failure. Strains of *H. pylori* that are apparently resistant to metronidazole are more common but still may be cleared by metronidazole-containing regimens, which have only slightly reduced efficacy. Assessment of antibiotic susceptibilities before treatment would be optimal but is not usually undertaken because endoscopy and mucosal biopsy are necessary to obtain *H. pylori* for culture and because most

TABLE 26-2

RECOMMENDED TREATMENT REGIMENS FOR *HELICOBACTER PYLORI*

REGIMEN (DURATION)	DRUG 1	DRUG 2	DRUG 3	DRUG 4
Regimen 1: OCM (7–14 days)[a]	Omeprazole[b] (20 mg bid)	Clarithromycin (500 mg bid)	Metronidazole (500 mg bid)	—
Regimen 2: OCA (7–14 days)[a]	Omeprazole[b] (20 mg bid)	Clarithromycin (500 mg bid)	Amoxicillin (1 g bid)	—
Regimen 3: OBTM (14 days)[c]	Omeprazole[b] (20 mg bid)	Bismuth subsalicylate (2 tabs qid)	Tetracycline HCl (500 mg qid)	Metronidazole (500 mg tid)
Regimen 4[d]: sequential (5 days + 5 days)	Omeprazole[b] (20 mg bid)	Amoxicillin 1 g bid		
	Omeprazole[b] (20 mg bid)	Clarithromycin (500 mg bid)	Tinidazole (500 mg bid)	
Regimen 5[e]: OAL (10 days)	Omeprazole[b] (20 mg bid)	Amoxicillin (1 g bid)	Levofloxacin (500 mg bid)	

[a]Meta-analyses show that a 14-day course of therapy is slightly superior to a 7-day course. However, in populations where 7-day treatment is known to have very high success rates, this shorter course is still often used.

[b]Omeprazole may be replaced with any proton pump inhibitor at an equivalent dosage or, in regimens 1 and 2, with ranitidine bismuth citrate (400 mg).

[c]Data supporting this regimen come mainly from Europe and are based on the use of bismuth subcitrate and metronidazole (400 mg tid). This is the most commonly used second-line regimen.

[d]Data supporting this regimen come from Europe. Although the two 5-day courses of different drugs have usually been given sequentially, recent evidence suggests no added benefit from this approach. Thus 10 days of the four drugs combined may be as good and may aid compliance.

[e]Data supporting this second- or third-line regimen come from Europe. This regimen may be less effective where rates of quinolone use are high. Theoretically, it may also be wise to avoid it in populations where *Clostridium difficile* infection is common after broad-spectrum antibiotic use.

microbiology laboratories are inexperienced in *H. pylori* culture. In the absence of susceptibility information, a history of the patient's (even distant) antibiotic use for other conditions should be obtained; use of the agent should then be avoided if possible, particularly in the case of clarithromycin (e.g., previous use for upper respiratory infection). If initial *H. pylori* treatment fails, one of two strategies may be used (Fig. 26-2). The more common approach is empirical re-treatment with another drug regimen, usually quadruple therapy (Table 26-2). The second approach is endoscopy, biopsy, and culture plus treatment based on documented antibiotic sensitivities. If re-treatment fails, susceptibility testing should ideally be performed, although empirical third-line therapies are often used.

Clearance of non-*H. pylori* gastric helicobacters can follow the use of bismuth compounds alone or of triple-drug regimens. However, in the absence of trials, it is unclear whether this outcome represents successful treatment or natural clearance of the bacterium.

PREVENTION

Carriage of *H. pylori* has considerable public health significance in developed countries, where it is associated with peptic ulcer disease and gastric adenocarcinoma, and in developing countries, where gastric adenocarcinoma may be an even more common cause of cancer death late in life. If mass prevention were contemplated, vaccination would be the most obvious method, and experimental immunization of animals has given promising results. However, given that *H. pylori* has co-evolved with its human host over millennia, preventing or eliminating colonization on a population basis may have distinct disadvantages. For example, lifelong absence of *H. pylori* is a risk factor for GERD complications, including esophageal adenocarcinoma. We have speculated that the disappearance of *H. pylori* may be associated with an increased risk of other emerging diseases reflecting aspects of the current Western lifestyle, such as asthma, obesity, and conceivably even type 2 diabetes mellitus.

CHAPTER 27

SALMONELLOSIS

David A. Pegues ■ Samuel I. Miller

Bacteria of the genus *Salmonella* are highly adapted for growth in both humans and animals and cause a wide spectrum of disease. The growth of serotypes *S. typhi* and *S. paratyphi* is restricted to human hosts, in whom these organisms cause enteric (typhoid) fever. The remaining serotypes (nontyphoidal *Salmonella*, or NTS) can colonize the gastrointestinal tracts of a broad range of animals, including mammals, reptiles, birds, and insects. More than 200 serotypes are pathogenic to humans, in whom they often cause gastroenteritis and can be associated with localized infections and/or bacteremia.

ETIOLOGY

This large genus of gram-negative bacilli within the family Enterobacteriaceae consists of two species: *S. enterica*, which contains six subspecies, and *S. bongori*. *S. enterica* subspecies I includes almost all the serotypes pathogenic for humans. According to the current *Salmonella* nomenclature system, the full taxonomic designation *S. enterica* subspecies *enterica* serotype *typhimurium* can be shortened to *Salmonella* serotype *typhimurium* or simply *S. typhimurium*.

Members of the seven *Salmonella* subspecies are classified into >2500 serotypes (serovars) according to the somatic O antigen (lipopolysaccharide [LPS] cell-wall components), the surface Vi antigen (restricted to *S. typhi* and *S. paratyphi* C), and the flagellar H antigen. For simplicity, most *Salmonella* serotypes are named for the city where they were identified, and the serotype is often used as the species designation.

Salmonellae are gram-negative, non-spore-forming, facultatively anaerobic bacilli that measure 2–3 by 0.4–0.6 μm. The initial identification of salmonellae in the clinical microbiology laboratory is based on growth characteristics. Salmonellae, like other Enterobacteriaceae, produce acid on glucose fermentation, reduce nitrates, and do not produce cytochrome oxidase. In addition, all salmonellae except *S. gallinarum-pullorum* are motile by means of peritrichous flagella, and all but *S. typhi* produce gas (H_2S) on sugar fermentation. Notably, only 1% of clinical isolates ferment lactose; a high level of suspicion must be maintained to detect these rare clinical lactose-fermenting isolates.

Although serotyping of all surface antigens can be used for formal identification, most laboratories perform a few simple agglutination reactions that define specific O-antigen serogroups, designated A, B, C_1, C_2, D, and E. Strains in these six serogroups cause ~99% of *Salmonella* infections in humans and other warm-blooded animals. Molecular typing methods, including pulsed-field gel electrophoresis and polymerase chain reaction (PCR) fingerprinting, are used in epidemiologic investigations to differentiate *Salmonella* strains of a common serotype.

PATHOGENESIS

All *Salmonella* infections begin with ingestion of organisms, most commonly in contaminated food or water. The infectious dose is 10^3–10^6 colony-forming units. Conditions that decrease either stomach acidity (an age of <1 year, antacid ingestion, or achlorhydric disease) or intestinal integrity (inflammatory bowel disease, prior gastrointestinal surgery, or alteration of the intestinal flora by antibiotic administration) increase susceptibility to *Salmonella* infection.

Once *S. typhi* and *S. paratyphi* reach the small intestine, they penetrate the mucus layer of the gut and traverse the intestinal layer through phagocytic microfold (M) cells that reside within Peyer's patches. Salmonellae can trigger the formation of membrane ruffles in normally nonphagocytic epithelial cells. These ruffles reach out and enclose adherent bacteria within large vesicles by a process referred to as *bacteria-mediated endocytosis* (BME). BME is dependent on the direct delivery of *Salmonella* proteins into the cytoplasm of epithelial

269

cells by a specialized bacterial secretion system (*type III secretion*). These bacterial proteins mediate alterations in the actin cytoskeleton that are required for *Salmonella* uptake.

After crossing the epithelial layer of the small intestine, *S. typhi* and *S. paratyphi,* which cause enteric (typhoid) fever, are phagocytosed by macrophages. These salmonellae survive the antimicrobial environment of the macrophage by sensing environmental signals that trigger alterations in regulatory systems of the phagocytosed bacteria. For example, PhoP/PhoQ (the best-characterized regulatory system) triggers the expression of outer-membrane proteins and mediates modifications in LPS so that the altered bacterial surface can resist microbicidal activities and potentially alter host cell signaling. In addition, salmonellae encode a second type III secretion system that directly delivers bacterial proteins across the phagosome membrane into the macrophage cytoplasm. This secretion system functions to remodel the *Salmonella*-containing vacuole, promoting bacterial survival and replication.

Once phagocytosed, typhoidal salmonellae disseminate throughout the body in macrophages via the lymphatics and colonize reticuloendothelial tissues (liver, spleen, lymph nodes, and bone marrow). Patients have relatively few or no signs and symptoms during this initial incubation stage. Signs and symptoms, including fever and abdominal pain, probably result from secretion of cytokines by macrophages and epithelial cells in response to bacterial products that are recognized by innate immune receptors when a critical number of organisms have replicated. Over time, the development of hepatosplenomegaly is likely to be related to the recruitment of mononuclear cells and the development of a specific acquired cell-mediated immune response to *S. typhi* colonization. The recruitment of additional mononuclear cells and lymphocytes to Peyer's patches during the several weeks after initial colonization/infection can result in marked enlargement and necrosis of the Peyer's patches, which may be mediated by bacterial products that promote cell death as well as the inflammatory response.

In contrast to enteric fever, which is characterized by an infiltration of mononuclear cells into the small-bowel mucosa, NTS gastroenteritis is characterized by massive polymorphonuclear leukocyte (PMN) infiltration into both the large- and small-bowel mucosa. This response appears to depend on the induction of interleukin (IL) 8, a strong neutrophil chemotactic factor, which is secreted by intestinal cells as a result of *Salmonella* colonization and translocation of bacterial proteins into host cell cytoplasm. The degranulation and release of toxic substances by neutrophils may result in damage to the intestinal mucosa, causing the inflammatory diarrhea observed with nontyphoidal gastroenteritis.

ENTERIC (TYPHOID) FEVER

Enteric (typhoid) fever is a systemic disease characterized by fever and abdominal pain and caused by dissemination of *S. typhi* or *S. paratyphi*. The disease was initially called *typhoid fever* because of its clinical similarity to typhus. However, in the early 1800s, typhoid fever was clearly defined pathologically as a unique illness on the basis of its association with enlarged Peyer's patches and mesenteric lymph nodes. In 1869, given the anatomic site of infection, the term *enteric fever* was proposed as an alternative designation to distinguish typhoid fever from typhus. However, to this day, the two designations are used interchangeably.

EPIDEMIOLOGY

In contrast to other *Salmonella* serotypes, the etiologic agents of enteric fever—*S. typhi* and *S. paratyphi* serotypes A, B, and C—have no known hosts other than humans. Most commonly, food-borne or waterborne transmission results from fecal contamination by ill or asymptomatic chronic carriers. Sexual transmission between male partners has been described. Health care workers occasionally acquire enteric fever after exposure to infected patients or during processing of clinical specimens and cultures.

With improvements in food handling and water/sewage treatment, enteric fever has become rare in developed nations. Worldwide, however, there are an estimated 22 million cases of enteric fever, with 200,000 deaths annually. The incidence is highest (>100 cases per 100,000 population per year) in south central and Southeast Asia; medium (10–100 cases per 100,000) in the rest of Asia, Africa, Latin America, and Oceania (excluding Australia and New Zealand); and low in other parts of the world (Fig. 27-1). A high incidence of enteric fever correlates with poor sanitation and lack of access to clean drinking water. In endemic regions, enteric fever is more common in urban than rural areas and among young children and adolescents. Risk factors include contaminated water or ice, flooding, food and drinks purchased from street vendors, raw fruits and vegetables grown in fields fertilized with sewage, ill household contacts, lack of hand washing and toilet access, and evidence of prior *Helicobacter pylori* infection (an association probably related to chronically reduced gastric acidity). It is estimated that there is one case of paratyphoid fever for every four cases of typhoid fever, but the incidence of infection associated with *S. paratyphi* A appears to be increasing, especially in India; this increase may be a result of vaccination for *S. typhi*.

Multidrug-resistant (MDR) strains of *S. typhi* emerged in 1989 in China and Southeast Asia and have since

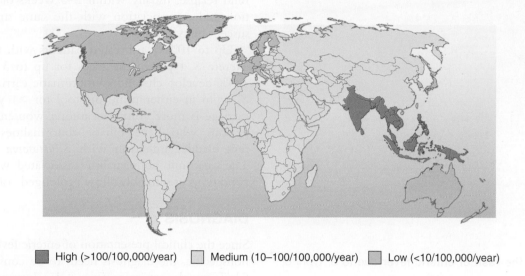

High (>100/100,000/year)   Medium (10–100/100,000/year)   Low (<10/100,000/year)

FIGURE 27-1
Annual incidence of typhoid fever per 100,000 population. (*Adapted from Crump JA et al: The global burden of typhoid fever. Bull World Health Organ 82:346, 2004.*)

disseminated widely. These strains contain plasmids encoding resistance to chloramphenicol, ampicillin, and trimethoprim—antibiotics long used to treat enteric fever. With the increased use of fluoroquinolones to treat MDR enteric fever in the 1990s, strains of *S. typhi* and *S. paratyphi* with reduced susceptibility to ciprofloxacin (minimal inhibitory concentration [MIC], 0.125–1 μg/mL) have emerged in the Indian subcontinent, southern Asia, and (most recently) sub-Saharan Africa and have been associated with clinical treatment failure. Testing of isolates for resistance to the first-generation quinolone nalidixic acid detects most but not all strains with reduced susceptibility to ciprofloxacin.

The incidence of enteric fever among U.S. travelers is estimated at 3–30 cases per 100,000. Of 1902 cases of *S. typhi*–associated enteric fever reported to the Centers for Disease Control and Prevention (CDC) in 1999–2006, 79% were associated with recent international travel, most commonly to India (47%), Pakistan (10%), Bangladesh (10%), Mexico (7%), and the Philippines (4%). Only 5% of travelers diagnosed with enteric fever had received *S. typhi* vaccine. Overall, 13% of *S. typhi* isolates in the United States were resistant to ampicillin, chloramphenicol, and trimethoprim-sulfamethoxazole (TMP-SMX), and the proportion of isolates resistant to nalidixic acid increased from 19% in 1999 to 58% in 2006. Infection with nalidixic acid–resistant (NAR) *S. typhi* was associated with travel to the Indian subcontinent. Of the 25–30% of reported cases of enteric fever in the United States that are domestically acquired, the majority are sporadic, but outbreaks linked to contaminated food products and previously unrecognized chronic carriers continue to occur.

CLINICAL COURSE

Enteric fever is a misnomer, in that the hallmark features of this disease—fever and abdominal pain—are variable. While fever is documented at presentation in >75% of cases, abdominal pain is reported in only 30–40%. Thus, a high index of suspicion for this potentially fatal systemic illness is necessary when a person presents with fever and a history of recent travel to a developing country.

The incubation period for *S. typhi* averages 10–14 days but ranges from 3–21 days, depending on the inoculum size and the host's health and immune status. The most prominent symptom is prolonged fever (38.8°–40.5°C; 101.8°–104.9°F), which can continue for up to 4 weeks if untreated. *S. paratyphi* A is thought to cause milder disease than *S. typhi*, with predominantly gastrointestinal symptoms. However, a prospective study of 669 consecutive cases of enteric fever in Kathmandu, Nepal, found that the infections were clinically indistinguishable. In this series, symptoms reported on initial medical evaluation included headache (80%), chills (35–45%), cough (30%), sweating (20–25%), myalgias (20%), malaise (10%), and arthralgia (2–4%). Gastrointestinal symptoms included anorexia (55%), abdominal pain (30–40%), nausea (18–24%), vomiting (18%), and diarrhea (22–28%) more commonly than constipation (13–16%). Physical findings included coated tongue (51–56%), splenomegaly (5–6%), and abdominal tenderness (4–5%).

Early physical findings of enteric fever include rash ("rose spots"; 30%), hepatosplenomegaly (3–6%), epistaxis, and relative bradycardia at the peak of high

FIGURE 27-2

"Rose spots," the rash of enteric fever due to *S. typhi* or *S. paratyphi*.

fever (<50%). Rose spots **(Fig. 27-2)** make up a faint, salmon-colored, blanching, maculopapular rash located primarily on the trunk and chest. The rash is evident in ~30% of patients at the end of the first week and resolves without a trace after 2–5 days. Patients can have two or three crops of lesions, and *Salmonella* can be cultured from punch biopsies of these lesions. The faintness of the rash makes it difficult to detect in highly pigmented patients.

The development of severe disease (which occurs in ~10–15% of patients) depends on host factors (immunosuppression, antacid therapy, previous exposure, and vaccination), strain virulence and inoculum, and choice of antibiotic therapy. Gastrointestinal bleeding (10–20%) and intestinal perforation (1–3%) most commonly occur in the third and fourth weeks of illness and result from hyperplasia, ulceration, and necrosis of the ileocecal Peyer's patches at the initial site of *Salmonella* infiltration. Both complications are life-threatening and require immediate fluid resuscitation and surgical intervention, with broadened antibiotic coverage for polymicrobial peritonitis (Chap. 25) and treatment of gastrointestinal hemorrhages, including bowel resection. Neurologic manifestations occur in 2–40% of patients and include meningitis, Guillain-Barré syndrome, neuritis, and neuropsychiatric symptoms (described as "muttering delirium" or "coma vigil"), with picking at bedclothes or imaginary objects.

Rare complications whose incidences are reduced by prompt antibiotic treatment include disseminated intravascular coagulation, hematophagocytic syndrome, pancreatitis, hepatic and splenic abscesses and granulomas, endocarditis, pericarditis, myocarditis, orchitis, hepatitis, glomerulonephritis, pyelonephritis and hemolytic-uremic syndrome, severe pneumonia, arthritis, osteomyelitis, and parotitis. Up to 10% of patients develop

mild relapse, usually within 2–3 weeks of fever resolution and in association with the same strain type and susceptibility profile.

Up to 10% of untreated patients with typhoid fever excrete *S. typhi* in the feces for up to 3 months, and 1–4% develop chronic asymptomatic carriage, shedding *S. typhi* in either urine or stool for >1 year. Chronic carriage is more common among women, infants, and persons who have biliary abnormalities or concurrent bladder infection with *Schistosoma haematobium*. The anatomic abnormalities associated with the latter conditions presumably allow prolonged colonization.

DIAGNOSIS

Since the clinical presentation of enteric fever is relatively nonspecific, the diagnosis needs to be considered in any febrile traveler returning from a developing region, especially the Indian subcontinent, the Philippines, or Latin America. Other diagnoses that should be considered in these travelers include malaria, hepatitis, bacterial enteritis, dengue fever, rickettsial infections, leptospirosis, amebic liver abscesses, and acute HIV infection. Other than a positive culture, no specific laboratory test is diagnostic for enteric fever. In 15–25% of cases, leukopenia and neutropenia are detectable. Leukocytosis is more common among children, during the first 10 days of illness, and in cases complicated by intestinal perforation or secondary infection. Other nonspecific laboratory findings include moderately elevated liver function tests and muscle enzyme levels.

The definitive diagnosis of enteric fever requires the isolation of *S. typhi* or *S. paratyphi* from blood, bone marrow, other sterile sites, rose spots, stool, or intestinal secretions. The sensitivity of blood culture is only 40–80%, probably because of high rates of antibiotic use in endemic areas and the small quantities of *S. typhi* (i.e., <15 organisms/mL) typically present in the blood. Since almost all *S. typhi* organisms in blood are associated with the mononuclear-cell/platelet fraction, centrifugation of blood and culture of the buffy coat can substantially reduce the time to isolation of the organism but do not increase sensitivity.

Bone marrow culture is 55–90% sensitive, and, unlike that of blood culture, its yield is not reduced by up to 5 days of prior antibiotic therapy. Culture of intestinal secretions (best obtained by a noninvasive duodenal string test) can be positive despite a negative bone marrow culture. If blood, bone marrow, and intestinal secretions are all cultured, the yield is >90%. Stool cultures, while negative in 60–70% of cases during the first week, can become positive during the third week of infection in untreated patients.

Several serologic tests, including the classic Widal test for "febrile agglutinins," are available. None of these tests is sufficiently sensitive or specific to replace culture-based methods for the diagnosis of enteric fever in developed countries. PCR and DNA probe assays to detect *S. typhi* in blood have been identified but have not yet been developed for clinical use.

TREATMENT ▸ Enteric (Typhoid) Fever

Prompt administration of appropriate antibiotic therapy prevents severe complications of enteric fever and results in a case-fatality rate of <1%. The initial choice of antibiotics depends on the susceptibility of the *S. typhi* and *S. paratyphi* strains in the area of residence or travel (Table 27-1). For treatment of drug-susceptible typhoid fever, fluoroquinolones are the most effective class of agents, with cure rates of ~98% and relapse and fecal carriage rates of <2%. Experience is most extensive with ciprofloxacin. Short-course ofloxacin therapy is similarly successful against infection caused by nalidixic acid–susceptible strains. However, the increased incidence of NAR *S. typhi* in Asia, which is probably related to the widespread availability of fluoroquinolones over the counter, is now limiting the use of this drug class for empirical therapy. Patients infected with NAR *S. typhi* strains should be treated with ceftriaxone, azithromycin, or high-dose ciprofloxacin. High-dose fluoroquinolone therapy for 7 days for NAR enteric fever has been associated with delayed resolution of fever and high rates of fecal carriage during convalescence. For NAR strains, 10–14 days of high-dose ciprofloxacin is preferred.

Ceftriaxone, cefotaxime, and (oral) cefixime are effective for treatment of MDR enteric fever, including NAR and fluoroquinolone-resistant strains. These agents clear fever in ~1 week, with failure rates of ~5–10%, fecal carriage rates of <3%, and relapse rates of 3–6%. Oral azithromycin results in defervescence in 4–6 days, with rates of relapse and convalescent stool carriage of <3%. Against NAR strains, azithromycin is associated with lower rates of treatment failure and shorter durations of hospitalization than are fluoroquinolones. Despite efficient in vitro killing of *Salmonella*, first- and second-generation cephalosporins as well as aminoglycosides are ineffective in the treatment of clinical infections.

Most patients with uncomplicated enteric fever can be managed at home with oral antibiotics and antipyretics. Patients with persistent vomiting, diarrhea, and/or abdominal distension should be hospitalized and given supportive therapy as well as a parenteral third-generation cephalosporin or fluoroquinolone, depending on the susceptibility profile. Therapy should be administered for at least 10 days or for 5 days after fever resolution.

In a randomized, prospective, double-blind study of critically ill patients with enteric fever (i.e., those with

TABLE 27-1

ANTIBIOTIC THERAPY FOR ENTERIC FEVER IN ADULTS

INDICATION	AGENT	DOSAGE (ROUTE)	DURATION, DAYS
Empirical Treatment			
	Ceftriaxone[a]	1–2 g/d (IV)	7–14
	Azithromycin	1 g/d (PO)	5
Fully Susceptible			
	Ciprofloxacin[b] (first line)	500 mg bid (PO) or 400 mg q12h (IV)	5–7
	Amoxicillin (second line)	1 g tid (PO) or 2 g q6h (IV)	14
	Chloramphenicol	25 mg/kg tid (PO or IV)	14–21
	Trimethoprim-sulfamethoxazole	160/800 mg bid (PO)	7–14
Multidrug-Resistant			
	Ciprofloxacin	500 mg bid (PO) or 400 mg q12h (IV)	5–7
	Ceftriaxone	2–3 g/d (IV)	7–14
	Azithromycin	1 g/d (PO)[c]	5
Nalidixic Acid–Resistant			
	Ceftriaxone	2–3 g/d (IV)	7–14
	Azithromycin	1 g/d (PO)	5
	High-dose ciprofloxacin	750 mg bid (PO) or 400 mg q8h (IV)	10–14

[a]Or another third-generation cephalosporin (e.g., cefotaxime, 2 g q8h [IV]; or cefixime, 400 mg bid [PO]).
[b]Or ofloxacin, 400 mg bid (PO) for 2–5 days.
[c]Or 1 g on day 1 followed by 500 mg/d PO for 6 days.

shock and obtundation) in Indonesia in the early 1980s, the administration of dexamethasone (an initial dose of 3 mg/kg followed by eight doses of 1 mg/kg every 6 h) with chloramphenicol was associated with a substantially lower mortality rate than was treatment with chloramphenicol alone (10% vs 55%). Although this study has not been repeated in the "post-chloramphenicol era," severe enteric fever remains one of the few indications for glucocorticoid treatment of an acute bacterial infection.

The 1–5% of patients who develop chronic carriage of *Salmonella* can be treated for 4–6 weeks with an appropriate oral antibiotic. Treatment with oral amoxicillin, TMP-SMX, ciprofloxacin, or norfloxacin is ~80% effective in eradicating chronic carriage of susceptible organisms. However, in cases of anatomic abnormality (e.g., biliary or kidney stones), eradication often requires both antibiotic therapy and surgical correction.

PREVENTION AND CONTROL

Theoretically, it is possible to eliminate the salmonellae that cause enteric fever since they survive only in human hosts and are spread by contaminated food and water. However, given the high prevalence of the disease in developing countries that lack adequate sewage disposal and water treatment, this goal is currently unrealistic. Thus, travelers to developing countries should be advised to monitor their food and water intake carefully and to consider vaccination.

Two typhoid vaccines are commercially available: (1) Ty21a, an oral live attenuated *S. typhi* vaccine (given on days 1, 3, 5, and 7, with a booster every 5 years); and (2) Vi CPS, a parenteral vaccine consisting of purified Vi polysaccharide from the bacterial capsule (given in one dose, with a booster every 2 years). The old parenteral whole-cell typhoid/paratyphoid A and B vaccine is no longer licensed, largely because of significant side effects (discussed later). An acetone-killed whole-cell vaccine is available only for use by the U.S. military. The minimal age for vaccination is 6 years for Ty21a and 2 years for Vi CPS. Currently, there is no licensed vaccine for paratyphoid fever.

A large-scale meta-analysis of vaccine trials comparing whole-cell vaccine, Ty21a, and Vi CPS in populations in endemic areas indicates that, while all three vaccines are similarly effective for the first year, the 3-year cumulative efficacy of the whole-cell vaccine (73%) exceeds that of both Ty21a (51%) and Vi CPS (55%). In addition, the heat-killed whole-cell vaccine maintains its efficacy for 5 years, whereas Ty21a and Vi CPS maintain their efficacy for 4 and 2 years, respectively. However, the whole-cell vaccine is associated with a much higher incidence of side effects (especially fever: 16% vs 1–2%) than the other two vaccines.

Vi CPS typhoid vaccine is poorly immunogenic in children <5 years of age because of T cell–independent properties. In the recently developed Vi-rEPA vaccine, Vi is bound to a nontoxic recombinant protein that is identical to *Pseudomonas aeruginosa* exotoxin A. In 2- to 4-year-olds, two injections of Vi-rEPA induced higher T cell responses and higher levels of serum IgG antibody to Vi than did Vi CPS in 5- to 14-year-olds. In a two-dose trial in 2- to 5-year-old children in Vietnam, Vi-rEPA provided 91% efficacy at 27 months and 88% efficacy at 43 months and was very well tolerated. This vaccine is not yet commercially available in the United States. At least three new live vaccines are in clinical development and may prove more efficacious and longer-lasting than previous live vaccines.

Typhoid vaccine is not required for international travel, but it is recommended for travelers to areas where there is a moderate to high risk of exposure to *S. typhi*, especially those who are traveling to southern Asia and other developing regions of Asia, Africa, the Caribbean, and Central and South America and who will be exposed to potentially contaminated food and drink. Typhoid vaccine should be considered even for persons planning <2 weeks of travel to high-risk areas. In addition, laboratory workers who deal with *S. typhi* and household contacts of known *S. typhi* carriers should be vaccinated. Because the protective efficacy of vaccine can be overcome by the high inocula that are commonly encountered in food-borne exposures, immunization is an adjunct and not a substitute for avoiding high-risk foods and beverages. Immunization is not recommended for adults residing in typhoid-endemic areas or for the management of persons who may have been exposed in a common-source outbreak.

Enteric fever is a notifiable disease in the United States. Individual health departments have their own guidelines for allowing ill or colonized food handlers or health care workers to return to their jobs. The reporting system enables public health departments to identify potential source patients and to treat chronic carriers in order to prevent further outbreaks. In addition, since 1–4% of patients with *S. typhi* infection become chronic carriers, it is important to monitor patients (especially child-care providers and food handlers) for chronic carriage and to treat this condition if indicated.

NONTYPHOIDAL SALMONELLOSIS

EPIDEMIOLOGY

In the United States, the incidence of NTS infection has doubled in the past 2 decades; the 2009 figure is ~14 million cases annually. In 2007, the incidence of NTS infection in this country was 14.9 per 100,000 persons—the highest rate among the 11 food-borne enteric pathogens under active surveillance. Five serotypes accounted for one-half of U.S. infections in 2007: *typhimurium* (19%), *enteritidis* (14%), Newport (9%), Javiana (5%), and Heidelberg (4%).

The incidence of nontyphoidal salmonellosis is highest during the rainy season in tropical climates and during the warmer months in temperate climates, coinciding with the peak in food-borne outbreaks. Rates of morbidity and mortality associated with NTS are highest among the elderly, infants, and immunocompromised individuals, including those with hemoglobinopathies, HIV infection, or infections that cause blockade of the reticuloendothelial system (e.g., bartonellosis, malaria, schistosomiasis, and histoplasmosis).

Unlike *S. typhi* and *S. paratyphi*, whose only reservoir is humans, NTS can be acquired from multiple animal reservoirs. Transmission is most commonly associated with animal food products, especially eggs, poultry, undercooked ground meat, dairy products, and fresh produce contaminated with animal waste.

S. enteritidis infection associated with chicken eggs emerged as a major cause of food-borne disease during the 1980s and 1990s. *S. enteritidis* infection of the ovaries and upper oviduct tissue of hens results in contamination of egg contents before shell deposition. Infection is spread to egg-laying hens from breeding flocks and through contact with rodents and manure. Of the 997 outbreaks of *S. enteritidis* with a confirmed source that were reported to the CDC in 1985–2003, 75% were associated with raw or undercooked eggs. After peaking at 3.9 cases per 100,000 U.S. population in 1995, the incidence of *S. enteritidis* infection declined substantially to 1.7 per 100,000 in 2003; this decrease probably reflected improved on-farm control measures, refrigeration, and education of consumers and food-service workers. Transmission via contaminated eggs can be prevented by cooking eggs until the yolk is solidified and through pasteurization of egg products.

 Centralization of food processing and widespread food distribution have contributed to the increased incidence of NTS in developed countries. Manufactured foods to which recent *Salmonella* outbreaks have been traced include peanut butter; milk products, including infant formula; and various processed foods, including packaged breakfast cereal, salsa, frozen prepared meals, and snack foods. Large outbreaks have also been linked to fresh produce, including alfalfa sprouts, cantaloupe, fresh-squeezed orange juice, and tomatoes; these items become contaminated by manure or water at a single site and then are widely distributed.

An estimated 6% of sporadic *Salmonella* infections in the United States are attributed to contact with reptiles and amphibians, especially iguanas, snakes, turtles, and lizards. Reptile-associated *Salmonella* infection more commonly leads to hospitalization and more frequently involves infants than do other *Salmonella* infections.

Other pets, including African hedgehogs, snakes, birds, rodents, baby chicks, ducklings, dogs, and cats, are also potential sources of NTS.

 Increasing antibiotic resistance in NTS species is a global problem and has been linked to the widespread use of antimicrobial agents in food animals and especially in animal feed. In the early 1990s, *S. typhimurium* definitive phage type 104 (DT104), characterized by resistance to ≥5 antibiotics (ampicillin, chloramphenicol, streptomycin, sulfonamides, and tetracyclines; R-type ACSSuT), emerged worldwide. In 2005, resistance to at least ACSSuT was the most common MDR phenotype among NTS isolates in the United States. Acquisition is associated with exposure to ill farm animals and to various meat products, including uncooked or undercooked ground beef. Although probably no more virulent than susceptible *S. typhimurium* strains, DT104 strains are associated with an increased risk of bloodstream infection and hospitalization. NAR and trimethoprim-resistant DT104 strains are emerging, especially in the United Kingdom.

Because of increased resistance to conventional antibiotics such as ampicillin and TMP-SMX, extended-spectrum cephalosporins and fluoroquinolones have emerged as the agents of choice for the treatment of MDR NTS infections. In 2005, 2% of all NTS strains and 12.6% of *S*. Newport strains were resistant to ceftriaxone. Most ceftriaxone-resistant isolates were from children <18 years of age, in whom ceftriaxone is the antibiotic of choice for treatment of invasive NTS infection. These strains contained plasmid-encoded AmpC β-lactamases that were probably acquired by horizontal genetic transfer from *Escherichia coli* strains in food-producing animals—an event linked to the widespread use of the veterinary cephalosporin ceftiofur.

Resistance to nalidixic acid and fluoroquinolones also has begun to emerge and is most commonly associated with point mutations in the DNA gyrase genes *gyr*A and *gyr*B. Nalidixic acid resistance is a good predictor of reduced susceptibility to clinically useful fluoroquinolones. From 1996–2005, the rate of NAR NTS isolates in the United States increased fivefold (from 0.5–2.4%). In Denmark, infection with NAR *S. typhimurium* DT104 has been linked to swine and associated with a threefold higher risk of invasive disease or death within 90 days. In Taiwan in 2000, a strain of ciprofloxacin-resistant (MIC, ≥4 μg/mL) *S. choleraesuis* caused a large outbreak of invasive infections that was linked to the use of enrofloxacin in swine feed.

CLINICAL MANIFESTATIONS
Gastroenteritis

Infection with NTS most often results in gastroenteritis indistinguishable from that caused by other enteric pathogens. Nausea, vomiting, and diarrhea occur 6–48 h after the ingestion of contaminated food or water. Patients often experience abdominal cramping and fever (38–39°C; 100.5–102.2°F). Diarrheal stools are usually loose, nonbloody, and of moderate volume. However, large-volume watery stools, bloody stools, or symptoms of dysentery may occur. Rarely, NTS causes pseudoappendicitis or an illness that mimics inflammatory bowel disease.

Gastroenteritis caused by NTS is usually self-limited. Diarrhea resolves within 3–7 days and fever within 72 h. Stool cultures remain positive for 4–5 weeks after infection and—in rare cases of chronic carriage (<1%)—for >1 year. Antibiotic treatment usually is not recommended and may prolong fecal carriage. Neonates, the elderly, and immunosuppressed patients (e.g., transplant recipients, HIV-infected persons) with NTS gastroenteritis are especially susceptible to dehydration and dissemination and may require hospitalization and antibiotic therapy. Acute NTS gastroenteritis was associated with a threefold increased risk of dyspepsia and irritable bowel syndrome at 1 year in a recent study from Spain.

Bacteremia and endovascular infections

Up to 8% of patients with NTS gastroenteritis develop bacteremia; of these, 5–10% develop localized infections. Bacteremia and metastatic infection are most common with *S. choleraesuis* and *S. Dublin* and among infants, the elderly, and immunocompromised patients. NTS endovascular infection should be suspected in high-grade or persistent bacteremia, especially with preexisting valvular heart disease, atherosclerotic vascular disease, prosthetic vascular graft, or aortic aneurysm. Arteritis should be suspected in elderly patients with prolonged fever and back, chest, or abdominal pain developing after an episode of gastroenteritis. Endocarditis and arteritis are rare (<1% of cases) but are associated with potentially fatal complications, including valve perforation, endomyocardial abscess, infected mural thrombus, pericarditis, mycotic aneurysms, aneurysm rupture, aortoenteric fistula, and vertebral osteomyelitis. In some areas of sub-Saharan Africa, NTS may be among the most common causes—or even the most common cause—of bacteremia in children. NTS bacteremia among these children is not associated with diarrhea and has been associated with nutritional status and HIV infection.

Localized infections

Intraabdominal infections

Intraabdominal infections due to NTS are rare and usually manifest as hepatic or splenic abscesses or as cholecystitis. Risk factors include hepatobiliary anatomic abnormalities (e.g., gallstones), abdominal malignancy, and sickle cell disease (especially with splenic abscesses). Eradication of the infection often requires surgical correction of abnormalities and percutaneous drainage of abscesses.

Central nervous system infections

NTS meningitis most commonly develops in infants 1–4 months of age. It often results in severe sequelae (including seizures, hydrocephalus, brain infarction, and mental retardation) with death in up to 60% of cases. Other rare central nervous system infections include ventriculitis, subdural empyema, and brain abscesses.

Pulmonary infections

NTS pulmonary infections usually present as lobar pneumonia, and complications include lung abscess, empyema, and bronchopleural fistula formation. The majority of cases occur in patients with lung cancer, structural lung disease, sickle cell disease, or glucocorticoid use.

Urinary and genital tract infections

Urinary tract infections caused by NTS present as either cystitis or pyelonephritis. Risk factors include malignancy, urolithiasis, structural abnormalities, HIV infection, and renal transplantation. NTS genital infections are rare and include ovarian and testicular abscesses, prostatitis, and epididymitis. Like other focal infections, both genital and urinary tract infections can be complicated by abscess formation.

Bone, joint, and soft tissue infections

Salmonella osteomyelitis most commonly affects the femur, tibia, humerus, or lumbar vertebrae and is most often seen in association with sickle cell disease, hemoglobinopathies, or preexisting bone disease (e.g., fractures). Prolonged antibiotic treatment is recommended to decrease the risk of relapse and chronic osteomyelitis. Septic arthritis occurs in the same patient population as osteomyelitis and usually involves the knee, hip, or shoulder joints. Reactive arthritis (Reiter's syndrome) can follow NTS gastroenteritis and is seen most frequently in persons with the HLA-B27 histocompatibility antigen. NTS rarely can cause soft tissue infections, usually at sites of local trauma in immunosuppressed patients.

DIAGNOSIS

The diagnosis of NTS infection is based on isolation of the organism from freshly passed stool or from blood or another ordinarily sterile body fluid. All salmonellae isolated in clinical laboratories should be sent to local public health departments for serotyping. Blood cultures should be done whenever a patient has prolonged or recurrent fever. Endovascular infection should be suspected if there is high-grade bacteremia (>50% of three or more positive blood cultures). Echocardiography, CT, and indium-labeled white cell scanning are used to identify localized infection. When another localized infection is suspected, joint fluid, abscess drainage, or cerebrospinal fluid should be cultured, as clinically indicated.

TREATMENT ▶ Nontyphoidal Salmonellosis

Antibiotics should not be used routinely to treat uncomplicated NTS gastroenteritis. The symptoms are usually self-limited, and the duration of fever and diarrhea is not significantly decreased by antibiotic therapy. In addition, antibiotic treatment has been associated with increased rates of relapse, prolonged gastrointestinal carriage, and adverse drug reactions. Dehydration secondary to diarrhea should be treated with fluid and electrolyte replacement.

Preemptive antibiotic treatment (Table 27-2) should be considered for patients at increased risk for invasive NTS infection, including neonates (probably up to 3 months of age); persons >50 years of age with suspected atherosclerosis; and patients with immunosuppression, cardiac valvular or endovascular abnormalities, or significant joint disease. Treatment should consist of an oral or IV antibiotic administered for 48–72 h or until the patient

TABLE 27-2

ANTIBIOTIC THERAPY FOR NONTYPHOIDAL *SALMONELLA* INFECTION IN ADULTS

INDICATION	AGENT	DOSAGE (ROUTE)	DURATION, DAYS
Preemptive Treatment[a]			
	Ciprofloxacin[b]	500 mg bid (PO)	2–3
Severe Gastroenteritis[c]			
	Ciprofloxacin	500 mg bid (PO) or 400 mg q12h (IV)	3–7
	Trimethoprim-sulfamethoxazole	160/800 mg bid (PO)	
	Amoxicillin	1 g tid (PO)	
	Ceftriaxone	1–2 g/d (IV)	
Bacteremia			
	Ceftriaxone[d]	2 g/d (IV)	7–14
	Ciprofloxacin	400 mg q12h (IV), then 500 mg bid (PO)	
Endocarditis or Arteritis			
	Ceftriaxone	2 g/d (IV)	42
	Ciprofloxacin	400 mg q8h (IV), then 750 mg bid (PO)	
	Ampicillin	2 g q4h (IV)	
Meningitis			
	Ceftriaxone	2 g q12 h (IV)	14–21
	Ampicillin	2 g q4h (IV)	
Other Localized Infection			
	Ceftriaxone	2 g/d (IV)	14–28
	Ciprofloxacin	500 mg bid (PO) or 400 mg q12h (IV)	
	Ampicillin	2 g q6h (IV)	

[a]Consider for neonates; persons >50 years of age with possible atherosclerotic vascular disease; and patients with immunosuppression, endovascular graft, or joint prosthesis.
[b]Or ofloxacin, 400 mg bid (PO).
[c]Consider on an individualized basis for patients with severe diarrhea and high fever who require hospitalization.
[d]Or cefotaxime, 2 g q8h (IV).

CHAPTER 27

Salmonellosis

becomes afebrile. Immunocompromised persons may require up to 7–14 days of therapy. The <1% of persons who develop chronic carriage of NTS should receive a prolonged antibiotic course, as described earlier for chronic carriage of *S. typhi*.

Because of the increasing prevalence of antibiotic resistance, empirical therapy for life-threatening NTS bacteremia or focal NTS infection should include a third-generation cephalosporin or a fluoroquinolone (Table 27-2). If the bacteremia is low-grade (<50% of positive blood cultures), the patient should be treated for 7–14 days. Patients with HIV/AIDS and NTS bacteremia should receive 1–2 weeks of IV antibiotic therapy followed by 4 weeks of oral therapy with a fluoroquinolone. Patients whose infections relapse after this regimen should receive long-term suppressive therapy with a fluoroquinolone or TMP-SMX, as indicated by bacterial sensitivities.

If the patient has endocarditis or arteritis, treatment for 6 weeks with an IV β-lactam antibiotic (such as ceftriaxone or ampicillin) is indicated. IV ciprofloxacin followed by prolonged oral therapy is an option, but published experience is limited. Early surgical resection of infected aneurysms or other infected endovascular sites is recommended. Patients with infected prosthetic vascular grafts that cannot be resected have been maintained successfully on chronic suppressive oral therapy. For extraintestinal nonvascular infections, a 2- to 4-week course of antibiotic therapy (depending on the infection site) is usually recommended. In chronic osteomyelitis, abscess, or urinary or hepatobiliary infection associated with anatomic abnormalities, surgical resection or drainage may be required in addition to prolonged antibiotic therapy for eradication of infection.

PREVENTION AND CONTROL

Despite widespread efforts to prevent or reduce bacterial contamination of animal-derived food products and to improve food-safety education and training, recent declines in the incidence of NTS in the United States have been modest compared with those of other food-borne pathogens. This observation probably reflects the complex epidemiology of NTS. Identifying effective risk-reduction strategies requires monitoring of every step of food production, from handling of raw animal or plant products to preparation of finished foods. Contaminated food can be made safe for consumption by pasteurization, irradiation, or proper cooking. All cases of NTS infection should be reported to local public health departments, since tracking and monitoring of these cases can identify the source(s) of infection and help authorities anticipate large outbreaks. Lastly, the prudent use of antimicrobial agents in both humans and animals is needed to limit the emergence of MDR *Salmonella*.

CHAPTER 28

SHIGELLOSIS

Philippe Sansonetti ■ Jean Bergounioux

The discovery of *Shigella* as the etiologic agent of dysentery—a clinical syndrome of fever, intestinal cramps, and frequent passage of small, bloody, mucopurulent stools—is attributed to the Japanese microbiologist Kiyoshi Shiga, who isolated the Shiga bacillus (now known as *Shigella dysenteriae* type 1) from patients' stools in 1897 during a large and devastating dysentery epidemic. *Shigella* cannot be distinguished from *Escherichia coli* by DNA hybridization and remains a separate species only on historical and clinical grounds.

DEFINITION

Shigella is a nonspore-forming, gram-negative bacterium that, unlike *E. coli*, is nonmotile and does not produce gas from sugars, decarboxylate lysine, or hydrolyze arginine. Some serovars produce indole, and occasional strains utilize sodium acetate. *S. dysenteriae*, *S. flexneri*, *S. boydii*, and *S. sonnei* (serogroups A, B, C, and D, respectively) can be differentiated on the basis of biochemical and serologic characteristics. Genome sequencing of *E. coli* K12, *S. flexneri* 2a, *S. sonnei*, *S. dysenteriae* type 1, and *S. boydii* has revealed that these species have ~93% of genes in common. The three major genomic "signatures" of *Shigella* are (1) a 215-kb virulence plasmid that carries most of the genes required for pathogenicity (particularly invasive capacity); (2) the lack or alteration of genetic sequences encoding products (e.g., lysine decarboxylase) that, if expressed, would attenuate pathogenicity; and (3) in *S. dysenteriae* type 1, the presence of genes encoding Shiga toxin, a potent cytotoxin.

EPIDEMIOLOGY

The human intestinal tract represents the major reservoir of *Shigella*, which is also found (albeit rarely) in the higher primates. Because excretion of shigellae is greatest in the acute phase of disease, the bacteria are transmitted most efficiently by the fecal-oral route via hand carriage; however, some outbreaks reflect food-borne or waterborne transmission. In impoverished areas, *Shigella* can be transmitted by flies. The high-level infectivity of *Shigella* is reflected by the very small inoculum required for experimental infection of volunteers (100 colony-forming units [CFU]), by the very high attack rates during outbreaks in day-care centers (33–73%), and by the high rates of secondary cases among family members of sick children (26–33%). Shigellosis can also be transmitted sexually.

Throughout history, *Shigella* epidemics have often occurred in settings of human crowding under conditions of poor hygiene—e.g., among soldiers in campaigning armies, inhabitants of besieged cities, groups on pilgrimages, and refugees in camps. Epidemics follow a cyclical pattern in areas such as the Indian subcontinent and sub-Saharan Africa. These devastating epidemics, which are most often caused by *S. dysenteriae* type 1, are characterized by high attack and mortality rates. In Bangladesh, for instance, an epidemic caused by *S. dysenteriae* type 1 was associated with a 42% increase in mortality rate among children 1–4 years of age. Apart from these epidemics, shigellosis is mostly an endemic disease, with 99% of cases occurring in the developing world and the highest prevalences in the most impoverished areas, where personal and general hygiene is below standard. *S. flexneri* isolates predominate in the least developed areas, whereas *S. sonnei* is more prevalent in economically emerging countries and in the industrialized world.

Prevalence in the developing world

In a review published under the auspices of the World Health Organization (WHO), the total annual number of cases in 1966–1997 was estimated at 165 million, and 69% of these cases occurred in children <5 years of age. In this review, the annual number of deaths was calculated to range between 500,000 and 1.1 million.

More recent data (2000–2004) from six Asian countries indicate that even though the incidence of shigellosis remains stable, mortality rates associated with this disease may have decreased significantly, possibly as a result of improved nutritional status. However, extensive and essentially uncontrolled use of antibiotics, which may also account for declining mortality rates, has increased the rate of emergence of multidrug-resistant *Shigella* strains. An often-overlooked complication of shigellosis is the short- and long-term impairment of the nutritional status of infected children in endemic areas. Combined with anorexia, the exudative enteropathy resulting from mucosal abrasions contributes to rapid deterioration of the patient's nutritional status. Shigellosis is thus a major contributor to stunted growth among children in developing countries.

Peaking in incidence in the pediatric population, endemic shigellosis is rare in young and middle-aged adults, probably because of naturally acquired immunity. Incidence then increases again in the elderly population.

Prevalence in the industrialized world

In pediatric populations, local outbreaks occur when proper and adapted hygiene policies are not implemented in group facilities like day-care centers and institutions for the mentally retarded. In adults, as in children, sporadic cases occur among travelers returning from endemic areas, and rare outbreaks of varying size can follow waterborne or food-borne infections.

PATHOGENESIS AND PATHOLOGY

Shigella infection occurs essentially through oral contamination via direct fecal-oral transmission, the organism being poorly adapted to survive in the environment. Resistance to low-pH conditions allows shigellae to survive passage through the gastric barrier, an ability that may explain in part why a small inoculum (as few as 100 CFU) is sufficient to cause infection.

The watery diarrhea that usually precedes the dysenteric syndrome is attributable to active secretion and abnormal water reabsorption—a secretory effect at the jejunal level described in experimentally infected rhesus monkeys. This initial purge is probably due to the combined action of an enterotoxin (ShET-1) and mucosal inflammation. The dysenteric syndrome, manifested by bloody and mucopurulent stools, reflects invasion of the mucosa.

The pathogenesis of *Shigella* is essentially determined by a large virulence plasmid of 214 kb comprising ~100 genes, of which 25 encode a type III secretion system that inserts into the membrane of the host cell to allow effectors to transit from the bacterial cytoplasm to the host cell cytoplasm **(Fig. 28-1)**. Bacteria are thereby able to invade intestinal epithelial cells by inducing their own uptake after the initial crossing of the epithelial barrier through M cells (the specialized translocating epithelial cells in the follicle-associated epithelium that covers mucosal lymphoid nodules). The organisms induce apoptosis of subepithelial resident macrophages. Once inside the cytoplasm of intestinal epithelial cells, *Shigella* effectors trigger the cytoskeletal rearrangements necessary to direct uptake of the organism into the epithelial cell. The *Shigella*-containing vacuole is then quickly lysed, releasing bacteria into the cytosol.

Intracellular shigellae next use cytoskeletal components to propel themselves inside the infected cell; when the moving organism and the host cell membrane come

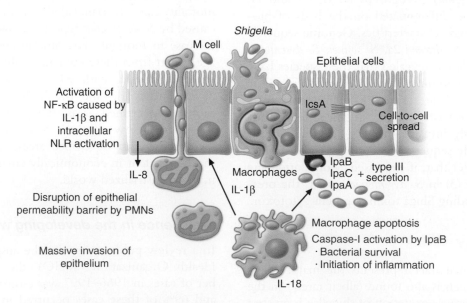

FIGURE 28-1

Invasive strategy of *Shigella flexneri*. IL, interleukin; NF-κB, nuclear factor κB; NLR, NOD-like receptor; PMN, polymorphonuclear leukocyte.

into contact, cellular protrusions form and are engulfed by neighboring cells. This series of events permits bacterial cell-to-cell spread.

Cytokines released by a growing number of infected intestinal epithelial cells attract increased numbers of immune cells (particularly polymorphonuclear leukocytes [PMNs]) to the infected site, thus further destabilizing the epithelial barrier, exacerbating inflammation, and leading to the acute colitis that characterizes shigellosis. Evidence indicates that some type III secretion system–injected effectors can control the extent of inflammation, thus facilitating bacterial survival.

Shiga toxin produced by *S. dysenteriae* type 1 increases disease severity. This toxin belongs to a group of A1-B5 protein toxins whose B subunit binds to the receptor globotriaosylceramide on the target cell surface and whose catalytic A subunit is internalized by receptor-mediated endocytosis and interacts with the subcellular machinery to inhibit protein synthesis by expressing RNA N-glycosidase activity on 28S ribosomal RNA. This process leads to inhibition of binding of the amino-acyl-tRNA to the 60S ribosomal subunit and thus to a general shutoff of cell protein biosynthesis. Shiga toxins are translocated from the bowel into the circulation. After binding of the toxins to target cells in the kidney, pathophysiologic alterations may result in hemolytic-uremic syndrome (HUS; discussed later).

CLINICAL MANIFESTATIONS

The presentation and severity of shigellosis depend to some extent on the infecting serotype but even more on the age and the immunologic and nutritional status of the host. Poverty and poor standards of hygiene are strongly related to the number and severity of diarrheal episodes, especially in children <5 years old who have been weaned.

Shigellosis typically evolves through four phases: incubation, watery diarrhea, dysentery, and the postinfectious phase. The incubation period usually lasts 1–4 days but may be as long as 8 days. Typical initial manifestations are transient fever, limited watery diarrhea, malaise, and anorexia. Signs and symptoms may range from mild abdominal discomfort to severe cramps, diarrhea, fever, vomiting, and tenesmus. The manifestations are usually exacerbated in children, with temperatures up to 40°–41°C (104.0°–105.8°F) and more severe anorexia and watery diarrhea. This initial phase may represent the only clinical manifestation of shigellosis, especially in developed countries. Otherwise, dysentery follows within hours or days and is characterized by uninterrupted excretion of small volumes of bloody mucopurulent stools with increased tenesmus and abdominal cramps. At this stage, *Shigella* produces acute colitis involving mainly the distal colon and the rectum.

Unlike most diarrheal syndromes, dysenteric syndromes rarely present with dehydration as a major feature. Endoscopy shows an edematous and hemorrhagic mucosa, with ulcerations and possibly overlying exudates resembling pseudomembranes. The extent of the lesions correlates with the number and frequency of stools and with the degree of protein loss by exudative mechanisms. Most episodes are self-limited and resolve without treatment in 1 week. With appropriate treatment, recovery takes place within a few days to a week, with no sequelae.

Acute life-threatening complications are seen most often in children <5 years of age (particularly those who are malnourished) and in elderly patients. Risk factors for death in a clinically severe case include nonbloody diarrhea, moderate to severe dehydration, bacteremia, absence of fever, abdominal tenderness, and rectal prolapse. Major complications are predominantly intestinal (e.g., toxic megacolon, intestinal perforations, rectal prolapse) or metabolic (e.g., hypoglycemia, hyponatremia, dehydration). Bacteremia is rare and is reported most frequently in severely malnourished and HIV-infected patients. Alterations of consciousness, including seizures, delirium, and coma, may occur, especially in children <5 years old, and are associated with a poor prognosis; fever and severe metabolic alterations are more often the major causes of altered consciousness than is meningitis or the Ekiri syndrome (toxic encephalopathy associated with bizarre posturing, cerebral edema, and fatty degeneration of viscera), which has been reported mostly in Japanese children. Pneumonia, vaginitis, and keratoconjunctivitis due to *Shigella* are rarely reported. In the absence of serious malnutrition, severe and very unusual clinical manifestations, such as meningitis, may be linked to genetic defects in innate immune functions (i.e., deficiency in interleukin 1 receptor–associated kinase 4 [IRAK-4]) and may require genetic investigation.

Two complications of particular importance are toxic megacolon and HUS. Toxic megacolon is a consequence of severe inflammation extending to the colonic smooth-muscle layer and causing paralysis and dilatation. The patient presents with abdominal distention and tenderness, with or without signs of localized or generalized peritonitis. The abdominal x-ray characteristically shows marked dilatation of the transverse colon (with the greatest distention in the ascending and descending segments); thumbprinting caused by mucosal inflammatory edema; and loss of the normal haustral pattern associated with pseudopolyps, often extending into the lumen. Pneumatosis coli is an occasional finding. If perforation occurs, radiographic signs of pneumoperitoneum may be apparent. Predisposing factors (e.g., hypokalemia and use of opioids, anticholinergics, loperamide, psyllium seeds, and antidepressants) should be investigated.

Shiga toxin produced by *S. dysenteriae* type 1 has been linked to HUS in developing countries but rarely in industrialized countries, where enterohemorrhagic *E. coli* (EHEC) predominates as the etiologic agent of this syndrome. HUS is an early complication that most often develops after several days of diarrhea. Clinical examination shows pallor, asthenia, and irritability and, in some cases, bleeding of the nose and gums, oliguria, and increasing edema. HUS is a nonimmune (Coombs test–negative) hemolytic anemia defined by a diagnostic triad: microangiopathic hemolytic anemia (hemoglobin level typically <80 g/L [<8 g/dL]), thrombocytopenia (mild to moderate in severity; typically <60,000 platelets/μL), and acute renal failure due to thrombosis of the glomerular capillaries (with markedly elevated creatinine levels). Anemia is severe, with fragmented red blood cells (schizocytes) in the peripheral smear, high serum concentrations of lactate dehydrogenase and free circulating hemoglobin, and elevated reticulocyte counts. Acute renal failure occurs in 55–70% of cases; however, renal function recovers in most of these cases (up to 70% in various series). Leukemoid reactions, with leukocyte counts of 50,000/μL, are sometimes noted in association with HUS.

The postinfectious immunologic complication known as reactive arthritis can develop weeks or months after shigellosis, especially in patients expressing the histocompatibility antigen HLA-B27. About 3% of patients infected with *S. flexneri* later develop this syndrome, with arthritis, ocular inflammation, and urethritis—a condition that can last for months or years and can progress to difficult-to-treat chronic arthritis. Postinfectious arthropathy occurs only after infection with *S. flexneri* and not after infection with the other *Shigella* serotypes.

LABORATORY DIAGNOSIS

The differential diagnosis in patients with a dysenteric syndrome depends on the clinical and environmental context. In developing areas, infectious diarrhea caused by other invasive pathogenic bacteria (*Salmonella*, *Campylobacter jejuni*, *Clostridium difficile*, *Yersinia enterocolitica*) or parasites (*Entamoeba histolytica*) should be considered. Only bacteriologic and parasitologic examinations of stool can truly differentiate among these pathogens. A first flare of inflammatory bowel disease, such as Crohn's disease or ulcerative colitis (Chap. 17), should be considered in patients in industrialized countries. Despite similar symptoms, anamnesis discriminates between shigellosis, which usually follows recent travel in an endemic zone, and these other conditions.

Microscopic examination of stool smears shows the presence of erythrophagocytic trophozoites with very few PMNs in *E. histolytica* infection, whereas bacterial enteroinvasive infections (particularly shigellosis) are characterized by high PMN counts in each microscopic field. However,

because shigellosis often manifests only as watery diarrhea, systematic attempts to isolate *Shigella* are necessary.

The "gold standard" for the diagnosis of *Shigella* infection remains the isolation and identification of the pathogen from fecal material. One major difficulty, particularly in endemic areas where laboratory facilities are not immediately available, is the fragility of *Shigella* and its common disappearance during transport, especially with rapid changes in temperature and pH. In the absence of a reliable enrichment medium, buffered glycerol saline or Cary-Blair medium can be used as a holding medium, but prompt inoculation onto isolation medium is essential. The probability of isolation is higher if the portion of stools that contains bloody and/or mucopurulent material is directly sampled. Rectal swabs can be used, as they offer the highest rate of successful isolation during the acute phase of disease. Blood cultures are positive in <5% of cases but should be done when a patient presents with a clinical picture of severe sepsis.

In addition to quick processing, the use of several media increases the likelihood of successful isolation: a nonselective medium such as bromocresol-purple agar lactose; a low-selectivity medium such as MacConkey or eosin-methylene blue; and a high-selectivity medium such as Hektoen, *Salmonella-Shigella*, or xylose-lysine-deoxycholate agar. After incubation on these media for 12–18 h at 37°C (98.6°F), shigellae appear as nonlactose-fermenting colonies that measure 0.5–1 mm in diameter and have a convex, translucent, smooth surface. Suspected colonies on nonselective or low-selectivity medium can be subcultured on a high-selectivity medium before being specifically identified or can be identified directly by standard commercial systems on the basis of four major characteristics: glucose positivity (usually without production of gas), lactose negativity, H_2S negativity, and lack of motility. The four *Shigella* serogroups (A–D) can then be differentiated by additional characteristics. This approach adds time and difficulty to the identification process; however, after presumptive diagnosis, the use of serologic methods (e.g., slide agglutination, with group- and then type-specific antisera) should be considered. Group-specific antisera are widely available; in contrast, because of the large number of serotypes and sub-serotypes, type-specific antisera are rare and more expensive and thus are often restricted to reference laboratories.

TREATMENT	Shigellosis

ANTIBIOTIC SUSCEPTIBILITY OF *SHIGELLA*

As an enteroinvasive disease, shigellosis requires antibiotic treatment. Since the mid-1960s, however, increasing resistance to multiple drugs has been a dominant factor in treatment decisions. Resistance rates are highly dependent on the geographic area. Clonal spread of particular strains and horizontal transfer of resistance determinants, particularly via plasmids and transposons, contribute to multidrug resistance. The current global status—i.e., high rates of resistance to classic first-line antibiotics such as amoxicillin—has led to a rapid switch to quinolones such as nalidixic acid. However, resistance to such early-generation quinolones has also emerged and spread quickly as a result of chromosomal mutations affecting DNA gyrase and topoisomerase IV; this resistance has necessitated the use of later-generation quinolones as first-line antibiotics in many areas. For instance, a review of the antibiotic resistance history of *Shigella* in India found that, after their introduction in the late 1980s, the second-generation quinolones norfloxacin, ciprofloxacin, and ofloxacin were highly effective in the treatment of shigellosis, including cases caused by multidrug-resistant strains of *S. dysenteriae* type 1. However, investigations of subsequent outbreaks in India and Bangladesh detected resistance to norfloxacin, ciprofloxacin, and ofloxacin in 5% of isolates. The incidence of multidrug resistance parallels the widespread, uncontrolled use of antibiotics and calls for the rational use of effective drugs.

ANTIBIOTIC TREATMENT OF SHIGELLOSIS

(Table 28-1) Because of the ready transmissibility of *Shigella*, current public health recommendations in the United States are that every case be treated with antibiotics. Ciprofloxacin is recommended as first-line treatment. A number of other drugs have been tested and shown to be effective, including ceftriaxone, azithromycin, pivmecillinam, and some fifth-generation quinolones. While infections caused by non-*dysenteriae Shigella* in immunocompetent individuals are routinely treated with a 3-day course of antibiotics, it is recommended that *S. dysenteriae* type 1 infections be treated for 5 days and that *Shigella* infections in immunocompromised patients be treated for 7–10 days.

Treatment for shigellosis must be adapted to the clinical context, with the recognition that the most fragile patients are children <5 years old, who represent two-thirds of all cases worldwide. There are few data on the use of quinolones in children, but *Shigella*-induced dysentery is a well-recognized indication for their use. The half-life of ciprofloxacin is longer in infants than in older individuals. The ciprofloxacin dose generally recommended for children is 30 mg/kg per day in two divided doses. Adults living in areas with high standards of hygiene are likely to develop milder, shorter-duration disease, whereas infants in endemic areas can develop severe, sometimes fatal dysentery. In the former setting, treatment will remain minimal and bacteriologic proof of infection will often come after symptoms have resolved; in the latter setting, antibiotic treatment and

TABLE 28-1

RECOMMENDED ANTIMICROBIAL THERAPY FOR SHIGELLOSIS

ANTIMICROBIAL AGENT	TREATMENT SCHEDULE		LIMITATIONS
	CHILDREN	ADULTS	
First line			
Ciprofloxacin	15 mg/kg 2 times per day for 3 days, PO	500 mg	
Second line			
Pivmecillinam	20 mg/kg 4 times per day for 5 days, PO	100 mg	Cost No pediatric formulation Frequent administration Resistance emerging
Ceftriaxone	50–100 mg/kg Once a day IM for 2–5 days	–	Efficacy not validated Must be injected
Azithromycin	6–20 mg/kg Once a day for 1–5 days, PO	1–1.5 g	Cost Efficacy not validated MIC near serum concentration Rapid emergence of resistance and spread to other bacteria

Source: WHO Library Cataloguing-in-Publication Data: Guidelines for the control of shigellosis, including epidemics due to *Shigella dysenteriae* type 1 (*www.searo. who.int/LinkFiles/CAH_Publications_ shigella.pdf*).

more aggressive measures, possibly including resuscitation, are often required.

REHYDRATION AND NUTRITION *Shigella* infection rarely causes significant dehydration. Cases requiring aggressive rehydration (particularly in industrialized countries) are uncommon. In developing countries, malnutrition remains the primary indicator for diarrhea-related death, highlighting the importance of nutrition in early management. Rehydration should be oral unless the patient is comatose or presents in shock. Because of the improved effectiveness of reduced-osmolarity oral rehydration solution (especially for children with acute noncholera diarrhea), the WHO and UNICEF now recommend a standard solution of

245 mOsm/L (sodium, 75 mmol/L; chloride, 65 mmol/L; glucose [anhydrous], 75 mmol/L; potassium, 20 mmol/L; citrate, 10 mmol/L). In shigellosis, the coupled transport of sodium to glucose may be variably affected, but oral rehydration therapy remains the easiest and most efficient form of rehydration, especially in severe cases.

Nutrition should be started as soon as possible after completion of initial rehydration. Early refeeding is safe, well tolerated, and clinically beneficial. Because breast-feeding reduces diarrheal losses and the need for oral rehydration in infants, it should be maintained in the absence of contraindications (e.g., maternal HIV infection).

NONSPECIFIC, SYMPTOM-BASED THERAPY

Antimotility agents have been implicated in prolonged fever in volunteers with shigellosis. These agents are suspected of increasing the risk of toxic megacolon and are thought to have been responsible for HUS in children infected by EHEC strains. For safety reasons, it is better to avoid antimotility agents in bloody diarrhea.

TREATMENT OF COMPLICATIONS There is no consensus regarding the best treatment for toxic megacolon. The patient should be assessed frequently by both medical and surgical teams. Anemia, dehydration, and electrolyte deficits (particularly hypokalemia) may aggravate colonic atony and should be actively treated. Nasogastric aspiration helps to deflate the colon. Parenteral nutrition has not been proven to be beneficial. Fever persisting beyond 48–72 h raises the possibility of local perforation or abscess. Most studies recommend colectomy if, after 48–72 h, colonic distention persists. However, some physicians recommend continuation of medical therapy for up to 7 days if the patient seems to be improving clinically despite persistent megacolon without free perforation. Intestinal perforation, either isolated or complicating toxic megacolon, requires surgical treatment and intensive medical support.

Rectal prolapse must be treated as soon as possible. With the health care provider using surgical gloves or a soft warm wet cloth and the patient in the knee-chest position, the prolapsed rectum is gently pushed back into place. If edema of the rectal mucosa is evident (rendering reintegration difficult), it can be osmotically reduced by applying gauze impregnated with a warm solution of saturated magnesium sulfate. Rectal prolapse often relapses but usually resolves along with the resolution of dysentery.

HUS must be treated by water restriction, including discontinuation of oral rehydration solution and potassium-rich alimentation. Hemofiltration is usually required.

PREVENTION

Hand washing after defecation or handling of children's feces and before handling of food is recommended. Stool decontamination (e.g., with sodium hypochlorite), together with a cleaning protocol for medical staff as well as for patients, has proven useful in limiting the spread of infection during *Shigella* outbreaks. Ideally, patients should have a negative stool culture before their infection is considered cured. Recurrences are rare if therapeutic and preventive measures are correctly implemented.

Although several live attenuated oral and subunit parenteral vaccine candidates have been produced and are undergoing clinical trials, no vaccine against shigellosis is currently available. Especially given the rapid progression of antibiotic resistance in *Shigella*, a vaccine is urgently needed.

CHAPTER 29

INFECTIONS DUE TO *CAMPYLOBACTER* AND RELATED ORGANISMS

Martin J. Blaser

DEFINITION

Bacteria of the genus *Campylobacter* and of the related genera *Arcobacter* and *Helicobacter* (Chap. 26) cause a variety of inflammatory conditions. Although acute diarrheal illnesses are most common, these organisms may cause infections in virtually all parts of the body, especially in compromised hosts, and these infections may have late nonsuppurative sequelae. The designation *Campylobacter* comes from the Greek for "curved rod" and refers to the organism's vibrio-like morphology.

ETIOLOGY

Campylobacters are motile, non-spore-forming, curved, gram-negative rods. Originally known as *Vibrio fetus*, these bacilli were reclassified as a new genus in 1973, after their dissimilarity to other vibrios was recognized. More than 15 species have since been identified. These species are currently divided into three genera: *Campylobacter*, *Arcobacter*, and *Helicobacter*. Not all of the species are pathogens of humans. The human pathogens fall into two major groups: those that primarily cause diarrheal disease and those that cause extraintestinal infection. The principal diarrheal pathogen is *C. jejuni*, which accounts for 80–90% of all cases of recognized illness due to campylobacters and related genera. Other organisms that cause diarrheal disease include *C. coli*, *C. upsaliensis*, *C. lari*, *C. hyointestinalis*, *C. fetus*, *A. butzleri*, *A. cryaerophilus*, *H. cinaedi*, and *H. fennelliae*. The two *Helicobacter* species causing diarrheal disease, *H. cinaedi* and *H. fennelliae*, are intestinal rather than gastric organisms; in terms of the clinical features of the illnesses they cause, these species most closely resemble *Campylobacter* rather than *H. pylori* (Chap. 26) and thus are considered in this chapter.

The major species causing extraintestinal illnesses is *C. fetus*. However, any of the diarrheal agents listed earlier may cause systemic or localized infection as well, especially in compromised hosts. Neither aerobes nor strict anaerobes, these microaerophilic organisms are adapted for survival in the gastrointestinal mucous layer. This chapter focuses on *C. jejuni* and *C. fetus* as the major pathogens in and prototypes for their groups. The key features of infection are listed by species (excluding *C. jejuni*, described in detail in the text in this chapter) in **Table 29-1**.

EPIDEMIOLOGY

Campylobacters are found in the gastrointestinal tract of many animals used for food (including poultry, cattle, sheep, and swine) and many household pets (including birds, dogs, and cats). These microorganisms usually do not cause illness in their animal hosts. In most cases, campylobacters are transmitted to humans in raw or undercooked food products or through direct contact with infected animals. In the United States and other developed countries, ingestion of contaminated poultry that has not been sufficiently cooked is the most common mode of acquisition (30–70% of cases). Other modes include ingestion of raw (unpasteurized) milk or untreated water, contact with infected household pets, travel to developing countries (campylobacters being among the leading causes of traveler's diarrhea; Chap. 23), oral-anal sexual contact, and (occasionally) contact with an index case who is incontinent of stool (e.g., a baby).

Campylobacter infections are common. Several studies indicate that, in the United States, diarrheal disease due to campylobacters is more common than that due to *Salmonella* and *Shigella* combined. Infections occur throughout the year, but their incidence peaks

TABLE 29-1

CLINICAL FEATURES ASSOCIATED WITH INFECTION DUE TO "ATYPICAL" *CAMPYLOBACTER* AND RELATED SPECIES IMPLICATED AS CAUSES OF HUMAN ILLNESS

SPECIES	COMMON CLINICAL FEATURES	LESS COMMON CLINICAL FEATURES	ADDITIONAL INFORMATION
Campylobacter coli	Fever, diarrhea, abdominal pain	Bacteremia[a]	Clinically indistinguishable from *C. jejuni*
Campylobacter fetus	Bacteremia,[a] sepsis, meningitis, vascular infections	Diarrhea, relapsing fevers	Not usually isolated from media containing cephalothin or incubated at 42°C
Campylobacter upsaliensis	Watery diarrhea, low-grade fever, abdominal pain	Bacteremia, abscesses	Difficult to isolate because of cephalothin susceptibility
Campylobacter lari	Abdominal pain, diarrhea	Colitis, appendicitis	Seagulls frequently colonized; organism often transmitted to humans via contaminated water
Campylobacter hyointestinalis	Watery or bloody diarrhea, vomiting, abdominal pain	Bacteremia	Causes proliferative enteritis in swine
Helicobacter fennelliae	Chronic mild diarrhea, abdominal cramps, proctitis	Bacteremia[a]	Best treated with fluoroquinolones
Helicobacter cinaedi	Chronic mild diarrhea, abdominal cramps, proctitis	Bacteremia[a]	Best treated with fluoroquinolones; identified in healthy hamsters
Campylobacter jejuni subspecies *doylei*	Diarrhea	Chronic gastritis, bacteremia[b]	Uncertain role as human pathogen
Arcobacter cryaerophilus	Diarrhea	Bacteremia	Cultured under aerobic conditions
Arcobacter butzleri	Fever, diarrhea, abdominal pain, nausea	Bacteremia, appendicitis	Cultured under aerobic conditions; enzootic in nonhuman primates
Campylobacter sputorum	Pulmonary, perianal, groin, and axillary abscesses; diarrhea	Bacteremia	Three clinically relevant biovars: *sputorum, fecalis,* and *paraureolyticus*

[a]In immunocompromised hosts, especially HIV-infected persons.
[b]In children.
Source: Adapted from BM Allos, MJ Blaser: Clin Infect Dis 20:1092, 1995.

during summer and early autumn. Persons of all ages are affected; however, attack rates for *C. jejuni* are highest among young children and young adults, while those for *C. fetus* are highest at the extremes of age. Systemic infections due to *C. fetus* (and to other *Campylobacter* and related species) are most common among compromised hosts. Persons at increased risk include those with AIDS, hypogammaglobulinemia, neoplasia, liver disease, diabetes mellitus, and generalized atherosclerosis as well as neonates and pregnant women. However, apparently healthy nonpregnant persons occasionally develop transient *Campylobacter* bacteremia as part of a gastrointestinal illness.

 In contrast, in many developing countries, *C. jejuni* infections are hyperendemic, with the highest rates among children <2 years old. Infection rates fall with age, as does the illness-to-infection ratio. These observations suggest that frequent exposure to *C. jejuni* leads to the acquisition of immunity.

PATHOLOGY AND PATHOGENESIS

C. jejuni infections may be subclinical, especially in hosts in developing countries who have had multiple prior infections and thus are partially immune. Symptomatic infections mostly occur within 2–4 days (range, 1–7 days) of exposure to the organism in food or water. The sites of tissue injury include the jejunum, ileum, and colon. Biopsies show an acute nonspecific inflammatory reaction, with neutrophils, monocytes, and eosinophils in the lamina propria, as well as damage to the epithelium, including loss of mucus, glandular degeneration, and crypt abscesses. Biopsy findings may be consistent with Crohn's disease or ulcerative colitis, but these "idiopathic" chronic inflammatory diseases should not be diagnosed unless infectious colitis, *specifically including* that due to infection with *Campylobacter* species and related organisms, has been ruled out.

The high frequency of *C. jejuni* infections and their severity and recurrence among hypogammaglobulinemic patients suggest that antibodies are important in protective immunity. The pathogenesis of infection is uncertain. Both the motility of the strain and its capacity to adhere to host tissues appear to favor disease, but classic enterotoxins and cytotoxins (although described and including cytolethal distending toxin, or CDT) appear not to play substantial roles in tissue injury or disease production. The organisms have been visualized within the epithelium, albeit in low numbers. The documentation of a significant tissue response and occasionally of *C. jejuni* bacteremia further suggests that tissue invasion is clinically significant, and in vitro studies are consistent with this pathogenetic feature.

The pathogenesis of *C. fetus* infections is better defined. Virtually all clinical isolates of *C. fetus* possess a proteinaceous capsule-like structure (an S-layer) that renders the organisms resistant to complement-mediated killing and opsonization. As a result, *C. fetus* can cause bacteremia and can seed sites beyond the intestinal tract. The ability of the organism to switch the S-layer proteins expressed—a phenomenon that results in antigenic variability—may contribute to the chronicity and high rate of recurrence of *C. fetus* infections in compromised hosts.

CLINICAL MANIFESTATIONS

The clinical features of infections due to *Campylobacter* and the related *Arcobacter* and intestinal *Helicobacter* species causing enteric disease appear to be highly similar. *C. jejuni* can be considered the prototype, in part because it is by far the most common enteric pathogen in the group. A prodrome of fever, headache, myalgia, and/or malaise often occurs 12–48 h before the onset of diarrheal symptoms. The most common signs and symptoms of the intestinal phase are diarrhea, abdominal pain, and fever. The degree of diarrhea varies from several loose stools to grossly bloody stools; most patients presenting for medical attention have ≥10 bowel movements on the worst day of illness. Abdominal pain usually consists of cramping and may be the most prominent symptom. Pain is usually generalized but may become localized; *C. jejuni* infection may cause pseudoappendicitis. Fever may be the only initial manifestation of *C. jejuni* infection, a situation mimicking the early stages of typhoid fever. Febrile young children may develop convulsions. *Campylobacter* enteritis is generally self-limited; however, symptoms persist for >1 week in 10–20% of patients seeking medical attention, and clinical relapses occur in 5–10% of such untreated patients. Studies of common-source epidemics indicate that milder illnesses or asymptomatic infections may commonly occur.

C. fetus may cause a diarrheal illness similar to that due to *C. jejuni*, especially in normal hosts. This organism also may cause either intermittent diarrhea or nonspecific abdominal pain without localizing signs. Sequelae are uncommon, and the outcome is benign. *C. fetus* may also cause a prolonged relapsing systemic illness (with fever, chills, and myalgias) that has no obvious primary source; this manifestation is especially common among compromised hosts. Secondary seeding of an organ (e.g., meninges, brain, bone, urinary tract, or soft tissue) complicates the course, which may be fulminant. *C. fetus* infections have a tropism for vascular sites: endocarditis, mycotic aneurysm, and septic thrombophlebitis may all occur. Infection during pregnancy often leads to fetal death. A variety of *Campylobacter* species and *H. cinaedi* can cause recurrent cellulitis with fever and bacteremia in immunocompromised hosts.

COMPLICATIONS

Except in infection with *C. fetus*, bacteremia is uncommon, developing most often in immunocompromised hosts and at the extremes of age. Three patterns of extraintestinal infection have been noted: (1) transient bacteremia in a normal host with enteritis (benign course, no specific treatment needed); (2) sustained bacteremia or focal infection in a normal host (bacteremia originating from enteritis, with patients responding well to antimicrobial therapy); and (3) sustained bacteremia or focal infection in a compromised host. Enteritis may not be clinically apparent. Antimicrobial therapy, possibly prolonged, is necessary for suppression or cure of the infection.

Campylobacter, *Arcobacter*, and intestinal *Helicobacter* infections in patients with AIDS or hypogammaglobulinemia may be severe, persistent, and extraintestinal; relapse after cessation of therapy is common. Hypogammaglobulinemic patients also may develop osteomyelitis and an erysipelas-like rash or cellulitis.

Local suppurative complications of infection include cholecystitis, pancreatitis, and cystitis; distant complications include meningitis, endocarditis, arthritis, peritonitis, cellulitis, and septic abortion. All these complications are rare, except in immunocompromised hosts. Hepatitis, interstitial nephritis, and the hemolytic-uremic syndrome occasionally complicate acute infection. Reactive arthritis and other rheumatologic complaints may develop several weeks after infection, especially in persons with the HLA-B27 phenotype. Guillain-Barré syndrome or its Miller Fisher (cranial polyneuropathy) variant follows *Campylobacter* infections uncommonly—i.e., in 1 of every 1000–2000 cases or, for certain *C. jejuni* serotypes (such as O19), in 1 of every 100–200 cases. Despite the low frequency of this complication, it is now estimated that *Campylobacter* infections, because of their high incidence, may trigger 20–40% of all cases of Guillain-Barré syndrome. Asymptomatic *Campylobacter* infection also may trigger this syndrome. Immunoproliferative small-intestinal disease (*alpha chain disease*), a form of lymphoma that originates in small-intestinal mucosa-associated lymphoid tissue, has been associated with *C. jejuni*; antimicrobial therapy has led to marked clinical improvement.

DIAGNOSIS

In patients with *Campylobacter* enteritis, peripheral leukocyte counts reflect the severity of the inflammatory process. However, stools from nearly all *Campylobacter*-infected patients presenting for medical attention in the United States contain leukocytes or erythrocytes. Gram- or Wright-stained fecal smears should be examined in all suspected cases. When the diagnosis of *Campylobacter* enteritis is suspected on the basis of findings indicating inflammatory diarrhea (fever, fecal leukocytes), clinicians can ask the microbiology laboratory to attempt the visualization of organisms with characteristic vibrioid morphology by direct microscopic examination of stools with Gram's staining or to use phase-contrast or dark-field microscopy to identify the organisms' characteristic "darting" motility. Confirmation of the diagnosis of *Campylobacter* infection is based on identification of an isolate from cultures of stool, blood, or another site. *Campylobacter*-specific media should be used to culture stools from all patients with inflammatory or bloody diarrhea. Since all *Campylobacter* species are fastidious, they will not be isolated unless selective media or other selective techniques are used. Not all media are equally useful for isolation of the broad array of campylobacters; therefore, failure to isolate campylobacters from stool does not entirely rule out their presence. The detection of the organisms in stool almost always implies infection; there is a brief period of postconvalescent fecal carriage and no obvious commensalism in humans. In contrast, *C. sputorum* and related organisms found in the oral cavity are commensals that only rarely have pathogenic significance. Because of the low levels of metabolic activity of *Campylobacter* species in standard blood culture media, *Campylobacter* bacteremia may be difficult to detect unless laboratorians check for low-positive results in quantitative assays.

DIFFERENTIAL DIAGNOSIS

The symptoms of *Campylobacter* enteritis are not sufficiently unusual to distinguish this illness from that due to *Salmonella*, *Shigella*, *Yersinia*, and other pathogens.

The combination of fever and fecal leukocytes or erythrocytes is indicative of inflammatory diarrhea, and definitive diagnosis is based on culture or demonstration of the characteristic organisms on stained fecal smears. Similarly, extraintestinal *Campylobacter* illness is diagnosed by culture. Infection due to *Campylobacter* should be suspected in the setting of septic abortion, and that due to *C. fetus* should be suspected specifically in the setting of septic thrombophlebitis. It is important to reiterate that (1) the presentation of *Campylobacter* enteritis may mimic that of ulcerative colitis or Crohn's disease, (2) *Campylobacter* enteritis is much more common than either of the latter (especially among young adults), and (3) biopsy may not distinguish among these entities. Thus a diagnosis of inflammatory bowel disease should not be made until *Campylobacter* infection has been ruled out, especially in persons with a history of foreign travel, significant animal contact, immunodeficiency, or exposure incurring a high risk of transmission.

TREATMENT *Campylobacter* Infection

Fluid and electrolyte replacement is central to the treatment of diarrheal illnesses (Chap. 23). Even among patients presenting for medical attention with *Campylobacter* enteritis, not all clearly benefit from specific antimicrobial therapy. Indications for therapy include high fever, bloody diarrhea, severe diarrhea, persistence for >1 week, and worsening of symptoms. A 5- to 7-day course of erythromycin (250 mg orally four times daily or—for children—30–50 mg/kg per day, in divided doses) is the regimen of choice. Both clinical trials and in vitro susceptibility testing indicate that other macrolides, including azithromycin (a 1- or 3-day regimen), also are useful therapeutic agents. An alternative regimen for adults is ciprofloxacin (500 mg orally twice daily) or another fluoroquinolone for 5–7 days, but resistance to this class of agents as well as to tetracyclines has been increasing. Patients infected with antibiotic-resistant strains are at increased risk of adverse outcomes. Use of antimotility agents, which may prolong the duration of symptoms and have been associated with toxic megacolon and with death, is not recommended.

For systemic infections, treatment with gentamicin (1.7 mg/kg IV every 8 h after a loading dose of 2 mg/kg), imipenem (500 mg IV every 6 h), or chloramphenicol (50 mg/kg IV each day in three or four divided doses) should be started empirically, but susceptibility testing should then be performed. Ciprofloxacin and amoxicillin/clavulanate are alternative agents for susceptible strains. In the absence of immunocompromise or endovascular infections, therapy should be administered for 14 days. For immunocompromised patients with systemic infections due to *C. fetus* and for patients with endovascular infections, prolonged therapy (for up to 4 weeks) is usually necessary. For recurrent infections in immunocompromised hosts, lifelong therapy/prophylaxis is sometimes necessary.

PROGNOSIS

Nearly all patients recover fully from *Campylobacter* enteritis, either spontaneously or after antimicrobial therapy. Volume depletion probably contributes to the few deaths that are reported. As stated earlier, occasional patients develop reactive arthritis or Guillain-Barré syndrome or its variants. Systemic infection with *C. fetus* is much more often fatal than that due to related species; this higher mortality rate reflects in part the population affected. Prognosis depends on the rapidity with which appropriate therapy is begun. Otherwise-healthy hosts usually survive *C. fetus* infections without sequelae. Compromised hosts often have recurrent and/or life-threatening infections due to a variety of *Campylobacter* species.

CHAPTER 30

CHOLERA AND OTHER VIBRIOSES

Matthew K. Waldor ■ Edward T. Ryan

Members of the genus *Vibrio* cause a number of important infectious syndromes. Classic among them is cholera, a devastating diarrheal disease caused by *V. cholerae* that has been responsible for seven global pandemics and much suffering over the past two centuries. Epidemic cholera remains a significant public health concern in the developing world today. Other vibrioses caused by other *Vibrio* species include syndromes of diarrhea, soft tissue infection, or primary sepsis. All *Vibrio* species are highly motile, facultatively anaerobic, curved gram-negative rods with one or more flagella. In nature, vibrios most commonly reside in tidal rivers and bays under conditions of moderate salinity. They proliferate in the summer months when water temperatures exceed 20°C. As might be expected, the illnesses they cause also increase in frequency during the warm months.

CHOLERA

DEFINITION

Cholera is an acute diarrheal disease that can, in a matter of hours, result in profound, rapidly progressive dehydration and death. Accordingly, cholera gravis (the severe form of cholera) is a much-feared disease, particularly in its epidemic presentation. Fortunately, prompt aggressive fluid repletion and supportive care can obviate the high mortality that cholera has historically wrought. While the term *cholera* has occasionally been applied to any severely dehydrating secretory diarrheal illness, whether infectious in etiology or not, it now refers to disease caused by *V. cholerae* serogroup O1 or O139—i.e., the serogroups with epidemic potential.

MICROBIOLOGY AND EPIDEMIOLOGY

The species *V. cholerae* is classified into more than 200 serogroups based on the carbohydrate determinants of their lipopolysaccharide (LPS) O antigens. Although some non-O1 *V. cholerae* serogroups (strains that do not agglutinate in antisera to the O1 group antigen) have occasionally caused sporadic outbreaks of diarrhea, serogroup O1 was, until the emergence of serogroup O139 in 1992, the exclusive cause of epidemic cholera. Two biotypes of *V. cholerae* O1, classical and El Tor, are distinguished. Each biotype is further subdivided into two serotypes, termed *Inaba* and *Ogawa*.

The natural habitat of *V. cholerae* is coastal salt water and brackish estuaries, where the organism lives in close relation to plankton. Humans become infected incidentally but, once infected, can act as vehicles for spread. Ingestion of water contaminated by human feces is the most common means of acquisition of *V. cholerae*. Consumption of contaminated food also can contribute to spread. There is no known animal reservoir. While the infectious dose is relatively high, it is markedly reduced in hypochlorhydric persons, in those using antacids, and when gastric acidity is buffered by a meal. Cholera is predominantly a pediatric disease in endemic areas, but it affects adults and children equally when newly introduced into a population. In endemic areas, the burden of disease is often greatest during "cholera seasons" associated with high temperatures, heavy rainfall, and flooding, but cholera can occur year-round. For unexplained reasons, susceptibility to cholera is significantly influenced by ABO blood group status; persons with type O blood are at greatest risk of severe disease if infected, while those with type AB are at least risk.

Cholera is native to the Ganges delta in the Indian subcontinent. Since 1817, seven global pandemics have occurred. The current (seventh) pandemic—the first due to the El Tor biotype—began in Indonesia in 1961 and spread throughout Asia as *V. cholerae* El Tor displaced the endemic classical biotype. In the early 1970s, El Tor cholera erupted in Africa, causing major epidemics before becoming a persistent endemic problem. Currently, >90% of cholera cases

FIGURE 30-1
World distribution of cholera in 2009. (*Adapted from WHO: Wkly Epidemiol Rec 84:309, 2009.*)

Countries reporting imported cases   Areas reporting outbreaks

reported annually to the World Health Organization (WHO) are from Africa (Fig. 30-1), but the true burden in Africa as well as in Asia is unknown since diagnosis is often syndromic and since many countries with endemic cholera do not report cholera to the WHO. It is possible that >3 million cases of cholera occur yearly (of which only ~200,000 are reported to the WHO), resulting in >100,000 deaths annually (of which <5000 are reported to the WHO).

The recent history of cholera has been punctuated by severe outbreaks, especially among impoverished or displaced persons. Such outbreaks are often precipitated by war or other circumstances that lead to the breakdown of public health measures. Such was the case in the camps for Rwandan refugees set up in 1994 around Goma, Zaire; in 2008–2009 in Zimbabwe; and in 2010 in Haiti. Since 1973, sporadic endemic infections due to *V. cholerae* O1 strains related to the seventh-pandemic strain have been recognized along the U.S. Gulf Coast of Louisiana and Texas. These infections are typically associated with the consumption of contaminated, locally harvested shellfish. Occasionally, cases in U.S. locations remote from the Gulf Coast have been linked to shipped-in Gulf Coast seafood.

After a century without cholera in Latin America, the current cholera pandemic reached Central and South America in 1991. Following an initial explosive spread that affected millions (Fig. 30-2), the burden of disease has markedly decreased in Latin America, although, as it did in Africa two decades earlier, the epidemic El Tor strain proved capable of establishing itself

in inland fresh waters rather than in its classic niche of coastal salt waters. In 2010, cholera reappeared in Haiti after a century-long absence.

In October 1992, a large-scale outbreak of clinical cholera caused by a new serogroup, O139, occurred in

Initial Epidemics January 1991
----- August 1991
—— February 1992
—— November 1994

FIGURE 30-2
Spread of *Vibrio cholerae* O1 in the Americas, 1991–1994. (*Courtesy of Dr. Robert V. Tauxe, Centers for Disease Control and Prevention, Atlanta; with permission.*)

FIGURE 30-3

Spread of *Vibrio cholerae* O139 in the Indian subcontinent and elsewhere in Asia, 1992–1994. (*Courtesy of Dr. Robert V. Tauxe, CDC, Atlanta; with permission.*)

Initial Epidemic, October 1992

March 1993

October 1994

southeastern India. The organism appears to be a derivative of El Tor O1 but has a distinct LPS and an immunologically related O-antigen polysaccharide capsule. (O1 organisms are not encapsulated.) After an initial spread across 11 Asian countries (Fig. 30-3), *V. cholerae* O139 has once again been largely replaced by O1, although O139 still causes a minority of cases in some Asian countries. The clinical manifestations of disease caused by *V. cholerae* O139 are indistinguishable from those of O1 cholera. Immunity to one, however, is not protective against the other.

PATHOGENESIS

In the final analysis, cholera is a toxin-mediated disease. The watery diarrhea characteristic of cholera is due to the action of cholera toxin, a potent protein enterotoxin elaborated by the organism in the small intestine. The toxin-coregulated pilus (TCP), so named because its synthesis is regulated in parallel with that of cholera toxin, is essential for *V. cholerae* to survive and multiply in (colonize) the small intestine. Cholera toxin, TCP, and several other virulence factors are coordinately regulated by ToxR. This protein modulates the expression of genes coding for virulence factors in response to environmental signals via a cascade of regulatory proteins. Additional regulatory processes, including bacterial responses to the density of the bacterial population (in a phenomenon known as *quorum sensing*), control the virulence of *V. cholerae*.

Once established in the human small bowel, the organism produces cholera toxin, which consists of a monomeric enzymatic moiety (the A subunit) and a pentameric binding moiety (the B subunit). The B pentamer binds to GM_1 ganglioside, a glycolipid on the surface of epithelial cells that serves as the toxin receptor and makes possible the delivery of the A subunit to its cytosolic target. The activated A subunit (A_1) irreversibly transfers ADP-ribose from nicotinamide adenine dinucleotide to its specific target protein, the GTP-binding regulatory component of adenylate cyclase. The ADP-ribosylated G protein upregulates the activity of adenylate cyclase; the result is the intracellular accumulation of high levels of cyclic AMP. In intestinal epithelial cells, cyclic AMP inhibits the absorptive sodium transport system in villus cells and activates the secretory chloride transport system in crypt cells, and these events lead to the accumulation of sodium chloride in the intestinal lumen. Since water moves passively to maintain osmolality, isotonic fluid accumulates in the lumen. When the volume of that fluid exceeds the capacity of the rest of the gut to resorb it, watery diarrhea results. Unless the wasted fluid and electrolytes are adequately replaced, shock (due to profound dehydration) and acidosis (due to loss of bicarbonate) follow. Although perturbation of the adenylate cyclase pathway is the primary mechanism by which cholera toxin causes excess fluid secretion, cholera toxin also enhances intestinal secretion via prostaglandins and/or neural histamine receptors.

The *V. cholerae* genome comprises two circular chromosomes. Lateral gene transfer has played a key role in the evolution of epidemic *V. cholerae*. The genes encoding cholera toxin (*ctxAB*) are part of the genome of a bacteriophage, CTXΦ. The receptor for this phage on the *V. cholerae* surface is the intestinal colonization factor TCP. Since *ctxAB* is part of a mobile genetic element (CTXΦ), horizontal transfer of this bacteriophage may account for the emergence of new toxigenic *V. cholerae* serogroups. Many of the other genes important for *V. cholerae* pathogenicity, including the genes encoding the biosynthesis of TCP, those encoding accessory colonization factors, and those regulating virulence gene expression, are clustered together in the *V. cholerae* pathogenicity island. Similar clustering of virulence genes is found in other bacterial pathogens. It is believed that pathogenicity islands are acquired by horizontal gene transfer. *V. cholerae* O139 is probably derived from an El Tor O1 strain that acquired the genes for O139 O-antigen synthesis by horizontal gene transfer.

CLINICAL MANIFESTATIONS

Individuals infected with *V. cholerae* O1 or O139 exhibit a range of clinical manifestations. Some individuals are asymptomatic or have only mild diarrhea; others present with the sudden onset of explosive and life-threatening diarrhea (*cholera gravis*). The reasons for the range in signs and symptoms of disease are incompletely understood but include the level of preexisting immunity, blood type, and nutritional status. In a nonimmune individual, after a 24- to 48-h incubation period, cholera characteristically begins with the sudden onset of painless watery diarrhea that may quickly become voluminous. Patients often vomit. In severe cases, volume loss can exceed 250 mL/kg in the first 24 h. If fluids and electrolytes are not replaced, hypovolemic shock and death may ensue. Fever is usually absent. Muscle cramps due to electrolyte disturbances are common. The stool has a characteristic appearance: a nonbilious, gray, slightly cloudy fluid with flecks of mucus, no blood, and a somewhat fishy, inoffensive odor. It has been called "rice-water" stool because of its resemblance to the water in which rice has been washed (**Fig. 30-4**). Clinical symptoms parallel volume contraction: At losses of <5% of normal body weight, thirst develops; at 5–10%, postural hypotension, weakness, tachycardia, and decreased skin turgor are documented; and at >10%, oliguria, weak or absent pulses,

FIGURE 30-4

Rice water cholera stool. Note floating mucus and gray watery appearance. (*Courtesy of Dr. ASG Faruque, International Centre for Diarrhoeal Disease Research, Dhaka; with permission.*)

sunken eyes (and, in infants, sunken fontanelles), wrinkled ("washerwoman") skin, somnolence, and coma are characteristic. Complications derive exclusively from the effects of volume and electrolyte depletion and include renal failure due to acute tubular necrosis. Thus, if the patient is adequately treated with fluid and electrolytes, complications are averted and the process is self-limited, resolving in a few days.

Laboratory data usually reveal an elevated hematocrit (due to hemoconcentration) in nonanemic patients; mild neutrophilic leukocytosis; elevated levels of blood urea nitrogen and creatinine consistent with prerenal azotemia; normal sodium, potassium, and chloride levels; a markedly reduced bicarbonate level (<15 mmol/L); and an elevated anion gap (due to increases in serum lactate, protein, and phosphate). Arterial pH is usually low (~7.2).

DIAGNOSIS

The clinical suspicion of cholera can be confirmed by the identification of *V. cholerae* in stool; however, the organism must be specifically sought. With experience, it can be detected directly by dark-field microscopy on a wet mount of fresh stool, and its serotype can be discerned by immobilization with specific antiserum. Laboratory isolation of the organism requires the use of a selective medium such as taurocholate-tellurite-gelatin (TTG) agar or thiosulfate–citrate–bile salts–sucrose (TCBS) agar. If a delay in sample processing is expected, Carey-Blair transport medium and/or alkaline-peptone water-enrichment medium may be used as well. In endemic areas, there is little need for biochemical confirmation and characterization, although these tasks may be worthwhile in places where *V. cholerae* is an uncommon isolate. Standard microbiologic biochemical testing for Enterobacteriaceae will suffice for identification of *V. cholerae*. All vibrios are oxidase-positive. A point-of-care antigen-detection cholera dipstick assay is now commercially available for use in the field or where laboratory facilities are lacking.

TREATMENT   **Cholera**

Death from cholera is due to hypovolemic shock; thus treatment of individuals with cholera first and foremost requires fluid resuscitation and management. In light of the level of dehydration (Table 30-1) and the patient's age and weight, euvolemia should first be rapidly restored, and adequate hydration should then be maintained to replace ongoing fluid losses (Table 30-2). Administration of oral rehydration solution (ORS) takes advantage of the hexose-Na⁺ co-transport mechanism to move Na⁺ across the gut mucosa

TABLE 30-1

ASSESSING THE DEGREE OF DEHYDRATION IN PATIENTS WITH CHOLERA	
DEGREE OF DEHYDRATION	**CLINICAL FINDINGS**
None or mild, but diarrhea	Thirst in some cases; <5% loss of total body weight
Moderate	Thirst, postural hypotension, weakness, tachycardia, decreased skin turgor, dry mouth/tongue, no tears; 5–10% loss of total body weight
Severe	Unconsciousness, lethargy, or "floppiness"; weak or absent pulse; inability to drink; sunken eyes (and, in infants, sunken fontanelles); >10% loss of total body weight

TABLE 30-2

TREATMENT OF CHOLERA, BASED ON DEGREE OF DEHYDRATION[a]	
DEGREE OF DEHYDRATION, PATIENT'S AGE (WEIGHT)	**TREATMENT**
None or Mild, but Diarrhea[b]	
<2 years	1/4–1/2 cup (50–100 mL) of ORS, to a maximum of 0.5 L/d
2–9 years	1/2–1 cup (100–200 mL) of ORS, to a maximum of 1 L/d
≥10 years	As much ORS as desired, to a maximum of 2 L/d
Moderate[b,c]	
<4 months (<5 kg)	200–400 mL of ORS
4–11 months (5–<8 kg)	400–600 mL of ORS
12–23 months (8–<11 kg)	600–800 mL of ORS
2–4 years (11–<16 kg)	800–1200 mL of ORS
5–14 years (16–<30 kg)	1200–2200 mL of ORS
≥15 years (≥30 kg)	2200–4000 mL of ORS
Severe[b]	
All ages and weights	IV fluid replacement with Ringer's lactate (or, if not available, normal saline): 100 mL/kg in first 3-h period (or first 6-h period for children <12 months old); start rapidly, then slow down; total of 200 mL/kg in first 24 h; continue until patient is awake, can ingest ORS, and no longer has a weak pulse

Note: Continue normal feeding during treatment.
[a]Adapted from World Health Organization: First steps for managing an outbreak of acute diarrhoea. Global Task Force on Cholera Control, 2009 (www.who.int/topics/cholera). ORS, oral rehydration solution.
[b]Reassess regularly; monitor stool and vomit output.
[c]Amounts of ORS listed should be given within the first 4 h.

together with an actively transported molecule such as glucose (or galactose). Cl⁻ and water follow. This transport mechanism remains intact even when cholera toxin is active. ORS may be made by adding safe water to prepackaged sachets containing salts and sugar or by adding 0.5 teaspoon of table salt (NaCl; 3.5 g) and 4 tablespoons of table sugar (glucose; 40 g) to 1 L of safe water. Potassium intake in bananas or green coconut water should be encouraged. A number of ORS formulations are available, and the WHO now recommends "low-osmolarity" ORS for treatment of individuals with dehydrating diarrhea of any cause (Table 30-3). If available, rice-based ORS is considered superior to standard ORS in the treatment of cholera. ORS can be administered via a nasogastric tube to individuals who cannot ingest fluid; however, optimal management of individuals with severe dehydration includes the administration of IV fluid and electrolytes. Because profound acidosis (pH <7.2) is common in this group, Ringer's lactate is the best choice among commercial products (Table 30-4). It must be used with additional potassium supplements, preferably given by mouth. The total fluid deficit in severely dehydrated patients (>10% of body weight) can be replaced safely within the first 3–6 h of therapy, half within the first hour. Transient muscle cramps and tetany are common. Thereafter, oral therapy can usually be initiated, with the goal of maintaining fluid intake equal to fluid output. However, patients with continued large-volume diarrhea may require prolonged IV treatment to match gastrointestinal fluid losses. Severe hypokalemia can develop but will respond to potassium given either IV or orally. In the absence of adequate staff to monitor the patient's progress, the oral route of rehydration and potassium replacement is safer than the IV route.

Although not necessary for cure, the use of an antibiotic to which the organism is susceptible diminishes the duration and volume of fluid loss and hastens clearance of the organism from the stool. The WHO recommends administration of antibiotics to cholera patients only if they are severely dehydrated, although wider use is often justifiable. Doxycycline (a single dose of 300 mg) or tetracycline (12.5 mg/kg four times a day for 3 days) may be effective in adults but is not recommended for children <8 years of age because of possible deposition in bone and developing teeth. Emerging drug resistance is an ever-present concern. For nonpregnant adults with cholera in areas where tetracycline resistance is prevalent, ciprofloxacin (either in a single dose [30 mg/kg, not to exceed a total dose of 1 g] or in a short

TABLE 30-3

COMPOSITION OF WORLD HEALTH ORGANIZATION REDUCED-OSMOLARITY ORAL REHYDRATION SOLUTION (ORS)[a,b]	
CONSTITUENT	**CONCENTRATION, mmol/L**
Na^+	75
K^+	20
Cl^-	65
Citrate[c]	10
Glucose	75
Total osmolarity	245

[a]Contains (per package, to be added to 1 L of drinking water): NaCl, 2.6 g; $Na_3C_6H_5O_7 \cdot 2H_2O$, 2.9 g; KCl, 1.5 g; and glucose (anhydrous), 13.5 g.

[b]If prepackaged ORS is unavailable, a simple homemade alternative can be prepared by combining 3.5 g (~1/2 teaspoon) of NaCl with either 50 g of precooked rice cereal or 40 g (4 tablespoons) of table sugar (sucrose) in 1 L of drinking water. In that case, potassium must be supplied separately (e.g., in orange juice or coconut water).

[c]10 mmol citrate per liter, which supplies 30 mmol HCO_3/L.

course [15 mg/kg bid for 3 days, not to exceed a total daily dose of 1 g]), erythromycin (40–50 mg/kg daily in three divided doses for 3 days), or azithromycin (a single 1-g dose) may be a clinically effective substitute. Pregnant women and children are usually treated with erythromycin or azithromycin (10 mg/kg in children).

PREVENTION

Provision of safe water and facilities for sanitary disposal of feces, improved nutrition, and attention to food preparation and storage in the household can significantly reduce the incidence of cholera.

Much effort has been devoted to the development of an effective cholera vaccine over the past few decades, with a particular focus on oral vaccine strains. Traditional killed cholera vaccine given intramuscularly

TABLE 30-4

ELECTROLYTE COMPOSITION OF CHOLERA STOOL AND OF INTRAVENOUS REHYDRATION SOLUTION				
	CONCENTRATION, mmol/L			
SUBSTANCE	**NA+**	**K+**	**CL-**	**BASE**
Stool				
Adult	135	15	100	45
Child	100	25	90	30
Ringer's lactate	130	4[a]	109	28

[a]Potassium supplements, preferably administered by mouth, are required to replace the usual potassium losses from stool.

provides little protection to nonimmune subjects and predictably causes adverse effects, including pain at the injection site, malaise, and fever. The vaccine's limited efficacy is due, at least in part, to its failure to induce a local immune response at the intestinal mucosal surface.

Two types of oral cholera vaccines have been developed. The first is a killed whole-cell (WC) vaccine. Two formulations of the killed WC vaccine have been prepared: one that also contains the nontoxic B subunit of cholera toxin (WC/BS) and one composed solely of killed bacteria. In placebo-controlled field trials in Bangladesh, both of the killed vaccines offered significant protection from cholera for the first 6 months after vaccination, with protection rates of ~58% for WC vaccine and 85% for WC/BS vaccine. Protective efficacy rates for both vaccines declined to ~50% by 3 years after vaccine administration. Immunity was relatively sustained in persons vaccinated at an age of >5 years but was not well sustained in younger vaccinees. The WC/BS vaccine proved effective in a trial conducted in a sub-Saharan African population with a high prevalence of HIV infection. Trials of locally produced killed WC vaccines have yielded promising results in Vietnam and in Kolkata (Calcutta), India. Killed oral vaccines also confer herd protection to unvaccinated individuals living in proximity to vaccinated individuals. The WHO now recommends that vaccination against cholera be part of a larger response plan for populations at risk for epidemic cholera. The oral killed vaccines are available in Europe and Asia but (like other cholera vaccines) are not available in the United States.

The second type of cholera vaccine under development involves the use of oral live attenuated vaccine strains developed, for example, by the isolation or creation of mutants lacking the genes encoding cholera toxin. One such vaccine, CVD 103-HgR, was safe and immunogenic in phase 1 and 2 studies but afforded minimal protection in a large field trial in Indonesia. Other live attenuated vaccine candidate strains have been prepared from El Tor and O139 *V. cholerae* and are now undergoing clinical trials. The development of effective and safe cholera vaccines and strategies that provide long-lasting protective mucosal immunity, especially among malnourished, impoverished, and potentially HIV-infected adults and children (the individuals most at risk for cholera), is a priority. As mentioned earlier, no cholera vaccine is commercially available in the United States.

OTHER *VIBRIO* SPECIES

The genus *Vibrio* includes several human pathogens that do not cause cholera. Abundant in coastal waters throughout the world, noncholera vibrios can reach high concentrations in the tissues of

CHAPTER 30 Cholera and Other Vibrioses

TABLE 30-5

FEATURES OF SELECTED NONCHOLERA VIBRIOSES			
ORGANISM	VEHICLE OR ACTIVITY	HOST AT RISK	SYNDROME
V. parahaemolyticus	Shellfish, seawater	Normal	Gastroenteritis
	Seawater	Normal	Wound infection
Non-O1/O139 *V. cholerae*	Shellfish, travel	Normal	Gastroenteritis
	Seawater	Normal	Wound infection, otitis media
V. vulnificus	Shellfish	Immunosuppressed[a]	Sepsis, secondary cellulitis
	Seawater	Normal, immunosuppressed[a]	Wound infection, cellulitis
V. alginolyticus	Seawater	Normal	Wound infection, cellulitis, otitis
	Seawater	Burned, other immunosuppressed	Sepsis

[a]Especially with liver disease or hemochromatosis.
Source: Table 161-3 in *Harrisons Principles of Internal Medicine,* 14th edition.

filter-feeding mollusks. As a result, human infection commonly follows the ingestion of seawater or of raw or undercooked shellfish **(Table 30-5)**. Most noncholera vibrios can be cultured on blood or MacConkey agar, which contains enough salt to support the growth of these halophilic species. In the microbiology laboratory, the species of noncholera vibrios are distinguished by standard biochemical tests. The most important of these organisms are *V. parahaemolyticus* and *V. vulnificus*.

The two major types of syndromes for which these species are responsible are gastrointestinal illness (due to *V. parahaemolyticus*, non-O1/O139 *V. cholerae*, *V. mimicus*, *V. fluvialis*, *V. hollisae*, and *V. furnissii*) and soft tissue infections (due to *V. vulnificus*, *V. alginolyticus*, and *V. damselae*). *V. vulnificus* is also a cause of primary sepsis in some compromised individuals.

SPECIES ASSOCIATED PRIMARILY WITH GASTROINTESTINAL ILLNESS

V. parahaemolyticus

Widespread in marine environments, the halophilic *V. parahaemolyticus* causes food-borne enteritis worldwide. This species was originally implicated in enteritis in Japan in 1953, accounting for 24% of reported cases in one study—a rate that presumably was due to the common practice of eating raw seafood in that country. In the United States, common-source outbreaks of diarrhea caused by this organism have been linked to the consumption of undercooked or improperly handled seafood or of other foods contaminated by seawater. Since the mid-1990s, the incidence of *V. parahaemolyticus* infections has increased in several countries, including the United States.

Serotypes O3:K6, O4:K68, and O1:K-untypable, which are genetically related to one another, account for this increase. The enteropathogenicity of *V. parahaemolyticus* is linked to its ability to cause hemolysis on Wagatsuma agar (i.e., the *Kanagawa phenomenon*). Although the mechanism by which the organism causes diarrhea remains unclear, the genome sequence of *V. parahaemolyticus* contains two type III secretion systems, which directly inject toxic bacterial proteins into host cells. *V. parahaemolyticus* should be considered a possible etiologic agent in all cases of diarrhea that can be linked epidemiologically to seafood consumption or to the sea itself.

Infections with *V. parahaemolyticus* can result in two distinct gastrointestinal presentations. The more common of the two presentations (including nearly all cases in North America) is characterized by watery diarrhea, usually occurring in conjunction with abdominal cramps, nausea, and vomiting and accompanied in ~25% of cases by fever and chills. After an incubation period of 4 h to 4 days, symptoms develop and persist for a median of 3 days. Dysentery, the less common presentation, is characterized by severe abdominal cramps, nausea, vomiting, and bloody or mucoid stools. *V. parahaemolyticus* also causes rare cases of wound infection and otitis and very rare cases of sepsis.

Most cases of *V. parahaemolyticus*–associated gastrointestinal illness, regardless of the presentation, are self-limited and require neither antimicrobial treatment nor hospitalization. Deaths are extremely rare among immunocompetent individuals. Severe infections are associated with underlying diseases, including diabetes, preexisting liver disease, iron-overload states, or immunosuppression. The occasional severe case should be treated with fluid replacement and antibiotics, as described earlier for cholera.

Non-O1/O139 (noncholera) V. cholerae

The heterogeneous non-O1/O139 *V. cholerae* organisms cannot be distinguished from *V. cholerae* O1 or O139 by routine biochemical tests but do not agglutinate in O1 or O139 antiserum. Non-O1/O139 strains have caused several well-studied food-borne outbreaks of gastroenteritis and have also been responsible for sporadic cases of otitis media, wound infection, and bacteremia; although gastroenteritis outbreaks can occur, non-O1/O139 *V. cholerae* strains do not cause epidemics of cholera. Like other vibrios, non-O1/O139 *V. cholerae* organisms are widely distributed in marine environments. In most instances, recognized cases in the United States have been associated with the consumption of raw oysters or with recent travel, typically to Mexico. The broad clinical spectrum of diarrheal illness caused by these organisms is probably due to the group's heterogeneous virulence attributes.

In the United States, about half of all non-O1/O139 *V. cholerae* isolates are from stool samples. The typical incubation period for gastroenteritis due to these organisms is <2 days, and the illness lasts for ~2–7 days. Patients' stools may be copious and watery or may be partly formed, less voluminous, and bloody or mucoid. Diarrhea can result in severe dehydration. Many cases include abdominal cramps, nausea, vomiting, and fever. Like those with cholera, patients who are seriously dehydrated should receive oral or IV fluids; the value of antibiotics is not clear.

Extraintestinal infections due to non-O1/O139 *V. cholerae* commonly follow occupational or recreational exposure to seawater. Around 10% of non-O1/O139 *V. cholerae* isolates come from cases of wound infection, 10% from cases of otitis media, and 20% from cases of bacteremia (which is particularly likely to develop in patients with liver disease). Extraintestinal infections should be treated with antibiotics. Information to guide antibiotic selection and dosing is limited, but most strains are sensitive in vitro to tetracycline, ciprofloxacin, and third-generation cephalosporins.

SPECIES ASSOCIATED PRIMARILY WITH SOFT TISSUE INFECTION OR BACTEREMIA

V. vulnificus

Infection with *V. vulnificus* is rare, but this organism is the most common cause of severe *Vibrio* infections in the United States. Like most vibrios, *V. vulnificus* proliferates in the warm summer months and requires a saline environment for growth. In this country, infections in humans typically occur in coastal states between May and October and most commonly affect men >40 years of age. *V. vulnificus* has been linked to two distinct syndromes: primary sepsis, which usually occurs in patients with underlying liver disease, and primary wound infection, which generally affects people without underlying disease. (*Vulnificus* is Latin for "wound maker.") Some authors have suggested that *V. vulnificus* also causes gastroenteritis independent of other clinical manifestations. *V. vulnificus* is endowed with a number of virulence attributes, including a capsule that confers resistance to phagocytosis and to the bactericidal activity of human serum as well as a cytolysin. Measured as the 50% lethal dose in mice, the organism's virulence is considerably increased under conditions of iron overload; this observation is consistent with the propensity of *V. vulnificus* to infect patients who have hemochromatosis.

Primary sepsis most often develops in patients who have cirrhosis or hemochromatosis. However, *V. vulnificus* bacteremia can also affect individuals who have hematopoietic disorders or chronic renal insufficiency, those who are using immunosuppressive medications or alcohol, or (in rare instances) those who have no known underlying disease. After a median incubation period of 16 h, the patient develops malaise, chills, fever, and prostration. One-third of patients develop hypotension, which is often apparent at admission. Cutaneous manifestations develop in most cases (usually within 36 h of onset) and characteristically involve the extremities (the lower more often than the upper). In a common sequence, erythematous patches are followed by ecchymoses, vesicles, and bullae. In fact, sepsis and hemorrhagic bullous skin lesions suggest the diagnosis in appropriate settings. Necrosis and sloughing may also be evident. Laboratory studies reveal leukopenia more often than leukocytosis, thrombocytopenia, or elevated levels of fibrin split products. *V. vulnificus* can be cultured from blood or cutaneous lesions. The mortality rate approaches 50%, with most deaths due to uncontrolled sepsis. Accordingly, prompt treatment is critical and should include empirical antibiotic administration, aggressive debridement, and general supportive care. *V. vulnificus* is sensitive in vitro to a number of antibiotics, including tetracycline, fluoroquinolones, and third-generation cephalosporins. Data from animal models suggest that either a fluoroquinolone or the combination of minocycline and cefotaxime should be used in the treatment of *V. vulnificus* septicemia.

V. vulnificus can infect either a fresh or an old wound that comes into contact with seawater; the patient may or may not have underlying disease. After a short incubation period (4 h to 4 days; mean, 12 h), the disease begins with swelling, erythema, and (in many cases) intense pain around the wound. These signs and symptoms are followed by cellulitis, which spreads rapidly and is sometimes accompanied by vesicular, bullous, or necrotic lesions. Metastatic events are uncommon. Most

297

CHAPTER 30 Cholera and Other Vibrioses

patients have a fever and leukocytosis. *V. vulnificus* can be cultured from skin lesions and occasionally from the blood. Prompt antibiotic therapy and debridement are usually curative.

V. alginolyticus

First identified as a pathogen of humans in 1973, *V. alginolyticus* occasionally causes eye, ear, and wound infections. This species is the most salt-tolerant of the vibrios and can grow in salt concentrations of >10%. Most clinical isolates come from superinfected wounds that presumably become contaminated at the beach.

Although its severity varies, *V. alginolyticus* infection tends not to be serious and generally responds well to antibiotic therapy and drainage. A few cases of otitis externa, otitis media, and conjunctivitis due to this pathogen have been described. Tetracycline treatment usually results in cure. *V. alginolyticus* is a rare cause of bacteremia in immunocompromised hosts.

ACKNOWLEDGMENT

The authors gratefully acknowledge the valuable contributions of Drs. Robert Deresiewicz and Gerald T. Keusch, coauthors of this chapter for previous editions of Harrison's Principles of Internal Medicine.

CHAPTER 31

VIRAL GASTROENTERITIS

Umesh D. Parashar ■ Roger I. Glass

Acute infectious gastroenteritis is a common illness that affects persons of all ages worldwide. It is a leading cause of mortality among children in developing countries, accounting for an estimated 1.8 million deaths each year, and is responsible for up to 10–12% of all hospitalizations among children in industrialized countries, including the United States. Elderly persons, especially those with debilitating health conditions, are also at risk of severe complications and death from acute gastroenteritis. Among healthy young adults, acute gastroenteritis is rarely fatal but incurs substantial medical and social costs, including those of time lost from work.

Several enteric viruses have been recognized as important etiologic agents of acute infectious gastroenteritis (Table 31-1, Fig. 31-1). Although most viral gastroenteritis is caused by RNA viruses, the DNA viruses that are occasionally involved (e.g., adenovirus types 40 and 41) are included in this chapter. Illness caused by these viruses is characterized by the acute onset of vomiting and/or diarrhea, which may be accompanied by fever, nausea, abdominal cramps, anorexia, and malaise. As shown in Table 31-2, several features can help distinguish gastroenteritis caused by viruses from that caused by bacterial agents. However, the distinction based on clinical and epidemiologic parameters alone is often difficult, and laboratory tests may be required to confirm the diagnosis.

HUMAN CALICIVIRUSES

Etiologic agent

The Norwalk virus is the prototype strain of a group of nonenveloped, small (27–40 nm), round, icosahedral viruses with relatively amorphous surface features on visualization by electron microscopy. These viruses have been difficult to classify because they have not been adapted to cell culture, they often are shed in low titers for only a few days, and no animal models are available.

TABLE 31-1

VIRAL CAUSES OF GASTROENTERITIS AMONG HUMANS					
VIRUS	**FAMILY**	**GENOME**	**PRIMARY AGE GROUP AT RISK**	**CLINICAL SEVERITY**	**DETECTION ASSAYS**
Group A rotavirus	Reoviridae	Double-strand segmented RNA	Children <5 years	+++	EM, EIA (commercial), PAGE, RT-PCR
Norovirus	Caliciviridae	Positive-sense single-strand RNA	All ages	++	EM, EIA, RT-PCR
Sapovirus	Caliciviridae	Positive-sense single-strand RNA	Children <5 years	+	EM, EIA, RT-PCR
Astrovirus	Astroviridae	Positive-sense single-strand RNA	Children <5 years	+	EM, EIA, RT-PCR
Adenovirus (types 40 and 41)	Adenoviridae	Double-strand DNA	Children <5 years	+/++	EM, EIA (commercial), PCR

Abbreviations: EIA, enzyme immunoassay; EM, electron microscopy; PAGE, polyacrylamide gel electrophoresis; PCR, polymerase chain reaction; RT-PCR, reverse-transcription PCR.

FIGURE 31-1
Viral agents of gastroenteritis. NV, norovirus; SV, sapovirus.

TABLE 31-2

CHARACTERISTICS OF GASTROENTERITIS CAUSED BY VIRAL AND BACTERIAL AGENTS

FEATURE	VIRAL GASTROENTERITIS	BACTERIAL GASTROENTERITIS
Setting	Incidence similar in developing and developed countries	More common in settings with poor hygiene and sanitation
Infectious dose	Low (10–100 viral particles) for most agents	High (>10^5 bacteria) for *Escherichia coli, Salmonella, Vibrio;* medium (10^2–10^5 bacteria) for *Campylobacter jejuni;* low (10–100 bacteria) for *Shigella*
Seasonality	In temperate climates, winter seasonality for most agents; year-round occurrence in tropical areas	More common in summer or rainy months, particularly in developing countries with a high disease burden
Incubation period	1–3 days for most agents; can be shorter for norovirus	1–7 days for common agents (e.g., *Campylobacter, E. coli, Shigella, Salmonella*); a few hours for bacteria producing preformed toxins (e.g., *Staphylococcus aureus, Bacillus cereus*)
Reservoir	Primarily humans	Depending on species, human (e.g., *Shigella, Salmonella*), animal (e.g., *Campylobacter, Salmonella, E. coli*), and water (e.g., *Vibrio*) reservoirs exist.
Fever	Common with rotavirus and norovirus; uncommon with other agents	Common with agents causing inflammatory diarrhea (e.g., *Salmonella, Shigella*)
Vomiting	Prominent and can be the only presenting feature, especially in children	Common with bacteria producing preformed toxins; less prominent in diarrhea due to other agents
Diarrhea	Common; nonbloody in almost all cases	Prominent and frequently bloody with agents causing inflammatory diarrhea
Duration	1–3 days for norovirus and sapovirus; 2–8 days for other viruses	1–2 days for bacteria producing preformed toxins; 2–8 days for most other bacteria
Diagnosis	This is often a diagnosis of exclusion in clinical practice. Commercial enzyme immunoassays are available for detection of rotavirus and adenovirus, but identification of other agents is limited to research and public health laboratories.	Fecal examination for leukocytes and blood is helpful in differential diagnosis. Culture of stool specimens, sometimes on special media, can identify several pathogens. Molecular techniques are useful epidemiologic tools but are not routinely used in most laboratories.
Treatment	Supportive therapy to maintain adequate hydration and nutrition should be given. Antibiotics and antimotility agents are contraindicated.	Supportive hydration therapy is adequate for most patients. Antibiotics are recommended for patients with dysentery caused by *Shigella* or *Vibrio cholerae* and for some patients with *Clostridium difficile* colitis.

Molecular cloning and characterization have demonstrated that the viruses have a single, positive-strand RNA genome ~7.5 kb in length and that they possess a single virion-associated protein—similar to that of typical caliciviruses—with a molecular mass of 60 kDa. On the basis of these molecular characteristics, these viruses are presently classified in two genera belonging to the family Caliciviridae: the *noroviruses* and the *sapoviruses* (previously called Norwalk-like viruses and Sapporo-like viruses, respectively).

Epidemiology

Infections with the Norwalk and related human caliciviruses are common worldwide, and most adults have antibodies to these viruses. Antibody is acquired at an earlier age in developing countries—a pattern consistent with the presumed fecal-oral mode of transmission. Infections occur year-round, although, in temperate climates, a distinct increase has been noted in cold-weather months. Noroviruses may be the most common infectious agents of mild gastroenteritis in the community and affect all age groups, whereas sapoviruses primarily cause gastroenteritis in children. Noroviruses also cause traveler's diarrhea, and outbreaks have occurred among military personnel deployed to various parts of the world. The limited data available indicate that norovirus may be the second most common viral agent (after rotavirus) among young children and the most common agent among older children and adults. For example, in a comprehensive evaluation of eight enteric pathogens in patients with gastroenteritis in England, three-fourths of patients had at least one pathogen detected in fecal specimens, and noroviruses were the most prevalent, detected in 36% of patients and 18% of healthy controls. Noroviruses are also recognized as the major cause of epidemics of gastroenteritis worldwide. In the United States, >90% of outbreaks of nonbacterial gastroenteritis are caused by noroviruses.

Virus is transmitted predominantly by the fecal-oral route but is also present in vomitus. Because an inoculum with very few viruses can be infectious, transmission can occur by aerosolization, by contact with contaminated fomites, and by person-to-person contact. Viral shedding and infectivity are greatest during the acute illness, but challenge studies with Norwalk virus in volunteers indicate that viral antigen may be shed by asymptomatically infected persons and also by symptomatic persons before the onset of symptoms and for several weeks after the resolution of illness.

Pathogenesis

The exact sites and cellular receptors for attachment of viral particles have not been determined. Data suggest that carbohydrates that are similar to human histo-blood group antigens and are present on the gastroduodenal epithelium of individuals with the secretor phenotype may serve as ligands for the attachment of Norwalk virus. Additional studies must more fully elucidate norovirus-carbohydrate interactions, including potential strain-specific variations. After the infection of volunteers, reversible lesions are noted in the upper jejunum, with broadening and blunting of the villi, shortening of the microvilli, vacuolization of the lining epithelium, crypt hyperplasia, and infiltration of the lamina propria by polymorphonuclear neutrophils and lymphocytes. The lesions persist for at least 4 days after the resolution of symptoms and are associated with malabsorption of carbohydrates and fats and a decreased level of brush-border enzymes. Adenylate cyclase activity is not altered. No histopathologic changes are seen in the stomach or colon, but gastric motor function is delayed, and this alteration is believed to contribute to the nausea and vomiting that are typical of this illness.

Clinical manifestations

Gastroenteritis caused by Norwalk and related human caliciviruses has a sudden onset, following an average incubation period of 24 h (range, 12–72 h). The illness generally lasts 12–60 h and is characterized by one or more of the following symptoms: nausea, vomiting, abdominal cramps, and diarrhea. Vomiting is more prevalent among children, whereas a greater proportion of adults develop diarrhea. Constitutional symptoms are common, including headache, fever, chills, and myalgias. The stools are characteristically loose and watery, without blood, mucus, or leukocytes. White cell counts are generally normal; rarely, leukocytosis with relative lymphopenia may be observed. Death is a rare outcome and usually results from severe dehydration in vulnerable persons (e.g., elderly patients with debilitating health conditions).

Immunity

Approximately 50% of persons challenged with Norwalk virus become ill and acquire short-term immunity against the infecting strain. Immunity to Norwalk virus appears to correlate inversely with level of antibody; i.e., persons with higher levels of preexisting antibody to Norwalk virus are more susceptible to illness. This observation suggests that some individuals have a genetic predisposition to illness. Specific ABO, Lewis, and secretor blood group phenotypes may influence susceptibility to norovirus infection.

Diagnosis

Cloning and sequencing of the genomes of Norwalk and several other human caliciviruses have allowed the development of assays based on polymerase chain reaction (PCR) for detection of virus in stool and vomitus. Virus-like particles produced by expression of capsid proteins in a recombinant baculovirus vector have been used to develop enzyme immunoassays (EIAs) for detection of virus in stool or a serologic response to a specific viral antigen. These newer diagnostic techniques are considerably more sensitive than previous detection methods, such as electron microscopy, immune electron microscopy, and EIAs based on reagents derived from humans. However, no currently available single assay can detect all human caliciviruses because of their great genetic and antigenic diversity. In addition, the assays are still cumbersome and are available primarily in research laboratories, although they are increasingly being adopted by public health laboratories for routine screening of fecal specimens from patients affected by outbreaks of gastroenteritis. Commercial EIA kits, which are available in some European countries and in Japan but not yet in the United States, have limited sensitivity and usefulness in clinical practice and are of greatest utility in outbreaks, in which many specimens are tested and only a few need be positive to identify norovirus as the cause.

TREATMENT	Infections with Norwalk and Related Human Caliciviruses

The disease is self-limited, and oral rehydration therapy is generally adequate. If severe dehydration develops, IV fluid therapy is indicated. No specific antiviral therapy is available.

Prevention

Epidemic prevention relies on situation-specific measures, such as control of contamination of food and water, exclusion of ill food handlers, and reduction of person-to-person spread through good personal hygiene and disinfection of contaminated fomites. The role of immunoprophylaxis is not clear, given the lack of long-term immunity from natural disease, but efforts to develop norovirus vaccines are ongoing.

ROTAVIRUS

Etiologic agent

Rotaviruses are members of the family Reoviridae. The viral genome consists of 11 segments of double-strand RNA that are enclosed in a triple-layered, nonenveloped, icosahedral capsid 75 nm in diameter. Viral protein 6 (VP6), the major structural protein, is the target of commercial immunoassays and determines the group specificity of rotaviruses. There are seven major groups of rotavirus (A through G); human illness is caused primarily by group A and, to a much lesser extent, by groups B and C. Two outer-capsid proteins, VP7 (G-protein) and VP4 (P-protein), determine serotype specificity, induce neutralizing antibodies, and form the basis for binary classification of rotaviruses (G and P types). The segmented genome of rotavirus allows genetic reassortment (i.e., exchange of genome segments between viruses) during co-infection—a property that may play a role in viral evolution and has been utilized in the development of reassortant animal-human rotavirus–based vaccines.

Epidemiology

Worldwide, nearly all children are infected with rotavirus by 3–5 years of age. Neonatal infections are common but are often asymptomatic or mild, presumably because of protection from maternal antibody or breast-feeding. First infections after 3 months of age are likely to be symptomatic, and the incidence of disease peaks among children 4–23 months of age. Reinfections are common, but the severity of disease decreases with each repeat infection. Therefore, severe rotavirus infections are relatively uncommon among older children and adults. Nevertheless, rotavirus can cause illness in parents and caretakers of children with rotavirus diarrhea, immunocompromised persons, travelers, and elderly individuals and should be considered in the differential diagnosis of gastroenteritis among adults.

In tropical settings, rotavirus disease occurs year-round, with less pronounced seasonal peaks than in temperate settings, where rotavirus disease occurs predominantly during the cooler fall and winter months. Before the introduction of rotavirus vaccine in the United States, the rotavirus season each year began in the Southwest during the autumn and early winter (October through December) and migrated across the continent, peaking in the Northeast during late winter and spring (March through May). The reasons for this characteristic pattern are not clear, but a recent study suggested a correlation with state-specific differences in birth rates, which could influence the rate of accumulation of susceptible infants after each rotavirus season. After the implementation of routine vaccination of U.S. infants against rotavirus in 2006, the onset of the 2007–2008 and 2008–2009 rotavirus seasons was delayed by 11 weeks and 6 weeks, respectively, and the seasons were shorter, lasting 14 and 17 weeks, respectively, in comparison with a median of 26 weeks in 2000–2006 (Fig. 31-2). These changes in seasonal patterns of rotavirus activity were accompanied by declines in the number of detections of rotavirus by 64% and 60% in 2007–2008 and 2008–2009, respectively, from the figures for 2000–2006, as collected by a national network of sentinel laboratories.

FIGURE 31-2

The maximal or minimal percentage of rotavirus-positive tests for 2000–2006 may have occurred during any of the six baseline seasons. The onset of rotavirus season was defined as the first of two consecutive weeks during which the percentage of stool specimens testing positive for rotavirus was ≥10%, and the end of the season was defined as the last of two consecutive weeks during which the percentage of stool specimens testing positive for rotavirus was ≥10%. At the top right, the dots bracket the rotavirus season from onset to end, and the diamond indicates the peak week during each period. (*Adapted from Centers for Disease Control and Prevention: MMWR Morb Mortal Wkly Rep 58:1146, 2009.*)

During episodes of rotavirus-associated diarrhea, virus is shed in large quantities in stool (10^7–10^{12}/g). Viral shedding detectable by EIA usually subsides within 1 week but may persist for >30 days in immunocompromised individuals. Viral shedding may be detected for longer periods by sensitive molecular assays, such as PCR. The virus is transmitted predominantly through the fecal-oral route. Spread through respiratory secretions, person-to-person contact, or contaminated environmental surfaces has also been postulated to explain the rapid acquisition of antibody in the first 3 years of life, regardless of sanitary conditions.

At least 10 different G serotypes of group A rotavirus have been identified in humans, but only five types (G1 through G4 and G9) are common. While human rotavirus strains that possess a high degree of genetic homology with animal strains have been identified, animal-to-human transmission appears to be uncommon. Group B rotaviruses have been associated with several large epidemics of severe gastroenteritis among adults in China since 1982 and have also been identified in India. Group C rotaviruses have been associated with a small proportion of pediatric gastroenteritis cases in several countries worldwide.

Pathogenesis

Rotaviruses infect and ultimately destroy mature enterocytes in the villous epithelium of the proximal small intestine. The loss of absorptive villous epithelium, coupled with the proliferation of secretory crypt cells, results in secretory diarrhea. Brush-border enzymes characteristic of differentiated cells are reduced, and this change leads to the accumulation of unmetabolized disaccharides and consequent osmotic diarrhea. Studies in mice indicate that a nonstructural rotavirus protein, NSP4, functions as an enterotoxin and contributes to secretory diarrhea by altering epithelial cell function and permeability. In addition, rotavirus may evoke fluid secretion through activation of the enteric nervous system in the intestinal wall. Recent data indicate that rotavirus antigenemia and viremia are common among children with acute rotavirus infection, although the antigen and RNA levels in serum are substantially lower than those in stool.

Clinical manifestations

The clinical spectrum of rotavirus infection ranges from subclinical infection to severe gastroenteritis leading to life-threatening dehydration. After an incubation period of 1–3 days, the illness has an abrupt onset, with vomiting frequently preceding the onset of diarrhea. Up to one-third of patients may have a temperature of >39°C. The stools are characteristically loose and watery and only infrequently contain red or white cells. Gastrointestinal symptoms generally resolve in 3–7 days.

Respiratory and neurologic features in children with rotavirus infection have been reported, but causal associations have not been proven. Moreover, rotavirus infection has been associated with a variety of other clinical conditions (e.g., sudden infant death syndrome, necrotizing enterocolitis, intussusception, Kawasaki's disease, and type 1 diabetes), but no causal relationship has been confirmed with any of these syndromes.

Rotavirus does not appear to be a major opportunistic pathogen in children with HIV infection. In severely immunodeficient children, rotavirus can cause protracted diarrhea with prolonged viral excretion and, in rare instances, can disseminate systemically. Persons who are immunosuppressed for bone marrow transplantation are also at risk for severe or even fatal rotavirus disease.

Immunity

Protection against rotavirus disease is correlated with the presence of virus-specific secretory IgA antibodies in the intestine and, to some extent, the serum. Because virus-specific IgA production at the intestinal surface is short lived, complete protection against disease is only temporary. However, each infection and subsequent reinfection confers progressively greater immunity; thus severe disease is most common among young children with first or second infections. Immunologic memory is believed to be important in the attenuation of disease severity upon reinfection.

Diagnosis

Illness caused by rotavirus is difficult to distinguish clinically from that caused by other enteric viruses. Because large quantities of virus are shed in feces, the diagnosis can usually be confirmed by a wide variety of commercially available EIAs or by techniques for detecting viral RNA, such as gel electrophoresis, probe hybridization, or PCR.

TREATMENT Rotavirus Infections

Rotavirus gastroenteritis can lead to severe dehydration. Thus appropriate treatment should be instituted early. Standard oral rehydration therapy is successful in most children who can take oral fluids, but IV fluid replacement may be required for patients who are severely dehydrated or are unable to tolerate oral therapy because of frequent vomiting. The therapeutic role of probiotics, bismuth subsalicylate, enkephalinase inhibitors, and nitazoxanide has been evaluated in clinical studies but is not clearly defined. Antibiotics and antimotility agents should be avoided. In immunocompromised

children with chronic symptomatic rotavirus disease, orally administered immunoglobulins or colostrum may result in the resolution of symptoms, but the best choices regarding agents and their doses have not been well studied, and treatment decisions are often empirical.

Prevention

Efforts to develop rotavirus vaccines were pursued because it was apparent—given the similar rates in less-developed and industrialized nations—that improvements in hygiene and sanitation were unlikely to reduce disease incidence. The first rotavirus vaccine licensed in the United States in 1998 was withdrawn from the market within 1 year because it was linked with intussusception, a severe bowel obstruction.

 In 2006, promising safety and efficacy results for two new rotavirus vaccines were reported from large clinical trials conducted in North America, Europe, and Latin America. Both vaccines are now recommended for routine immunization of all U.S. infants, and their use has rapidly led to a decline in rotavirus hospitalizations and emergency department visits at hospitals across the United States. In Mexico, a decline in deaths from childhood diarrhea following introduction of rotavirus vaccines has been documented. Furthermore, postmarketing surveillance information has not revealed an association of these vaccines with any serious adverse events (including intussusception), although a risk of low magnitude cannot be excluded on the basis of available data.

Global considerations

Rotavirus is ubiquitous and infects nearly all children worldwide by 5 years of age. However, compared with rotavirus disease in industrialized countries, disease in developing countries occurs at a younger age, is less seasonal, and is more frequently caused by uncommon rotavirus strains. Moreover, because of suboptimal access to hydration therapy, rotavirus is a leading cause of diarrheal death among children in the developing world, with the highest mortality rates among children in sub-Saharan Africa and southern Asia (Fig. 31-3).

The different epidemiology of rotavirus disease and the greater prevalence of co-infection with other enteric pathogens, of comorbidities, and of malnutrition in developing countries may adversely affect the performance of oral rotavirus vaccines, as is the case with oral vaccines against poliomyelitis, cholera, and typhoid in these regions. Therefore, evaluation of the efficacy of rotavirus vaccines in resource-poor settings of Africa and Asia was specifically recommended, and these trials have now been completed. As anticipated, the efficacy

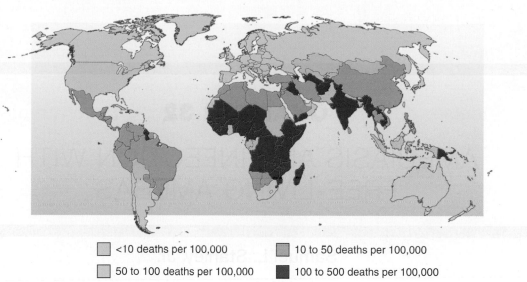

FIGURE 31-3

Rotavirus mortality rates by country, per 100,000 children <5 years of age. (*Reproduced with permission from UD Parashar et al: J Infect Dis 200:S9, 2009.*)

of rotavirus vaccines was moderate (50–75%) in these settings when compared with that in industrialized countries. Nevertheless, even a moderately efficacious rotavirus vaccine would be likely to have substantial public health benefits in these areas with a high disease burden. Given these considerations, in April 2009 the World Health Organization recommended the use of rotavirus vaccines in all countries worldwide.

OTHER VIRAL AGENTS OF GASTROENTERITIS

Enteric *adenoviruses* of serotypes 40 and 41 belonging to subgroup F are 70- to 80-nm viruses with double-strand DNA that cause ~2–12% of all diarrhea episodes in young children. Unlike adenoviruses that cause respiratory illness, enteric adenoviruses are difficult to cultivate in cell lines, but they can be detected with commercially available EIAs.

Astroviruses, 28- to 30-nm viruses with a characteristic icosahedral structure, contain a positive-sense, single-strand RNA. At least seven serotypes have been identified, of which serotype 1 is most common. Astroviruses are primarily pediatric pathogens, causing ~2–10% of cases of mild to moderate gastroenteritis in children. The availability of simple immunoassays to detect virus in fecal specimens and of molecular methods to confirm and characterize strains will permit more comprehensive assessment of the etiologic role of these agents.

Toroviruses are 100- to 140-nm, enveloped, positive-strand RNA viruses that are recognized as causes of gastroenteritis in horses (Berne virus) and cattle (Breda virus). Their role as a cause of diarrhea in humans is still unclear, but studies from Canada have demonstrated associations between torovirus excretion and both nosocomial gastroenteritis and necrotizing enterocolitis in neonates. These associations require further evaluation.

Picobirnaviruses are small, bisegmented, double-strand RNA viruses that cause gastroenteritis in a variety of animals. Their role as primary causes of gastroenteritis in humans remains unclear, but several studies have found an association between picobirnaviruses and gastroenteritis in HIV-infected adults.

Several other viruses (e.g., enteroviruses, reoviruses, pestiviruses, and parvovirus B) have been identified in the feces of patients with diarrhea, but their etiologic role in gastroenteritis has not been proven. Diarrhea has also been noted as a manifestation of infection with recently recognized viruses that primarily cause severe respiratory illness: the severe acute respiratory syndrome–associated coronavirus (SARS-CoV), influenza A/H5N1 virus, and the current pandemic strain of influenza A/H1N1 virus.

CHAPTER 32

AMEBIASIS AND INFECTION WITH FREE-LIVING AMEBAS

Samuel L. Stanley, Jr.

AMEBIASIS

DEFINITION

Amebiasis is infection with the parasitic intestinal protozoan *Entamoeba histolytica* (the "tissue-lysing ameba"). Most infections are probably asymptomatic, but *E. histolytica* can cause disease ranging from dysentery to extraintestinal infections, including liver abscesses.

LIFE CYCLE AND TRANSMISSION

E. histolytica exists in two stages: a hardy multinucleate cyst form (**Fig. 32-1**) and the motile trophozoite stage (**Fig. 32-2**). Infection (of which humans are the natural hosts) is acquired by ingestion of cysts contained in fecally contaminated food or water or, more rarely, through oral-anal sexual contact. Cysts survive stomach

FIGURE 32-2
***E. histolytica* trophozoite with ingested red blood cells.** Note the single nucleus with central nucleolus. (*Courtesy of the Centers for Disease Control and Prevention.*)

acidity and excyst within the small intestine to form the 20- to 50-μm trophozoite stage. Trophozoites can live within the large-bowel lumen without causing disease or can invade the intestinal mucosa, causing amebic colitis. In some cases, *E. histolytica* trophozoites invade through the mucosa and into the bloodstream, traveling through the portal circulation to reach the liver and causing amebic liver abscesses. Motile trophozoites may be excreted into the stool—a diagnostically important event—but are rapidly killed upon exposure to air or stomach acid and therefore are not infectious. Trophozoite cysts within the large bowel are excreted in the stool, continuing the life cycle.

FIGURE 32-1
***Entamoeba* cyst.** Three of the four nuclei are clearly visible. (*Courtesy of Dr. George Healy, Centers for Disease Control and Prevention.*)

EPIDEMIOLOGY

Molecular diagnostics continue to clarify what was once a confusing picture of the true incidence and prevalence of *E. histolytica* infection and disease. It was a staple of most textbooks that 10% of the world's population was infected with *E. histolytica*. We now know that most asymptomatic individuals harboring amebic trophozoites or cysts in their stools are infected with a noninvasive species: *Entamoeba dispar* or *Entamoeba moshkovskii*. *E. dispar* appears not to cause disease, even in the most profoundly immunosuppressed individuals; furthermore, at this time, there is little evidence to suggest that *E. moshkovskii* causes disease, although epidemiologic studies of this species are in their infancy. In contrast, *E. histolytica* infection can cause disease, although not all patients develop symptoms. It remains unclear how frequently people infected with *E. histolytica* do develop symptoms; in one study in a highly endemic area, only 10% of infected patients developed symptoms over a 1-year observation period. A remarkable feature of amebiasis is its more common occurrence in men than in women, although the prevalence of infection with *E. histolytica* does not appear to differ between the sexes. This pattern is particularly pronounced for amebic liver abscess, whose prevalence is ~7 times higher among men than among women. The explanation for this difference remains unknown, but less efficient complement-mediated killing of amebic trophozoites by serum from men than by serum from women has been reported.

 E. histolytica infections are most common in areas of the world where poor sanitation and crowding compromise the barriers to contamination of food and drinking water with human feces. Endemic areas include parts of Mexico, India, and nations in the tropical regions of Africa, South and Central America, and Asia. *E. histolytica* was present in ~2.1% of individuals presenting with diarrhea in a large series from Bangladesh and in 1.4% of the asymptomatic control group. In 2007, amebiasis was listed as the sixth most common cause of disease in Mexico, with an incidence of ~544 cases per 100,000 population. In the United States and other developed countries, disease is unusual and is found almost exclusively in travelers or immigrants from endemic areas. Rarely, outbreaks take place in institutionalized populations, and infections have been documented with increased frequency among men who have sex with men; however, most of the latter cases have been asymptomatic and probably represent *E. dispar* infections.

PATHOGENESIS AND PATHOLOGY

E. histolytica trophozoites possess a potent repertoire of adhesins, proteinases, pore-forming proteins, and other effector molecules that enable them to lyse cells and tissue, induce both cellular necrosis and apoptosis, and resist both innate and adaptive immune defenses. Disease begins when *E. histolytica* trophozoites adhere to colonic mucosal epithelial cells. Disruption of the colonic mucin barrier is seen in pathologic sections from the diseased colon, but it is not clear whether this disruption is caused by the parasite, facilitating its adherence to mucosal cells, or occurs as a consequence of the adhesion event, with subsequent mucosal damage. Adherence is mediated primarily by a family of surface lectin molecules capable of binding to galactose and *N*-acetylgalactosamine residues. *E. histolytica* can lyse host cells upon contact through a family of amphipathic peptides called *amoebapores* that form barrel-stave pores in target cell membranes. Both cellular necrosis and apoptosis can occur after *E. histolytica* comes into contact with host cells, and which outcome predominates may relate to inherent characteristics of the target cell or the tissue environment. One consistent and unequivocal finding is the important role played by amebic cysteine proteinases in the disease process. *E. histolytica* possesses a large family of cysteine proteinases that are capable of lysing the extracellular matrix between host cells (thus detaching cells and facilitating invasion) and cleaving host defense molecules (including complement components and antibodies). Studies in animal models, including chimeric mice with human intestinal xenografts, have shown that inhibition of *E. histolytica* cysteine proteinase activity, via either direct gene targeting or chemical inhibitors, significantly reduces disease. The ultimate effect of all these amebic virulence factors on the human colon is the production of small ulcers that have heaped borders and contain focal areas of epithelial cell loss, a modest inflammatory response, and mucosal hemorrhage. The intervening mucosa is usually normal, but diffuse hyperemia is sometimes seen. *E. histolytica* trophozoites can then invade laterally through the submucosal layer, creating the classic flask-shaped ulcers that appear on pathologic examination as narrow-necked lesions, broadening in the submucosal region, with *E. histolytica* trophozoites at the margins between dead and live tissues (**Fig. 32-3**). Ulcers tend to stop at the muscularis layer, and full-thickness lesions and colonic perforation are unusual. Amebomas, a rare complication of intestinal disease, are granulomatous mass lesions protruding into the bowel lumen, with a thickened edematous and hemorrhagic bowel wall that can cause obstructive symptoms.

In some individuals with *E. histolytica* colonic infection, trophozoites invade the portal venous system and reach the liver, where they cause amebic liver abscesses. *E. histolytica* trophozoites must resist lysis by serum complement to survive in the bloodstream. Amebic liver abscesses have a characteristic appearance on pathologic examination: the roughly circular abscesses contain a large necrotic center resembling anchovy paste that is surrounded by a narrow ring of a few inflammatory cells, fibrosis, and occasionally a few amebic trophozoites. The adjacent liver parenchyma

FIGURE 32-3

E. histolytica **flask-shaped intestinal ulceration** from a kitten. (*Courtesy of Dr. Mae Melvin, Centers for Disease Control and Prevention.*)

is usually completely normal. Results in experimental rodent models of amebic liver abscess suggest that initial lesions may have more inflammatory cells and that lysis of neutrophils by *E. histolytica* trophozoites may contribute to tissue damage. In murine models of disease, apoptosis is a prominent component of hepatocyte death and the blockade of caspase activity can significantly reduce liver abscess formation, but whether any of these factors is applicable to human disease is unclear.

The role of innate and adaptive immunity in preventing *E. histolytica* infection or controlling disease needs further clarification. Studies of children in a highly endemic area have suggested that prior *E. histolytica* intestinal infection may stimulate mucosal IgA antibodies to amebic antigens, thereby reducing the likelihood of subsequent infections; this protection is relatively short lived. In contrast, among individuals in an area of Vietnam with a high prevalence of amebic liver abscess, a prior episode of disease did not reduce the risk of a second case, despite the presence of serum antibodies. Studies of animal models suggest that cell-mediated immunity may play a role in host defense, and glucocorticoid use has been associated with worse outcomes in patients with amebic colitis. However, individuals with HIV/AIDS do not appear to be at increased risk for infection with *E. histolytica*, and there is no evidence that they develop more severe disease than do immunocompetent hosts.

CLINICAL SYNDROMES

Intestinal amebiasis

Most patients harboring *Entamoeba* species are asymptomatic, but individuals with *E. histolytica* infection can develop disease. Symptoms of amebic colitis generally appear 2–6 weeks after ingestion of the cyst form of the parasite. Diarrhea (classically heme-positive) and lower abdominal pain are the most common symptoms. Malaise and weight loss may be noted as disease progresses. Severe dysentery, with 10–12 small-volume, blood- and mucus-containing stools daily, may develop, but only ~40% of patients are febrile. Fulminant amebic colitis, with even more profuse diarrhea, severe abdominal pain (including peritoneal signs), fever, and pronounced leukocytosis are rare, disproportionately affecting young children, pregnant women, individuals being treated with glucocorticoids, and possibly individuals with diabetes or alcoholism. Paralytic ileus and colonic mucosal sloughing may be seen; intestinal perforation occurs in >75% of patients with this fulminant form of disease. Mortality rates from fulminant amebic colitis exceed 40% in some series. Recognized complications of amebic colitis also include toxic megacolon (documented in ~0.5% of patients with colitis), with severe bowel dilation and intramural air, and the aforementioned ameboma, which presents as an abdominal mass that may be confused with colon cancer.

Amebic liver abscess

Just a century ago, amebic liver abscess—the most common extraintestinal manifestation of amebiasis—was almost always fatal; however, with current rapid diagnostic methods and effective medical treatment, mortality rates are now 1–3%. Disease begins when *E. histolytica* trophozoites penetrate through the colonic mucosa, travel through the portal circulation, and reach the liver. Most individuals with amebic liver abscess do not have concurrent signs or symptoms of colitis, and most do not have *E. histolytica* trophozoites in their stools. The exceptions are individuals with fulminant amebic colitis, in which concurrent amebic liver abscess is not uncommon. Disease can arise from months to years after travel to or residence in an endemic area; therefore, a careful travel history is key in making the diagnosis. The classic presentations of amebic liver abscess are right-upper-quadrant pain, fever, and hepatic tenderness. The pace of disease is usually acute, with symptoms lasting <10 days. However, a more chronic presentation, with weight loss and anorexia as prominent accompanying features, does occur. Jaundice is unusual, but dullness and rales at the right lung base (secondary to pleural effusion) are common. The most common laboratory findings are leukocytosis (without eosinophilia), an elevated alkaline phosphatase level, mild anemia, and an elevated erythrocyte sedimentation rate.

Other extraintestinal complications of amebiasis

Right-sided pleural effusions and atelectasis are common in cases of amebic liver abscess and generally require no treatment. However, the abscess ruptures through the diaphragm in ~10% of patients, causing pleuropulmonary amebiasis. Suggestive symptoms are sudden-onset cough, pleuritic chest pain, and shortness of breath. In some patients, pleuropulmonary amebiasis is the presenting manifestation of amebic liver abscess and may be confused with bacterial pneumonia and empyema. A dramatic complication is the development of a hepatobronchial fistula, in which patients can cough up the contents of the liver abscess—copious amounts of brown sputum that may contain *E. histolytica* trophozoites. In ~1–3% of cases, the amebic liver abscess ruptures into the peritoneum, and peritoneal signs and shock develop. Even rarer is rupture of an amebic liver abscess into the pericardium; the signs and symptoms are those commonly seen with pericarditis (chest pain, pericardial rub, dyspnea, tachypnea, or cardiac tamponade), and nearly 30% of cases end in death. Cerebral abscesses complicate <0.1% of cases of amebic liver abscess and are associated with the sudden onset of headache, vomiting, seizures, and mental status changes and a high mortality rate. Cutaneous amebiasis (which usually involves the anal and perianal regions), genital disease (including rectovaginal fistulas), and urinary tract lesions are rare but reported complications of amebiasis.

DIAGNOSTIC TESTS

The diagnosis of amebic colitis has traditionally been based on the demonstration of *E. histolytica* trophozoites or cysts in the stool or colonic mucosa of patients with diarrhea. However, the inability of microscopy to differentiate between *E. histolytica* and other *Entamoeba* species, such as *E. dispar* and *E. moshkovskii*, limits its effectiveness as a sole diagnostic method. Examination of three stool samples improves sensitivity for the detection of *Entamoeba* species, and it has been argued that the presence of amebic trophozoites containing red blood cells in a diarrheal stool is highly suggestive of *E. histolytica* infection. However, because trophozoites containing red blood cells are not found in most patients with *E. histolytica* infection, the applicability of this finding is limited.

 Despite these inherent limitations, microscopy, often combined with serologic testing, remains the standard diagnostic approach in many hospitals and clinics worldwide. Culture of stools for *E. histolytica* trophozoites serves as a research tool but is generally not available for clinical use. PCR assay for DNA in stool samples is currently the most sensitive and specific method for identifying *E. histolytica* infection and has become a valuable epidemiologic and research tool; probes can be configured to detect *E. dispar* and *E. moshkovskii* as well. While significant advances are being made in reducing the costs of PCR-based diagnostics, this method still is not feasible for clinical diagnosis in most endemic areas. Commercially available tests that use enzyme-linked immunosorbent assays (ELISAs) or immunochromatographic techniques to detect *Entamoeba* antigens are less expensive and more easily performed and are being used with increasing frequency. Greater sensitivity than microscopy and the ability to detect *E. histolytica* specifically are claimed by some of the leading kits, representing significant advantages over microscopy. Unfortunately, not all clinical studies have supported these claims, concerns have been raised about the specificity of the tests in nonendemic areas, and the ELISAs are less sensitive and specific than are PCR-based diagnostics. At this point, antigen detection–based ELISAs that can specifically identify *E. histolytica* in stool probably represent the best choice in endemic areas; however, the results of any of these diagnostic tests need to be interpreted in light of clinical presentation, and a second confirmatory test (e.g., microscopy and/or amebic serology) may be prudent. In instances in which amebiasis is suspected on clinical grounds in a patient with acute colitis but initial stool samples are negative, colonoscopy with examination of brushings or mucosal biopsies for *E. histolytica* trophozoites may be helpful in making the diagnosis or in identifying other diseases, such as inflammatory bowel disease or pseudomembranous colitis.

The diagnosis of amebic liver abscess is based on the detection (generally by ultrasound or CT; **Fig. 32-4**) of one or more space-occupying lesions in the liver and a positive serologic test for antibodies to *E. histolytica* antigens. As has been noted, amebiasis can present

FIGURE 32-4

Large amebic abscess in the right lobe of the liver visualized by CT. (*Courtesy of Dr. M. M. Reeder, International Registry of Tropical Imaging.*)

months or years after travel to or residence in an endemic area, and so a careful travel history is mandatory when anyone presents with a liver abscess. Amebic liver abscesses are classically described as single, large, and located in the right lobe of the liver, but sensitive imaging techniques have shown that multiple abscesses are more common than previously suspected. When a patient has a space-occupying lesion of the liver, a positive amebic serology is highly sensitive (>94%) and highly specific (>95%) for the diagnosis of amebic liver abscess. False-negative serologic tests have been reported when serum samples were obtained very early in the course of abscess (within 7–10 days of onset), but repeat tests are almost always positive.

DIFFERENTIAL DIAGNOSIS

The differential diagnosis of amebic colitis includes bacterial dysentery (e.g., *Shigella* and *Campylobacter* infections), schistosomiasis, *Balantidium coli* infection, pseudomembranous colitis, inflammatory bowel disease, and ischemic colitis. Stool cultures for bacterial pathogens, microscopic examination of stools, and amebic serology help differentiate amebic colitis from these other entities. Amebomas may be confused with colonic carcinoma; several case reports describe instances in which amebomas and associated liver abscesses were initially considered to be colon cancer with liver metastases. Amebic liver abscess must be distinguished from pyogenic liver abscess, echinococcal cysts, and primary or metastatic liver tumors. It is difficult to differentiate pyogenic from amebic liver abscesses on purely clinical grounds, but amebic serology is usually the key test in excluding or diagnosing amebic liver abscess. Abscesses that rupture into the pleural space may be accompanied by cough, sputum production, and dyspnea and may initially be diagnosed as bronchopneumonia.

TREATMENT   Amebiasis

The nitroimidazole compounds tinidazole and metronidazole are the drugs of choice for the treatment of amebic colitis and amebic liver abscess (Table 32-1). To date, *E. histolytica* has not demonstrated resistance to any of the commonly used agents—a situation that greatly simplifies treatment. Tinidazole appears to be better tolerated and slightly more effective than metronidazole for amebic colitis and amebic liver abscess. Metronidazole is available as a parenteral formulation for patients who cannot take oral medications. Whenever possible, fulminant amebic colitis is managed conservatively, even in the presence of perforation, with the addition

TABLE 32-1

RECOMMENDED THERAPEUTIC DOSAGES OF ANTIAMEBIC DRUGS

DRUG	DOSAGE	DURATION, DAYS
Amebic Colitis or Amebic Liver Abscess		
Tinidazole	2 g/d PO with food	3
Metronidazole	750 mg tid PO or IV	5–10
***Entamoeba histolytica* Luminal Infection**		
Paromomycin	30 mg/kg qd PO in 3 divided doses	5–10
Iodoquinol	650 mg PO tid	20

of antibiotics to treat gut bacteria and percutaneous catheter drainage of fluid collections if needed.

Remarkably, given the large size of amebic liver abscesses, treatment with tinidazole or metronidazole in the same doses used for amebic colitis is almost always successful. More than 90% of patients respond with a decrease in abdominal pain and fever within 72 h of the initiation of therapy. Drainage of amebic liver abscesses is rarely needed; in one large series, neither time to becoming afebrile nor length of hospitalization was significantly different for patients who underwent percutaneous radiography-guided aspiration of the abscess accompanied by medical therapy than for those who received medical therapy alone. Aspiration should be reserved for individuals in whom pyogenic abscess or a bacterial superinfection is suspected but whose diagnosis is uncertain, for patients failing to respond to tinidazole or metronidazole (i.e., those who have persistent fever or abdominal pain after 4 days of treatment), for individuals with large liver abscesses in the left lobe (because of the risk of rupture into the pericardium), and for patients whose large abscesses and accelerated clinical course raise concerns about imminent rupture. In contrast, aspiration and/or percutaneous catheter drainage improves outcomes in patients with pleuropulmonary amebiasis and empyema (where amebic liver abscesses have ruptured into the pleural space), and percutaneous catheter or surgical drainage is absolutely indicated for cases of amebic pericarditis. Rupture of an amebic liver abscess into the peritoneum is generally managed conservatively, with medical therapy and percutaneous catheter drainage of fluid collections as needed.

Neither metronidazole nor tinidazole reaches high levels in the gut lumen; therefore, patients with amebic colitis or amebic liver abscess should also receive treatment with a luminal agent (paromomycin or iodoquinol) to ensure eradication of the infection (Table 32-1). Paromomycin is the preferred agent. Asymptomatic individuals with documented *E. histolytica* infection should be treated because of the risks of developing amebic colitis or amebic liver abscess in the future and of transmitting the infection to others. Paromomycin or iodoquinol in the doses listed in the table should be used in these cases.

Nitazoxanide, a broad-spectrum antiparasitic drug, is efficacious against *E. histolytica* trophozoites in both tissue and gut lumen and may become an important addition to the therapeutic repertoire. However, clinical experience with nitazoxanide for the treatment of *E. histolytica* infection remains limited at this point.

PREVENTION

Avoidance of the ingestion of food and water contaminated with human feces is the only way to prevent *E. histolytica* infection. Travelers to endemic areas should exercise the same measures used to reduce the risk of travelers' diarrhea. Treatment of asymptomatic persons who pass *E. histolytica* cysts in the stool may help reduce opportunities for disease transmission. There is no evidence for any effective prophylaxis, and no vaccine is available.

INFECTION WITH FREE-LIVING AMEBAS

In contrast to the trophozoites of the parasitic *E. histolytica*, which can survive only in humans and some other primate hosts, free-living amebas of the genera *Naegleria*, *Acanthamoeba*, and *Balamuthia* live in brackish or freshwater habitats around the world (including lakes, tap water, swimming pools, and air conditioning and heating ducts) and are accidental and opportunistic agents of disease.

NAEGLERIA INFECTIONS

Naegleria (the "brain-eating ameba") is the causative agent of primary amebic meningoencephalitis (PAM). Nearly always fatal but quite rare, cases of PAM have been reported from 15 countries and from all continents except Antarctica; 35 cases were reported in the United States between 1998 and 2009. *Naegleria* prefers warm freshwater, and most cases occur in otherwise healthy children, who usually have swum in lakes or swimming pools during the previous 2 weeks. *Naegleria* enters the central nervous system via water inhaled or splashed into the nose, with trophozoites disrupting the olfactory mucosa, invading through the cribriform plate, and ascending via the olfactory nerves into the brain. The earliest manifestations are anosmia (usually perceived as alterations in taste), headache, fever, photophobia, nausea, and vomiting. Cranial nerve palsies, especially of the third, fourth, and sixth

FIGURE 32-5
***Naegleria* in a section of human brain tissue** from a patient with primary amebic meningoencephalitis. (*Courtesy of Dr. George Healy, Centers for Disease Control and Prevention.*)

nerves, are documented, and rapid progression of disease, with seizures, coma, and death within 7–10 days of the onset of symptoms, is common. Pathologic examination reveals hemorrhagic necrosis of brain tissue (often most prominent in the olfactory bulbs), evidence of increased intracranial pressure, scant purulent material that may contain a few amebas, and marked leptomeningitis (**Fig. 32-5**).

The diagnosis of PAM is based on the finding of motile *Naegleria* trophozoites in wet mounts of freshly obtained cerebrospinal fluid (CSF). Laboratory findings in the CSF resemble those in bacterial meningitis, with high opening pressures, low glucose levels, high protein concentrations, and elevated polymorphonuclear cell–predominant white blood cell counts. PAM should be suspected in any patient who has an appropriate history and purulent meningoencephalitis with negative gram stains, negative antigen detection and PCR tests for other pathogens, and negative bacterial cultures. Unfortunately, the prognosis for PAM is dismal. The few survivors who have been reported were treated with high-dose amphotericin B and rifampin in combination.

ACANTHAMOEBA INFECTIONS

Acanthamoeba species are free-living amebas that cause two major clinical syndromes: granulomatous amebic encephalitis and keratitis. Granulomatous amebic encephalitis occurs in debilitated, chronically ill, and immunosuppressed individuals who may be undergoing chemotherapy, receiving glucocorticoids, or suffering from lymphoproliferative diseases, systemic lupus erythematosus, or AIDS. It is believed that *Acanthamoeba* reaches the central nervous system through the bloodstream, traveling from a primary site of infection in the nares, skin, sinuses, or lungs. The pace of infection is

312

FIGURE 32-6

Acanthamoeba **cyst in brain tissue** from a patient with granulomatous amebic encephalitis. (*Courtesy of Dr. George Healy, Centers for Disease Control and Prevention.*)

indolent compared with that of PAM. Granulomatous amebic encephalitis tends to present as a space-occupying lesion in the brain. Common symptoms include altered mental status, stiff neck, and headache along with focal findings including hemiparesis, ataxia, and cranial nerve palsies. Seizures and coma often precede death. Pathologic findings in the brain include cerebral edema and multiple areas of necrosis and hemorrhage. Amebic trophozoites and cysts are scattered throughout the tissue and are often located near blood vessels **(Fig. 32-6).** Multinucleated giant cells forming granulomas give the syndrome its name but are seen less often in highly immunocompromised patients. The diagnosis is usually made by detection of *Acanthamoeba* trophozoites or cysts in biopsy specimens; a fluorescein-labeled antiserum is available from the Centers for Disease Control and Prevention (CDC) to help identify *Acanthamoeba* in microscopic sections. *Acanthamoeba* trophozoites and cysts are occasionally seen in CSF, but samples from most patients with granulomatous amebic encephalitis show mild lymphocyte-predominant pleocytosis, slightly elevated protein levels, and normal or slightly depressed glucose concentrations without the presence of amebas. CT findings vary, with hypodense lesions that resemble infarcts in some patients and multiple enhancing lesions that resemble toxoplasmosis in others. Unfortunately, there are no therapies with proven efficacy against this disease, and almost all cases have ended in death. There have been case reports of survivors treated with multidrug combinations

that included pentamidine, sulfadiazine, flucytosine, rifampin, and fluconazole.

Acanthamoeba keratitis is associated with corneal injuries complicated by exposure to water or soil and with the wearing of contact lenses. In contact lens–associated infection, extended wear, breaches in hygiene and disinfection procedures, swimming with contact lenses in place, and the use of homemade saline solutions contaminated with *Acanthamoeba* are important risk factors. The incidence of *Acanthamoeba* keratitis varies from 1.65–2.01 cases per million contact lens users in the United States to 17.53–19.5 cases per million users in the United Kingdom. Unilateral photophobia, excessive tearing, redness, and foreign-body sensation are the earliest signs and symptoms; disease is bilateral in some contact lens users. *Acanthamoeba* keratitis can progress rapidly; abscesses, hypopyon, scleritis, and corneal perforation with vision loss can develop within weeks. The disease may be diagnosed by identification of the polygonal cyst form in corneal scrapings or biopsy material, by culture of biopsy samples or contact lenses on *Escherichia coli*–seeded agar plates, by confocal microscopy, and by PCR. The differential diagnosis includes bacterial, fungal, mycobacterial, and viral (particularly herpetic) causes. Current therapy involves topical administration of a cationic antiseptic agent such as a biguanide or chlorhexidine, with or without a diamidine agent. The persistence of the cyst form of *Acanthamoeba* complicates treatment, and long durations of therapy (6 months to 1 year) are required. In severe cases, particularly when vision is threatened or already diminished, penetrating keratoplasty may be indicated.

BALAMUTHIA INFECTIONS

Balamuthia mandrillaris is a free-living ameba that causes meningoencephalitis in both immunosuppressed and immunocompetent hosts, particularly children and the elderly. The disease presents similarly to granulomatous amebic encephalitis caused by *Acanthamoeba*, and essentially all of the points made earlier with regard to the latter organism—in terms of clinical presentation, pathologic findings, and lack of proven therapies—apply to *Balamuthia* infections as well. Most cases are identified post mortem; the few cases identified before death have been found during histologic examination of brain biopsy specimens. A specific antiserum is available from the CDC to aid in identifying *B. mandrillaris* in clinical specimens.

SECTION IV Infections of the Alimentary Tract

CHAPTER 33

PROTOZOAL INTESTINAL INFECTIONS AND TRICHOMONIASIS

Peter F. Weller

PROTOZOAL INFECTIONS

GIARDIASIS

Giardia intestinalis (also known as *G. lamblia* or *G. duodenalis*) is a cosmopolitan protozoal parasite that inhabits the small intestines of humans and other mammals. Giardiasis is one of the most common parasitic diseases in both developed and developing countries worldwide, causing both endemic and epidemic intestinal disease and diarrhea.

Life cycle and epidemiology

(Fig. 33–1) Infection follows the ingestion of environmentally hardy cysts, which excyst in the small intestine, releasing flagellated trophozoites (Fig. 33–2) that multiply by binary fission. *Giardia* remains a pathogen of the proximal small bowel and does not disseminate hematogenously. Trophozoites remain free in the lumen or attach to the mucosal epithelium by means of a ventral sucking disk. As a trophozoite encounters altered conditions, it forms a morphologically distinct cyst, which is the stage of the parasite usually found in the feces. Trophozoites may be present and even predominate in loose or watery stools, but it is the resistant cyst that survives outside the body and is responsible for transmission. Cysts do not tolerate heating, desiccation, or continued exposure to feces but do remain viable for months in cold fresh water. The number of cysts excreted varies widely but can approach 10^7 per gram of stool.

Ingestion of as few as 10 cysts is sufficient to cause infection in humans. Because cysts are infectious when excreted, person-to-person transmission occurs where fecal hygiene is poor. Giardiasis (symptomatic or asymptomatic) is especially prevalent in day-care centers; person-to-person spread also takes place in other institutional settings with poor fecal hygiene and during

Excystation follows exposure to stomach acid and intestinal proteases, releasing trophozoite forms that multiply by binary fission and reside in the upper small bowel adherent to enterocytes.

Causes: Asymptomatic infection, acute diarrhea, or chronic diarrhea and malabsorption. Small bowel may demonstrate villous blunting, crypt hypertrophy, and mucosal inflammation.

Encystation occurs under conditions of bile salt concentration changes and alkaline pH.
Smooth-walled cysts can contain two trophozoites.

Cysts are ingested (10-25 cysts) in contaminated water or food or by direct fecal-oral transmission (as in day-care centers).

Cysts can survive in the environment (up to several weeks in cold water). They may also infect nonhuman mammalian species.

Cysts and trophozoites are passed in the stool into the environment.

FIGURE 33-1

Life cycle of *Giardia*. *(Reprinted from RL Guerrant et al: Tropical Infectious Disease: Principles, Pathogens and Practice, 2nd ed, 2006, p 987, with permission from Elsevier Science.)*

FIGURE 33-2
Flagellated, binucleate *Giardia* trophozoites.

anal-oral contact. If food is contaminated with *Giardia* cysts after cooking or preparation, food-borne transmission can occur. Waterborne transmission accounts for episodic infections (e.g., in campers and travelers) and for major epidemics in metropolitan areas. Surface water, ranging from mountain streams to large municipal reservoirs, can become contaminated with fecally derived *Giardia* cysts; outmoded water systems are subject to cross-contamination from leaking sewer lines. The efficacy of water as a means of transmission is enhanced by the small infectious inoculum of *Giardia*, the prolonged survival of cysts in cold water, and the resistance of cysts to killing by routine chlorination methods that are adequate for controlling bacteria. Viable cysts can be eradicated from water by either boiling or filtration. In the United States, *Giardia* (like *Cryptosporidium*; discussed later) is a common cause of waterborne epidemics of gastroenteritis.

Giardia is common in developing countries, and infections may be acquired by travelers.

Giardia parasites genotypically similar to those in humans are found in many mammals, including beavers from reservoirs implicated in epidemics. The importance of dogs and cats as sources of infection for humans is unclear.

Giardiasis, like cryptosporidiosis, creates a significant economic burden because of the costs incurred in the installation of water filtration systems required to prevent waterborne epidemics, in the management of epidemics that involve large communities, and in the evaluation and treatment of endemic infections.

Pathophysiology

The reasons that some, but not all, infected patients develop clinical manifestations and the mechanisms by which *Giardia* causes alterations in small-bowel function are largely unknown. Although trophozoites adhere to the epithelium, they do not cause invasive or locally destructive alterations. The lactose intolerance and, in a minority of infected adults and children, significant malabsorption that develop are clinical signs of the loss of brush-border enzyme activities. In most infections, the morphology of the bowel is unaltered; however, in a few cases (usually in chronically infected, symptomatic patients), the histopathologic findings (including flattened villi) and the clinical manifestations resemble those of tropical sprue and gluten-sensitive enteropathy. The pathogenesis of diarrhea in giardiasis is not known.

The natural history of *Giardia* infection varies markedly. Infections may be aborted, transient, recurrent, or chronic. Parasite as well as host factors may be important in determining the course of infection and disease. Both cellular and humoral responses develop in human infections, but their precise roles in the control of infection and/or disease are unknown. Because patients with hypogammaglobulinemia suffer from prolonged, severe infections that are poorly responsive to treatment, humoral immune responses appear to be important. The greater susceptibility of the young than of the old and of newly exposed persons than of chronically exposed populations suggests that at least partial protective immunity may develop. *Giardia* isolates vary genotypically, biochemically, and biologically, and variations among isolates may contribute to different courses of infection.

Clinical manifestations

Disease manifestations of giardiasis range from asymptomatic carriage to fulminant diarrhea and malabsorption. Most infected persons are asymptomatic, but in epidemics the proportion of symptomatic cases may be higher. Symptoms may develop suddenly or gradually. In persons with acute giardiasis, symptoms develop after an incubation period that lasts at least 5–6 days and usually 1–3 weeks. Prominent early symptoms include diarrhea, abdominal pain, bloating, belching, flatus, nausea, and vomiting. Although diarrhea is common, upper intestinal manifestations such as nausea, vomiting, bloating, and abdominal pain may predominate. The duration of acute giardiasis is usually >1 week, although diarrhea often subsides. Individuals with chronic giardiasis may present with or without having experienced an antecedent acute symptomatic episode. Diarrhea is not necessarily prominent, but increased flatus, loose stools, sulfurous belching, and (in some instances) weight loss occur. Symptoms may be continual or episodic and can persist for years. Some persons who have relatively mild symptoms for long periods recognize the extent of their discomfort only in retrospect. Fever, the presence of blood and/or mucus in the stools, and other signs and symptoms of colitis are uncommon and suggest a different diagnosis or a concomitant illness. Symptoms tend to be intermittent yet recurring and gradually debilitating, in contrast with the acute disabling symptoms associated with many enteric bacterial infections. Because

TABLE 33-1

DIAGNOSIS OF INTESTINAL PROTOZOAL INFECTIONS

PARASITE	STOOL O+P[a]	FECAL ACID-FAST STAIN	STOOL ANTIGEN IMMUNOASSAYS	OTHER
Giardia	+		+	
Cryptosporidium	−	+	+	
Isospora	−	+		
Cyclospora	−	+		
Microsporidia	−			Special fecal stains, tissue biopsies

[a]O+P, ova and parasites.

of the less severe illness and the propensity for chronic infections, patients may seek medical advice late in the course of the illness; however, disease can be severe, resulting in malabsorption, weight loss, growth retardation, and dehydration. A number of extraintestinal manifestations have been described, such as urticaria, anterior uveitis, and arthritis; whether these are caused by giardiasis or concomitant processes is unclear.

Giardiasis can be severe in patients with hypogammaglobulinemia and can complicate other preexisting intestinal diseases, such as that occurring in cystic fibrosis. In patients with AIDS, *Giardia* can cause enteric illness that is refractory to treatment.

Diagnosis

(Table 33-1) Giardiasis is diagnosed by detection of parasite antigens in the feces or by identification of cysts in the feces or of trophozoites in the feces or small intestines. Cysts are oval, measure 8–12 μm × 7–10 μm, and characteristically contain four nuclei. Trophozoites are pear-shaped, dorsally convex, flattened parasites with two nuclei and four pairs of flagella (Fig. 33-2). The diagnosis is sometimes difficult to establish. Direct examination of fresh or properly preserved stools as well as concentration methods should be used. Because cyst excretion is variable and may be undetectable at times, repeated examination of stool, sampling of duodenal fluid, and biopsy of the small intestine may be required to detect the parasite. Tests for parasitic antigens in stool are at least as sensitive and specific as good microscopic examinations and are easier to perform. All of these methods occasionally yield false-negative results.

TREATMENT ▶ **Giardiasis**

Cure rates with metronidazole (250 mg thrice daily for 5 days) are usually >90%. Tinidazole (2 g once by mouth) is reportedly more effective than metronidazole.

Nitazoxanide (500 mg twice daily for 3 days) is an alternative agent for treatment of giardiasis. Paromomycin, an oral aminoglycoside that is not well absorbed, can be given to symptomatic pregnant patients, although information is limited on how effectively this agent eradicates infection.

Almost all patients respond to therapy and are cured, although some with chronic giardiasis experience delayed resolution of symptoms after eradication of *Giardia*. For many of the latter patients, residual symptoms probably reflect delayed regeneration of intestinal brush-border enzymes. Continued infection should be documented by stool examinations before treatment is repeated. Patients who remain infected after repeated treatments should be evaluated for reinfection through family members, close personal contacts, and environmental sources as well as for hypogammaglobulinemia. In cases refractory to multiple treatment courses, prolonged therapy with metronidazole (750 mg thrice daily for 21 days) has been successful.

Prevention

Although giardiasis is extremely infectious, disease can be prevented by consumption of noncontaminated food and water and by personal hygiene when caring for infected children. Boiling or filtering potentially contaminated water prevents infection.

CRYPTOSPORIDIOSIS

The coccidian parasite *Cryptosporidium* causes diarrheal disease that is self-limited in immunocompetent human hosts but can be severe in persons with AIDS or other forms of immunodeficiency. Two species of *Cryptosporidium*, *C. hominis* and *C. parvum*, cause most human infections.

Life cycle and epidemiology

 Cryptosporidium species are widely distributed in the world. Cryptosporidiosis is acquired by the consumption of oocysts (50% infectious dose:

~132 oocysts in nonimmune individuals), which excyst to liberate sporozoites that in turn enter and infect intestinal epithelial cells. The parasite's further development involves both asexual and sexual cycles, which produce forms capable of infecting other epithelial cells and of generating oocysts that are passed in the feces. *Cryptosporidium* species infect a number of animals, and *C. parvum* can spread from infected animals to humans. Since oocysts are immediately infectious when passed in feces, person-to-person transmission takes place in day-care centers and among household contacts and medical providers. Waterborne transmission (especially that of *C. hominis*) accounts for infections in travelers and for common-source epidemics. Oocysts are quite hardy and resist killing by routine chlorination. Both drinking water and recreational water (e.g., pools, waterslides) have been increasingly recognized as sources of infection.

Pathophysiology

Although intestinal epithelial cells harbor cryptosporidia in an intracellular vacuole, the means by which secretory diarrhea is elicited remain uncertain. No characteristic pathologic changes are found by biopsy. The distribution of infection can be spotty within the principal site of infection, the small bowel. Cryptosporidia are found in the pharynx, stomach, and large bowel of some patients and at times in the respiratory tract. Especially in patients with AIDS, involvement of the biliary tract can cause papillary stenosis, sclerosing cholangitis, or cholecystitis.

Clinical manifestations

Asymptomatic infections can occur in both immunocompetent and immunocompromised hosts. In immunocompetent persons, symptoms develop after an incubation period of ~1 week and consist principally of watery nonbloody diarrhea, sometimes in conjunction with abdominal pain, nausea, anorexia, fever, and/or weight loss. In these hosts, the illness usually subsides after 1–2 weeks. In contrast, in immunocompromised hosts (especially those with AIDS and CD4+ T cell counts <100/μL), diarrhea can be chronic, persistent, and remarkably profuse, causing clinically significant fluid and electrolyte depletion. Stool volumes may range from 1 to 25 L/d. Weight loss, wasting, and abdominal pain may be severe. Biliary tract involvement can manifest as midepigastric or right-upper-quadrant pain.

Diagnosis

(Table 33-1) Evaluation starts with fecal examination for small oocysts, which are smaller (4–5 μm in diameter) than the fecal stages of most other parasites.

Because conventional stool examination for ova and parasites does not detect *Cryptosporidium*, specific testing must be requested. Detection is enhanced by evaluation of stools (obtained on multiple days) by several techniques, including modified acid-fast and direct immunofluorescent stains and enzyme immunoassays. Cryptosporidia can also be identified by light and electron microscopy at the apical surfaces of intestinal epithelium from biopsy specimens of the small bowel and, less frequently, the large bowel.

TREATMENT   Cryptosporidiosis

Nitazoxanide is approved by the U.S. Food and Drug Administration for the treatment of cryptosporidiosis and is available in tablet form for adults (500 mg twice daily for 3 days) and as an elixir for children. To date, however, this agent has not been effective for the treatment of HIV-infected patients, in whom improved immune status due to antiretroviral therapy can lead to amelioration of cryptosporidiosis. Otherwise, treatment includes supportive care with replacement of fluids and electrolytes and administration of antidiarrheal agents. Biliary tract obstruction may require papillotomy or T-tube placement. Prevention requires minimizing exposure to infectious oocysts in human or animal feces. Use of submicron water filters may minimize acquisition of infection from drinking water.

ISOSPORIASIS

The coccidian parasite *Isospora belli* causes human intestinal disease. Infection is acquired by the consumption of oocysts, after which the parasite invades intestinal epithelial cells and undergoes both sexual and asexual cycles of development. Oocysts excreted in stool are not immediately infectious but must undergo further maturation.

Although *I. belli* infects many animals, little is known about the epidemiology or prevalence of this parasite in humans. It appears to be most common in tropical and subtropical countries. Acute infections can begin abruptly with fever, abdominal pain, and watery nonbloody diarrhea and can last for weeks or months. In patients who have AIDS or are immunocompromised for other reasons, infections often are not self-limited but rather resemble cryptosporidiosis, with chronic, profuse watery diarrhea. Eosinophilia, which is not found in other enteric protozoan infections, may be detectable. The diagnosis (Table 33-1) is usually made by detection of the large (~25-μm) oocysts in stool by modified acid-fast staining. Oocyst excretion may be low-level and intermittent; if repeated stool examinations are unrevealing, sampling of duodenal contents by aspiration or small-bowel biopsy (often with electron-microscopic examination) may be necessary.

TREATMENT **Isosporiasis**

Trimethoprim-sulfamethoxazole (TMP-SMX, 160/800 mg four times daily for 10 days; and for HIV-infected patients, then three times daily for 3 weeks) is effective. For patients intolerant of sulfonamides, pyrimethamine (50–75 mg/d) can be used. Relapses can occur in persons with AIDS and necessitate maintenance therapy with TMP-SMX (160/800 mg three times per week).

CYCLOSPORIASIS

Cyclospora cayetanensis, a cause of diarrheal illness, is globally distributed: illness due to *C. cayetanensis* has been reported in the United States, Asia, Africa, Latin America, and Europe. The epidemiology of this parasite has not yet been fully defined, but waterborne transmission and food-borne transmission by basil and imported raspberries have been recognized. The full spectrum of illness attributable to *Cyclospora* has not been delineated. Some patients may harbor the infection without symptoms, but many have diarrhea, flulike symptoms, and flatulence and belching. The illness can be self-limited, can wax and wane, or in many cases can involve prolonged diarrhea, anorexia, and upper gastrointestinal symptoms, with sustained fatigue and weight loss in some instances. Diarrheal illness may persist for >1 month. *Cyclospora* can cause enteric illness in patients infected with HIV.

The parasite is detectable in epithelial cells of small-bowel biopsy samples and elicits secretory diarrhea by unknown means. The absence of fecal blood and leukocytes indicates that disease due to *Cyclospora* is not caused by destruction of the small-bowel mucosa. The diagnosis (Table 33-1) can be made by detection of spherical 8- to 10-μm oocysts in the stool, although routine stool ova and parasite (O+P) examinations are not sufficient. Specific fecal examinations must be requested to detect the oocysts, which are variably acid-fast and are fluorescent when viewed with ultraviolet light microscopy. Cyclosporiasis should be considered in the differential diagnosis of prolonged diarrhea, with or without a history of travel by the patient to other countries.

TREATMENT **Cyclosporiasis**

Cyclosporiasis is treated with TMP-SMX (160/800 mg twice daily for 7 days). HIV-infected patients may experience relapses after such treatment and thus may require longer-term suppressive maintenance therapy.

MICROSPORIDIOSIS

Microsporidia are obligate intracellular spore-forming protozoa that infect many animals and cause disease in humans, especially as opportunistic pathogens in AIDS. Microsporidia are members of a distinct phylum, Microspora, which contains dozens of genera and hundreds of species. The various microsporidia are differentiated by their developmental life cycles, ultrastructural features, and molecular taxonomy based on ribosomal RNA. The complex life cycles of the organisms result in the production of infectious spores (Fig. 33-3). Currently, eight genera of microsporidia—*Encephalitozoon*, *Pleistophora*, *Nosema*, *Vittaforma*, *Trachipleistophora*, *Brachiola*, *Microsporidium*, and *Enterocytozoon*—are recognized as causes of human disease. Although some microsporidia are probably prevalent causes of self-limited or asymptomatic infections in immunocompetent patients, little is known about how microsporidiosis is acquired.

Microsporidiosis is most common among patients with AIDS, less common among patients with other types of immunocompromise, and rare among immunocompetent hosts. In patients with AIDS, intestinal infections with *Enterocytozoon bieneusi* and *Encephalitozoon* (formerly *Septata*) *intestinalis* are recognized to contribute to chronic diarrhea and wasting; these infections are found in 10–40% of patients with chronic diarrhea. Both organisms have been found in the biliary tracts of patients with cholecystitis. *E. intestinalis* may also disseminate to cause fever, diarrhea, sinusitis, cholangitis, and bronchiolitis. In patients with AIDS, *Encephalitozoon hellem* has caused superficial keratoconjunctivitis as well as sinusitis, respiratory tract disease, and disseminated infection. Myositis due to *Pleistophora* has been documented. *Nosema*, *Vittaforma*, and *Microsporidium* have caused stromal keratitis associated with trauma in immunocompetent patients.

Microsporidia are small gram-positive organisms with mature spores measuring 0.5–2 μm × 1–4 μm. Diagnosis of microsporidial infections in tissue often requires electron microscopy, although intracellular spores can be visualized by light microscopy with hematoxylin and eosin, Giemsa, or tissue Gram's stain. For the diagnosis of intestinal microsporidiosis, modified trichrome or chromotrope 2R-based staining and Uvitex 2B or calcofluor fluorescent staining reveal spores in smears of feces or duodenal aspirates. Definitive therapies for microsporidial infections remain to be established. For superficial keratoconjunctivitis due to *E. hellem*, topical therapy with fumagillin suspension has shown promise. For enteric infections with *E. bieneusi* and *E. intestinalis* in HIV-infected patients, therapy with albendazole may be efficacious.

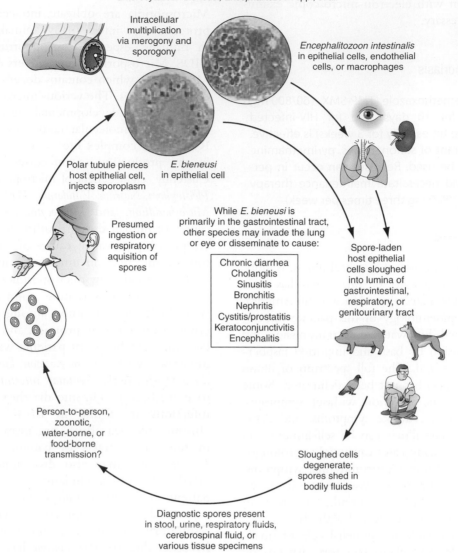

Microsporidia
Enterocytozoon bieneusi, Encephalitozoon spp., et al.

Intracellular multiplication via merogony and sporogony

Encephalitozoon intestinalis in epithelial cells, endothelial cells, or macrophages

Polar tubule pierces host epithelial cell, injects sporoplasm

E. bieneusi in epithelial cell

Presumed ingestion or respiratory aquisition of spores

While *E. bieneusi* is primarily in the gastrointestinal tract, other species may invade the lung or eye or disseminate to cause:

Chronic diarrhea
Cholangitis
Sinusitis
Bronchitis
Nephritis
Cystitis/prostatitis
Keratoconjunctivitis
Encephalitis

Spore-laden host epithelial cells sloughed into lumina of gastrointestinal, respiratory, or genitourinary tract

Person-to-person, zoonotic, water-borne, or food-borne transmission?

Sloughed cells degenerate; spores shed in bodily fluids

Diagnostic spores present in stool, urine, respiratory fluids, cerebrospinal fluid, or various tissue specimens

FIGURE 33-3

Life cycle of microsporidia. (*Reprinted from RL Guerrant et al: Tropical Infectious Disease: Principles, Pathogens and Practice, 2nd ed, 2006, p 1128, with permission from Elsevier Science.*)

OTHER INTESTINAL PROTOZOA

Balantidiasis

Balantidium coli is a large ciliated protozoal parasite that can produce a spectrum of large-intestinal disease analogous to amebiasis. The parasite is widely distributed in the world. Since it infects pigs, cases in humans are more common where pigs are raised. Infective cysts can be transmitted from person to person and through water, but many cases are due to the ingestion of cysts derived from porcine feces in association with slaughtering, with use of pig feces for fertilizer, or with contamination of water supplies by pig feces.

Ingested cysts liberate trophozoites, which reside and replicate in the large bowel. Many patients remain asymptomatic, but some have persisting intermittent

diarrhea, and a few develop more fulminant dysentery. In symptomatic individuals, the pathology in the bowel—both gross and microscopic—is similar to that seen in amebiasis, with varying degrees of mucosal invasion, focal necrosis, and ulceration. Balantidiasis, unlike amebiasis, does not spread hematogenously to other organs. The diagnosis is made by detection of the trophozoite stage in stool or sampled colonic tissue. Tetracycline (500 mg four times daily for 10 days) is an effective therapeutic agent.

Blastocystis hominis *infection*

B. hominis, while believed by some to be a protozoan capable of causing intestinal disease, remains an organism of uncertain pathogenicity. Some patients who pass

B. hominis in their stools are asymptomatic, whereas others have diarrhea and associated intestinal symptoms. Diligent evaluation reveals other potential bacterial, viral, or protozoal causes of diarrhea in some but not all patients with symptoms. Because the pathogenicity of B. hominis is uncertain and because therapy for *Blastocystis* infection is neither specific nor uniformly effective, patients with prominent intestinal symptoms should be fully evaluated for other infectious causes of diarrhea. If diarrheal symptoms associated with *Blastocystis* are prominent, either metronidazole (750 mg thrice daily for 10 days) or TMP-SMX (160 mg/800 mg twice daily for 7 days) can be used.

Dientamoeba fragilis *infection*

D. fragilis is unique among intestinal protozoa in that it has a trophozoite stage but not a cyst stage. How trophozoites survive to transmit infection is not known. When symptoms develop in patients with D. fragilis infection, they are generally mild and include intermittent diarrhea, abdominal pain, and anorexia. The diagnosis is made by the detection of trophozoites in stool; the lability of these forms accounts for the greater yield when fecal samples are preserved immediately after collection. Since fecal excretion rates vary, examination of several samples obtained on alternate days increases the rate of detection. Iodoquinol (650 mg three times daily for 20 days), paromomycin (25–35 mg/kg per day in three doses for 7 days), metronidazole (500–750 mg three times daily for 10 days), or tetracycline (500 mg four times daily for 10 days) is appropriate for treatment.

TRICHOMONIASIS

Various species of trichomonads can be found in the mouth (in association with periodontitis) and occasionally in the gastrointestinal tract. *Trichomonas vaginalis*—one of the most prevalent protozoal parasites in the United States—is a pathogen of the genitourinary tract and a major cause of symptomatic vaginitis.

Life cycle and epidemiology

T. vaginalis is a pear-shaped, actively motile organism that measures about 10×7 μm, replicates by binary fission, and inhabits the lower genital tract of females and the urethra and prostate of males. In the United States, it accounts for ~3 million infections per year in women. While the organism can survive for a few hours in moist environments and could be acquired by direct contact, person-to-person venereal transmission accounts for virtually all cases of trichomoniasis. Its prevalence is greatest among persons with multiple sexual partners and among those with other sexually transmitted diseases.

Clinical manifestations

Many men infected with T. vaginalis are asymptomatic, although some develop urethritis and a few have epididymitis or prostatitis. In contrast, infection in women, which has an incubation period of 5–28 days, is usually symptomatic and manifests with malodorous vaginal discharge (often yellow), vulvar erythema and itching, dysuria or urinary frequency (in 30–50% of patients), and dyspareunia. These manifestations, however, do not clearly distinguish trichomoniasis from other types of infectious vaginitis.

Diagnosis

Detection of motile trichomonads by microscopic examination of wet mounts of vaginal or prostatic secretions has been the conventional means of diagnosis. Although this approach provides an immediate diagnosis, its sensitivity for the detection of T. vaginalis is only ~50–60% in routine evaluations of vaginal secretions. Direct immunofluorescent antibody staining is more sensitive (70–90%) than wet-mount examinations. T. vaginalis can be recovered from the urethra of both males and females and is detectable in males after prostatic massage. Culture of the parasite is the most sensitive means of detection; however, facilities for culture are not generally available, and detection of the organism takes 3–7 days.

TREATMENT   Trichomoniasis

Metronidazole, given either as a single 2-g dose or in 500-mg doses twice daily for 7 days, is usually effective. Tinidazole (a single 2-g dose) is also effective. All sexual partners must be treated concurrently to prevent reinfection, especially from asymptomatic males. In males with persistent symptomatic urethritis after therapy for nongonococcal urethritis, metronidazole therapy should be considered for possible trichomoniasis. Alternatives to metronidazole for treatment during pregnancy are not readily available, although use of 100-mg clotrimazole vaginal suppositories nightly for 2 weeks may cure some infections in pregnant women. Reinfection often accounts for apparent treatment failures, but strains of T. vaginalis exhibiting high-level resistance to metronidazole have been encountered. Treatment of these resistant infections with higher oral doses, parenteral doses, or concurrent oral and vaginal doses of metronidazole or with tinidazole has been successful.

CHAPTER 34
INTESTINAL NEMATODE INFECTIONS

Peter F. Weller ■ Thomas B. Nutman

More than a billion persons worldwide are infected with one or more species of intestinal nematodes. Table 34-1 summarizes biologic and clinical features of infections due to the major intestinal parasitic nematodes. These parasites are most common in regions with poor fecal sanitation, particularly in resource-poor countries in the tropics and subtropics, but they have also been seen with increasing frequency among immigrants and refugees to resource-rich countries. Although nematode infections are not usually fatal, they contribute to malnutrition and diminished work capacity. It is interesting that these helminth infections may protect some individuals from allergic disease. Humans may on occasion be infected with nematode parasites that ordinarily infect animals; these zoonotic infections produce diseases such as trichostrongyliasis, anisakiasis, capillariasis, and abdominal angiostrongyliasis.

Intestinal nematodes are roundworms; they range in length from 1 mm to many centimeters when mature (Table 34-1). Their life cycles are complex and highly varied; some species, including *Strongyloides stercoralis* and *Enterobius vermicularis*, can be transmitted directly from person to person, while others, such as *Ascaris lumbricoides*, *Necator americanus*, and *Ancylostoma duodenale*, require a soil phase for development. Because most helminth parasites do not self-replicate, the acquisition of a heavy burden of adult worms requires repeated exposure to the parasite in its infectious stage, whether larval or egg. Hence, clinical disease, as opposed to asymptomatic infection, generally develops only with prolonged residence in an endemic area and is typically related to infection intensity. In persons with marginal nutrition, intestinal helminth infections may impair growth and development. Eosinophilia and elevated serum IgE levels are features of many helminth infections and, when unexplained, should always prompt a search for intestinal helminths. Significant protective immunity to intestinal nematodes appears not to develop in humans, although mechanisms of parasite immune evasion and host immune responses to these infections have not been elucidated in detail.

ASCARIASIS

A. lumbricoides is the largest intestinal nematode parasite of humans, reaching up to 40 cm in length. Most infected individuals have low worm burdens and are asymptomatic. Clinical disease arises from larval migration in the lungs or effects of the adult worms in the intestines.

Life cycle

Adult worms live in the lumen of the small intestine. Mature female *Ascaris* worms are extraordinarily fecund, each producing up to 240,000 eggs a day, which pass with the feces. Ascarid eggs, which are remarkably resistant to environmental stresses, become infective after several weeks of maturation in the soil and can remain infective for years. After infective eggs are swallowed, larvae hatched in the intestine invade the mucosa, migrate through the circulation to the lungs, break into the alveoli, ascend the bronchial tree, and return—through swallowing—to the small intestine, where they develop into adult worms. Between 2 and 3 months elapse between initial infection and egg production. Adult worms live for 1–2 years.

Epidemiology

Ascaris is widely distributed in tropical and subtropical regions as well as in other humid areas, including the rural southeastern United States. Transmission typically occurs through fecally contaminated soil and is due either to a lack of sanitary facilities or to the use of human feces as fertilizer. With their propensity for hand-to-mouth fecal carriage, younger

320

TABLE 34-1

MAJOR HUMAN INTESTINAL PARASITIC NEMATODES

	PARASITIC NEMATODE				
FEATURE	ASCARIS LUMBRICOIDES (ROUNDWORM)	NECATOR AMERICANUS, ANCYLOSTOMA DUODENALE (HOOKWORM)	STRONGYLOIDES STERCORALIS	TRICHURIS TRICHIURA (WHIPWORM)	ENTEROBIUS VERMICULARIS (PINWORM)
Global prevalence in humans (millions)	807	576	100	604	209
Endemic areas	Worldwide	Hot, humid regions	Hot, humid regions	Worldwide	Worldwide
Infective stage	Egg	Filariform larva	Filariform larva	Egg	Egg
Route of infection	Oral	Percutaneous	Percutaneous or autoinfection	Oral	Oral
Gastrointestinal location of worms	Jejunal lumen	Jejunal mucosa	Small-bowel mucosa	Cecum, colonic mucosa	Cecum, appendix
Adult worm size	15–40 cm	7–12 mm	2 mm	30–50 mm	8–13 mm (female)
Pulmonary passage of larvae	Yes	Yes	Yes	No	No
Incubation period[a] (days)	60–75	40–100	17–28	70–90	35–45
Longevity	1 y	N. americanus: 2–5 y A. duodenale: 6–8 y	Decades (owing to autoinfection)	5 y	2 months
Fecundity (eggs/day/worm)	240,000	N. americanus: 4000–10,000 A. duodenale: 10,000–25,000	5000–10,000	3000–7000	2000
Principal symptoms	Rarely gastrointestinal or biliary obstruction	Iron-deficiency anemia in heavy infection	Gastrointestinal symptoms; malabsorption or sepsis in hyperinfection	Gastrointestinal symptoms, anemia	Perianal pruritus
Diagnostic stage	Eggs in stool	Eggs in fresh stool, larvae in old stool	Larvae in stool or duodenal aspirate; sputum in hyperinfection	Eggs in stool	Eggs from perianal skin on cellulose acetate tape
Treatment	Mebendazole Albendazole Pyrantel pamoate Ivermectin Nitazoxanide	Mebendazole Pyrantel pamoate Albendazole	1. Ivermectin 2. Albendazole	Mebendazole Albendazole Ivermectin	Mebendazole Pyrantel pamoate Albendazole

[a]Time from infection to egg production by mature female worm.

children are most affected. Infection outside endemic areas, though uncommon, can occur when eggs on transported vegetables are ingested.

Clinical features

During the lung phase of larval migration, ~9–12 days after egg ingestion, patients may develop an irritating nonproductive cough and burning substernal discomfort that is aggravated by coughing or deep inspiration. Dyspnea and blood-tinged sputum are less common. Fever is usually reported. Eosinophilia develops during this symptomatic phase and subsides slowly over weeks. Chest x-rays may reveal evidence of eosinophilic pneumonitis (Löffler's syndrome), with rounded infiltrates a few millimeters to several centimeters in size. These infiltrates may be transient and intermittent, clearing after several weeks. Where there is seasonal transmission of the parasite, seasonal pneumonitis with eosinophilia may develop in previously infected and sensitized hosts.

In established infections, adult worms in the small intestine usually cause no symptoms. In heavy infections, particularly in children, a large bolus of entangled worms can cause pain and small-bowel obstruction, sometimes complicated by perforation, intussusception, or volvulus. Single worms may cause disease when they migrate into aberrant sites. A large worm can enter and occlude the biliary tree, causing biliary colic, cholecystitis, cholangitis, pancreatitis, or (rarely) intrahepatic abscesses. Migration of an adult worm up the esophagus can provoke coughing and oral expulsion of the worm. In highly endemic areas, intestinal and biliary ascariasis can rival acute appendicitis and gallstones as causes of surgical acute abdomen.

Laboratory findings

Most cases of ascariasis can be diagnosed by microscopic detection of characteristic *Ascaris* eggs (65 by 45 μm) in fecal samples. Occasionally, patients present after passing an adult worm—identifiable by its large size and smooth cream-colored surface—in the stool or through the mouth or nose. During the early transpulmonary migratory phase, when eosinophilic pneumonitis occurs, larvae can be found in sputum or gastric aspirates before diagnostic eggs appear in the stool. The eosinophilia that is prominent during this early stage usually decreases to minimal levels in established infection. Adult worms may be visualized, occasionally serendipitously, on contrast studies of the gastrointestinal tract. A plain abdominal film may reveal masses of worms in gas-filled loops of bowel in patients with intestinal obstruction. Pancreaticobiliary worms can be detected by ultrasound and endoscopic retrograde cholangiopancreatography; the latter method also has been used to extract biliary *Ascaris* worms.

TREATMENT Ascariasis

Ascariasis should always be treated to prevent potentially serious complications. Albendazole (400 mg once), mebendazole (100 g twice daily for 3 days or 500 mg once), or ivermectin (150–200 μg/kg once) is effective. These medications are contraindicated in pregnancy, however. Pyrantel pamoate (11 mg/kg once; maximum, 1 g) is safe in pregnancy. Nitazoxanide (7.5 mg/kg once; maximum, 500 mg) has also been used in ascariasis. Mild diarrhea and abdominal pain are uncommon side effects of these agents. Partial intestinal obstruction should be managed with nasogastric suction, IV fluid administration, and instillation of piperazine through the nasogastric tube, but complete obstruction and its severe complications require immediate surgical intervention.

HOOKWORM

Two hookworm species (*A. duodenale* and *N. americanus*) are responsible for human infections. Most infected individuals are asymptomatic. Hookworm disease develops from a combination of factors—a heavy worm burden, a prolonged duration of infection, and an inadequate iron intake—and results in iron-deficiency anemia and, on occasion, hypoproteinemia.

Life cycle

Adult hookworms, which are ~1 cm long, use buccal teeth (*Ancylostoma*) or cutting plates (*Necator*) to attach to the small-bowel mucosa and suck blood (0.2 mL/d per *Ancylostoma* adult) and interstitial fluid. The adult hookworms produce thousands of eggs daily. The eggs are deposited with feces in soil, where rhabditiform larvae hatch and develop over a 1-week period into infectious filariform larvae. Infective larvae penetrate the skin and reach the lungs by way of the bloodstream. There they invade alveoli and ascend the airways before being swallowed and reaching the small intestine. The prepatent period from skin invasion to appearance of eggs in the feces is ~6–8 weeks, but it may be longer with *A. duodenale*. Larvae of *A. duodenale*, if swallowed, can survive and develop directly in the intestinal mucosa. Adult hookworms may survive over a decade but usually live ~6–8 years for *A. duodenale* and 2–5 years for *N. americanus*.

Epidemiology

A. duodenale is prevalent in southern Europe, North Africa, and northern Asia, and *N. americanus* is the predominant species in the Western Hemisphere and equatorial Africa. The two species overlap in many tropical regions, particularly Southeast Asia. In most areas, older children have the highest incidence and greatest intensity of hookworm infection. In rural areas where fields are fertilized with human feces, older working adults also may be heavily infected.

Clinical features

Most hookworm infections are asymptomatic. Infective larvae may provoke pruritic maculopapular dermatitis ("ground itch") at the site of skin penetration as well as serpiginous tracks of subcutaneous migration (similar to those of cutaneous larva migrans) in previously sensitized hosts. Larvae migrating through the lungs occasionally cause mild transient pneumonitis, but this condition develops less frequently in hookworm infection than in ascariasis. In the early intestinal phase, infected persons may develop epigastric pain (often with postprandial accentuation), inflammatory diarrhea, or other abdominal symptoms accompanied by eosinophilia. The major consequence of chronic hookworm infection is iron deficiency. Symptoms are minimal if iron intake is adequate, but marginally nourished individuals develop symptoms of progressive iron-deficiency anemia and hypoproteinemia, including weakness and shortness of breath.

Laboratory findings

The diagnosis is established by the finding of characteristic 40- by 60-μm oval hookworm eggs in the feces. Stool-concentration procedures may be required to detect light infections. Eggs of the two species are indistinguishable by light microscopy. In a stool sample that is not fresh, the eggs may have hatched to release rhabditiform larvae, which need to be differentiated from those of *S. stercoralis*. Hypochromic microcytic anemia, occasionally with eosinophilia or hypoalbuminemia, is characteristic of hookworm disease.

TREATMENT ► Hookworm Infection

Hookworm infection can be eradicated with several safe and highly effective antihelminthic drugs, including albendazole (400 mg once), mebendazole (500 mg once), and pyrantel pamoate (11 mg/kg for 3 days). Mild iron-deficiency anemia can often be treated with oral iron alone. Severe hookworm disease with protein loss and malabsorption necessitates nutritional support and oral iron replacement along with deworming. There is some concern that the benzimidazoles (mebendazole and albendazole) are becoming less effective against human hookworms than in the past.

Ancylostoma caninum *and* Ancylostoma braziliense

A. caninum, the canine hookworm, has been identified as a cause of human eosinophilic enteritis, especially in northeastern Australia. In this zoonotic infection, adult hookworms attach to the small intestine (where they may be visualized by endoscopy) and elicit abdominal pain and intense local eosinophilia. Treatment with mebendazole (100 mg twice daily for 3 days) or albendazole (400 mg once) or endoscopic removal is effective. Both of these animal hookworm species can cause cutaneous larva migrans ("creeping eruption").

STRONGYLOIDIASIS

S. stercoralis is distinguished by its ability—unique among helminths (except for *Capillaria*; discussed later)—to replicate in the human host. This capacity permits ongoing cycles of autoinfection as infective larvae are internally produced. Strongyloidiasis can thus persist for decades without further exposure of the host to exogenous infective larvae. In immunocompromised hosts, large numbers of invasive *Strongyloides* larvae can disseminate widely and can be fatal.

Life cycle

In addition to a parasitic cycle of development, *Strongyloides* can undergo a free-living cycle of development in the soil (**Fig. 34-1**). This adaptability facilitates the parasite's survival in the absence of mammalian hosts. Rhabditiform larvae passed in feces can transform into infectious filariform larvae either directly or after a free-living phase of development. Humans acquire strongyloidiasis when filariform larvae in fecally contaminated soil penetrate the skin or mucous membranes. The larvae then travel through the bloodstream to the lungs, where they break into the alveolar spaces, ascend the bronchial tree, are swallowed, and thereby reach the small intestine. There the larvae mature into adult worms that penetrate the mucosa of the proximal small bowel. The minute (2-mm-long) parasitic adult female worms reproduce by parthenogenesis; adult males do not exist. Eggs hatch in the intestinal mucosa, releasing rhabditiform larvae that migrate to the lumen and pass with the feces into soil. Alternatively, rhabditiform larvae in the bowel can develop directly into filariform larvae that penetrate the colonic wall or perianal skin and enter the circulation to repeat the migration that establishes ongoing internal reinfection. This autoinfection cycle allows strongyloidiasis to persist for decades.

Epidemiology

S. stercoralis is spottily distributed in tropical areas and other hot, humid regions and is particularly common in Southeast Asia, sub-Saharan Africa, and Brazil. In the United States, the parasite is endemic in parts of the Southeast and is found in immigrants, refugees, travelers, and military personnel who have lived in endemic areas.

Clinical features

In uncomplicated strongyloidiasis, many patients are asymptomatic or have mild cutaneous and/or abdominal symptoms. Recurrent urticaria, often involving the buttocks and wrists, is the most common cutaneous manifestation. Migrating larvae can elicit a pathognomonic serpiginous eruption, *larva currens* ("running larva"). This pruritic, raised, erythematous lesion advances as rapidly as 10 cm/h along the course of larval migration. Adult parasites burrow into the duodenojejunal mucosa and can cause abdominal (usually midepigastric) pain, which resembles peptic ulcer pain except that it is

324

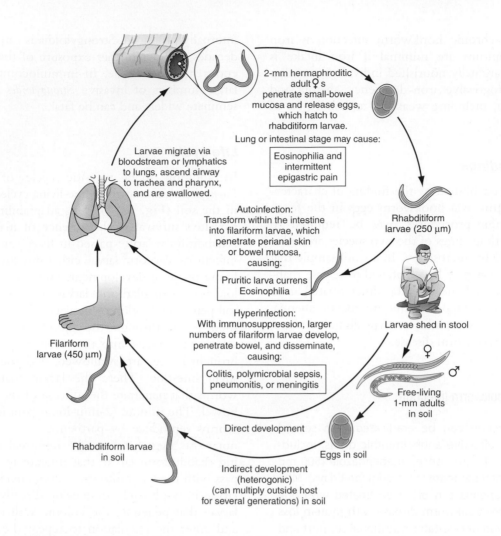

FIGURE 34-1

Life cycle of *Strongyloides stercoralis*. *(Adapted from Guerrant RL et al [eds]: Tropical Infectious Diseases: Principles, Pathogens and Practice, 2nd ed, p 1276. © 2006, with permission from Elsevier Science.)*

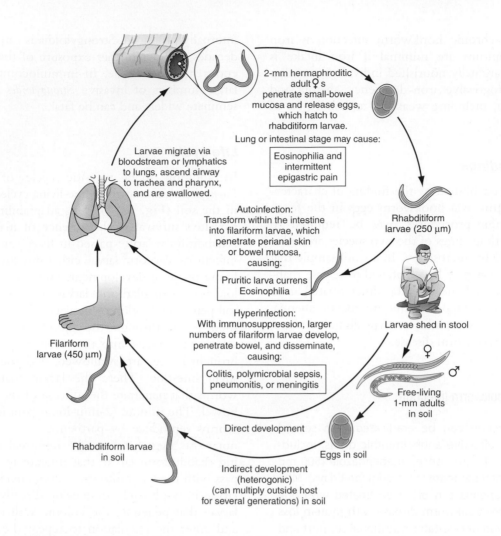

Within the figure:

- 2-mm hermaphroditic adult ♀s penetrate small-bowel mucosa and release eggs, which hatch to rhabditiform larvae.
- Lung or intestinal stage may cause: Eosinophilia and intermittent epigastric pain
- Larvae migrate via bloodstream or lymphatics to lungs, ascend airway to trachea and pharynx, and are swallowed.
- Autoinfection: Transform within the intestine into filariform larvae, which penetrate perianal skin or bowel mucosa, causing: Pruritic larva currens, Eosinophilia
- Hyperinfection: With immunosuppression, larger numbers of filariform larvae develop, penetrate bowel, and disseminate, causing: Colitis, polymicrobial sepsis, pneumonitis, or meningitis
- Rhabditiform larvae (250 μm)
- Larvae shed in stool
- Free-living 1-mm adults in soil
- Eggs in soil
- Indirect development (heterogonic) (can multiply outside host for several generations) in soil
- Direct development
- Rhabditiform larvae in soil
- Filariform larvae (450 μm)

aggravated by food ingestion. Nausea, diarrhea, gastrointestinal bleeding, mild chronic colitis, and weight loss can occur. Small-bowel obstruction may develop with early, heavy infection. Pulmonary symptoms are rare in uncomplicated strongyloidiasis. Eosinophilia is common, with levels fluctuating over time.

The ongoing autoinfection cycle of strongyloidiasis is normally constrained by unknown factors of the host's immune system. Abrogation of host immunity, especially with glucocorticoid therapy and much less commonly with other immunosuppressive medications, leads to hyperinfection, with the generation of large numbers of filariform larvae. Colitis, enteritis, or malabsorption may develop. In disseminated strongyloidiasis, larvae may invade not only gastrointestinal tissues and the lungs but also the central nervous system, peritoneum, liver, and kidneys. Moreover, bacteremia may develop because of the passage of enteric flora through disrupted mucosal barriers. Gram-negative sepsis, pneumonia, or meningitis may complicate or dominate the clinical

course. Eosinophilia is often absent in severely infected patients. Disseminated strongyloidiasis, particularly in patients with unsuspected infection who are given glucocorticoids, can be fatal. Strongyloidiasis is a frequent complication of infection with human T cell lymphotropic virus type I, but disseminated strongyloidiasis is not common among patients infected with HIV-1.

Diagnosis

In uncomplicated strongyloidiasis, the finding of rhabditiform larvae in feces is diagnostic. Rhabditiform larvae are ~250 μm long, with a short buccal cavity that distinguishes them from hookworm larvae. In uncomplicated infections, few larvae are passed and single stool examinations detect only about one-third of cases. Serial examinations and the use of the agar plate detection method improve the sensitivity of stool diagnosis. In uncomplicated strongyloidiasis (but not in hyperinfection), stool examinations may be repeatedly negative. *Strongyloides* larvae may also be found by sampling of the duodenojejunal contents by aspiration or biopsy. An enzyme-linked immunosorbent assay for serum antibodies to antigens of *Strongyloides* is a sensitive method of diagnosing uncomplicated infections. Such serologic testing should be performed for patients whose geographic histories indicate potential exposure, especially those who exhibit eosinophilia and/or are candidates for glucocorticoid treatment of other conditions. In disseminated strongyloidiasis, filariform larvae should be sought in stool as well as in samples obtained from sites of potential larval migration, including sputum, bronchoalveolar lavage fluid, or surgical drainage fluid.

TREATMENT Strongyloidiasis

Even in the asymptomatic state, strongyloidiasis must be treated because of the potential for subsequent fatal hyperinfection. Ivermectin (200 mg/kg daily for 2 days) is more effective than albendazole (400 mg daily for 3 days). For disseminated strongyloidiasis, treatment with ivermectin should be extended for at least 5–7 days or until the parasites are eradicated.

TRICHURIASIS

Most infections with *Trichuris trichiura* are asymptomatic, but heavy infections may cause gastrointestinal symptoms. Like the other soil-transmitted helminths, whipworm is distributed globally in the tropics and subtropics and is most common among poor children from resource-poor regions of the world.

Life cycle

Adult *Trichuris* worms reside in the colon and cecum, the anterior portions threaded into the superficial mucosa. Thousands of eggs laid daily by adult female worms pass with the feces and mature in the soil. After ingestion, infective eggs hatch in the duodenum, releasing larvae that mature before migrating to the large bowel. The entire cycle takes ~3 months, and adult worms may live for several years.

Clinical features

Tissue reactions to *Trichuris* are mild. Most infected individuals have no symptoms or eosinophilia. Heavy infections may result in abdominal pain, anorexia, and bloody or mucoid diarrhea resembling inflammatory bowel disease. Rectal prolapse can result from massive infections in children, who often suffer from malnourishment and other diarrheal illnesses. Moderately heavy *Trichuris* burdens also contribute to growth retardation.

Diagnosis and treatment

The characteristic 50- by 20-μm lemon-shaped *Trichuris* eggs are readily detected on stool examination. Adult worms, which are 3–5 cm long, are occasionally seen on proctoscopy. Mebendazole (500 mg once) or albendazole (400 mg daily for 3 doses) is safe and moderately effective for treatment, with cure rates of 70–90%. Ivermectin (200 mg/kg daily for 3 doses) is also safe but is not quite as efficacious as the benzimidazoles.

ENTEROBIASIS (PINWORM)

E. vermicularis is more common in temperate countries than in the tropics. In the United States, ~40 million persons are infected with pinworms, with a disproportionate number of cases among children.

Life cycle and epidemiology

Enterobius adult worms are ~1 cm long and dwell in the cecum. Gravid female worms migrate nocturnally into the perianal region and release up to 10,000 immature eggs each. The eggs become infective within hours and are transmitted by hand-to-mouth passage. From ingested eggs, larvae hatch and mature into adults. This life cycle takes ~1 month, and adult worms survive for ~2 months. Self-infection results from perianal scratching and transport of infective eggs on the hands or under the nails to the mouth. Because of the ease of person-to-person spread, pinworm infections are common among family members.

Clinical features

Most pinworm infections are asymptomatic. Perianal pruritus is the cardinal symptom. The itching, which is often worse at night as a result of the nocturnal migration of the female worms, may lead to excoriation and bacterial superinfection. Heavy infections have been claimed to cause abdominal pain and weight loss. On rare occasions, pinworms invade the female genital tract, causing vulvovaginitis and pelvic or peritoneal granulomas. Eosinophilia is uncommon.

Diagnosis

Since pinworm eggs are not released in feces, the diagnosis cannot be made by conventional fecal ova and parasite tests. Instead, eggs are detected by the application of clear cellulose acetate tape to the perianal region in the morning. After the tape is transferred to a slide, microscopic examination will detect pinworm eggs, which are oval, measure 55 by 25 μm, and are flattened along one side.

TREATMENT	Enterobiasis

Infected children and adults should be treated with mebendazole (100 mg once), albendazole (400 mg once), or pyrantel pamoate (11 mg/kg once; maximum, 1 g), with the same treatment repeated after 2 weeks. Treatment of household members is advocated to eliminate asymptomatic reservoirs of potential reinfection.

TRICHOSTRONGYLIASIS

Trichostrongylus species, which are normally parasites of herbivorous animals, occasionally infect humans, particularly in Asia and Africa. Humans acquire the infection by accidentally ingesting *Trichostrongylus* larvae on contaminated leafy vegetables. The larvae do not migrate in humans but mature directly into adult worms in the small bowel. These worms ingest far less blood than hookworms; most infected persons are asymptomatic, but heavy infections may give rise to mild anemia and eosinophilia. *Trichostrongylus* eggs in stool examinations resemble those of hookworms but are larger (85 by 115 μm). Treatment consists of mebendazole or albendazole.

ANISAKIASIS

Anisakiasis is a gastrointestinal infection caused by the accidental ingestion in uncooked saltwater fish of nematode larvae belonging to the family Anisakidae. The incidence of anisakiasis in the United States has increased as a result of the growing popularity of raw fish dishes. Most cases occur in Japan, the Netherlands, and Chile, where raw fish—sashimi, pickled green herring, and ceviche, respectively—are national culinary staples. Anisakid nematodes parasitize large sea mammals such as whales, dolphins, and seals. As part of a complex parasitic life cycle involving marine food chains, infectious larvae migrate to the musculature of a variety of fish. Both *Anisakis simplex* and *Pseudoterranova decipiens* have been implicated in human anisakiasis, but an identical gastric syndrome may be caused by the red larvae of eustrongylid parasites of fish-eating birds.

When humans consume infected raw fish, live larvae may be coughed up within 48 h. Alternatively, larvae may immediately penetrate the mucosa of the stomach. Within hours, violent upper abdominal pain accompanied by nausea and occasionally vomiting ensues, mimicking an acute abdomen. The diagnosis can be established by direct visualization on upper endoscopy, outlining of the worm by contrast radiographic studies, or histopathologic examination of extracted tissue. Extraction of the burrowing larvae during endoscopy is curative. In addition, larvae may pass to the small bowel, where they penetrate the mucosa and provoke a vigorous eosinophilic granulomatous response. Symptoms may appear 1–2 weeks after the infective meal, with intermittent abdominal pain, diarrhea, nausea, and fever resembling the manifestations of Crohn's disease. The diagnosis may be suggested by barium studies and confirmed by curative surgical resection of a granuloma in which the worm is embedded. Anisakid eggs are not found in the stool, since the larvae do not mature in humans. Serologic tests have been developed but are not widely available.

Anisakid larvae in saltwater fish are killed by cooking to 60°C, freezing at −20°C for 3 days, or commercial blast freezing, but not usually by salting, marinating, or cold smoking. No medical treatment is available; surgical or endoscopic removal should be undertaken.

CAPILLARIASIS

Intestinal capillariasis is caused by ingestion of raw fish infected with *Capillaria philippinensis*. Subsequent autoinfection can lead to a severe wasting syndrome. The disease occurs in the Philippines and Thailand and, on occasion, elsewhere in Asia. The natural cycle of *C. philippinensis* involves fish from fresh and brackish water. When humans eat infected raw fish, the larvae mature in the intestine into adult worms, which produce invasive larvae that cause intestinal inflammation and villus loss. Capillariasis has an insidious onset with nonspecific abdominal pain and watery diarrhea. If untreated, progressive autoinfection can lead to protein-losing enteropathy, severe malabsorption, and ultimately death from cachexia, cardiac failure, or superinfection. The diagnosis is established by identification of the characteristic peanut-shaped (20- by 40-μm) eggs on stool examination. Severely ill patients require hospitalization and supportive therapy in addition to prolonged antihelminthic treatment with albendazole (200 mg twice daily for 10 days).

ABDOMINAL ANGIOSTRONGYLIASIS

Abdominal angiostrongyliasis is found in Latin America and Africa. The zoonotic parasite *Angiostrongylus costaricensis* causes eosinophilic ileocolitis after the ingestion of contaminated vegetation. *A. costaricensis* normally parasitizes the cotton rat and other rodents, with slugs and snails serving as intermediate hosts. Humans become infected by accidentally ingesting infective larvae in mollusk slime deposited on fruits and vegetables; children are at highest risk. The larvae penetrate the gut wall and migrate to the mesenteric artery, where they develop into adult worms. Eggs deposited in the gut wall provoke an intense eosinophilic granulomatous reaction, and adult worms may cause mesenteric arteritis, thrombosis, or frank bowel infarction. Symptoms may mimic those of appendicitis, including abdominal pain and tenderness,

fever, vomiting, and a palpable mass in the right iliac fossa. Leukocytosis and eosinophilia are prominent. CT with contrast medium typically shows inflamed bowel, often with concomitant obstruction, but a definitive diagnosis is usually made surgically with partial bowel resection. Pathologic study reveals a thickened bowel wall with eosinophilic granulomas surrounding the *Angiostrongylus* eggs. In nonsurgical cases, the diagnosis rests solely on clinical grounds because larvae and eggs cannot be detected in the stool. Medical therapy for abdominal angiostrongyliasis is of uncertain efficacy. Careful observation and surgical resection for severe symptoms are the mainstays of treatment.

SECTION V

EVALUATION OF THE PATIENT WITH LIVER DISEASE

CHAPTER 35

APPROACH TO THE PATIENT WITH LIVER DISEASE

Marc Ghany ■ Jay H. Hoofnagle

A diagnosis of liver disease usually can be made accurately by a careful history, physical examination, and application of a few laboratory tests. In some circumstances, radiologic examinations are helpful or, indeed, diagnostic. Liver biopsy is considered the criterion standard in evaluation of liver disease but is now needed less for diagnosis than for grading and staging of disease. This chapter provides an introduction to diagnosis and management of liver disease, briefly reviewing the structure and function of the liver; the major clinical manifestations of liver disease; and the use of clinical history, physical examination, laboratory tests, imaging studies, and liver biopsy.

LIVER STRUCTURE AND FUNCTION

The liver is the largest organ of the body, weighing 1–1.5 kg and representing 1.5–2.5% of the lean body mass. The size and shape of the liver vary and generally match the general body shape—long and lean or squat and square. The liver is located in the right upper quadrant of the abdomen under the right lower rib cage against the diaphragm and projects for a variable extent into the left upper quadrant. The liver is held in place by ligamentous attachments to the diaphragm, peritoneum, great vessels, and upper gastrointestinal organs. It receives a dual blood supply; ~20% of the blood flow is oxygen-rich blood from the hepatic artery, and 80% is nutrient-rich blood from the portal vein arising from the stomach, intestines, pancreas, and spleen.

The majority of cells in the liver are hepatocytes, which constitute two-thirds of the mass of the liver. The remaining cell types are Kupffer cells (members of the reticuloendothelial system), stellate (Ito or fat-storing) cells, endothelial cells and blood vessels, bile ductular cells, and supporting structures. Viewed by light microscopy, the liver appears to be organized in lobules,

with portal areas at the periphery and central veins in the center of each lobule. However, from a functional point of view, the liver is organized into acini, with both hepatic arterial and portal venous blood entering the acinus from the portal areas (zone 1) and then flowing through the sinusoids to the terminal hepatic veins (zone 3); the intervening hepatocytes constituting zone 2. The advantage of viewing the acinus as the physiologic unit of the liver is that it helps to explain the morphologic patterns and zonality of many vascular and biliary diseases not explained by the lobular arrangement.

Portal areas of the liver consist of small veins, arteries, bile ducts, and lymphatics organized in a loose stroma of supporting matrix and small amounts of collagen. Blood flowing into the portal areas is distributed through the sinusoids, passing from zone 1 to zone 3 of the acinus and draining into the terminal hepatic veins ("central veins"). Secreted bile flows in the opposite direction, in a countercurrent pattern from zone 3 to zone 1. The sinusoids are lined by unique endothelial cells that have prominent fenestrae of variable size, allowing the free flow of plasma but not cellular elements. The plasma is thus in direct contact with hepatocytes in the subendothelial space of Disse.

Hepatocytes have distinct polarity. The basolateral side of the hepatocyte lines the space of Disse and is richly lined with microvilli; it demonstrates endocytotic and pinocytotic activity, with passive and active uptake of nutrients, proteins, and other molecules. The apical pole of the hepatocyte forms the canalicular membranes through which bile components are secreted. The canaliculi of hepatocytes form a fine network, which fuses into the bile ductular elements near the portal areas. Kupffer cells usually lie within the sinusoidal vascular space and represent the largest group of fixed macrophages in the body. The stellate cells are located in the space of Disse but are not usually prominent unless activated, when they produce collagen and matrix. Red blood cells stay in the sinusoidal space as blood flows through the lobules, but white blood cells can migrate through or around endothelial cells into the space of Disse and from there to portal areas, where they can return to the circulation through lymphatics.

Hepatocytes perform numerous and vital roles in maintaining homeostasis and health. These functions include the synthesis of most essential serum proteins (albumin, carrier proteins, coagulation factors, many hormonal and growth factors), the production of bile and its carriers (bile acids, cholesterol, lecithin, phospholipids), the regulation of nutrients (glucose, glycogen, lipids, cholesterol, amino acids), and metabolism and conjugation of lipophilic compounds (bilirubin, anions, cations, drugs) for excretion in the bile or urine. Measurement of these activities to assess liver function is complicated by the multiplicity and variability of these functions. The most commonly used liver "function" tests are measurements of serum bilirubin, albumin, and prothrombin time. The serum bilirubin level is a measure of hepatic conjugation and excretion, and the serum albumin level and prothrombin time are measures of protein synthesis. Abnormalities of bilirubin, albumin, and prothrombin time are typical of hepatic dysfunction. Frank liver failure is incompatible with life, and the functions of the liver are too complex and diverse to be subserved by a mechanical pump; dialysis membrane; or concoction of infused hormones, proteins, and growth factors.

LIVER DISEASES

While there are many causes of liver disease (Table 35-1), they generally present clinically in a few distinct

TABLE 35-1

LIVER DISEASES

Inherited hyperbilirubinemia
  Gilbert's syndrome
  Crigler-Najjar syndrome, types I and II
  Dubin-Johnson syndrome
  Rotor syndrome

Viral hepatitis
  Hepatitis A
  Hepatitis B
  Hepatitis C
  Hepatitis D
  Hepatitis E
  Others (mononucleosis, herpes, adenovirus hepatitis)
  Cryptogenic hepatitis

Immune and autoimmune liver diseases
  Primary biliary cirrhosis
  Autoimmune hepatitis
  Sclerosing cholangitis
  Overlap syndromes
  Graft-versus-host disease
  Allograft rejection

Genetic liver diseases
  α_1 Antitrypsin deficiency
  Hemochromatosis
  Wilson's disease
  Benign recurrent intrahepatic cholestasis (BRIC)
  Progressive familial intrahepatic cholestasis (PFIC), types I–III
  Others (galactosemia, tyrosinemia, cystic fibrosis, Newman-Pick disease, Gaucher's disease)

Alcoholic liver disease
  Acute fatty liver
  Acute alcoholic hepatitis
  Laënnec's cirrhosis

Nonalcoholic fatty liver
  Steatosis
  Steatohepatitis

Acute fatty liver of pregnancy

Liver involvement in systemic diseases
  Sarcoidosis
  Amyloidosis
  Glycogen storage diseases
  Celiac disease
  Tuberculosis
  Mycobacterium avium intracellulare

Cholestatic syndromes
  Benign postoperative cholestasis
  Jaundice of sepsis
  Total parenteral nutrition (TPN)-induced jaundice
  Cholestasis of pregnancy
  Cholangitis and cholecystitis
  Extrahepatic biliary obstruction (stone, stricture, cancer)
  Biliary atresia
  Caroli's disease
  Cryptosporidiosis

Drug-induced liver disease
  Hepatocellular patterns (isoniazid, acetaminophen)
  Cholestatic patterns (methyltestosterone)
  Mixed patterns (sulfonamides, phenytoin)
  Micro- and macrovesicular steatosis (methotrexate, fialuridine)

Vascular injury
  Venoocclusive disease
  Budd-Chiari syndrome
  Ischemic hepatitis
  Passive congestion
  Portal vein thrombosis
  Nodular regenerative hyperplasia

Mass lesions
  Hepatocellular carcinoma
  Cholangiocarcinoma
  Adenoma
  Focal nodular hyperplasia
  Metastatic tumors
  Abscess
  Cysts
  Hemangioma

patterns, usually classified as hepatocellular, cholestatic (obstructive), or mixed. In *hepatocellular diseases* (such as viral hepatitis or alcoholic liver disease), features of liver injury, inflammation, and necrosis predominate. In *cholestatic diseases* (such as gallstone or malignant obstruction, primary biliary cirrhosis, some drug-induced liver diseases), features of inhibition of bile flow predominate. In a mixed pattern, features of both hepatocellular and cholestatic injury are present (such as in cholestatic forms of viral hepatitis and many drug-induced liver diseases). The pattern of onset and prominence of symptoms can rapidly suggest a diagnosis, particularly if major risk factors are considered such as the age and sex of the patient and a history of exposure or risk behaviors.

Typical presenting symptoms of liver disease include jaundice, fatigue, itching, right upper quadrant pain, nausea, poor appetite, abdominal distention, and intestinal bleeding. At present, however, many patients are diagnosed with liver disease who have no symptoms and who have been found to have abnormalities in biochemical liver tests as a part of a routine physical examination or screening for blood donation or for insurance or employment. The wide availability of batteries of liver tests makes it relatively simple to demonstrate the presence of liver injury as well as to rule it out in someone suspected of liver disease.

Evaluation of patients with liver disease should be directed at (1) establishing the etiologic diagnosis, (2) estimating the disease severity (grading), and (3) establishing the disease stage (staging). *Diagnosis* should focus on the category of disease such as hepatocellular, cholestatic, or mixed injury, as well as on the specific etiologic diagnosis. *Grading* refers to assessing the severity or activity of disease—active or inactive, and mild, moderate, or severe. *Staging* refers to estimating the place in the course of the natural history of the disease, whether acute or chronic; early or late; precirrhotic, cirrhotic, or end-stage.

The goal of this chapter is to introduce general, salient concepts in the evaluation of patients with liver disease that help lead to the diagnoses discussed in subsequent chapters.

CLINICAL HISTORY

The clinical history should focus on the symptoms of liver disease—their nature, patterns of onset, and progression—and on potential risk factors for liver disease. The symptoms of liver disease include constitutional symptoms such as fatigue, weakness, nausea, poor appetite, and malaise and the more liver-specific symptoms of jaundice, dark urine, light stools, itching, abdominal pain, and bloating. Symptoms can also suggest the presence of cirrhosis, end-stage liver disease, or complications of cirrhosis such as portal hypertension.

Generally, the constellation of symptoms and their patterns of onset rather than a specific symptom points to an etiology.

Fatigue is the most common and most characteristic symptom of liver disease. It is variously described as lethargy, weakness, listlessness, malaise, increased need for sleep, lack of stamina, and poor energy. The fatigue of liver disease typically arises after activity or exercise and is rarely present or severe in the morning after adequate rest (afternoon versus morning fatigue). Fatigue in liver disease is often intermittent and variable in severity from hour to hour and day to day. In some patients, it may not be clear whether fatigue is due to the liver disease or to other problems such as stress, anxiety, sleep disturbance, or a concurrent illness.

Nausea occurs with more severe liver disease and may accompany fatigue or be provoked by odors of food or eating fatty foods. Vomiting can occur but is rarely persistent or prominent. Poor appetite with weight loss occurs commonly in acute liver diseases but is rare in chronic disease, except when cirrhosis is present and advanced. Diarrhea is uncommon in liver disease, except with severe jaundice, where lack of bile acids reaching the intestine can lead to steatorrhea.

Right upper quadrant discomfort or ache ("liver pain") occurs in many liver diseases and is usually marked by tenderness over the liver area. The pain arises from stretching or irritation of Glisson's capsule, which surrounds the liver and is rich in nerve endings. Severe pain is most typical of gallbladder disease, liver abscess, and severe venoocclusive disease but is an occasional accompaniment of acute hepatitis.

Itching occurs with acute liver disease, appearing early in obstructive jaundice (from biliary obstruction or drug-induced cholestasis) and somewhat later in hepatocellular disease (acute hepatitis). Itching also occurs in chronic liver diseases, typically the cholestatic forms such as primary biliary cirrhosis and sclerosing cholangitis where it is often the presenting symptom, occurring before the onset of jaundice. However, itching can occur in any liver disease, particularly once cirrhosis is present.

Jaundice is the hallmark symptom of liver disease and perhaps the most reliable marker of severity. Patients usually report darkening of the urine before they notice scleral icterus. Jaundice is rarely detectable with a bilirubin level <43 μmol/L (2.5 mg/dL). With severe cholestasis there will also be lightening of the color of the stools and steatorrhea. Jaundice without dark urine usually indicates indirect (unconjugated) hyperbilirubinemia and is typical of hemolytic anemia and the genetic disorders of bilirubin conjugation, the common and benign form being Gilbert's syndrome and the rare and severe form being Crigler-Najjar syndrome. Gilbert's syndrome affects up to 5% of the population; the jaundice is more noticeable after fasting and with stress.

Major risk factors for liver disease that should be sought in the clinical history include details of alcohol use, medications (including herbal compounds, birth control pills, and over-the-counter medications), personal habits, sexual activity, travel, exposure to jaundiced or other high-risk persons, injection drug use, recent surgery, remote or recent transfusion with blood and blood products, occupation, accidental exposure to blood or needlestick, and familial history of liver disease.

For assessing the risk of viral hepatitis, a careful history of sexual activity is of particular importance and should include the number of lifetime sexual partners and, for men, a history of having sex with men. Sexual exposure is a common mode of spread of hepatitis B but is rare for hepatitis C. A family history of hepatitis, liver disease, and liver cancer is also important. Maternal-infant transmission occurs with both hepatitis B and C. Vertical spread of hepatitis B can now be prevented by passive and active immunization of the infant at birth. Vertical spread of hepatitis C is uncommon, but there are no reliable means of prevention. Transmission is more common in HIV-co-infected mothers and is also linked to prolonged and difficult labor and delivery, early rupture of membranes, and internal fetal monitoring. A history of injection drug use, even in the remote past, is of great importance in assessing the risk for hepatitis B and C. Injection drug use is now the single most common risk factor for hepatitis C. Transfusion with blood or blood products is no longer an important risk factor for acute viral hepatitis. However, blood transfusions received before the introduction of sensitive enzyme immunoassays for antibody to hepatitis C virus (anti-HCV) in 1992 is an important risk factor for chronic hepatitis C. Blood transfusion before 1986, when screening for antibody to hepatitis B core antigen (anti-HBc) was introduced, is also a risk factor for hepatitis B. Travel to an underdeveloped area of the world, exposure to persons with jaundice, and exposure to young children in day-care centers are risk factors for hepatitis A. Hepatitis E is one of the more common causes of jaundice in Asia and Africa but is uncommon in developed nations, although mild cases have been associated with eating raw or undercooked pork or game (deer and wild boars). Tattooing and body piercing (for hepatitis B and C) and eating shellfish (for hepatitis A) are frequently mentioned but are actually quite rare types of exposure for acquiring hepatitis.

A history of alcohol intake is important in assessing the cause of liver disease and also in planning management and recommendations. In the United States, for example, at least 70% of adults drink alcohol to some degree, but significant alcohol intake is less common; in population-based surveys, only 5% have more than two drinks per day, the average drink representing 11–15 g alcohol. Alcohol consumption associated with an increased rate of alcoholic liver disease is probably more than two drinks (22–30 g) per day in women and three drinks (33–45 g) in men. Most patients with alcoholic cirrhosis have a much higher daily intake and have drunk excessively for ≥10 years before onset of liver disease. In assessing alcohol intake, the history should also focus on whether alcohol abuse or dependence is present. Alcoholism is usually defined by the behavioral patterns and consequences of alcohol intake, not on the basis of the amount of alcohol intake. *Abuse* is defined by a repetitive pattern of drinking alcohol that has adverse effects on social, family, occupational, or health status. *Dependence* is defined by alcohol-seeking behavior, despite its adverse effects. Many alcoholics demonstrate both dependence and abuse, and dependence is considered the more serious and advanced form of alcoholism. A clinically helpful approach to diagnosis of alcohol dependence and abuse is the use of the CAGE questionnaire (Table 35-2), which is recommended in all medical history-taking.

Family history can be helpful in assessing liver disease. Familial causes of liver disease include Wilson's disease; hemochromatosis and α_1 antitrypsin (α_1AT) deficiency; and the more uncommon inherited pediatric liver diseases of familial intrahepatic cholestasis, benign recurrent intrahepatic cholestasis, and Alagille's syndrome. Onset of severe liver disease in childhood or adolescence with a family history of liver disease or neuropsychiatric disturbance should lead to investigation for Wilson's disease. A family history of cirrhosis, diabetes, or endocrine failure and the appearance of liver disease in adulthood should suggest hemochromatosis and lead to investigation of iron status. Adult patients with abnormal iron studies warrant genotyping of the *HFE* gene for the C282Y and H63D mutations typical of genetic hemochromatosis. In children and adolescents with iron overload, other non-*HFE* causes of hemochromatosis should be sought. A family history

TABLE 35-2

CAGE QUESTIONS*

ACRONYM	QUESTION
C	Have you ever felt you ought to *Cut* down on your drinking?
A	Have people *Annoyed* you by criticizing your drinking?
G	Have you ever felt *Guilty* or bad about your drinking?
E	Have you ever had a drink first thing in the morning to steady your nerves or get rid of a hangover (*Eye*-opener)?

*One "yes" response should raise suspicion of an alcohol use problem, and more than one is a strong indication that abuse or dependence exists.

of emphysema should provoke investigation of α_1AT levels and, if low, for Pi genotype.

PHYSICAL EXAMINATION

The physical examination rarely demonstrates evidence of liver dysfunction in a patient without symptoms or laboratory findings, nor are most signs of liver disease specific to one diagnosis. Thus, the physical examination complements rather than replaces the need for other diagnostic approaches. In many patients, the physical examination is normal unless the disease is acute or severe and advanced. Nevertheless, the physical examination is important in that it can be the first evidence for the presence of hepatic failure, portal hypertension, and liver decompensation. In addition, the physical examination can reveal signs that point to a specific diagnosis, either in risk factors or in associated diseases or findings.

Typical physical findings in liver disease are icterus, hepatomegaly, hepatic tenderness, splenomegaly, spider angiomata, palmar erythema, and excoriations. Signs of advanced disease include muscle wasting, ascites, edema, dilated abdominal veins, hepatic fetor, asterixis, mental confusion, stupor, and coma. In males with cirrhosis, particularly when related to alcohol, signs of hyperestrogenemia such as gynecomastia, testicular atrophy, and loss of male-pattern hair distribution may be found.

Icterus is best appreciated by inspecting the sclera under natural light. In fair-skinned individuals, a yellow color of the skin may be obvious. In dark-skinned individuals, the mucous membranes below the tongue can demonstrate jaundice. Jaundice is rarely detectable if the serum bilirubin level is <43 μmol/L (2.5 mg/dL) but may remain detectable below this level during recovery from jaundice (because of protein and tissue binding of conjugated bilirubin).

Spider angiomata and palmar erythema occur in both acute and chronic liver disease and may be especially prominent in persons with cirrhosis, but they can occur in normal individuals and are frequently present during pregnancy. Spider angiomata are superficial, tortuous arterioles and, unlike simple telangiectases, typically fill from the center outward. Spider angiomata occur only on the arms, face, and upper torso; they can be pulsatile and may be difficult to detect in dark-skinned individuals.

Hepatomegaly is not a very reliable sign of liver disease, because of the variability of the size and shape of the liver and the physical impediments to assessing liver size by percussion and palpation. Marked hepatomegaly is typical of cirrhosis, venoocclusive disease, infiltrative disorders such as amyloidosis, metastatic or primary cancers of the liver, and alcoholic hepatitis. Careful assessment of the liver edge may also demonstrate unusual firmness, irregularity of the surface, or frank nodules. Perhaps the most reliable physical finding in examining the liver is hepatic tenderness. Discomfort on touching or pressing on the liver should be carefully sought with percussive comparison of the right and left upper quadrants.

Splenomegaly occurs in many medical conditions but can be a subtle but significant physical finding in liver disease. The availability of ultrasound (US) assessment of the spleen allows for confirmation of the physical finding.

Signs of advanced liver disease include muscle-wasting and weight loss as well as hepatomegaly, bruising, ascites, and edema. Ascites is best appreciated by attempts to detect shifting dullness by careful percussion. US examination will confirm the finding of ascites in equivocal cases. Peripheral edema can occur with or without ascites. In patients with advanced liver disease, other factors frequently contribute to edema formation, including hypoalbuminemia, venous insufficiency, heart failure, and medications.

Hepatic failure is defined as the occurrence of signs or symptoms of hepatic encephalopathy in a person with severe acute or chronic liver disease. The first signs of hepatic encephalopathy can be subtle and nonspecific—change in sleep patterns, change in personality, irritability, and mental dullness. Thereafter, confusion, disorientation, stupor, and eventually coma supervene. In acute liver failure, excitability and mania may be present. Physical findings include asterixis and flapping tremors of the body and tongue. *Fetor hepaticus* refers to the slightly sweet, ammoniacal odor that can occur in patients with liver failure, particularly if there is portal-venous shunting of blood around the liver. Other causes of coma and disorientation should be excluded, mainly electrolyte imbalances, sedative use, and renal or respiratory failure. The appearance of hepatic encephalopathy during acute hepatitis is the major criterion for diagnosis of fulminant hepatitis and indicates a poor prognosis. In chronic liver disease, encephalopathy is usually triggered by a medical complication such as gastrointestinal bleeding, over-diuresis, uremia, dehydration, electrolyte imbalance, infection, constipation, or use of narcotic analgesics.

A helpful measure of hepatic encephalopathy is a careful mental status examination and use of the trail-making test, which consists of a series of 25 numbered circles that the patient is asked to connect as rapidly as possible using a pencil. The normal range for the connect-the-dot test is 15–30 s; it is considerably delayed in patients with early hepatic encephalopathy. Other tests include drawing abstract objects or comparison of a signature to previous examples. More sophisticated testing such as with electroencephalography and visual evoked potentials can detect mild forms of encephalopathy, but are rarely clinically useful.

Other signs of advanced liver disease include umbilical hernia from ascites, hydrothorax, prominent veins over the abdomen, and *caput medusa*, which consists of collateral veins seen radiating from the umbilicus and resulting from the recanulation of the umbilical vein. Widened pulse pressure and signs of a hyperdynamic circulation can occur in patients with cirrhosis as a result of fluid and sodium retention, increased cardiac output, and reduced peripheral resistance. Patients with long-standing cirrhosis and portal hypertension are prone to develop the hepatopulmonary syndrome, defined by the triad of liver disease, hypoxemia, and pulmonary arteriovenous shunting. The hepatopulmonary syndrome is characterized by platypnea and orthodeoxia, representing shortness of breath and oxygen desaturation that occur paradoxically upon assuming an upright position. Measurement of oxygen saturation by pulse oximetry is a reliable screening test for the presence of hepatopulmonary syndrome.

Several skin disorders and changes occur commonly in liver disease. Hyperpigmentation is typical of advanced chronic cholestatic diseases such as primary biliary cirrhosis and sclerosing cholangitis. In these same conditions, xanthelasma and tendon xanthomata occur as a result of retention and high serum levels of lipids and cholesterol. A slate-gray pigmentation to the skin also occurs with hemochromatosis if iron levels are high for a prolonged period. Mucocutaneous vasculitis with palpable purpura, especially on the lower extremities, is typical of cryoglobulinemia of chronic hepatitis C but can also occur in chronic hepatitis B.

Some physical signs point to specific liver diseases. Kayser-Fleischer rings occur in Wilson's disease and consist of a golden-brown copper pigment deposited in Descemet's membrane at the periphery of the cornea; they are best seen by slit-lamp examination. Dupuytren contracture and parotid enlargement are suggestive of chronic alcoholism and alcoholic liver disease. In metastatic liver disease or primary hepatocellular carcinoma, signs of cachexia and wasting may be prominent, as well as firm hepatomegaly and a hepatic bruit.

LABORATORY TESTING

Diagnosis in liver disease is greatly aided by the availability of reliable and sensitive tests of liver injury and function. A typical battery of blood tests used for initial assessment of liver disease includes measuring levels of serum alanine and aspartate aminotransferases (ALT and AST), alkaline phosphatase (AlkP), direct and total serum bilirubin, and albumin and assessing prothrombin time. The pattern of abnormalities generally points to hepatocellular versus cholestatic liver disease and will help to decide whether the disease is acute or chronic and whether cirrhosis and hepatic failure are present. Based on these results, further testing over time may be necessary. Other laboratory tests may be helpful, such as γ-glutamyl transpeptidase (gGT) to define whether alkaline phosphatase elevations are due to liver disease; hepatitis serology to define the type of viral hepatitis; and autoimmune markers to diagnose primary biliary cirrhosis (antimitochondrial antibody; AMA), sclerosing cholangitis (perinuclear antineutrophil cytoplasmic antibody; P-ANCA), and autoimmune hepatitis (antinuclear, smooth-muscle, and liver-kidney microsomal antibody). A simple delineation of laboratory abnormalities and common liver diseases is given in Table 35-3.

The use and interpretation of liver function tests is summarized in Chap. 36.

TABLE 35-3

IMPORTANT DIAGNOSTIC TESTS IN COMMON LIVER DISEASES

DISEASE	DIAGNOSTIC TEST
Hepatitis A	Anti-HAV IgM
Hepatitis B	
Acute	HBsAg and anti-HBc IgM
Chronic	HBsAg and HBeAg and/or HBV DNA
Hepatitis C	Anti-HCV and HCV RNA
Hepatitis D (delta)	HBsAg and anti-HDV
Hepatitis E	Anti-HEV
Autoimmune hepatitis	ANA or SMA, elevated IgG levels, and compatible histology
Primary biliary cirrhosis	Mitochondrial antibody, elevated IgM levels, and compatible histology
Primary sclerosing cholangitis	P-ANCA, cholangiography
Drug-induced liver disease	History of drug ingestion
Alcoholic liver disease	History of excessive alcohol intake and compatible histology
Nonalcoholic steatohepatitis	Ultrasound or CT evidence of fatty liver and compatible histology
α_1 Antitrypsin disease	Reduced α_1 antitrypsin levels, phenotypes PiZZ or PiSZ
Wilson's disease	Decreased serum ceruloplasmin and increased urinary copper; increased hepatic copper level
Hemochromatosis	Elevated iron saturation and serum ferritin; genetic testing for *HFE* gene mutations
Hepatocellular cancer	Elevated α-fetoprotein level >500; US or CT image of mass

Abbreviations: HAV, HBV, HCV, HDV, HEV: hepatitis A, B, C, D, or E virus; HBsAg, hepatitis B surface antigen; anti-HBc, antibody to hepatitis B core (antigen); HBeAg, hepatitis e antigen; ANA, antinuclear antibodies; SMA, smooth-muscle antibody; P-ANCA, perinuclear antineutrophil cytoplasmic antibody.

DIAGNOSTIC IMAGING

There have been great advances made in hepatic imaging, although no method is suitably accurate in demonstrating underlying cirrhosis. There are many modalities available for imaging the liver. US, CT, and MRI are the most commonly employed and are complementary to each other. In general, US and CT have a high sensitivity for detecting biliary duct dilatation and are the first-line options for investigating the patient with suspected obstructive jaundice. All three modalities can detect a fatty liver, which appears bright on imaging studies. Modifications of CT and MRI can be used to quantify liver fat, which may ultimately be valuable in monitoring therapy in patients with fatty liver disease. Magnetic resonance cholangiopancreatography (MRCP) and endoscopic retrograde cholangiopancreatography (ERCP) are the procedures of choice for visualization of the biliary tree. MRCP offers several advantages over ERCP; there is no need for contrast media or ionizing radiation, images can be acquired faster, it is less operator dependent, and it carries no risk of pancreatitis. MRCP is superior to US and CT for detecting choledocholithiasis but less specific. It is useful in the diagnosis of bile duct obstruction and congenital biliary abnormalities, but ERCP is more valuable in evaluating ampullary lesions and primary sclerosing cholangitis. ERCP allows for biopsy, direct visualization of the ampulla and common bile duct, and intraductal ultrasonography. It also provides several therapeutic options in patients with obstructive jaundice such as sphincterotomy, stone extraction, and placement of nasobiliary catheters and biliary stents. Doppler US and MRI are used to assess hepatic vasculature and hemodynamics and to monitor surgically or radiologically placed vascular shunts such as transjugular intrahepatic portosystemic shunts. CT and MRI are indicated for the identification and evaluation of hepatic masses, staging of liver tumors, and preoperative assessment. With regard to mass lesions, sensitivity of hepatic imaging continues to increase; unfortunately, specificity remains a problem, and often two and sometimes three studies are needed before a diagnosis can be reached. Recently, methods using elastography have been developed to measure hepatic stiffness as a means of assessing hepatic fibrosis. US and MR elastrography are now undergoing evaluation for their ability to detect different degrees of hepatic fibrosis and to obviate the need for liver biopsy in assessing disease stage. If found to be reliable, hepatic elastography may be an appropriate means of monitoring fibrosis and disease progression. Finally, interventional radiologic techniques allow the biopsy of solitary lesions, performance of radiofrequency ablation and chemoembolization of cancerous lesions, insertion of drains into hepatic abscesses, measurement of portal pressure, and creation of vascular shunts in patients with portal hypertension. Which modality to use depends on factors such as availability, cost, and experience of the radiologist with each technique.

LIVER BIOPSY

Liver biopsy remains the criterion standard in the evaluation of patients with liver disease, particularly in patients with chronic liver diseases. In selected instances, liver biopsy is necessary for diagnosis but is more often useful in assessing the severity (grade) and stage of liver damage, in predicting prognosis, and in monitoring response to treatment. The size of the liver biopsy is an important determinant of its reliability; a length of 1.5–2 cm being necessary for accurate assessment of fibrosis. In the future, noninvasive means of assessing disease activity (batteries of blood tests) and fibrosis (elastography and fibrosis markers) may replace liver biopsy in assessing stage and grade of disease.

DIAGNOSIS OF LIVER DISEASE

The major causes of liver disease and key diagnostic features are outlined in Table 35-3, and an algorithm for evaluation of the patient with suspected liver disease is given in Fig. 35-1. Specifics of diagnosis are discussed in later chapters. The most common causes of acute liver disease are viral hepatitis (particularly hepatitis A, B, and C), drug-induced liver injury, cholangitis, and alcoholic liver disease. Liver biopsy is usually not needed in the diagnosis and management of acute liver disease, exceptions being situations where the diagnosis remains unclear despite thorough clinical and laboratory investigation. Liver biopsy can be helpful in the diagnosis of drug-induced liver disease and in establishing the diagnosis of acute alcoholic hepatitis.

The most common causes of chronic liver disease in general order of frequency are chronic hepatitis C, alcoholic liver disease, nonalcoholic steatohepatitis, chronic hepatitis B, autoimmune hepatitis, sclerosing cholangitis, primary biliary cirrhosis, hemochromatosis, and Wilson's disease. Strict diagnostic criteria have not been developed for most liver diseases, but liver biopsy plays an important role in the diagnosis of autoimmune hepatitis, primary biliary cirrhosis, nonalcoholic and alcoholic steatohepatitis, and Wilson's disease (with a quantitative hepatic copper level).

GRADING AND STAGING OF LIVER DISEASE

Grading refers to an assessment of the severity or activity of liver disease, whether acute or chronic; active or inactive; and mild, moderate, or severe. Liver biopsy is the most accurate means of assessing severity,

EVALUATION OF ABNORMAL LIVER TESTS

Suspected Liver Disease
↓
Abnormal liver tests

Acute < 6 months

Hepatitic: ⇈⇈ALT
Mixed: ↑ALT, ↑AlkP

Diagnostic evaluation
1. IgM Anti-HAV
2. HBsAg
3. IgM Anti-HBc
4. Anti-HCV
5. ANA, SMA
6. Monospot, heterophile
7. Ceruloplasmin
8. Alcohol history
9. Drug history

Cholestatic: ⇈⇈AlkP, ⇈⇈gGT, ↑ALT

Diagnostic evaluation
1. AMA
2. Drug history
3. Ultrasound/MRI
4. MRCP/ERCP

Liver biopsy in acute liver disease: Reserved for patients in whom the diagnosis remains unclear despite medical evaluation

Chronic > 6 months

Hepatitic: ⇈⇈ALT
Mixed: ↑ALT, ↑AlkP

Diagnostic evaluation
1. HBsAg
2. Anti-HCV
3. Fe saturation, ferritin
4. Ceruloplasmin
5. α_1AT
6. ANA, SMA
7. Ultrasound
8. Alcohol history

Cholestatic: ⇈⇈AlkP, ⇈⇈gGT, ↑ALT

Diagnostic evaluation
1. Drug history
2. AMA
3. P-ANCA
4. Ultrasound
5. MRCP/ERCP

Liver biopsy in chronic liver disease: Often valuable for diagnosis as well as staging and grading liver disease

FIGURE 35-1

Algorithm for evaluation of abnormal liver tests. For patients with suspected liver disease, an appropriate approach to evaluation is initial testing for routine liver tests such as bilirubin, albumin, alanine aminotransferase (ALT), aspartate aminotransferase (AST), and alkaline phosphatase (AlkP). These results (sometimes complemented by testing of γ-glutamyl transpeptidase; gGT) will establish whether the pattern of abnormalities is hepatic, cholestatic, or mixed. In addition, the duration of symptoms or abnormalities will show whether the disease is acute or chronic. If the disease is acute and if history, laboratory tests, and imaging studies do not reveal a diagnosis, liver biopsy is appropriate to help establish the diagnosis. If the disease is chronic, liver biopsy can be helpful not only for diagnosis but also to grade the activity and stage the progression of disease. This approach is largely applicable to patients without immune deficiency. In patients with HIV infection or after bone marrow or solid organ transplantation, diagnostic evaluation should also include evaluation of opportunistic infections (adenovirus, cytomegalovirus, coccidioidomycosis, etc.) as well as vascular and immunologic conditions (venoocclusive disease, graft-versus-host disease). HAV, HCV: hepatitis A or C virus; HBsAg, hepatitis B surface antigen; anti-HBc, antibody to hepatitis B core (antigen); ANA, antinuclear antibodies; SMA, smooth-muscle antibody; MRCP, magnetic resonance cholangiopancreatography; ERCP, endoscopic retrograde cholangiopancreatography; α_1AT, α_1 antitrypsin; AMA; antimitochondrial antibody; P-ANCA, perinuclear antineutrophil cytoplasmic antibody.

particularly in chronic liver disease. Serum aminotransferase levels are used as convenient and noninvasive means to follow disease activity, but aminotransferase levels are not always reliable in reflecting disease severity. Thus, normal serum aminotransferase levels in patients with hepatitis B surface antigen (HBsAg) in serum may indicate the inactive HBsAg carrier state or may reflect mild chronic hepatitis B or hepatitis B with fluctuating disease activity. Serum testing for hepatitis B e antigen and hepatitis B virus DNA can help resolve these different patterns, but these markers can also fluctuate and change over time. Similarly, in chronic hepatitis C, serum aminotransferase levels can be normal despite moderate activity of disease. Finally, in both alcoholic and nonalcoholic steatohepatitis, aminotransferase levels are quite unreliable in reflecting severity. In these conditions, liver biopsy is helpful in guiding management and recommending therapy, particularly if therapy is difficult, prolonged, and expensive as is often the case in chronic viral hepatitis. There are several well-verified numerical scales for grading activity in chronic liver disease, the most common being the histology activity index and the Ishak histology scale.

Liver biopsy is also the most accurate means of assessing stage of disease as early or advanced, precirrhotic, and cirrhotic. Staging of disease pertains largely to chronic liver diseases in which progression to cirrhosis and end-stage liver disease can occur, but which may require years or decades to develop. Clinical features, biochemical tests, and hepatic imaging studies are helpful in assessing stage but generally become abnormal only in the middle to late stages of cirrhosis. Noninvasive tests that suggest advanced fibrosis include mild elevations of bilirubin, prolongation of prothrombin time, slight decreases in serum albumin, and mild thrombocytopenia (which is often the first indication of worsening fibrosis). Combinations of blood test results have been used to create models for predicting advanced liver disease, but these are not reliable enough to use on a regular basis and they only separate advanced from early disease. Recently, elastography and noninvasive breath tests using ^{13}C-labeled compounds have been proposed as a means of detecting early stages of fibrosis and liver dysfunction, but their reliability and reproducibility remain to be proven. Thus, at present, mild to moderate stages of hepatic fibrosis are detectable only by liver biopsy. In assessing stage, the degree of fibrosis is usually used as its quantitative measure. The amount of fibrosis is generally staged on a 0 to 4+ (Metavir scale) or 0 to 6+ scale (Ishak scale). The importance of staging relates primarily to prognosis and to guiding management of complications. Patients with cirrhosis are candidates for screening and surveillance for esophageal varices and hepatocellular carcinoma. Patients without advanced fibrosis need not undergo screening.

Cirrhosis can also be staged clinically. A reliable staging system is the modified Child-Pugh classification with a scoring system of 5–15: scores of 5 and 6 being Child-Pugh class A (consistent with "compensated cirrhosis"), scores of 7–9 indicating class B, and 10–15 indicating class C (Table 35-4). This scoring system was initially devised to stratify patients into risk groups prior to undergoing portal decompressive surgery. The Child-Pugh score is a reasonably reliable predictor of survival in many liver diseases and predicts the likelihood of major complications of cirrhosis such as bleeding from varices and spontaneous bacterial peritonitis. It was used to assess prognosis in cirrhosis and to provide the standard criteria for listing liver transplantation (Child-Pugh class B). Recently the Child-Pugh system has been replaced by the Model for End-Stage Liver Disease (MELD) score for assessing the need for liver transplantation. The MELD score is a prospectively

TABLE 35-4

CHILD-PUGH CLASSIFICATION OF CIRRHOSIS

FACTOR	UNITS	1	2	3
Serum bilirubin	μmol/L	<34	34-51	>51
	mg/dL	<2.0	2.0-3.0	>3.0
Serum albumin	g/L	>35	30-35	<30
	g/dL	>3.5	3.0-3.5	<3.0
Prothrombin time	seconds prolonged	0-4	4-6	>6
	INR	<1.7	1.7-2.3	>2.3
Ascites		None	Easily controlled	Poorly controlled
Hepatic encephalopathy		None	Minimal	Advanced

Note: The Child-Pugh score is calculated by adding the scores of the five factors and can range from 5 to 15. Child-Pugh class can be A (a score of 5-6), B (7-9), or C (10 or above). Decompensation indicates cirrhosis with a Child-Pugh score of ≥7 (class B). This level has been the accepted criterion for listing liver transplantation.

derived scoring system designed to predict prognosis of patients with liver disease and portal hypertension. It is calculated using three noninvasive variables—the prothrombin time expressed as international normalized ratio (INR), serum bilirubin, and serum creatinine (http://www.unos.org/resources/meldPeldCalculator.asp).

MELD provides a more objective means of assessing disease severity and has less center-to-center variation than the Child-Pugh score and has a wider range of values. MELD is currently used to establish priority listing for liver transplantation in the United States. A similar system using bilirubin, INR, serum albumin, age, and nutritional status is used for children below the age of 12 years (pediatric end-stage liver disease [PELD]).

Thus, liver biopsy is helpful not only in diagnosis but also in management of chronic liver disease and assessment of prognosis. Because liver biopsy is an invasive procedure and not without complications, it should be used only when it will contribute materially to management and therapeutic decisions.

NONSPECIFIC ISSUES IN MANAGEMENT OF PATIENTS WITH LIVER DISEASE

Specifics on management of different forms of acute or chronic liver disease are given in subsequent chapters, but certain issues are applicable to any patient with liver disease. These include advice regarding alcohol use, medications, vaccination, and surveillance for complications of liver disease. Alcohol should be used sparingly, if at all, by patients with liver disease. Abstinence from alcohol should be encouraged for all patients with alcohol-related liver disease and in patients with cirrhosis and those receiving interferon-based therapy for hepatitis B or C. Regarding vaccinations, all patients with liver disease should receive hepatitis A vaccine and those with risk factors should receive hepatitis B vaccination as well. Influenza and pneumococcal vaccination should also be encouraged. Patients with liver disease should be careful using any medications, other than the most necessary. Drug-induced hepatotoxicity can mimic many forms of liver disease and can cause exacerbations of chronic hepatitis and cirrhosis; drugs should be suspected in any situation in which the cause of exacerbation is unknown. Finally, consideration should be given to surveillance for complications of chronic liver disease such as variceal hemorrhage and hepatocellular carcinoma. Patients with cirrhosis warrant upper endoscopy to assess the presence of varices and should be given chronic therapy with beta blockers or offered endoscopic obliteration if large varices are found. Patients with cirrhosis also warrant screening and long-term surveillance for development of hepatocellular carcinoma. While the optimal regimen for such surveillance has not been established, an appropriate approach is US of the liver at 6- to 12-month intervals.

CHAPTER 36

EVALUATION OF LIVER FUNCTION

Daniel S. Pratt ■ Marshall M. Kaplan

Several biochemical tests are useful in the evaluation and management of patients with hepatic dysfunction. These tests can be used to (1) detect the presence of liver disease, (2) distinguish among different types of liver disorders, (3) gauge the extent of known liver damage, and (4) follow the response to treatment.

Liver tests have shortcomings. They can be normal in patients with serious liver disease and abnormal in patients with diseases that do not affect the liver. Liver tests rarely suggest a specific diagnosis; rather, they suggest a general category of liver disease, such as hepatocellular or cholestatic, which then further directs the evaluation.

The liver carries out thousands of biochemical functions, most of which cannot be easily measured by blood tests. Laboratory tests measure only a limited number of these functions. In fact, many tests, such as the aminotransferases or alkaline phosphatase, do not measure liver function at all. Rather, they detect liver cell damage or interference with bile flow. Thus, no one test enables the clinician to accurately assess the liver's total functional capacity.

To increase both the sensitivity and the specificity of laboratory tests in the detection of liver disease, it is best to use them as a battery. Tests usually employed in clinical practice include the bilirubin, aminotransferases, alkaline phosphatase, albumin, and prothrombin time tests. When more than one of these tests provide abnormal findings or the findings are persistently abnormal on serial determinations, the probability of liver disease is high. When all test results are normal, the probability of missing occult liver disease is low.

When evaluating patients with liver disorders, it is helpful to group these tests into general categories. The classification we have found most useful is discussed later in this chapter.

TESTS BASED ON DETOXIFICATION AND EXCRETORY FUNCTIONS

Serum bilirubin

(See also Chap. 8) Bilirubin, a breakdown product of the porphyrin ring of heme-containing proteins, is found in the blood in two fractions—conjugated and unconjugated. The unconjugated fraction, also termed the *indirect fraction*, is insoluble in water and is bound to albumin in the blood. The conjugated (direct) bilirubin fraction is water soluble and can therefore be excreted by the kidney. When measured by modifications of the original van den Bergh method, normal values of total serum bilirubin are reported between 1 and 1.5 mg/dL with 95% of a normal population falling between 0.2 and 0.9 mg/dL. If the direct-acting fraction is less than 15% of the total, the bilirubin can be considered to all be indirect. The most frequently reported upper limit of normal for conjugated bilirubin is 0.3 mg/dL.

Elevation of the unconjugated fraction of bilirubin is rarely due to liver disease. An isolated elevation of unconjugated bilirubin is seen primarily in hemolytic disorders and in a number of genetic conditions such as Crigler-Najjar and Gilbert's syndromes (Chap. 8). Isolated unconjugated hyperbilirubinemia (bilirubin elevated but <15% direct) should prompt a workup for hemolysis (Fig. 36-1). In the absence of hemolysis, an isolated, unconjugated hyperbilirubinemia in an otherwise healthy patient can be attributed to Gilbert's syndrome, and no further evaluation is required.

In contrast, conjugated hyperbilirubinemia almost always implies liver or biliary tract disease. The rate-limiting step in bilirubin metabolism is not conjugation of bilirubin, but rather the transport of conjugated bilirubin into the bile canaliculi. Thus, elevation of the conjugated fraction may be seen in any type of

EVALUATION OF CHRONICALLY ABNORMAL LIVER TESTS

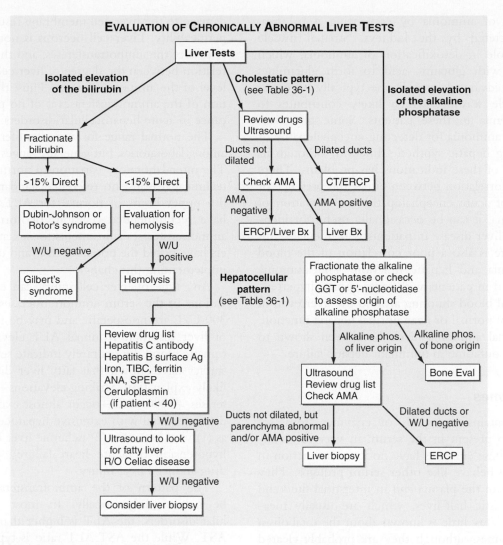

FIGURE 36-1

Algorithm for the evaluation of chronically abnormal liver tests. ERCP, endoscopic retrograde cholangiopancreatography; CT, computed tomography; AMA, antimitochondrial antibody; ANA, antinuclear antibody; SPEP, serum protein electrophoresis; TIBC, total iron-binding capacity; GGT, γ-glutamyl transpeptidase; W/U, work up.

liver disease. In most liver diseases, both conjugated and unconjugated fractions of the bilirubin tend to be elevated. Except in the presence of a purely unconjugated hyperbilirubinemia, fractionation of the bilirubin is rarely helpful in determining the cause of jaundice.

While the degree of elevation of the serum bilirubin has not been critically assessed as a prognostic marker, it important in a number of conditions. In viral hepatitis, the higher the serum bilirubin, the greater the hepatocellular damage. Total serum bilirubin correlates with poor outcomes in alcoholic hepatitis. It is also a critical component of the Model for Endstage Liver Disease (MELD) score, a tool used to estimate survival of patients with end-stage liver disease. An elevated total serum bilirubin in patients with drug-induced liver disease indicates more severe injury.

Urine bilirubin

Unconjugated bilirubin always binds to albumin in the serum and is not filtered by the kidney. Therefore, any bilirubin found in the urine is conjugated bilirubin; the presence of bilirubinuria implies the presence of liver disease. A urine dipstick test can theoretically give the same information as fractionation of the serum bilirubin. This test is almost 100% accurate. Phenothiazines may give a false-positive reading with the Ictotest tablet. In patients recovering from jaundice, the urine bilirubin clears prior to the serum bilirubin.

Blood ammonia

Ammonia is produced in the body during normal protein metabolism and by intestinal bacteria, primarily those in the colon. The liver plays a role in the detoxification of ammonia by converting it to urea, which is excreted by the kidneys. Striated muscle also plays a role in detoxification of ammonia, which is combined with glutamic acid to form glutamine. Patients with advanced liver disease typically have significant muscle wasting, which likely contributes to hyperammonemia in these patients. Some physicians use the blood ammonia for detecting encephalopathy or for monitoring hepatic synthetic function, although its use for either of these indications has problems. There is very poor correlation between either the presence or the severity of acute encephalopathy and elevation of blood ammonia; it can be occasionally useful for identifying occult liver disease in patients with mental status changes. There is also a poor correlation of the blood serum ammonia and hepatic function. The ammonia can be elevated in patients with severe portal hypertension and portal blood shunting around the liver even in the presence of normal or near-normal hepatic function. Elevated arterial ammonia levels have been shown to correlate with outcome in fulminant hepatic failure.

Serum enzymes

The liver contains thousands of enzymes, some of which are also present in the serum in very low concentrations. These enzymes have no known function in the serum and behave like other serum proteins. They are distributed in the plasma and in interstitial fluid and have characteristic half-lives, which are usually measured in days. Very little is known about the catabolism of serum enzymes, although they are probably cleared by cells in the reticuloendothelial system. The elevation of a given enzyme activity in the serum is thought to primarily reflect its increased rate of entrance into serum from damaged liver cells.

Serum enzyme tests can be grouped into three categories: (1) enzymes whose elevation in serum reflects damage to hepatocytes, (2) enzymes whose elevation in serum reflects cholestasis, and (3) enzyme tests that do not fit precisely into either pattern.

Enzymes that reflect damage to hepatocytes
The aminotransferases (transaminases) are sensitive indicators of liver cell injury and are most helpful in recognizing acute hepatocellular diseases such as hepatitis. They include the aspartate aminotransferase (AST) and the alanine aminotransferase (ALT). AST is found in the liver, cardiac muscle, skeletal muscle, kidneys, brain, pancreas, lungs, leukocytes, and erythrocytes in decreasing order of concentration. ALT is found primarily in the liver and is therefore a more specific indicator of liver injury. The aminotransferases are normally present in the serum in low concentrations. These enzymes are released into the blood in greater amounts when there is

damage to the liver cell membrane resulting in increased permeability. Liver cell necrosis is not required for the release of the aminotransferases, and there is a poor correlation between the degree of liver cell damage and the level of the aminotransferases. Thus, the absolute elevation of the aminotransferases is of no prognostic significance in acute hepatocellular disorders.

The normal range for aminotransferases varies widely among laboratories, but generally ranges from 10-40 U/L. The inter-laboratory variation in normal range is due to technical reasons; no reference standards exist to establish upper limits of normal for ALT and AST. Some have recommended revisions of normal limits of the aminotransferases adjustments for sex and BMI, but others have noted the potential costs and unclear benefits of implementing this change.

Any type of liver cell injury can cause modest elevations in the serum aminotransferases. Levels of up to 300 U/L are nonspecific and may be found in any type of liver disorder. Minimal ALT elevations in asymptomatic blood donors rarely indicate severe liver disease; studies have shown that fatty liver disease is the most likely explanation. Striking elevations—i.e., aminotransferases >1000 U/L—occur almost exclusively in disorders associated with extensive hepatocellular injury such as (1) viral hepatitis, (2) ischemic liver injury (prolonged hypotension or acute heart failure), or (3) toxin- or drug-induced liver injury.

The pattern of the aminotransferase elevation can be helpful diagnostically. In most acute hepatocellular disorders, the ALT is higher than or equal to the AST. While the AST:ALT ratio is typically less than 1 in patients with chronic viral hepatitis and nonalcoholic fatty liver disease, a number of groups have noted that as cirrhosis develops this ratio rises to greater than 1. An AST:ALT ratio >2:1 is suggestive, while a ratio >3:1 is highly suggestive of alcoholic liver disease. The AST in alcoholic liver disease is rarely >300 U/L, and the ALT is often normal. A low level of ALT in the serum is due to an alcohol-induced deficiency of pyridoxal phosphate.

The aminotransferases are usually not greatly elevated in obstructive jaundice. One notable exception occurs during the acute phase of biliary obstruction caused by the passage of a gallstone into the common bile duct. In this setting, the aminotransferases can briefly be in the 1000–2000 U/L range. However, aminotransferase levels decrease quickly, and the liver-function tests rapidly evolve into one typical of cholestasis.

Enzymes that reflect cholestasis
The activities of three enzymes—alkaline phosphatase, 5′-nucleotidase, and γ-glutamyl transpeptidase (GGT)—are usually elevated in cholestasis. Alkaline phosphatase and 5′-nucleotidase are found in or near the bile

canalicular membrane of hepatocytes, while GGT is located in the endoplasmic reticulum and in bile duct epithelial cells. Reflecting its more diffuse localization in the liver, GGT elevation in serum is less specific for cholestasis than are elevations of alkaline phosphatase or 5′-nucleotidase. Some have advocated the use of GGT to identify patients with occult alcohol use. Its lack of specificity makes its use in this setting questionable.

The normal serum alkaline phosphatase consists of many distinct isoenzymes found in the liver; bone; placenta; and, less commonly, small intestine. Patients over age 60 can have a mildly elevated alkaline phosphatase (1–1½ times normal), while individuals with blood types O and B can have an elevation of the serum alkaline phosphatase after eating a fatty meal due to the influx of intestinal alkaline phosphatase into the blood. It is also nonpathologically elevated in children and adolescents undergoing rapid bone growth, because of bone alkaline phosphatase, and late in normal pregnancies due to the influx of placental alkaline phosphatase.

Elevation of liver-derived alkaline phosphatase is not totally specific for cholestasis, and a less than threefold elevation can be seen in almost any type of liver disease. Alkaline phosphatase elevations greater than four times normal occur primarily in patients with cholestatic liver disorders, infiltrative liver diseases such as cancer and amyloidosis, and bone conditions characterized by rapid bone turnover (e.g., Paget's disease). In bone diseases, the elevation is due to increased amounts of the bone isoenzymes. In liver diseases, the elevation is almost always due to increased amounts of the liver isoenzyme.

If an elevated serum alkaline phosphatase is the only abnormal finding in an apparently healthy person, or if the degree of elevation is higher than expected in the clinical setting, identification of the source of elevated isoenzymes is helpful (Fig. 36-1). This problem can be approached in several ways. First, and most precise, is the fractionation of the alkaline phosphatase by electrophoresis. The second approach is based on the observation that alkaline phosphatases from individual tissues differ in susceptibility to inactivation by heat. The finding of an elevated serum alkaline phosphatase level in a patient with a heat-stable fraction strongly suggests that the placenta or a tumor is the source of the elevated enzyme in serum. Susceptibility to inactivation by heat increases, respectively, for the intestinal, liver, and bone alkaline phosphatases, bone being by far the most sensitive. The third, best substantiated, and most available approach involves the measurement of serum 5′-nucleotidase or GGT. These enzymes are rarely elevated in conditions other than liver disease.

In the absence of jaundice or elevated aminotransferases, an elevated alkaline phosphatase of liver origin often, but not always, suggests early cholestasis and, less often, hepatic infiltration by tumor or granulomata. Other conditions that cause isolated elevations of the alkaline phosphatase include Hodgkin's disease, diabetes, hyperthyroidism, congestive heart failure, amyloidosis, and inflammatory bowel disease.

The level of serum alkaline phosphatase elevation is not helpful in distinguishing between intrahepatic and extrahepatic cholestasis. There is essentially no difference among the values found in obstructive jaundice due to cancer, common duct stone, sclerosing cholangitis, or bile duct stricture. Values are similarly increased in patients with intrahepatic cholestasis due to drug-induced hepatitis; primary biliary cirrhosis; rejection of transplanted livers; and, rarely, alcohol-induced steatohepatitis. Values are also greatly elevated in hepatobiliary disorders seen in patients with AIDS (e.g., AIDS cholangiopathy due to cytomegalovirus or cryptosporidial infection and tuberculosis with hepatic involvement).

TESTS THAT MEASURE BIOSYNTHETIC FUNCTION OF THE LIVER

Serum albumin

Serum albumin is synthesized exclusively by hepatocytes. Serum albumin has a long half-life: 18–20 days, with ~4% degraded per day. Because of this slow turnover, the serum albumin is not a good indicator of acute or mild hepatic dysfunction; only minimal changes in the serum albumin are seen in acute liver conditions such as viral hepatitis, drug-related hepatoxicity, and obstructive jaundice. In hepatitis, albumin levels <3 g/dL should raise the possibility of chronic liver disease. Hypoalbuminemia is more common in chronic liver disorders such as cirrhosis and usually reflects severe liver damage and decreased albumin synthesis. One exception is the patient with ascites in whom synthesis may be normal or even increased, but levels are low because of the increased volume of distribution. However, hypoalbuminemia is not specific for liver disease and may occur in protein malnutrition of any cause, as well as protein-losing enteropathies, nephrotic syndrome, and chronic infections that are associated with prolonged increases in levels of serum interleukin 1 and/or tumor necrosis factor, cytokines that inhibit albumin synthesis. Serum albumin should not be measured for screening in patients in whom there is no suspicion of liver disease. A general medical clinic study of consecutive patients in whom no indications were present for albumin measurement showed that while 12% of patients had abnormal test results, the finding was of clinical importance in only 0.4%.

Serum globulins

Serum globulins are a group of proteins made up of γ globulins (immunoglobulins) produced by B lymphocytes and α and β globulins produced primarily in hepatocytes. γ Globulins are increased in chronic liver disease, such as chronic hepatitis and cirrhosis. In cirrhosis, the increased serum γ globulin concentration is due to the increased synthesis of antibodies, some of which are directed against intestinal bacteria. This occurs because the cirrhotic liver fails to clear bacterial antigens that normally reach the liver through the hepatic circulation.

Increases in the concentration of specific isotypes of γ globulins are often helpful in the recognition of certain chronic liver diseases. Diffuse polyclonal increases in IgG levels are common in autoimmune hepatitis; increases >100% should alert the clinician to this possibility. Increases in the IgM levels are common in primary biliary cirrhosis, while increases in the IgA levels occur in alcoholic liver disease.

COAGULATION FACTORS

With the exception of factor VIII, which is produced by vascular endothelial cells, the blood clotting factors are made exclusively in hepatocytes. Their serum half-lives are much shorter than albumin, ranging from 6 h for factor VII to 5 days for fibrinogen. Because of their rapid turnover, measurement of the clotting factors is the single best acute measure of hepatic synthetic function and helpful in both the diagnosis and assessing the prognosis of acute parenchymal liver disease. Useful for this purpose is the *serum prothrombin time*, which collectively measures factors II, V, VII, and X. Biosynthesis of factors II, VII, IX, and X depends on vitamin K. The international normalized ratio (INR) is used to express the degree of anticoagulation on warfarin therapy. The INR standardizes prothrombin time measurement according to the characteristics of the thromboplastin reagent used in a particular lab, which is expressed as an International Sensitivity Index (ISI); the ISI is then used in calculating the INR. Because the ISI is validated only for patients on vitamin K antagonists, there has been concern regarding the validity of using it for patients with chronic liver disease.

The prothrombin time may be elevated in hepatitis and cirrhosis as well as in disorders that lead to vitamin K deficiency such as obstructive jaundice or fat malabsorption of any kind. Marked prolongation of the prothrombin time, >5 s above control and not corrected by parenteral vitamin K administration, is a poor prognostic sign in acute viral hepatitis and other acute and chronic liver diseases. The INR, along with the total serum bilirubin and creatinine, are components of the MELD score, which is used to allocate organs for liver transplantation.

OTHER DIAGNOSTIC TESTS

While tests may direct the physician to a category of liver disease, additional radiologic testing and procedures are often necessary to make the proper diagnosis, as shown in Fig. 36-1. The two most commonly used ancillary tests are reviewed here.

Percutaneous liver biopsy

Percutaneous biopsy of the liver is a safe procedure that can be easily performed at the bedside with local anesthesia and ultrasound guidance. Liver biopsy is of proven value in the following situations: (1) hepatocellular disease of uncertain cause, (2) prolonged hepatitis with the possibility of chronic active hepatitis, (3) unexplained hepatomegaly, (4) unexplained splenomegaly, (5) hepatic filling defects by radiologic imaging, (6) fever of unknown origin, and (7) staging of malignant lymphoma. Liver biopsy is most accurate in disorders causing diffuse changes throughout the liver and is subject to sampling error in focal infiltrative disorders such as hepatic metastases. Liver biopsy should not be the initial procedure in the diagnosis of cholestasis. The biliary tree should first be assessed for signs of obstruction. Contraindications to performing a percutaneous liver biopsy include significant ascites and prolonged INR. Under these circumstances, the biopsy can be performed via the transjugular approach.

Ultrasonography

Ultrasonography is the first diagnostic test to use in patients whose liver tests suggest cholestasis, to look for the presence of a dilated intrahepatic or extrahepatic biliary tree or to identify gallstones. In addition, it shows space-occupying lesions within the liver, enables the clinician to distinguish between cystic and solid masses, and helps direct percutaneous biopsies. Ultrasound with Doppler imaging can detect the patency of the portal vein, hepatic artery, and hepatic veins and determine the direction of blood flow. This is the first test ordered in patients suspected of having Budd-Chiari syndrome.

USE OF LIVER TESTS

As previously noted, the best way to increase the sensitivity and specificity of laboratory tests in the detection of liver disease is to employ a battery of tests that includes the aminotransferases, alkaline phosphatase,

TABLE 36-1

LIVER TEST PATTERNS IN HEPATOBILIARY DISORDERS

TYPE OF DISORDER	BILIRUBIN	AMINOTRANSFERASES	ALKALINE PHOSPHATASE	ALBUMIN	PROTHROMBIN TIME
Hemolysis/Gilbert's syndrome	Normal to 86 μmol/L (5 mg/dL) 85% due to indirect fractions No bilirubinuria	Normal	Normal	Normal	Normal
Acute hepatocellular necrosis (viral and drug hepatitis, hepatotoxins, acute heart failure)	Both fractions may be elevated Peak usually follows aminotransferases Bilirubinuria	Elevated, often >500 IU ALT >AST	Normal to <3 times normal elevation	Normal	Usually normal. If >5 times above control and not corrected by parenteral vitamin K, suggests poor prognosis
Chronic hepatocellular disorders	Both fractions may be elevated Bilirubinuria	Elevated, but usually <300 IU	Normal to <3 times normal elevation	Often decreased	Often prolonged Fails to correct with parenteral vitamin K
Alcoholic hepatitis Cirrhosis	Both fractions may be elevated Bilirubinuria	AST:ALT > 2 suggests alcoholic hepatitis or cirrhosis	Normal to <3 times normal elevation	Often decreased	Often prolonged Fails to correct with parenteral vitamin K
Intra- and extrahepatic cholestasis (Obstructive jaundice)	Both fractions may be elevated Bilirubinuria	Normal to moderate elevation Rarely >500 IU	Elevated, often >4 times normal elevation	Normal, unless chronic	Normal If prolonged, will correct with parenteral vitamin K
Infiltrative diseases (tumor, granulomata); partial bile duct obstruction	Usually normal	Normal to slight elevation	Elevated, often >4 times normal elevation Fractionate, or confirm liver origin with 5′-nucleotidase or γ-glutamyl transpeptidase	Normal	Normal

bilirubin, albumin, and prothrombin time along with the judicious use of the other tests described in this chapter. Table 36-1 shows how patterns of liver tests can lead the clinician to a category of disease that will direct further evaluation. However, it is important to remember that no single set of liver tests will necessarily provide a diagnosis. It is often necessary to repeat these tests on several occasions over days to weeks for a diagnostic pattern to emerge. Figure 36-1 is an algorithm for the evaluation of chronically abnormal liver tests.

SECTION VI

DISORDERS OF
THE LIVER AND
BILIARY TREE

CHAPTER 37

THE HYPERBILIRUBINEMIAS

Allan W. Wolkoff

BILIRUBIN METABOLISM

The details of bilirubin metabolism are presented in Chap. 8. However, the hyperbilirubinemias are best understood in terms of perturbations of specific aspects of bilirubin metabolism and transport, and these will be briefly reviewed here as depicted in **Fig. 37-1**.

Bilirubin is the end product of heme degradation. Some 70–90% of bilirubin is derived from degradation of the hemoglobin of senescent red blood cells. Bilirubin produced in the periphery is transported to the liver within the plasma, where, due to its insolubility in

FIGURE 37-1

Hepatocellular bilirubin transport. Albumin-bound bilirubin in sinusoidal blood passes through endothelial cell fenestrae to reach the hepatocyte surface, entering the cell by both facilitated and simple diffusional processes. Within the cell it is bound to glutathione-S-transferases and conjugated by bilirubin-UDP-glucuronosyltransferase (UGT1A1) to mono- and diglucuronides, which are actively transported across the canalicular membrane into the bile. ALB, albumin; BDG, bilirubin diglucuronide; BMG, bilirubin monoglucuronide; BT, proposed bilirubin transporter; GST, glutathione-S-transferase; MRP2, multidrug resistance–associated protein 2; UCB, unconjugated bilirubin; UGT1A1, bilirubin-UDP-glucuronosyltransferase.

aqueous solutions, it is tightly bound to albumin. Under normal circumstances, bilirubin is removed from the circulation rapidly and efficiently by hepatocytes. Transfer of bilirubin from blood to bile involves four distinct but interrelated steps (Fig. 37-1).

1. *Hepatocellular uptake:* Uptake of bilirubin by the hepatocyte has carrier-mediated kinetics. Although a number of candidate bilirubin transporters have been proposed, the actual transporter remains elusive.

2. *Intracellular binding:* Within the hepatocyte, bilirubin is kept in solution by binding as a nonsubstrate ligand to several of the glutathione-S-transferases, formerly called ligandins.

3. *Conjugation:* Bilirubin is conjugated with one or two glucuronic acid moieties by a specific UDP-glucuronosyltransferase to form bilirubin mono- and diglucuronide, respectively. Conjugation disrupts the internal hydrogen bonding that limits aqueous solubility of bilirubin, and the resulting glucuronide conjugates are highly soluble in water. Conjugation is obligatory for excretion of bilirubin across the bile canalicular membrane into bile. The UDP-glucuronosyltransferases have been classified into gene families based on the degree of homology among the mRNAs for the various isoforms. Those that conjugate bilirubin and certain other substrates have been designated the *UGT1* family. These are expressed from a single gene complex by alternative promoter usage. This gene complex contains multiple substrate-specific first exons, designated A1, A2, etc. **(Fig. 37-2)**, each with its own promoter and each encoding the amino-terminal half of a specific isoform. In addition, there are four common exons (exons 2–5) that encode the shared carboxyl-terminal half of all of the *UGT1* isoforms. The various first exons encode the specific aglycone substrate binding sites for each isoform, while the shared exons encode the binding site for the sugar donor, UDP-glucuronic acid, and the transmembrane

FIGURE 37-2

Structural organization of the human *UGT1* gene complex. This large complex on chromosome 2 contains at least 13 substrate-specific first exons (A1, A2, etc.). Since four of these are pseudogenes, nine UGT1 isoforms with differing substrate specificities are expressed. Each exon 1 has its own promoter and encodes the amino-terminal substrate-specific ~286 amino acids of the various *UGT1*-encoded isoforms, and common exons 2–5 that encode the

245 carboxyl-terminal amino acids common to all of the isoforms. mRNAs for specific isoforms are assembled by splicing a particular first exon such as the bilirubin-specific exon A1 to exons 2 to 5. The resulting message encodes a complete enzyme, in this particular case bilirubin-UDP-glucuronosyltransferase (UGT1A1). Mutations in a first exon affect only a single isoform. Those in exons 2–5 affect all enzymes encoded by the UGT1 complex.

domain. Exon A1 and the four common exons, collectively designated the *UGT1A1* gene (Fig. 37-2), encode the physiologically critical enzyme bilirubin-UDP-glucuronosyltransferase (UGT1A1). A functional corollary of the organization of the *UGT1* gene is that a mutation in one of the first exons will affect only a single enzyme isoform. By contrast, a mutation in exons 2–5 will alter all isoforms encoded by the *UGT1* gene complex.

4. *Biliary excretion:* Bilirubin mono- and diglucuronides are excreted across the canalicular plasma membrane into the bile canaliculus by an ATP-dependent transport process mediated by a canalicular membrane protein called *multidrug resistance–associated protein 2* (MRP2). Mutations of MRP2 result in the Dubin-Johnson syndrome (discussed later).

EXTRAHEPATIC ASPECTS OF BILIRUBIN DISPOSITION

Bilirubin in the gut

Following secretion into bile, conjugated bilirubin reaches the duodenum and passes down the gastrointestinal tract without reabsorption by the intestinal mucosa. An appreciable fraction is converted by bacterial metabolism in the gut to the water-soluble colorless compound urobilinogen. Urobilinogen undergoes enterohepatic cycling. Urobilinogen not taken up by the liver reaches the systemic circulation, from which some is cleared by the kidneys. Unconjugated bilirubin ordinarily does not reach the gut except in neonates or, by ill-defined alternative pathways, in the presence of severe unconjugated hyperbilirubinemia (e.g., Crigler-Najjar

syndrome, type I [CN-I]). Unconjugated bilirubin that reaches the gut is partly reabsorbed, amplifying any underlying hyperbilirubinemia. Recent reports suggest that oral administration of calcium phosphate with or without the lipase inhibitor orlistat may be an efficient means to interrupt bilirubin enterohepatic cycling to reduce serum bilirubin levels in this situation. Although orlistat administration for 4–6 weeks to 16 patients with Crigler-Najjar syndrome was associated with a 10-20% decrease in serum bilirubin in 7 patients, the cost and side effects (i.e., diarrhea) may obviate the small benefit achievable with this treatment.

Renal excretion of bilirubin conjugates

Unconjugated bilirubin is not excreted in urine, as it is too tightly bound to albumin for effective glomerular filtration and there is no tubular mechanism for its renal secretion. In contrast, the bilirubin conjugates are readily filtered at the glomerulus and can appear in urine in disorders characterized by increased bilirubin conjugates in the circulation.

DISORDERS OF BILIRUBIN METABOLISM LEADING TO UNCONJUGATED HYPERBILIRUBINEMIA

INCREASED BILIRUBIN PRODUCTION

Hemolysis

Increased destruction of erythrocytes leads to increased bilirubin turnover and unconjugated hyperbilirubinemia; the hyperbilirubinemia is usually modest in the presence of normal liver function. In particular, the bone marrow is only capable of a sustained eight-fold increase in erythrocyte production in response to a hemolytic stress. Therefore, hemolysis alone cannot result in a sustained hyperbilirubinemia of more than ~68 μmol/L (4 mg/dL). Higher values imply concomitant hepatic dysfunction. When hemolysis is the only abnormality in an otherwise healthy individual, the result is a purely unconjugated hyperbilirubinemia, with the direct-reacting fraction as measured in a typical clinical laboratory being ≤15% of the total serum bilirubin. In the presence of systemic disease, which may include a degree of hepatic dysfunction, hemolysis may produce a component of conjugated hyperbilirubinemia in addition to an elevated unconjugated bilirubin concentration. Prolonged hemolysis may lead to the precipitation of bilirubin salts within the gallbladder or biliary tree, resulting in the formation of gallstones in which bilirubin, rather than cholesterol, is the major component. Such pigment stones may lead to acute or chronic cholecystitis, biliary obstruction, or any other biliary tract consequence of calculous disease.

Ineffective erythropoiesis

During erythroid maturation, small amounts of hemoglobin may be lost at the time of nuclear extrusion, and a fraction of developing erythroid cells is destroyed within the marrow. These processes normally account for a small proportion of bilirubin that is produced. In various disorders, including thalassemia major, megaloblastic anemias due to folate or vitamin B_{12} deficiency, congenital erythropoietic porphyria, lead poisoning, and various congenital and acquired dyserythropoietic anemias, the fraction of total bilirubin production derived from ineffective erythropoiesis is increased, reaching as much as 70% of the total. This may be sufficient to produce modest degrees of unconjugated hyperbilirubinemia.

Miscellaneous

Degradation of the hemoglobin of extravascular collections of erythrocytes, such as those seen in massive tissue infarctions or large hematomas, may lead transiently to unconjugated hyperbilirubinemia.

DECREASED HEPATIC BILIRUBIN CLEARANCE

Decreased hepatic uptake

Decreased hepatic bilirubin uptake is believed to contribute to the unconjugated hyperbilirubinemia of Gilbert's syndrome (GS), although the molecular basis for this finding remains unclear (discussed later). Several

drugs, including flavaspidic acid, novobiocin, and rifampin, as well as various cholecystographic contrast agents, have been reported to inhibit bilirubin uptake. The resulting unconjugated hyperbilirubinemia resolves with cessation of the medication.

Impaired conjugation

Physiologic neonatal jaundice

Bilirubin produced by the fetus is cleared by the placenta and eliminated by the maternal liver. Immediately after birth, the neonatal liver must assume responsibility for bilirubin clearance and excretion. However, many hepatic physiologic processes are incompletely developed at birth. Levels of UGT1A1 are low, and alternative excretory pathways allow passage of unconjugated bilirubin into the gut. Since the intestinal flora that convert bilirubin to urobilinogen are also undeveloped, an enterohepatic circulation of unconjugated bilirubin ensues. As a consequence, most neonates develop mild unconjugated hyperbilirubinemia between days 2 and 5 after birth. Peak levels are typically <85–170 μmol/L (5–10 mg/dL) and decline to normal adult concentrations within 2 weeks, as mechanisms required for bilirubin disposition mature. Prematurity, often associated with more profound immaturity of hepatic function and hemolysis, can result in higher levels of unconjugated hyperbilirubinemia. A rapidly rising unconjugated bilirubin concentration, or absolute levels >340 μmol/L (20 mg/dL), puts the infant at risk for bilirubin encephalopathy, or kernicterus. Under these circumstances, bilirubin crosses an immature blood-brain barrier and precipitates in the basal ganglia and other areas of the brain. The consequences range from appreciable neurologic deficits to death. Treatment options include phototherapy, which converts bilirubin into water-soluble photoisomers that are excreted directly into bile, and exchange transfusion. The canalicular mechanisms responsible for bilirubin excretion are also immature at birth, and their maturation may lag behind that of UGT1A1; this can lead to transient conjugated neonatal hyperbilirubinemia, especially in infants with hemolysis.

Acquired conjugation defects

A modest reduction in bilirubin-conjugating capacity may be observed in advanced hepatitis or cirrhosis. However, in this setting, conjugation is better preserved than other aspects of bilirubin disposition, such as canalicular excretion. Various drugs, including pregnanediol, novobiocin, chloramphenicol, and gentamicin, may produce unconjugated hyperbilirubinemia by inhibiting UGT1A1 activity. Bilirubin conjugation may be inhibited by certain fatty acids that are present in breast milk but not serum of mothers whose infants have excessive neonatal hyperbilirubinemia (*breast milk jaundice*). Alternatively, there may be increased enterohepatic circulation of bilirubin in these infants. A recent study has correlated epidermal growth factor (EGF) content of breast milk with elevated bilirubin levels in these infants; however, a cause and effect relationship remains to be established. The pathogenesis of breast milk jaundice appears to differ from that of transient familial neonatal hyperbilirubinemia (Lucey-Driscoll syndrome), in which there is a UGT1A1 inhibitor in maternal serum.

HEREDITARY DEFECTS IN BILIRUBIN CONJUGATION

Three familial disorders characterized by differing degrees of unconjugated hyperbilirubinemia have long been recognized. The defining clinical features of each are described in the following sections (Table 37-1). While these disorders have been recognized for decades to reflect differing degrees of deficiency in the ability to conjugate bilirubin, recent advances in the molecular biology of the *UGT1* gene complex have elucidated their interrelationships and clarified previously puzzling features.

Crigler-Najjar syndrome, type I

CN-I is characterized by striking unconjugated hyperbilirubinemia of about 340–765 µmol/L (20–45 mg/dL) that appears in the neonatal period and persists for life. Other conventional hepatic biochemical tests such as serum aminotransferases and alkaline phosphatase are normal, and there is no evidence of hemolysis. Hepatic

histology is also essentially normal except for the occasional presence of bile plugs within canaliculi. Bilirubin glucuronides are virtually absent from the bile, and there is no detectable constitutive expression of UGT1A1 activity in hepatic tissue. Neither UGT1A1 activity nor the serum bilirubin concentration responds to administration of phenobarbital or other enzyme inducers. In the absence of conjugation, unconjugated bilirubin accumulates in plasma, from which it is eliminated very slowly by alternative pathways that include direct passage into the bile and small intestine. These account for the small amounts of urobilinogen found in feces. No bilirubin is found in the urine. First described in 1952, the disorder is rare (estimated prevalence, 0.6–1.0 per million). Many patients are from geographically or socially isolated communities in which consanguinity is common, and pedigree analyses show an autosomal recessive pattern of inheritance. The majority of patients (type IA) exhibit defects in the glucuronide conjugation of a spectrum of substrates in addition to bilirubin, including various drugs and other xenobiotics. These individuals have mutations in one of the common exons (2–5) of the *UGT1* gene (Fig. 37-2). In a smaller subset (type IB), the defect is limited largely to bilirubin conjugation, and the causative mutation is in the bilirubin-specific exon A1. Estrogen glucuronidation is mediated by UGT1A1 and is defective in all CN-I patients. More than 30 different genetic lesions of *UGT1A1* responsible for CN-I have been identified, including deletions, insertions, alterations in intron splice donor and

TABLE 37-1

PRINCIPAL DIFFERENTIAL CHARACTERISTICS OF GILBERT'S AND CRIGLER-NAJJAR SYNDROMES			
	CRIGLER-NAJJAR SYNDROME		
FEATURE	TYPE I	TYPE II	GILBERT'S SYNDROME
Total serum bilirubin, µmol/L (mg/dL)	310–755 (usually >345) (18–45 [usually >20])	100–430 (usually ≤345) (6–25 [usually ≤20])	Typically ≤70 µmol/L (≤4 mg/dL) in absence of fasting or hemolysis
Routine liver tests	Normal	Normal	Normal
Response to phenobarbital	None	Decreases bilirubin by >25%	Decreases bilirubin to normal
Kernicterus	Usual	Rare	No
Hepatic histology	Normal	Normal	Usually normal; increased lipofuscin pigment in some
Bile characteristics			
Color	Pale or colorless	Pigmented	Normal dark color
Bilirubin fractions	>90% unconjugated	Largest fraction (mean: 57%) monoconjugates	Mainly diconjugates but monoconjugates increased (mean: 23%)
Bilirubin UDP-glucuronosyltransferase activity	Typically absent; traces in some patients	Markedly reduced: 0–10% of normal	Reduced: typically 10–33% of normal
Inheritance (all autosomal)	Recessive	Predominantly recessive	Promoter mutation: recessive Missense mutations: 7 of 8 dominant; 1 reportedly recessive

acceptor sites, exon skipping, and point mutations that introduce premature stop codons or alter critical amino acids. Their common feature is that they all encode proteins with absent or, at most, traces of bilirubin-UDP-glucuronosyltransferase enzymatic activity.

Prior to the availability of phototherapy, most patients with CN-I died of bilirubin encephalopathy (*kernicterus*) in infancy or early childhood. A few lived as long as early adult life without overt neurologic damage, although more subtle testing usually indicated mild but progressive brain damage. In the absence of liver transplantation, death eventually supervened from late-onset bilirubin encephalopathy, which often followed a nonspecific febrile illness. Although isolated hepatocyte transplantation has been used in a small number of cases of CN-I, early liver transplantation (Chap. 46) remains the best hope to prevent brain injury and death.

Crigler-Najjar syndrome, type II (CN-II)

This condition was recognized as a distinct entity in 1962 and is characterized by marked unconjugated hyperbilirubinemia in the absence of abnormalities of other conventional hepatic biochemical tests, hepatic histology, or hemolysis. It differs from CN-I in several specific ways (Table 37-1): (1) Although there is considerable overlap, average bilirubin concentrations are lower in CN-II; (2) accordingly, CN-II is only infrequently associated with kernicterus; (3) bile is deeply colored, and bilirubin glucuronides are present, with a striking, characteristic increase in the proportion of monoglucuronides; (4) UGT1A1 in liver is usually present at reduced levels (typically ≤10% of normal) but may be undetectable by older, less sensitive assays; (5) while typically detected in infancy, hyperbilirubinemia was not recognized in some cases until later in life and, in one instance, at age 34. As with CN-I, most CN-II cases exhibit abnormalities in the conjugation of other compounds, such as salicylamide and menthol, but in some instances the defect appears limited to bilirubin. Reduction of serum bilirubin concentrations by >25% in response to enzyme inducers such as phenobarbital distinguishes CN-II from CN-I, although this response may not be elicited in early infancy and often is not accompanied by measurable UGT1A1 induction. Bilirubin concentrations during phenobarbital administration do not return to normal but are typically in the range of 51–86 μmol/L (3–5 mg/dL). Although the incidence of kernicterus in CN-II is low, instances have occurred, not only in infants but also in adolescents and adults, often in the setting of an intercurrent illness, fasting, or another factor that temporarily raises the serum bilirubin concentration above baseline and reduces serum albumin levels. For this reason, phenobarbital therapy is widely recommended, a single bedtime dose often sufficing to maintain clinically safe plasma bilirubin concentrations.

Over 77 different mutations in the *UGT1* gene have been identified as causing CN-I or CN-II. It was found that missense mutations are more common in CN-II patients, as would be expected in this less severe phenotype. Their common feature is that they encode for a bilirubin-UDP-glucuronosyltransferase with markedly reduced, but detectable, enzymatic activity. The spectrum of residual enzyme activity explains the spectrum of phenotypic severity of the resulting hyperbilirubinemia. Molecular analysis has established that a large majority of CN-II patients are either homozygotes or compound heterozygotes for CN-II mutations and that individuals carrying one mutated and one entirely normal allele have normal bilirubin concentrations.

Gilbert's syndrome

This syndrome is characterized by mild unconjugated hyperbilirubinemia, normal values for standard hepatic biochemical tests, and normal hepatic histology other than a modest increase of lipofuscin pigment in some patients. Serum bilirubin concentrations are most often <51 μmol/L (<3 mg/dL), although both higher and lower values are frequent. The clinical spectrum of hyperbilirubinemia fades into that of CN-II at serum bilirubin concentrations of 86–136 μmol/L (5–8 mg/dL). At the other end of the scale, the distinction between mild cases of GS and a normal state is often blurred. Bilirubin concentrations may fluctuate substantially in any given individual, and at least 25% of patients will exhibit temporarily normal values during prolonged follow-up. More elevated values are associated with stress, fatigue, alcohol use, reduced caloric intake, and intercurrent illness, while increased caloric intake or administration of enzyme-inducing agents produces lower bilirubin levels. GS is most often diagnosed at or shortly after puberty or in adult life during routine examinations that include multichannel biochemical analyses. UGT1A1 activity is typically reduced to 10–35% of normal, and bile pigments exhibit a characteristic increase in bilirubin monoglucuronides. Studies of radiobilirubin kinetics indicate that hepatic bilirubin clearance is reduced to an average of one-third of normal. Administration of phenobarbital normalizes both the serum bilirubin concentration and hepatic bilirubin clearance; however, failure of UGT1A1 activity to improve in many such instances suggests the possible coexistence of an additional defect. Compartmental analysis of bilirubin kinetic data suggests that GS patients have a defect in bilirubin uptake as well as in conjugation. Defect(s) in the hepatic uptake of other organic anions that at least partially share an uptake mechanism with bilirubin, such as sulfobromophthalein and indocyanine green (ICG), are observed in a minority of patients. The metabolism and transport of bile acids that do not utilize the bilirubin uptake mechanism, are normal. The magnitude of changes in the plasma bilirubin concentration induced by provocation tests such as 48 h of fasting or the IV administration of nicotinic acid have been reported to be of help in separating GS patients from normal individuals. Other studies dispute this assertion. Moreover, on theoretical grounds, the results of such studies should provide no more information than simple measurements of the baseline plasma bilirubin concentration. Family studies indicate that GS and hereditary hemolytic anemias such as hereditary spherocytosis, glucose-6-phosphate dehydrogenase deficiency, and β-thalassemia trait sort independently. Reports of hemolysis in up to 50% of GS patients are believed to reflect better case finding, since patients with both GS and hemolysis have higher bilirubin concentrations, and are more likely to be jaundiced, than patients with either defect alone.

GS is common, with many series placing its prevalence at ≥8%. Males predominate over females by reported ratios ranging from 1.5:1 to >7:1. However, these ratios may have a large artifactual component since normal males have higher mean bilirubin levels than normal females, but the diagnosis of GS is often based on comparison to normal ranges established in men. The high prevalence of GS in the general population may explain the reported frequency of mild unconjugated hyperbilirubinemia in liver transplant recipients. The disposition of most xenobiotics metabolized by glucuronidation appears to be normal in GS, as is oxidative drug metabolism in the majority of reported studies. The principal exception is the metabolism of the antitumor agent irinotecan (CPT-11), whose active metabolite (SN-38) is glucuronidated specifically by bilirubin-UDP-glucuronosyltransferase. Administration of CPT-11 to patients with GS has resulted in several toxicities, including intractable diarrhea and myelosuppression. Some reports also suggest abnormal disposition of menthol, estradiol benzoate, acetaminophen, tolbutamide, and rifamycin SV. Although some of these studies have been disputed, and there have been no reports of clinical complications from use of these agents in GS, prudence should be exercised in prescribing them, or any agents metabolized primarily by glucuronidation, in this condition. It should also be noted that the HIV protease inhibitors indinavir and atazanavir can inhibit UGT1A1, resulting in hyperbilirubinemia that is most pronounced in patients with preexisting GS.

Most older pedigree studies of GS were consistent with autosomal dominant inheritance with variable expressivity. However, studies of the UGT1 gene in GS have indicated a variety of molecular genetic bases

for the phenotypic picture and several different patterns of inheritance. Studies in Europe and the United States found that nearly all patients had normal coding regions for UGT1A1 but were homozygous for the insertion of an extra TA (i.e., A[TA]₇TAA rather than A[TA]₆TAA) in the promoter region of the first exon. This appeared to be necessary, but not sufficient, for clinically expressed GS, since 15% of normal controls were also homozygous for this variant. While normal by standard criteria, these individuals had somewhat higher bilirubin concentrations than the rest of the controls studied. Heterozygotes for this abnormality had bilirubin concentrations identical to those homozygous for the normal A[TA]₆TAA allele. The prevalence of the A[TA]₇TAA allele in a general Western population is 30%, in which case 9% would be homozygotes. This is slightly higher than the prevalence of GS based on purely phenotypic parameters. It was suggested that additional variables, such as mild hemolysis or a defect in bilirubin uptake, might be among the factors enhancing phenotypic expression of the defect.

Phenotypic expression of GS due solely to the A[TA]₇TAA promoter abnormality is inherited as an autosomal recessive trait. A number of CN-II kindreds have been identified in whom there is also an allele containing a normal coding region but the A[TA]₇TAA promoter abnormality. CN-II heterozygotes who have the A[TA]₆TAA promoter are phenotypically normal, whereas those with the A[TA]₇TAA promoter express the phenotypic picture of GS. GS in such kindreds may also result from homozygosity for the A[TA]₇TAA promoter abnormality. Seven different missense mutations in the UGT1 gene that reportedly cause GS with dominant inheritance have been found in Japanese individuals. Another Japanese patient with mild unconjugated hyperbilirubinemia was homozygous for a missense mutation in exon 5. GS in her family appeared to be recessive. Missense mutations causing GS have not been reported outside of certain Asian populations.

DISORDERS OF BILIRUBIN METABOLISM LEADING TO MIXED OR PREDOMINANTLY CONJUGATED HYPERBILIRUBINEMIA

In hyperbilirubinemia due to acquired liver disease (e.g., acute hepatitis, common bile duct stone), there are usually elevations in the serum concentrations of both conjugated and unconjugated bilirubin. Although biliary tract obstruction or hepatocellular cholestatic injury may present on occasion with a predominantly conjugated hyperbilirubinemia, it is generally not possible to differentiate intrahepatic from extrahepatic causes of jaundice based on the serum levels or relative proportions of unconjugated and conjugated bilirubin. The major reason for determining the amounts of conjugated and unconjugated bilirubin in the serum is for the initial differentiation of hepatic parenchymal and obstructive disorders (mixed conjugated and unconjugated hyperbilirubinemia) from the inheritable and hemolytic disorders discussed earlier that are associated with unconjugated hyperbilirubinemia.

FAMILIAL DEFECTS IN HEPATIC EXCRETORY FUNCTION

Dubin-Johnson syndrome (DJS)

This benign, relatively rare disorder is characterized by low-grade, predominantly conjugated hyperbilirubinemia (Table 37-2). Total bilirubin concentrations are typically between 34 and 85 μmol/L (2 and 5 mg/dL) but on occasion can be in the normal range or as high as 340–430 μmol/L (20–25 mg/dL) and can fluctuate widely in any given patient. The degree of hyperbilirubinemia may be increased by intercurrent illness, oral contraceptive use, and pregnancy. As the hyperbilirubinemia is due to a predominant rise in conjugated bilirubin, bilirubinuria is characteristically present. Aside from elevated serum bilirubin levels, other routine laboratory tests are normal. Physical examination is usually normal except for jaundice, although an occasional patient may have hepatosplenomegaly.

Patients with DJS are usually asymptomatic, although some may have vague constitutional symptoms. These latter patients have usually undergone extensive and

often unnecessary diagnostic examinations for unexplained jaundice and have high levels of anxiety. In women, the condition may be subclinical until the patient becomes pregnant or receives oral contraceptives, at which time chemical hyperbilirubinemia becomes frank jaundice. Even in these situations, other routine liver function tests, including serum alkaline phosphatase and transaminase activities, are normal.

A cardinal feature of DJS is the accumulation in the lysosomes of centrilobular hepatocytes of dark, coarsely granular pigment. As a result, the liver may be grossly black in appearance. This pigment is thought to be derived from epinephrine metabolites that are not excreted normally. The pigment may disappear during bouts of viral hepatitis, only to reaccumulate slowly after recovery.

Biliary excretion of a number of anionic compounds is compromised in DJS. These include various cholecystographic agents, as well as sulfobromophthalein (Bromsulphalein, BSP), a synthetic dye formerly used in a test of liver function. In this test, the rate of disappearance of BSP from plasma was determined following bolus IV administration. BSP is conjugated with glutathione in the hepatocyte; the resulting conjugate is normally excreted rapidly into the bile canaliculus. Patients with DJS exhibit characteristic rises in plasma concentrations at 90 min after injection, due to reflux of conjugated BSP into the circulation from the hepatocyte. Dyes such as ICG that are taken up by hepatocytes but are not further metabolized prior to biliary excretion do not show this reflux phenomenon. Continuous BSP infusion studies suggest a reduction in the t_{max} for

TABLE 37-2

PRINCIPAL DIFFERENTIAL CHARACTERISTICS OF INHERITABLE DISORDERS OF BILE CANALICULAR FUNCTION

	DJS	ROTOR	PFIC1	BRIC1	PFIC2	BRIC2	PFIC3
Gene	ABCCA	?	ATP8B1	ATP8B1	ABCB11	ABCB11	ABCB4
Protein	MRP2	?	FIC1	FIC1	BSEP	BSEP	MDR3
Cholestasis	No	No	Yes	Episodic	Yes	Episodic	Yes
Serum γ-GT	Normal	Normal	Normal	Normal	Normal	Normal	↑↑
Serum bile acids	Normal	Normal	↑↑	↑↑ during episodes	↑↑	↑↑ during episodes	↑↑
Clinical features	Mild conjugated hyperbilirubinemia; otherwise normal liver function; dark pigment in liver; characteristic pattern of urinary coproporphyrins	Mild conjugated hyperbilirubinemia; otherwise normal liver function; liver without abnormal pigmentation	Severe cholestasis beginning in childhood	Recurrent episodes of cholestasis beginning at any age	Severe cholestasis beginning in childhood	Recurrent episodes of cholestasis beginning at any age	Severe cholestasis beginning in childhood; decreased phospholipids in bile

Abbreviations: BRIC, benign recurrent intrahepatic cholestasis; BSEP, bile salt excretory protein; DJS, Dubin-Johnson syndrome; γ-GT, γ-glutamyltransferase; MRP2, multidrug resistance–associated protein 2; PFIC, progressive familial intrahepatic cholestasis; ↑↑, increased.

biliary excretion. Bile acid disposition, including hepatocellular uptake and biliary excretion, is normal in DJS. These patients have normal serum and biliary bile acid concentrations and do not have pruritus.

By analogy with findings in several mutant rat strains, the selective defect in biliary excretion of bilirubin conjugates and certain other classes of organic compounds, but not of bile acids, that characterizes DJS in humans was found to reflect defective expression of MRP2, an ATP-dependent canalicular membrane transporter. Several different mutations in the *MRP2* gene produce the Dubin-Johnson phenotype, which has an autosomal recessive pattern of inheritance. Although MRP2 is undoubtedly important in the biliary excretion of conjugated bilirubin, the fact that this pigment is still excreted in the absence of MRP2 suggests that other, as yet uncharacterized, transport proteins may serve in a secondary role in this process.

Patients with DJS also have a diagnostic abnormality in urinary coproporphyrin excretion. There are two naturally occurring coproporphyrin isomers, I and III. Normally, ~75% of the coproporphyrin in urine is isomer III. In urine from DJS patients, total coproporphyrin content is normal, but >80% is isomer I. Heterozygotes for the syndrome show an intermediate pattern. The molecular basis for this phenomenon remains unclear.

Rotor syndrome

This benign, autosomal recessive disorder is clinically similar to DJS (Table 37-2), although it is seen even less frequently. A major phenotypic difference is that the liver in patients with Rotor syndrome has no increased pigmentation and appears totally normal. The only abnormality in routine laboratory tests is an elevation of total serum bilirubin, due to a predominant rise in conjugated bilirubin. This is accompanied by bilirubinuria. Several additional features differentiate Rotor syndrome from DJS. In Rotor syndrome, the gallbladder is usually visualized on oral cholecystography, in contrast to the nonvisualization that is typical of DJS. The pattern of urinary coproporphyrin excretion also differs. The pattern in Rotor syndrome resembles that of many acquired disorders of hepatobiliary function, in which coproporphyrin I, the major coproporphyrin isomer in bile, refluxes from the hepatocyte back into the circulation and is excreted in urine. Thus, total urinary coproporphyrin excretion is substantially increased in Rotor syndrome, in contrast to the normal levels seen in DJS. Although the fraction of coproporphyrin I in urine is elevated, it is usually <70% of the total, compared with ≥80% in DJS. The disorders also can be distinguished by their patterns of BSP excretion. Although clearance of BSP from plasma is delayed in Rotor syndrome, there is no reflux of conjugated BSP back into the circulation

as seen in DJS. Kinetic analysis of plasma BSP infusion studies suggests the presence of a defect in intrahepatocellular storage of this compound. This has never been demonstrated directly, and the molecular basis of Rotor syndrome remains unknown.

Benign recurrent intrahepatic cholestasis (BRIC)

This rare disorder is characterized by recurrent attacks of pruritus and jaundice. The typical episode begins with mild malaise and elevations in serum aminotransferase levels, followed rapidly by rises in alkaline phosphatase and conjugated bilirubin and onset of jaundice and itching. The first one or two episodes may be misdiagnosed as acute viral hepatitis. The cholestatic episodes, which may begin in childhood or adulthood, can vary in duration from several weeks to months, followed by a complete clinical and biochemical resolution. Intervals between attacks may vary from several months to years. Between episodes, physical examination is normal, as are serum levels of bile acids, bilirubin, transaminases, and alkaline phosphatase. The disorder is familial and has an autosomal recessive pattern of inheritance. BRIC is considered a benign disorder in that it does not lead to cirrhosis or end-stage liver disease. However, the episodes of jaundice and pruritus can be prolonged and debilitating, and some patients have undergone liver transplantation to relieve the intractable and disabling symptoms. Treatment during the cholestatic episodes is symptomatic; there is no specific treatment to prevent or shorten the occurrence of episodes.

A gene termed *FIC1* was recently identified and found to be mutated in patients with BRIC. Curiously, this gene is expressed strongly in the small intestine but only weakly in the liver. The protein encoded by *FIC1* shows little similarity to those that have been shown to play a role in bile canalicular excretion of various compounds. Rather, it appears to be a member of a P-type ATPase family that transports aminophospholipids from the outer to the inner leaflet of a variety of cell membranes. Its relationship to the pathobiology of this disorder remains unclear. A second phenotypically identical form of BRIC, termed BRIC type 2, has been described resulting from mutations in the bile salt excretory protein (BSEP), the protein that is defective in progressive familial intrahepatic cholestasis type 2 (Table 37-2). How some mutations in this protein result in the episodic BRIC phenotype is unknown.

Progressive familial intrahepatic cholestasis (FIC)

This name is applied to three phenotypically related syndromes (Table 37-2). Progressive FIC type 1 (Byler disease) presents in early infancy as cholestasis that may be initially episodic. However, in contrast to BRIC, Byler's disease progresses to malnutrition, growth retardation, and end-stage liver disease during childhood. This disorder is also a consequence of an *FIC1* mutation. The functional relationship of the FIC1 protein to the pathogenesis of cholestasis in these disorders is unknown. Two other types of progressive FIC (types 2 and 3) have been described. Progressive FIC type 2 is associated with a mutation in the protein named *sister of p-glycoprotein*, which is the major bile canalicular exporter of bile acids and is also known as *bile salt*

excretory protein. As noted earlier, some mutations of this protein are associated with BRIC type 2, rather than the progressive FIC type 2 phenotype. Progressive FIC type 3 has been associated with a mutation of MDR3, a protein that is essential for normal hepatocellular excretion of phospholipids across the bile canaliculus. Although all three types of progressive FIC have similar clinical phenotypes, only type 3 is associated with high serum levels of γ-glutamyltransferase activity. In contrast, activity of this enzyme is normal or only mildly elevated in symptomatic BRIC and progressive FIC types 1 and 2.

CHAPTER 38

ACUTE VIRAL HEPATITIS

Jules L. Dienstag

Acute viral hepatitis is a systemic infection affecting the liver predominantly. Almost all cases of acute viral hepatitis are caused by one of five viral agents: hepatitis A virus (HAV), hepatitis B virus (HBV), hepatitis C virus (HCV), the HBV-associated delta agent or hepatitis D virus (HDV), and hepatitis E virus (HEV). Other transfusion-transmitted agents (e.g., "hepatitis G" virus and "TT" virus) have been identified but do not cause hepatitis. All these human hepatitis viruses are RNA viruses, except for hepatitis B, which is a DNA virus. Although these agents can be distinguished by their molecular and antigenic properties, all types of viral hepatitis produce clinically similar illnesses. These range from asymptomatic and inapparent to fulminant and fatal acute infections common to all types, on the one hand, and from subclinical persistent infections to rapidly progressive chronic liver disease with cirrhosis and even hepatocellular carcinoma, common to the blood-borne types (HBV, HCV, and HDV), on the other.

VIROLOGY AND ETIOLOGY

Hepatitis A

Hepatitis A virus is a nonenveloped 27-nm, heat-, acid-, and ether-resistant RNA virus in the *Hepatovirus* genus of the picornavirus family **(Fig. 38-1)**. Its virion contains four capsid polypeptides, designated VP1 to VP4, which are cleaved posttranslationally from the polyprotein product of a 7500-nucleotide genome. Inactivation of viral activity can be achieved by boiling for 1 min, by contact with formaldehyde and chlorine, or by ultraviolet irradiation. Despite nucleotide sequence variation of up to 20% among isolates of HAV, and despite the recognition of four genotypes affecting humans, all strains of this virus are immunologically indistinguishable and belong to one serotype. Hepatitis A has an incubation period of ~4 weeks. Its replication is limited to the liver, but the virus is present in the liver, bile, stools, and blood during the late

FIGURE 38-1
Electron micrographs of hepatitis A virus particles and serum from a patient with hepatitis B. *Left:* 27-nm hepatitis A virus particles purified from stool of a patient with acute hepatitis A and aggregated by antibody to hepatitis A virus. ***Right:*** Concentrated serum from a patient with hepatitis B, demonstrating the 42-nm virions, tubular forms, and spherical 22-nm particles of hepatitis B surface antigen. 132,000×. (Hepatitis D resembles 42-nm virions of hepatitis B but is smaller, 35–37 nm; hepatitis E resembles hepatitis A virus but is slightly larger, 32–34 nm; hepatitis C has been visualized as a 55-nm particle.)

FIGURE 38-2
Scheme of typical clinical and laboratory features of hepatitis A.

incubation period and acute preicteric phase of illness. Despite persistence of virus in the liver, viral shedding in feces, viremia, and infectivity diminish rapidly once jaundice becomes apparent. HAV can be cultivated reproducibly in vitro.

Antibodies to HAV (anti-HAV) can be detected during acute illness when serum aminotransferase activity is elevated and fecal HAV shedding is still occurring. This early antibody response is predominantly of the IgM class and persists for several months, rarely for 6–12 months. During convalescence, however, anti-HAV of the IgG class becomes the predominant antibody (Fig. 38-2). Therefore, the diagnosis of hepatitis A is made during acute illness by demonstrating anti-HAV of the IgM class. After acute illness, anti-HAV of the IgG class remains detectable indefinitely, and patients with serum anti-HAV are immune to reinfection. Neutralizing antibody activity parallels the appearance of anti-HAV, and the IgG anti-HAV present in immune globulin accounts for the protection it affords against HAV infection.

Hepatitis B

Hepatitis B virus is a DNA virus with a remarkably compact genomic structure; despite its small, circular, 3200-bp size, HBV DNA codes for four sets of viral products with a complex, multiparticle structure. HBV achieves its genomic economy by relying on an efficient strategy of encoding proteins from four overlapping genes: S, C, P, and X (Fig. 38-3), as detailed later. Once thought to be unique among viruses, HBV is now recognized as one of a family of animal viruses, hepadnaviruses (hepatotropic DNA viruses), and is classified as hepadnavirus type 1. Similar viruses infect certain species of woodchucks, ground and tree squirrels, and Pekin ducks, to mention the most carefully characterized. Like HBV, all have the same distinctive three morphologic forms, have counterparts to the envelope and nucleocapsid virus antigens of HBV, replicate in the

FIGURE 38-3
Compact genomic structure of HBV. This structure, with overlapping genes, permits HBV to code for multiple proteins. The S gene codes for the "major" envelope protein, HBsAg. Pre-S1 and pre-S2, upstream of S, combine with S to code for two larger proteins, "middle" protein, the product of pre-S2 + S, and "large" protein, the product of pre-S1 + pre-S2 + S. The largest gene, P, codes for DNA polymerase. The C gene codes for two nucleocapsid proteins, HBeAg, a soluble, secreted protein (initiation from the pre-C region of the gene), and HBcAg, the intracellular core protein (initiation after pre-C). The X gene codes for HBxAg, which can transactivate the transcription of cellular and viral genes; its clinical relevance is not known, but it may contribute to carcinogenesis by binding to p53.

liver but exist in extrahepatic sites, contain their own endogenous DNA polymerase, have partially double-strand and partially single-strand genomes, are associated with acute and chronic hepatitis and hepatocellular carcinoma, and rely on a replicative strategy unique among DNA viruses but typical of retroviruses. Instead of DNA replication directly from a DNA template, hepadnaviruses rely on reverse transcription (effected by the DNA polymerase) of minus-strand DNA from a "pregenomic" RNA intermediate. Then plus-strand DNA is transcribed from the minus-strand DNA template by the DNA-dependent DNA polymerase and converted in the hepatocyte nucleus to a covalently closed circular DNA, which serves as a template for messenger RNA and pregenomic RNA. Viral proteins are translated by the messenger RNA, and the proteins and genome are packaged into virions and secreted from the hepatocyte. Although HBV is difficult to cultivate in vitro in the conventional sense from clinical material, several cell lines have been transfected with HBV DNA. Such transfected cells support in vitro replication of the intact virus and its component proteins.

Viral proteins and particles

Of the three particulate forms of HBV (Table 38-1), the most numerous are the 22-nm particles, which

TABLE 38-1

NOMENCLATURE AND FEATURES OF HEPATITIS VIRUSES

HEPATITIS TYPE	VIRUS PARTICLE, nm	MORPHOLOGY	GENOME[a]	CLASSIFICATION	ANTIGEN(S)	ANTIBODIES	REMARKS
HAV	27	Icosahedral nonenveloped	7.5-kb RNA, linear, ss, +	Hepatovirus	HAV	Anti-HAV	Early fecal shedding Diagnosis: IgM anti-HAV Previous infection: IgG anti-HAV
HBV	42	Double-shelled virion (surface and core) spherical	3.2-kb DNA, circular, ss/ds	Hepadnavirus	HBsAg HBcAg HBeAg	Anti-HBs Anti-HBc Anti-HBe	Bloodborne virus; carrier state Acute diagnosis: HBsAg, IgM anti-HBc Chronic diagnosis: IgG anti-HBc, HBsAg Markers of replication: HBeAg, HBV DNA Liver, lymphocytes, other organs
	27	Nucleocapsid core			HBcAg HBeAg	Anti-HBc Anti-HBe	Nucleocapsid contains DNA and DNA polymerase; present in hepatocyte nucleus; HBcAg does not circulate; HBeAg (soluble, nonparticulate) and HBV DNA circulate—correlate with infectivity and complete virions
	22	Spherical and filamentous; represents excess virus coat material			HBsAg	Anti-HBs	HBsAg detectable in >95% of patients with acute hepatitis B; found in serum, body fluids, hepatocyte cytoplasm; anti-HBs appears following infection—protective antibody
HCV	Approx. 40–60	Enveloped	9.4-kb RNA, linear, ss, +	Hepacivirus	HCV C100-3 C33c C22-3 NS5	Anti-HCV	Bloodborne agent, formerly labeled non-A, non-B hepatitis Acute diagnosis: anti-HCV (C33c, C22-3, NS5), HCV RNA Chronic diagnosis: anti-HCV (C100-3, C33c, C22-3, NS5) and HCV RNA; cytoplasmic location in hepatocytes
HDV	35–37	Enveloped hybrid particle with HBsAg coat and HDV core	1.7-kb RNA, circular, ss, –	Resembles viroids and plant satellite viruses	HBsAg HDV antigen	Anti-HBs Anti-HDV	Defective RNA virus, requires helper function of HEV (hepadnaviruses); HDV antigen present in hepatocyte nucleus Diagnosis: anti-HDV, HDV RNA; HBV/HDV coinfection—IgM anti-HBc and anti-HDV; HDV superinfection—IgG anti-HBc and anti-HDV
HEV	32–34	Nonenveloped icosahedral	7.6-kb RNA, linear, ss, +	Hepevirus	HEV antigen	Anti-HEV	Agent of enterically transmitted hepatitis; rare in USA; occurs in Asia, Mediterranean countries, Central America Diagnosis: IgM/IgG anti-HEV (assays not routinely available); virus in stool, bile, hepatocyte cytoplasm

[a]ss, single-strand; ss/ds, partially single-strand, partially double-strand; –, minus-strand; +, plus-strand.

appear as spherical or long filamentous forms; these are antigenically indistinguishable from the outer surface or envelope protein of HBV and are thought to represent excess viral envelope protein. Outnumbered in serum by a factor of 100 or 1000 to 1 compared with the spheres and tubules are large, 42-nm, double-shelled spherical particles, which represent the intact hepatitis B virion (Fig. 38-1). The envelope protein expressed on the outer surface of the virion and on the smaller spherical and tubular structures is referred to as *hepatitis B surface antigen* (HBsAg). The concentration of HBsAg and virus particles in the blood may reach 500 μg/mL and 10 trillion particles per milliliter, respectively. The envelope protein, HBsAg, is the product of the S gene of HBV.

A number of different HBsAg subdeterminants have been identified. There is a common group-reactive antigen, *a*, shared by all HBsAg isolates. In addition, HBsAg may contain one of several subtype-specific antigens—namely, *d* or *y*, *w* or *r*—as well as other more recently characterized specificities. Hepatitis B isolates fall into one of at least eight subtypes and eight genotypes (A–H). Geographic distribution of genotypes and subtypes varies; genotypes A (corresponding to subtype *adw*) and D (*ayw*) predominate in the United States and Europe, while genotypes B (*adw*) and C (*adr*) predominate in Asia. Clinical course and outcome are independent of subtype, but preliminary reports suggest that genotype B is associated with less rapidly progressive liver disease and a lower likelihood, or delayed appearance, of hepatocellular carcinoma than genotype C. Patients with genotype A appear to be more likely to clear circulating viremia and to achieve HBsAg seroconversion, both spontaneously and in response to antiviral therapy. In addition, "precore" mutations are favored by certain genotypes (discussed later).

Upstream of the S gene are the pre-S genes (Fig. 38-3), which code for pre-S gene products, including receptors on the HBV surface for polymerized human serum albumin and for hepatocyte membrane proteins. The pre-S region actually consists of both pre-S1 and pre-S2. Depending on where translation is initiated, three potential HBsAg gene products are synthesized. The protein product of the S gene is HBsAg (*major protein*), the product of the S region plus the adjacent pre-S2 region is the *middle protein*, and the product of the pre-S1 plus pre-S2 plus S regions is the *large protein*. Compared with the smaller spherical and tubular particles of HBV, complete 42-nm virions are enriched in the large protein. Both pre-S proteins and their respective antibodies can be detected during HBV infection, and the period of pre-S antigenemia appears to coincide with other markers of virus replication, as detailed later.

The intact 42-nm virion contains a 27-nm nucleocapsid core particle. Nucleocapsid proteins are coded for by the C gene. The antigen expressed on the surface of the nucleocapsid core is referred to as *hepatitis B core antigen* (HBcAg), and its corresponding antibody is anti-HBc. A third HBV antigen is *hepatitis B e antigen* (HBeAg), a soluble, nonparticulate, nucleocapsid protein that is immunologically distinct from intact HBcAg but is a product of the same C gene. The C gene has two initiation codons, a precore and a core region (Fig. 38-3). If translation is initiated at the precore region, the protein product is HBeAg, which has a signal peptide that binds it to the smooth endoplasmic reticulum and leads to its secretion into the circulation. If translation begins with the core region, HBcAg is the protein product; it has no signal peptide, it is not secreted, but it assembles into nucleocapsid particles, which bind to and incorporate RNA, and which, ultimately, contain HBV DNA. Also packaged within the nucleocapsid core is a DNA polymerase, which directs replication and repair of HBV DNA. When packaging within viral proteins is complete, synthesis of the incomplete plus strand stops; this accounts for the single-strand gap and for differences in the size of the gap. HBcAg particles remain in the hepatocyte, where they are readily detectable by immunohistochemical staining, and are exported after encapsidation by an envelope of HBsAg. Therefore, naked core particles do not circulate in the serum. The secreted nucleocapsid protein, HBeAg, provides a convenient, readily detectable, qualitative marker of HBV replication and relative infectivity.

HBsAg-positive serum containing HBeAg is more likely to be highly infectious and to be associated with the presence of hepatitis B virions (and detectable HBV DNA, discussed later) than HBeAg-negative or anti-HBe-positive serum. For example, HBsAg carrier mothers who are HBeAg-positive almost invariably (>90%) transmit hepatitis B infection to their offspring, whereas HBsAg carrier mothers with anti-HBe rarely (10–15%) infect their offspring.

Early during the course of acute hepatitis B, HBeAg appears transiently; its disappearance may be a harbinger of clinical improvement and resolution of infection. Persistence of HBeAg in serum beyond the first three months of acute infection may be predictive of the development of chronic infection, and the presence of HBeAg during chronic hepatitis B is associated with ongoing viral replication, infectivity, and inflammatory liver injury.

The third of the HBV genes is the largest, the P gene (Fig. 38-3), which codes for the DNA polymerase; as noted earlier, this enzyme has both DNA-dependent DNA polymerase and RNA-dependent reverse transcriptase activities. The fourth gene, X, codes for a small, nonparticulate protein, *hepatitis B x antigen* (HBxAg), that is capable of transactivating the transcription of both viral and cellular genes (Fig. 38-3). In the cytoplasm, HBxAg effects calcium release (possibly from mitochondria), which activates signal-transduction pathways that lead to stimulation of HBV reverse transcription and HBV DNA replication. Such transactivation may enhance the replication of HBV, leading to the clinical association observed between the expression of HBxAg and antibodies to it in patients with severe chronic hepatitis and hepatocellular carcinoma. The transactivating activity can enhance the transcription and replication of other viruses besides HBV, such as HIV. Cellular processes transactivated by X include the human interferon γ gene and class I major histocompatibility genes; potentially, these effects could contribute to enhanced susceptibility of HBV-infected hepatocytes to cytolytic T cells. The expression of X can also induce programmed cell death (apoptosis).

Serologic and virologic markers

After a person is infected with HBV, the first virologic marker detectable in serum within 1–12 weeks, usually between 8–12 weeks, is HBsAg **(Fig. 38-4)**. Circulating HBsAg precedes elevations of serum aminotransferase activity and clinical symptoms by 2–6 weeks and remains detectable during the entire icteric or symptomatic phase of acute hepatitis B and beyond. In typical cases, HBsAg becomes undetectable 1–2 months after the onset of jaundice and rarely persists beyond 6 months. After HBsAg disappears, antibody to HBsAg (anti-HBs) becomes detectable in serum and remains detectable indefinitely thereafter. Because HBcAg is intracellular and, when in the serum, sequestered within an HBsAg coat, naked core particles do not circulate in serum and, therefore, HBcAg is not detectable routinely in the serum of patients with HBV infection. By contrast, anti-HBc is readily demonstrable in serum, beginning within the first 1–2 weeks after the appearance of HBsAg and preceding detectable levels of anti-HBs by

weeks to months. Because variability exists in the time of appearance of anti-HBs after HBV infection, occasionally a gap of several weeks or longer may separate the disappearance of HBsAg and the appearance of anti-HBs. During this "gap" or "window" period, anti-HBc may represent the only serologic evidence of current or recent HBV infection, and blood containing anti-HBc in the absence of HBsAg and anti-HBs has been implicated in the development of transfusion-associated hepatitis B. In part because the sensitivity of immunoassays for HBsAg and anti-HBs has increased, however, this window period is rarely encountered. In some persons, years after HBV infection, anti-HBc may persist in the circulation longer than anti-HBs. Therefore, isolated anti-HBc does not necessarily indicate active virus replication; most instances of isolated anti-HBc represent hepatitis B infection in the remote past. Rarely, however, isolated anti-HBc represents low-level hepatitis B viremia, with HBsAg below the detection threshold; occasionally, isolated anti-HBc represents a cross-reacting or false-positive immunologic specificity. Recent and remote HBV infections can be distinguished by determination of the immunoglobulin class of anti-HBc. Anti-HBc of the IgM class (IgM anti-HBc) predominates during the first 6 months after acute infection, whereas IgG anti-HBc is the predominant class of anti-HBc beyond 6 months. Therefore, patients with current or recent acute hepatitis B, including those in the anti-HBc window, have IgM anti-HBc in their serum. In patients who have recovered from hepatitis B in the remote past as well as those with chronic HBV infection, anti-HBc is predominantly of the IgG class. Infrequently, in ≤1–5% of patients with acute HBV infection, levels of HBsAg are too low to be detected; in such cases, the presence of IgM anti-HBc establishes the diagnosis of acute hepatitis B. When isolated anti-HBc occurs in the rare patient with chronic hepatitis B whose HBsAg level is below the sensitivity threshold of contemporary immunoassays (a low-level carrier), the anti-HBc is of the IgG class. Generally, in persons who have recovered from hepatitis B, anti-HBs and anti-HBc persist indefinitely.

The temporal association between the appearance of anti-HBs and resolution of HBV infection as well as the observation that persons with anti-HBs in serum are protected against reinfection with HBV suggests that *anti-HBs is the protective antibody*. Therefore, strategies for prevention of HBV infection are based on providing susceptible persons with circulating anti-HBs (discussed later). Occasionally, in 10–20% of patients with chronic hepatitis B, low-level, low-affinity anti-HBs can be detected. This antibody is directed against a subtype determinant different from that represented by the patient's HBsAg; its presence is thought to reflect the stimulation of a related clone of antibody-forming cells, but it has no clinical relevance and does not signal

FIGURE 38-4
Scheme of typical clinical and laboratory features of acute hepatitis B.

imminent clearance of hepatitis B. These patients with HBsAg and such nonneutralizing anti-HBs should be categorized as having chronic HBV infection.

The other readily detectable serologic marker of HBV infection, HBeAg, appears concurrently with or shortly after HBsAg. Its appearance coincides temporally with high levels of virus replication and reflects the presence of circulating intact virions and detectable HBV DNA (with the notable exception of patients with precore mutations who cannot synthesize HBeAg—see "Molecular Variants"). Pre-S1 and pre-S2 proteins are also expressed during periods of peak replication, but assays for these gene products are not routinely available. In self-limited HBV infections, HBeAg becomes undetectable shortly after peak elevations in aminotransferase activity, before the disappearance of HBsAg, and anti-HBe then becomes detectable, coinciding with a period of relatively lower infectivity (Fig. 38-4). Because markers of HBV replication appear transiently during acute infection, testing for such markers is of little clinical utility in typical cases of acute HBV infection. In contrast, markers of HBV replication provide valuable information in patients with protracted infections.

Departing from the pattern typical of acute HBV infections, in chronic HBV infection, HBsAg remains detectable beyond 6 months, anti-HBc is primarily of the IgG class, and anti-HBs is either undetectable or detectable at low levels (see "Laboratory Features") **(Fig. 38-5)**. During early chronic HBV infection, HBV DNA can be detected both in serum and in hepatocyte nuclei, where it is present in free or episomal form. This *replicative stage* of HBV infection is the time of maximal infectivity and liver injury; HBeAg is a qualitative marker and HBV DNA a quantitative marker of this replicative phase, during which all three forms of HBV circulate, including intact virions. Over time, the replicative phase of chronic HBV infection gives way to a relatively *nonreplicative phase*. This occurs at a rate of ~10% per year and is accompanied by seroconversion from HBeAg-positive to anti-HBe-positive. In most cases, this seroconversion coincides with a transient, acute hepatitis-like elevation in aminotransferase activity, believed to reflect cell-mediated immune clearance of virus-infected hepatocytes. In the nonreplicative phase of chronic infection, when HBV DNA is demonstrable in hepatocyte nuclei, it tends to be integrated into the host genome. In this phase, only spherical and tubular forms of HBV, *not intact virions*, circulate, and liver injury tends to subside. Most such patients would be characterized as *inactive HBV carriers*. In reality, the designations *replicative* and *nonreplicative* are only relative; even in the so-called nonreplicative phase, HBV replication can be detected at levels of ~$\leq 10^3$ virions with highly sensitive amplification probes such as the polymerase chain reaction (PCR); below this replication

FIGURE 38-5
Scheme of typical laboratory features of wild-type chronic hepatitis B. HBeAg and HBV DNA can be detected in serum during the *replicative phase* of chronic infection, which is associated with infectivity and liver injury. Seroconversion from the replicative phase to the *nonreplicative phase* occurs at a rate of ~10% per year and is heralded by an acute hepatitis–like elevation of ALT activity; during the nonreplicative phase, infectivity and liver injury are limited. In HBeAg-negative chronic hepatitis B associated with mutations in the precore region of the HBV genome, replicative chronic hepatitis B occurs in the absence of HBeAg.

threshold, liver injury and infectivity of HBV are limited to negligible. Still, the distinctions are pathophysiologically and clinically meaningful. Occasionally, nonreplicative HBV infection converts back to replicative infection. Such spontaneous reactivations are accompanied by re-expression of HBeAg and HBV DNA, and sometimes of IgM anti-HBc, as well as by exacerbations of liver injury. Because high-titer IgM anti-HBc can reappear during acute exacerbations of chronic hepatitis B, relying on IgM anti-HBc versus IgG anti-HBc to distinguish between acute and chronic hepatitis B infection, respectively, may not always be reliable; in such cases, patient history is invaluable in helping to distinguish de novo acute hepatitis B infection from acute exacerbation of chronic hepatitis B infection.

Molecular variants

Variation occurs throughout the HBV genome, and clinical isolates of HBV that do not express typical viral proteins have been attributed to mutations in individual or even multiple gene locations. For example, variants have been described that lack nucleocapsid proteins, envelope proteins, or both. Two categories of naturally occurring HBV variants have attracted the most attention. One of these was identified initially in Mediterranean countries among patients with an unusual serologic clinical profile. They have severe chronic HBV infection and detectable HBV DNA but with anti-HBe instead of HBeAg. These patients were found to be infected with an HBV mutant that contained an alteration in the precore region rendering the virus incapable of encoding HBeAg. Although several potential mutation sites exist in the pre-C region, the region of the C gene necessary for the expression of HBeAg (see "Virology and Etiology"), the most commonly encountered in such patients is a single base substitution, from G to A, which occurs in the second to last codon of the pre-C gene at nucleotide 1896. This substitution results in the replacement of the TGG tryptophan codon by a stop codon (TAG), which prevents the translation of HBeAg. Another mutation, in the core-promoter region, prevents transcription of the coding region for HBeAg and yields an HBeAg-negative phenotype. Patients with such mutations in the precore region and who are unable to secrete HBeAg tend to have severe liver disease that progresses more rapidly to cirrhosis or, alternatively, they are identified clinically later in the course of the natural history of chronic hepatitis B, when the disease is more advanced. Both "wild-type" HBV and precore-mutant HBV can coexist in the same patient, or mutant HBV may arise late during wild-type HBV infection. In addition, clusters of fulminant hepatitis B in Israel and Japan have been attributed to common-source infection with a precore mutant. Fulminant hepatitis B in North America and western Europe, however, occurs in patients infected with wild-type HBV, in the absence of precore mutants, and both precore mutants and other mutations throughout the HBV genome occur commonly, even in patients with typical, self-limited, milder forms of HBV infection. HBeAg-negative chronic hepatitis with mutations in the precore region is now the most frequently encountered form of hepatitis B in Mediterranean countries and in Europe. In the United States, where HBV genotype A (less prone to G1896A mutation) is prevalent, precore-mutant HBV is much less common; however, as a result of immigration from Asia and Europe, the proportion of HBeAg-negative hepatitis B–infected individuals has increased in the United States, and they now represent approximately one-third of patients with chronic hepatitis B. Characteristic of such HBeAg-negative chronic hepatitis B are lower levels of HBV DNA (usually $\leq 10^5$ copies/mL) and one of several patterns of aminotransferase activity—persistent elevations, periodic fluctuations above the normal range, and periodic fluctuations between the normal and elevated range.

The second important category of HBV mutants consists of *escape mutants*, in which a single amino acid substitution, from glycine to arginine, occurs at position 145 of the immunodominant *a* determinant common to all subtypes of HBsAg. This change in HBsAg leads to a critical conformational change that results in a loss of neutralizing activity by anti-HBs. This specific HBV/*a* mutant has been observed in two situations, active and

passive immunization, in which humoral immunologic pressure may favor evolutionary change ("escape") in the virus—in a small number of hepatitis B vaccine recipients who acquired HBV infection despite the prior appearance of neutralizing anti-HBs and in liver transplant recipients who underwent the procedure for hepatitis B and who were treated with a high-potency human monoclonal anti-HBs preparation. Although such mutants have not been recognized frequently, their existence raises a concern that may complicate vaccination strategies and serologic diagnosis.

Different types of mutations emerge during antiviral therapy of chronic hepatitis B with nucleoside analogues; such "YMDD" and similar mutations in the polymerase motif of HBV are described in Chap. 40.

Extrahepatic sites

Hepatitis B antigens and HBV DNA have been identified in extrahepatic sites, including lymph nodes, bone marrow, circulating lymphocytes, spleen, and pancreas. Although the virus does not appear to be associated with tissue injury in any of these extrahepatic sites, its presence in these "remote" reservoirs has been invoked (but is not necessary) to explain the recurrence of HBV infection after orthotopic liver transplantation. A more complete understanding of the clinical relevance of extrahepatic HBV remains to be defined.

Hepatitis D

The delta hepatitis agent, or HDV, the only member of the genus *Deltavirus*, is a defective RNA virus that coinfects with and requires the helper function of HBV (or other hepadnaviruses) for its replication and expression. Slightly smaller than HBV, delta is a formalin-sensitive, 35- to 37-nm virus with a hybrid structure. Its nucleocapsid expresses delta antigen, which bears no antigenic homology with any of the HBV antigens, and contains the virus genome. The delta core is "encapsidated" by an outer envelope of HBsAg, indistinguishable from that of HBV except in its relative compositions of major, middle, and large HBsAg component proteins. The genome is a small, 1700-nucleotide, circular, single-strand RNA of negative polarity that is nonhomologous with HBV DNA (except for a small area of the polymerase gene) but that has features and the rolling circle model of replication common to genomes of plant satellite viruses or viroids. HDV RNA contains many areas of internal complementarity; therefore, it can fold on itself by internal base pairing to form an unusual, very stable, rodlike structure that contains a very stable, self-cleaving and self-ligating ribozyme. HDV RNA requires host RNA polymerase II for its replication via RNA-directed RNA synthesis by transcription of genomic RNA to a complementary antigenomic (plus strand) RNA; the antigenomic RNA, in turn, serves as a template for subsequent genomic RNA synthesis. HDV RNA has only one open reading frame, and delta antigen (HDAg), a product of the antigenomic strand is the only known HDV protein; HDAg exists in two forms: a small, 195-amino-acid species, which plays a role in facilitating HDV RNA replication, and a large, 214-amino-acid species, which appears to suppress replication but is required for assembly of the antigen into virions. Delta antigens have been shown to bind directly to RNA polymerase II, resulting in stimulation of transcription. Although complete hepatitis D virions and liver injury require the cooperative helper function of HBV, intracellular replication of HDV RNA can occur without HBV. Genomic heterogeneity among HDV isolates has been described; however, pathophysiologic and clinical consequences of this genetic diversity have not been recognized. The clinical spectrum of hepatitis D is common to all seven genotypes identified, the predominant of which is genotype 1.

HDV can either infect a person simultaneously with HBV (*co-infection*) or superinfect a person already infected with HBV (*superinfection*); when HDV infection is transmitted from a donor with one HBsAg subtype to an HBsAg-positive recipient with a different subtype, the HDV agent assumes the HBsAg subtype of the recipient, rather than the donor. Because HDV relies absolutely on HBV, the duration of HDV infection is determined by the duration of (and cannot outlast) HBV infection. HDV antigen is expressed primarily in hepatocyte nuclei and is occasionally detectable in serum. During acute HDV infection, anti-HDV of the IgM class predominates, and 30–40 days may elapse after symptoms appear before anti-HDV can be detected. In self-limited infection, anti-HDV is low-titer and transient, rarely remaining detectable beyond the clearance of HBsAg and HDV antigen. In chronic HDV infection, anti-HDV circulates in high titer, and both IgM and IgG anti-HDV can be detected. HDV antigen in the liver and HDV RNA in serum and liver can be detected during HDV replication.

Hepatitis C

Hepatitis C virus, which, before its identification was labeled "non-A, non-B hepatitis," is a linear, single-strand, positive-sense, 9600-nucleotide RNA virus, the genome of which is similar in organization to that of flaviviruses and pestiviruses; HCV is the only member of the genus *Hepacivirus* in the family Flaviviridae. The HCV genome contains a single, large open reading frame (gene) that codes for a virus polyprotein of ~3000 amino acids, which is cleaved after translation to yield 10 viral proteins. The 5′ end of the genome consists of an untranslated region (containing an internal ribosomal entry site) adjacent to the genes for four structural proteins, the nucleocapsid core protein, C; two envelope glycoproteins, E1 and E2; and a membrane protein p7. The 5′ untranslated region and core gene are highly conserved among genotypes, but the envelope proteins are coded for by the hypervariable region, which varies from isolate to isolate and may allow the virus to evade host immunologic containment directed at accessible virus-envelope proteins. The 3′ end of the genome also includes an untranslated region and contains the genes for six nonstructural (NS) proteins NS2, NS3, NS4A, NS4B, NS5A, and NS5B. The NS2 cysteine protease cleaves NS3 from NS2, and the NS3-4A serine protease cleaves all the downstream proteins from the polyprotein. Important NS proteins involved in virus replication include the NS3 helicase, NS3-NS4A serine protease, and the NS5B RNA-dependent RNA polymerase (**Fig. 38-6**). Because HCV does not replicate via a

FIGURE 38-6

Organization of the hepatitis C virus genome and its associated, 3000 amino-acid (AA) proteins. The three structural genes at the 5′ end are the core region, C, which codes for the nucleocapsid, and the envelope regions, E1 and E2, which code for envelope glycoproteins. The 5′ untranslated region and the C region are highly conserved among isolates, while the envelope domain E2 contains the hypervariable region. Adjacent to the structural proteins is p7, a membrane protein that appears to function as an ion channel. At the 3′ end are six nonstructural (NS) regions, NS2, which codes for a cysteine protease; NS3, which codes for a serine protease and an RNA helicase; NS4 and NS4B; NS5A; and NS5B, which codes for an RNA-dependent RNA polymerase. After translation of the entire polyprotein, individual proteins are cleaved by both host and viral proteases.

DNA intermediate, it does not integrate into the host genome. Because HCV tends to circulate in relatively low titer, 10^3–10^7 virions/mL, visualization of virus particles, estimated to be 40–60 nm in diameter, remains difficult. Still, the replication rate of HCV is very high, 10^{12} virions per day; its half-life is 2.7 h. The chimpanzee is a helpful but cumbersome animal model. Although a robust, reproducible, small animal model is lacking, HCV replication has been documented in an immunodeficient mouse model containing explants of human liver and in transgenic mouse and rat models. Although in vitro replication has been difficult, hepatocellular carcinoma–derived cell lines have been described (replicon systems) that support replication of genetically manipulated, truncated, or full-length HCV RNA (but not intact virions). Recently, complete replication of HCV and intact 55-nm virions have been described in cell culture systems. HCV gains entry into the hepatocyte via the nonliver-specific CD81 receptor and the liver-specific tight junction protein claudin-1. Relying on the same assembly and secretion pathway as low-density lipoproteins (LPLs), HCV masquerades as a lipoprotein, which may limit its visibility to the adaptive immune system and which may explain its ability to evade immune containment and clearance.

At least six distinct major genotypes, as well as >50 subtypes within genotypes, of HCV have been identified by nucleotide sequencing. Genotypes differ one from another in sequence homology by ≥30%. Because divergence of HCV isolates within a genotype or subtype and, within the same host, may vary insufficiently to define a distinct genotype, these intragenotypic differences are referred to as *quasispecies* and differ in sequence homology by only a few percent. The genotypic and quasispecies diversity of HCV, resulting from its high mutation rate, interferes with effective humoral immunity. Neutralizing antibodies to HCV have been demonstrated, but they tend to be short lived, and HCV infection does not induce lasting immunity against reinfection with different virus isolates or even the same virus isolate. Thus, neither *heterologous* nor *homologous* immunity appears to develop commonly after acute HCV infection. Some HCV genotypes are distributed worldwide, while others are more geographically confined (see "Epidemiology and Global Features"). In addition, differences exist among genotypes in responsiveness to antiviral therapy; however, early reports of differences in pathogenicity among genotypes have not been corroborated.

Currently available, third-generation immunoassays, which incorporate proteins from the core, NS3, and NS5 regions, detect anti-HCV antibodies during acute infection. The most sensitive indicator of HCV infection is the presence of HCV RNA, which requires molecular amplification by PCR or transcription-mediated amplification (TMA) (**Fig. 38-7**). To allow

FIGURE 38-7
Scheme of typical laboratory features during acute hepatitis C progressing to chronicity. HCV RNA is the first detectable event, preceding alanine aminotransferase (ALT) elevation and the appearance of anti-HCV.

standardization of the quantification of HCV RNA among laboratories and commercial assays, HCV RNA is reported as international units (IUs) per milliliter; quantitative assays are available that allow detection of HCV RNA with a sensitivity as low as 5 IU/mL. HCV RNA can be detected within a few days of exposure to HCV—well before the appearance of anti-HCV—and tends to persist for the duration of HCV infection; however, occasionally in patients with chronic HCV infection, HCV RNA may be detectable only intermittently. Application of sensitive molecular probes for HCV RNA has revealed the presence of replicative HCV in peripheral blood lymphocytes of infected persons; however, as is the case for HBV in lymphocytes, the clinical relevance of HCV lymphocyte infection is not known.

Hepatitis E

Previously labeled *epidemic* or *enterically transmitted non-A, non-B hepatitis*, HEV is an enterically transmitted virus that occurs primarily in India, Asia, Africa, and Central America; in those geographic areas, HEV is the most common cause of acute hepatitis. This agent, with epidemiologic features resembling those of hepatitis A, is a 32- to 34-nm, nonenveloped, HAV-like virus with a 7600-nucleotide, single-strand, positive-sense RNA genome. HEV has three open reading frames (ORF) (genes), the largest of which, *ORF1*, encodes nonstructural proteins involved in virus replication. A middle-sized gene, *ORF2*, encodes the nucleocapsid protein, the major nonstructural protein, and the smallest, *ORF3*, encodes a structural protein whose function remains undetermined. All HEV isolates appear to belong to a single serotype, despite genomic heterogeneity of up to 25% and the existence of five genotypes, only four of which have been detected in humans; genotypes 1 and 2 appear to be more virulent, while genotypes 3 and 4 are more attenuated and account for subclinical infections. Contributing to the perpetuation of this virus are animal reservoirs, most notably in swine. There is no genomic or antigenic homology, however, between HEV and HAV or other picornaviruses; and HEV, although resembling caliciviruses, is sufficiently distinct from any known agent to merit a new classification of its own as a unique genus, *Hepevirus*, within the family Hepeviridae. The virus has been detected in stool, bile, and liver and is excreted in the stool during the late incubation period; immune responses to viral antigens occur very early during the course of acute infection. Both IgM anti-HEV and IgG anti-HEV can be detected, but both fall rapidly after acute infection, reaching low levels within 9–12 months. Currently, serologic testing for HEV infection is not available routinely.

PATHOGENESIS

Under ordinary circumstances, none of the hepatitis viruses is known to be directly cytopathic to hepatocytes. Evidence suggests that the clinical manifestations and outcomes after acute liver injury associated with viral hepatitis are determined by the immunologic responses of the host. Among the viral hepatitides, the immunopathogenesis of hepatitis B and C has been studied most extensively.

Hepatitis B

For HBV, the existence of inactive hepatitis B carriers with normal liver histology and function suggests that the virus is not directly cytopathic. The fact that patients with defects in cellular immune competence are more likely to remain chronically infected rather than to clear HBV supports the role of cellular immune responses in the pathogenesis of hepatitis B–related liver injury. The model that has the most experimental support involves cytolytic T cells sensitized specifically to recognize host and hepatitis B viral antigens on the liver cell surface. Nucleocapsid proteins (HBcAg and possibly HBeAg), present on the cell membrane in minute quantities, are the viral target antigens that, with host antigens, invite cytolytic T cells to destroy HBV-infected hepatocytes. Differences in the robustness and broad polyclonality of CD8+ cytolytic T cell responsiveness and in the elaboration of antiviral cytokines by T cells have been invoked to explain differences in outcomes between those who recover after acute hepatitis, and those who progress to chronic hepatitis, or between those with mild and those with severe (fulminant) acute HBV infection.

Although a robust cytolytic T cell response occurs and eliminates virus-infected liver cells during acute hepatitis B, >90% of HBV DNA has been found in

experimentally infected chimpanzees to disappear from the liver and blood before maximal T cell infiltration of the liver and before most of the biochemical and histologic evidence of liver injury. This observation suggests that components of the innate immune system and inflammatory cytokines, independent of cytopathic antiviral mechanisms, participate in the early immune response to HBV infection; this effect has been shown to represent elimination of HBV replicative intermediates from the cytoplasm and covalently closed circular viral DNA from the nucleus of infected hepatocytes. Ultimately, HBV-HLA-specific cytolytic T cell responses of the adaptive immune system are felt to be responsible for recovery from HBV infection.

Debate continues over the relative importance of viral and host factors in the pathogenesis of HBV-associated liver injury and its outcome. As noted earlier, precore genetic mutants of HBV have been associated with the more severe outcomes of HBV infection (severe chronic and fulminant hepatitis), suggesting that, under certain circumstances, relative pathogenicity is a property of the virus, not the host. The fact that concomitant HDV and HBV infections are associated with more severe liver injury than HBV infection alone and the fact that cells transfected in vitro with the gene for HDV (delta) antigen express HDV antigen and then become necrotic in the absence of any immunologic influences are also consistent with a viral effect on pathogenicity. Similarly, in patients who undergo liver transplantation for end-stage chronic hepatitis B, occasionally, rapidly progressive liver injury appears in the new liver. This clinical pattern is associated with an unusual histologic pattern in the new liver, *fibrosing cholestatic hepatitis*, which, ultrastructurally, appears to represent a choking of the cell with overwhelming quantities of HBsAg. This observation suggests that, under the influence of the potent immunosuppressive agents required to prevent allograft rejection, HBV may have a direct cytopathic effect on liver cells, independent of the immune system.

Although the precise mechanism of liver injury in HBV infection remains elusive, studies of nucleocapsid proteins have shed light on the profound immunologic tolerance to HBV of babies born to mothers with highly replicative (HBeAg-positive), chronic HBV infection. In HBeAg-expressing transgenic mice, in utero exposure to HBeAg, which is sufficiently small to traverse the placenta, induces T cell tolerance to both nucleocapsid proteins. This, in turn, may explain why, when infection occurs so early in life, immunologic clearance does not occur, and protracted, lifelong infection ensues.

An important distinction should be drawn between HBV infection acquired at birth, common in endemic areas, such as the Far East, and infection acquired in adulthood, common in the West. Infection in the neonatal period is associated with the acquisition of immunologic tolerance to HBV, absence of an acute hepatitis illness, but the almost invariable establishment of chronic, often lifelong infection. Neonatally acquired HBV infection can culminate decades later in cirrhosis and hepatocellular carcinoma (see "Complications and Sequelae"). In contrast, when HBV infection is acquired during adolescence or early adulthood, the host immune response to HBV infected hepatocytes tends to be robust, an acute hepatitis-like illness is the rule, and failure to recover is the exception. After adulthood acquired infection, chronicity is uncommon, and the risk of hepatocellular carcinoma is very low. Based on these observations, some authorities categorize HBV infection into an "immunotolerant" phase, an "immunoreactive" phase, and an "inactive" phase. This somewhat simplistic formulation does not apply at all to the typical adult in the west with self-limited acute hepatitis B, in whom no period of immunologic tolerance occurs. Even among those with neonatally acquired HBV infection, in whom immunologic tolerance is established definitively, intermittent bursts of hepatic necroinflammatory activity punctuate the period during the early decades of life during which liver injury appears to be quiescent (labeled by some as the "immunotolerant" phase). In addition, even when clinically apparent, liver injury and progressive fibrosis emerge during later decades (the so-called immunoreactive, or immunointolerant phase), the level of immunologic tolerance to HBV remains substantial. More accurately, in patients with neonatally acquired HBV infection, a dynamic equilibrium exists between tolerance and intolerance, the outcome of which determines the clinical expression of chronic infection. Those individuals who are infected as neonates tend to have a relatively higher level of immunologic tolerance during the early decades of life and a relatively lower level (but only rarely a loss) of tolerance in the later decades of life.

Hepatitis C

Cell-mediated immune responses and elaboration by T cells of antiviral cytokines contribute to the containment of infection and pathogenesis of liver injury associated with hepatitis C. Perhaps HCV infection of lymphoid cells plays a role in moderating immune responsiveness to the virus, as well. Intrahepatic HLA class I restricted cytolytic T cells directed at nucleocapsid, envelope, and nonstructural viral protein antigens have been demonstrated in patients with chronic hepatitis C; however, such virus-specific cytolytic T cell responses do not correlate adequately with the degree of liver injury or with recovery. Yet, a consensus has emerged supporting a role in the pathogenesis of HCV-associated liver injury of virus-activated CD4 helper T cells that stimulate, via the cytokines they elaborate,

HCV-specific CD8 cytotoxic T cells. These responses appear to be more robust (higher in number, more diverse in viral antigen specificity, more functionally effective, and more long lasting) in those who recover from HCV than in those who have chronic infection. Several HLA alleles have been linked with self-limited hepatitis C, the most convincing of which is the C/C haplotype of the IL28B gene. Although attention has focused on adaptive immunity, HCV proteins have been shown to interfere with innate immunity by resulting in blocking of type 1 interferon responses and inhibition of interferon signaling and effector molecules in the interferon signaling cascade. Also shown to contribute to limiting HCV infection are natural killer cells of the innate immune system that function when HLA class 1 molecules required for successful adaptive immunity are underexpressed. Of note, the emergence of substantial viral quasispecies diversity and HCV sequence variation allow the virus to evade attempts by the host to contain HCV infection by both humoral and cellular immunity.

Finally, cross-reactivity between viral antigens (HCV NS3 and NS5A) and host autoantigens (cytochrome P450 2D6) has been invoked to explain the association between hepatitis C and a subset of patients with autoimmune hepatitis and antibodies to liver-kidney microsomal (LKM) antigen (anti-LKM) (Chap. 40).

EXTRAHEPATIC MANIFESTATIONS

Immune complex–mediated tissue damage appears to play a pathogenetic role in the extrahepatic manifestations of acute hepatitis B. The occasional prodromal serum sickness–like syndrome observed in acute hepatitis B appears to be related to the deposition in tissue blood vessel walls of HBsAg-anti-HBs circulating immune complexes, leading to activation of the complement system and depressed serum complement levels.

In patients with chronic hepatitis B, other types of immune-complex disease may be seen. Glomerulonephritis with the nephrotic syndrome is observed occasionally; HBsAg, immunoglobulin, and C3 deposition has been found in the glomerular basement membrane. While generalized vasculitis (polyarteritis nodosa) develops in considerably fewer than 1% of patients with chronic HBV infection, 20–30% of patients with polyarteritis nodosa have HBsAg in serum. In these patients, the affected small- and medium-size arterioles contain HBsAg, immunoglobulins, and complement components. Another extrahepatic manifestation of viral hepatitis, essential mixed cryoglobulinemia (EMC), was reported initially to be associated with hepatitis B. The disorder is characterized clinically by arthritis; cutaneous vasculitis (palpable purpura); and, occasionally, with glomerulonephritis and serologically by the presence of circulating cryoprecipitable immune complexes of more than one immunoglobulin class. Many patients with this syndrome have chronic liver disease, but the association with HBV infection is limited; instead, a substantial proportion has chronic HCV infection, with circulating immune complexes containing HCV RNA. Immune-complex glomerulonephritis is another recognized extrahepatic manifestation of chronic hepatitis C.

PATHOLOGY

The typical morphologic lesions of all types of viral hepatitis are similar and consist of panlobular infiltration with mononuclear cells, hepatic cell necrosis, hyperplasia of Kupffer cells, and variable degrees of cholestasis. Hepatic cell regeneration is present, as evidenced by numerous mitotic figures, multinucleated cells, and "rosette" or "pseudoacinar" formation. The mononuclear infiltration consists primarily of small lymphocytes, although plasma cells and eosinophils occasionally are present. Liver cell damage consists of hepatic cell degeneration and necrosis, cell dropout, ballooning of cells, and acidophilic degeneration of hepatocytes (forming so-called Councilman or apoptotic bodies). Large hepatocytes with a ground-glass appearance of the cytoplasm may be seen in chronic but not in acute HBV infection; these cells contain HBsAg and can be identified histochemically with orcein or aldehyde fuchsin. In uncomplicated viral hepatitis, the reticulin framework is preserved.

In hepatitis C, the histologic lesion is often remarkable for a relative paucity of inflammation, a marked increase in activation of sinusoidal lining cells, lymphoid aggregates, the presence of fat (more frequent in genotype 3 and linked to increased fibrosis), and, occasionally, bile duct lesions in which biliary epithelial cells appear to be piled up without interruption of the basement membrane. Occasionally, microvesicular steatosis occurs in hepatitis D. In hepatitis E, a common histologic feature is marked cholestasis. A cholestatic variant of slowly resolving acute hepatitis A also has been described.

A more severe histologic lesion, *bridging hepatic necrosis*, also termed *subacute* or *confluent necrosis* or *interface hepatitis*, is observed occasionally in acute hepatitis. "Bridging" between lobules results from large areas of hepatic cell dropout, with collapse of the reticulin framework. Characteristically, the bridge consists of condensed reticulum, inflammatory debris, and degenerating liver cells that span adjacent portal areas, portal to central veins, or central vein to central vein. This lesion had been thought to have prognostic significance; in many of the originally described patients with this lesion, a subacute course terminated in death within several weeks to months, or severe chronic hepatitis and

cirrhosis developed; however, the association between bridging necrosis and a poor prognosis in patients with acute hepatitis has not been upheld. Therefore, although demonstration of this lesion in patients with chronic hepatitis has prognostic significance (Chap. 40), its demonstration during acute hepatitis is less meaningful, and liver biopsies to identify this lesion are no longer undertaken routinely in patients with acute hepatitis. In *massive hepatic necrosis* (fulminant hepatitis, "acute yellow atrophy"), the striking feature at postmortem examination is the finding of a small, shrunken, soft liver. Histologic examination reveals massive necrosis and dropout of liver cells of most lobules with extensive collapse and condensation of the reticulin framework. When histologic documentation is required in the management of fulminant or very severe hepatitis, a biopsy can be done by the angiographically guided transjugular route, which permits the performance of this invasive procedure in the presence of severe coagulopathy.

Immunohistochemical and electron-microscopic studies have localized HBsAg to the cytoplasm and plasma membrane of infected liver cells. In contrast, HBcAg predominates in the nucleus, but, occasionally, scant amounts are also seen in the cytoplasm and on the cell membrane. HDV antigen is localized to the hepatocyte nucleus, while HAV, HCV, and HEV antigens are localized to the cytoplasm.

EPIDEMIOLOGY AND GLOBAL FEATURES

Before the availability of serologic tests for hepatitis viruses, all viral hepatitis cases were labeled either as "infectious" or "serum" hepatitis. Modes of transmission overlap, however, and *a clear distinction among the different types of viral hepatitis cannot be made solely on the basis of clinical or epidemiologic features* (Table 38-2). The most accurate means to distinguish the various types of viral hepatitis involves specific serologic testing.

Hepatitis A

This agent is transmitted almost exclusively by the fecal-oral route. Person-to-person spread of HAV is enhanced by poor personal hygiene and overcrowding; large outbreaks as well as sporadic cases have been traced to contaminated food, water, milk, frozen raspberries and strawberries, green onions imported from Mexico, and shellfish. Intrafamily and intrainstitutional spread are also common. Early epidemiologic observations supported a predilection for hepatitis A to occur in late fall and early winter. In temperate zones, epidemic waves have been recorded every 5–20 years as new segments of nonimmune population appeared; however, in developed

TABLE 38-2

CLINICAL AND EPIDEMIOLOGIC FEATURES OF VIRAL HEPATITIS

FEATURE	HAV	HBV	HCV	HDV	HEV
Incubation (days)	15–45, mean 30	30–180, mean 60–90	15–160, mean 50	30–180, mean 60–90	14–60, mean 40
Onset	Acute	Insidious or acute	Insidious	Insidious or acute	Acute
Age preference	Children, young adults	Young adults (sexual and percutaneous), babies, toddlers	Any age, but more common in adults	Any age (similar to HBV)	Young adults (20–40 years)
Transmission					
Fecal-oral	+++	–	–	–	+++
Percutaneous	Unusual	+++	+++	+++	–
Perinatal	–	+++	±[a]	+	–
Sexual	±	++	±[a]	++	–
Clinical					
Severity	Mild	Occasionally severe	Moderate	Occasionally severe	Mild
Fulminant	0.1%	0.1–1%	0.1%	5–20%[b]	1–2%[e]
Progression to chronicity	None	Occasional (1–10%) (90% of neonates)	Common (85%)	Common[d]	None
Carrier	None	0.1–30%[c]	1.5–3.2%	Variable[f]	None
Cancer	None	+ (Neonatal infection)	+	±	None
Prognosis	Excellent	Worse with age, debility	Moderate	Acute, good Chronic, poor	Good
Prophylaxis	IG, inactivated vaccine	HBIG, recombinant vaccine	None	HBV vaccine (none for HBV carriers)	Vaccine
Therapy	None	Interferon Lamivudine Adefovir Pegylated interferon Entecavir Telbivudine Tenofovir	Pegylated interferon plus ribavirin Telaprevir Boceprevir	Interferon or pegylated interferon (efficacy moderate)	None

[a]Primarily with HIV co-infection and high-level viremia in index case; risk ~5%.
[b]Up to 5% in acute HBV/HDV co-infection; up to 20% in HDV superinfection of chronic HBV infection.
[c]Varies considerably throughout the world and in subpopulations within countries; see text.
[d]In acute HBV/HDV co-infection, the frequency of chronicity is the same as that for HBV; in HDV superinfection, chronicity is invariable.
[e]10–20% in pregnant women.
[f]Common in Mediterranean countries, rare in North America and western Europe.
Abbreviation: HBIG, hepatitis B immunoglobulin.

countries, the incidence of hepatitis A has been declining, presumably as a function of improved sanitation, and these cyclic patterns are no longer observed. No HAV carrier state has been identified after acute hepatitis A; perpetuation of the virus in nature depends presumably on nonepidemic, inapparent subclinical infection, ingestion of contaminated food or water in, or imported from, endemic areas, and/or contamination linked to environmental reservoirs.

In the general population, anti-HAV, a marker for previous HAV infection, increases in prevalence as a function of increasing age and of decreasing socioeconomic status. In the 1970s, serologic evidence of prior hepatitis A infection occurred in ~40% of urban populations in the United States, most of whose members

never recalled having had a symptomatic case of hepatitis. In subsequent decades, however, the prevalence of anti-HAV has been declining in the United States. In developing countries, exposure, infection, and subsequent immunity are almost universal in childhood. As the frequency of subclinical childhood infections declines in developed countries, a susceptible cohort of adults emerges. Hepatitis A tends to be more symptomatic in adults; therefore, paradoxically, as the frequency of HAV infection declines, the likelihood of clinically apparent, even severe, HAV illnesses increases in the susceptible adult population. Travel to endemic areas is a common source of infection for adults from nonendemic areas. More recently recognized epidemiologic foci of HAV infection include child-care centers, neonatal intensive care units, promiscuous men who have sex with men, and injection drug users. Although hepatitis A is rarely bloodborne, several outbreaks have been recognized in recipients of clotting-factor concentrates. In the United States, the introduction of hepatitis A vaccination programs among children from high-incidence states has resulted in a >70% reduction in the annual incidence of new HAV infections and has shifted the burden of new infections from children to young adults.

Hepatitis B

Percutaneous inoculation has long been recognized as a major route of hepatitis B transmission, but the outmoded designation "serum hepatitis" is an inaccurate label for the epidemiologic spectrum of HBV infection recognized today. As detailed later, most of the hepatitis transmitted by blood transfusion is not caused by HBV; moreover, in approximately two-thirds of patients with acute type B hepatitis, no history of an identifiable percutaneous exposure can be elicited. We now recognize that many cases of hepatitis B result from less obvious modes of nonpercutaneous or covert percutaneous transmission. HBsAg has been identified in almost every body fluid from infected persons, and at least some of these body fluids—most notably semen and saliva—are infectious, albeit less so than serum, when administered percutaneously or nonpercutaneously to experimental animals. Among the nonpercutaneous modes of HBV transmission, oral ingestion has been documented as a potential but inefficient route of exposure. By contrast, the two nonpercutaneous routes considered to have the greatest impact are intimate (especially sexual) contact and perinatal transmission.

In sub-Saharan Africa, intimate contact among toddlers is considered instrumental in contributing to the maintenance of the high frequency of hepatitis B in the population. Perinatal transmission occurs primarily in infants born to HBsAg carrier mothers or mothers with acute hepatitis B during the third trimester of pregnancy or during the early postpartum period. Perinatal transmission is uncommon in North America and western Europe but occurs with great frequency and is the most important mode of HBV perpetuation in the Far East and developing countries. Although the precise mode of perinatal transmission is unknown, and although ~10% of infections may be acquired in utero, epidemiologic evidence suggests that most infections occur approximately at the time of delivery and are not related to breast-feeding. The likelihood of perinatal transmission of HBV correlates with the presence of HBeAg and high-level viral replication; 90% of HBeAg-positive mothers but only 10–15% of anti-HBe-positive mothers transmit HBV infection to their offspring. In most cases,

acute infection in the neonate is clinically asymptomatic, but the child is very likely to remain chronically infected.

The >350–400 million HBsAg carriers in the world constitute the main reservoir of hepatitis B in human beings. Whereas serum HBsAg is infrequent (0.1–0.5%) in normal populations in the United States and western Europe, a prevalence of up to 5–20% has been found in the Far East and in some tropical countries; in persons with Down's syndrome, lepromatous leprosy, leukemia, Hodgkin's disease, and polyarteritis nodosa; in patients with chronic renal disease on hemodialysis; and in injection drug users.

Other groups with high rates of HBV infection include spouses of acutely infected persons; sexually promiscuous persons (especially promiscuous men who have sex with men); health care workers exposed to blood; persons who require repeated transfusions especially with pooled blood-product concentrates (e.g., hemophiliacs); residents and staff of custodial institutions for the developmentally handicapped; prisoners; and, to a lesser extent, family members of chronically infected patients. In volunteer blood donors, the prevalence of anti-HBs, a reflection of previous HBV infection, ranges from 5–10%, but the prevalence is higher in lower socioeconomic strata, older age groups, and persons—including those mentioned earlier—exposed to blood products. Because of highly sensitive virologic screening of donor blood, the risk of acquiring HBV infection from a blood transfusion is 1 in 230,000.

Prevalence of infection, modes of transmission, and human behavior conspire to mold geographically different epidemiologic patterns of HBV infection. In the Far East and Africa, hepatitis B, a disease of the newborn and young children, is perpetuated by a cycle of maternal-neonatal spread. In North America and western Europe, hepatitis B is primarily a disease of adolescence and early adulthood, the time of life when intimate sexual contact as well as recreational and occupational percutaneous exposures tend to occur. To some degree, however, this dichotomy between high-prevalence and low-prevalence geographic regions has been minimized by immigration from high-prevalence to low-prevalence areas. The introduction of hepatitis B vaccine in the early 1980s and adoption of universal childhood vaccination policies in many countries resulted in a dramatic, ~90%, decline in the incidence of new HBV infections in those countries as well as in the dire consequences of chronic infection, including hepatocellular carcinoma. Populations and groups for whom HBV-infection screening is recommended are listed in Table 38-3.

Hepatitis D

Infection with HDV has a worldwide distribution, but two epidemiologic patterns exist. In Mediterranean

TABLE 38-3

HIGH-RISK POPULATIONS FOR WHICH HBV-INFECTION SCREENING IS RECOMMENDED

Persons born in countries/regions with a high (>8%) and intermediate (>2%) prevalence of HBV infection including immigrants and adopted children and including persons born in the United States who were not vaccinated as infants and whose parents immigrated from areas of high HBV endemicity

Household and sexual contacts of persons with hepatitis B

Persons who have used injection drugs

Persons with multiple sexual contacts or a history of sexually transmitted disease

Men who have sex with men

Inmates of correctional facilities

Persons with elevated alanine or aspartate aminotransferase levels

Persons with HCV or HIV infection

Hemodialysis patients

Pregnant women

Persons who require immunosuppressive or cytotoxic therapy

countries (northern Africa, southern Europe, the Middle East), HDV infection is endemic among those with hepatitis B, and the disease is transmitted predominantly by nonpercutaneous means, especially close personal contact. In nonendemic areas, such as the United States and northern Europe, HDV infection is confined to persons exposed frequently to blood and blood products, primarily injection drug users and hemophiliacs. HDV infection can be introduced into a population through drug users or by migration of persons from endemic to nonendemic areas. Thus, patterns of population migration and human behavior facilitating percutaneous contact play important roles in the introduction and amplification of HDV infection. Occasionally, the migrating epidemiology of hepatitis D is expressed in explosive outbreaks of severe hepatitis, such as those that have occurred in remote South American villages as well as in urban centers in the United States. Ultimately, such outbreaks of hepatitis D—either of co-infections with acute hepatitis B or of superinfections in those already infected with HBV—may blur the distinctions between endemic and nonendemic areas. On a global scale, HDV infection declined at the end of the 1990s. Even in Italy, an HDV-endemic area, public health measures introduced to control HBV infection resulted during the 1990s in a 1.5%/year reduction in the prevalence of HDV infection. Still, the frequency of HDV infection during the first decade of the twenty-first century has not fallen below levels reached during the 1990s; the reservoir has been sustained by survivors infected during 1970–1980 and recent immigrants from still-endemic to less-endemic countries.

Hepatitis C

Routine screening of blood donors for HBsAg and the elimination of commercial blood sources in the early 1970s reduced the frequency of, but did not eliminate, transfusion-associated hepatitis. During the 1970s, the likelihood of acquiring hepatitis after transfusion of voluntarily donated, HBsAg-screened blood was ~10% per patient (up to 0.9% per unit transfused); 90–95% of these cases were classified, based on serologic exclusion of hepatitis A and B, as "non-A, non-B" hepatitis. For patients requiring transfusion of pooled products, such as clotting factor concentrates, the risk was even higher, up to 20–30%.

During the 1980s, voluntary self-exclusion of blood donors with risk factors for AIDS and then the introduction of donor screening for anti-HIV reduced further the likelihood of transfusion-associated hepatitis to <5%. During the late 1980s and early 1990s, the introduction first of "surrogate" screening tests for non-A, non-B hepatitis (alanine aminotransferase [ALT] and anti-HBc, both shown to identify blood donors with a higher likelihood of transmitting non-A, non-B hepatitis to recipients) and, subsequently, after the discovery of HCV, first-generation immunoassays for anti-HCV reduced the frequency of transfusion-associated hepatitis even further. A prospective analysis of transfusion-associated hepatitis conducted between 1986 and 1990 showed that the frequency of transfusion-associated hepatitis at one urban university hospital fell from a baseline of 3.8% per patient (0.45% per unit transfused) to 1.5% per patient (0.19% per unit) after the introduction of surrogate testing and to 0.6% per patient (0.03% per unit) after the introduction of first-generation anti-HCV assays. The introduction of second-generation anti-HCV assays reduced the frequency of transfusion-associated hepatitis C to almost imperceptible levels—1 in 100,000—and these gains were reinforced by the application of third-generation anti-HCV assays and of automated PCR testing of donated blood for HCV RNA, which has resulted in a reduction in the risk of transfusion-associated HCV infection to 1 in 2.3 million transfusions.

In addition to being transmitted by transfusion, hepatitis C can be transmitted by other percutaneous routes, such as injection drug use. In addition, this virus can be transmitted by occupational exposure to blood, and the likelihood of infection is increased in hemodialysis units. Although the frequency of transfusion-associated hepatitis C fell as a result of blood-donor screening, the overall frequency of hepatitis C remained the same until the early 1990s, when the overall frequency fell by 80%, in parallel with a reduction in the number of new cases in injection drug users. After the exclusion of anti-HCV-positive plasma units from the donor pool, rare, sporadic instances have occurred of hepatitis C among recipients of immunoglobulin (IG) preparations for intravenous (but not intramuscular) use.

Serologic evidence for HCV infection occurs in 90% of patients with a history of transfusion-associated hepatitis (almost all occurring before 1992, when second-generation HCV-screening tests were introduced); hemophiliacs and others treated with clotting factors; injection drug users; 60–70% of patients with sporadic "non-A, non-B" hepatitis who lack identifiable risk factors; 0.5% of volunteer blood donors; and, in the most recent survey conducted in the United States between 1999 and 2000, 1.6% of the general population in the United States, which translates into 4.1 million persons (3.2 million with viremia). Comparable frequencies of HCV infection occur in most countries around the world, with 170 million persons infected worldwide, but extraordinarily high prevalences of HCV infection occur in certain countries such as Egypt, where >20% of the population in some cities is infected. The high frequency in Egypt is attributable to contaminated equipment used for medical procedures and unsafe injection practices in the 1970s. In the United States, African Americans and Mexican Americans have higher frequencies of HCV infection than whites. Between 1988 and 1994, 30- to 40-year-old adult males had the highest prevalence of HCV infection; however, in a survey conducted between 1999 and 2000, the peak age decile had shifted to those age 40–49 years; an increase in hepatitis C–related mortality has paralleled this secular trend, increasing since 1995 predominantly in the 55- to 64-year age group. Thus, despite an 80% reduction in new HCV infections during the 1990s, the prevalence of HCV infection in the population was sustained by an aging cohort that had acquired their infections 2 to 3 decades earlier, during the 1960s and 1970s, as a result predominantly of self-inoculation with recreational drugs. Hepatitis C accounts for 40% of chronic liver disease, is the most frequent indication for liver transplantation, and is estimated to account for 8000–10,000 deaths per year in the United States.

The distribution of HCV genotypes varies in different parts of the world. Worldwide, genotype 1 is the most common. In the United States, genotype 1 accounts for 70% of HCV infections, while genotypes 2 and3 account for the remaining 30%; among African Americans, the frequency of genotype 1 is even higher (i.e., 90%). Genotype 4 predominates in Egypt; genotype 5 is localized to South Africa, and genotype 6 to Hong Kong.

Most asymptomatic blood donors found to have anti-HCV and ~20–30% of persons with reported cases of acute hepatitis C do not fall into a recognized risk group; however, many such blood donors do recall risk-associated behaviors when questioned carefully.

As a bloodborne infection, HCV potentially can be transmitted sexually and perinatally; however, both of these modes of transmission are inefficient for hepatitis C.

Although 10–15% of patients with acute hepatitis C report having potential sexual sources of infection, most studies have failed to identify sexual transmission of this agent. The chances of sexual and perinatal transmission have been estimated to be ~5%, well below comparable rates for HIV and HBV infections. Moreover, sexual transmission appears to be confined to such subgroups as persons with multiple sexual partners and sexually transmitted diseases; transmission of HCV infection is rare between stable, monogamous sexual partners. Breast-feeding does not increase the risk of HCV infection between an infected mother and her infant. Infection of health workers is not dramatically higher than among the general population; however, health workers are more likely to acquire HCV infection through accidental needle punctures, the efficiency of which is ~3%. Infection of household contacts is rare as well.

Other groups with an increased frequency of HCV infection include patients who require hemodialysis and organ transplantation, those who require transfusions in the setting of cancer chemotherapy, HIV-infected persons, and persons with unexplained serum aminotransferase elevations. In immunosuppressed individuals, levels of anti-HCV may be undetectable, and a diagnosis may require testing for HCV RNA. Although new acute cases of hepatitis C are rare, newly diagnosed cases are common among otherwise healthy persons who experimented briefly with injection drugs, as noted earlier, 2 or 3 decades earlier. Such instances usually remain unrecognized for years, until unearthed by laboratory screening for routine medical examinations, insurance applications, and attempted blood donation. Populations groups for whom HCV-infection screening is recommended are listed in Table 38-4.

Hepatitis E

This type of hepatitis, identified in India, Asia, Africa, the Middle East, and Central America, resembles hepatitis A

TABLE 38-4

HIGH-RISK POPULATIONS FOR WHICH HCV-INFECTION SCREENING IS RECOMMENDED
Persons who have used injection drugs or those who have used illicit drugs by noninjection routes
Persons with HIV infection
Hemophiliacs treated with clotting factor concentrates prior to 1987
Hemodialysis patients
Persons with unexplained elevations of aminotransferase levels
Transfusion or transplantation recipients prior to July 1992
Children born to women with hepatitis C
Health care, public safety, and emergency medical personnel following needle injury or mucosal exposure to HCV-contaminated blood
Sexual partners of persons with hepatitis C infection

in its primarily enteric mode of spread. The commonly recognized cases occur after contamination of water supplies such as after monsoon flooding, but sporadic, isolated cases occur. An epidemiologic feature that distinguishes HEV from other enteric agents is the rarity of secondary person-to-person spread from infected persons to their close contacts. Infections arise in populations that are immune to HAV and favor young adults. In endemic areas, the prevalence of antibodies to HEV is ≤40%. In nonendemic areas of the world, such as the United States, clinically apparent acute hepatitis E is extremely rare; however, the prevalence of antibodies to HEV can be as high as 20% in such areas. In nonendemic areas, HEV does not account for any of the sporadic "non-A, non-B" cases of hepatitis; however, cases imported from endemic areas have been found in the United States. Several reports suggest a zoonotic reservoir for HEV in swine.

CLINICAL AND LABORATORY FEATURES

Symptoms and signs

Acute viral hepatitis occurs after an incubation period that varies according to the responsible agent. Generally, incubation periods for hepatitis A range from 15–45 days (mean, 4 weeks), for hepatitis B and D from 30–180 days (mean, 8–12 weeks), for hepatitis C from 15–160 days (mean, 7 weeks), and for hepatitis E from 14–60 days (mean, 5–6 weeks). The *prodromal symptoms* of acute viral hepatitis are systemic and quite variable. Constitutional symptoms of anorexia, nausea and vomiting, fatigue, malaise, arthralgias, myalgias, headache, photophobia, pharyngitis, cough, and coryza may precede the onset of jaundice by 1–2 weeks. The nausea, vomiting, and anorexia are frequently associated with alterations in olfaction and taste. A low-grade fever between 38° and 39°C (100°–102°F) is more often present in hepatitis A and E than in hepatitis B or C, except when hepatitis B is heralded by a serum sickness–like syndrome; rarely, a fever of 39.5°–40°C (103°–104°F) may accompany the constitutional symptoms. Dark urine and clay-colored stools may be noticed by the patient from 1–5 days before the onset of clinical jaundice.

With the onset of *clinical jaundice*, the constitutional prodromal symptoms usually diminish, but in some patients mild weight loss (2.5–5 kg) is common and may continue during the entire icteric phase. The liver becomes enlarged and tender and may be associated with right upper quadrant pain and discomfort. Infrequently, patients present with a cholestatic picture, suggesting extrahepatic biliary obstruction. Splenomegaly and cervical adenopathy are present in 10–20% of patients with acute hepatitis. Rarely, a few spider angiomas appear during the icteric phase and disappear during convalescence. During the *recovery phase*, constitutional symptoms disappear, but usually some

liver enlargement and abnormalities in liver biochemical tests are still evident. The duration of the posticteric phase is variable, ranging 2–12 weeks, and is usually more prolonged in acute hepatitis B and C. Complete clinical and biochemical recovery is to be expected 1–2 months after all cases of hepatitis A and E and 3–4 months after the onset of jaundice in three-quarters of uncomplicated, self-limited cases of hepatitis B and C (among healthy adults, acute hepatitis B is self-limited in 95–99% while hepatitis C is self-limited in only ~15%). In the remainder, biochemical recovery may be delayed. A substantial proportion of patients with viral hepatitis never become icteric.

Infection with HDV can occur in the presence of acute or chronic HBV infection; the duration of HBV infection determines the duration of HDV infection. When acute HDV and HBV infection occur simultaneously, clinical and biochemical features may be indistinguishable from those of HBV infection alone, although occasionally they are more severe. As opposed to patients with *acute* HBV infection, patients with *chronic* HBV infection can support HDV replication indefinitely. This can happen when acute HDV infection occurs in the presence of a nonresolving acute HBV infection. More commonly, acute HDV infection becomes chronic when it is superimposed on an underlying chronic HBV infection. In such cases, the HDV superinfection appears as a clinical exacerbation or an episode resembling acute viral hepatitis in someone already chronically infected with HBV. Superinfection with HDV in a patient with chronic hepatitis B often leads to clinical deterioration (discussed later).

In addition to superinfections with other hepatitis agents, acute hepatitis-like clinical events in persons with chronic hepatitis B may accompany spontaneous HBeAg to anti-HBe seroconversion or spontaneous reactivation (i.e., reversion from nonreplicative to replicative infection). Such reactivations can occur as well in therapeutically immunosuppressed patients with chronic HBV infection when cytotoxic/immunosuppressive drugs are withdrawn; in these cases, restoration of immune competence is thought to allow resumption of previously checked cell-mediated immune cytolysis of HBV-infected hepatocytes. Occasionally, acute clinical exacerbations of chronic hepatitis B may represent the emergence of a precore mutant (see "Virology and Etiology"), and the subsequent course in such patients may be characterized by periodic exacerbations.

Laboratory features

The serum aminotransferases aspartate aminotransferase (AST) and ALT (previously designated SGOT and SGPT) show a variable increase during the prodromal phase of acute viral hepatitis and precede the rise in bilirubin level (Figs. 38-2 and 38-4). The acute level of these enzymes, however, does not correlate well with the degree of liver cell damage. Peak levels vary from 400–4000 IU or more; these levels are usually reached at the time the patient is clinically icteric and diminish progressively during the recovery phase of acute hepatitis. The diagnosis of anicteric hepatitis is based on clinical features and on aminotransferase elevations.

Jaundice is usually visible in the sclera or skin when the serum bilirubin value is >43 μmol/L (2.5 mg/dL). When jaundice appears, the serum bilirubin typically rises to levels ranging from 85–340 μmol/L (5–20 mg/dL). The serum bilirubin may continue to rise despite falling serum aminotransferase levels. In most instances, the total bilirubin is equally divided between the conjugated and unconjugated fractions. Bilirubin levels >340 μmol/L (20 mg/dL) extending and persisting late into the course of viral hepatitis are more likely to be associated with severe disease. In certain patients with underlying hemolytic anemia, however, such as glucose-6-phosphate dehydrogenase deficiency and sickle cell anemia, a high serum bilirubin level is common, resulting from superimposed hemolysis. In such patients, bilirubin levels >513 μmol/L (30 mg/dL) have been observed and are not necessarily associated with a poor prognosis.

Neutropenia and lymphopenia are transient and are followed by a relative lymphocytosis. Atypical lymphocytes (varying between 2 and 20%) are common during the acute phase. Measurement of the prothrombin time (PT) is important in patients with acute viral hepatitis, for a prolonged value may reflect a severe hepatic synthetic defect, signify extensive hepatocellular necrosis, and indicate a worse prognosis. Occasionally, a prolonged PT may occur with only mild increases in the serum bilirubin and aminotransferase levels. Prolonged nausea and vomiting, inadequate carbohydrate intake, and poor hepatic glycogen reserves may contribute to hypoglycemia noted occasionally in patients with severe viral hepatitis. Serum alkaline phosphatase may be normal or only mildly elevated, while a fall in serum albumin is uncommon in uncomplicated acute viral hepatitis. In some patients, mild and transient steatorrhea has been noted as well as slight microscopic hematuria and minimal proteinuria.

A diffuse but mild elevation of the γ globulin fraction is common during acute viral hepatitis. Serum IgG and IgM levels are elevated in about one-third of patients during the acute phase of viral hepatitis, but the serum IgM level is elevated more characteristically during acute hepatitis A. During the acute phase of viral hepatitis, antibodies to smooth muscle and other cell constituents may be present, and low titers of rheumatoid factor, nuclear antibody, and heterophil antibody can also be found occasionally. In hepatitis C and D, antibodies to LKM may occur; however, the species of LKM antibodies in the two types of hepatitis are different from each other as well as from the LKM antibody species characteristic of autoimmune hepatitis type 2 (Chap. 40). The autoantibodies in viral hepatitis are nonspecific and can also be associated with other viral and systemic diseases. In contrast, virus-specific antibodies, which appear during and after hepatitis virus infection, are serologic markers of diagnostic importance.

As described earlier, serologic tests are available with which to establish a diagnosis of hepatitis A, B, D, and C. Tests for fecal or serum HAV are not routinely available. Therefore, a diagnosis of hepatitis A is based on detection of IgM anti-HAV during acute illness (Fig. 38-2). Rheumatoid factor can give rise to false-positive results in this test.

A diagnosis of HBV infection can usually be made by detection of HBsAg in serum. Infrequently, levels of HBsAg are too low to be detected during acute HBV infection, even with contemporary, highly sensitive immunoassays. In such cases, the diagnosis can be established by the presence of IgM anti-HBc.

The titer of HBsAg bears little relation to the severity of clinical disease. Indeed, an inverse correlation exists between the serum concentration of HBsAg and the degree of liver cell damage. For example, titers are highest in immunosuppressed patients, lower in patients with chronic liver disease (but higher in mild chronic than in severe chronic hepatitis), and very low in patients with acute fulminant hepatitis. These observations suggest that, in hepatitis B, the degree of liver cell damage and the clinical course are related to variations in the patient's immune response to HBV rather than to the amount of circulating HBsAg. In immunocompetent persons, however, a correlation exists between markers of HBV *replication* and liver injury (discussed later).

Another serologic marker that may be of value in patients with hepatitis B is HBeAg. Its principal clinical usefulness is as an indicator of relative infectivity. Because HBeAg is invariably present during early acute hepatitis B, HBeAg testing is indicated primarily during follow-up of chronic infection.

In patients with hepatitis B surface antigenemia of unknown duration (e.g., blood donors found to be HBsAg-positive and referred to a physician for evaluation), testing for IgM anti-HBc may be useful to distinguish between acute or recent infection (IgM anti-HBc-positive) and chronic HBV infection (IgM anti-HBc-negative, IgG anti-HBc-positive). A false-positive test for IgM anti-HBc may be encountered in patients with high-titer rheumatoid factor.

Anti-HBs is rarely detectable in the presence of HBsAg in patients with *acute* hepatitis B, but 10–20% of persons with *chronic* HBV infection may harbor low-level anti-HBs. This antibody is directed not against the common group determinant, *a*, but against the heterotypic subtype determinant (e.g., HBsAg of subtype *ad* with anti-HBs of subtype *y*). In most cases, this serologic pattern cannot be attributed to infection with two different HBV subtypes, and the presence of this antibody is not a harbinger of imminent HBsAg clearance. When such antibody is detected, its presence is of no recognized clinical significance (see "Virology and Etiology").

After immunization with hepatitis B vaccine, which consists of HBsAg alone, anti-HBs is the only serologic marker to appear. The commonly encountered serologic patterns of hepatitis B and their interpretations are summarized in Table 38-5. Tests for the detection of HBV DNA in liver and serum are now available. Like HBeAg, serum HBV DNA is an indicator of HBV replication, but tests for HBV DNA are more sensitive and quantitative. First-generation hybridization assays for HBV DNA had a sensitivity of 10^5–10^6 virions/mL, a relative threshold below which infectivity and liver injury are limited and HBeAg is usually undetectable. Currently, testing for HBV DNA has shifted from insensitive hybridization assays to amplification assays (e.g., the PCR-based assay, which can detect as few as 10 or 100 virions/mL); among the commercially available PCR assays, the most useful are those with the highest sensitivity (5–10 IU/mL) and the largest dynamic range (10^0–10^9 IU/mL). With increased sensitivity, amplification assays remain reactive well below the threshold for infectivity and liver injury. These markers are useful in following the course of HBV replication in patients with chronic hepatitis B receiving antiviral chemotherapy (e.g., with interferon or nucleoside analogues) (Chap. 40). In immunocompetent persons with chronic hepatitis B, a general correlation does appear to exist between the level of HBV replication, as reflected by the level of HBV DNA in serum, and the degree of liver injury. High-serum HBV DNA levels, increased expression of viral antigens, and necroinflammatory activity in the liver go hand in hand unless immunosuppression interferes with cytolytic T cell responses to virus-infected cells; reduction of HBV replication with antiviral drugs tends to be accompanied by an improvement in liver histology. Among patients with chronic hepatitis B, high levels of HBV DNA increase the risk of cirrhosis, hepatic decompensation, and hepatocellular carcinoma (see "Complications and Sequelae").

In patients with hepatitis C, an episodic pattern of aminotransferase elevation is common. A specific serologic diagnosis of hepatitis C can be made by demonstrating the presence in serum of anti-HCV. When contemporary immunoassays are used, anti-HCV can be detected in acute hepatitis C during the initial phase of elevated aminotransferase activity. This antibody may never become detectable in 5–10% of patients with acute hepatitis C, and levels of anti-HCV may become undetectable after recovery (albeit rare) from acute hepatitis C. In patients with chronic hepatitis C, anti-HCV is detectable in >95% of cases. Nonspecificity can confound immunoassays for anti-HCV, especially in persons with a low prior probability of infection, such as volunteer blood donors, or in persons with circulating rheumatoid factor, which can bind nonspecifically to assay reagents; testing for HCV RNA can be used in such settings to distinguish between true-positive and false-positive anti-HCV determinations. Assays for HCV RNA are the most sensitive tests for HCV infection and represent the "gold standard" in establishing a diagnosis of hepatitis C. HCV RNA can be detected even before acute elevation of aminotransferase activity and before the appearance of anti-HCV in patients with acute hepatitis C.

TABLE 38-5

COMMONLY ENCOUNTERED SEROLOGIC PATTERNS OF HEPATITIS B INFECTION

HBsAg	ANTI-HBs	ANTI-HBc	HBeAg	ANTI-HBe	INTERPRETATION
+	–	IgM	+	–	Acute hepatitis B, high infectivity
+	–	IgG	+	–	Chronic hepatitis B, high infectivity
+	–	IgG	–	+	1. Late acute or chronic hepatitis B, low infectivity 2. HBeAg–negative ("precore–mutant") hepatitis B (chronic or, rarely, acute)
+	+	+	+/–	+/–	1. HBsAg of one subtype and heterotypic anti–HBs (common) 2. Process of seroconversion from HBsAg to anti–HBs (rare)
–	–	IgM	+/–	+/–	1. Acute hepatitis B 2. Anti–HBc "window"
–	–	IgG	–	+/–	1. Low–level hepatitis B carrier 2. Hepatitis B in remote past
–	+	IgG	–	+/–	Recovery from hepatitis B
–	+	–	–	–	1. Immunization with HBsAg (after vaccination) 2. Hepatitis B in the remote past (?) 3. False–positive

In addition, HCV RNA remains detectable indefinitely, continuously in most but intermittently in some, in patients with chronic hepatitis C (detectable as well in some persons with normal liver tests (i.e., inactive carriers). In the small minority of patients with hepatitis C who lack anti-HCV, a diagnosis can be supported by detection of HCV RNA. If all these tests are negative and the patient has a well-characterized case of hepatitis after percutaneous exposure to blood or blood products, a diagnosis of hepatitis caused by an unidentified agent can be entertained.

Amplification techniques are required to detect HCV RNA, and two types are available. One is a branched-chain complementary DNA (bDNA) assay, in which the detection signal (a colorimetrically detectable enzyme bound to a complementary DNA probe) is amplified. The other involves target amplification (i.e., synthesis of multiple copies of the viral genome). This can be done by PCR or TMA, in which the viral RNA is reverse transcribed to complementary DNA and then amplified by repeated cycles of DNA synthesis. Both can be used as quantitative assays and a measurement of relative "viral load"; PCR and TMA, with a sensitivity of $10–10^2$ IU/mL, are more sensitive than bDNA, with a sensitivity of 10^3 IU/mL; assays are available with a wide dynamic range ($10–10^7$ IU/mL). Determination of HCV RNA level is not a reliable marker of disease severity or prognosis but is helpful in predicting relative responsiveness to antiviral therapy. The same is true for determinations of HCV genotype (Chap. 40).

A proportion of patients with hepatitis C have isolated anti-HBc in their blood, a reflection of a common risk in certain populations of exposure to multiple bloodborne hepatitis agents. The anti-HBc in such cases is almost invariably of the IgG class and usually represents HBV infection in the remote past (HBV DNA undetectable), rarely current HBV infection with low-level virus carriage.

The presence of HDV infection can be identified by demonstrating intrahepatic HDV antigen or, more practically, an anti-HDV seroconversion (a rise in titer of anti-HDV or de novo appearance of anti-HDV). Circulating HDV antigen, also diagnostic of acute infection, is detectable only briefly, if at all. Because anti-HDV is often undetectable once HBsAg disappears, retrospective serodiagnosis of acute self-limited, simultaneous HBV and HDV infection is difficult. Early diagnosis of acute infection may be hampered by a delay of up to 30–40 days in the appearance of anti-HDV.

When a patient presents with acute hepatitis and has HBsAg and anti-HDV in serum, determination of the class of anti-HBc is helpful in establishing the relationship between infection with HBV and HDV. Although IgM anti-HBc does not distinguish *absolutely* between acute and chronic HBV infection, its presence is a reliable indicator of recent infection and its absence a reliable indicator of infection in the remote past. In simultaneous acute HBV and HDV infections, IgM anti-HBc will be detectable, while in acute HDV infection superimposed on chronic HBV infection, anti-HBc will be of the IgG class.

Tests for the presence of HDV RNA are useful for determining the presence of ongoing HDV replication and relative infectivity. Diagnostic tests for hepatitis E are commercially available in several countries outside the United States; in the United States, diagnostic assays can be performed at the Centers for Disease Control and Prevention.

Liver biopsy is rarely necessary or indicated in acute viral hepatitis, except when the diagnosis is questionable or when clinical evidence suggests a diagnosis of chronic hepatitis.

A diagnostic algorithm can be applied in the evaluation of cases of acute viral hepatitis. A patient with acute hepatitis should undergo four serologic tests, HBsAg, IgM anti-HAV, IgM anti-HBc, and anti-HCV (Table 38-6). The presence of HBsAg, with or without IgM anti-HBc, represents HBV infection. If IgM anti-HBc is present, the HBV infection is considered acute; if IgM anti-HBc is absent, the HBV infection is

TABLE 38-6

SIMPLIFIED DIAGNOSTIC APPROACH IN PATIENTS PRESENTING WITH ACUTE HEPATITIS

SEROLOGIC TESTS OF PATIENT'S SERUM

HBsAg	IgM ANTI-HAV	IgM ANTI-HBc	ANTI-HCV	DIAGNOSTIC INTERPRETATION
+	−	+	−	Acute hepatitis B
+	−	−	−	Chronic hepatitis B
+	+	−	−	Acute hepatitis A superimposed on chronic hepatitis B
+	+	+	−	Acute hepatitis A and B
−	+	−	−	Acute hepatitis A
−	+	+	−	Acute hepatitis A and B (HBsAg below detection threshold)
−	−	+	−	Acute hepatitis B (HBsAg below detection threshold)
−	−	−	+	Acute hepatitis C

considered chronic. A diagnosis of acute hepatitis B can be made in the absence of HBsAg when IgM anti-HBc is detectable. A diagnosis of acute hepatitis A is based on the presence of IgM anti-HAV. If IgM anti-HAV coexists with HBsAg, a diagnosis of simultaneous HAV and HBV infections can be made; if IgM anti-HBc (with or without HBsAg) is detectable, the patient has simultaneous acute hepatitis A and B, and if IgM anti-HBc is undetectable, the patient has acute hepatitis A superimposed on chronic HBV infection. The presence of anti-HCV supports a diagnosis of acute hepatitis C. Occasionally, testing for HCV RNA or repeat anti-HCV testing later during the illness is necessary to establish the diagnosis. Absence of all serologic markers is consistent with a diagnosis of "non-A, non-B, non-C" hepatitis, if the epidemiologic setting is appropriate.

In patients with chronic hepatitis, initial testing should consist of HBsAg and anti-HCV. Anti-HCV supports and HCV RNA testing establishes the diagnosis of chronic hepatitis C. If a serologic diagnosis of chronic hepatitis B is made, testing for HBeAg and anti-HBe is indicated to evaluate relative infectivity. Testing for HBV DNA in such patients provides a more quantitative and sensitive measure of the level of virus replication and, therefore, is very helpful during antiviral therapy (Chap. 40). In patients with chronic hepatitis B and normal aminotransferase activity in the absence of HBeAg, serial testing over time is often required to distinguish between inactive carriage and HBeAg-negative chronic hepatitis B with fluctuating virologic and necroinflammatory activity. In persons with hepatitis B, testing for anti-HDV is useful in those with severe and fulminant disease, with severe chronic disease, with chronic hepatitis B and acute hepatitis-like exacerbations, with frequent percutaneous exposures, and from areas where HDV infection is endemic.

PROGNOSIS

Virtually all previously healthy patients with hepatitis A recover completely with no clinical sequelae. Similarly, in acute hepatitis B, 95–99% of previously healthy adults have a favorable course and recover completely. Certain clinical and laboratory features, however, suggest a more complicated and protracted course. Patients of advanced age and with serious underlying medical disorders may have a prolonged course and are more likely to experience severe hepatitis. Initial presenting features such as ascites, peripheral edema, and symptoms of hepatic encephalopathy suggest a poorer prognosis. In addition, a prolonged PT, low-serum albumin level, hypoglycemia, and very high-serum bilirubin values suggest severe hepatocellular disease. Patients with these clinical and laboratory features deserve prompt hospital admission. The case fatality rate in hepatitis A and B is very low (~0.1%) but is increased by advanced age

and underlying debilitating disorders. Among patients ill enough to be hospitalized for acute hepatitis B, the fatality rate is 1%. Hepatitis C is less severe during the acute phase than hepatitis B and is more likely to be anicteric; fatalities are rare, but the precise case fatality rate is not known. In outbreaks of waterborne hepatitis E in India and Asia, the case fatality rate is 1–2% and up to 10–20% in pregnant women. Patients with simultaneous acute hepatitis B and hepatitis D do not necessarily experience a higher mortality rate than do patients with acute hepatitis B alone; however, in several recent outbreaks of acute simultaneous HBV and HDV infection among injection drug users, the case fatality rate has been ~5%. In the case of HDV superinfection of a person with chronic hepatitis B, the likelihood of fulminant hepatitis and death is increased substantially. Although the case fatality rate for hepatitis D has not been defined adequately, in outbreaks of severe HDV superinfection in isolated populations with a high hepatitis B carrier rate, the mortality rate has been recorded in excess of 20%.

COMPLICATIONS AND SEQUELAE

A small proportion of patients with hepatitis A experience *relapsing hepatitis* weeks to months after apparent recovery from acute hepatitis. Relapses are characterized by recurrence of symptoms, aminotransferase elevations, occasionally jaundice, and fecal excretion of HAV. Another unusual variant of acute hepatitis A is *cholestatic hepatitis*, characterized by protracted cholestatic jaundice and pruritus. Rarely, liver test abnormalities persist for many months, even up to a year. Even when these complications occur, hepatitis A remains self-limited and does not progress to chronic liver disease. During the prodromal phase of acute hepatitis B, a serum sickness-like syndrome characterized by arthralgia or arthritis, rash, angioedema, and rarely, hematuria and proteinuria may develop in 5–10% of patients. This syndrome occurs before the onset of clinical jaundice, and these patients are often diagnosed erroneously as having rheumatologic diseases. The diagnosis can be established by measuring serum aminotransferase levels, which are almost invariably elevated, and serum HBsAg. As noted earlier, EMC is an immune-complex disease that can complicate chronic hepatitis C and is part of a spectrum of B cell lymphoproliferative disorders, which, in rare instances, can evolve to B cell lymphoma. Attention has been drawn as well to associations between hepatitis C and such cutaneous disorders as porphyria cutanea tarda and lichen planus. A mechanism for these associations is unknown. Finally, related to the reliance of HCV on lipoprotein secretion and assembly pathways and on interactions of HCV with glucose metabolism, HCV infection may be complicated by hepatic steatosis, hypercholesterolemia, insulin resistance (and other manifestations of the metabolic syndrome), and type 2 diabetes mellitus; both hepatic steatosis and insulin resistance appear to accelerate hepatic fibrosis and blunt responsiveness to antiviral therapy (Chap. 40).

The most feared complication of viral hepatitis is *fulminant hepatitis* (massive hepatic necrosis); fortunately, this is a rare event. Fulminant hepatitis is primarily seen in hepatitis B and D, as well as hepatitis E, but rare fulminant cases of hepatitis A occur primarily in older adults and in persons with underlying chronic liver disease, including, according to some reports, chronic hepatitis B and C. Hepatitis B accounts for >50% of fulminant cases of viral hepatitis, a sizable proportion of which are associated with HDV infection and another proportion with underlying chronic hepatitis C. Fulminant hepatitis is hardly ever seen in hepatitis C, but hepatitis E, as noted earlier, can be complicated by fatal fulminant hepatitis in 1–2% of all cases and in up to 20% of cases in pregnant women. Patients usually present with signs and symptoms of encephalopathy that may evolve to deep coma. The liver is usually small and the PT excessively prolonged. The combination of rapidly shrinking liver size, rapidly rising bilirubin level, and marked prolongation of the PT, even as aminotransferase levels fall, together with clinical signs of confusion, disorientation, somnolence, ascites, and edema, indicates that the patient has hepatic failure with encephalopathy. Cerebral edema is common; brainstem compression, gastrointestinal bleeding, sepsis, respiratory failure, cardiovascular collapse, and renal failure are terminal events. The mortality rate is exceedingly high (>80% in patients with deep coma), but patients who survive may have a complete biochemical and histologic recovery. If a donor liver can be located in time, liver transplantation may be life-saving in patients with fulminant hepatitis (Chap. 46).

Documenting the disappearance of HBsAg after apparent clinical recovery from acute hepatitis B is particularly important. Before laboratory methods were available to distinguish between acute hepatitis and acute hepatitis-like exacerbations (*spontaneous reactivations*) of chronic hepatitis B, observations suggested that ~10% of previously healthy patients remained HBsAg-positive for >6 months after the onset of clinically apparent acute hepatitis B. One-half of these persons cleared the antigen from their circulations during the next several years, but the other 5% remained chronically HBsAg-positive. More recent observations suggest that the true rate of chronic infection after clinically apparent acute hepatitis B is as low as 1% in normal, immunocompetent, young adults. Earlier, higher estimates may have been confounded by inadvertent inclusion of acute exacerbations in chronically infected patients; these patients, chronically HBsAg-positive before exacerbation, were unlikely to seroconvert to

HBsAg-negative thereafter. Whether the rate of chronicity is 10% or 1%, such patients have anti-HBc in serum; anti-HBs is either undetected or detected at low titer against the opposite subtype specificity of the antigen (see "Laboratory Features"). These patients may (1) be inactive carriers; (2) have low-grade, mild chronic hepatitis; or (3) have moderate to severe chronic hepatitis with or without cirrhosis. The likelihood of remaining chronically infected after acute HBV infection is especially high among neonates, persons with Down's syndrome, chronically hemodialyzed patients, and immunosuppressed patients, including persons with HIV infection.

Chronic hepatitis is an important late complication of acute hepatitis B occurring in a small proportion of patients with acute disease but more common in those who present with chronic infection without having experienced an acute illness, as occurs typically after neonatal infection or after infection in an immunosuppressed host (Chap. 40). Certain clinical and laboratory features suggest progression of acute hepatitis to chronic hepatitis: (1) lack of complete resolution of clinical symptoms of anorexia, weight loss, fatigue, and the persistence of hepatomegaly; (2) the presence of bridging/interface or multilobular hepatic necrosis on liver biopsy during protracted, severe acute viral hepatitis; (3) failure of the serum aminotransferase, bilirubin, and globulin levels to return to normal within 6–12 months after the acute illness; and (4) the persistence of HBeAg for >3 months or HBsAg for >6 months after acute hepatitis.

Although acute hepatitis D infection does not increase the likelihood of chronicity of simultaneous acute hepatitis B, hepatitis D has the potential for contributing to the severity of chronic hepatitis B. Hepatitis D superinfection can transform inactive or mild chronic hepatitis B into severe, progressive chronic hepatitis and cirrhosis; it also can accelerate the course of chronic hepatitis B. Some HDV superinfections in patients with chronic hepatitis B lead to fulminant hepatitis. As defined in longitudinal studies over 3 decades, the annual rates of cirrhosis and hepatocellular carcinoma in patients with chronic hepatitis D are 4% and 2.8%, respectively. Although HDV and HBV infections are associated with severe liver disease, mild hepatitis and even inactive carriage have been identified in some patients, and the disease may become indolent beyond the early years of infection.

After acute HCV infection, the likelihood of remaining chronically *infected* approaches 85–90%. Although many patients with chronic hepatitis C have no symptoms, cirrhosis may develop in as many as 20% within 10–20 years of acute illness; in some series of cases reported by referral centers, cirrhosis has been reported in as many as 50% of patients with chronic hepatitis C. Although chronic hepatitis C accounts for at least 40% of cases of chronic liver disease and of patients undergoing liver transplantation for end-stage liver disease in the United States and Europe, in the majority of patients with chronic hepatitis C, morbidity and mortality are limited during the initial 20 years after the onset of infection. Progression of chronic hepatitis C may be influenced by age of acquisition, duration of infection, immunosuppression, coexisting excessive alcohol use, concomitant hepatic steatosis, other hepatitis virus infection, or HIV co-infection. In fact, instances of severe and rapidly progressive chronic hepatitis B and C are being recognized with increasing frequency in patients with HIV infection. In contrast, neither HAV nor HEV causes chronic liver disease.

Rare complications of viral hepatitis include pancreatitis, myocarditis, atypical pneumonia, aplastic anemia, transverse myelitis, and peripheral neuropathy. Persons with chronic hepatitis B, particularly those infected in infancy or early childhood and especially those with HBeAg and/or high-level HBV DNA, have an enhanced risk of hepatocellular carcinoma. The risk of hepatocellular carcinoma is increased as well in patients with chronic hepatitis C, almost exclusively in patients with cirrhosis, and almost always after at least several decades, usually after 3 decades of disease (Chap. 50). In children, hepatitis B may present rarely with anicteric hepatitis, a nonpruritic papular rash of the face, buttocks, and limbs, and lymphadenopathy (papular acrodermatitis of childhood or Gianotti-Crosti syndrome).

Rarely, autoimmune hepatitis (Chap. 40) can be triggered by a bout of otherwise self-limited acute hepatitis, as reported after acute hepatitis A, B, and C.

DIFFERENTIAL DIAGNOSIS

Viral diseases such as infectious mononucleosis; those due to cytomegalovirus, herpes simplex, and coxsackieviruses; and toxoplasmosis may share certain clinical features with viral hepatitis and cause elevations in serum aminotransferase and, less commonly, in serum bilirubin levels. Tests such as the differential heterophile and serologic tests for these agents may be helpful in the differential diagnosis if HBsAg, anti-HBc, IgM anti-HAV, and anti-HCV determinations are negative. Aminotransferase elevations can accompany almost any systemic viral infection; other rare causes of liver injury confused with viral hepatitis are infections with *Leptospira, Candida, Brucella, Mycobacteria,* and *Pneumocystis.* A complete drug history is particularly important, for many drugs and certain anesthetic agents can produce a picture of either acute hepatitis or cholestasis (Chap. 39). Equally important is a past history of unexplained "repeated episodes" of acute hepatitis. This history should alert the physician to the possibility that the underlying disorder is chronic hepatitis. Alcoholic hepatitis must also be considered, but usually the serum aminotransferase levels are not as markedly elevated and

other stigmata of alcoholism may be present. The finding on liver biopsy of fatty infiltration, a neutrophilic inflammatory reaction, and "alcoholic hyaline" would be consistent with alcohol-induced rather than viral liver injury. Because acute hepatitis may present with right upper quadrant abdominal pain, nausea and vomiting, fever, and icterus, it is often confused with acute cholecystitis, common duct stone, or ascending cholangitis. Patients with acute viral hepatitis may tolerate surgery poorly; therefore, it is important to exclude this diagnosis, and in confusing cases, a percutaneous liver biopsy may be necessary before laparotomy. Viral hepatitis in the elderly is often misdiagnosed as obstructive jaundice resulting from a common duct stone or carcinoma of the pancreas. Because acute hepatitis in the elderly may be quite severe and the operative mortality high, a thorough evaluation including biochemical tests, radiographic studies of the biliary tree, and even liver biopsy may be necessary to exclude primary parenchymal liver disease. Another clinical constellation that may mimic acute hepatitis is right ventricular failure with passive hepatic congestion or hypoperfusion syndromes, such as those associated with shock, severe hypotension, and severe left ventricular failure. Also included in this general category is any disorder that interferes with venous return to the heart, such as right atrial myxoma, constrictive pericarditis, hepatic vein occlusion (Budd-Chiari syndrome), or veno-occlusive disease. Clinical features are usually sufficient to distinguish among these vascular disorders and viral hepatitis. Acute fatty liver of pregnancy, cholestasis of pregnancy, eclampsia, and the HELLP (*h*emolysis, *e*levated *l*iver tests, and *l*ow *p*latelets) syndrome can be confused with viral hepatitis during pregnancy. Very rarely, malignancies metastatic to the liver can mimic acute or even fulminant viral hepatitis. Occasionally, genetic or metabolic liver disorders (e.g., Wilson's disease, α_1 antitrypsin deficiency) as well as nonalcoholic fatty liver disease are confused with viral hepatitis.

TREATMENT   Acute Viral Hepatitis

In hepatitis B, among previously healthy adults who present with clinically apparent acute hepatitis, recovery occurs in ~99%; therefore, antiviral therapy is not likely to improve the rate of recovery and is not required. In rare instances of severe acute hepatitis B, treatment with a nucleoside analogue at oral doses used to treat chronic hepatitis B (Chap. 40) has been attempted successfully. Although clinical trials have not been done to establish the efficacy of this approach, although severe acute hepatitis B is not an approved indication for therapy, and although the duration of therapy has not been determined, nonetheless, most authorities would recommend institution of antiviral therapy with a nucleoside analogue for severe, but not mild–moderate, acute hepatitis B. In typical cases of acute hepatitis C, recovery is rare, progression to chronic hepatitis is the rule, and meta-analyses of small clinical trials suggest that antiviral therapy with interferon alfa monotherapy (3 million units SC three times a week) is beneficial, reducing the rate of chronicity considerably by inducing sustained responses in 30–70% of patients. In a German multicenter study of 44 patients with acute symptomatic hepatitis C, initiation of intensive interferon alfa therapy (5 million units SC daily for 4 weeks, then three times a week for another 20 weeks) within an average of 3 months after infection resulted in a sustained virologic response rate of 98%. Although treatment of acute hepatitis C is recommended, the optimum regimen, duration of therapy, and time to initiate therapy remain to be determined. Many authorities now opt for a 24-week course (beginning within 2–3 months after onset) of the best regimen identified for the treatment of chronic hepatitis C, long-acting pegylated interferon plus the nucleoside analogue ribavirin, although the value of adding ribavirin has not been demonstrated (see Chap. 40 for doses). Because of the marked reduction over the past 2 decades in the frequency of acute hepatitis C, opportunities to identify and treat patients with acute hepatitis C are rare, except in injection drug users. Hospital epidemiologists, however, will encounter health workers who sustain hepatitis C-contaminated needle sticks; when monitoring for ALT elevations and HCV, RNA after these accidents identifies acute hepatitis C (risk only ~3%), therapy should be initiated.

Notwithstanding these specific therapeutic considerations, in most cases of typical acute viral hepatitis, specific treatment generally is not necessary. Although hospitalization may be required for clinically severe illness, most patients do not require hospital care. Forced and prolonged bed rest is not essential for full recovery, but many patients will feel better with restricted physical activity. A high-calorie diet is desirable, and because many patients may experience nausea late in the day, the major caloric intake is best tolerated in the morning. Intravenous feeding is necessary in the acute stage if the patient has persistent vomiting and cannot maintain oral intake. Drugs capable of producing adverse reactions such as cholestasis and drugs metabolized by the liver should be avoided. If severe pruritus is present, the use of the bile salt-sequestering resin cholestyramine is helpful. Glucocorticoid therapy has no value in acute viral hepatitis, even in severe cases associated with *bridging necrosis*, and may be deleterious, even increasing the risk of chronicity (e.g., of acute hepatitis B).

Physical isolation of patients with hepatitis to a single room and bathroom is rarely necessary except in the case of fecal incontinence for hepatitis A and E or uncontrolled, voluminous bleeding for hepatitis B (with or without concomitant hepatitis D) and hepatitis C. Because most patients hospitalized with hepatitis A excrete little, if any, HAV, the likelihood of HAV transmission from these patients during their hospitalization is low. Therefore, burdensome *enteric precautions are no longer recommended*. Although gloves should be worn when the bedpans or fecal material of patients with hepatitis A are handled, these precautions do not represent a departure from sensible procedure and contemporary universal precautions for all hospitalized patients. For patients with hepatitis B and hepatitis C, emphasis should be placed on blood precautions (i.e., avoiding direct, ungloved hand contact with blood and other body fluids). Enteric precautions are unnecessary. The importance of simple hygienic precautions such as hand washing cannot be overemphasized. Universal precautions that have been adopted for all patients apply to patients with viral hepatitis.

Hospitalized patients may be discharged following substantial symptomatic improvement, a significant downward trend in the serum aminotransferase and bilirubin values, and a return to normal of the PT. Mild aminotransferase elevations should not be considered contraindications to the gradual resumption of normal activity.

In *fulminant hepatitis*, the goal of therapy is to support the patient by maintenance of fluid balance, support of circulation and respiration, control of bleeding, correction of hypoglycemia, and treatment of other complications of the comatose state in anticipation of liver regeneration and repair. Protein intake should be restricted, and oral lactulose or neomycin administered. Glucocorticoid therapy has been shown in controlled trials to be ineffective. Likewise, exchange transfusion, plasmapheresis, human cross-circulation, porcine liver cross-perfusion, hemoperfusion, and extracorporeal liver-assist devices have not been proven to enhance survival. Meticulous intensive care that includes prophylactic antibiotic coverage is the one factor that does appear to improve survival. Orthotopic liver transplantation is resorted to with increasing frequency, with excellent results, in patients with fulminant hepatitis (Chap. 46).

PROPHYLAXIS

Because application of therapy for acute viral hepatitis is limited and because antiviral therapy for chronic viral hepatitis is cumbersome and costly but effective in only a proportion of patients (Chap. 40), emphasis is placed on prevention through immunization. The prophylactic approach differs for each of the types of viral hepatitis.

In the past, immunoprophylaxis relied exclusively on passive immunization with antibody-containing globulin preparations purified by cold ethanol fractionation from the plasma of hundreds of normal donors. Currently, for hepatitis A and B, active immunization with vaccines is the preferable approach to prevention.

Hepatitis A

Both passive immunization with IG and active immunization with killed vaccines are available. All preparations of IG contain anti-HAV concentrations sufficient to be protective. When administered before exposure or during the early incubation period, IG is effective in preventing clinically apparent hepatitis A. For postexposure prophylaxis of intimate contacts (household, sexual, institutional) of persons with hepatitis A, the administration of 0.02 mL/kg is recommended as early after exposure as possible; it may be effective even when administered as late as 2 weeks after exposure. Prophylaxis is not necessary for those who have already received hepatitis A vaccine, casual contacts (office, factory, school, or hospital), for most elderly persons, who are very likely to be immune, or for those known to have anti-HAV in their serum. In day-care centers, recognition of hepatitis A in children or staff should provide a stimulus for immunoprophylaxis in the center and in the children's family members. By the time most common-source outbreaks of hepatitis A are recognized, it is usually too late in the incubation period for IG to be effective; however, prophylaxis may limit the frequency of secondary cases. For travelers to tropical countries, developing countries, and other areas outside standard tourist routes, IG prophylaxis had been recommended before a vaccine became available. When such travel lasted <3 months, 0.02 mL/kg was given; for longer travel or residence in these areas, a dose of 0.06 mL/kg every 4–6 months was recommended. Administration of plasma-derived globulin is safe; all contemporary lots of IG are subjected to viral inactivation steps and must be free of HCV RNA as determined by PCR testing. Administration of IM lots of IG has not been associated with transmission of HBV, HCV, or HIV.

Formalin-inactivated vaccines made from strains of HAV attenuated in tissue culture have been shown to be safe, immunogenic, and effective in preventing hepatitis A. Hepatitis A vaccines are approved for use in persons who are at least one year old and appear to provide adequate protection beginning 4 weeks after a primary inoculation. If it can be given within 4 weeks of an expected exposure, such as by travel to an endemic area, hepatitis A vaccine is the preferred approach to *pre-exposure* immunoprophylaxis. If travel is more imminent, IG (0.02 mL/kg) should be administered at a different injection site, along with the first dose of vaccine. Because vaccination provides long-lasting protection

(protective levels of anti-HAV should last 20 years after vaccination), persons whose risk will be sustained (e.g., frequent travelers or those remaining in endemic areas for prolonged periods) should be vaccinated, and vaccine should supplant the need for repeated IG injections. Shortly after its introduction, hepatitis A vaccine was recommended for children living in communities with a high incidence of HAV infection; in 1999, this recommendation was extended to include all children living in states, counties, and communities with high rates of HAV infection. As of 2006, the Advisory Committee on Immunization Practices of the U.S. Public Health Service recommended *routine hepatitis A vaccination of all children*. Other groups considered to be at increased risk for HAV infection and who are candidates for hepatitis A vaccination include military personnel, populations with cyclic outbreaks of hepatitis A (e.g., Alaskan natives), employees of day-care centers, primate handlers, laboratory workers exposed to hepatitis A or fecal specimens, and patients with chronic liver disease. Because of an increased risk of fulminant hepatitis A—observed in some experiences but not confirmed in others—among patients with chronic hepatitis C, patients with chronic hepatitis C are candidates for hepatitis A vaccination, as are persons with chronic hepatitis B. Other populations whose recognized risk of hepatitis A is increased should be vaccinated, including men who have sex with men, injection drug users, persons with clotting disorders who require frequent administration of clotting-factor concentrates, persons traveling from the United States to countries with high or intermediate hepatitis A endemicity, postexposure prophylaxis for contacts of persons with hepatitis A, and household members and other close contacts of adopted children arriving from countries with high and moderate hepatitis A endemicity. Recommendations for dose and frequency differ for the two approved vaccine preparations (Table 38-7); all injections are IM. Hepatitis A vaccine has been reported to be effective in preventing secondary household cases of acute hepatitis A, but its role in other instances of postexposure prophylaxis remains to be demonstrated. In the United States, reported mortality resulting from hepatitis A declined in parallel with hepatitis A vaccine-associated reductions in the annual incidence of new infections.

Hepatitis B

Until 1982, prevention of hepatitis B was based on *passive* immunoprophylaxis either with standard IG, containing modest levels of anti-HBs, or hepatitis B immunoglobulin (HBIG), containing high-titer anti-HBs. The efficacy of standard IG has never been established and remains questionable; even the efficacy of HBIG, demonstrated in several clinical trials, has been challenged, and its contribution appears to be in reducing

TABLE 38-7

HEPATITIS A VACCINATION SCHEDULES

AGE, YEARS	NO. OF DOSES	DOSE	SCHEDULE, MONTHS
HAVRIX (GlaxoSmithKline)[a]			
1–18	2	720 ELU[b] (0.5 mL)	0, 6–12
≥19	2	1440 ELU (1 mL)	0, 6–12
VAQTA (Merck)			
1–18	2	25 units (0.5 mL)	0, 6–18
≥19	2	50 units (1 mL)	0, 6–18

[a]A combination of this hepatitis A vaccine and hepatitis B vaccine, TWINRIX, is licensed for simultaneous protection against both of these viruses among adults (age ≥18 years). Each 1-mL dose contains 720 ELU of hepatitis A vaccine and 20 μg of hepatitis B vaccine. These doses are recommended at months 0, 1, and 6.
[b]Enzyme-linked immunoassay units.
Abbreviation: ELU, enzyme-linked immunoassay unit.

the frequency of clinical *illness*, not in preventing *infection*. The first vaccine for *active* immunization, introduced in 1982, was prepared from purified, noninfectious 22-nm spherical forms of HBsAg derived from the plasma of healthy HBsAg carriers. In 1987, the plasma-derived vaccine was supplanted by a genetically engineered vaccine derived from recombinant yeast. The latter vaccine consists of HBsAg particles that are nonglycosylated but are otherwise indistinguishable from natural HBsAg; two recombinant vaccines are licensed for use in the United States. Current recommendations can be divided into those for pre-exposure and postexposure prophylaxis.

For *pre-exposure* prophylaxis against hepatitis B in settings of frequent exposure (health workers exposed to blood; hemodialysis patients and staff; residents and staff of custodial institutions for the developmentally handicapped; injection drug users; inmates of long-term correctional facilities; persons with multiple sexual partners; persons such as hemophiliacs who require long-term, high-volume therapy with blood derivatives; household and sexual contacts of HBsAg carriers; persons living in or traveling extensively in endemic areas; unvaccinated children under the age of 18; and unvaccinated children who are Alaskan natives, Pacific Islanders, or residents in households of first-generation immigrants from endemic countries), three IM (deltoid, not gluteal) injections of hepatitis B vaccine are recommended at 0, 1, and 6 months (other, optional schedules are summarized in Table 38-8). Pregnancy is *not* a contraindication to vaccination. In areas of low HBV endemicity such as the United States, despite the availability of safe and effective hepatitis B vaccines, a strategy of vaccinating persons in high-risk groups has not been effective. The incidence of new hepatitis B cases continued to increase in the United States after the introduction

of vaccines; <10% of all targeted persons in high-risk groups have actually been vaccinated, and ~30% of persons with sporadic acute hepatitis B do not fall into any high-risk-group category. Therefore, to have an impact on the frequency of HBV infection in an area of low endemicity such as the United States, universal hepatitis B vaccination in childhood has been recommended. For unvaccinated children born after the implementation of universal infant vaccination, vaccination during early adolescence, at age 11–12 years, was recommended, and this recommendation has been extended to include all unvaccinated children age 0–19 years. In HBV-hyperendemic areas (e.g., Asia), universal vaccination of children has resulted in a marked 10- to 15-year decline in hepatitis B and its complications, including hepatocellular carcinoma.

The two available recombinant hepatitis B vaccines are comparable, one containing 10 μg of HBsAg (Recombivax-HB) and the other containing 20 μg of HBsAg (Engerix-B), and recommended doses for each injection vary for the two preparations (Table 38-8). Combinations of hepatitis B vaccine with other childhood vaccines are available as well (Table 38-8).

For unvaccinated persons sustaining an exposure to HBV, *postexposure* prophylaxis with a combination of HBIG (for rapid achievement of high-titer circulating anti-HBs) and hepatitis B vaccine (for achievement of long-lasting immunity as well as its apparent efficacy in attenuating clinical illness after exposure) is recommended. For *perinatal* exposure of infants born to HBsAg-positive mothers, a single dose of HBIG, 0.5 mL, should be administered IM in the thigh *immediately after birth*, followed by a complete course of three injections of recombinant hepatitis B vaccine (see doses earlier) to be started within the first 12 h of life. For those experiencing a direct percutaneous inoculation or transmucosal exposure to HBsAg-positive blood or body fluids (e.g., accidental *needle stick*, other mucosal penetration, or ingestion), a single IM dose of HBIG, 0.06 mL/kg, administered as soon after exposure as possible, is followed by a complete course of hepatitis B vaccine to begin within the first week. For those exposed by *sexual* contact to a patient with acute hepatitis B, a single IM dose of HBIG, 0.06 mL/kg, should be given within 14 days of exposure, to be followed by a complete course of hepatitis B vaccine. When both HBIG and hepatitis B vaccine are recommended, they may be given at the same time but at separate sites.

The precise duration of protection afforded by hepatitis B vaccine is unknown; however, ~80–90% of immunocompetent vaccinees retain protective levels of anti-HBs for at least 5 years, and 60–80% for 10 years. Thereafter and even after anti-HBs becomes undetectable, protection persists against clinical hepatitis B, hepatitis B surface antigenemia, and chronic HBV infection. Currently, *booster* immunizations are not

TABLE 38-8

PRE-EXPOSURE HEPATITIS B VACCINATION SCHEDULES

TARGET GROUP	NO. OF DOSES	DOSE	SCHEDULE, MONTHS
RECOMBIVAX-HB (Merck)[a]			
Infants, children (<1–10 years)	3	5 µg (0.5 mL)	0, 1–2, 4–6
Adolescents (11–19 years)	3 or 4	5 µg (0.5 mL)	0–2, 1–4, 4–6 or 0, 12, 24 or 0, 1, 2, 12
	or 2	10 µg (1 mL)	0, 4–6 (age 11–15)
Adults (≥20 years)	3	10 µg (1 mL)	0–2, 1–4, 4–6
Hemodialysis patients[b]			
<20 years	3	5 µg (0.5 mL)	0, 1, 6
≥20 years	3	40 µg (4 mL)	0, 1, 6
ENGERIX-B (GlaxoSmithKline)[c]			
Infants, children (<1–10 years)	3 or 4	10 µg (0.5 mL)	0, 1–2, 4–6 or 0, 1, 2,12
Adolescents (10–19 years)	3 or 4	10 µg (0.5 mL)	0, 1–2, 4–6 or 0, 12, 24 or 0, 1, 2, 12
Adults (≥20 years)	3 or 4	20 µg (1 mL)	0–2, 1–4, 4–6 or 0, 1, 2, 12
Hemodialysis patients[b]			
<20 years	4	10 µg (0.5 mL)	0, 1, 2, 6
≥20 years	4	40 µg (2 mL)	0, 1, 2, 6

[a]This manufacturer produces a licensed combination of hepatitis B vaccine and vaccines against *Haemophilus influenzae* type b and *Neisseria meningitides*, Comvax, for use in infants and young children. Please consult product insert for dose and schedule.

[b]This group also includes other immunocompromised persons.

[c]This manufacturer produces two licensed combination hepatitis B vaccines: (1) Twinrix, recombinant hepatitis B vaccine plus inactivated hepatitis A vaccine, is licensed for simultaneous protection against both of these viruses among adults (age ≥18 years). Each 1-mL dose contains 720 ELU of hepatitis A vaccine and 20 µg of hepatitis B vaccine. These doses are recommended at months 0, 1, and 6. (2) Pediatrix, recombinant hepatitis B vaccine plus diphtheria and tetanus toxoid, pertussis, and inactivated poliovirus, is licensed for use in infants and young children. Please consult product insert for doses and schedules.

recommended routinely, except in immunosuppressed persons who have lost detectable anti-HBs or immunocompetent persons who sustain percutaneous HBsAg-positive inoculations after losing detectable antibody. Specifically, for hemodialysis patients, annual anti-HBs testing is recommended after vaccination; booster doses are recommended when anti-HBs levels fall to <10 mIU/mL. As noted earlier, for persons at risk of both hepatitis A and B, a combined vaccine is available containing 720 enzyme-linked immunoassay units (ELUs) of inactivated HAV and 20 µg of recombinant HBsAg (at 0, 1, and 6 months).

Hepatitis D

Infection with hepatitis D can be prevented by vaccinating susceptible persons with hepatitis B vaccine. No product is available for immunoprophylaxis to prevent HDV superinfection in HBsAg carriers; for them, avoidance of percutaneous exposures and limitation of intimate contact with persons who have HDV infection are recommended.

Hepatitis C

IG is ineffective in preventing hepatitis C and is no longer recommended for postexposure prophylaxis in cases of perinatal, needle stick, or sexual exposure. Although prototype vaccines that induce antibodies to HCV envelope proteins have been developed, currently, hepatitis C vaccination is not feasible practically. Genotype and quasispecies viral heterogeneity, as well as rapid evasion of neutralizing antibodies by this rapidly mutating virus, conspire to render HCV a difficult target for immunoprophylaxis with a vaccine. Prevention of transfusion-associated hepatitis C has been accomplished by the following successively introduced measures: exclusion of commercial blood donors and reliance on a volunteer blood supply; screening donor blood with surrogate markers such as ALT (no longer recommended) and anti-HBc, markers that identify segments of the blood donor population with an increased risk of bloodborne infections; exclusion of blood donors in high-risk groups for AIDS and the introduction of anti-HIV screening tests; and progressively sensitive serologic and virologic screening tests for HCV infection.

In the absence of active or passive immunization, prevention of hepatitis C includes behavior changes and precautions to limit exposures to infected persons. Recommendations designed to identify patients with clinically inapparent hepatitis as candidates for medical management have as a secondary benefit the identification of persons whose contacts could be at risk of becoming infected. A so-called look-back program has been recommended to identify persons who were transfused before 1992 with blood from a donor found subsequently to have hepatitis C. In addition, anti-HCV testing is recommended for anyone who received a blood transfusion or a transplanted organ before the introduction of second-generation screening tests in 1992, those who ever used injection drugs (or took other illicit drugs by noninjection routes), chronically hemodialyzed patients, persons with clotting disorders who received clotting factors made before 1987 from pooled blood products, persons with elevated aminotransferase levels, health workers exposed to HCV-positive blood or contaminated needles, persons with HIV infection, health care and public safety personnel following a needle-stick or other nonpercutaneous exposure to HCV-infected material, sexual partners of persons with hepatitis C, and children born to HCV-positive mothers (Table 38-4).

For stable, monogamous sexual partners, sexual transmission of hepatitis C is unlikely, and sexual barrier precautions are not recommended. For persons with multiple sexual partners or with sexually transmitted diseases, the risk of sexual transmission of hepatitis C is increased, and barrier precautions (latex condoms) are

recommended. A person with hepatitis C should avoid sharing such items as razors, toothbrushes, and nail clippers with sexual partners and family members. No special precautions are recommended for babies born to mothers with hepatitis C, and breast-feeding does not have to be restricted.

Hepatitis E

Whether IG prevents hepatitis E remains undetermined. A safe and effective recombinant vaccine has been developed and is available in endemic areas but not in the United States.

CHAPTER 39

TOXIC AND DRUG-INDUCED HEPATITIS

Jules L. Dienstag

Liver injury may follow the inhalation, ingestion, or parenteral administration of a number of pharmacologic and chemical agents. These include industrial toxins (e.g., carbon tetrachloride, trichloroethylene, and yellow phosphorus); the heat-stable toxic bicyclic octapeptides of certain species of *Amanita* and *Galerina* (hepatotoxic mushroom poisoning); and, more commonly, pharmacologic agents used in medical therapy. Among patients with acute liver failure, drug-induced liver injury is the cause in a majority of all cases, and liver toxicity accounts for the abandonment of many new drugs during their development. It is essential that any patient presenting with jaundice or altered biochemical liver tests be questioned carefully about exposure to chemicals used in work or at home, drugs taken by prescription or bought over the counter, and herbal or alternative medicines. Hepatotoxic drugs can injure the hepatocyte directly (e.g., via a free-radical or metabolic intermediate that causes peroxidation of membrane lipids and that results in liver cell injury). Alternatively, the drug or its metabolite can distort cell membranes or other cellular molecules, bind covalently to intracellular proteins, activate apoptotic pathways, interfere with bile salt export proteins, or block biochemical pathways or cellular integrity (Fig. 39-1). Interference with bile canalicular pumps can allow endogenous bile acids, which can injure the liver, to accumulate. Such injuries, in turn, may lead to necrosis of hepatocytes; injure bile ducts, producing cholestasis; or block pathways of lipid movement, inhibit protein synthesis, or impair mitochondrial oxidation of fatty acids, resulting in lactic acidosis and intracellular triglyceride accumulation (expressed histologically as microvesicular steatosis). In some cases, drug metabolites sensitize hepatocytes to toxic cytokines, and differences between susceptible and nonsusceptible drug recipients may be attributable to polymorphisms in elaboration of competing, protective cytokines, as has been suggested for acetaminophen hepatotoxicity (discussed later). Immunologically mediated liver injury has been postulated to represent another mechanism of drug hepatotoxicity (discussed later). In addition, a role has been shown for activation of nuclear transporters, such as the constitutive androstane receptor (CAR), in the induction of drug hepatotoxicity.

Most drugs, which are water-insoluble, undergo a series of hepatic metabolic transformation steps, culminating in a water-soluble form appropriate for renal or biliary excretion. This process begins with oxidation or methylation initially mediated by the microsomal mixed-function oxygenases cytochrome P450 (phase I reaction) followed by glucuronidation or sulfation (phase II reaction) or inactivation by glutathione. Most drug hepatotoxicity is mediated by a phase I toxic metabolite, but glutathione depletion, precluding inactivation of harmful compounds by glutathione S-transferase, can contribute as well.

In general, two major types of chemical hepatotoxicity have been recognized: (1) direct toxic and (2) idiosyncratic. As shown in Table 39-1, direct toxic hepatitis occurs with predictable regularity in individuals exposed to the offending agent and is dose-dependent. The latent period between exposure and liver injury is usually short (often several hours), although clinical manifestations may be delayed for 24–48 h. Agents producing toxic hepatitis are generally systemic poisons or are converted in the liver to toxic metabolites. The direct hepatotoxins result in morphologic abnormalities that are reasonably characteristic and reproducible for each toxin. For example, carbon tetrachloride and trichloroethylene characteristically produce a centrilobular zonal necrosis, whereas yellow phosphorus poisoning typically results in periportal injury. The hepatotoxic octapeptides of *Amanita phalloides* usually produce massive hepatic necrosis; the lethal dose of the toxin is ~10 mg, the amount found in a single death-cap mushroom. Tetracycline, when administered in IV doses >1.5 g daily, leads to microvesicular fat deposits in the liver. Liver injury, which is often only one facet of

Six Mechanisms of Liver Injury

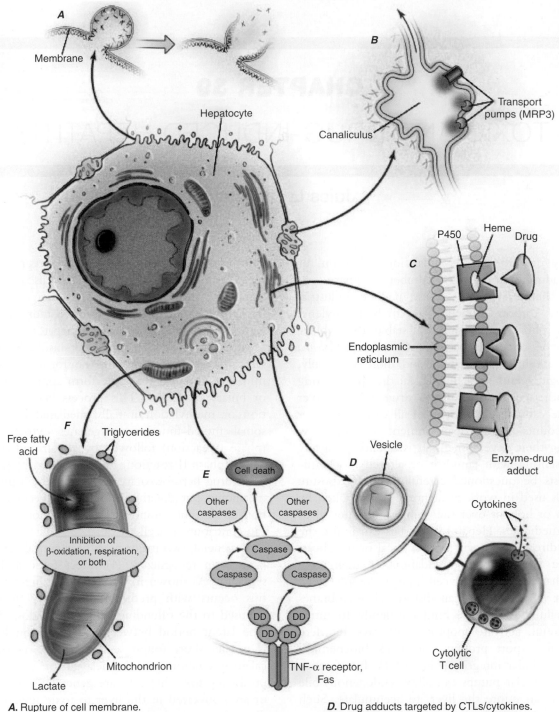

A. Rupture of cell membrane.
B. Injury of bile canaliculus (disruption of transport pumps).
C. P450-drug covalent binding (drug adducts).
D. Drug adducts targeted by CTLs/cytokines.
E. Activation of apoptotic pathway by TNFα/Fas.
F. Inhibition of mitochondrial function.

FIGURE 39-1

Potential mechanisms of drug-induced liver injury. The normal hepatocyte may be affected adversely by drugs through **A.** disruption of intracellular calcium homeostasis that leads to the disassembly of actin fibrils at the surface of the hepatocyte, resulting in blebbing of the cell membrane, rupture, and cell lysis; **B.** disruption of actin filaments next to the canaliculus (the specialized portion of the cell responsible for bile excretion), leading to loss of villous processes and interruption of transport pumps such as multidrug resistance–associated protein 3 (MRP3), which, in turn, prevents the excretion of bilirubin and other organic compounds; **C.** covalent binding of the heme-containing cytochrome P450 enzyme to the drug, thus creating nonfunctioning adducts; **D.** migration of these enzyme-drug adducts to the cell surface in vesicles to serve as target immunogens for cytolytic attack by T cells, stimulating an immune response involving cytolytic T cells and cytokines; **E.** activation of apoptotic pathways by tumor necrosis factor α (TNFα) receptor or

TABLE 39-1

SOME FEATURES OF TOXIC AND DRUG-INDUCED HEPATIC INJURY

| FEATURES | DIRECT TOXIC EFFECT* | | IDIOSYNCRATIC* | | | OTHER[a] |
	(CARBON TETRACHLORIDE)	(ACETAMINOPHEN)	(HALOTHANE)	(ISONIAZID)	(CHLORPROMAZINE)	(ORAL CONTRACEPTIVE AGENTS)
Predictable and dose-related toxicity	+	+	0	0	0	+
Latent period	Short	Short	Variable	Variable	Variable	Variable
Arthralgia, fever, rash, eosinophilia	0	0	+	0	+	0
Liver morphology	Necrosis, fatty infiltration	Centrilobular necrosis	Similar to viral hepatitis	Similar to viral hepatitis	Cholestasis *with* portal inflammation	Cholestasis *without* portal inflammation, vascular lesions

[a]The drugs listed are typical samples.

the toxicity produced by the direct hepatotoxins, may go unrecognized until jaundice appears.

In idiosyncratic drug reactions, the occurrence of hepatitis is usually infrequent (1 in 10^3–10^5 patients) and unpredictable; the response is not as clearly dose-dependent as is injury associated with direct hepatotoxins, and liver injury may occur at any time during or shortly after exposure to the drug. Adding to the difficulty of predicting or identifying idiosyncratic drug hepatotoxicity is the occurrence of mild, transient, nonprogressive serum aminotransferase elevations that resolve with continued drug use. Such "adaptation," the mechanism of which is unknown, occurs in such drugs as isoniazid, valproate, phenytoin, and HMG-CoA reductase inhibitors (statins). Extrahepatic manifestations of hypersensitivity, such as rash, arthralgias, fever, leukocytosis, and eosinophilia, occur in about one-quarter of patients with idiosyncratic hepatotoxic drug reactions; this observation and the unpredictability of idiosyncratic drug hepatotoxicity contributed to the hypothesis that this category of drug reactions is immunologically mediated. More recent evidence, however, suggests that, in most cases, even idiosyncratic reactions represent direct hepatotoxicity but are caused by drug

metabolites rather than by the intact compound. Even the prototypes of idiosyncratic hepatotoxicity reactions, halothane hepatitis and isoniazid hepatotoxicity, associated frequently with hypersensitivity manifestations, are now recognized to be mediated by toxic metabolites that damage liver cells directly. Currently, most idiosyncratic reactions are thought to result from differences in metabolic reactivity to specific agents; host susceptibility is mediated by the kinetics of toxic metabolite generation, which differs among individuals, probably mediated by genetic polymorphisms in drug-metabolizing pathways (e.g., differences in cytochrome P450 enzyme isotypes or in acetylation). Associations between certain HLA haplotypes have been drawn with hepatotoxicity of such drugs as amoxicillin/clavulanate, statins, halothane, nitrofurantoin, chlorpromazine, and flucloxacillin. Occasionally, however, the clinical features of an allergic reaction (prominent tissue eosinophilia, autoantibodies, etc.) are difficult to ignore. In vitro models have been described in which lymphocyte cytotoxicity can be demonstrated against rabbit hepatocytes altered by incubation with the potential offending drug. Furthermore, several instances of drug hepatotoxicity are associated with the appearance of autoantibodies, including

Fas (DD denotes death domain), triggering the cascade of intercellular caspases, resulting in programmed cell death; or *F.* inhibition of mitochondrial function by a dual effect on both β-oxidation and the respiratory-chain enzymes, leading to failure of free fatty acid metabolism, a lack of aerobic respiration, and accumulation of lactate and reactive

oxygen species (which may disrupt mitochondrial DNA). Toxic metabolites excreted in bile may damage bile-duct epithelium (not shown). CTLs, cytolytic T lymphocytes. (*Reproduced from WM Lee: Drug-induced hepatotoxicity. N Engl J Med 349:474, 2003, with permission.*)

CHAPTER 39 Toxic and Drug-Induced Hepatitis

a class of antibodies to liver-kidney microsomes, anti-LKM2, directed against a cytochrome P450 enzyme. Similarly, in selected cases, a drug or its metabolite has been shown to bind to a host cellular component forming a hapten; the immune response to this "neoantigen" is postulated to play a role in the pathogenesis of liver injury. Therefore, some authorities subdivide idiosyncratic drug hepatotoxicity into hypersensitivity (allergic) and "metabolic" categories. Several unusual exceptions notwithstanding, true drug allergy is difficult to support in most cases of idiosyncratic drug-induced liver injury.

Idiosyncratic reactions lead to a morphologic pattern that is more variable than those produced by direct toxins; a single agent is often capable of causing a variety of lesions, although certain patterns tend to predominate. Depending on the agent involved, idiosyncratic hepatitis may result in a clinical and morphologic picture indistinguishable from that of viral hepatitis (e.g., halothane) or may simulate extrahepatic bile duct obstruction clinically with morphologic evidence of cholestasis. Drug-induced cholestasis ranges from mild to increasingly severe: (1) bland cholestasis with limited hepatocellular injury (e.g., estrogens, 17,α-substituted androgens); (2) inflammatory cholestasis (e.g., phenothiazines, amoxicillin-clavulanic acid [the most frequently implicated antibiotic among cases of drug-induced liver injury], oxacillin, erythromycin estolate); (3) sclerosing cholangitis (e.g., after intrahepatic infusion of the chemotherapeutic agent floxuridine for hepatic metastases from a primary colonic carcinoma); (4) disappearance of bile ducts, "ductopenic" cholestasis, similar to that observed in chronic rejection following liver transplantation (e.g., carbamazepine, chlorpromazine, tricyclic antidepressant agents). Cholestasis may result from binding of drugs to canalicular membrane transporters, accumulation of toxic bile acids resulting from canalicular pump failure, or genetic defects in canalicular transporter proteins. Morphologic alterations may also include bridging hepatic necrosis (e.g., methyldopa), or, infrequently, hepatic granulomas (e.g., sulfonamides). Some drugs result in macrovesicular or microvesicular steatosis or steatohepatitis, which, in some cases, has been linked to mitochondrial dysfunction and lipid peroxidation. Severe hepatotoxicity associated with steatohepatitis, most likely a result of mitochondrial toxicity, is being recognized with increasing frequency among patients receiving antiretroviral therapy with reverse transcriptase inhibitors (e.g., zidovudine, didanosine) or protease inhibitors (e.g., indinavir, ritonavir) for HIV infection. Generally, such mitochondrial hepatotoxicity of these antiretroviral agents is reversible, but dramatic, nonreversible hepatotoxicity associated with mitochondrial injury (inhibition of DNA polymerase γ) was the cause of acute liver failure encountered during early clinical trials of now-abandoned fialuridine, a fluorinated pyrimidine analogue with potent antiviral activity against hepatitis B virus. Another potential target for idiosyncratic drug hepatotoxicity is sinusoidal lining cells; when these are injured, such as by high-dose chemotherapeutic agents (e.g., cyclophosphamide, melphalan, busulfan) administered prior to bone marrow transplantation, venoocclusive disease can result.

Not all adverse hepatic drug reactions can be classified as either toxic or idiosyncratic in type. For example, oral contraceptives, which combine estrogenic and progestational compounds, may result in impairment of hepatic tests and, occasionally, jaundice; however, they do not produce necrosis or fatty change, manifestations of hypersensitivity are generally absent, and susceptibility to the development of oral contraceptive–induced cholestasis appears to be genetically determined. Such estrogen-induced cholestasis is more common in women with cholestasis of pregnancy, a disorder linked to genetic defects in multidrug resistance–associated canalicular transporter proteins. Other instances of genetically determined drug hepatotoxicity have been identified. For example, ~10% of the population have an autosomal recessive trait associated with the absence of cytochrome P450 enzyme 2D6 and have impaired debrisoquine-4-hydroxylase enzyme activity. As a result, they cannot metabolize, and are at increased risk of hepatotoxicity resulting from certain compounds such as desipramine, propranolol, and quinidine.

Some forms of drug hepatotoxicity are so rare (e.g., occurring in <1:10,000 recipients), that they do not become apparent during clinical trials, involving only several thousand recipients, conducted to obtain drug registration. An example of such rare, but serious, idiosyncratic drug hepatotoxicity followed the approval and generalized use of troglitazone, a peroxisomal, proliferator activator–receptor γ agonist, the first introduced example of a thiazolidinedione insulin-sensitizing agent. This instance of drug hepatotoxicity was not recognized until well after the drug was introduced, underlining the importance of postmarketing surveillance in identifying toxic drugs and in leading to their withdrawal from use. Fortunately, such hepatotoxicity is not characteristic of the second-generation thiazolidinedione insulin-sensitizing agents rosiglitazone and pioglitazone; in clinical trials, the frequency of aminotransferase elevations in patients treated with these medications did not differ from that in placebo recipients, and isolated reports of liver injury among recipients are extremely rare.

Because drug-induced hepatitis is often a presumptive diagnosis and many other disorders produce a similar clinicopathologic picture, evidence of a causal relationship between the use of a drug and subsequent liver injury may be difficult to establish. The relationship is most convincing for the direct hepatotoxins, which lead to a high frequency of hepatic impairment after a short latent period. Idiosyncratic reactions may be reproduced, in some instances, when rechallenge, after an asymptomatic period, results in a recurrence of signs, symptoms, and morphologic and biochemical abnormalities. Rechallenge, however, is often ethically unfeasible, because severe reactions may occur. Causality-assessment methodologies (scoring systematically based on a checklist of such variables as index of suspicion, time of onset, clinical-biochemical features, type of injury [direct, idiosyncratic], extrahepatic features, course, histologic features, drug serum levels, genetic markers and polymorphisms, and exclusion of other potential causes) have been adopted to add objectivity to diagnoses of drug-induced liver injury; however, even these approaches have their limitations and yield residual uncertainty.

Generally, drug hepatotoxicity is not more frequent in persons with underlying chronic liver disease. Reported exceptions include hepatotoxicity of aspirin, methotrexate, isoniazid (only in certain experiences), and antiretroviral therapy for HIV infection.

TREATMENT   Toxic and Drug-Induced Hepatic Disease

Treatment is largely supportive, except in acetaminophen hepatotoxicity (discussed later). In patients with fulminant hepatitis resulting from drug hepatotoxicity, liver transplantation may be lifesaving (Chap. 46). Withdrawal of the suspected agent is indicated at the first sign of an adverse reaction. In the case of the direct toxins, liver involvement should not divert attention from renal or other organ involvement, which may also threaten survival. Glucocorticoids for drug hepatotoxicity with allergic features, silibinin for hepatotoxic mushroom poisoning, and ursodeoxycholic acid for cholestatic drug hepatotoxicity have never been shown to be effective and are not recommended.

In **Table 39-2**, several classes of chemical agents are listed together with examples of the pattern of liver injury produced by them. Certain drugs appear to be responsible for the development of chronic as well as acute hepatic injury. For example, oxyphenisatin, methyldopa, and isoniazid have been associated with moderate to severe chronic hepatitis, and halothane and methotrexate have been implicated in the development of cirrhosis. A syndrome resembling primary biliary cirrhosis has been described following treatment with chlorpromazine, methyl testosterone, tolbutamide, and other drugs. Portal hypertension in the absence of cirrhosis may result from alterations in hepatic architecture produced by vitamin A or arsenic intoxication, industrial exposure to vinyl chloride, or administration of

thorium dioxide. The latter three agents have also been associated with angiosarcoma of the liver. Oral contraceptives have been implicated in the development of hepatic adenoma and, rarely, hepatocellular carcinoma and hepatic vein occlusion (Budd-Chiari syndrome). Another unusual lesion, peliosis hepatis (blood cysts of the liver), has been observed in some patients treated with anabolic steroids. The existence of these hepatic disorders expands the spectrum of liver injury induced by chemical agents and emphasizes the need for a thorough drug history in all patients with liver dysfunction.

The following are patterns of adverse hepatic reactions for some prototypic agents.

ACETAMINOPHEN HEPATOTOXICITY (DIRECT TOXIN)

Acetaminophen can cause severe centrilobular hepatic necrosis when ingested in large amounts in suicide attempts or accidentally by children. In the United States and England, acetaminophen hepatotoxicity is the most common culprit among patients presenting with acute liver failure and the leading indication for liver transplantation among patients with drug-induced liver failure. A single dose of 10–15 g, occasionally less, may produce clinical evidence of liver injury. Fatal fulminant disease is usually (although not invariably) associated with ingestion of ≥25 g. Blood levels of acetaminophen correlate with the severity of hepatic injury (levels >300 μg/mL 4 h after ingestion are predictive of the development of severe damage; levels <150 μg/mL suggest that hepatic injury is highly unlikely). Nausea, vomiting, diarrhea, abdominal pain, and shock are early manifestations occurring 4–12 h after ingestion. Then 24–48 h later, when these features are abating, hepatic injury becomes apparent. Maximal abnormalities and hepatic failure may not be evident until 4–6 days after ingestion, and aminotransferase levels approaching 10,000 units are not uncommon (i.e., levels far exceeding those in patients with viral hepatitis). Renal failure and myocardial injury may be present.

Acetaminophen is metabolized predominantly by a phase II reaction to innocuous sulfate and glucuronide metabolites; however, a small proportion of acetaminophen is metabolized by a phase I reaction to a hepatotoxic metabolite formed from the parent compound by the cytochrome P450 CYP2E1. This metabolite, N-acetyl-benzoquinone-imine (NAPQI), is detoxified by binding to "hepatoprotective" glutathione to become harmless, water-soluble mercapturic acid, which undergoes renal excretion. When excessive amounts of NAPQI are formed, or when glutathione levels are low, glutathione levels are depleted and overwhelmed, permitting covalent binding to nucleophilic hepatocyte macromolecules forming acetaminophen-protein "adducts." These adducts, which can be measured

TABLE 39-2

PRINCIPAL ALTERATIONS OF HEPATIC MORPHOLOGY PRODUCED BY SOME COMMONLY USED DRUGS AND CHEMICALS[a]

PRINCIPAL MORPHOLOGIC CHANGE	CLASS OF AGENT	EXAMPLE
Cholestasis	Anabolic steroid	Methyl testosterone
	Antibiotic	Erythromycin estolate, nitrofurantoin, rifampin, amoxicillinclavulanic acid, oxacillin
	Anticonvulsant	Carbamazine
	Antidepressant	Duloxetine, mirtazapine, tricyclic antidepressants
	Anti-inflammatory	Sulindac
	Antiplatelet	Clopidogrel
	Antihypertensive	Irbesartan, fosinopril
	Antithyroid	Methimazole
	Calcium channel blocker	Nifedipine, verapamil
	Immunosuppressive	Cyclosporine
	Lipid-lowering	Ezetimibe
	Oncotherapeutic	Anabolic steroids, busulfan, tamoxifen, irinotecan, cytarabine
	Oral contraceptive	Norethynodrel with mestranol
	Oral hypoglycemic	Chlorpropamide
	Tranquilizer	Chlorpromazine[b]
Fatty liver	Antiarrhythmic	Amiodarone
	Antibiotic	Tetracycline (high-dose, IV)
	Anticonvulsant	Valproic acid
	Antiviral	Dideoxynucleosides (e.g., zidovudine), protease inhibitors (e.g., indinavir, ritonavir)
	Oncotherapeutic	Asparaginase, methotrexate
Hepatitis	Anesthetic	Halothane[c]
	Antiandrogen	Flutamide
	Antibiotic	Isoniazid,[c] rifampicin, nitrofurantoin, telithromycin, minocycline,[d] pyrazinamide, trovafloxacin[e]
	Anticonvulsant	Phenytoin, carbamazine, valproic acid, phenobarbital
	Antidepressant	Iproniazid, amitriptyline, imipramine, trazodone, venlafaxine, fluoxetine, paroxetine, duloxetine, sertraline, nefazodone,[e] bupropion
	Antifungal	Ketoconazole, fluconazole, itraconazole
	Antihypertensive	Methyldopa,[c] captopril, enalapril, lisinopril, losartan
	Anti-inflammatory	Ibuprofen, indomethacin, diclofenac, sulindac, bromfenac
	Antipsychotic	Risperidone
	Antiviral	Zidovudine, didanosine, stavudine, nevirapine, ritonavir, indinavir, tipranavir, zalcitabine
	Calcium channel blocker	Nifedipine, verapamil, diltiazem
	Cholinesterase inhibitor	Tacrine
	Diuretic	Chlorothiazide
	Laxative	Oxyphenisatin[c,e]
	Norepinephrine-reuptake inhibitor	Atomoxetine
	Oral hypoglycemic	Troglitazone,[e] acarbose
Mixed hepatitis/ cholestatic	Antibiotic	Amoxicillin-clavulanic acid, trimethoprim-sulfamethoxazole
	Antibacterial	Clindamycin
	Antifungal	Terbinafine
	Antihistamine	Cyproheptadine
	Immunosuppressive	Azathioprine
	Lipid-lowering	Nicotinic acid, lovastatin, ezetimide

(continued)

TABLE 39-2

PRINCIPAL ALTERATIONS OF HEPATIC MORPHOLOGY PRODUCED BY SOME COMMONLY USED DRUGS AND CHEMICALS[a] (*CONTINUED*)

PRINCIPAL MORPHOLOGIC CHANGE	CLASS OF AGENT	EXAMPLE
Toxic (necrosis)	Analgesic	Acetaminophen
	Hydrocarbon	Carbon tetrachloride
	Metal	Yellow phosphorus
	Mushroom	*Amanita phalloides*
	Solvent	Dimethylformamide
Granulomas	Antiarrhythmic	Quinidine, diltiazem
	Antibiotic	Sulfonamides
	Anticonvulsant	Carbamazine
	Anti-inflammatory	Phenylbutazone
	Xanthine oxidase inhibitor	Allopurinol

[a]Several agents cause more than one type of liver lesion and appear under more than one category.
[b]Rarely associated with primary biliary cirrhosis-like lesion.
[c]Occasionally associated with chronic hepatitis or bridging hepatic necrosis or cirrhosis.
[d]Associated with an autoimmune hepatitis-like syndrome.
[e]Withdrawn from use because of severe hepatotoxicity.

in serum by high-performance liquid chromatography, hold promise as diagnostic markers of acetaminophen hepatotoxicity. The binding of acetaminophen to hepatocyte macromolecules is believed to lead to hepatocyte necrosis; the precise sequence and mechanism are unknown. Hepatic injury may be potentiated by prior administration of alcohol, phenobarbital, isoniazid, or other drugs; by conditions that stimulate the mixed-function oxidase system; or by conditions such as starvation that reduce hepatic glutathione levels. The xenobiotic (environmental, exogenous substance) receptor CAR has been shown in a mouse model of acetaminophen hepatotoxicity to induce acetaminophen-metabolizing enzymes and, thereby, regulate and increase hepatotoxicity. Cimetidine, which inhibits P450 enzymes, has the potential to reduce generation of the toxic metabolite. Alcohol induces cytochrome P450 CYP2E1; consequently, increased levels of the toxic metabolite NAPQI are produced in chronic alcoholics after acetaminophen ingestion. In addition, alcohol suppresses hepatic glutathione production. Therefore, in chronic alcoholics, the toxic dose of acetaminophen may be as low as 2 g, and alcoholic patients should be warned specifically about the dangers of even standard doses of this commonly used drug. Such "therapeutic misadventures" also occur occasionally in patients with severe, febrile illnesses or pain syndromes; in such a setting, several days of anorexia and near-fasting coupled with regular administration of extra-strength acetaminophen formulations result in a combination of glutathione depletion and relatively high NAPQI levels in the absence of a history of recognized acetaminophen overdose. In a 2006 study, aminotransferase elevations

were identified in 31–44% of normal subjects treated for 14 days with the maximal recommended dose of acetaminophen, 4 g daily (administered alone or as part of an acetaminophen/opioid combination); because these changes were transient and never associated with bilirubin elevation, the clinical relevance of these findings remains to be determined. Although underlying HCV infection was found to be associated with an increased risk of acute liver injury in patients hospitalized for acetaminophen overdose, generally, in patients with nonalcoholic liver disease, acetaminophen taken in recommended doses, may be the safest analgesic/antipyretic. In this vein, acetaminophen use in cirrhotic patients has not been associated with hepatic decompensation. On the other hand, because of the link between acetaminophen use and liver injury, and because of the limited safety margin between safe and toxic doses, the Food and Drug Administration (FDA) has recommended that the daily dose of acetaminophen be reduced from 4 g to 3.25 g (even lower for persons with chronic alcohol use), that all acetaminophen-containing products be labeled prominently as containing acetaminophen, and that the potential for liver injury be prominent in the packaging of acetaminophen and acetaminophen-containing products.

TREATMENT ▶ Acetaminophen Overdosage

Treatment includes gastric lavage, supportive measures, and oral administration of activated charcoal or cholestyramine to prevent absorption of residual drug.

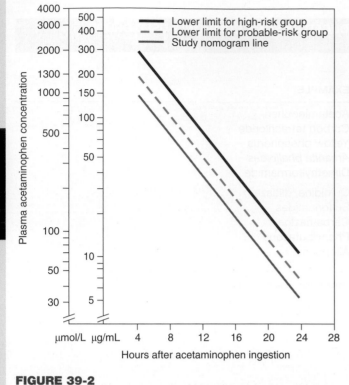

FIGURE 39-2

Nomogram to define risk of acetaminophen hepatotoxicity according to initial plasma acetaminophen concentration. (*After BH Rumack, H Matthew: Pediatrics 55:871, 1975.*)

Neither charcoal nor cholestyramine appears to be effective if given >30 min after acetaminophen ingestion; if they are used, the stomach lavage should be done before other agents are administered orally. The chances of possible, probable, and high-risk hepatotoxicity can be derived from a nomogram plot (Fig. 39-2), readily available in emergency departments as a function of measuring acetaminophen plasma levels 8 h after ingestion. In patients with high acetaminophen blood levels (>200 μg/mL measured at 4 h or >100 μg/mL at 8 h after ingestion), the administration of sulfhydryl compounds (e.g., cysteamine, cysteine, or *N*-acetylcysteine) reduces the severity of hepatic necrosis. These agents appear to act by providing a reservoir of sulfhydryl groups to bind the toxic metabolites or by stimulating synthesis and repletion of hepatic glutathione. Therapy should be begun within 8 h of ingestion but may be effective even if given as late as 24–36 h after overdose. Later administration of sulfhydryl compounds is of uncertain value. Routine use of *N*-acetylcysteine has substantially reduced the occurrence of fatal acetaminophen hepatotoxicity. When given orally, *N*-acetylcysteine is diluted to yield a 5% solution. A loading dose of 140 mg/kg is given, followed by 70 mg/kg every 4 h for 15–20 doses. Whenever a patient with potential acetaminophen hepatotoxicity is encountered,

a local poison control center should be contacted. Treatment can be stopped when plasma acetaminophen levels indicate that the risk of liver damage is low. If signs of hepatic failure (e.g., progressive jaundice, coagulopathy, confusion) occur despite *N*-acetylcysteine therapy for acetaminophen hepatotoxicity, liver transplantation may be the only option. Early arterial blood lactate levels among such patients with acute liver failure may distinguish patients highly likely to require liver transplantation (lactate levels >3.5 mmol/L) from those likely to survive without liver replacement.

Survivors of acute acetaminophen overdose usually have no hepatic sequelae. In a few patients, prolonged or repeated administration of acetaminophen in therapeutic doses appears to have led to the development of chronic hepatitis and cirrhosis.

HALOTHANE HEPATOTOXICITY (IDIOSYNCRATIC REACTION)

Although, currently, halothane anesthesia is administered in only rare situations, halothane hepatotoxicity was one of the prototypical, and most intensively studied, examples of idiosyncratic drug hepatotoxicity. Administration of halothane, a nonexplosive fluorinated hydrocarbon anesthetic agent that is structurally similar to chloroform, results in severe hepatic necrosis in a small number of individuals, many of whom have previously been exposed to this agent. The failure to produce similar hepatic lesions reliably in animals, the rarity of hepatic impairment in human beings, and the delayed appearance of hepatic injury suggest that halothane is not a direct hepatotoxin but rather a sensitizing agent; however, manifestations of hypersensitivity are seen in <25% of cases. A genetic predisposition leading to an idiosyncratic metabolic reactivity has been postulated and appears to be the most likely mechanism of halothane hepatotoxicity. Adults (rather than children), obese people, and women appear to be particularly susceptible. Fever, moderate leukocytosis, and eosinophilia may occur in the first week following halothane administration. Jaundice is usually noted 7–10 days after exposure but may occur earlier in previously exposed patients. Nausea and vomiting may precede the onset of jaundice. Hepatomegaly is often mild, but liver tenderness is common, and serum aminotransferase levels are elevated. The pathologic changes at autopsy are indistinguishable from massive hepatic necrosis resulting from viral hepatitis. The case–fatality rate of halothane hepatitis is not known but may vary from 20–40% in cases with severe liver involvement. Patients in whom unexplained spiking fever, especially delayed fever, or jaundice develops after halothane anesthesia should not receive this agent again. Because cross-reactions between halothane and methoxyflurane have been reported, the latter agent should not be used after halothane reactions. Later-generation halogenated hydrocarbon anesthetics that have supplanted halothane except in rare instances (e.g., certain types of thoracic surgery) are believed to be associated with a lower risk of hepatotoxicity.

METHYLDOPA HEPATOTOXICITY (TOXIC AND IDIOSYNCRATIC REACTION)

Minor alterations in liver tests are reported in ~5% of patients treated with this antihypertensive agent. These trivial abnormalities typically resolve despite continued drug administration. In <1% of patients, acute liver injury resembling viral or chronic hepatitis or, rarely, a cholestatic reaction is seen 1–20 weeks after methyldopa is started. In 50% of cases the interval is <4 weeks. A prodrome of fever, anorexia, and malaise may be noted for a few days before the onset of jaundice. Rash, lymphadenopathy, arthralgia, and eosinophilia are rare. Serologic markers of autoimmunity are detected infrequently, and <5% of patients have a Coombs-positive hemolytic anemia. In ~15% of patients with methyldopa hepatotoxicity, the clinical, biochemical, and histologic features are those of moderate to severe chronic hepatitis, with or without bridging necrosis and macronodular cirrhosis. With discontinuation of the drug, the disorder usually resolves. Although methyldopa is currently used infrequently, its hepatotoxicity is very well characterized. Among the currently popular antihypertensive agents, angiotensin-converting enzyme (ACE) inhibitors, such as captopril and enalapril, have been blamed, albeit rarely, for hepatotoxicity (primarily cholestasis and cholestatic hepatitis, but also hepatocellular injury). Angiotensin-II receptor antagonists, such as losartan, are unlikely hepatotoxins, although rare reports of liver injury in their recipients have appeared.

ISONIAZID HEPATOTOXICITY (TOXIC AND IDIOSYNCRATIC REACTION)

In ~10% of adults treated with the antituberculosis agent isoniazid, elevated serum aminotransferase levels develop during the first few weeks of therapy; this appears to represent an adaptive response to a toxic metabolite of the drug. Whether or not isoniazid is continued, these values (usually <200 units) return to normal in a few weeks. In ~1% of treated patients, an illness develops that is indistinguishable from viral hepatitis; approximately one-half of these cases occur within the first 2 months of treatment; in the remainder, clinical disease may be delayed for many months.

Liver biopsy reveals morphologic changes similar to those of viral hepatitis or bridging hepatic necrosis. The disease may be severe, with a case-fatality rate of 10%. Important liver injury appears to be age-related, increasing substantially after age 35; the highest frequency is in patients over age 50, the lowest under the age of 20. Even for patients >50 years of age monitored carefully during therapy, hepatotoxicity occurs in only ~2%, well below the risk estimate derived from earlier experiences. Isoniazid hepatotoxicity is enhanced by alcohol, rifampin, and pyrazinamide. Fever, rash, eosinophilia, and other manifestations of drug allergy are distinctly unusual. A reactive metabolite of acetylhydrazine, a metabolite of isoniazid, may be responsible for liver injury, and patients who are rapid acetylators would be more prone to such injury. Counterintuitively, in some reports, the opposite is true; slow acetylators are more likely to experience hepatotoxicity and more severe hepatotoxicity than rapid acetylators. Contrary to past reports, more recent studies suggest that hepatotoxicity due to isoniazid as well as to combination antituberculous therapy that includes isoniazid is more likely in patients with underlying chronic hepatitis B. A picture resembling chronic hepatitis has been observed in a few patients. Careful liver-test monitoring is advisable in patients being treated with isoniazid.

SODIUM VALPROATE HEPATOTOXICITY (TOXIC AND IDIOSYNCRATIC REACTION)

Sodium valproate, an anticonvulsant useful in the treatment of petit mal and other seizure disorders, has been associated with the development of severe hepatic toxicity and, rarely, fatalities, predominantly in children but also in adults. Among children listed as candidates for liver transplantation, valproate is the most common antiepileptic drug implicated. Asymptomatic elevations of serum aminotransferase levels have been recognized in as many as 45% of treated patients. These "adaptive" changes, however, appear to have no clinical importance, because major hepatotoxicity is not seen in the majority of patients despite continuation of drug therapy. In the rare patients in whom jaundice, encephalopathy, and evidence of hepatic failure are found, examination of liver tissue reveals microvesicular fat and bridging hepatic necrosis, predominantly in the centrilobular zone. Bile duct injury may also be apparent. Most likely, sodium valproate is not directly hepatotoxic, but its metabolite, 4-pentenoic acid, may be responsible for hepatic injury. Valproate hepatotoxicity is more common in persons with mitochondrial enzyme deficiencies and may be ameliorated by IV administration of carnitine, which valproate therapy can deplete.

PHENYTOIN HEPATOTOXICITY (IDIOSYNCRATIC REACTION)

Phenytoin, formerly diphenylhydantoin, a mainstay in the treatment of seizure disorders, has been associated in rare instances with the development of severe hepatitis-like liver injury leading to fulminant hepatic failure. In many patients, the hepatitis is associated with striking fever, lymphadenopathy, rash (Stevens-Johnson syndrome or exfoliative dermatitis), leukocytosis, and eosinophilia, suggesting an immunologically mediated hypersensitivity mechanism. Despite these observations, evidence suggests that metabolic idiosyncrasy may be responsible for hepatic injury. In the liver, phenytoin is converted by cytochrome P450 to metabolites, including the highly reactive electrophilic arene oxides. These metabolites are normally metabolized further by epoxide hydrolases. A defect (genetic or acquired) in epoxide hydrolase activity could permit covalent binding of arene oxides to hepatic macromolecules, thereby leading to hepatic injury. Hepatic injury is usually manifest within the first 2 months after beginning phenytoin therapy. With the exception of an abundance of eosinophils in the liver, the clinical, biochemical, and histologic picture resembles that of viral hepatitis. In rare instances, bile duct injury may be the salient feature of phenytoin hepatotoxicity, with striking features of intrahepatic cholestasis. Asymptomatic elevations of aminotransferase and alkaline phosphatase levels have been observed in a sizable proportion of patients receiving long-term phenytoin therapy. These liver changes are believed by some authorities to represent the potent hepatic enzyme-inducing properties of phenytoin and are accompanied histologically by swelling of hepatocytes in the absence of necroinflammatory activity or evidence of chronic liver disease.

AMIODARONE HEPATOTOXICITY (TOXIC AND IDIOSYNCRATIC REACTION)

Therapy with this potent antiarrhythmic drug is accompanied in 15–50% of patients by modest elevations of serum aminotransferase levels that may remain stable or diminish despite continuation of the drug. Such abnormalities may appear days to many months after beginning therapy. A proportion of those with elevated aminotransferase levels have detectable hepatomegaly, and clinically important liver disease develops in <5% of patients. Features that represent a direct effect of the drug on the liver and that are common to the majority of long-term recipients are ultrastructural phospholipidosis, unaccompanied by clinical liver disease, and interference with hepatic mixed-function oxidase metabolism of other drugs. The cationic amphiphilic drug and its major metabolite desethylamiodarone accumulate in hepatocyte lysosomes and mitochondria and in bile duct epithelium. The relatively common elevations in aminotransferase levels are also considered a predictable, dose-dependent, direct hepatotoxic effect. On the other hand, in the rare patient with clinically apparent, symptomatic liver disease, liver injury resembling that seen in alcoholic liver disease is observed. The so-called pseudoalcoholic liver injury can range from steatosis to alcoholic hepatitis-like neutrophilic infiltration and Mallory's hyaline to cirrhosis. Electron-microscopic demonstration of phospholipid-laden lysosomal lamellar bodies can help to distinguish amiodarone hepatotoxicity from typical alcoholic hepatitis. This category of liver injury appears to be a metabolic idiosyncrasy that allows hepatotoxic metabolites to be generated. Rarely, an acute idiosyncratic hepatocellular injury resembling viral hepatitis or cholestatic hepatitis occurs. Hepatic granulomas have occasionally been observed. Because amiodarone has a long half-life, liver injury may persist for months after the drug is stopped.

ERYTHROMYCIN HEPATOTOXICITY (CHOLESTATIC IDIOSYNCRATIC REACTION)

The most important adverse effect associated with erythromycin, more common in children than adults, is the infrequent occurrence of a cholestatic reaction. Although most of these reactions have been associated with erythromycin estolate, other erythromycins may also be responsible. The reaction usually begins during the first 2 or 3 weeks of therapy and includes nausea, vomiting, fever, right upper quadrant abdominal pain, jaundice, leukocytosis, and moderately elevated aminotransferase and alkaline phosphatase levels. The clinical picture can resemble acute cholecystitis or bacterial cholangitis. Liver biopsy reveals variable cholestasis; portal inflammation comprising lymphocytes, polymorphonuclear leukocytes, and eosinophils; and scattered foci of hepatocyte necrosis. Symptoms and laboratory findings usually subside within a few days of drug withdrawal, and evidence of chronic liver disease has not been found on follow-up. The precise mechanism remains ill-defined.

ORAL CONTRACEPTIVE HEPATOTOXICITY (CHOLESTATIC REACTION)

The administration of oral contraceptive combinations of estrogenic and progestational steroids leads to intrahepatic cholestasis with pruritus and jaundice in a small number of patients weeks to months after taking these agents. Especially susceptible seem to be patients with recurrent idiopathic jaundice of pregnancy, severe pruritus of pregnancy, or a family history of these disorders. With the exception of liver biochemical tests, laboratory studies are normal, and extrahepatic manifestations of hypersensitivity are absent. Liver biopsy reveals cholestasis with bile plugs in dilated canaliculi and striking bilirubin staining of liver cells. In contrast to chlorpromazine-induced cholestasis, portal inflammation is absent. The lesion is reversible on withdrawal of the agent. The two steroid components appear to act synergistically on hepatic function, although the estrogen may be primarily responsible. Oral contraceptives are contraindicated in patients with a history of recurrent jaundice of pregnancy. Primarily benign, but rarely malignant, neoplasms of the liver, hepatic vein occlusion, and peripheral sinusoidal dilatation have also been associated with oral contraceptive therapy. Focal nodular hyperplasia of the liver is not more frequent among users of oral contraceptives.

17, α-ALKYL-SUBSTITUTED ANABOLIC STEROIDS (CHOLESTATIC REACTION)

In the majority of patients receiving these agents, used therapeutically mainly in the treatment of bone marrow failure but used surreptitiously and without medical indication (or unknowingly when included in nutritional supplements) by athletes to improve their performance, mild hepatic dysfunction develops. Impaired excretory function is the predominant defect, but the precise mechanism is uncertain. Jaundice, which appears to be dose-related, develops in only a minority of patients and may be the sole clinical manifestation of hepatotoxicity, although anorexia, nausea, and malaise may occur. Pruritus is not a prominent feature. Serum aminotransferase levels are usually <100 units, and serum alkaline phosphatase levels are normal; mildly elevated; or, in <5% of patients, three or more times the upper limit of normal. Examination of liver tissue reveals cholestasis without inflammation or necrosis. Hepatic sinusoidal dilatation and peliosis hepatis have been found in a few patients. The cholestatic disorder is usually reversible on cessation of treatment, although fatalities have been linked to peliosis. An association with hepatic adenoma and hepatocellular carcinoma has been reported.

TRIMETHOPRIM-SULFAMETHOXAZOLE HEPATOTOXICITY (IDIOSYNCRATIC REACTION)

This antibiotic combination is used routinely for urinary tract infections in immunocompetent persons and for prophylaxis against and therapy of *Pneumocystis carinii* pneumonia in immunosuppressed persons (transplant recipients, patients with AIDS). With its increasing use, its occasional hepatotoxicity is being recognized with growing frequency. Its likelihood is unpredictable, but when it occurs, trimethoprim-sulfamethoxazole hepatotoxicity follows a relatively uniform latency period of several weeks and is often accompanied by eosinophilia, rash, and other features of a hypersensitivity reaction.

Biochemically and histologically, acute hepatocellular necrosis predominates, but cholestatic features are quite frequent. Occasionally, cholestasis without necrosis occurs, and, very rarely, a severe cholangiolytic pattern of liver injury is observed. In most cases, liver injury is self-limited, but rare fatalities have been recorded. The hepatotoxicity is attributable to the sulfamethoxazole component of the drug and is similar in features to that seen with other sulfonamides; tissue eosinophilia and granulomas may be seen. The risk of trimethoprim-sulfamethoxazole hepatotoxicity is increased in persons with HIV infection.

HMG-COA REDUCTASE INHIBITORS (STATINS) (IDIOSYNCRATIC MIXED HEPATOCELLULAR AND CHOLESTATIC REACTION)

Between 1 and 2% of patients taking lovastatin, simvastatin, pravastatin, fluvastatin, or one of the newer statin drugs for the treatment of hypercholesterolemia experience asymptomatic, reversible elevations (>threefold) of aminotransferase activity. Acute hepatitis-like histologic changes, centrilobular necrosis, and centrilobular cholestasis have been described in several cases. In a larger proportion, minor aminotransferase elevations appear during the first several weeks of therapy. Careful laboratory monitoring can distinguish between patients with minor, transitory changes; who may continue therapy; and those with more profound and sustained abnormalities, who should discontinue therapy. Because clinically meaningful aminotransferase elevations are so rare after statin use and do not differ in meta-analyses from the frequency of such laboratory abnormalities in placebo recipients, a panel of liver experts recommended to the National Lipid Association's Safety Task Force that liver-test monitoring was not necessary in patients treated with statins and that statin therapy need not be discontinued in patients found to have asymptomatic isolated aminotransferase elevations during therapy. Statin hepatotoxicity is not increased in patients with chronic hepatitis C, hepatic steatosis, or other underlying liver diseases, and statins can be used safely in these patients.

TOTAL PARENTERAL NUTRITION (STEATOSIS, CHOLESTASIS)

Total parenteral nutrition (TPN) is often complicated by cholestatic hepatitis attributable to either steatosis, cholestasis, or gallstones (or gallbladder sludge). Steatosis or steatohepatitis may result from the excess carbohydrate calories in these nutritional supplements and is the predominant form of TPN-associated liver disorder in adults. The frequency of this complication has been reduced substantially by the introduction of balanced

TPN formulas that rely on lipid as an alternative caloric source. Cholestasis and cholelithiasis, caused by the absence of stimulation of bile flow and secretion resulting from the lack of oral intake, are the predominant forms of TPN-associated liver disease in infants, especially in premature neonates. Often, cholestasis in such neonates is multifactorial, contributed to by other factors such as sepsis, hypoxemia, and hypotension; occasionally, TPN-induced cholestasis in neonates culminates in chronic liver disease and liver failure. When TPN-associated liver-test abnormalities occur in adults, balancing the TPN formula with more lipid is the intervention of first recourse. In infants with TPN-associated cholestasis, the addition of oral feeding may ameliorate the problem. Therapeutic interventions suggested, but not shown, to be of proven benefit, include cholecystokinin, ursodeoxycholic acid, S-adenosyl methionine, and taurine.

"ALTERNATIVE AND COMPLEMENTARY MEDICINES" (IDIOSYNCRATIC HEPATITIS, STEATOSIS)

The misguided popularity of herbal medications that are of scientifically unproven efficacy and that lack prospective safety oversight by regulatory agencies has resulted in occasional instances of hepatotoxicity. Included among the herbal remedies associated with toxic hepatitis are Jin Bu Huan, xiao-chai-hu-tang, germander, chaparral, senna, mistletoe, skullcap, gentian, comfrey (containing pyrrolizidine alkaloids), Ma huang, bee pollen, valerian root, pennyroyal oil, kava, celandine, Impila (Callilepsis laureaola), LipoKinetix, Hyroxycut, herbal nutritional supplements, and herbal teas. Well characterized are the acute hepatitis-like histologic lesions following Jin Bu Huan use: focal hepatocellular necrosis, mixed mononuclear portal tract infiltration, coagulative necrosis, apoptotic hepatocyte degeneration, tissue eosinophilia, and microvesicular steatosis. Megadoses of vitamin A can injure the liver, as can pyrrolizidine alkaloids, which often contaminate Chinese herbal preparations and can cause a venoocclusive injury leading to sinusoidal hepatic vein obstruction. Because some alternative medicines induce toxicity via active metabolites, alcohol and drugs that stimulate cytochrome P450 enzymes may enhance the toxicity of some of these products. Conversely, some alternative medicines also stimulate cytochrome P450 and may result in or amplify the toxicity of recognized drug hepatotoxins. Given the widespread use of such poorly defined herbal preparations, hepatotoxicity is likely to be encountered with increasing frequency; therefore, a drug history in patients with acute and chronic liver disease should include use of "alternative medicines" and other non-prescription preparations sold in so-called health food stores.

HIGHLY ACTIVE ANTIRETROVIRAL THERAPY (HAART) FOR HIV INFECTION (MITOCHONDRIAL TOXIC, IDIOSYNCRATIC, STEATOSIS; HEPATOCELLULAR, CHOLESTATIC, AND MIXED)

The recognition of drug hepatotoxicity in persons with HIV infection is complicated in this population by the many alternative causes of liver injury (chronic viral hepatitis, fatty infiltration, infiltrative disorders, mycobacterial infection, etc.), but drug hepatotoxicity associated with HAART is an emerging and common type of liver injury in HIV-infected persons. Although no one antiviral agent is recognized as a potent hepatotoxin, combination regimens including reverse transcriptase and protease inhibitors cause hepatotoxicity in ~10% of treated patients. Implicated most frequently are combinations including nucleoside analogue reverse transcriptase inhibitors zidovudine, didanosine, and, to a lesser extent, stavudine; protease inhibitors ritonavir and indinavir (and amprenavir when used together with ritonavir) as well as tipranavir; and nonnucleoside reverse transcriptase inhibitors nevirapine and, to a lesser extent, efavirenz. These drugs cause predominantly hepatocellular injury but cholestatic injury as well, and prolonged (>6 months) use of reverse transcriptase inhibitors has been associated with mitochondrial injury, steatosis, and lactic acidosis. Indirect hyperbilirubinemia, resulting from direct inhibition of bilirubin-conjugating activity by UDP-glucuronosyltransferase, usually without elevation of aminotransferase or alkaline phosphatase activities, occurs in ~10% of patients treated with the protease inhibitor indinavir. Distinguishing the impact of HAART hepatotoxicity in patients with HIV and hepatitis virus co-infection is made challenging by the following: (1) both chronic hepatitis B and hepatitis C can affect the natural history of HIV infection and the response to HAART, and (2) HAART can have an impact on chronic viral hepatitis. For example, immunologic reconstitution with HAART can result in immunologically mediated liver-cell injury in patients with chronic hepatitis B co-infection if treatment with an antiviral agent for hepatitis B, e.g., the nucleoside analogue lamivudine, is withdrawn or if nucleoside analogue resistance emerges. Infection with HIV, especially with low CD4+ T cell counts, has been reported to increase the rate of hepatic fibrosis associated with chronic hepatitis C, and HAART therapy can increase levels of serum aminotransferases and hepatitis C virus RNA in patients with hepatitis C co-infection. Didanosine or stavudine should not be used with ribavirin in patients with HIV/hepatitis C virus co-infection, because of an increased risk of severe mitochondrial toxicity and lactic acidosis.

ACKNOWLEDGEMENT

Kurt J. Isselbacher, MD, contributed to this chapter in previous editions of Harrison's Principles of Internal Medicine.

CHAPTER 40

CHRONIC HEPATITIS

Jules L. Dienstag

Chronic hepatitis represents a series of liver disorders of varying causes and severity in which hepatic inflammation and necrosis continue for at least 6 months. Milder forms are nonprogressive or only slowly progressive, while more severe forms may be associated with scarring and architectural reorganization, which, when advanced, lead ultimately to cirrhosis. Several categories of chronic hepatitis have been recognized. These include chronic viral hepatitis, drug-induced chronic hepatitis (Chap. 39), and autoimmune chronic hepatitis. In many cases, clinical and laboratory features are insufficient to allow assignment into one of these three categories; these "idiopathic" cases are also believed to represent autoimmune chronic hepatitis. Finally, clinical and laboratory features of chronic hepatitis are observed occasionally in patients with such hereditary/metabolic disorders as Wilson's disease (copper overload) (Chap. 42) and nonalcoholic fatty liver disease (Chap. 44) and even occasionally in patients with alcoholic liver injury (Chap. 41). Although all types of chronic hepatitis share certain clinical, laboratory, and histopathologic features, chronic viral and chronic autoimmune hepatitis are sufficiently distinct to merit separate discussions. For discussion of acute hepatitis, see Chap. 38.

CLASSIFICATION OF CHRONIC HEPATITIS

Common to all forms of chronic hepatitis are histopathologic distinctions based on localization and extent of liver injury. These vary from the milder forms, previously labeled *chronic persistent hepatitis* and *chronic lobular hepatitis*, to the more severe form, formerly called *chronic active hepatitis*. When first defined, these designations were believed to have prognostic implications, which have been challenged by more recent observations. Categorization of chronic hepatitis based primarily on histopathologic features has been replaced by a more informative classification based on a combination of clinical, serologic, and histologic variables. Classification of chronic hepatitis is based on (1) its *cause*; (2) its histologic activity, or *grade*; and (3) its degree of progression, or *stage*. Thus, neither clinical features alone nor histologic features—requiring liver biopsy—alone are sufficient to characterize and distinguish among the several categories of chronic hepatitis.

CLASSIFICATION BY CAUSE

Clinical and serologic features allow the establishment of a diagnosis of *chronic viral hepatitis*, caused by hepatitis B, hepatitis B plus D, or hepatitis C; *autoimmune hepatitis*, including several subcategories, I and II (perhaps III), based on serologic distinctions; *drug-associated chronic hepatitis*; and a category of unknown cause, or *cryptogenic chronic hepatitis* (Table 40-1). These are addressed in more detail later in this chapter.

CLASSIFICATION BY GRADE

Grade, a histologic assessment of necroinflammatory activity, is based on examination of the liver biopsy. An assessment of important histologic features includes the degree of *periportal necrosis* and the disruption of the limiting plate of periportal hepatocytes by inflammatory cells (so-called *piecemeal necrosis* or *interface hepatitis*); the degree of confluent necrosis that links or forms bridges between vascular structures—between portal tract and portal tract or even more important bridges between portal tract and central vein—referred to as *bridging necrosis*; the degree of hepatocyte degeneration and focal necrosis within the lobule; and the degree of *portal inflammation*. Several scoring systems that take these histologic features into account have been devised, and the most popular are the histologic activity index (HAI), used commonly in the United States, and the METAVIR score, used in Europe (Table 40-2). Based on the presence and degree of these features of histologic activity, chronic hepatitis can be graded as mild, moderate, or severe.

TABLE 40-1

CLINICAL AND LABORATORY FEATURES OF CHRONIC HEPATITIS

TYPE OF HEPATITIS	DIAGNOSTIC TEST(S)	AUTOANTIBODIES	THERAPY
Chronic hepatitis B	HBsAg, IgG anti-HBc, HBeAg, HBV DNA	Uncommon	IFN-α, PEG IFN-α Lamivudine Adefovir Entecavir Telbivudine Tenofovir
Chronic hepatitis C	Anti-HCV, HCV RNA	Anti-LKM1[a]	PEG IFN-α plus ribavirin PEG IFN-α plus ribavirin plus telaprevir (genotype I) PEG IFN-α plus ribavirin plus boceprevir (genotype I)
Chronic hepatitis D	Anti-HDV, HDV RNA, HBsAg, IgG anti-HBc	Anti-LKM3	IFN-α, PEG IFN-α[c]
Autoimmune hepatitis	ANA[b] (homogeneous), anti-LKM1 (±) Hyperglobulinemia	ANA, anti-LKM1 anti-SLA[d]	Prednisone, azathioprine
Drug-associated	—	Uncommon	Withdraw drug
Cryptogenic	All negative	None	Prednisone (?), azathioprine (?)

[a]Antibodies to liver-kidney microsomes type 1 (autoimmune hepatitis type II and some cases of hepatitis C).
[b]Antinuclear antibody (autoimmune hepatitis type I).
[c]Clinical trials suggest benefit of IFN-α therapy; PEG IFN-α is as effective, if not more so.
[d]Antibodies to soluble liver antigen (autoimmune hepatitis type III).
Abbreviations: HBc, hepatitis B core; HBeAg, hepatitis B e antigen; HBsAg, hepatitis B surface antigen; HBV, hepatitis B virus; HCV, hepatitis C virus; HDV, hepatitis D virus; IFN-α, interferon-α; IgG, immunoglobulin G; LKM, liver-kidney microsome; IFN-α, PEG pegylated interferon-α; SLA, soluble liver antigen.

CLASSIFICATION BY STAGE

The stage of chronic hepatitis, which reflects the level of progression of the disease, is based on the degree of hepatic fibrosis. When fibrosis is so extensive that fibrous septa surround parenchymal nodules and alter the normal architecture of the liver lobule, the histologic lesion is defined as *cirrhosis*. Staging is based on the degree of fibrosis as categorized on a numerical scale from 0–6 (HAI) or 0–4 (METAVIR) (Table 40-2).

CHRONIC VIRAL HEPATITIS

Both the enterically transmitted forms of viral hepatitis, hepatitis A and E, are self-limited and do not cause chronic hepatitis (rare reports notwithstanding in which acute hepatitis A serves as a trigger for the onset of autoimmune hepatitis in genetically susceptible patients). In contrast, the entire clinicopathologic spectrum of chronic hepatitis occurs in patients with chronic viral hepatitis B and C as well as in patients with chronic hepatitis D superimposed on chronic hepatitis B.

CHRONIC HEPATITIS B

The likelihood of chronicity after acute hepatitis B varies as a function of age. Infection at birth is associated

with clinically silent acute infection but a 90% chance of chronic infection, while infection in young adulthood in immunocompetent persons is typically associated with clinically apparent acute hepatitis but a risk of chronicity of only approximately 1%. Most cases of chronic hepatitis B among adults, however, occur in patients who never had a recognized episode of clinically apparent acute viral hepatitis. The degree of liver injury (grade) in patients with chronic hepatitis B is variable, ranging from none in inactive carriers to mild to moderate to severe. Among adults with chronic hepatitis B, histologic features are of prognostic importance. In one long-term study of patients with chronic hepatitis B, investigators found a 5-year survival rate of 97% for patients with mild chronic hepatitis, 86% for patients with moderate to severe chronic hepatitis, and only 55% for patients with chronic hepatitis and postnecrotic cirrhosis. The 15-year survival in these cohorts was 77, 66, and 40%, respectively. On the other hand, more recent observations do not allow us to be so sanguine about the prognosis in patients with mild chronic hepatitis; among such patients followed for 1–13 years, progression to more severe chronic hepatitis and cirrhosis has been observed in more than a quarter of cases.

More important to consider than histology alone in patients with chronic hepatitis B is the degree of hepatitis B virus (HBV) replication. As reviewed in

TABLE 40-2

HISTOLOGIC GRADING AND STAGING OF CHRONIC HEPATITIS

HISTOLOGIC FEATURE	HISTOLOGIC ACTIVITY INDEX (HAI)[a]		METAVIR[b]	
	SEVERITY	SCORE	SEVERITY	SCORE
Necroinflammatory Activity (grade)				
Periportal necrosis, including piecemeal necrosis and/or bridging necrosis (BN)	None	0	None	0
	Mild	1	Mild	1
	Mild/Moderate	2	Moderate	2
	Moderate	3	Severe	3
	Severe	4		
			Bridging necrosis	Yes No
Intralobular necrosis — Confluent	—none	0	None or mild	0
	—focal	1	Moderate	1
	—Zone 3 some	2	Severe	2
	—Zone 3 most	3		
	—Zone 3 + BN few	4		
	—Zone 3 + BN multiple	5		
	—Panacinar/multiacinar	6		
Focal	—none	0		
	—≤1 focus/10x field	1		
	—2–4 foci/10x field	2		
	—5–10 foci/10x field	3		
	—>10 foci/10x field	4		
Portal Inflammation	None	0		
	Mild	1		
	Moderate	2		
	Moderate/marked	3		
	Marked	4		
	Total	0–18		A0–A3[c]
Fibrosis (stage)				
None		0		F0
Portal fibrosis—some		1		F1
Portal fibrosis—most		2		F1
Bridging fibrosis—few		3		F2
Bridging fibrosis—many		4		F3
Incomplete cirrhosis		5		F4
Cirrhosis		6		F4
	Total	6		4

[a]J Hepatol 22:696, 1995.
[b]Hepatology 24:289, 1996.
[c]Necroinflammatory grade: A0 = none; A1 = mild; A2 = moderate; A3 = severe.

Chap. 38, chronic HBV infection can occur in the presence or absence of serum hepatitis B e antigen (HBeAg), and generally, for both HBeAg-reactive and HBeAg-negative chronic hepatitis B, the level of HBV DNA correlates with the level of liver injury and risk of progression. In *HBeAg-reactive chronic hepatitis B*, two phases have been recognized based on the relative level of HBV replication. The relatively *replicative phase* is characterized by the presence in the serum of HBeAg and HBV DNA levels well in excess of 10^5–10^6 virions/mL, by the presence in the liver of detectable intrahepatocyte nucleocapsid antigens [primarily hepatitis B core antigen (HBcAg)], by high infectivity, and by accompanying liver injury. In contrast, the relatively *nonreplicative*

phase is characterized by the absence of the conventional serum marker of HBV replication (HBeAg), the appearance of anti-HBe, levels of HBV DNA below a threshold of ~10^3 virions/mL, the absence of intrahepatocytic HBcAg, limited infectivity, and minimal liver injury. Those patients in the replicative phase tend to have more severe chronic hepatitis, while those in the nonreplicative phase tend to have minimal or mild chronic hepatitis or to be inactive hepatitis B carriers; however, distinctions in HBV replication and in histologic category do not always coincide. The likelihood in a patient with HBeAg-reactive chronic hepatitis B of converting spontaneously from relatively replicative to nonreplicative infection is approximately 10–15% per year.

In patients with HBeAg-reactive chronic HBV infection, especially when acquired at birth or in early childhood, as recognized commonly in Asian countries, a dichotomy is common between very high levels of HBV replication and negligible levels of liver injury. Yet despite the relatively immediate, apparently benign nature of liver disease for many decades in this population, patients with childhood-acquired HBV infection are the ones at ultimately increased risk later in life of cirrhosis and hepatocellular carcinoma (HCC) (Chap. 50). A discussion of the pathogenesis of liver injury in patients with chronic hepatitis B appears in Chap. 38.

HBeAg-negative chronic hepatitis B [i.e., chronic HBV infection with active virus replication, readily detectable HBV DNA but without HBeAg (anti-HBe-reactive)], is more common than HBeAg-reactive chronic hepatitis B in Mediterranean and European countries and in Asia (and, correspondingly, in HBV genotypes other than A). Compared to patients with HBeAg-reactive chronic hepatitis B, patients with HBeAg-negative chronic hepatitis B have levels of HBV DNA that are several orders of magnitude lower (no more than 10^5–10^6 virions/mL) than those observed in the HBeAg-reactive subset. Most such cases represent precore or core-promoter mutations acquired late in the natural history of the disease (mostly early-life onset; age range 40–55 years, older than that for HBeAg-reactive chronic hepatitis B); these mutations prevent translation of HBeAg from the precore component of the HBV genome (precore mutants) or are characterized by down-regulated transcription of precore mRNA (core-promoter mutants; Chap. 38). Although their levels of HBV DNA tend to be lower than among patients with HBeAg-reactive chronic hepatitis B, patients with HBeAg-negative chronic hepatitis B can have progressive liver injury (complicated by cirrhosis and HCC) and experience episodic reactivation of liver disease reflected in fluctuating levels of aminotransferase activity ("flares"). The biochemical and histologic activity of HBeAg-negative disease tends to correlate closely with levels of HBV replication, unlike the case mentioned earlier of Asian patients with HBeAg-reactive chronic hepatitis B during the early decades of their HBV infection. An important point worth reiterating is the observation that the level of HBV replication is the most important risk factor for the ultimate development of cirrhosis and HCC in both HBeAg-reactive and HBeAg-negative patients. Although levels of HBV DNA are lower and more readily suppressed by therapy to undetectable levels in HBeAg-negative (compared to HBeAg-reactive) chronic hepatitis B, achieving sustained responses that permit discontinuation of antiviral therapy is less likely in HBeAg-negative patients (discussed later). Inactive carriers are patients with circulating hepatitis B surface antigen (HBsAg), normal serum aminotransferase levels, undetectable HBeAg, and levels of HBV DNA that are either undetectable or present at levels ≤10^3 virions/mL. This serologic profile can occur not only in inactive carriers but also in patients with HBeAg-negative chronic hepatitis B during periods of relative inactivity; distinguishing between the two requires sequential biochemical and virologic monitoring over many months.

The spectrum of *clinical features* of chronic hepatitis B is broad, ranging from asymptomatic infection to debilitating disease or even end-stage, fatal hepatic failure. As noted earlier, the onset of the disease tends to be insidious in most patients, with the exception of the very few in whom chronic disease follows failure of resolution of clinically apparent acute hepatitis B. The clinical and laboratory features associated with progression from acute to chronic hepatitis B are discussed in Chap. 38.

Fatigue is a common symptom, and persistent or intermittent *jaundice* is a common feature in severe or advanced cases. Intermittent deepening of jaundice and recurrence of malaise and anorexia, as well as worsening fatigue, are reminiscent of acute hepatitis; such exacerbations may occur spontaneously, often coinciding with evidence of virologic reactivation; may lead to progressive liver injury; and, when superimposed on well-established cirrhosis, may cause hepatic decompensation. Complications of cirrhosis occur in end-stage chronic hepatitis and include ascites, edema, bleeding gastroesophageal varices, hepatic encephalopathy, coagulopathy, or hypersplenism. Occasionally, these complications bring the patient to initial clinical attention. Extrahepatic complications of chronic hepatitis B, similar to those seen during the prodromal phase of acute hepatitis B, are associated with deposition of circulating hepatitis B antigen–antibody immune complexes. These include arthralgias and arthritis, which are common, and the more rare purpuric cutaneous lesions (leukocytoclastic vasculitis), immune-complex glomerulonephritis, and generalized vasculitis (polyarteritis nodosa) (Chap. 38).

Laboratory features of chronic hepatitis B do not distinguish adequately between histologically mild and severe hepatitis. Aminotransferase elevations tend to be modest for chronic hepatitis B but may fluctuate in the range of 100–1000 units. As is true for acute viral hepatitis B, alanine aminotransferase (ALT) tends to be more elevated than aspartate aminotransferase (AST); however, once cirrhosis is established, AST tends to exceed ALT. Levels of alkaline phosphatase activity tend to be normal or only marginally elevated. In severe cases, moderate elevations in serum bilirubin [51.3–171 μmol/L (3–10 mg/dL)] occur. Hypoalbuminemia and prolongation of the prothrombin time occur in severe or end-stage cases. Hyperglobulinemia and detectable circulating autoantibodies are distinctly absent in chronic hepatitis B (in contrast to autoimmune hepatitis). Viral markers of chronic HBV infection are discussed in Chap. 38.

TREATMENT Chronic Hepatitis B

Although progression to cirrhosis is more likely in severe than in mild or moderate chronic hepatitis B, all forms of chronic hepatitis B can be progressive, and progression occurs primarily in patients with active HBV replication. Moreover, in populations of patients with chronic hepatitis B who are at risk for HCC (Chap. 50), the risk is highest for those with continued, high-level HBV replication and lower for persons in whom initially high-level HBV DNA falls spontaneously over time. Therefore, management of chronic hepatitis B is directed at suppressing the level of virus replication. Although clinical trials tend to focus on clinical endpoints achieved over 1–2 years (e.g., suppression of HBV DNA to undetectable levels, loss of HBeAg/HBsAg, improvement in histology, normalization of ALT), these short-term gains translate into reductions in the risk of clinical progression, hepatic decompensation, and death. To date, seven drugs have been approved for treatment of chronic hepatitis B: injectable interferon (IFN) α pegylated interferon [long-acting IFN bound to polyethylene glycol (PEG), known as *PEG IFN*]; and the oral agents lamivudine, adefovir dipivoxil, entecavir, telbivudine, and tenofovir.

Antiviral therapy for hepatitis B has evolved rapidly since the mid-1990s, as has the sensitivity of tests for HBV DNA. When IFN and lamivudine were evaluated in clinical trials, HBV DNA was measured by insensitive hybridization assays with detection thresholds of 10^5–10^6 virions/mL; when adefovir, entecavir, telbivudine, tenofovir, and PEG IFN were studied in clinical trials, HBV DNA was measured by sensitive amplification assays [polymerase chain reaction (PCR)] with detection thresholds of 10^1–10^3 virions/mL. Recognition of these distinctions is helpful when comparing results of clinical trials that established the efficacy of these therapies (reviewed later in chronological order of publication of these efficacy trials).

INTERFERON IFN-α was the first approved therapy for chronic hepatitis B. Although it is no longer used to treat hepatitis B, standard IFN is important historically, having provided important lessons about antiviral therapy in general. For immunocompetent adults with HBeAg-reactive chronic hepatitis B [who tend to have high-level HBV DNA (>10^5–10^6 virions/mL) and histologic evidence of chronic hepatitis on liver biopsy], a 16-week course of IFN given subcutaneously at a daily dose of 5 million units, or three times a week at a dose of 10 million units, results in a loss of HBeAg and hybridization-detectable HBV DNA (i.e., a reduction to levels below 10^5–10^6 virions/mL) in ~30% of patients, with a concomitant improvement in liver histology. Seroconversion from HBeAg to anti-HBe occurs in approximately 20%, and, in early trials, approximately 8% lost HBsAg. Successful IFN therapy and seroconversion are often accompanied by an acute hepatitis-like elevation in aminotransferase activity, which has been postulated to result from enhanced cytolytic T cell clearance of HBV-infected hepatocytes. Relapse after successful therapy is rare (1 or 2%). The likelihood of responding to IFN is higher in patients with lower levels of HBV DNA and substantial elevations of ALT. Although children can respond as well as adults, IFN therapy has not been effective in very young children infected at birth. Similarly, IFN therapy has not been effective in immunosuppressed persons, Asian patients with minimal-to-mild ALT elevations, or patients with decompensated chronic hepatitis B (in whom such therapy can actually be detrimental, sometimes precipitating decompensation, often associated with severe adverse effects). Among patients with HBeAg loss during therapy, long-term follow-up has demonstrated that 80% experience eventual loss of HBsAg (i.e., all serologic markers of infection, and normalization of ALT over a 9-year post-treatment period). In addition, improved long-term and complication-free survival as well as a reduction in the frequency of HCC have been documented among interferon responders, supporting the conclusion that successful interferon therapy improves the natural history of chronic hepatitis B.

Initial trials of brief-duration IFN therapy in patients with *HBeAg-negative chronic hepatitis B* were disappointing, suppressing HBV replication transiently during therapy but almost never resulting in sustained antiviral responses. In subsequent IFN trials among patients with HBeAg-negative chronic hepatitis B, however, more protracted courses, lasting up to 1.5 years, have been reported to result in sustained remissions documented to last for several years, with suppressed HBV DNA and aminotransferase activity, in ~20%.

Complications of IFN therapy include systemic "flu-like" symptoms; marrow suppression; emotional lability (irritability, depression, anxiety); autoimmune reactions (especially autoimmune thyroiditis); and miscellaneous side effects such as alopecia, rashes, diarrhea, and numbness and tingling of the extremities. With the possible exception of autoimmune thyroiditis, all these side effects are reversible upon dose lowering or cessation of therapy.

Although no longer competitive with the newer generation of antivirals, IFN did represent the first successful antiviral approach and set a standard against which to measure subsequent drugs in the achievement of durable virologic, serologic, biochemical, and histologic responses; consolidation of virologic and biochemical benefit in the ensuing years after therapy; and improvement in the natural history of chronic hepatitis B. Standard IFN has been supplanted by long-acting PEG IFN (discussed later), and IFN nonresponders are now treated with one of the newer oral nucleoside analogues.

LAMIVUDINE The first of the nucleoside analogues to be approved, the dideoxynucleoside lamivudine, inhibits reverse transcriptase activity of both HIV and HBV and is a potent and effective agent for patients with chronic hepatitis B. Although generally superseded by newer, more potent agents, lamivudine is still used in regions of the world where newer agents are not yet approved are or not affordable. In clinical trials among patients with HBeAg-reactive chronic hepatitis B, lamivudine therapy at daily doses of 100 mg for 48–52 weeks suppressed HBV DNA by a median of approximately 5.5 $\log_{10}$ copies/mL and to undetectable levels, as measured by PCR amplification assays, in approximately 40% of patients. Therapy was associated with HBeAg loss in 32–33%; HBeAg seroconversion (i.e., conversion from HBeAg-reactive to anti-HBe-reactive) in 16–21%; normalization of ALT in 40–75%; improvement in histology in 50–60%; retardation in fibrosis in 20–30%; and prevention of progression to cirrhosis. HBeAg responses can occur even in subgroups who are resistant to IFN (e.g., those with high-level HBV DNA) or who failed in the past to respond to it. As is true for IFN therapy of chronic hepatitis B, patients with near-normal ALT activity tend not to experience HBeAg responses (despite suppression of HBV DNA), and those with ALT levels exceeding five times the upper limit of normal can expect 1-year HBeAg seroconversion rates of 50–60%. Generally, HBeAg seroconversions are confined to patients who achieve suppression of HBV DNA to <10^4 genomes/mL. Among patients who undergo HBeAg responses during a year-long course of therapy and in whom the response is sustained for 4–6 months after cessation of therapy, the response is durable thereafter in the vast majority, >80%; therefore, the achievement of an HBeAg response represents a viable stopping point in therapy. Reduced durability has been reported in some Asian experiences; however, in most Western and Asian patient study populations, long-term durability of HBeAg responses is the rule, which, at least in Western patients, is accompanied by a post-treatment HBsAg seroconversion rate comparable to that seen after IFN-induced HBeAg responses. To support the durability of HBeAg responses, patients receive a period of consolidation therapy (at least 6 months in Western patients, at least 1 year in Asian patients) after HBeAg seroconversion; close posttreatment monitoring is necessary to identify HBV reactivation promptly and to resume therapy. If HBeAg is unaffected by lamivudine therapy, the current approach is to continue therapy until an HBeAg response occurs, but long-term therapy may be required to suppress HBV replication and, in turn, limit liver injury; HBeAg seroconversions can increase to a level of 50% after 5 years of therapy. Histologic improvement continues to accrue with therapy

beyond the first year; after a cumulative course of 3 years of lamivudine therapy, necroinflammatory activity is reduced in the majority of patients, and even cirrhosis has been shown to regress to precirrhotic stages.

Losses of HBsAg have been few during the first year of lamivudine therapy, and this observation had been cited as an advantage of IFN-based over lamivudine therapy; however, in head-to-head comparisons between standard IFN and lamivudine monotherapy, HBsAg losses were rare in both groups. Trials in which lamivudine and IFN were administered in combination failed to show a benefit of combination therapy over lamivudine monotherapy for either treatment-naïve patients or prior IFN nonresponders.

In patients with *HBeAg-negative chronic hepatitis B* (i.e., in those with precore and core-promoter HBV mutations), 1 year of lamivudine therapy results in HBV DNA suppression and normalization of ALT in three-quarters of patients and in histologic improvement in approximately two-thirds. Therapy has been shown to suppress HBV DNA by approximately 4.5 $\log_{10}$ copies/mL (baseline HBV DNA levels are lower than in patients with HBeAg-reactive hepatitis B) and to undetectable levels in approximately 70%, as measured by sensitive PCR amplification assays. Lacking HBeAg at the outset, patients with HBeAg-negative chronic hepatitis B cannot achieve an HBeAg response—a stopping point in HBeAg-reactive patients; almost invariably, when therapy is discontinued, reactivation is the rule. Therefore, these patients require long-term therapy; with successive years, the proportion with suppressed HBV DNA and normal ALT increases.

Clinical and laboratory side effects of lamivudine are negligible, indistinguishable from those observed in placebo recipients. Still, lamivudine doses should be reduced in patients with reduced creatinine clearance. During lamivudine therapy, transient ALT elevations, resembling those seen during IFN therapy and during spontaneous HBeAg-to-anti-HBe seroconversions, occur in one-fourth of patients. These ALT elevations may result from restored cytolytic T cell activation permitted by suppression of HBV replication. Similar ALT elevations, however, occur at an identical frequency in placebo recipients, but ALT elevations associated with HBeAg seroconversion are confined to lamivudine-treated patients. When therapy is stopped after a year of therapy, two- to threefold ALT elevations occur in 20–30% of lamivudine-treated patients, representing renewed liver-cell injury as HBV replication returns. Although these posttreatment flares are almost always transient and mild, rare severe exacerbations, especially in cirrhotic patients, have been observed, mandating close and careful clinical and virologic monitoring after discontinuation of treatment. Many authorities caution against discontinuing therapy in patients with cirrhosis, in whom posttreatment flares could precipitate decompensation.

Long-term monotherapy with lamivudine is associated with methionine-to-valine (M204V) or methionine-to-isoleucine (M204I) mutations, primarily at amino acid 204 in the tyrosine-methionine-aspartate-aspartate (YMDD) motif of HBV DNA polymerase, analogous to mutations that occur in HIV-infected patients treated with this drug. During a year of therapy, YMDD mutations occur in 15–30% of patients; the frequency increases with each year of therapy, reaching 70% at year 5. Ultimately, patients with YMDD mutants experience degradation of clinical, biochemical, and histologic responses; therefore, if treatment is begun with lamivudine monotherapy, the emergence of lamivudine resistance, reflected clinically by a breakthrough from suppressed levels of HBV DNA and ALT, is managed by adding another antiviral to which YMDD variants are sensitive (e.g., adefovir, tenofovir; discussed later).

Currently, although lamivudine is very safe and still used widely in other parts of the world, in the United States and Europe, lamivudine has been eclipsed by more potent antivirals that have superior resistance profiles (discussed later). Still, as the first successful oral antiviral agent for use in hepatitis B, lamivudine has provided proof of the concept that polymerase inhibitors can achieve virologic, serologic, biochemical, and histologic benefits. In addition, lamivudine has been shown to be effective in the treatment of patients with decompensated hepatitis B (for whom IFN is contraindicated), in some of whom decompensation can be reversed. Moreover, among patients with cirrhosis or advanced fibrosis, lamivudine has been shown to be effective in reducing the risk of progression to hepatic decompensation and, marginally, the risk of HCC.

Because lamivudine monotherapy can result universally in the rapid emergence of YMDD variants in persons with HIV infection, patients with chronic hepatitis B should be tested for anti-HIV prior to therapy; if HIV infection is identified, lamivudine monotherapy at the HBV daily dose of 100 mg is contraindicated. These patients should be treated for both HIV and HBV with an HIV drug regimen that includes or is supplemented by at least two drugs active against HBV; highly active antiretroviral therapy (HAART) often contains two drugs with antiviral activity against HBV (e.g., tenofovir and emtricitabine), but if lamivudine is part of the regimen, the daily dose should be 300 mg. The safety of lamivudine during pregnancy has not been established; however, the drug is not teratogenic in rodents and has been used safely in pregnant women with HIV infection and with HBV infection. Limited data even suggest that administration of lamivudine during the last months of pregnancy to mothers with high-level hepatitis B viremia ($\geq 10^8$ IU/mL) can reduce the likelihood of perinatal transmission of hepatitis B.

ADEFOVIR DIPIVOXIL At an oral daily dose of 10 mg, the acyclic nucleotide analogue adefovir dipivoxil, the prodrug of adefovir, reduces HBV DNA by approximately 3.5–4 $\log_{10}$ copies/mL and is equally effective in treatment-naïve patients and IFN nonresponders. In HBeAg-reactive chronic hepatitis B, a 48 week course of adefovir dipivoxil was shown to achieve histologic improvement (and reduce the progression of fibrosis) and normalization of ALT in just over one-half of patients, HBeAg seroconversion in 12%, HBeAg loss in 23%, and suppression to an undetectable level of HBV DNA in 13–21%, as measured by PCR. Similar to IFN and lamivudine, adefovir dipivoxil is more likely to achieve an HBeAg response in patients with high baseline ALT (e.g., among adefovir-treated patients with ALT level >5 times the upper limit of normal), HBeAg seroconversions occurred in 25%. The durability of adefovir-induced HBeAg responses is high (91% in one study); therefore, HBeAg response can be relied upon as a stopping point for adefovir therapy, after a period of consolidation therapy, as outlined earlier. Although data on the impact of additional therapy beyond 1 year are limited, biochemical, serologic, and virologic outcomes improve progressively as therapy is continued.

In patients with *HBeAg-negative chronic hepatitis B*, a 48-week course of 10 mg/d of adefovir dipivoxil resulted in histologic improvement in two-thirds, normalization of ALT in three-fourths, and suppression of HBV DNA to PCR-undetectable levels in one-half to two-thirds. As was true for lamivudine, because HBeAg responses—a potential stopping point—cannot be achieved in this group, reactivation is the rule when adefovir therapy is discontinued, and indefinite, long-term therapy is required. Treatment beyond the first year consolidates the gain of the first year; after 5 years of therapy, improvement in hepatic inflammation and regression of fibrosis was observed in three-fourths of patients, ALT was normal in 70%, and HBV DNA was undetectable in almost 70%.

Adefovir contains a flexible acyclic linker instead of the L-nucleoside ring of lamivudine, avoiding steric hindrance by mutated amino acids. In addition, the molecular structure of phosphorylated adefovir is very similar to that of its natural substrate; therefore mutations to adefovir would also affect binding of the natural substrate, dATP. Hypothetically, these are among the reasons that resistance to adefovir dipivoxil is much less likely than resistance to lamivudine; no resistance was encountered in 1 year of clinical-trial therapy. In subsequent years, however, adefovir resistance begins to emerge [asparagine to threonine at amino acid 236 (N236T) and alanine to valine or threonine at amino acid 181 (A181V/T), primarily], occurring in 2.5% after 2 years, but in 29% after 5 years of therapy (reported in HBeAg-negative patients). Among patients coinfected with HBV and HIV and who have normal CD4+ T cell counts, adefovir dipivoxil is effective in suppressing HBV dramatically (by 5 logs$_{10}$ in one study). Moreover, adefovir dipivoxil is effective in lamivudine-resistant, YMDD-mutant HBV and can be used when such lamivudine-induced variants emerge. When lamivudine resistance occurs, adding adefovir (i.e., maintaining lamivudine to preempt the emergence of adefovir resistance), is superior to switching to adefovir. Almost invariably, patients with adefovir-mutant HBV respond to lamivudine (or newer agents, such as entecavir, discussed later). When, in the past, adefovir had been evaluated as therapy for HIV infection, doses of 60–120 mg were required to suppress HIV, and, at these doses, the drug was nephrotoxic. Even at 30 mg/d, creatinine elevations of 44 μmol/L (0.5 mg/dL) occur in 10% of patients; however, at the HBV-effective dose of 10 mg, such elevations of creatinine are rarely encountered. If any nephrotoxicity does occur, it rarely appears before 6–8 months of therapy. Although renal tubular injury is a rare potential side effect, and although creatinine monitoring is recommended during treatment, the therapeutic index of adefovir dipivoxil is high, and the nephrotoxicity observed in clinical trials at higher doses was reversible. For patients with underlying renal disease, frequency of administration of adefovir dipivoxil should be reduced to every 48 h for creatinine clearances of 20–49 mL/min; to every 72 h for creatinine clearances of 10–19 mL/min; and once a week, following dialysis, for patients undergoing hemodialysis. Adefovir dipivoxil is very well tolerated, and ALT elevations during and after withdrawal of therapy are similar to those observed and described earlier in clinical trials of lamivudine. An advantage of adefovir is its relatively favorable resistance profile; however, it is not as potent as the other approved oral agents, it does not suppress HBV DNA as rapidly or as uniformly as the others, it is the least likely of all agents to result in HBeAg seroconversion, and 20–50% of patients fail to suppress HBV DNA by 2 log$_{10}$ ("primary nonresponders"). For these reasons, adefovir has been supplanted in both treatment-naïve and lamivudine-resistant patients by the more potent, less resistance-prone nucleotide analogue tenofovir (discussed later).

PEGYLATED INTERFERON After long-acting PEG IFN was shown to be effective in the treatment of hepatitis C (discussed later), this more convenient drug was evaluated in the treatment of chronic hepatitis B. Once-a-week PEG IFN is more effective than the more frequently administered, standard IFN, and several large-scale trials of PEG IFN versus oral nucleoside analogues have been conducted among patients with HBeAg-reactive and HBeAg-negative chronic hepatitis B.

In HBeAg-reactive chronic hepatitis B, two large-scale studies were done, one with PEG IFN-α 2b (100 μg weekly for 32 weeks, then 50 μg weekly for another 20 weeks for a total of 52 weeks, with a comparison arm of combination PEG IFN with oral lamivudine) in 307 subjects; the other involved PEG IFN-α 2a (180 μg weekly for 48 weeks) in 814 primarily Asian patients, three-fourths of whom had ALT ≥2 × the upper limit of normal, with comparison arms of lamivudine monotherapy and combination PEG IFN plus lamivudine. At the end of therapy (48–52 weeks) in the PEG IFN monotherapy arms, HBeAg loss occurred in approximately 30%, HBeAg seroconversion in 22–27%, undetectable HBV DNA (<400 copies/mL by PCR) in 10–25%, normal ALT in 34–39%, and a mean reduction in HBV DNA of 2 log$_{10}$ copies/mL (PEG IFN-α 2b) to 4.5 log$_{10}$ copies/mL (PEG IFN-α 2a). Six months after completing PEG IFN monotherapy in these trials, HBeAg losses were present in approximately 35%, HBeAg seroconversion in approximately 30%, undetectable HBV DNA in 7–14%, normal ALT in 32–41%, and a mean reduction in HBV DNA of 2–2.4 log$_{10}$ copies/mL. Although the combination of PEG IFN and lamivudine was superior at the end of therapy in one or more serologic, virologic, or biochemical outcomes, neither the combination arm (in both studies) nor the lamivudine monotherapy arm (in the PEG IFN-α 2a trial) demonstrated any benefit compared to the PEG IFN monotherapy arms 6 months after therapy. Moreover, HBsAg seroconversion occurred in 3–7% of PEG IFN recipients (with or without lamivudine); some of these seroconversions were identified by the end of therapy, but many were identified during the posttreatment follow-up period. The likelihood of HBeAg loss in PEG IFN–treated HBeAg-reactive patients is associated with HBV genotype A > B > C > D (shown for PEG IFN α-2b but not for α-2a).

Based on these results, some authorities concluded that PEG IFN monotherapy should be the first-line therapy of choice in HBeAg-reactive chronic hepatitis B; however, this conclusion has been challenged. Although a finite, 1-year course of PEG IFN results in a higher rate of sustained response (6 months after treatment) than is achieved with oral nucleoside/nucleotide analogue therapy, the comparison is confounded by the fact that oral agents are not discontinued at the end of 1 year. Instead, taken orally and free of side effects, therapy with oral agents is extended indefinitely or until after the occurrence of an HBeAg response. The rate of HBeAg responses after 2 years of oralagent nucleoside analogue therapy is at least as high as, if not higher

TABLE 40-3

407

COMPARISON OF PEGYLATED INTERFERON (PEG IFN), LAMIVUDINE, ADEFOVIR, ENTECAVIR, TELBIVUDINE, AND TENOFOVIR THERAPY FOR CHRONIC HEPATITIS B[a]

FEATURE	PEG IFN[b]	LAMIVUDINE	ADEFOVIR	ENTECAVIR	TELBIVUDINE	TENOFOVIR
Route of administration	Subcutaneous Injection	Oral	Oral	Oral	Oral	Oral
Duration of therapy[c]	48–52 weeks	≥52 weeks	≥48 weeks	≥48 weeks	≥52 weeks	≥48 weeks
Tolerability	Poorly tolerated	Well tolerated	Well tolerated; creatinine monitoring recommended	Well tolerated	Well tolerated	Well tolerated; creatinine monitoring recommended
HBeAg seroconversion						
1 yr Rx	18–20%	16–21%	12%	21%	22%	21%
>1 yr Rx	NA	up to 50% @ 5 yrs	43% @ 3 yrs[d]	31% @ 2 yrs 39% @ 3 yrs	30% @ 2 yrs	27% @ 2 yrs
Log₁₀ HBV DNA reduction (mean copies/mL)						
HBeAg-reactive	4.5	5.5	median 3.5–5	6.9	6.4	6.2
HBeAg-negative	4.1	4.4–4.7	median 3.5–3.9	5.0	5.2	4.6
HBV DNA PCR negative (<300–400 copies/mL; <1000 copies/mL for adefovir) end of yr 1						
HBeAg-reactive	10–25%	36–44%	13–21%	67% (91% @ 4 yrs)	60%	76%
HBeAg-negative	63%	60–73%	48–77%	90%	88%	93%
ALT normalization at end of yr 1						
HBeAg-reactive	39%	41–75%	48–61%	68%	77%	68%
HBeAg-negative	34–38%	62–79%	48–77%	78%	74%	76%
HBsAg loss yr 1	3–4%	≥1%	0%	2%	<1%	3%
yr 2	12% 5 yr after 1 yr of Rx	no data	5% at yr 5	5%	no data	6%
Histologic improvement (≥2 point reduction in HAI) at yr 1						
HBeAg-reactive	38% 6 months after	49–62%	53–68%	72%	65%	74%
HBeAg-negative	48% 6 months after	61–66%	64%	70%	67%	72%
Viral resistance	None	15-30% @ 1 yr 70% @ 5 yrs	None @ 1 yr 29% at 5 yrs	≤1% @ 1 yr[e] 1.2% @ 5 yr[e]	up to 5% @ yr 1 up to 22% @ yr 2	0% @ yr 1 0% through yr 3
Cost (US$) for 1 yr	~$18,000	~$2,500	~$6,500	~$8,700[f]	~$6,000	~$6,000

[a]Generally, these comparisons are based on data on each drug tested individually versus placebo in registration clinical trials; because, with rare exception, these comparisons are not based on head-to-head testing of these drugs, relative advantages and disadvantages should be interpreted cautiously.

[b]Although standard interferon α administered daily or three times a week is approved as therapy for chronic hepatitis B, it has been supplanted by PEG IFN, which is administered once a week and is more effective. Standard interferon has no advantages over PEG IFN.

[c]Duration of therapy in clinical efficacy trials; use in clinical practice may vary.

[d]Because of a computer-generated randomization error that resulted in misallocation of drug versus placebo during the second year of clinical-trial treatment, the frequency of HBeAg seroconversion beyond the first year is an estimate (Kaplan-Meier analysis) based on the small subset in whom adefovir was administered correctly.

[e]7% during a year of therapy (43% at year 4) in lamivudine-resistant patients.

[f]$17,400 for lamivudine-refractory patients.

Abbreviations: ALT, alanine aminotransferase; HAI, histologic activity index; HBeAg, hepatitis B e antigen; HBsAg, hepatitis B surface antigen; HBV, hepatitis B virus; NA, not applicable; PCR, polymerase chain reaction; PEG IFN, pegylated interferon; Rx, therapy; yr, year.

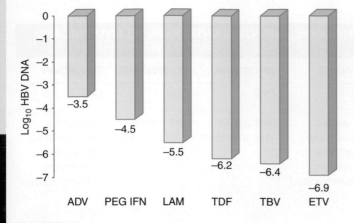

FIGURE 40-1

Relative potency of antiviral drugs for hepatitis B, as reflected by median log₁₀ HBV DNA reduction in HBeAg-positive chronic hepatitis B. These data are from individual reports of large, randomized controlled registration trials that were the basis for approval of the drugs. In most instances, these data do not represent direct comparisons among the drugs, because study populations were different, baseline patient variables were not always uniform, and the sensitivity and dynamic range of the HBV DNA assays used in the trials varied. ADV, adefovir dipivoxil; PEG IFN, pegylated interferon α-2a; LAM, lamivudine; TDF, tenofovir disoproxil fumarate; TBV, telbivudine; ETV, entecavir.

chronic hepatitis B; the most authoritative and updated (and free of financial support by pharmaceutical companies) are those of the American Association for the Study of Liver Diseases (AASLD) and of the European Association for the Study of the Liver (EASL). Although the recommendations differ slightly, a consensus has emerged on most of the important points (Table 40-4). No treatment is recommended or available for inactive "nonreplicative" hepatitis B carriers (undetectable HBeAg with normal ALT and HBV DNA ≤10³ IU/mL documented serially over time). In patients with detectable HBeAg and HBV DNA levels >2 × 10⁴ IU/mL, treatment is recommended by the AASLD for those with ALT levels above 2 × the upper limit of normal. (The EASL recommends treatment in HBeAg-positive patients for HBV DNA levels >2 × 10³ IU/mL and ALT above the upper limit of normal.) For HBeAg-positive patients with ALT ≤2 × the upper limit of normal, in whom sustained responses are not likely and who would require multi-year therapy, antiviral therapy is not recommended currently. This pattern is common during the early decades of life among Asian patients infected at birth; even in this group, therapy would be considered for those >40 years of age, ALT persistently at the high end of the two-fold range, and/or with a family history of hepatocellular carcinoma, especially if the liver biopsy shows moderate to severe necroinflammatory activity or fibrosis. In this

group, when, eventually, ALT becomes elevated later in life, antiviral therapy should be instituted. For patients with HBeAg-negative chronic hepatitis B, ALT >2 × the upper limit of normal (above the upper limit of normal according to EASL) and HBV DNA >2 × 10³ IU/mL, antiviral therapy is recommended. If HBV DNA is >2 × 10³ IU/mL and ALT is 1 to >2 × the upper limit of normal, liver biopsy should be considered to help in arriving at a decision to treat if substantial liver injury is present (treatment in this subset would be recommended according to EASL guidelines, because ALT is elevated).

For patients with compensated cirrhosis, because antiviral therapy has been shown to retard clinical progression, treatment is recommended regardless of HBeAg status and ALT as long as HBV DNA is detectable at >2 × 10³ IU/mL (detectable at any level according to the EASL); monitoring without therapy is recommended for those with HBV DNA <2 × 10³ IU/mL, unless ALT is elevated. For patients with decompensated cirrhosis, treatment is recommended regardless of serologic and biochemical status, as long as HBV DNA is detectable. Patients with decompensated cirrhosis should be evaluated as candidates for liver transplantation.

Among the seven available drugs for hepatitis B, PEG IFN has supplanted standard IFN, entecavir has supplanted lamivudine, and tenofovir has supplanted adefovir. PEG IFN, entecavir, or tenofovir are recommended as first-line therapy (Table 40-3). PEG IFN requires finite-duration therapy, achieves the highest rate of HBeAg responses after a year of therapy, and does not support viral mutations, but it requires subcutaneous injections and is associated with inconvenience and intolerability. Oral nucleoside analogues require long-term therapy in most patients, and when used alone, lamivudine and telbivudine foster the emergence of viral mutations, adefovir somewhat less so, and entecavir (except in lamivudine-experienced patients) and tenofovir rarely at all. Oral agents do not require injections, are very well tolerated, lead to improved histology in 50–90% of patients, suppress HBV DNA more profoundly than PEG IFN, and are effective even in patients who fail to respond to IFN-based therapy. Although oral agents are less likely to result in HBeAg responses during the first year of therapy, as compared to PEG IFN, treatment with oral agents tends to be extended beyond the first year and, by the end of the second year, yields HBeAg responses (and even HBsAg responses) comparable in frequency to those achieved after 1 year of PEG IFN (and without the associated side effects) (Table 40-5). Although adefovir and tenofovir are safe, creatinine monitoring is recommended. Substantial experience with lamivudine during pregnancy (discussed earlier) has identified no teratogenicity. Although interferons do not appear to cause congenital anomalies, interferons

TABLE 40-4

409

CHAPTER 40

Chronic Hepatitis

RECOMMENDATIONS FOR TREATMENT OF CHRONIC HEPATITIS B[a]

HBeAg STATUS	CLINICAL	HBV DNA (IU/mL)	ALT	RECOMMENDATION
HBeAg-reactive	[b]	$>2 \times 10^4$	$\leq 2 \times$ ULN[c]	No treatment; monitor. In patients >40, with family history of hepatocellular carcinoma, and/or ALT persistently at the high end of the twofold range, liver biopsy may help in decision to treat
	Chronic hepatitis	$>2 \times 10^{4d}$	$>2 \times$ ULN[d]	Treat[e]
	Cirrhosis compensated	$>2 \times 10^3$	< or > ULN	Treat[e] with oral agents, not PEG IFN
		$<2 \times 10^3$	>ULN	Consider treatment[f]
	Cirrhosis decompensated	Detectable	< or > ULN	Treat[e] with oral agents[g], not PEG IFN; refer for liver transplantation
		Undetectable	< or > ULN	Observe; refer for liver transplantation
HBeAg-negative	[b]	$\leq 2 \times 10^3$	$\leq$ULN	Inactive carrier; treatment not necessary
	Chronic hepatitis	$>10^3$	1->2 $\times$ ULN[d]	Consider liver biopsy; treat[h] if biopsy shows moderate to severe inflammation or fibrosis
	Chronic hepatitis	$>10^4$	$>2 \times$ ULN[d]	Treat[h,i]
	Cirrhosis compensated	$>2 \times 10^3$	< or > ULN	Treat[e] with oral agents, not PEG IFN
		$<2 \times 10^3$	>ULN	Consider treatment[f]
	Cirrhosis decompensated	Detectable	< or > ULN	Treat[h] with oral agents[g], not PEG IFN; refer for liver transplantation
		Undetectable	< or > ULN	Observe; refer for liver transplantation

[a]Based on practice guidelines of the American Association for the Study of Liver Diseases (AASLD). Except as indicated in footnotes, these guidelines are similar to those issued by the European Association for the Study of the Liver (EASL).

[b]Liver disease tends to be mild or inactive clinically; most such patients do not undergo liver biopsy.

[c]This pattern is common during early decades of life in Asian patients infected at birth.

[d]According to the EASL guidelines, treat if HBV DNA is $>2 \times 10^3$ IU/mL and ALT >ULN.

[e]One of the potent oral drugs with a high barrier to resistance (entecavir or tenofovir) or PEG IFN can be used as first-line therapy (see text). These oral agents, but not PEG IFN, should be used for interferon-refractory/intolerant and immunocompromised patients. PEG IFN is administered weekly by subcutaneous injection for a year; the oral agents are administered daily for at least a year and continued indefinitely or until at least 6 months after HBeAg seroconversion.

[f]According to EASL guidelines, patients with compensated cirrhosis and detectable HBV DNA at any level, even with normal ALT, are candidates for therapy. Most authorities would treat indefinitely, even in HBeAg-positive disease after HBeAg seroconversion.

[g]Because the emergence of resistance can lead to loss of antiviral benefit and further deterioration in decompensated cirrhosis, a low-resistance regimen is recommended-entecavir or tenofovir monotherapy or combination therapy with the more resistance-prone lamivudine (or telbivudine) plus adefovir. Therapy should be instituted urgently.

[h]Because HBeAg seroconversion is not an option, the goal of therapy is to suppress HBV DNA and maintain a normal ALT. PEG IFN is administered by subcutaneous injection weekly for a year; caution is warranted in relying on a 6-month posttreatment interval to define a sustained response, because the majority of such responses are lost thereafter. Oral agents, entecavir or tenofovir, are administered daily, usually indefinitely or, until as very rarely occurs, virologic and biochemical responses are accompanied by HBsAg seroconversion.

[i]For older patients and those with advanced fibrosis, consider lowering the HBV DNA threshold to $>2 \times 10^3$ IU/mL.

Abbreviations: ALT, alanine aminotransferase; AASLD, American Association for the Study of Liver Diseases; EASL, European Association for the Study of the Liver; HBeAg, hepatitis B e antigen; HBsAg, hepatitis B surface antigen; HBV, hepatitis B virus; PEG IFN, pegylated interferon; ULN, upper limits of normal.

have antiproliferative properties and should not be used during pregnancy. Adefovir during pregnancy has not been associated with birth defects; however, there may be an increased risk of spontaneous abortion. Data on the safety of entecavir during pregnancy have not been published. Sufficient data in animals and limited data in humans suggest that telbivudine and tenofovir can be used safely during pregnancy. In general, except perhaps for lamivudine, and until additional data become available, the other antivirals for hepatitis B should be avoided or used with extreme caution during pregnancy.

As noted earlier, some physicians prefer to begin with PEG IFN, while other physicians and patients prefer oral agents as first-line therapy. For patients with decompensated cirrhosis, the emergence of resistance can result in further deterioration and loss of antiviral effectiveness. Therefore, in this patient subset, the threshold for

TABLE 40-5

PEGYLATED INTERFERON VERSUS ORAL NUCLEOSIDE ANALOGUES FOR THE TREATMENT OF CHRONIC HEPATITIS B

	PEG IFN	NUCLEOSIDE ANALOGUES
Administration	Weekly injection	Daily, orally
Tolerability	Poorly tolerated, intensive monitoring	Well tolerated, limited monitoring
Duration of therapy	Finite 48 weeks	≥1 year, indefinite in most patients
Maximum mean HBV DNA suppression	4.5 $\log_{10}$	6.9 $\log_{10}$
Effective in high-level HBV DNA (≥10^9 IU/mL)	No	Yes
HBeAg seroconversion		
During 1 year of therapy	~30%	~20%
During >1 year of therapy	Not applicable	30% (year 2)–50% (year 5)
HBeAg-negative posttreatment HBV DNA suppression	17% @ 5 years	7% @ 4 years (lamivudine)
HBsAg loss		
During 1 year of therapy	3–4%	0–3%
During >1 year of therapy	Not applicable	3–6% @ 2 years of therapy
After 1 year of therapy– HBeAg-negative	12% @ 5 years	3.5% @ 5 years
Antiviral resistance	None	Lamivudine: ~30% year 1, ~70% year 5 Adefovir: 0% year 1, ~30% year 5 Telbivudine: up to 4% year 1, 22% year 2 Entecavir: ≤1.2% through year 5 Tenofovir: 0% through year 3
Use in cirrhosis, transplantation, immuno-suppressed	No	Yes
Cost, 1 year of therapy	++++	+ to ++

Abbreviations: HBV, hepatitis B virus; HBeAg, hepatitis B e antigen; HBsAg, hepatitis B surface antigen; IU/mL, international units per milliliter; PEG IFN, pegylated interferon.

relying on therapy with a very favorable resistance profile (e.g., entecavir or tenofovir) or on combination therapy (e.g., lamivudine or telbivudine with adefovir) is low. PEG IFN should not be used in patients with compensated or decompensated cirrhosis.

For patients with end-stage chronic hepatitis B who undergo liver transplantation, reinfection of the new liver is almost universal in the absence of antiviral therapy. The majority of patients become high-level viremic carriers with minimal liver injury. Before the availability of antiviral therapy, an unpredictable proportion experienced severe hepatitis B–related liver injury, sometimes a fulminant-like hepatitis, sometimes a rapid recapitulation of the original severe chronic hepatitis B (Chap. 38). Currently, however, prevention of recurrent hepatitis B after liver transplantation has been achieved definitively by *combining* hepatitis B immune globulin with one of the oral nucleoside or nucleotide analogues (Chap. 46).

For patients treated with the more resistance-prone (lamivudine, telbivudine) or less potent (adefovir) oral agents, assessment of response at 24 weeks (48 weeks for adefovir) can identify those at high risk for inadequate response and breakthrough resistance (i.e., the presence of residual detectable viremia). When such inadequate responses are identified, a second, noncross-resistant agent can be added or the initial agent can be replaced by a more potent agent. This "roadmap" approach has been rendered irrelevant by the use of the current generation of highly potent, low-resistant agents entecavir and tenofovir. Still, at 24 weeks, if HBV DNA exceeds 2×10^3 IU/mL, switching to a different agent or adding a second agent is advisable.

Patients with HBV-HIV co-infection can have progressive HBV-associated liver disease and, occasionally, a severe exacerbation of hepatitis B resulting from immunologic reconstitution following highly active antiretroviral therapy. Lamivudine should never be used as monotherapy in patients with HBV-HIV infection because HIV resistance emerges rapidly to both viruses. Adefovir has been used successfully to treat chronic hepatitis B in HBV-HIV co-infected patients but is no longer considered a first-line agent for HBV. Entecavir has low-level activity against HIV and can result in selection of HIV resistance; therefore, it should be avoided in HBV-HIV co-infection. Tenofovir and the combination of tenofovir and emtricitabine in one pill are approved therapies for HIV and represent excellent choices for treating HBV infection in HBV-HIV co-infected patients. Generally, even for HBV-HIV co-infected patients who do not yet meet treatment criteria for HIV infection, treating for both HBV and HIV is recommended.

Patients with chronic hepatitis B who undergo cytotoxic chemotherapy for treatment of malignancies as well as patients treated with immunosuppressive, anticytokine, or antitumor necrosis factor therapies experience enhanced HBV replication and viral expression on hepatocyte membranes during chemotherapy coupled with suppression of cellular immunity. When chemotherapy is withdrawn, such patients are at risk for reactivation of hepatitis B, often severe and occasionally fatal. Such rebound reactivation represents restoration of cytolytic T cell function against a target organ enriched in HBV expression. Preemptive treatment with lamivudine prior to the initiation of chemotherapy has been shown to reduce the risk of such reactivation. In all likelihood, the newer, more potent oral antiviral agents will work as well and with a lower risk of antiviral drug resistance. The optimal duration of antiviral therapy after completion of chemotherapy is not known, but a suggested approach is 6 months for inactive hepatitis B carriers and longer-duration therapy in patients with baseline HBV DNA levels $>2 \times 10^3$ IU/mL, until standard clinical endpoints are met (Table 40-4).

CHRONIC HEPATITIS D (DELTA HEPATITIS)

Chronic hepatitis D (HDV) may follow acute co-infection with HBV but at a rate no higher than the rate of chronicity of acute hepatitis B. That is, although HDV co-infection can increase the severity of acute hepatitis B, HDV does not increase the likelihood of progression to chronic hepatitis B. When, however, HDV superinfection occurs in a person who is already chronically infected with HBV, long-term HDV infection is the rule and a worsening of the liver disease the expected consequence. Except for severity, chronic hepatitis B plus D has similar clinical and laboratory features to those seen in chronic hepatitis B alone. Relatively severe and progressive chronic hepatitis, with or without cirrhosis, is the rule, and mild chronic hepatitis is the exception. Occasionally, mild hepatitis or even, rarely, inactive carriage occurs in patients with chronic hepatitis B plus D, and the disease may become indolent after several years of infection. A distinguishing serologic feature of chronic hepatitis D is the presence in the circulation of antibodies to liver-kidney microsomes (anti-LKM); however, the anti-LKM seen in hepatitis D, anti-LKM3, are directed against uridine diphosphate glucuronosyltransferase and are distinct from anti-LKM1 seen in patients with autoimmune hepatitis and in a subset of patients with chronic hepatitis C (discussed next). The clinical and laboratory features of chronic HDV infection are summarized in Chap. 38.

TREATMENT   Chronic Hepatitis D

Management is not well defined. Glucocorticoids are ineffective and are not used. Preliminary experimental trials of IFN-α suggested that conventional doses and durations of therapy lower levels of HDV RNA and aminotransferase activity only transiently during treatment but have no impact on the natural history of the disease. In contrast, high-dose IFN-α (9 million units three times a week) for 12 months may be associated with a sustained loss of HDV replication and clinical improvement in up to 50% of patients. Moreover, the beneficial impact of treatment has been observed to persist for 15 years and to be associated with a reduction in grade of hepatic necrosis and inflammation, reversion of advanced fibrosis (improved stage), and clearance of HDV RNA in some patients. A suggested approach to therapy has been high-dose, long-term IFN for at least a year and, in responders, extension of therapy until HDV RNA and HBsAg clearance. PEG IFN has also been shown to be effective in the treatment of chronic hepatitis D and is likely to become a more convenient replacement for standard IFN. None of the nucleoside analogue antiviral agents for hepatitis B is effective in hepatitis D. In patients with end-stage liver disease secondary to chronic hepatitis D, liver transplantation has been effective. If hepatitis D recurs in the new liver without the expression of hepatitis B (an unusual serologic profile in immunocompetent persons but common in transplant patients), liver injury is limited. In fact, the outcome of transplantation for chronic hepatitis D is superior to that for chronic hepatitis B; in such patients, combination hepatitis B immune globulin and nucleoside analogue therapy for hepatitis B is indicated (Chap. 46).

CHRONIC HEPATITIS C

Regardless of the epidemiologic mode of acquisition of hepatitis C virus (HCV) infection, chronic hepatitis follows acute hepatitis C in 50–70% of cases; chronic infection is common even in those with a return to normal in aminotransferase levels after acute hepatitis C, adding up to an 85% likelihood of chronic HCV infection after acute hepatitis C. Few clues had emerged to explain host differences associated with chronic infection until recently, when variation in a single nucleotide polymorphism (SNP) on chromosome 19, IL28B (which codes for interferon-λ3), was identified that distinguished between responders and nonresponders to antiviral therapy (discussed later). The same variants correlated with spontaneous resolution after acute infection: 53% in genotype C/C, 30% in genotype C/T, but only 23% in genotype T/T.

In patients with chronic hepatitis C followed for 20 years, progression to cirrhosis occurs in about

20–25%. Such is the case even for patients with relatively clinically mild chronic hepatitis, including those without symptoms, with only modest elevations of aminotransferase activity and with mild chronic hepatitis on liver biopsy. Even in cohorts of well-compensated patients with chronic hepatitis C referred for clinical research trials (no complications of chronic liver disease and with normal hepatic synthetic function), the prevalence of cirrhosis may be as high as 50%. Most cases of hepatitis C are identified initially in asymptomatic patients who have no history of acute hepatitis C (e.g., those discovered while attempting to donate blood, while undergoing lab testing as part of an application for life insurance, or as a result of routine laboratory tests). The source of HCV infection in many of these cases is not defined, although a long-forgotten percutaneous exposure in the remote past can be elicited in a substantial proportion and probably accounts for most infections; most of these infections were acquired in the 1960s and 1970s, coming to clinical attention decades later.

Approximately one-third of patients with chronic hepatitis C have normal or near-normal aminotransferase activity; although one-third to one-half of these patients have chronic hepatitis on liver biopsy, the grade of liver injury and stage of fibrosis tend to be mild in the vast majority. In some cases, more severe liver injury has been reported—even, rarely, cirrhosis, most likely the result of previous histologic activity. Among patients with persistent normal aminotransferase activity sustained over ≥5–10 years, histologic progression has been shown to be rare; however, approximately one-fourth of patients with normal aminotransferase activity experience subsequent aminotransferase elevations, and histologic injury can be progressive once abnormal biochemical activity resumes. Therefore, continued clinical monitoring is indicated, even for patients with normal aminotransferase activity.

Despite this substantial rate of progression of chronic hepatitis C, and despite the fact that liver failure can result from end-stage chronic hepatitis C, the long-term prognosis for chronic hepatitis C in a majority of patients is relatively benign. Mortality over 10–20 years among patients with transfusion-associated chronic hepatitis C has been shown not to differ from mortality in a matched population of transfused patients in whom hepatitis C did not develop. Although death in the hepatitis group is more likely to result from liver failure, and although hepatic decompensation may occur in ~15% of such patients over the course of a decade, the majority (almost 60%) of patients remain asymptomatic and well compensated, with no clinical sequelae of chronic liver disease. Overall, chronic hepatitis C tends to be very slowly and insidiously progressive, if at all, in the vast majority of patients, while in approximately one-fourth of cases, chronic hepatitis C will progress eventually to end-stage cirrhosis. In fact,

because HCV infection is so prevalent, and because a proportion of patients progress inexorably to end-stage liver disease, hepatitis C is the most frequent indication for liver transplantation (Chap. 46). Referral bias may account for the more severe outcomes described in cohorts of patients reported from tertiary care centers (20-year progression of ≥20%) versus the more benign outcomes in cohorts of patients monitored from initial blood-product-associated acute hepatitis or identified in community settings (20-year progression of only 4–7%). Still unexplained, however, are the wide ranges in reported progression to cirrhosis, from 2% over 17 years in a population of women with hepatitis C infection acquired from contaminated anti-D immune globulin to 30% over ≤11 years in recipients of contaminated intravenous immune globulin.

Progression of liver disease in patients with chronic hepatitis C has been reported to be more likely in patients with older age, longer duration of infection, advanced histologic stage and grade, genotype 1, more complex quasispecies diversity, increased hepatic iron, concomitant other liver disorders (alcoholic liver disease, chronic hepatitis B, hemochromatosis, α_1-antitrypsin deficiency, and steatohepatitis), HIV infection, and obesity. Among these variables, however, duration of infection appears to be one of the most important, and some of the others probably reflect disease duration to some extent (e.g., quasispecies diversity, hepatic iron accumulation). No other epidemiologic or clinical features of chronic hepatitis C (e.g., severity of acute hepatitis, level of aminotransferase activity, level of HCV RNA, presence or absence of jaundice during acute hepatitis) are predictive of eventual outcome. Despite the relatively benign nature of chronic hepatitis C over time in many patients, cirrhosis following chronic hepatitis C has been associated with the late development, after several decades, of HCC; the annual rate of HCC in cirrhotic patients with hepatitis C is 1–4%, occurring primarily in patients who have had HCV infection for 30 years or more.

Perhaps the best prognostic indicator in chronic hepatitis C is liver histology; the rate of hepatic fibrosis may be slow, moderate, or rapid. Patients with mild necrosis and inflammation as well as those with limited fibrosis have an excellent prognosis and limited progression to cirrhosis. In contrast, among patients with moderate to severe necroinflammatory activity or fibrosis, including septal or bridging fibrosis, progression to cirrhosis is highly likely over the course of 10–20 years. Among patients with compensated cirrhosis associated with hepatitis C, the 10-year survival rate is close to 80%; mortality occurs at a rate of 2–6% per year; decompensation at a rate of 4–5% per year; and, as noted earlier, HCC at a rate of 1–4% per year. A discussion of the pathogenesis of liver injury in patients with chronic hepatitis C appears in Chap. 38.

Clinical features of chronic hepatitis C are similar to those described earlier for chronic hepatitis B. Generally, fatigue is the most common symptom; jaundice is rare. Immune complex–mediated extrahepatic complications of chronic hepatitis C are less common than in chronic hepatitis B (despite the fact that assays for immune complexes are often positive in patients with chronic hepatitis C), with the exception of essential mixed cryoglobulinemia (Chap. 38), which is linked to cutaneous vasculitis and membranoproliferative glomerulonephritis as well as lymphoproliferative disorders such as B-cell lymphoma and unexplained monoclonal gammopathy. In addition, chronic hepatitis C has been associated with extrahepatic complications unrelated to immune-complex injury. These include Sjögren's syndrome, lichen planus, porphyria cutanea tarda, type 2 diabetes mellitus, and the metabolic syndrome (including insulin resistance and steatohepatitis).

Laboratory features of chronic hepatitis C are similar to those in patients with chronic hepatitis B, but aminotransferase levels tend to fluctuate more (the characteristic episodic pattern of aminotransferase activity) and to be lower, especially in patients with long-standing disease. An interesting and occasionally confusing finding in patients with chronic hepatitis C is the presence of autoantibodies. Rarely, patients with autoimmune hepatitis (discussed later) and hyperglobulinemia have false-positive immunoassays for anti-HCV. On the other hand, some patients with serologically confirmable chronic hepatitis C have circulating anti-LKM. These antibodies are anti-LKM1, as seen in patients with autoimmune hepatitis type 2 (discussed later), and are directed against a 33-aminoacid sequence of cytochrome P450 IID6. The occurrence of anti-LKM1 in some patients with chronic hepatitis C may result from the partial sequence homology between the epitope recognized by anti-LKM1 and two segments of the HCV polyprotein. In addition, the presence of this autoantibody in some patients with chronic hepatitis C suggests that autoimmunity may be playing a role in the pathogenesis of chronic hepatitis C.

Histopathologic features of chronic hepatitis C, especially those that distinguish hepatitis C from hepatitis B, are described in Chap. 38.

TREATMENT | Chronic Hepatitis C

Therapy for chronic hepatitis C has evolved substantially in the two decades since IFN-α was introduced for this indication. The therapeutic armamentarium has grown to include pegylated IFN (PEG IFN) with ribavirin and most recently the introduction of protease inhibitors telaprevir and boceprevir used in combination with PEG IFN and ribavirin in patients with HCV genotype 1.

INTERFERON, PEGYLATED INTERFERON, AND RIBAVIRIN When first approved, IFN-α was administered via subcutaneous injection three times a week for 6 months but achieved a sustained virologic response (SVR) (Fig. 40-2) (a reduction of HCV RNA to undetectable levels by PCR when measured ≥6 months after completion of therapy) below 10%. Doubling the duration of therapy—but not increasing the dose or changing IFN preparations—increased the SVR rate to ~20%, and addition to the regimen of daily ribavirin, an oral guanosine nucleoside, increased the SVR rate to 40%. When used alone, ribavirin is ineffective and does not reduce HCV RNA levels, but ribavirin enhances the efficacy of IFN by reducing the likelihood of virologic relapse after the achievement of an end-treatment response (ETR) (Fig. 40-2) (response measured during, and maintained to the end of, treatment). Proposed mechanisms to explain the role of ribavirin include subtle direct reduction of HCV replication, inhibition of

FIGURE 40-2

Virologic responses during a 48-week course of antiviral therapy in patients with hepatitis C, genotype 1 or 4 (for genotypes 2 or 3, the course would be 24 weeks). Nonresponders can be classified as null responders (HCV RNA reduction of <2 log₁₀ IU/mL) or partial responders (HCV RNA reduction ≥2 log₁₀ IU/mL but not suppressed to undetectable) by week 24 of therapy. In responders, HCV RNA can become undetectable, as shown with sensitive amplification assays, within 4 weeks (RVR, rapid virologic response); can be reduced by ≥2 log₁₀ IU/mL within 12 weeks (early virologic response, EVR; if HCV RNA is undetectable at 12 weeks, the designation is "complete" EVR); or at the end of therapy, 48 weeks (ETR, end-treatment response). In responders, if HCV RNA remains undetectable for 24 weeks after ETR, week 72, the patient has a sustained virologic response (SVR), but if HCV RNA becomes detectable again, the patient is considered to have relapsed. (*Reproduced with permission, courtesy of Marc G. Ghany, National Institute of Diabetes and Digestive and Kidney Diseases, National Institutes of Health and the American Association for the Study of Liver Diseases. Hepatology 49:1335, 2009.*)

host inosine monophosphate dehydrogenase activity (and associated depletion of guanosine pools), immune modulation, induction of virologic mutational catastrophe, and enhancement of interferon-stimulated gene expression. Interferon therapy results in activation of the JAK-STAT signal transduction pathway, which culminates in the intracellular elaboration of genes and their protein products that have antiviral properties. Hepatitis C proteins inhibit JAK-STAT signaling at several steps along the pathway, and exogenous interferon restores expression of interferon-stimulated genes and their antiviral effects.

Treatment with the combination of PEG IFN and ribavirin increased responsiveness (frequency of SVR) to as high as 55% overall, to >40% in genotypes 1 and 4, and to >80% in genotypes 2 and 3. Still, many important lessons about antiviral therapy for chronic hepatitis C were learned from the experience with IFN monotherapy and combination IFN-ribavirin therapy. Even in the absence of biochemical and virologic responses, histologic improvement occurs in approximately three-fourths of all treated patients. In chronic hepatitis C, unlike the case in hepatitis B, responses to therapy are not accompanied by transient, acute hepatitis-like aminotransferase elevations. Instead, ALT levels fall precipitously during therapy. Up to 90% of virologic responses are achieved within the first 12 weeks of therapy; responses thereafter are rare. Most relapses occur within the first 12 weeks after treatment. Sustained virologic responses are very durable; normal ALT, improved histology, and absence of HCV RNA in serum and liver have been documented a decade after successful therapy, and "relapses" 2 years after sustained responses are almost unheard of. Thus, an SVR to antiviral therapy of chronic hepatitis C is tantamount to a cure.

Patient variables that tend to correlate with sustained virologic responsiveness to IFN-based therapy include favorable genotype (genotypes 2 and 3 as opposed to genotypes 1 and 4), low baseline HCV RNA level (<2 million copies/mL, which is equivalent to <800,000 IU/mL, the current convention of quantitation), histologically mild hepatitis and minimal fibrosis, age <40, absence of obesity as well as insulin resistance and type 2 diabetes mellitus, and female gender. Patients with cirrhosis can respond, but they are less likely to do so. For patients treated with combination IFN-ribavirin, in those with genotype 1, therapy should last a full 48 weeks, while in those with genotypes 2 and 3, a 24-week course of therapy suffices (although refined tailoring of treatment duration may be indicated based on rapidity of response or associated cofactors, discussed later). The response rate in African Americans is disappointingly low for reasons that are not fully understood. Potentially contributing to, but not explaining entirely, low responsiveness in African Americans are

a higher proportion with genotype 1, slower early viral kinetics during therapy, impaired HCV-specific immunity, and recently recognized host genetic differences in IL28B alleles, described later. The response rate in Latino patients is also low, despite the fact that the frequency of the favorable IL28B C allele is as common in Hispanic patients as in whites. Moreover, the likelihood of a sustained response is best if adherence to the treatment regimen is high (i.e., if patients receive ≥80% of the IFN and ribavirin doses and if they continue treatment for ≥80% of the anticipated duration of therapy). Other variables reported to correlate with increased responsiveness include brief duration of infection, low HCV quasispecies diversity, immunocompetence, absence of hepatic steatosis and insulin resistance, and low liver iron levels. High levels of HCV RNA, more histologically advanced liver disease, and high quasispecies diversity all go hand in hand with advanced duration of infection, which may be the single most important clinical variable determining IFN responsiveness. The ironic fact, then, is that patients whose disease is least likely to progress are the ones *most* likely to respond to interferon and vice versa.

Genetic changes in the virus may explain differences in treatment responsiveness in some patients (e.g., among patients with genotype 1b, responsiveness to IFN is enhanced in those with amino-acid-substitution mutations in the nonstructural protein 5A gene). As described earlier in the discussion of spontaneous recovery from acute hepatitis C, interferon gene variants discovered recently in gene-wide association studies have been shown to have a substantial impact on responsiveness of patients with genotype 1 to antiviral therapy. In studies of patients treated with PEG IFN and ribavirin, variants of the IL28B SNP that code for IFN-λ3 (a type-3 IFN, the receptors for which are more discretely distributed than IFN-α receptors and more concentrated in hepatocytes) correlate significantly with responsiveness. Patients homozygous for the C allele at this locus have the highest frequency of achieving an SVR (~80%), those homozygous for the T allele at this locus are least likely to achieve an SVR (~25%), and those heterozygous at this locus (C/T) have an intermediate level of responsiveness (SVRs in ~35%). The fact that C/C is common in whites of European ancestry and even more so in Japanese persons but rare in African Americans helps explain the differences in observed responsiveness among these population groups.

Side effects of IFN therapy are described earlier in the section on treatment of chronic hepatitis B. The most pronounced side effect of ribavirin therapy is hemolysis; a reduction in hemoglobin of up to 2–3 g or in hematocrit of 5–10% can be anticipated. A small, unpredictable proportion of patients experience profound, brisk hemolysis, resulting in symptomatic anemia; therefore, close monitoring of blood counts is crucial, and ribavirin should be avoided in patients with anemia or hemoglobinopathies and in patients with coronary artery disease or cerebrovascular disease, in whom anemia can precipitate an ischemic event. When symptomatic anemia occurs, ribavirin dose reductions or addition of erythropoietin to boost red blood cell levels may be required; erythropoietin has been shown to improve patients' quality of life but not the likelihood of achieving an SVR. If ribavirin is stopped during therapy, SVR rates fall, but responsiveness can be maintained as long as the ribavirin is not stopped and the total ribavirin dose exceeds 60% of the planned dose. In addition, ribavirin, which is renally excreted, should not be used in patients with renal insufficiency; the drug is teratogenic, precluding its use during pregnancy and mandating the scrupulous use of efficient contraception during therapy (interferons, too, because of their antiproliferative properties, are contraindicated during pregnancy).

Ribavirin can also cause nasal and chest congestion, pruritus, and precipitation of gout. Combination IFN-ribavirin therapy is more difficult to tolerate than IFN monotherapy. In one large clinical trial of combination therapy versus monotherapy, among those in the 1-year treatment group, 21% of the combination group (but only 14% of the monotherapy group) had to discontinue treatment, while 26% of the combination group (but only 9% of the monotherapy group) required dose reductions.

Studies of viral kinetics have shown that despite a virion half-life in serum of only 2–3 h, the level of HCV is maintained by a high replication rate of 10^{12} hepatitis C virions per day. IFN-α blocks virion production or release with an efficacy that increases with increasing drug doses; moreover, the calculated death rate for infected cells during IFN therapy is inversely related to viral load; patients with the most rapid death rate of infected hepatocytes are more likely to achieve undetectable HCV RNA at 3 months; in practice, failure to achieve an early virologic response (EVR), a ≥ 2-$\log_{10}$ reduction in HCV RNA by week 12, predicts failure to experience a subsequent SVR. Similarly, patients in whom HCV RNA becomes undetectable within 4 weeks [i.e., who achieve a rapid virologic response (RVR)] have a very high likelihood of achieving a sustained virologic response (Fig. 40-2). Therefore, to achieve rapid viral clearance from serum and the liver, *high-dose induction therapy* has been advocated. In practice, however, high-dose induction with IFN-based therapy has not yielded higher sustained response rates.

For the treatment of chronic hepatitis C, standard IFNs were supplanted by PEG IFNs. These have elimination times up to sevenfold longer than standard IFNs (i.e., a substantially longer half-life) and achieve prolonged concentrations, permitting administration once (rather than three times) a week. Instead of the frequent drug peaks (linked to side effects) and troughs (when drug is absent) associated with frequent administration of short-acting IFNs, administration of PEG IFNs results in drug concentrations that are more stable and sustained over time. Once-a-week PEG IFN monotherapy is twice as effective as monotherapy with its standard IFN counterpart, approaches the efficacy of combination standard IFN plus ribavirin, and is as well tolerated as standard IFNs, without more difficult-to-manage thrombocytopenia and leukopenia than standard IFNs.

Two PEG IFNs are available: PEG IFN-α2b and -α2a. PEG IFN-α2b consists of a 12-kD, linear PEG molecule bound to IFN-α2b, while PEG IFN-α2a consists of a larger, 40-kD, branched PEG molecule bound to IFN-α2a; because of its larger size and smaller volume of extravascular distribution, PEG IFN-α2a can be given at a uniform dose independent of weight, while the dose of the smaller PEG IFN-α2b, which has a much wider volume distribution, must be weight-based (Table 40-6). In the registration trial for PEG IFN-α2b plus ribavirin, the best regimen was 48 weeks of 1.5 µg/kg of PEG IFN once a week plus 800 mg of ribavirin daily. A post hoc analysis suggested that weight-based dosing of ribavirin would have been more effective than the fixed 800-mg dose used in the study (a broader dose/weight range was approved subsequently [see later]). In the first registration trial for PEG IFN-α2a plus ribavirin, the best regimen was 48 weeks of 180 µg of PEG IFN plus 1000 mg (for patients <75 kg) to 1200 mg (for patients $\geq$75 kg) of ribavirin. Sustained virologic responses of 54 and 56% were reported in these two studies, respectively. A subsequent study of PEG IFN-α2a plus ribavirin showed that, for patients with genotypes 2 and 3, a duration of 24 weeks and a ribavirin dose of 800 mg was sufficient. Among the three studies, for patients in the optimal treatment arm, SVR rates for patients with genotype 1 were 42–51%, and for patients with genotypes, 2 and 3, rates were 76–82%. Between genotypes 2 and 3, genotype 3 is somewhat more refractory, and some authorities would extend therapy for a full 48 weeks in patients with genotype 3, especially if they have advanced hepatic fibrosis or cirrhosis and/or high-level HCV RNA.

In the initial registration trials for combination PEG IFN plus ribavirin, both combination PEG IFN regimens were compared to standard IFN-α2b plus ribavirin. Side effects of the combination PEG IF-α2b regimen were comparable to those for the combination standard IFN regimen; however, when the combination PEG IFN-α2a regimen was compared to the combination standard IFN-α2b regimen, flu-like symptoms and depression were less common in the combination PEG IFN group. Although ascertainment of side effects differed between studies of the two drugs, when each was tested against standard IFN-α2b plus ribavirin, combination PEG IFN-α2a plus ribavirin appeared to be

TABLE 40-6

PEGYLATED INTERFERON α-2a AND α-2b FOR CHRONIC HEPATITIS C

	PEG IFN α-2b	PEG IFN α-2a
PEG size	12 kD linear	40 kD branched
Elimination half-life	54 h	65 h
Clearance	725 mL/h	60 mL/h
Dose	1.5 μg/kg (weight-based)	180 μg
Storage	Room temperature	Refrigerated
Ribavirin dose		
Genotype 1	800–1400 mg[a]	1000–1200 mg[b]
Genotype 2/3	800 mg	800 mg
Duration of therapy		
Genotype 1	48 weeks	48 weeks
Genotype 2/3	48 weeks[c]	24 weeks
Efficacy of combination Rx[d]	54%	56%
Genotype 1	40–42%	41–51%
Genotype 2/3	82%	76–78%

[a]In the registration trial for PEG IFN α-2b plus ribavirin, the optimal regimen was 1.5 μg of PEG IFN plus 800 mg of ribavirin; however, a posthoc analysis of this study suggested that higher ribavirin doses are better. In subsequent trials of PEG IFN α-2b with ribavirin in patients with genotype 1, the following daily ribavirin doses have been validated: 800 mg for patients weighing <65 kg, 1000 mg for patients weighing >65–85 kg, 1200 for patients weighing >85–105 kg, and 1400 mg for patients weighing >105 kg.

[b]1000 mg for patients weighing <75 kg; 1200 mg for patients weighing ≥75 kg.

[c]In the registration trial for PEG IFN α-2b plus ribavirin, all patients were treated for 48 weeks; however, data from other trials of standard interferons and the other PEG IFN demonstrated that 24 weeks suffices for patients with genotypes 2 and 3. For patients with genotype 3 who have advanced fibrosis/cirrhosis and/or high-level HCV RNA, a full 48 weeks is preferable.

[d]Attempts to compare the two PEG IFN preparations based on the results of registration clinical trials are confounded by differences between trials of the two agents in methodological details (different ribavirin doses, different methods for recording depression, and other side effects) and study-population composition (different proportion with bridging fibrosis/cirrhosis, proportion from the United States versus international, mean weight, proportion with genotype 1, and proportion with high-level HCV RNA). In the head-to-head comparison of the two PEG IFN preparations in the "IDEAL" trial reported in 2009, the two drugs were comparable in tolerability and efficacy. PEG IFN α-2b was administered at a weekly weight-based dose of 1.0 μg/kg or 1.5 μg/kg, and PEG IFN α-2a was administered at a weekly fixed dose of 180 μg. For PEG IFN α-2b, daily ribavirin weight-based doses ranged between 800–1400 mg based on weight criteria (see footnote a, above), while for PEG IFN α-2a, daily ribavirin weight-based doses ranged between 1000–1200 mg (footnote b, above). For the two PEG IFN α-2b study arms, ribavirin dose reductions for ribavirin-associated adverse effects were done in 200–400-mg decrements; for PEG IFN α-2a, the ribavirin dose was reduced to 600 mg for intolerance. Sustained virologic responses occurred in 38.0% of the low-dose PEG IFN α-2b group, 39.8% of the standard, full-dose PEG IFN α-2b group, and 40.9% of the PEG IFN α-2a group.

Abbreviations: PEG, polyethylene glycol; PEG IFN, pegylated interferon; HCV RNA, hepatitis C virus RNA.

better tolerated. In a head-to-head trial of the two PEG IFNs (the "IDEAL" trial), the two PEG IFNs were found to be comparable in efficacy (achievement of SVR) (Fig. 40-3) and tolerability, although headache, nausea, fever, myalgia, depression, and drug discontinuation for any reason were less frequent in patients treated with PEG IFN-α2a than standard-dose PEG IFN-α2b. In contrast, neutropenia and rash were more frequent in patients treated with PEG IFN-α2a than standard dose PEG IFN-α2b. In two subsequent head-to-head trials and a systematic review of randomized trials, PEG IFN-α2a was more effective than IFN-α2b (SVR in genotype 1-4: 48–55% versus 32–40%, respectively). In trials of PEG IFN-α2b among patients with HCV genotype 1, a broader range of weight-based daily ribavirin doses has been validated: 800 mg for weight <65 kg, 1000 mg for weight 65–85 kg, 1200 mg for weight >85–105 kg, and 1400 mg for weight >105 kg. Recommended doses for the two PEG IFNs plus ribavirin and other comparisons between the two therapies are shown in Table 40-6.

Until the 2011 introduction of protease inhibitors, unless ribavirin was contraindicated (see earlier discussion), combination PEG IFN plus ribavirin was the recommended course of therapy—24 weeks for genotypes 2 and 3 and 48 weeks for genotype 1. For patients with genotype 1, the standard of care now includes protease inhibitors (discussed later); however, PEG IFN/ribavirin remain the standard of care for patients with other genotypes. Similarly, PEG IFN/ribavirin continue to be used in patients for whom protease inhibitors are not available or contraindicated. For patients treated with combination PEG IFN/ribavirin, measurement of quantitative HCV RNA levels at 12 weeks is helpful in guiding therapy; if a 2-$\log_{10}$ drop in HCV RNA has not been achieved by this time, chances for an SVR are negligible, and additional therapy is futile. If the 12-week HCV RNA has fallen by two $\log_{10}$s (EVR), the chances for an SVR at the end of therapy are approximately two-thirds; if the 12-week HCV RNA is undetectable ("complete" EVR), the chances for a sustained virologic response exceed 80% (Fig. 40-2). Because absence of an EVR is such a strong predictor of the absence of an ultimate sustained virologic response, therapy is discontinued for failure to achieve a 12-week 2-$\log_{10}$ drop in HCV RNA (EVR).

Studies have suggested that the frequency of an SVR to PEG IFN/ribavirin therapy can be increased in patients with baseline variables weighing against a response (e.g., HCV RNA >8 × 10^5 IU/mL, weight >85 kg) by raising the dose of PEG IFN (e.g., to as high as 270 μg of PEG IFN-α2a) and/or the dose of ribavirin to as high as 1600 mg daily (if tolerated or supplemented by erythropoietin) or by tailoring treatment based on viral response to prolong the duration of viral clearance before discontinuing therapy, i.e., extending therapy from 48 to

FIGURE 40-3

Head-to-head comparison of standard-dose PEG IFN α-2b 1.5 µg/kg weekly and PEG IFN α-2a 180 µg weekly administered with daily ribavirin in the "IDEAL" trial. Percent achieving treatment milestones for PEG IFN α-2b (green boxes) and PEG IFN α-2a (orange boxes). RVR, rapid virologic response, HCV RNA undetectable at week 4; EVR, early virologic response, HCV RNA undetectable at week 12; ETR, end-treatment response, HCV RNA undetectable at end of treatment week 48; SVR, sustained virologic response, HCV RNA remaining undetectable 24 weeks after completing 48 weeks of therapy. Relapse, reappearance of detectable HCV RNA by week 72 in patients with an end-treatment response at week 48. PEG IFN α-2a suppressed HCV RNA in a higher proportion of patients at weeks 12 and 48 but, because of a higher relapse rate at week 72, resulted in the same SVR rate as PEG IFN α-2b.

72 weeks for patients with genotype 1 and a slow virologic response, i.e., those whose HCV RNA has not fallen rapidly to undetectable levels within 4 weeks (absence of "rapid virologic response"). Tailoring therapy based on the kinetics of HCV RNA reduction has also been applied to abbreviating the duration of therapy in patients with genotype 1 (and 4). The results of several clinical trials suggest that, in patients with genotype 1 (and 4) who have a 4-week RVR (which occurs in ≤20%), especially in the subset with low baseline HCV RNA, 24 weeks of therapy with PEG IFN and weight-based ribavirin suffices, yielding SVR rates of ~90% and comparable to those achieved in this cohort with 48 weeks of therapy. Although initial reports suggested that, for patients with genotype 2 and (somewhat less so) genotype 3, in rapid virologic responders with undetectable HCV RNA at week 4, the total duration of therapy required to achieve an SVR could be as short as 12–16 weeks, a very sizable, definitive subsequent trial showed that relapse is increased if treatment duration is curtailed and that a full 24 weeks is superior for these genotypes (except for the minority with very low baseline levels of HCV RNA).

Persons with chronic HCV infection have been shown to suffer increased liver-related mortality. On the other hand, successful antiviral therapy of chronic hepatitis C resulting in an SVR has been shown to improve survival, to lower the risk of liver failure and liver-related death and all-cause deaths, to slow the progression of chronic hepatitis C, and to reverse fibrosis and even cirrhosis. Although successful treatment reduces mortality in cirrhotic patients (and those with advanced fibrosis) and reduces the likelihood of hepatocellular carcinoma, the risk of decompensation, death, and liver cancer persists, albeit at a much reduced level, necessitating continued clinical monitoring and cancer surveillance after SVR in cirrhotics. On the other hand, in the absence of an SVR, routine-dose/duration IFN-based therapy does not reduce the risk of hepatocellular carcinoma. Similarly, for nonresponders to PEG IFN/ribavirin therapy, three trials of long-term maintenance therapy with PEG IFN have shown no benefit in reducing the risk of histologic progression or clinical decompensation, including the development of hepatocellular carcinoma. For PEG IFN/ribavirin nonresponders who have had a full, adequate course of therapy, the benefit of retreatment—with higher doses or a longer course of the original PEG IFN regimen or the alternative PEG IFN regimen or with a different type of IFN preparation (e.g., consensus IFN)—is marginal at best. Fortunately, such nonresponders can now be retreated with protease inhibitor-based therapy (see following).

PROTEASE INHIBITORS The HCV RNA genome encodes a single polyprotein, which is cleaved during and after translation by host and viral-encoded proteases. One protease involved in the cleavage of the viral polyprotein is an NS3-4A viral protein that has serine protease activity. Telaprevir and boceprevir are serine protease inhibitors that target NS3-4A. In 2011, telaprevir and boceprevir used in combination with PEG IFN and ribavirin were FDA-approved for the treatment of hepatitis C genotype 1 in adults with stable liver disease, both in patients who have not been treated before or who have failed previous treatment. Because the presently available HCV protease inhibitors have not been studied in patients with genotypes other than 1, their use in these populations is not recommended.

Because resistance develops rapidly, both telaprevir and boceprevir must be used in combination with a PEG IFN and ribavirin-based regimen and should never be used alone. Ribavirin in particular appears to reduce relapse rates significantly in protease inhibitor-based regimens, such that those who cannot take or are intolerant to ribavirin are unlikely to benefit from the addition of these agents. All current telaprevir and boceprevir regimens consist of periods of triple therapy (protease inhibitor plus PEG IFN plus ribavirin) and periods of dual therapy (PEG IFN plus ribavirin). Teleprevir regimens begin with 12 weeks of triple therapy followed by dual therapy of a duration based upon HCV RNA status at weeks 4 and 12 and prior treatment status. Boceprevir-based regimens consist of a 4-week lead-in period of dual (PEG IFN, ribavirin) therapy followed by triple therapy and in some instances a further extension of dual therapy, with duration based upon HCV RNA status at weeks 4, 8, and 24 and prior treatment status (Table 40-7).

For patients with HCV genotype 1, protease inhibitors have significantly improved the frequency of rapid and sustained viral responses as compared to PEG IFN plus ribavirin alone. In treatment-naïve patients treated with telaprevir, a sustained viral response was seen in up to 79% of patients who received 12 weeks of triple therapy followed by 12 weeks of dual therapy, and among those with early virologic responses (undetectable HCV RNA at weeks 4 and 12), the rate of sustained virologic responses was 83–89%. In studies with boceprevir in treatment-naïve patients, sustained virologic responses were seen in 59–66% of patients, and among those with an undetectable HCV RNA level at 8 weeks, the sustained virologic response rate rose to 86–88%.

Protease inhibitors have also been studied in patients previously treated unsuccessfully with PEG IFN plus ribavirin. In studies with telaprevir, sustained viral responses were seen in 83–88% who had a previous relapse, 54–59% of partial responders (HCV RNA reduced by ≥2 $\log_{10}$ IU/mL), and 29–33% of null responders (HCV RNA reduced by <2 $\log_{10}$ IU/mL). With boceprevir, sustained virologic responses occurred in 75% of prior relapsers and in 40–52% of previous partial responders; response rates in null responders are similar to those achieved with telaprevir-based therapy.

Both protease inhibitors have potential toxicities. Telaprevir is associated with a severe rash in ~5% of treated patients. Other common side effects include pruritus, rectal burning, nausea, diarrhea, fatigue, and anemia, which may be relatively refractory, occasionally requiring transfusion. Complete blood counts should be obtained at baseline and then at 2, 4, 8, and 12 weeks

after starting telaprevir. Anemia can occur in half of boceprevir treated patients, as can a lower frequency of neutropenia and thrombocytopenia. Complete blood counts should be obtained at baseline and then at 4, 8, and 12 weeks after starting boceprevir. Other side effects of boceprevir include fatigue, nausea, headache, dysgeusia (altered or unpleasant taste), dry mouth, vomiting, and diarrhea.

Use of protease inhibitors is further complicated by numerous drug-drug interactions. As telaprevir and boceprevir are both eliminated by and inhibit CYP3A4, these agents should not be administered with other medications that induce CYP3A4 or are dependent upon CYP3A4 for elimination. Care should be taken to examine for any potential interactions between protease inhibitors and other medications the patient may be taking, as serious adverse events can occur.

TREATMENT RECOMMENDATIONS Prior to therapy, HCV genotype should be determined, as the genotype dictates the duration of therapy and potentially the agents to be used. PEG IFN plus ribavirin represents the foundation of treatment for all HCV genotypes; patients infected with genotype 1 should also receive a protease inhibitor (telaprevir or boceprevir) when these are available and not contraindicated (Table 40-7). For chronic HCV genotype 1 infection, the American Association for the Study of Liver Diseases (AASLD) and the European Association for the Study of the Liver (EASL) published treatment guidelines in 2011, and, in 2012, UK and French consensus guidelines were published.

Monitoring of HCV plasma RNA is crucial in assessing response to therapy. The goal of treatment is to eradicate HCV RNA, which is predicted by the absence of HCV RNA by polymerase chain reaction 6 months after stopping treatment (sustained viral response). When therapy relied on PEG IFN and ribavirin, failure to achieve a 2-$\log_{10}$ drop in HCV RNA by week 12 of therapy (early virologic response) rendered it unlikely that further therapy would result in a sustained virologic response. When PEG IFN/ribavirin are part of a protease inhibitor regimen, HCV RNA should be measured at baseline and at weeks 4, 8 (for boceprevir), 12, and 24 to assess response to treatment and to aid in decisions regarding treatment duration as well as 12 and 24 weeks after therapy. Stopping rules are important to prevent the emergence of resistance; if HCV RNA is >1000 IU/mL at 4 or 12 weeks of telaprevir (or still detectable at week 24), or if HCV RNA is ≥100 IU/mL at week 12 of boceprevir (or detectable at week 24), all treatment should be stopped.

Indications for Antiviral Therapy Patients with chronic hepatitis C who have detectable HCV RNA in serum, whether or not aminotransferase levels are

TABLE 40-7

INDICATIONS AND RECOMMENDATIONS FOR ANTIVIRAL THERAPY OF CHRONIC HEPATITIS C

Standard Indications for Therapy

Detectable HCV RNA (with or without elevated ALT)
Portal/bridging fibrosis or moderate to severe hepatitis on liver biopsy

Retreatment Recommended

Genotype 1
Relapsers, partial responders, or nonresponders after a previous course of standard interferon monotherapy or combination standard interferon/ribavirin therapy or PEG IFN/ribavirin
   A course of PEG-IFN/ribavirin plus protease inhibitor as below
Genotypes 2, 3, 4
   Relapsers after a previous course of standard interferon monotherapy or combination standard interferon/ribavirin therapy
    A course of PEG IFN plus ribavirin
   Nonresponders to a previous course of standard IFN monotherapy or combination standard IFN/ribavirin therapy
   A course of PEG IFN plus ribavirin—more likely to achieve a sustained virologic response in Caucasian patients without previous ribavirin therapy, with low baseline HCV RNA levels, with a $\geq$2-$\log_{10}$ reduction in HCV RNA during previous therapy, with genotypes 2 and 3, and without reduction in ribavirin dose.

Antiviral Therapy Management Decisions Made on an Individual Basis

Children (age <18 years) – protease inhibitors not recommended
Age >70 (in protease inhibitor trials, telaprevir trials included patients aged 18–70; boceprevir trials included patients >18 years of age (no upper age cutoff)
Mild hepatitis on liver biopsy
Persons with severe renal insufficiency (require reduced doses of PEG IFN and ribavirin)

Long-Term Maintenance Therapy Recommended

Cryoglobulinemic vasculitis associated with chronic hepatitis C

Long-Term Maintenance Therapy in Nonresponders Not Recommended

Antiviral Therapy Not Recommended

Decompensated cirrhosis
Pregnancy (teratogenicity of ribavirin)
Contraindications to medications

Therapeutic Regimens

HCV genotype 1
TREATMENT-NAÏVE
PEG IFN-α2a 180 μg weekly plus weight-based ribavirin 1000 mg/d (<75 kg) to 1200 mg/d ($\geq$75 kg) or
PEG IFN-α2b 1.5 μg/kg weekly plus weight-based ribavirin 800 mg/d ($\leq$65 kg), 1000 mg/d (>65–85 kg), 1200 mg/d (>85–105 kg), to 1400 mg/d (>105 kg)
Plus response-guided therapy with a protease inhibitor consisting of either:
Boceprevir 800 mg three times daily with food started after a lead-in treatment of 4 weeks with PEG IFN/ribavirin
- Patients with undetectable HCV RNA at 8 and 24 weeks should receive triple therapy (PEG-IFN/ribavirin, boceprevir) through week 28 (4 weeks of PEG IFN/ribavirin then 24 weeks of triple therapy). If HCV RNA is detectable at 4 weeks, continuing therapy through 48 weeks (4 weeks of PEG IFN/ribavirin then 44 weeks of triple therapy) may increase the sustained response rate.
- Patients with detectable HCV RNA at 8 weeks and undetectable at 24 weeks should receive triple therapy (PEG-IFN/ribavirin, boceprevir) through week 36 (4 weeks of PEG IFN/ribavirin then 32 weeks of triple therapy) followed by a return to PEG IFN/ribavirin for 12 more weeks, for a total treatment duration of 48 weeks.
- Patients with cirrhosis who are treatment-naive and have undetectable HCV RNA at week 8 and 24 should continue triple therapy (PEG IFN/ribavirin, boceprevir) through 48 weeks (4 weeks of PEG IFN/ribavirin then 44 weeks of triple therapy).
- Stopping rules for futility: HCV RNA $\geq$100 IU/mL at week 12 or any detectable HCV RNA at week 24
Telapravir 750 mg three times daily with fatty food started at the beginning of therapy without a PEG IFN/ribavirin lead-in.
- Patients with undetectable HCV RNA at 4 and 12 weeks should receive triple therapy (PEG IFN/ribavirin, telapravir) for 12 weeks then PEG IFN and ribavirin for another 12 weeks, for a total of 24 weeks.
- Patients with detectable HCV RNA at 4 or 12 weeks and undetectable at 24 weeks should receive triple therapy (PEG-IFN/ribavirin, telapravir) for 12 weeks, then PEG IFN/ribavirin for another 36 weeks, for a total treatment duration of 48 weeks.
- Patients with cirrhosis who are treatment-naïve and have undetectable HCV RNA at 4 and 12 weeks should receive triple therapy for 12 weeks then PEG-IFN, ribavirin for another 36 weeks, for a total treatment duration of 48 weeks.
- Stopping rules for futility: HCV RNA >1000 IU/mL at week 4 or 12 or any detectable HCV RNA at week 24

TREATMENT-EXPERIENCED
PEG IFN-α2a 180 μg weekly plus weight-based ribavirin 1000 mg/d (<75 kg) to 1200 mg/d ($\geq$75 kg) or
PEG IFN-α2b 1.5 μg/kg weekly plus weight-based ribavirin 800 mg/d ($\leq$65 kg), 1000 mg/d (>65–85 kg), 1200 mg/d (>85–105 kg), to 1400 mg/d (>105 kg)
Plus a protease inhibitor consisting of either:
Response-guided therapy with boceprevir 800 mg three times daily with food started after a lead-in treatment of 4 weeks with PEG IFN/ribavirin

(continued)

TABLE 40-7

INDICATIONS AND RECOMMENDATIONS FOR ANTIVIRAL THERAPY OF CHRONIC HEPATITIS C (*CONTINUED*)

- For prior relapsers and partial responders (HCV RNA reduction of ≥ 2 $\log_{10}$ during previous therapy), follow the response-guided algorithm below; for prior null responders (HCV RNA reduction <2 $\log_{10}$ during previous therapy), a full 48-week course of therapy (4-week PEG IFN/ribavirin lead-in, followed by 44 weeks of triple-drug therapy (PEG IFN/ribavirin, boceprevir) is recommended.
- Patients with undetectable HCV RNA at 8 and 24 weeks should receive triple therapy: PEG-IFN/ribavirin, boceprevir) through week 36 (4 weeks of PEG IFN/ribavirin then 32 weeks of triple therapy). If HCV RNA is detectable at 4 weeks, continuing therapy through 48 weeks (4 weeks of PEG IFN/ribavirin then 44 weeks of triple therapy) may increase the sustained response rate.
- Patients with detectable HCV RNA at 8 weeks and undetectable at week 24 should receive triple therapy (PEG-IFN/ribavirin, boceprevir) through week 36 (4 weeks of PEG IFN/ribavirin then 32 weeks of triple therapy), followed by a return to PEG IFN/ribavirin for 12 more weeks, for a total treatment duration of 48 weeks.
- Patients with cirrhosis who are treatment-experienced and have undetectable HCV RNA at weeks 8 and 24 should continue triple therapy (PEG IFN/ribavirin, boceprevir) through 48 weeks (4 weeks of PEG IFN/ribavirin then 44 weeks of triple therapy).
- Stopping rules for futility: HCV RNA ≥ 100 IU/mL at week 12 or any detectable HCV RNA at week 24

Telaprevir 750 mg three times daily with fatty food started at the beginning of therapy without a PEG IFN/ribavirin lead-in and without a response-guided approach, i.e., all patients received a full 48-week course, independent of early responsiveness.

- For prior relapsers, follow guidelines for treatment-naïve patients above.
- Prior partial responders and null responders should receive triple therapy (PEG IFN/ribavirin, telaprevir) for 12 weeks then PEG IFN and ribavirin for another 36 weeks, for a total of 48 weeks.
- Stopping rules for futility: HCV RNA >1000 IU/mL at week 4 or 12 or any detectable HCV RNA at week 24

HCV genotype I but protease inhibitors unavailable or contraindicated: 48 weeks of therapy
PEG IFN-α2a 180 µg weekly plus weight-based ribavirin 1000 mg/d (<75 kg) to 1200 mg/d (≥ 75 kg) or
PEG IFN-α2b 1.5 µg/kg weekly plus weight-based ribavirin 800 mg/d (≤ 65 kg), 1000 mg/d (>65–85 kg), 1200 mg/d (>85–105 kg), to 1400 mg/d (>105 kg)

HCV genotype 4: 48 weeks of PEG IFN/ribavirin therapy
PEG IFN-α2a 180 µg weekly plus weight-based ribavirin 1000 mg/d (<75 kg) to 1200 mg/d (≥ 75 kg) or
PEG IFN-α2b 1.5 µg/kg weekly plus weight-based ribavirin 800 mg/d (≤ 65 kg), 1000 mg/d (>65–85 kg), 1200 mg/d (>85–105 kg), to 1400 mg/d (>105 kg)

- Treatment should be discontinued in patients who do not achieve an early virologic response at week 12
- Patients who do achieve an early virologic response should be retested at week 24 and treatment should be discontineud if HCV RNA remains detectable

HCV genotypes 2 and 3: 24 weeks of therapy
PEG IFN-α2a 180 µg weekly plus ribavirin 800 mg/d or
PEG IFN-α2b 1.5 µg/kg weekly plus ribavirin 800 mg/d (for patients with genotype 3 who have advanced fibrosis and/or high-level HCV RNA, a full 48 weeks of therapy may be preferable)

For HCV-HIV co-infected patients: 48 weeks, regardless of genotype, of weekly PEG IFN-α2a (180 µg) or PEG IFN-α2b (1.5 µg/kg) plus a daily ribavirin dose of at least 600–800 mg, up to full weight-based 1000–1400 mg dosing if tolerated. Protease inhibitors may be used for genotype 1; however, because of potential drug-drug interactions between HCV protease inhibitors and HIV antiretroviral drugs, HCV protease inhibitors should be used cautiously in HCV/HIV-coinfected patients. If protease inhibitors are used, a full 48-week course is recommended without response-guided therapy: For boceprevir, 4 weeks of PEG IFN/ribavirin lead-in, followed by 44 weeks of triple-drug therapy (PEG IFN, ribavirin, boceprevir). For telaprevir, 12 weeks of triple-drug therapy (PEG IFN, ribavirin, telaprevir), followed by 36 weeks of PEG IFN/ribavirin therapy. Stopping rules for futility are as noted above.

Features Associated with Reduced Responsiveness

Single nucleotide polymorphism (SNP) T allele (as opposed to C allele) at IL28B locus
Genotype 1a (compared to 1b)
High-level HCV RNA ($>800,000$ IU/mL)[a]
Advanced fibrosis (bridging fibrosis, cirrhosis)
Long-duration disease
Age >40*
High HCV quasispecies diversity
Immunosuppression
African-American ethnicity

Latino ethnicity
Obesity
Hepatic steatosis
Insulin resistance, type 2 diabetes mellitus[a]
Reduced adherence (lower drug doses and reduced duration of therapy)
For boceprevir, <1 $\log_{10}$ reduction in HCV RNA during 4-week PEG IFN/ribavirin lead-in
For protease inhibitor therapy, absence of extended rapid virologic response (eRVR), i.e., detectable HCV RNA, at weeks 4 and 12 for telaprevir; at weeks 8 and 24 for boceprevir

[a]Less influential in patients treated with protease inhibitors

Abbreviations: ALT, alanine aminotransferase; HCV, hepatitis C virus; IFN, interferon; IU, international units (1 IU/mL is equivalent to ~2.5 copies/mL); PEG IFN, pegylated interferon.

increased, and chronic hepatitis of at least moderate grade and stage (portal or bridging fibrosis) are candidates for antiviral therapy. Most authorities recommend 800 mg of ribavirin for patients with genotypes 2 and 3 for both types of PEG IFN and weight-based 1000–1200 mg (when used with PEG IFN-α2a) or 800–1400 mg (when used with PEG IFN-α2b) ribavirin for patients with genotype 1 (and 4), unless ribavirin is contraindicated (Table 40-7). These PEG IFN and ribavirin doses are used with protease inhibitors for patients with genotype 1 (Table 40-7). Although patients with persistently normal ALT activity tend to progress histologically very slowly or not at all, they respond to antiviral therapy just as well as do patients with elevated ALT levels; therefore, while observation without therapy is an option, such patients are potential candidates for antiviral therapy. As noted earlier, therapy with IFN has been shown to improve survival and complication-free survival and to slow progression of fibrosis.

HCV genotype determines the duration of PEG IFN and ribavirin therapy: 24 weeks for those with genotypes 2 and 3 and 48 weeks for patients with genotypes 4 and 1 (in patients for whom protease inhibitors are not available or contraindicated). For patients with genotype 4, treatment should be discontinued in patients who do not achieve an early virologic response at week 12; for patients with genotypes 2 and 3, a full, 24-week course is most effective, although the duration may be increased to 48 weeks for patients with genotype 3 who have advanced fibrosis and/or a high baseline level of viremia. As noted earlier, the absence of a 2-$\log_{10}$ drop in HCV RNA at week 12 (EVR) weighs heavily against the likelihood of a sustained virologic response; therefore, measuring HCV RNA at 12 weeks is recommended routinely (Fig. 40-2), and therapy can be discontinued if an EVR is not achieved. Among genotype 4 patients with an EVR (≥2-$\log_{10}$ HCV RNA reduction) but with HCV RNA still detectable at week 24, a sustained virologic response is unlikely, and therapy can be discontinued. Although response rates are lower in patients with certain pretreatment variables, selection for treatment should not be based on symptoms, genotype, HCV RNA level, mode of acquisition of hepatitis C, or advanced hepatic fibrosis. Patients with cirrhosis can respond and should not be excluded as candidates for therapy.

Patients who have relapsed after, or failed to respond to (Fig. 40-2), a course of IFN monotherapy are potential candidates for retreatment with PEG IFN plus ribavirin (i.e., a more effective treatment regimen is required), and this approach remains current for patients with genotypes 2, 3, or 4; however, for patients with genotype 1, combination protease inhibitor/PEG IFN/ribavirin therapy is indicated. For patients with genotypes 2, 3, or 4 who were nonresponders to a prior course of IFN monotherapy, retreatment with IFN monotherapy or combination IFN plus ribavirin therapy is unlikely to achieve a sustained virologic response; however, a trial of combination PEG IFN plus ribavirin may be worthwhile, although a sustained virologic response is the outcome in <15–20% of patients. Sustained virologic responses to retreatment of nonresponders are more frequent in those who had never received ribavirin in the past, those with low pretreatment HCV RNA levels, and noncirrhotics, but less frequent in African Americans, those who failed to achieve a substantial reduction in HCV RNA during their previous course of therapy (null responders, Fig. 40-2), and those who required ribavirin dose reductions. Potential approaches to improving responsiveness to PEG IFN/ribavirin in prior nonresponders include longer duration of treatment; higher doses of either PEG IFN, ribavirin, or both; and switching to a different IFN preparation; however, as noted earlier, none of these approaches achieves more than a marginal benefit. Treatment with a protease inhibitor-based regimen should be pursued in patients with genotype 1 who have relapsed after or not responded to prior treatment with IFN monotherapy or PEG IFN plus ribavirin, unless these protease inhibitors are not available or contraindicated (Table 40-7).

Early treatment is indicated for persons with acute hepatitis C (Chap. 38). In patients with biochemically and histologically mild chronic hepatitis C, the rate of progression is slow, and monitoring without therapy is an option; however, such patients respond just as well to combination PEG IFN plus ribavirin therapy or triple-drug, protease-based therapy as those with elevated ALT and more histologically severe hepatitis. Therefore, therapy for these patients should be considered and the decision made based on such factors as patient motivation, genotype, stage of fibrosis, age, and comorbid conditions. A pretreatment liver biopsy to assess histologic grade and stage provides substantial information about progression of hepatitis C in the past, has prognostic value for future progression, and can identify such histologic factors as steatosis and stage of fibrosis, which can influence responsiveness to therapy. As therapy has improved for patients with a broad range of histologic severity, and as noninvasive laboratory markers and imaging correlates of fibrosis have gained popularity, some authorities, especially in Europe, place less value on, and do not recommend, pretreatment liver biopsies. On the other hand, serum markers of fibrosis are not considered sufficiently accurate, and histologic findings provide important prognostic information to physician and patient. Therefore, although the contemporary role of a pretreatment liver biopsy commands less of a consensus, a pretreatment liver biopsy still provides useful information and should be considered.

Patients with compensated cirrhosis can respond to therapy, although their likelihood of a sustained response is lower than in noncirrhotics; moreover, survival has been shown to improve after successful antiviral therapy in cirrhotics. Similarly, although several retrospective studies have suggested that antiviral therapy in cirrhotics with chronic hepatitis C, independent of treatment outcome per se, reduces the frequency of HCC, less advanced disease in the treated cirrhotics, not treatment itself (i.e., lead-time bias), may have accounted for the reduced frequency of HCC observed in the treated cohorts in these reports; prospective studies to address this question have failed to demonstrate benefit, unless a sustained virologic response is achieved. Patients with decompensated cirrhosis are not candidates for IFN-based antiviral therapy but should be referred for liver transplantation. Some liver-transplantation centers have evaluated progressively escalated, low-dose antiviral therapy in an attempt to eradicate hepatitis C viremia prior to transplantation; however, such therapy has been shown to reduce but not to prevent the risk of HCV reinfection after transplantation. After liver transplantation for end-stage liver disease caused by hepatitis C, recurrent hepatitis C is the rule, and the pace of disease progression is more accelerated than in immunocompetent patients (Chap. 46). Current therapy with PEG IFN and ribavirin after liver transplantation is unsatisfactory in most patients, but attempts to minimize immunosuppression are beneficial. Early experience with protease inhibitor-based therapy is encouraging, but inhibition of CYP3A4 by protease inhibitors can lead to markedly increased levels of immunosuppressive calcineurin inhibitors (especially tacrolimus), which requires intensive monitoring and can be very challenging. The cutaneous and renal vasculitis of HCV-associated essential mixed cryoglobulinemia (Chap. 38) may respond to antiviral therapy, but sustained responses are rare after discontinuation of therapy; therefore, prolonged, perhaps indefinite, therapy (as reported with interferon-based therapy) is recommended in this group (no indication for prolonged protease inhibitor therapy exists currently). Anecdotal reports suggest that antiviral therapy may be effective in porphyria cutanea tarda or lichen planus associated with hepatitis C.

In patients with HCV/HIV co-infection, hepatitis C is more progressive and severe than in HCV-monoinfected patients. Although patients with HCV/HIV co-infection respond to antiviral therapy for hepatitis C, they do not respond as well as patients with HCV infection alone. Four large national and international trials of antiviral therapy among patients with HCV/HIV co-infection have shown that PEG IFN (both α2a and α2b) plus ribavirin (daily doses ranging from flat-dosed 600–800 mg to weight-based 1000/1200 mg) is superior to standard IFN regimens; however, SVR rates were lower than in HCV-monoinfected patients, ranging from 14 to 38% for patients with genotypes 1 and 4 and from 44 to 73% for patients with genotypes 2 and 3. In the three largest trials, all patients, including those with genotypes 2 and 3, were treated for a full 48 weeks. In addition, tolerability of therapy was lower than in HCV monoinfected patients; therapy was discontinued because of side effects in 12–39% of patients in these clinical trials. Based on these trials, weekly PEG IFN plus daily ribavirin at a daily dose of at least 600–800 mg, up to full weight-based doses, at doses recommended for HCV-monoinfected patients, if tolerated, is recommended for a full 48 weeks, regardless of genotype. An alternative recommendation for ribavirin doses was issued by a European Consensus Conference and consisted of standard, weight-based 1000–1200 mg for genotypes 1 and 4, but 800 mg for genotypes 2 and 3. A head-to-head trial of combination PEG IFN/ribavirin therapy in HCV/HIV co-infection demonstrated statistically indistinguishable efficacy of the two types of PEG IFN, despite a small advantage for PEG IFN-α2a: for PEG IFN-α2b and -α2a, sustained virologic responses occurred in 28% versus 32%, respectively, of patients with genotypes 1 and 4 and in 62% versus 71%, respectively, of patients with genotypes 2 and 3.

Although data are limited and recommendations pending, protease inhibitors may be used for genotype 1; however, because of potential drug-drug interactions between HCV protease inhibitors and HIV antiretroviral drugs, HCV protease inhibitors should be used cautiously in HCV/HIV co-infected patients. If protease inhibitors are used, a full 48-week course is recommended without response-guided therapy: for boceprevir, 4 weeks of PEG IFN/ribavirin lead-in, followed by 44 weeks of triple-drug therapy (PEG IFN, ribavirin, boceprevir); for telaprevir, 12 weeks of triple-drug therapy (PEG IFN, ribavirin, telaprevir), followed by 36 weeks of PEG IFN/ribavirin therapy.

In HCV/HIV-infected patients, ribavirin can potentiate the toxicity of didanosine (e.g., lactic acidosis) and the lipoatrophy of stavudine, and zidovudine can exacerbate ribavirin-associated hemolytic anemia; therefore, these drug combinations should be avoided. Patients with a history of injection-drug use and alcoholism can be treated successfully for chronic hepatitis C, preferably in conjunction with drug- and alcohol-treatment programs. Because ribavirin is excreted renally, patients with end-stage renal disease, including those undergoing dialysis (which does not clear ribavirin), are not ideal candidates for ribavirin therapy. Rare reports suggest that reduced-dose ribavirin can be used, but the frequency of anemia is very high and data on efficacy are limited. If patients with renal failure (glomerular filtration rate <60 mL/min) are treated, the PEG IFN-α2a dose should be reduced from 180 to 135 μg weekly and the

PEG IFN-α2b dose reduced from 1.5 to 1 μg/kg weekly; similarly, the daily ribavirin dose in this population should be reduced to 200–800 mg (but not used or used cautiously at very low doses) if hemodialysis is required. Neither the optimal regimen nor the efficacy of therapy is well established in this population.

NOVEL ANTIVIRALS To date, attempts to develop better-tolerated ribavirin successors or improved types of IFN-α or longer acting IFNs than PEG IFN have not been successful. The demonstration that responsiveness to antiviral therapy is influenced by genetic variation in IL28B, which codes for IFN-λ (as noted earlier), raises the possibility that IFN-λ might be an effective or even more effective IFN for treating hepatitis C; early trials are in progress. Beyond telaprevir and boceprevir, other direct antivirals that target HCV polymerase, protease, or NS5A (required for replication assembly) are being investigated as well as agents that can target host-encoded proteins. The pace of successful trials of all-oral regimens has accelerated. Combinations of a protease inhibitor plus an NS5A inhibitor; of a polymerase inhibitor plus ribavirin; of a protease inhibitor plus a polymerase inhibitor plus an NS5A inhibitor; and of a polymerase inhibitor plus an NS5A inhibitor have been studied in clinical trials, with sustained virologic responses exceeding 90%, even approaching 100%, for both treatment-naïve and treatment-experienced patients. Potentially, as early as 2014 or 2015, such combinations of direct antiviral agents will be used in drug cocktails that may replace IFN-based regimens entirely.

AUTOIMMUNE HEPATITIS

DEFINITION

Autoimmune hepatitis is a chronic disorder characterized by continuing hepatocellular necrosis and inflammation, usually with fibrosis, which can progress to cirrhosis and liver failure. When fulfilling criteria of severity, this type of chronic hepatitis, when untreated, may have a 6-month mortality of as high as 40%. Based on contemporary estimates of the natural history of treated autoimmune hepatitis, the 10-year survival is 80–90%. The prominence of extrahepatic features of autoimmunity as well as seroimmunologic abnormalities in this disorder supports an autoimmune process in its pathogenesis; this concept is reflected in the labels *lupoid, plasma cell,* or *autoimmune hepatitis.* Autoantibodies and other typical features of autoimmunity, however, do not occur in all cases; among the broader categories of "idiopathic" or cryptogenic chronic hepatitis, many, perhaps the majority, are probably autoimmune in origin. Cases in which hepatotropic viruses, metabolic/genetic derangements, and hepatotoxic drugs have been excluded represent a spectrum of heterogeneous liver disorders of unknown cause, a proportion of which are most likely autoimmune hepatitis.

IMMUNOPATHOGENESIS

The weight of evidence suggests that the progressive liver injury in patients with autoimmune hepatitis is the result of a cell-mediated immunologic attack directed against liver cells. In all likelihood, predisposition to autoimmunity is inherited, while the liver specificity of this injury is triggered by environmental (e.g., chemical or viral) factors. For example, patients have been described in whom apparently self-limited cases of acute hepatitis A, B, or C led to autoimmune hepatitis, presumably because of genetic susceptibility or predisposition. Evidence to support an autoimmune pathogenesis in this type of hepatitis includes the following: (1) In the liver, the histopathologic lesions are composed predominantly of cytotoxic T cells and plasma cells; (2) circulating autoantibodies (nuclear, smooth muscle, thyroid, etc.; discussed later), rheumatoid factor, and hyperglobulinemia are common; (3) other autoimmune disorders—such as thyroiditis, rheumatoid arthritis, autoimmune hemolytic anemia, ulcerative colitis, membranoproliferative glomerulonephritis, juvenile diabetes mellitus, celiac disease, and Sjögren's syndrome—occur with increased frequency in patients and in their relatives who have autoimmune hepatitis; (4) histocompatibility haplotypes associated with autoimmune diseases, such as HLA-B1, –B8, –DR3, and –DR4 as well as extended haplotype DRB1 alleles, are common in patients with autoimmune hepatitis; and (5) this type of chronic hepatitis is responsive to glucocorticoid/immunosuppressive therapy, effective in a variety of autoimmune disorders.

Cellular immune mechanisms appear to be important in the pathogenesis of autoimmune hepatitis. In vitro studies have suggested that in patients with this disorder, lymphocytes are capable of becoming sensitized to hepatocyte membrane proteins and of destroying liver cells. Abnormalities of immunoregulatory control over cytotoxic lymphocytes (impaired regulatory CD4+CD25+ T cell influences) may play a role as well. Studies of genetic predisposition to autoimmune hepatitis demonstrate that certain haplotypes are associated with the disorder, as enumerated earlier. The precise triggering factors, genetic influences, and cytotoxic and immunoregulatory mechanisms involved in this type of liver injury remain incompletely defined.

Intriguing clues into the pathogenesis of autoimmune hepatitis come from the observation that circulating autoantibodies are prevalent in patients with this disorder. Among the autoantibodies described in these patients are antibodies to nuclei [so-called antinuclear antibodies (ANAs), primarily in a homogeneous pattern] and smooth muscle (so-called anti-smooth-muscle antibodies, directed at actin), anti-LKM (discussed later), antibodies to "soluble liver antigen/liver pancreas antigen" (directed against a uracil-guanineadenine transfer RNA suppressor protein), as well as antibodies to the liver-specific asialoglycoprotein receptor (or "hepatic lectin") and other hepatocyte membrane proteins. Although some of these provide helpful diagnostic markers, their involvement in the pathogenesis of autoimmune hepatitis has not been established.

Humoral immune mechanisms have been shown to play a role in the extrahepatic manifestations of autoimmune and idiopathic hepatitis. Arthralgias, arthritis, cutaneous vasculitis, and glomerulonephritis occurring in patients with autoimmune hepatitis appear to be mediated by the deposition of circulating immune complexes in affected tissue vessels, followed by complement activation, inflammation, and tissue injury. While specific viral antigen-antibody complexes can be identified in acute and chronic viral hepatitis, the nature of the immune complexes in autoimmune hepatitis has not been defined.

Many of the *clinical features* of autoimmune hepatitis are similar to those described for chronic viral hepatitis. The onset of disease may be insidious or abrupt; the disease may present initially like, and be confused with, acute viral hepatitis; a history of recurrent bouts of what had been labeled *acute hepatitis* is not uncommon. A subset of patients with autoimmune hepatitis has distinct features. Such patients are predominantly young to middle-aged women with marked hyperglobulinemia and high-titer circulating ANAs. This is the group with positive lupus erythematosus (LE) preparations (initially labeled "lupoid" hepatitis) in whom other autoimmune features are common. Fatigue, malaise, anorexia, amenorrhea, acne, arthralgias, and jaundice are common. Occasionally arthritis, maculopapular eruptions (including cutaneous vasculitis), erythema nodosum, colitis, pleurisy, pericarditis, anemia, azotemia, and sicca syndrome (keratoconjunctivitis, xerostomia) occur. In some patients, complications of cirrhosis, such as ascites and edema (associated with hypoalbuminemia), encephalopathy, hypersplenism, coagulopathy, or variceal bleeding may bring the patient to initial medical attention.

The course of autoimmune hepatitis may be variable. In those with mild disease or limited histologic lesions (e.g., piecemeal necrosis without bridging), progression to cirrhosis is limited. In those with severe symptomatic autoimmune hepatitis (aminotransferase levels >10 times normal, marked hyperglobulinemia, "aggressive" histologic lesions—bridging necrosis or

multilobular collapse, cirrhosis), the 6-month mortality without therapy may be as high as 40%. Such severe disease accounts for only 20% of cases; the natural history of milder disease is variable, often accentuated by spontaneous remissions and exacerbations. Especially poor prognostic signs include the presence histologically of multilobular collapse at the time of initial presentation and failure of the bilirubin to improve after 2 weeks of therapy. Death may result from hepatic failure, hepatic coma, other complications of cirrhosis (e.g., variceal hemorrhage), and intercurrent infection. In patients with established cirrhosis, HCC may be a late complication (Chap. 50) but occurs less frequently than in cirrhosis associated with viral hepatitis.

Laboratory features of autoimmune hepatitis are similar to those seen in chronic viral hepatitis. Liver biochemical tests are invariably abnormal but may not correlate with the clinical severity or histopathologic features in individual cases. Many patients with autoimmune hepatitis have normal serum bilirubin, alkaline phosphatase, and globulin levels with only minimal aminotransferase elevations. Serum AST and ALT levels are increased and fluctuate in the range of 100–1000 units. In severe cases, the serum bilirubin level is moderately elevated [51–171 μmol/L (3–10 mg/dL)]. Hypoalbuminemia occurs in patients with very active or advanced disease. Serum alkaline phosphatase levels may be moderately elevated or near normal. In a small proportion of patients, marked elevations of alkaline phosphatase activity occur; in such patients, clinical and laboratory features overlap with those of primary biliary cirrhosis (Chap. 42). The prothrombin time is often prolonged, particularly late in the disease or during active phases.

Hypergammaglobulinemia (>2.5 g/dL) is common in autoimmune hepatitis. Rheumatoid factor is common as well. As noted earlier, circulating autoantibodies are also prevalent. The most characteristic are ANAs in a homogeneous staining pattern. Smooth-muscle antibodies are less specific, seen just as frequently in chronic viral hepatitis. Because of the high levels of globulins achieved in the circulation of some patients with autoimmune hepatitis, occasionally the globulins may bind nonspecifically in solid-phase binding immunoassays for viral antibodies. This has been recognized most commonly in tests for antibodies to hepatitis C virus, as noted earlier. In fact, studies of autoantibodies in autoimmune hepatitis have led to the recognition of new categories of autoimmune hepatitis. *Type I autoimmune hepatitis* is the classic syndrome occurring in young women, associated with marked hyperglobulinemia, lupoid features, circulating ANAs, and HLA-DR3 or HLA-DR4 (especially B8-DRB1*03). Also associated with type I autoimmune hepatitis are autoantibodies against actin as well as atypical perinuclear antineutrophilic cytoplasmic antibodies (pANCA).

Type II autoimmune hepatitis, often seen in children, more common in Mediterranean populations, and linked to HLA-DRB1 and HLA-DQB1 haplotypes, is associated not with ANA but with anti-LKM. Actually, anti-LKM represent a heterogeneous group of antibodies. In type II autoimmune hepatitis, the antibody is anti-LKM1, directed against cytochrome P450 2D6. This is the same anti-LKM seen in some patients with chronic hepatitis C. Anti-LKM2 is seen in drug-induced hepatitis, and anti-LKM3 is seen in patients with chronic hepatitis D. Another autoantibody observed in type II autoimmune hepatitis is directed against liver cytosol formiminotransferase cyclodeaminase (anti-liver cytosol 1). More controversial is whether or not a third category of autoimmune hepatitis exists, *type III autoimmune hepatitis*. These patients lack ANA and anti-LKM1 but have circulating antibodies to soluble liver antigen/liver pancreas antigen. Most of these patients are women and have clinical features similar to, perhaps more severe than, those of patients with type I autoimmune hepatitis. Type III autoimmune hepatitis does not appear to represent a distinct category but, instead, is part of the spectrum of type I autoimmune hepatitis; this subcategory has not been adopted by a consensus of international experts.

Liver biopsy abnormalities are similar to those described for chronic viral hepatitis. Expanding portal tracts and extending beyond the plate of periportal hepatocytes into the parenchyma (designated *interface hepatitis* or *piecemeal necrosis*) is a mononuclear cell infiltrate that, in autoimmune hepatitis, may include the presence of plasma cells. Necroinflammatory activity characterizes the lobular parenchyma, and evidence of hepatocellular regeneration is reflected by "rosette" formation, the occurrence of thickened liver cell plates, and regenerative "pseudolobules." Septal fibrosis, bridging fibrosis, and cirrhosis are frequent. Bile duct injury and granulomas are uncommon; however, a subgroup of patients with autoimmune hepatitis has histologic, biochemical, and serologic features overlapping those of primary biliary cirrhosis (Chap. 42).

DIAGNOSTIC CRITERIA

An international group has suggested a set of criteria for establishing a diagnosis of autoimmune hepatitis. Exclusion of liver disease caused by genetic disorders, viral hepatitis, drug hepatotoxicity, and alcohol are linked with such inclusive diagnostic criteria as hyperglobulinemia, autoantibodies, and characteristic histologic features. This international group has also suggested a comprehensive diagnostic scoring system that, rarely required for typical cases, may be helpful when typical features are not present. Factors that weigh in favor of the diagnosis include female gender; predominant aminotransferase elevation; presence and level of globulin elevation; presence of nuclear, smooth-muscle, LKM1, and other autoantibodies; concurrent other autoimmune diseases; characteristic histologic features (interface hepatitis, plasma cells, rosettes); HLA DR3 or DR4 markers; and response to treatment (discussed later). Weighing against the diagnosis are predominant alkaline phosphatase elevation, mitochondrial antibodies, markers of viral hepatitis, history of hepatotoxic drugs or excessive alcohol, histologic evidence of bile duct injury, or such atypical histologic features as fatty infiltration, iron overload, and viral inclusions.

DIFFERENTIAL DIAGNOSIS

Early during the course of chronic hepatitis, autoimmune hepatitis may resemble typical *acute viral hepatitis* (Chap. 38). Without histologic assessment, severe chronic hepatitis cannot be readily distinguished based on clinical or biochemical criteria from mild chronic hepatitis. In adolescence, *Wilson's disease* (Chap. 42) may present with features of chronic hepatitis long before neurologic manifestations become apparent and before the formation of Kayser-Fleischer rings. In this age group, serum ceruloplasmin and serum and urinary copper determinations plus measurement of liver copper levels will establish the correct diagnosis. *Postnecrotic* or *cryptogenic cirrhosis* and *primary biliary cirrhosis* (Chap. 42) share clinical features with autoimmune hepatitis, and both alcoholic hepatitis (Chap. 41) and nonalcoholic steatohepatitis (Chap. 44) may present with many features common to autoimmune hepatitis; historic, biochemical, serologic, and histologic assessments are usually sufficient to allow these entities to be distinguished from autoimmune hepatitis. Of course, the distinction between autoimmune and chronic viral hepatitis is not always straightforward, especially when viral antibodies occur in patients with autoimmune disease or when autoantibodies occur in patients with viral disease. Furthermore, the presence of extrahepatic features such as arthritis, cutaneous vasculitis, or pleuritis—not to mention the presence of circulating autoantibodies—may cause confusion with *rheumatologic disorders* such as rheumatoid arthritis and systemic lupus erythematosus. The existence of clinical and biochemical features of progressive necroinflammatory liver disease distinguishes chronic hepatitis from these other disorders, which are not associated with severe liver disease.

Finally, occasionally, features of autoimmune hepatitis overlap with features of autoimmune biliary disorders such as primary biliary cirrhosis, primary sclerosing cholangitis (Chaps. 42 and 45), or, even more rarely, mitochondrial antibody-negative autoimmune cholangitis. Such overlap syndromes are difficult to categorize, and often response to therapy may be the distinguishing factor that establishes the diagnosis.

TREATMENT ▶ Autoimmune Hepatitis

The mainstay of management in autoimmune hepatitis is glucocorticoid therapy. Several controlled clinical trials have documented that such therapy leads to symptomatic, clinical, biochemical, and histologic improvement as well as increased survival. A therapeutic response can be expected in up to 80% of patients. Unfortunately, therapy has not been shown to prevent ultimate progression to cirrhosis; however, instances of reversal of fibrosis and cirrhosis have been reported in patients responding to treatment. Although some advocate the use of prednisolone (the hepatic metabolite of prednisone), prednisone is just as effective and is favored by most authorities. Therapy may be initiated at 20 mg/d, but a popular regimen in the United States relies on an initiation dose of 60 mg/d. This high dose is tapered successively over the course of a month down to a maintenance level of 20 mg/d. An alternative, but equally effective, approach is to begin with half the prednisone dose (30 mg/d) along with azathioprine (50 mg/d). With azathioprine maintained at 50 mg/d, the prednisone dose is tapered over the course of a month down to a maintenance level of 10 mg/d. The advantage of the combination approach is a reduction, over the span of an 18-month course of therapy, in serious, life-threatening complications of steroid therapy from 66% down to under 20%. In combination regimens, 6-mercaptopurine may be substituted for its prodrug azathioprine, but this is rarely required. Azathioprine alone, however, is not effective in achieving remission, nor is alternate-day glucocorticoid therapy. Limited experience with budesonide in noncirrhotic patients suggests that this steroid side effect–sparing drug may be effective. Although therapy has been shown to be effective for severe autoimmune hepatitis (AST ≥10 times the upper limit of normal or ≥5 times the upper limit of normal in conjunction with serum globulin greater than or equal to twice normal; bridging necrosis or multilobular necrosis on liver biopsy; presence of symptoms), therapy is not indicated for mild forms of chronic hepatitis, and the efficacy of therapy in mild or asymptomatic autoimmune hepatitis has not been established.

Improvement of fatigue, anorexia, malaise, and jaundice tends to occur within days to several weeks; biochemical improvement occurs over the course of several weeks to months, with a fall in serum bilirubin and globulin levels and an increase in serum albumin.

Serum aminotransferase levels usually drop promptly, but improvements in AST and ALT alone do not appear to be reliable markers of recovery in individual patients; histologic improvement, characterized by a decrease in mononuclear infiltration and in hepatocellular necrosis, may be delayed for 6–24 months. Still, if interpreted cautiously, aminotransferase levels are valuable indicators of relative disease activity, and many authorities do *not* advocate for serial liver biopsies to assess therapeutic success or to guide decisions to alter or stop therapy. Rapidity of response is more common in older patients (≥69 years) and those with HLA DBR1*04; although rapid responders may progress less slowly to cirrhosis and liver transplantation, they are no less likely than slower responders to relapse after therapy. Therapy should continue for at least 12–18 months. After tapering and cessation of therapy, the likelihood of relapse is at least 50%, even if posttreatment histology has improved to show mild chronic hepatitis, and the majority of patients require therapy at maintenance doses indefinitely. Continuing azathioprine alone (2 mg/kg body weight daily) after cessation of prednisone therapy may reduce the frequency of relapse.

In medically refractory cases, an attempt should be made to intensify treatment with high-dose glucocorticoid monotherapy (60 mg daily) or combination glucocorticoid (30 mg daily) plus high-dose azathioprine (150 mg daily) therapy. After a month, doses of prednisone can be reduced by 10 mg a month, and doses of azathioprine can be reduced by 50 mg a month toward ultimate, conventional maintenance doses. Patients refractory to this regimen may be treated with cyclosporine, tacrolimus, or mycophenolate mofetil; however, to date, only limited anecdotal reports support these approaches. If medical therapy fails, or when chronic hepatitis progresses to cirrhosis and is associated with life-threatening complications of liver decompensation, liver transplantation is the only recourse (Chap. 46); failure of the bilirubin to improve after 2 weeks of therapy should prompt early consideration of the patient for liver transplantation. Recurrence of autoimmune hepatitis in the new liver occurs rarely in most experiences but in as many as 35–40% of cases in others.

ACKNOWLEDGMENT

Kurt J. Isselbacher, MD, contributed to this chapter in previous editions of Harrison's Principles of Internal Medicine.

CHAPTER 41

ALCOHOLIC LIVER DISEASE

Mark E. Mailliard ■ Michael F. Sorrell

Chronic and excessive alcohol ingestion is one of the major causes of liver disease. Per capita, alcohol consumption and cirrhosis have risen in the last decade in United Kingdom and Russia but has decreased in many developed countries including the United States. The pathology of alcoholic liver disease consists of three major lesions, with the injury rarely existing in a pure form: (1) fatty liver, (2) alcoholic hepatitis, and (3) cirrhosis. Fatty liver is present in >90% of binge and chronic drinkers. A much smaller percentage of heavy drinkers will progress to alcoholic hepatitis, thought to be a precursor to cirrhosis. The prognosis of severe alcoholic liver disease is dismal; the mortality of patients with alcoholic hepatitis concurrent with cirrhosis is nearly 60% at 4 years. Although alcohol is considered a direct hepatotoxin, only between 10 and 20% of alcoholics will develop alcoholic hepatitis. The explanation for this apparent paradox is unclear but involves the complex interaction of facilitating factors, such as intake frequency, diet, and gender.

ETIOLOGY AND PATHOGENESIS

Quantity and duration of alcohol intake are the most important risk factors involved in the development of alcoholic liver disease (Table 41-1). The roles of beverage type(s), i.e. wine, beer, or spirits, and pattern of drinking (daily versus binge drinking) are less clear. Progress of the hepatic injury beyond the fatty liver stage seems to require additional risk factors that remain incompletely defined. Although there are genetic predispositions for alcoholism, and candidate genes for liver steatosis and fibrosis, gender is a strong determinant for alcoholic liver disease. Women are more susceptible to alcoholic liver injury when compared to men. They develop advanced liver disease with substantially less alcohol intake. In general, the time it takes to develop liver disease is directly related to the amount of alcohol consumed. It is useful in estimating alcohol

TABLE 41-1

RISK FACTORS FOR ALCOHOLIC LIVER DISEASE	
RISK FACTOR	COMMENT
Quantity	In men, 40–80 g/d of ethanol produces fatty liver; 160 g/d for 10–20 years causes hepatitis or cirrhosis. Only 15% of alcoholics develop alcoholic liver disease.
Gender	Women exhibit increased susceptibility to alcoholic liver disease at amounts >20 g/d; two drinks per day is probably safe.
Hepatitis C	HCV infection concurrent with alcoholic liver disease is associated with younger age for severity, more advanced histology, decreased survival.
Genetics	Gene polymorphisms may include alcohol dehydrogenase, cytochrome P4502E1, and those associated with alcoholism (twin studies).
Malnutrition	Alcohol injury does not require malnutrition, but obesity and fatty liver from the effect of carbohydrate on the transcriptional control of lipid synthesis and transport may be factors. Patients should receive vigorous attention to nutritional support.

consumption to understand that one beer, four ounces of wine, or one ounce of 80% spirits all contain ~12 g of alcohol. The threshold for developing alcoholic liver disease in men is an intake of >60–80 g/d of alcohol for 10 years, while women are at increased risk for developing similar degrees of liver injury by consuming 20–40 g/d. Ingestion of 160 g/d is associated with a 25-fold increased risk of developing alcoholic cirrhosis. Gender-dependent differences result from poorly understood effects of estrogen and the metabolism of alcohol. Diet, particularly an increase in liver injury from high fat or the protective effect of coffee, has been postulated to play a part in the development of the pathogenic process.

Chronic infection with hepatitis C (HCV) (Chap. 40) is an important comorbidity in the progression of alcoholic liver disease to cirrhosis in chronic and excessive drinkers. Even moderate alcohol intake of 20–50 g/d increases the risk of cirrhosis and hepatocellular cancer in HCV-infected individuals. Patients with both alcoholic liver injury and HCV infection develop decompensated liver disease at a younger age and have poorer overall survival. Increased liver iron stores and, rarely, porphyria cutanea tarda can occur as a consequence of the overlapping injurious processes secondary to alcohol abuse and HCV infection. In addition, alcohol intake of >50 g/d by HCV-infected patients decreases the efficacy of interferon-based antiviral therapy.

Our understanding of the pathogenesis of alcoholic liver injury is incomplete. Alcohol is a direct hepatotoxin, but ingestion of alcohol initiates a variety of metabolic responses that influence the final hepatotoxic response. The initial concept of malnutrition as the major pathogenic mechanism has been replaced by the understanding that the hepatic metabolism of alcohol initiates a pathogenic process including the production of toxic protein-aldehyde adducts, the generation of reducing equivalents that promotes lipogenesis, and the inhibition of fatty-acid oxidation. Endotoxins, oxidative stress, immunologic activity, and pro-inflammatory cytokine release contribute to the resulting liver injury **(Fig. 41-1)**. The complex interaction of intestinal and hepatic cells is crucial to alcohol-mediated liver injury. Tumor necrosis factor α (TNF-α) and intestine-derived endotoxemia facilitate hepatocyte apoptosis and necrosis. Stellate cell activation and collagen production are key events in hepatic fibrogenesis. The resulting fibrosis determines the architectural derangement of the liver following chronic alcohol ingestion.

PATHOLOGY

The liver has a limited repertoire in response to injury. Fatty liver is the initial and most common histologic response to hepatotoxic stimuli, including excessive alcohol ingestion. The accumulation of fat within the perivenular hepatocytes coincides with the location of alcohol dehydrogenase, the major enzyme responsible for alcohol metabolism. Continuing alcohol ingestion results in fat accumulation throughout the entire hepatic lobule. Despite extensive fatty change and distortion of the hepatocytes with macrovesicular fat, the cessation of drinking results in normalization of hepatic architecture and fat content within the liver. Alcoholic fatty liver has traditionally been regarded as entirely benign, but similar to the spectrum of nonalcoholic fatty-liver disease (Chap. 44), the appearance of steatohepatitis and certain

FIGURE 41-1
Biomedical and cellular pathogenesis of liver injury secondary to chronic ethanol ingestion. MAA, malondialdehyde-acetaldehyde; TNF, tumor necrosis factor; TGF, transforming growth factor; IL, interleukin; PPAR, peroxisome proliferator-activated receptor; RXR, retinoid X receptor.

pathologic features such as giant mitochondria, perivenular fibrosis, and macrovesicular fat may be associated with progressive liver injury.

The transition between fatty liver and the development of alcoholic hepatitis is blurred. The hallmark of alcoholic hepatitis is hepatocyte injury characterized by ballooning degeneration, spotty necrosis, polymorphonuclear infiltrate, and fibrosis in the perivenular and perisinusoidal space of Disse. Mallory bodies are often present in florid cases but are neither specific nor necessary to establishing the diagnosis. Alcoholic hepatitis is thought to be a precursor to the development of cirrhosis. However, like fatty liver, it is potentially reversible with cessation of drinking. Cirrhosis is present in up to 50% of patients with biopsy-proven alcoholic hepatitis and its regression is uncertain, even with abstention.

CLINICAL FEATURES

The clinical manifestations of alcoholic fatty liver are subtle and characteristically detected as a consequence of the patient's visit for a seemingly unrelated matter.

Previously unsuspected hepatomegaly is often the only clinical finding. Occasionally, patients with fatty liver will present with right upper quadrant discomfort, nausea, and, rarely, jaundice. Differentiation of alcoholic fatty liver from nonalcoholic fatty liver is difficult unless an accurate drinking history is ascertained. In every instance where liver disease is present, a thoughtful and sensitive drinking history should be obtained. Standard, validated questions accurately detect alcohol-related problems. Alcoholic hepatitis is associated with a wide gamut of clinical features. Fever, spider nevi, jaundice, and abdominal pain simulating an acute abdomen represent the extreme end of the spectrum, while many patients will be entirely asymptomatic. Portal hypertension, ascites, or variceal bleeding can occur in the absence of cirrhosis. Recognition of the clinical features of alcoholic hepatitis is central to the initiation of an effective and appropriate diagnostic and therapeutic strategy. It is important to recognize that patients with alcoholic cirrhosis often exhibit clinical features identical to other causes of cirrhosis.

LABORATORY FEATURES

Patients with alcoholic liver disease are often identified through routine screening tests. The typical laboratory abnormalities seen in fatty liver are nonspecific and include modest elevations of the aspartate aminotransferase (AST), alanine aminotransferase (ALT), and γ-glutamyl transpeptidase (GGTP), accompanied by hypertriglyceridemia, hypercholesterolemia, and, occasionally, hyperbilirubinemia. In alcoholic hepatitis and in contrast to other causes of fatty liver, the AST and ALT are usually elevated two- to sevenfold. They are rarely >400 U/L, and the AST/ALT ratio is >1 **(Table 41-2)**.

TABLE 41-2

LABORATORY DIAGNOSIS OF ALCOHOLIC FATTY LIVER AND ALCOHOLIC HEPATITIS	
TEST	**COMMENT**
AST	Increased two- to sevenfold, <400 U/L, greater than ALT
ALT	Increased two- to sevenfold, <400 U/L
AST/ALT	Usually >1
GGTP	Not specific to alcohol, easily inducible, elevated in all forms of fatty liver
Bilirubin	May be markedly increased in alcoholic hepatitis despite modest elevation in alkaline phosphatase
PMN	If >5500/μL, predicts severe alcoholic hepatitis when discriminant function >32

Abbreviations: AST, aspartate aminotransferase; ALT, alanine aminotransferase; GGTP, gamma-glutamyl transpeptidase; PMN, polymorphonuclear cells.

Hyperbilirubinemia is common and is accompanied by modest increases in the alkaline phosphatase level. Derangement in hepatocyte synthetic function indicates more serious disease. Hypoalbuminemia and coagulopathy are common in advanced liver injury. Ultrasonography is useful in detecting fatty infiltration of the liver and determining liver size. The demonstration by ultrasound of portal vein flow reversal, ascites, and intraabdominal collaterals indicates serious liver injury with less potential for complete reversal of liver disease.

PROGNOSIS

Critically ill patients with alcoholic hepatitis have short-term (30-day) mortality rates >50%. Severe alcoholic hepatitis is heralded by coagulopathy (prothrombin time increased >5 s), anemia, serum albumin concentrations <25 g/L (2.5 mg/dL), serum bilirubin levels >137 μmol/L (8 mg/dL), renal failure, and ascites. A discriminant function calculated as 4.6 × [the prolongation of the prothrombin time above control (seconds)] + serum bilirubin (mg/dL) can identify patients with a poor prognosis (discriminant function >32). A Model for End-Stage Liver Disease score (MELD, Chap. 46) ≥21 also is associated with significant mortality in alcoholic hepatitis. The presence of ascites, variceal hemorrhage, deep encephalopathy, or hepatorenal syndrome predicts a dismal prognosis. The pathologic stage of the injury can be helpful in predicting prognosis. Liver biopsy should be performed whenever possible to confirm the diagnosis, to establish potential reversibility of the liver disease, and to guide the therapeutic decisions.

TREATMENT   Alcoholic Liver Disease

Complete abstinence from alcohol is the cornerstone in the treatment of alcoholic liver disease. Improved survival and the potential for reversal of histologic injury regardless of the initial clinical presentation are associated with total avoidance of alcohol ingestion. Referral of patients to experienced alcohol counselors and/or alcohol treatment programs should be routine in the management of patients with alcoholic liver disease. Attention should be directed to the nutritional and psychosocial states during the evaluation and treatment periods. Because of data suggesting that the pathogenic mechanisms in alcoholic hepatitis involve cytokine release and the perpetuation of injury by immunologic processes, glucocorticoids have been extensively evaluated in the treatment of alcoholic hepatitis. Patients with severe alcoholic hepatitis, defined as a discriminant function >32 or MELD >20, should be given prednisone, 40 mg/d, or prednisolone, 32 mg/d, for

FIGURE 41-2

Effect of glucocorticoid therapy of severe alcoholic hepatitis on short-term survival: the result of a meta-analysis of individual data from three studies. Prednisolone, solid line; placebo, dotted line. (*Adapted from P Mathurin et al: J Hepatol 36:480, 2002, with permission from Elsevier Science.*)

4 weeks, followed by a steroid taper (Fig. 41-2). Exclusion criteria include active gastrointestinal bleeding, renal failure, or pancreatitis. Women with encephalopathy from severe alcoholic hepatitis may be particularly good candidates for glucocorticoids. A Lille score >0.45, at *http://www.lillemodel.com*, uses pretreatment variables plus the change in total bilirubin at day 7 of glucocorticoids to identify patients unresponsive to therapy.

The role of TNF-α expression and receptor activity in alcoholic liver injury has led to an examination of TNF inhibition as an alternative to glucocorticoids for severe alcoholic hepatitis. The nonspecific TNF inhibitor, pentoxifylline, demonstrated improved survival in the therapy of severe alcoholic hepatitis (Fig. 41-3). Monoclonal

FIGURE 41-3

Treatment algorithm for alcoholic hepatitis. As identified by a calculated discriminant function >32 (see text), patients with severe alcoholic hepatitis, without the presence of gastrointestinal bleeding or infection, would be candidates for either glucocorticoids or pentoxifylline administration.

antibodies that neutralize serum TNF-α should not be used in alcoholic hepatitis because of recent studies reporting increased deaths secondary to infection and renal failure. Because of inordinate surgical mortality and the high rates of recidivism following transplantation, patients with alcoholic hepatitis are not candidates for immediate liver transplantation. The transplant candidacy of these patients should be reevaluated after a defined period of sobriety.

CHAPTER 42
CIRRHOSIS AND ITS COMPLICATIONS

Bruce R. Bacon

Cirrhosis is a condition that is defined histopathologically and has a variety of clinical manifestations and complications, some of which can be life-threatening. In the past, it has been thought that cirrhosis was never reversible; however, it has become apparent that when the underlying insult that has caused the cirrhosis has been removed, there can be reversal of fibrosis. This is most apparent with the successful treatment of chronic hepatitis C; however, reversal of fibrosis is also seen in patients with hemochromatosis who have been successfully treated and in patients with alcoholic liver disease who have discontinued alcohol use.

Regardless of the cause of cirrhosis, the pathologic features consist of the development of fibrosis to the point that there is architectural distortion with the formation of regenerative nodules. This results in a decrease in hepatocellular mass, and thus function, and an alteration of blood flow. The induction of fibrosis occurs with activation of hepatic stellate cells, resulting in the formation of increased amounts of collagen and other components of the extracellular matrix.

Clinical features of cirrhosis are the result of pathologic changes and mirror the severity of the liver disease. Most hepatic pathologists provide an assessment of grading and staging when evaluating liver biopsy samples. These grading and staging schemes vary between disease states and have been developed for most conditions, including chronic viral hepatitis, nonalcoholic fatty liver disease, and primary biliary cirrhosis. Advanced fibrosis usually includes bridging fibrosis with nodularity designated as stage 3 and cirrhosis designated as stage 4. Patients who have cirrhosis have varying degrees of compensated liver function, and clinicians need to differentiate between those who have stable, compensated cirrhosis and those who have decompensated cirrhosis. Patients who have developed complications of their liver disease and have become decompensated should be considered for liver transplantation. Many of the complications of cirrhosis will require specific therapy. *Portal hypertension*

TABLE 42-1

CAUSES OF CIRRHOSIS	
Alcoholism	Cardiac cirrhosis
Chronic viral hepatitis	Inherited metabolic liver
Hepatitis B	disease
Hepatitis C	Hemochromatosis
Autoimmune hepatitis	Wilson's disease
Nonalcoholic steatohepatitis	α_1 Antitrypsin deficiency
Biliary cirrhosis	Cystic fibrosis
Primary biliary cirrhosis	Cryptogenic cirrhosis
Primary sclerosing	
cholangitis	
Autoimmune	
cholangiopathy	

is a significant complicating feature of decompensated cirrhosis and is responsible for the development of ascites and bleeding from esophagogastric varices, two complications that signify decompensated cirrhosis. Loss of hepatocellular function results in jaundice, coagulation disorders, and hypoalbuminemia and contributes to the causes of portosystemic encephalopathy. The complications of cirrhosis are basically the same regardless of the etiology. Nonetheless, it is useful to classify patients by the cause of their liver disease (Table 42-1); patients can be divided into broad groups with alcoholic cirrhosis, cirrhosis due to chronic viral hepatitis, biliary cirrhosis, and other, less-common causes such as cardiac cirrhosis, cryptogenic cirrhosis, and other miscellaneous causes.

ALCOHOLIC CIRRHOSIS

Excessive chronic alcohol use can cause several different types of chronic liver disease, including alcoholic fatty liver, alcoholic hepatitis, and alcoholic cirrhosis.

Furthermore, use of excessive alcohol can contribute to liver damage in patients with other liver diseases, such as hepatitis C, hemochromatosis, and those patients who have fatty liver disease related to obesity. Chronic alcohol use can produce fibrosis in the absence of accompanying inflammation and/or necrosis. Fibrosis can be centrilobular, pericellular, or periportal. When fibrosis reaches a certain degree, there is disruption of the normal liver architecture and replacement of liver cells by regenerative nodules. In alcoholic cirrhosis, the nodules are usually <3 mm in diameter; this form of cirrhosis is referred to as *micronodular*. With cessation of alcohol use, larger nodules may form, resulting in a mixed micronodular and macronodular cirrhosis.

Pathogenesis

Alcohol is the most commonly used drug in the United States, and more than two-thirds of adults drink alcohol each year. Thirty percent have had a binge within the past month, and over 7% of adults regularly consume more than two drinks per day. Unfortunately, more than 14 million adults in the United States meet the diagnostic criteria for alcohol abuse or dependence. In the United States, chronic liver disease is the tenth most common cause of death in adults, and alcoholic cirrhosis accounts for approximately 40% of deaths due to cirrhosis.

Ethanol is mainly absorbed by the small intestine and, to a lesser degree, through the stomach. Gastric alcohol dehydrogenase (ADH) initiates alcohol metabolism. Three enzyme systems account for metabolism of alcohol in the liver. These include cytosolic ADH, the microsomal ethanol oxidizing system (MEOS), and peroxisomal catalase. The majority of ethanol oxidation occurs via ADH to form acetaldehyde, which is a highly reactive molecule that may have multiple effects. Ultimately, acetaldehyde is metabolized to acetate by aldehyde dehydrogenase (ALDH). Intake of ethanol increases intracellular accumulation of triglycerides by increasing fatty acid uptake and by reducing fatty acid oxidation and lipoprotein secretion. Protein synthesis, glycosylation, and secretion are impaired. Oxidative damage to hepatocyte membranes occurs due to the formation of reactive oxygen species; acetaldehyde is a highly reactive molecule that combines with proteins to form protein-acetaldehyde adducts. These adducts may interfere with specific enzyme activities, including microtubular formation and hepatic protein trafficking. With acetaldehyde-mediated hepatocyte damage, certain reactive oxygen species can result in Kupffer cell activation. As a result, profibrogenic cytokines are produced that initiate and perpetuate stellate cell activation, with the resultant production of excess collagen and extracellular matrix. Connective tissue appears in both periportal and pericentral zones and eventually connects portal triads with central veins forming regenerative nodules. Hepatocyte loss occurs, and with increased collagen production and deposition, together with continuing hepatocyte destruction, the liver contracts and shrinks in size. This process generally takes from years to decades to occur and requires repeated insults.

Clinical features

The diagnosis of alcoholic liver disease requires an accurate history regarding both amount and duration of alcohol consumption. Patients with alcoholic liver disease can present with nonspecific symptoms such as vague right upper quadrant pain, fever, nausea and vomiting, diarrhea, anorexia, and malaise. Alternatively, they may present with more specific complications of chronic liver disease, including ascites, edema, or upper gastrointestinal (GI) hemorrhage. Many cases present incidentally at the time of autopsy or elective surgery. Other clinical manifestations include the development of jaundice or encephalopathy. The abrupt onset of any of these complications may be the first event prompting the patient to seek medical attention. Other patients may be identified in the course of an evaluation of routine laboratory studies that are found to be abnormal. On physical examination, the liver and spleen may be enlarged, with the liver edge being firm and nodular. Other frequent findings include scleral icterus, palmar erythema **(Fig. 42-1)**, spider angiomas **(Fig. 42-2)**, parotid gland enlargement, digital clubbing, muscle wasting, or the development of edema and ascites. Men may have decreased body hair and gynecomastia as well as testicular atrophy, which may be a consequence of hormonal abnormalities or a direct toxic effect of alcohol on the testes. In women with advanced alcoholic cirrhosis, menstrual irregularities usually occur, and

FIGURE 42-1
Palmar erythema. This figure shows palmar erythema in a patient with alcoholic cirrhosis. The erythema is peripheral over the palm with central pallor.

FIGURE 42-2
Spider angioma. This figure shows a spider angioma in a patient with hepatitis C cirrhosis. With release of central compression, the arteriole fills from the center and spreads out peripherally.

some women may be amenorrheic. These changes are often reversible following cessation of alcohol.

Laboratory tests may be completely normal in patients with early compensated alcoholic cirrhosis. Alternatively, in advanced liver disease, many abnormalities usually are present. Patients may be anemic either from chronic GI blood loss, nutritional deficiencies, or hypersplenism related to portal hypertension, or as a direct suppressive effect of alcohol on the bone marrow. A unique form of hemolytic anemia (with spur cells and acanthocytes) called *Zieve's syndrome* can occur in patients with severe alcoholic hepatitis. Platelet counts are often reduced early in the disease, reflective of portal hypertension with hypersplenism. Serum total bilirubin can be normal or elevated with advanced disease. Direct bilirubin is frequently mildly elevated in patients with a normal total bilirubin, but the abnormality typically progresses as the disease worsens. Prothrombin times are often prolonged and usually do not respond to administration of parenteral vitamin K. Serum sodium levels are usually normal unless patients have ascites and then can be depressed, largely due to ingestion of excess free water. Serum alanine and aspartate aminotransferases (ALT, AST) are typically elevated, particularly in patients who continue to drink, with AST levels being higher than ALT levels, usually by a 2:1 ratio.

Diagnosis

Patients who have any of the previously-mentioned clinical features, physical examination findings, or laboratory studies should be considered to have alcoholic liver disease. The diagnosis, however, requires accurate knowledge that the patient is continuing to use and abuse alcohol. Furthermore, other forms of chronic liver disease (e.g., chronic viral hepatitis or metabolic or autoimmune liver diseases) must be considered or ruled out or, if present, an estimate of relative causality along with the alcohol use should be determined. Liver biopsy can be helpful to confirm a diagnosis, but generally when patients present with alcoholic hepatitis and are still drinking, liver biopsy is withheld until abstinence has been maintained for at least 6 months to determine residual, nonreversible disease.

In patients who have had complications of cirrhosis and who continue to drink, there is a <50% 5-year survival. In contrast, in those patients who are able to remain abstinent, the prognosis is significantly improved. In patients with advanced liver disease, the prognosis remains poor; however, in those individuals who are able to remain abstinent, liver transplantation is a viable option.

TREATMENT Alcoholic Cirrhosis

Abstinence is the cornerstone of therapy for patients with alcoholic liver disease. In addition, patients require good nutrition and long-term medical supervision to manage underlying complications that may develop. Complications such as the development of ascites and edema, variceal hemorrhage, or portosystemic encephalopathy all require specific management and treatment. Glucocorticoids are occasionally used in patients with severe alcoholic hepatitis in the absence of infection. Survival has been shown to improve in certain studies. Treatment is restricted to patients with a discriminant function (DF) value of >32. The DF is calculated as the serum total bilirubin plus the difference in the patient's prothrombin time compared to control (in seconds) multiplied by 4.6. In patients for whom this value is >32, there is improved survival at 28 days with the use of glucocorticoids.

Other therapies that have been used include oral pentoxifylline, which decreases the production of tumor necrosis factor α (TNF-α) and other proinflammatory cytokines. In contrast to glucocorticoids, with which complications can occur, pentoxifylline is relatively easy to administer and has few if any side effects. A variety of nutritional therapies have been tried with either parenteral or enteral feedings; however, it is unclear whether any of these modalities have significantly improved survival.

Recent studies have used parenterally administered inhibitors of TNF-α such as infliximab or etanercept. Early results have shown no adverse events; however, there was no clear-cut improvement in survival. Anabolic steroids, propylthiouracil, antioxidants, colchicine, and penicillamine have all been used but do not show clear-cut benefits and are not recommended.

As mentioned earlier, the cornerstone to treatment is cessation of alcohol use. Recent experience with medications that reduce craving for alcohol such as acamprosate calcium has been favorable. Patients may take other necessary medications even in the presence of cirrhosis. Acetaminophen use is often discouraged in patients with liver disease; however, if no more than 2 g of acetaminophen per day are consumed, there generally are no problems.

CIRRHOSIS DUE TO CHRONIC VIRAL HEPATITIS B OR C

Of patients exposed to the hepatitis C virus (HCV), approximately 80% develop chronic hepatitis C, and of those, about 20–30% will develop cirrhosis over 20–30 years. Many of these patients have had concomitant alcohol use, and the true incidence of cirrhosis due to hepatitis C alone is unknown. Nonetheless, this represents a significant number of patients. It is expected that an even higher percentage will go on to develop cirrhosis over longer periods of time. In the United States, approximately 5 million people have been exposed to the hepatitis C virus, with about 3.5 to 4 million who are chronically viremic. Worldwide, about 170 million individuals have hepatitis C, with some areas of the world (e.g., Egypt) having up to 15% of the population infected. HCV is a noncytopathic virus, and liver damage is probably immune-mediated. Progression of liver disease due to chronic hepatitis C is characterized by portal-based fibrosis with bridging fibrosis and nodularity developing, ultimately culminating in the development of cirrhosis. In cirrhosis due to chronic hepatitis C, the liver is small and shrunken with characteristic features of a mixed micro- and macronodular cirrhosis seen on liver biopsy. In addition to the increased fibrosis that is seen in cirrhosis due to hepatitis C, an inflammatory infiltrate is found in portal areas with interface hepatitis and occasionally some lobular hepatocellular injury and inflammation. In patients with HCV genotype 3, steatosis is often present.

Similar findings are seen in patients with cirrhosis due to chronic hepatitis B. Of adult patients exposed to hepatitis B, about 5% develop chronic hepatitis B, and about 20% of those patients will go on to develop cirrhosis. Special stains for hepatitis B core (HBc) and hepatitis B surface (HBs) antigen will be positive, and ground-glass hepatocytes signifying hepatitis B surface antigen (HBsAg) may be present. In the United States, there are about 2 million carriers of hepatitis B, whereas in other parts of the world where hepatitis B virus (HBV) is endemic (i.e., Asia, Southeast Asia, sub-Saharan Africa), up to 15% of the population may be infected having acquired the infection vertically at the time of birth. Thus, over 300–400 million individuals are thought to have hepatitis B worldwide. Approximately 25% of these individuals may ultimately develop cirrhosis.

Clinical features and diagnosis

Patients with cirrhosis due to either chronic hepatitis C or B can present with the usual symptoms and signs of chronic liver disease. Fatigue, malaise, vague right upper quadrant pain, and laboratory abnormalities are frequent presenting features. Diagnosis requires a thorough laboratory evaluation, including quantitative HCV RNA testing and analysis for HCV genotype, or hepatitis B serologies to include HBsAg, anti-HBs, HBeAg (hepatitis B e antigen), anti-HBe, and quantitative HBV DNA levels.

TREATMENT Cirrhosis Due to Chronic Viral Hepatitis B or C

Management of complications of cirrhosis revolves around specific therapy for treatment of whatever complications occur, whether they be esophageal variceal hemorrhage, development of ascites and edema, or encephalopathy. In patients with chronic hepatitis B, numerous studies have shown beneficial effects of antiviral therapy, which is effective at viral suppression, as evidenced by reducing aminotransferase levels and HBV DNA levels, and improving histology by reducing inflammation and fibrosis. Several clinical trials and case series have demonstrated that patients with decompensated liver disease can become compensated with the use of antiviral therapy directed against hepatitis B. Currently available therapy includes lamivudine, adefovir, telbivudine, entecavir, and tenofovir. Interferon α can also be used for treating hepatitis B, but it should not be used in cirrhotics.

Treatment of patients with cirrhosis due to hepatitis C is a little more difficult because the side effects of pegylated interferon and ribavirin therapy are oftentimes difficult to manage. Dose-limiting cytopenias (platelets, white blood cells, red blood cells) or severe side effects can result in discontinuation of treatment. Nonetheless, if patients can tolerate treatment, and if it is successful, the benefit is great and disease progression is reduced.

CIRRHOSIS FROM AUTOIMMUNE HEPATITIS AND NONALCOHOLIC FATTY LIVER DISEASE

Other causes of posthepatitic cirrhosis include autoimmune hepatitis and cirrhosis due to nonalcoholic steatohepatitis. Many patients with autoimmune hepatitis (AIH) present with cirrhosis that is already established. Typically, these patients will not benefit from immunosuppressive therapy with glucocorticoids or azathioprine because the AIH is "burned out." In this situation, liver biopsy does not show a significant inflammatory infiltrate. Diagnosis in this setting requires positive autoimmune markers such as antinuclear antibody (ANA) or anti-smooth-muscle antibody (ASMA). When patients with AIH present with cirrhosis and active inflammation accompanied by elevated liver enzymes, there can be considerable benefit from the use of immunosuppressive therapy.

Patients with nonalcoholic steatohepatitis are increasingly being found to have progressed to cirrhosis. With the epidemic of obesity that continues in Western countries, more and more patients are identified with nonalcoholic fatty liver disease. Of these, a significant subset have nonalcoholic steatohepatitis and can progress to increased fibrosis and cirrhosis. Over the past several years, it has been increasingly recognized that many patients who were thought to have cryptogenic cirrhosis in fact have nonalcoholic steatohepatitis. As their cirrhosis progresses, they become catabolic and then lose the telltale signs of steatosis seen on biopsy. Management of complications of cirrhosis due to either AIH or nonalcoholic steatohepatitis is similar to that for other forms of cirrhosis.

BILIARY CIRRHOSIS

Biliary cirrhosis has pathologic features that are different from either alcoholic cirrhosis or posthepatitic cirrhosis, yet the manifestations of end-stage liver disease are the same. Cholestatic liver disease may result from necroinflammatory lesions, congenital or metabolic processes, or external bile duct compression. Thus, two broad categories reflect the anatomic sites of abnormal bile retention: *intrahepatic* and *extrahepatic*. The distinction is important for obvious therapeutic reasons. Extrahepatic obstruction may benefit from surgical or endoscopic biliary tract decompression, whereas intrahepatic cholestatic processes will not improve with such interventions and require a different approach.

The major causes of chronic cholestatic syndromes are primary biliary cirrhosis (PBC), autoimmune cholangitis (AIC), primary sclerosing cholangitis (PSC), and idiopathic adulthood ductopenia. These syndromes are usually clinically distinguished from each other by antibody testing, cholangiographic findings, and clinical presentation. However, they all share the histopathologic features of chronic cholestasis, such as cholate stasis; copper deposition; xanthomatous transformation of hepatocytes; and irregular, so-called biliary fibrosis. In addition, there may be chronic portal inflammation, interface activity, and chronic lobular inflammation. Ductopenia is a result of this progressive disease as patients develop cirrhosis.

PRIMARY BILIARY CIRRHOSIS

PBC is seen in about 100–200 individuals per million, with a strong female preponderance and a median age of around 50 years at the time of diagnosis. The cause of PBC is unknown; it is characterized by portal inflammation and necrosis of cholangiocytes in small- and medium-sized bile ducts. Cholestatic features prevail, and biliary cirrhosis is characterized by an elevated bilirubin level and progressive liver failure. Liver transplantation is the treatment of choice for patients with decompensated cirrhosis due to PBC. A variety of therapies have been proposed, but ursodeoxycholic acid (UDCA) is the only approved treatment that has some degree of efficacy by slowing the rate of progression of the disease.

Antimitochondrial antibodies (AMA) are present in about 90% of patients with PBC. These autoantibodies recognize intermitochondrial membrane proteins that are enzymes of the pyruvate dehydrogenase complex (PDC), the branched-chain 2-oxoacid dehydrogenase complex, and the 2-oxogluterate dehydrogenase complex. Most relate to pyruvate dehydrogenase. These autoantibodies are not pathogenic but rather are useful markers for making a diagnosis of PBC.

Pathology

Histopathologic analyses of liver biopsies of patients with PBC have resulted in identifying four distinct stages of the disease as it progresses. The earliest lesion is termed *chronic nonsuppurative destructive cholangitis* and is a necrotizing inflammatory process of the portal tracts. Medium and small bile ducts are infiltrated with lymphocytes and undergo duct destruction. Mild fibrosis and sometimes bile stasis can occur. With progression, the inflammatory infiltrate becomes less prominent, but the number of bile ducts is reduced and there is proliferation of smaller bile ductules. Increased fibrosis ensues with the expansion of periportal fibrosis to bridging fibrosis. Finally, cirrhosis, which may be micronodular or macronodular, develops.

Clinical features

Currently, most patients with PBC are diagnosed well before the end-stage manifestations of the disease are present, and, as such, most patients are actually asymptomatic. When symptoms are present, they most prominently include a significant degree of fatigue out of proportion to what would be expected for either the severity of the liver disease or the age of the patient. Pruritus is seen in approximately 50% of patients at the time of diagnosis, and it can be debilitating. It might be intermittent and usually is most bothersome in the evening. In some patients, pruritus can develop toward the end of pregnancy, and there are examples of patients having been diagnosed with cholestasis of pregnancy rather than PBC. Pruritus that presents prior to the development of jaundice indicates severe disease and a poor prognosis.

Physical examination can show jaundice and other complications of chronic liver disease, including hepatomegaly, splenomegaly, ascites, and edema. Other features that are unique to PBC include hyperpigmentation, xanthelasma, and xanthomata, which are related to the altered cholesterol metabolism seen in this disease. Hyperpigmentation is evident on the trunk and the arms and is seen in areas of exfoliation and lichenification associated with progressive scratching related to the pruritus. Bone pain resulting from osteopenia or osteoporosis is occasionally seen at the time of diagnosis.

Laboratory findings

Laboratory findings in PBC show cholestatic liver enzyme abnormalities with an elevation in γ-glutamyl transpeptidase and alkaline phosphatase (ALP) along with mild elevations in aminotransferases (ALT and AST). Immunoglobulins, particularly IgM, are typically increased. Hyperbilirubinemia usually is seen once cirrhosis has developed. Thrombocytopenia, leukopenia, and anemia may be seen in patients with portal hypertension and hypersplenism. Liver biopsy shows characteristic features as described earlier and should be evident to any experienced hepatopathologist. Up to 10% of patients with characteristic PBC will have features of AIH as well and are defined as having "overlap" syndrome. These patients are treated as PBC patients and may progress to cirrhosis with the same frequency as typical PBC patients.

Diagnosis

PBC should be considered in patients with chronic cholestatic liver enzyme abnormalities. It is most often seen in middle-aged women. AMA testing may be negative, and it should be remembered that as many as 10% of patients with PBC may be AMA-negative. Liver biopsy is most important in this setting of AMA-negative PBC. In patients who are AMA-negative with cholestatic liver enzymes, PSC should be ruled out by way of cholangiography.

TREATMENT   Primary Biliary Cirrhosis

Treatment of the typical manifestations of cirrhosis are no different for PBC than for other forms of cirrhosis. UDCA has been shown to improve both biochemical and histologic features of the disease. Improvement is greatest when therapy is initiated early; the likelihood of significant improvement with UDCA is low in patients with PBC who present with manifestations of cirrhosis. UDCA is given in doses of 13–15 mg/kg per day; the medication is usually well-tolerated, although some patients have worsening pruritus with initiation of therapy. A small proportion of patients may have diarrhea or headache as a side effect of the drug. UDCA has been shown to slow the rate of progression of PBC, but it does not reverse or cure the disease. Patients with PBC require long-term follow-up by a physician experienced with the disease. Certain patients may need to be considered for liver transplantation should their liver disease decompensate.

The main symptoms of PBC are fatigue and pruritus, and symptom management is important. Several therapies have been tried for treatment of fatigue, but none of them have been successful; frequent naps should be encouraged. Pruritus is treated with antihistamines, narcotic receptor antagonists (naltrexone), and rifampin. Cholestyramine, a bile salt–sequestering agent, has been helpful in some patients but is somewhat tedious and difficult to take. Plasmapheresis has been used rarely in patients with severe intractable pruritus. There is an increased incidence of osteopenia and osteoporosis in patients with cholestatic liver disease, and bone density testing should be performed. Treatment with a bisphosphonate should be instituted when bone disease is identified.

PRIMARY SCLEROSING CHOLANGITIS

As in PBC, the cause of PSC remains unknown. PSC is a chronic cholestatic syndrome that is characterized by diffuse inflammation and fibrosis involving the entire biliary tree, resulting in chronic cholestasis. This pathologic process ultimately results in obliteration of both the intra- and extrahepatic biliary tree, leading to biliary cirrhosis, portal hypertension, and liver failure. The cause of PSC remains unknown despite extensive investigation into various mechanisms related to bacterial and viral infections, toxins, genetic predisposition, and immunologic mechanisms, all of which have been postulated to contribute to the pathogenesis and progression of this syndrome.

Pathologic changes that can occur in PSC show bile duct proliferation as well as ductopenia and fibrous cholangitis (pericholangitis). Often, liver biopsy changes in PSC are not pathognomonic, and establishing the diagnosis of PSC must involve imaging of the biliary tree. Periductal fibrosis is occasionally seen on biopsy specimens and can be quite helpful in making the diagnosis. As the disease progresses, biliary cirrhosis is the final, end-stage manifestation of PSC.

Clinical features

The usual clinical features of PSC are those found in cholestatic liver disease, with fatigue, pruritus, steatorrhea, deficiencies of fat-soluble vitamins, and the associated consequences. As in PBC, the fatigue is profound and nonspecific. Pruritus can often be debilitating and is related to the cholestasis. The severity of pruritus does not correlate with the severity of the disease. Metabolic bone disease, as seen in PBC, can occur with PSC and should be treated (discussed earlier).

Laboratory findings

Patients with PSC typically are identified in the course of an evaluation of abnormal liver enzymes. Most patients have at least a twofold increase in ALP and may have elevated aminotransferases as well. Albumin levels may be decreased, and prothrombin times are prolonged in a substantial proportion of patients at the time of diagnosis. Some degree of correction of a prolonged prothrombin time may occur with parenteral vitamin K. A small subset of patients have aminotransferase elevations greater than five times the upper limit of normal and may have features of AIH on biopsy. These individuals are thought to have an overlap syndrome between PSC and AIH. Autoantibodies are frequently positive in patients with the overlap syndrome but are typically negative in patients who only have PSC. One autoantibody, the perinuclear antineutrophil cytoplasmic antibody (p-ANCA), is positive in about 65% of patients with PSC. Over 50% of patients with PSC also have ulcerative colitis (UC); accordingly, once a diagnosis of PSC is established, colonoscopy should be performed to look for evidence of UC.

Diagnosis

The definitive diagnosis of PSC requires cholangiographic imaging. Over the last several years, MRI with magnetic resonance cholangiopancreatography (MRCP) has been used as the imaging technique of choice for initial evaluation. Once patients are screened in this manner, some investigators feel that endoscopic retrograde cholangiopancreatography (ERCP) should also be performed to be certain whether or not a dominant stricture is present. Typical cholangiographic findings in PSC are multifocal stricturing and beading involving both the intrahepatic and extrahepatic biliary tree. However, though involvement may be of the intrahepatic bile ducts alone or of the extrahepatic bile ducts alone, more commonly, both are involved. These strictures are typically short and with intervening segments of normal or slightly dilated bile ducts that are distributed diffusely, producing the classic beaded appearance. The gallbladder and cystic duct can be involved in up to 15% of cases. Patients with high-grade, diffuse stricturing of the intrahepatic bile ducts have an overall poor prognosis. Gradually, biliary cirrhosis develops, and patients will progress to decompensated liver disease with all the manifestations of ascites, esophageal variceal hemorrhage, and encephalopathy.

TREATMENT | Primary Sclerosing Cholangitis

There is no specific proven treatment for PSC, although studies are currently ongoing using high-dose (20 mg/kg per day) UDCA to determine its benefit. Endoscopic dilatation of dominant strictures can be helpful, but the ultimate treatment is liver transplantation. A dreaded complication of PSC is the development of cholangiocarcinoma, which is a relative contraindication to liver transplantation. Symptoms of pruritus are common, and the approach is as mentioned previously for this problem in patients with PBC (discussed earlier).

CARDIAC CIRRHOSIS

Definition

Patients with long-standing right-sided congestive heart failure may develop chronic liver injury and cardiac cirrhosis. This is an increasingly uncommon, if not rare, cause of chronic liver disease given the advances made in the care of patients with heart failure.

Etiology and pathology

In the case of long-term right-sided heart failure, there is an elevated venous pressure transmitted via the inferior vena cava and hepatic veins to the sinusoids of the liver, which become dilated and engorged with blood. The liver becomes enlarged and swollen, and with long-term passive congestion and relative ischemia due to poor circulation, centrilobular hepatocytes can become necrotic, leading to pericentral fibrosis. This fibrotic pattern can extend to the periphery of the lobule outward until a unique pattern of fibrosis causing cirrhosis can occur.

Clinical features

Patients typically have signs of congestive heart failure and will manifest an enlarged firm liver on physical examination. ALP levels are characteristically elevated, and aminotransferases may be normal or slightly increased with AST usually higher than ALT. It is unlikely that patients will develop variceal hemorrhage or encephalopathy.

Diagnosis

The diagnosis is usually made in someone with clear-cut cardiac disease who has an elevated ALP and an enlarged liver. Liver biopsy shows a pattern of fibrosis that can be recognized by an experienced hepato-pathologist. Differentiation from Budd-Chiari syndrome (BCS) can be made by seeing extravasation of red blood cells in BCS, but not in cardiac hepatopathy. Venoocclusive disease can also affect hepatic outflow and has characteristic features on liver biopsy. Venoocclusive disease can be seen under the circumstances of conditioning for bone marrow transplant with radiation and chemotherapy; it can also be seen with the ingestion of certain herbal teas as well as pyrrolizidine alkaloids. This is typically seen in Caribbean countries and rarely in the United States. Treatment is based on management of the underlying cardiac disease.

OTHER TYPES OF CIRRHOSIS

There are several other less-common causes of chronic liver disease that can progress to cirrhosis. These include inherited metabolic liver diseases such as hemochromatosis, Wilson's disease, α_1 antitrypsin (α_1AT) deficiency, and cystic fibrosis. For all of these disorders, the manifestations of cirrhosis are similar, with some minor variations, to those seen in other patients with other causes of cirrhosis.

Hemochromatosis is an inherited disorder of iron metabolism that results in a progressive increase in hepatic iron deposition, which, over time, can lead to a portal-based fibrosis progressing to cirrhosis, liver failure, and hepatocellular cancer. While the frequency of hemochromatosis is relatively common, with genetic susceptibility occurring in 1 in 250 individuals, the frequency of end-stage manifestations due to the disease is relatively low, and fewer than 5% of those patients who are genotypically susceptible will go on to develop severe liver disease from hemochromatosis. Diagnosis is made with serum iron studies showing an elevated transferrin saturation and an elevated ferritin level, along with abnormalities identified by *HFE* mutation analysis. Treatment is straightforward, with regular therapeutic phlebotomy.

Wilson's disease is an inherited disorder of copper homeostasis with failure to excrete excess amounts of copper, leading to an accumulation in the liver. This disorder is relatively uncommon, affecting 1 in 30,000 individuals. Wilson's disease typically affects adolescents and young adults. Prompt diagnosis before end-stage manifestations become irreversible can lead to significant clinical improvement. Diagnosis requires determination of ceruloplasmin levels, which are low; 24-hour urine copper levels, which are elevated; typical physical examination findings, including Kayser-Fleischer corneal rings; and characteristic liver biopsy findings. Treatment consists of copper-chelating medications.

α_1AT *deficiency* results from an inherited disorder that causes abnormal folding of the α_1AT protein, resulting in failure of secretion of that protein from the liver. It is unknown how the retained protein leads to liver disease. Patients with α_1AT deficiency at greatest risk for developing chronic liver disease have the ZZ phenotype, but only about 10–20% of such individuals will develop chronic liver disease. Diagnosis is made by determining α_1AT levels and phenotype. Characteristic periodic acid–Schiff (PAS)-positive, diastase-resistant globules are seen on liver biopsy. The only effective treatment is liver transplantation, which is curative.

Cystic fibrosis is an uncommon inherited disorder affecting Caucasians of Northern European descent. A biliary-type cirrhosis can occur, and some patients derive benefit from the chronic use of UDCA.

MAJOR COMPLICATIONS OF CIRRHOSIS

The clinical course of patients with advanced cirrhosis is often complicated by a number of important sequelae that can occur regardless of the underlying cause of the liver disease. These include portal hypertension and its consequences of gastroesophageal variceal hemorrhage, splenomegaly, ascites, hepatic encephalopathy, spontaneous bacterial peritonitis (SBP), hepatorenal syndrome, and hepatocellular carcinoma (Table 42-2).

PORTAL HYPERTENSION

Portal hypertension is defined as the elevation of the hepatic venous pressure gradient (HVPG) to >5 mmHg. Portal hypertension is caused by a combination of

TABLE 42-2

COMPLICATIONS OF CIRRHOSIS	
Portal hypertension	Coagulopathy
Gastroesophageal varices	Factor deficiency
Portal hypertensive gastropathy	Fibrinolysis
Splenomegaly, hypersplenism	Thrombocytopenia
Ascites	Bone disease
Spontaneous bacterial	Osteopenia
peritonitis	Osteoporosis
Hepatorenal syndrome	Osteomalacia
Type 1	Hematologic
Type 2	abnormalities
Hepatic encephalopathy	Anemia
Hepatopulmonary syndrome	Hemolysis
Portopulmonary hypertension	Thrombocytopenia
Malnutrition	Neutropenia

two simultaneously occurring hemodynamic processes: (1) increased intrahepatic resistance to the passage of blood flow through the liver due to cirrhosis and regenerative nodules, and (2) increased splanchnic blood flow secondary to vasodilation within the splanchnic vascular bed. Portal hypertension is directly responsible for the two major complications of cirrhosis: variceal hemorrhage and ascites. *Variceal hemorrhage* is an immediate life-threatening problem with a 20–30% mortality rate associated with each episode of bleeding. The portal venous system normally drains blood from the stomach, intestines, spleen, pancreas, and gallbladder, and the portal vein is formed by the confluence of the superior mesenteric and splenic veins. Deoxygenated blood from the small bowel drains into the superior mesenteric vein along with blood from the head of the pancreas, the ascending colon, and part of the transverse colon. Conversely, the splenic vein drains the spleen and the pancreas and is joined by the inferior mesenteric vein, which brings blood from the transverse and descending colon as well as from the superior two-thirds of the rectum. Thus, the portal vein normally receives blood from almost the entire GI tract.

The causes of portal hypertension are usually subcategorized as prehepatic, intrahepatic, and posthepatic (Table 42-3). Prehepatic causes of portal hypertension are those affecting the portal venous system before it enters the liver; they include portal vein thrombosis and splenic vein thrombosis. Posthepatic causes encompass those affecting the hepatic veins and venous drainage to the heart; they include BCS, venoocclusive disease, and chronic right-sided cardiac congestion. Intrahepatic

causes account for over 95% of cases of portal hypertension and are represented by the major forms of cirrhosis. Intrahepatic causes of portal hypertension can be further subdivided into presinusoidal, sinusoidal, and postsinusoidal causes. Postsinusoidal causes include venoocclusive disease, while presinusoidal causes include congenital hepatic fibrosis and schistosomiasis. Sinusoidal causes are related to cirrhosis from various causes.

Cirrhosis is the most common cause of portal hypertension in the United States, and clinically significant portal hypertension is present in >60% of patients with cirrhosis. Portal vein obstruction may be idiopathic or can occur in association with cirrhosis or with infection, pancreatitis, or abdominal trauma.

Coagulation disorders that can lead to the development of portal vein thrombosis include polycythemia vera; essential thrombocytosis; deficiencies in protein C, protein S, antithrombin 3, and factor V Leiden; and abnormalities in the gene-regulating prothrombin production. Some patients may have a subclinical myeloproliferative disorder.

Clinical features

The three primary complications of portal hypertension are gastroesophageal varices with hemorrhage, ascites, and hypersplenism. Thus, patients may present with upper GI bleeding, which, on endoscopy, is found to be due to esophageal or gastric varices, with the development of ascites along with peripheral edema, or with an enlarged spleen with associated reduction in platelets and white blood cells on routine laboratory testing.

Esophageal varices
Over the last decade, it has become common practice to screen known cirrhotics with endoscopy to look for esophageal varices. Such screening studies have shown that approximately one-third of patients with histologically confirmed cirrhosis have varices. Approximately 5–15% of cirrhotics per year develop varices, and it is estimated that the majority of patients with cirrhosis will develop varices over their lifetimes. Furthermore, it is anticipated that roughly one-third of patients with varices will develop bleeding. Several factors predict the risk of bleeding, including the severity of cirrhosis (Child's class, MELD score); the height of wedged-hepatic vein pressure; the size of the varix; the location of the varix; and certain endoscopic stigmata, including red wale signs, hematocystic spots, diffuse erythema, bluish color, cherry red spots, or white-nipple spots. Patients with tense ascites are also at increased risk for bleeding from varices.

Diagnosis

In patients with cirrhosis who are being followed chronically, the development of portal hypertension is

TABLE 42-3

CLASSIFICATION OF PORTAL HYPERTENSION

Prehepatic
  Portal vein thrombosis
  Splenic vein thrombosis
  Massive splenomegaly (Banti's syndrome)

Hepatic
  Presinusoidal
    Schistosomiasis
    Congenital hepatic fibrosis
  Sinusoidal
    Cirrhosis—many causes
    Alcoholic hepatitis
  Postsinusoidal
    Hepatic sinusoidal obstruction (venoocclusive syndrome)

Posthepatic
  Budd-Chiari syndrome
  Inferior vena caval webs
  Cardiac causes
    Restrictive cardiomyopathy
    Constrictive pericarditis
    Severe congestive heart failure

usually revealed by the presence of thrombocytopenia; the appearance of an enlarged spleen; or the development of ascites, encephalopathy, and/or esophageal varices with or without bleeding. In previously undiagnosed patients, any of these features should prompt further evaluation to determine the presence of portal hypertension and liver disease. Varices should be identified by endoscopy. Abdominal imaging, either by CT or MRI, can be helpful in demonstrating a nodular liver and in finding changes of portal hypertension with intraabdominal collateral circulation. If necessary, interventional radiologic procedures can be performed to determine wedged and free hepatic vein pressures that will allow for the calculation of a wedged-to-free gradient, which is equivalent to the portal pressure. The average normal wedged-to-free gradient is 5 mmHg, and patients with a gradient >12 mmHg are at risk for variceal hemorrhage.

TREATMENT   Variceal Hemorrhage

Treatment for variceal hemorrhage as a complication of portal hypertension is divided into two main categories: (1) primary prophylaxis and (2) prevention of re-bleeding once there has been an initial variceal hemorrhage. Primary prophylaxis requires routine screening by endoscopy of all patients with cirrhosis. Once varices that are at increased risk for bleeding are identified, primary prophylaxis can be achieved either through nonselective beta blockade or by variceal band ligation. Numerous placebo-controlled clinical trials of either propranolol or nadolol have been reported in the literature. The most rigorous studies were those that only included patients with significantly enlarged varices or with hepatic vein pressure gradients >12 mmHg. Patients treated with beta blockers have a lower risk of variceal hemorrhage than those treated with placebo over 1 and 2 years of follow-up. There is also a decrease in mortality related to variceal hemorrhage. Unfortunately, overall survival was improved in only one study. Further studies have demonstrated that the degree of reduction of portal pressure is a significant feature to determine success of therapy. Therefore, it has been suggested that repeat measurements of hepatic vein pressure gradients may be used to guide pharmacologic therapy; however, this may be cost-prohibitive. Several studies have evaluated variceal band ligation and variceal sclerotherapy as methods for providing primary prophylaxis.

Endoscopic variceal ligation (EVL) has achieved a level of success and comfort with most gastroenterologists who see patients with these complications of portal hypertension. Thus, in patients with cirrhosis who are screened for portal hypertension and are found to have large varices, it is recommended that they receive either beta blockade or primary prophylaxis with EVL.

The approach to patients once they have had a variceal bleed is first to treat the acute bleed, which can be life-threatening, and then to prevent further bleeding. Prevention of further bleeding is usually accomplished with repeated variceal band ligation until varices are obliterated. Treatment of acute bleeding requires both fluid and blood-product replacement as well as prevention of subsequent bleeding with EVL.

The medical management of acute variceal hemorrhage includes the use of vasoconstricting agents, usually somatostatin or octreotide. Vasopressin was used in the past but is no longer commonly used. Balloon tamponade (Sengstaken-Blakemore tube or Minnesota tube) can be used in patients who cannot get endoscopic therapy immediately or who need stabilization prior to endoscopic therapy. Control of bleeding can be achieved in the vast majority of cases; however, bleeding recurs in the majority of patients if definitive endoscopic therapy has not been instituted. Octreotide, a direct splanchnic vasoconstrictor, is given at dosages of 50–100 µg/h by continuous infusion. Endoscopic intervention is employed as first-line treatment to control bleeding acutely. Some endoscopists will use variceal injection therapy (sclerotherapy) as initial therapy, particularly when bleeding is vigorous. Variceal band ligation is used to control acute bleeding in over 90% of cases and should be repeated until obliteration of all varices is accomplished. When esophageal varices extend into the proximal stomach, band ligation is less successful. In these situations, when bleeding continues from gastric varices, consideration for transjugular intrahepatic portosystemic shunt (TIPS) should be made. This technique creates a portosystemic shunt by a percutaneous approach using an expandable metal stent, which is advanced under angiographic guidance to the hepatic veins and then through the substance of the liver to create a direct portocaval shunt. This offers an alternative to surgery for acute decompression of portal hypertension. Encephalopathy can occur in as many as 20% of patients after TIPS and is particularly problematic in elderly patients and in those patients with preexisting encephalopathy. TIPS should be reserved for those individuals who fail endoscopic or medical management or who are poor surgical risks. TIPS can sometimes be used as a bridge to transplantation. Surgical esophageal transsection is a procedure that is rarely used and generally is associated with a poor outcome.

PREVENTION OF RECURRENT BLEEDING

(Fig. 42-3) Once patients have had an acute bleed and have been managed successfully, attention should be paid to preventing recurrent bleeding. This usually requires repeated variceal band ligation until varices are

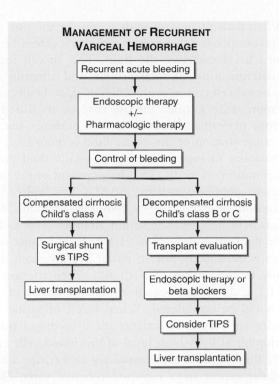

MANAGEMENT OF RECURRENT VARICEAL HEMORRHAGE

Recurrent acute bleeding

Endoscopic therapy +/− Pharmacologic therapy

Control of bleeding

Compensated cirrhosis Child's class A → Surgical shunt vs TIPS → Liver transplantation

Decompensated cirrhosis Child's class B or C → Transplant evaluation → Endoscopic therapy or beta blockers → Consider TIPS → Liver transplantation

FIGURE 42-3

Management of recurrent variceal hemorrhage. This algorithm describes an approach to management of patients who have recurrent bleeding from esophageal varices. Initial therapy is generally with endoscopic therapy often supplemented by pharmacologic therapy. With control of bleeding, a decision needs to be made as to whether patients should go on to a surgical shunt or TIPS (if they are Child's class A) and be considered for transplant, or if they should have TIPS and be considered for transplant (if they are Child's class B or C). TIPS, transjugular intrahepatic portosystemic shunt.

obliterated. Beta blockade may be of adjunctive benefit in patients who are having recurrent variceal band ligation; however, once varices have been obliterated, the need for beta blockade is lessened. Despite successful variceal obliteration, many patients will still have portal hypertensive gastropathy from which bleeding can occur. Nonselective beta blockade may be helpful to prevent further bleeding from portal hypertensive gastropathy once varices have been obliterated.

Portosystemic shunt surgery is less commonly performed with the advent of TIPS; nonetheless, this procedure should be considered for patients with good hepatic synthetic function who could benefit by having portal decompressive surgery.

SPLENOMEGALY AND HYPERSPLENISM

Congestive splenomegaly is common in patients with portal hypertension. Clinical features include the presence of an enlarged spleen on physical examination and the development of thrombocytopenia and leukopenia in patients who have cirrhosis. Some patients will have fairly significant left-sided and left upper quadrant abdominal pain related to an enlarged and engorged spleen. Splenomegaly itself usually requires no specific treatment, although splenectomy can be successfully performed under very special circumstances.

Hypersplenism with the development of thrombocytopenia is a common feature of patients with cirrhosis and is usually the first indication of portal hypertension.

ASCITES

Definition

Ascites is the accumulation of fluid within the peritoneal cavity. Overwhelmingly, the most common cause of ascites is portal hypertension related to cirrhosis; however, clinicians should remember that malignant or infectious causes of ascites can be present as well, and careful differentiation of these other causes are obviously important for patient care.

Pathogenesis

The presence of portal hypertension contributes to the development of ascites in patients who have cirrhosis (Fig. 42-4). There is an increase in intrahepatic resistance, causing increased portal pressure, but there

DEVELOPMENT OF ASCITES IN CIRRHOSIS

Cirrhosis → Portal hypertension → Splanchnic vasodilation

↑ Splanchnic pressure → Lymph formation → Formation of ascites

Arterial underfilling → Activation of vasoconstrictors and antinatriuretic factors* → Sodium retention → Plasma volume expansion

FIGURE 42-4

Development of ascites in cirrhosis. This flow diagram illustrates the importance of portal hypertension with splanchnic vasodilation in the development of ascites. *Antinatriuretic factors include the renin-angiotensin-aldosterone system and the sympathetic nervous system.

is also vasodilation of the splanchnic arterial system, which, in turn, results in an increase in portal venous inflow. Both of these abnormalities result in increased production of splanchnic lymph. Vasodilating factors such as nitric oxide are responsible for the vasodilatory effect. These hemodynamic changes result in sodium retention by causing activation of the renin-angiotensin-aldosterone system with the development of hyperaldosteronism. The renal effects of increased aldosterone leading to sodium retention also contribute to the development of ascites. Sodium retention causes fluid accumulation and expansion of the extracellular fluid volume, which results in the formation of peripheral edema and ascites. Sodium retention is the consequence of a homeostatic response caused by underfilling of the arterial circulation secondary to arterial vasodilation in the splanchnic vascular bed. Because the retained fluid is constantly leaking out of the intravascular compartment into the peritoneal cavity, the sensation of vascular filling is not achieved, and the process continues. Hypoalbuminemia and reduced plasma oncotic pressure also contribute to the loss of fluid from the vascular compartment into the peritoneal cavity. Hypoalbuminemia is due to decreased synthetic function in a cirrhotic liver.

Clinical features

Patients typically note an increase in abdominal girth that is often accompanied by the development of peripheral edema. The development of ascites is often insidious, and it is surprising that some patients wait so long and become so distended before seeking medical attention. Patients usually have at least 1–2 L of fluid in the abdomen before they are aware that there is an increase. If ascitic fluid is massive, respiratory function can be compromised, and patients will complain of shortness of breath. Hepatic hydrothorax may also occur in this setting, contributing to respiratory symptoms. Patients with massive ascites are often malnourished and have muscle wasting and excessive fatigue and weakness.

Diagnosis

Diagnosis of ascites is by physical examination and is often aided by abdominal imaging. Patients will have bulging flanks, may have a fluid wave, or may have the presence of shifting dullness. This is determined by taking patients from a supine position to lying on either their left or right side and noting the movement of the dullness to percussion. Subtle amounts of ascites can be detected by ultrasound or CT scanning. Hepatic hydrothorax is more common on the right side and implicates a rent in the diaphragm with free flow of ascitic fluid into the thoracic cavity.

When patients present with ascites for the first time, it is recommended that a diagnostic paracentesis be performed to characterize the fluid. This should include the determination of total protein and albumin content, blood cell counts with differential, and cultures. In the appropriate setting, amylase may be measured and cytology performed. In patients with cirrhosis, the protein concentration of the ascitic fluid is quite low, with the majority of patients having an ascitic fluid protein concentration <1 g/dL. The development of the serum ascites-to-albumin gradient (SAAG) has replaced the description of exudative or transudative fluid. When the gradient between the serum albumin level and the ascitic fluid albumin level is >1.1 g/dL, the cause of the ascites is most likely due to portal hypertension; this is usually in the setting of cirrhosis. When the gradient is <1.1 g/dL, infectious or malignant causes of ascites should be considered. When levels of ascitic fluid proteins are very low, patients are at increased risk for developing SBP. A high level of red blood cells in the ascitic fluid signifies a traumatic tap or perhaps a hepatocellular cancer or a ruptured omental varix. When the absolute level of polymorphonuclear leukocytes is >250/μL, the question of ascitic fluid infection should be strongly considered. Ascitic fluid cultures should be obtained using bedside inoculation of culture media.

TREATMENT   Ascites

Patients with small amounts of ascites can usually be managed with dietary sodium restriction alone. Most average diets in the United States contain 6 to 8 g of sodium per day, and if patients eat at restaurants or fast-food outlets, the amount of sodium in their diet can exceed this amount. Thus, it is often extremely difficult to get patients to change their dietary habits to ingest <2 g of sodium per day, which is the recommended amount. Patients are frequently surprised to realize how much sodium is in the standard U.S. diet; thus, it is important to make educational pamphlets available to the patient. Often, a simple recommendation is to eat fresh or frozen foods, avoiding canned or processed foods, which are usually preserved with sodium. When a moderate amount of ascites is present, diuretic therapy is usually necessary. Traditionally, spironolactone at 100–200 mg/d as a single dose is started, and furosemide may be added at 40–80 mg/d, particularly in patients who have peripheral edema. In patients who have never received diuretics before, the failure of the previously-mentioned dosages suggests that they are not being compliant with a low-sodium diet. If compliance is confirmed and ascitic fluid is not being mobilized, spironolactone can be increased to 400–600 mg/d and furosemide increased to 120–160 mg/d. If ascites is

TREATMENT OF REFRACTORY ASCITES

- Refractory ascites
- Large-volume paracentesis (LVP) + albumin
- Dietary sodium restriction + diuretics
- Ascites reaccumulation
  - Consider TIPS
  - Continue LVP with albumin as needed
  - Consider liver transplantation

FIGURE 42-5

Treatment of refractory ascites. In patients who develop azotemia in the course of receiving diuretics in the management of their ascites, some will require repeated large-volume paracentesis (LVP), some may be considered for transjugular intrahepatic portosystemic shunt (TIPS), and some would be good candidates for liver transplantation. These decisions are all individualized.

still present with these dosages of diuretics in patients who are compliant with a low-sodium diet, then they are defined as having *refractory ascites*, and alternative treatment modalities including repeated large-volume paracentesis or a TIPS procedure should be considered (Fig. 42-5). Recent studies have shown that TIPS, while managing the ascites, does not improve survival in these patients. Unfortunately, TIPS is often associated with an increased frequency of hepatic encephalopathy and must be considered carefully on a case-by-case basis. The prognosis for patients with cirrhosis with ascites is poor, and some studies have shown that <50% of patients survive 2 years after the onset of ascites. Thus, there should be consideration for liver transplantation in patients with the onset of ascites.

SPONTANEOUS BACTERIAL PERITONITIS

SBP is a common and severe complication of ascites characterized by spontaneous infection of the ascitic fluid without an intraabdominal source. In patients with cirrhosis and ascites severe enough for hospitalization, SBP can occur in up to 30% of individuals and can have a 25% in-hospital mortality rate. Bacterial translocation is the presumed mechanism for development of SBP, with gut flora traversing the intestine into mesenteric lymph nodes, leading to bacteremia and seeding of the ascitic fluid. The most common organisms are *Escherichia coli* and other gut bacteria; however, gram-positive bacteria, including *Streptococcus viridans, Staphylococcus aureus*, and *Enterococcus* sp., can also be found.

If more than two organisms are identified, secondary bacterial peritonitis due to a perforated viscus should be considered. The diagnosis of SBP is made when the fluid sample has an absolute neutrophil count >250/μL. Bedside cultures should be obtained when ascitic fluid is tapped. Patients with ascites may present with fever, altered mental status, elevated white blood cell count, and abdominal pain or discomfort, or they may present without any of these features. Therefore, it is necessary to have a high degree of clinical suspicion, and peritoneal taps are important for making the diagnosis. Treatment is with a second-generation cephalosporin, with cefotaxime being the most commonly used antibiotic. In patients with variceal hemorrhage, the frequency of SBP is significantly increased, and prophylaxis against SBP is recommended when a patient presents with upper GI bleeding. Furthermore, in patients who have had an episode(s) of SBP and recovered, once-weekly administration of antibiotics is used as prophylaxis for recurrent SBP.

HEPATORENAL SYNDROME

The hepatorenal syndrome (HRS) is a form of functional renal failure without renal pathology that occurs in about 10% of patients with advanced cirrhosis or acute liver failure. There are marked disturbances in the arterial renal circulation in patients with HRS; these include an increase in vascular resistance accompanied by a reduction in systemic vascular resistance. The reason for renal vasoconstriction is most likely multifactorial and is poorly understood. The diagnosis is made usually in the presence of a large amount of ascites in patients who have a stepwise progressive increase in creatinine. Type 1 HRS is characterized by a progressive impairment in renal function and a significant reduction in creatinine clearance within 1–2 weeks of presentation. Type 2 HRS is characterized by a reduction in glomerular filtration rate with an elevation of serum creatinine level, but it is fairly stable and is associated with a better outcome than that of type 1 HRS.

HRS is often seen in patients with refractory ascites and requires exclusion of other causes of acute renal failure. Treatment has, unfortunately, been difficult, and in the past, dopamine or prostaglandin analogues were used as renal vasodilating medications. Carefully performed studies have failed to show clear-cut benefit from these therapeutic approaches. Currently, patients are treated with midodrine, an α-agonist, along with octreotide and intravenous albumin. The best therapy for HRS is liver transplantation; recovery of renal function is typical in this setting. In patients with either type 1 or type 2 HRS, the prognosis is poor unless transplant can be achieved within a short period of time.

HEPATIC ENCEPHALOPATHY

Portosystemic encephalopathy is a serious complication of chronic liver disease and is broadly defined as an alteration in mental status and cognitive function occurring in the presence of liver failure. In acute liver injury with fulminant hepatic failure, the development of encephalopathy is a requirement for a diagnosis of fulminant failure. Encephalopathy is much more commonly seen in patients with chronic liver disease. Gut-derived neurotoxins that are not removed by the liver because of vascular shunting and decreased hepatic mass get to the brain and cause the symptoms that we know of as hepatic encephalopathy. Ammonia levels are typically elevated in patients with hepatic encephalopathy, but the correlation between severity of liver disease and height of ammonia levels is often poor, and most hepatologists do not rely on ammonia levels to make a diagnosis. Other compounds and metabolites that may contribute to the development of encephalopathy include certain false neurotransmitters and mercaptans.

Clinical features

In acute liver failure, changes in mental status can occur within weeks to months. Brain edema can be seen in these patients, with severe encephalopathy associated with swelling of the gray matter. Cerebral herniation is a feared complication of brain edema in acute liver failure, and treatment is meant to decrease edema with mannitol and judicious use of intravenous fluids.

In patients with cirrhosis, encephalopathy is often found as a result of certain precipitating events such as hypokalemia, infection, an increased dietary protein load, or electrolyte disturbances. Patients may be confused or exhibit a change in personality. They may actually be quite violent and difficult to manage; alternatively, patients may be very sleepy and difficult to rouse. Because precipitating events are so commonly found, they should be sought carefully. If patients have ascites, this should be tapped to rule out infection. Evidence of GI bleeding should be sought, and patients should be appropriately hydrated. Electrolytes should be measured and abnormalities corrected. In patients presenting with encephalopathy, asterixis is often present. Asterixis can be elicited by having patients extend their arms and bend their wrists back. In this maneuver, patients who are encephalopathic have a "liver flap"—i.e., a sudden forward movement of the wrist. This requires patients to be able to cooperate with the examiner and obviously cannot be elicited in patients who are severely encephalopathic or in hepatic coma.

The diagnosis of hepatic encephalopathy is clinical and requires an experienced clinician to recognize and put together all of the various features. Often when patients have encephalopathy for the first time, they are unaware of what is transpiring, but once they have been through the experience for the first time, they can identify when this is developing in subsequent situations and can often self-medicate to impair the development or worsening of encephalopathy.

TREATMENT Hepatic Encephalopathy

Treatment is multifactorial and includes management of the previously mentioned precipitating factors. Sometimes hydration and correction of electrolyte imbalance is all that is necessary. In the past, restriction of dietary protein was considered for patients with encephalopathy; however, the negative impact of that maneuver on overall nutrition is thought to outweigh the benefit when treating encephalopathy, and it is thus discouraged. There may be some benefit to replacing animal-based protein with vegetable-based protein in some patients with encephalopathy that is difficult to manage. The mainstay of treatment for encephalopathy, in addition to correcting precipitating factors, is to use lactulose, a nonabsorbable disaccharide, which results in colonic acidification. Catharsis ensues, contributing to the elimination of nitrogenous products in the gut that are responsible for the development of encephalopathy. The goal of lactulose therapy is to promote 2–3 soft stools per day. Patients are asked to titrate their amount of ingested lactulose to achieve the desired effect. Poorly absorbed antibiotics are often used as adjunctive therapies for patients who have had a difficult time with lactulose. The alternating administration of neomycin and metronidazole has commonly been employed to reduce the individual side effects of each: neomycin for renal insufficiency and ototoxicity and metronidazole for peripheral neuropathy. More recently, rifaximin at 550 mg twice daily has been very effective in treating encephalopathy without the known side effects of neomycin or metronidazole. Zinc supplementation is sometimes helpful in patients with encephalopathy and is relatively harmless. The development of encephalopathy in patients with chronic liver disease is a poor prognostic sign, but this complication can be managed in the vast majority of patients.

MALNUTRITION IN CIRRHOSIS

Because the liver is principally involved in the regulation of protein and energy metabolism in the body, it is not surprising that patients with advanced liver disease are commonly malnourished. Once patients become cirrhotic, they are more catabolic, and muscle protein is metabolized. There are multiple factors that contribute to the malnutrition of cirrhosis, including poor dietary intake, alterations in gut nutrient absorption, and alterations in protein metabolism. Dietary supplementation for patients with cirrhosis is helpful in preventing patients from becoming catabolic.

ABNORMALITIES IN COAGULATION

Coagulopathy is almost universal in patients with cirrhosis. There is decreased synthesis of clotting factors and impaired clearance of anticoagulants. In addition, patients may have thrombocytopenia from hypersplenism due to portal hypertension. Vitamin K–dependent clotting factors are factors II, VII, IX, and X. Vitamin K requires biliary excretion for its subsequent absorption; thus, in patients with chronic cholestatic syndromes, vitamin K absorption is frequently diminished. Intravenous or intramuscular vitamin K can quickly correct this abnormality. More commonly, the synthesis of vitamin K–dependent clotting factors is diminished because of a decrease in hepatic mass, and, under these circumstances, administration of parenteral vitamin K does not improve the clotting factors or the prothrombin time. Platelet function is often abnormal in patients with chronic liver disease, in addition to decreases in platelet levels due to hypersplenism.

BONE DISEASE IN CIRRHOSIS

Osteoporosis is common in patients with chronic cholestatic liver disease because of malabsorption of vitamin D and decreased calcium ingestion. The rate of bone resorption exceeds that of new bone formation in patients with cirrhosis resulting in bone loss. Dual x-ray absorptiometry (DEXA) is a useful method for determining osteoporosis or osteopenia in patients with chronic liver disease. When a DEXA scan shows decreased bone mass, treatment should be administered with bisphosphonates that are effective at inhibiting resorption of bone and efficacious in the treatment of osteoporosis.

HEMATOLOGIC ABNORMALITIES IN CIRRHOSIS

Numerous hematologic manifestations of cirrhosis are present, including anemia from a variety of causes including hypersplenism, hemolysis, iron deficiency, and perhaps folate deficiency from malnutrition. Macrocytosis is a common abnormality in red blood cell morphology seen in patients with chronic liver disease, and neutropenia may be seen as a result of hypersplenism.

CHAPTER 43
ATLAS OF LIVER BIOPSIES

Jules L. Dienstag ■ Atul K. Bhan

Although clinical and laboratory features yield clues to the extent of inflammatory processes (disease grade), the degree of scarring and architectural distortion (disease stage), and the nature of the disease process, the liver biopsy is felt to represent the gold standard for assessing the degree of liver injury and fibrosis. Examination of liver histology provides not only a basis for quantitative scoring of disease activity and progression but also a wealth of qualitative information that can direct and inform diagnosis and management.

A normal liver lobule consists of portal (zone 1), lobular (midzonal or zone 2), and central (zone 3) zones. The portal tract contains the hepatic artery (HA) and portal vein (PV), which represent the dual vascular supply to the liver, as well as the bile duct (BD). The lobular area contains cords of liver cells surrounded by vascular sinusoids, and the central zone consists of the central vein (CV), the terminal branch of the hepatic vein (see figure below).

Included in this atlas of liver biopsies are examples of common morphologic features of acute and chronic liver disorders, some involving the lobular areas (e.g., the lobular inflammatory changes of acute hepatitis, apoptotic hepatocyte degeneration in acute and chronic hepatitis, virus antigen localization in hepatocyte cytoplasm and/or nuclei, viral inclusion bodies, copper or iron deposition, other inclusion bodies), and others involving the portal tracts (e.g., the portal mononuclear infiltrate

that expands and spills over beyond the border of periportal hepatocytes in chronic hepatitis C, autoimmune hepatitis, and liver allograft rejection) or centrizonal areas (e.g., acute acetaminophen hepatotoxicity). Other histologic features of importance include hepatic steatosis (observed in alcoholic liver injury, in nonalcoholic fatty liver disorders, in metabolic disorders—including mitochondrial injury—and in patients with chronic viral hepatitis); injury of bile ducts in the portal tract, an important diagnostic hallmark of primary biliary cirrhosis, primary sclerosing cholangitis, as well as of liver allograft rejection; cholestasis in intrahepatic or extrahepatic biliary obstruction or in infiltrative disorders; ductular proliferation in the setting of marked hepatocellular necrosis; plasma cell infiltration common in autoimmune hepatitis; portal inflammation affecting portal veins ("endothelialitis") in liver allograft rejection; and mild-to-severe fibrosis, in varying distribution and pattern, as a consequence of liver injury common to many disorders. (All magnifications reflect the objective lens used.)

FIGURE 43-1

Acute hepatitis with lobular inflammation and hepatocellular ballooning (H&E, 10×).

446

FIGURE 43-2
Acute hepatitis, higher magnification, showing lobular inflammation, hepatocellular ballooning, and acidophilic bodies (*arrows*) (H&E, 20×).

FIGURE 43-3
Chronic hepatitis C with portal lymphoid infiltrate and lymphoid follicle containing germinal center (H&E, 10×).

FIGURE 43-4
Chronic hepatitis C with portal and lobular inflammation and steatosis (H&E, 10×).

FIGURE 43-5
Chronic hepatitis C with portal inflammation and interface hepatitis (erosion of the limiting plate of periportal hepatocytes by infiltrating mononuclear cells) (H&E, 20×).

FIGURE 43-6
Lobular inflammation with acidophilic body (apoptotic body) surrounded by lymphoid cells (H&E, 40×).

FIGURE 43-7
Chronic hepatitis B with hepatocellular cytoplasmic staining for hepatitis B surface antigen (immunoperoxidase, 20×).

FIGURE 43-8
Chronic hepatitis B with hepatocellular nuclear staining for hepatitis B core antigen (immunoperoxidase, 20×).

FIGURE 43-9
Autoimmune hepatitis with portal and lobular inflammation, interface hepatitis, and cholestasis (H&E, 10×).

FIGURE 43-10
Autoimmune hepatitis, higher magnification, showing dense plasma cell infiltrate in the portal and periportal regions (H&E, 40×).

FIGURE 43-11
Primary biliary cirrhosis with degenerating bile duct epithelium ("florid ductular lesion") (arrow) surrounded by epithelioid granulomatous reaction and lymphoplasmacytic infiltrate (H&E, 40×).

FIGURE 43-12
Chronic hepatitis C with bridging fibrosis (arrow) (Masson trichrome, 10×).

FIGURE 43-13
Cirrhosis with architectural alteration resulting from fibrosis and nodular hepatocellular regeneration (Masson trichrome, 2×).

FIGURE 43-14
Acute cellular rejection of orthotopic liver allograft demonstrating a mixed inflammatory cell infiltrate (lymphoid cells, eosinophils, neutrophils) of the portal tract as well as endothelialitis of the portal vein (*arrow*) and bile duct injury (H&E, 10×).

FIGURE 43-15
Liver allograft with cytomegalovirus infection showing hepatocytes with nuclear inclusions (*arrows*) surrounded by a neutrophilic and lymphoid infiltrate (H&E, 10×).

FIGURE 43-16
Combined acetaminophen hepatotoxicity and alcoholic liver injury with extensive centrilobular areas of necrosis (H&E, 4×).

FIGURE 43-17
Combined acetaminophen hepatotoxicity and alcoholic liver injury at higher magnification showing necrotic centrilobular area with Mallory bodies (H&E 20×).

FIGURE 43-18
α₁ **Antitrypsin deficiency** with cytoplasmic periodic acid–Schiff (PAS)-positive, diastase-resistant globules in many hepatocytes, predominantly at the periphery of a cirrhotic nodule (PAS, 20×).

FIGURE 43-19
α₁ **Antitrypsin deficiency** with higher magnification of PAS-positive, diastase-resistant globules (PAS, 40×).

FIGURE 43-20

Cirrhosis secondary to hemochromatosis with hepato-cellular carcinoma; brown hemosiderin pigment (iron) is present in the cirrhotic liver, while the hepatocellular carcinoma nodules are hemosiderin-free (H&E, 4×).

FIGURE 43-21

Cirrhosis secondary to hemochromatosis with hepato-cellular carcinoma at higher magnification, demonstrating nodules of large malignant cells with highly disorganized architecture (H&E, 10×).

FIGURE 43-22

Hemochromatosis with iron stain demonstrating extensive iron deposition and characteristic pattern of pericanalicular distribution of iron (iron stain, 10×).

FIGURE 43-23

Primary sclerosing cholangitis showing cirrhosis and periductular fibrosis (Masson trichrome, 4×).

FIGURE 43-24

Primary sclerosing cholangitis showing the extrahepatic bile duct (in a liver explant obtained at the time of hepatectomy for orthotopic liver transplantation) with marked mural chronic inflammation and fibrosis as well as peribiliary glands (H&E, 2×).

FIGURE 43-25

Primary sclerosing cholangitis showing peripheral cholestasis (*green*) and cytoplasmic red granular staining of hepatocytes for copper (rhodanine copper stain, 20×).

FIGURE 43-26
Nonalcoholic steatohepatitis (NASH) showing steatosis, ballooned hepatocytes, and Mallory bodies with surrounding polymorphonuclear leukocytes (*arrow*) (H&E, 20×).

FIGURE 43-27
Nonalcoholic steatohepatitis (NASH) showing steatosis with perisinusoidal and pericellular fibrosis (H&E, 20×).

FIGURE 43-28
Acute hepatitis with submassive hepatic necrosis with marked parenchymal collapse, remnant islands of surviving hepatocytes, and a marked ductular reaction (H&E, 10×).

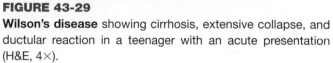

FIGURE 43-29
Wilson's disease showing cirrhosis, extensive collapse, and ductular reaction in a teenager with an acute presentation (H&E, 4×).

FIGURE 43-30
Wilson's disease showing extensive hepatocyte cytoplasmic red granular staining for copper in a cirrhotic nodule (rhodanine copper stain, 20×).

CHAPTER 44

GENETIC, METABOLIC, AND INFILTRATIVE DISEASES AFFECTING THE LIVER

Bruce R. Bacon

There are a number of disorders of the liver that fit within the categories of genetic, metabolic, and infiltrative disorders. Inherited disorders include hemochromatosis, Wilson's disease, α_1 antitrypsin (α_1AT) deficiency, and cystic fibrosis (CF). Hemochromatosis is the most common inherited disorder affecting Caucasian populations, with the genetic susceptibility for the disease being identified in 1 in 250 individuals. Over the past 15 years, it has become increasingly apparent that nonalcoholic fatty liver disease (NAFLD) is the most common cause of elevated liver enzymes found in the U.S. population. With the obesity epidemic in the United States, it is estimated that 20% of the population may have abnormal liver enzymes on the basis of NAFLD and 3% may have nonalcoholic steatohepatitis (NASH). Infiltrative disorders of the liver are relatively rare.

GENETIC LIVER DISEASES

Hereditary hemochromatosis

Hereditary hemochromatosis (HH) is a common inherited disorder of iron metabolism. Our knowledge of the disease and its phenotypic expression has changed since 1996, when the gene for HH, called *HFE*, was identified, allowing for genetic testing for the two major mutations (C282Y and H63D) that are responsible for *HFE*-related HH. Subsequently, several additional genes/proteins involved in the regulation of iron homeostasis have been identified, contributing to a better understanding of cellular iron uptake and release and the characterization of additional causes of inherited iron overload (Table 44-1).

Most patients with HH are asymptomatic; however, when patients present with symptoms, they are frequently nonspecific and include weakness, fatigue, lethargy, and weight loss. Specific, organ-related symptoms include abdominal pain, arthralgias, and symptoms and signs of chronic liver disease. Increasingly, most

patients are now identified before they have symptoms, either through family studies or from the performance of screening iron studies. Several prospective population studies have shown that C282Y homozygosity is found in about 1 in 250 individuals of Northern European descent, with the heterozygote frequency seen in approximately 1 in 10 individuals. It is important to consider HH in patients who present with the symptoms and signs known to occur in established HH. When confronted with abnormal serum iron studies,

TABLE 44-1

CLASSIFICATION OF IRON OVERLOAD SYNDROMES

Hereditary Hemochromatosis (HH)

HFE-related (type 1)
  C282Y/C282Y
  C282Y/H63D
  Other *HFE* mutations

Non-*HFE*-related
  Juvenile HH
    HJV—hemojuvelin (type 2a)
    HAMP—hepcidin (type 2b)
  TfR2-related HH (type 3)
  Ferroportin-related HH (type 4)
  African iron overload

Secondary Iron Overload

Iron-loading anemias
Parenteral iron overload
Chronic liver disease

Miscellaneous

Neonatal iron overload
Aceruloplasminemia
Congenital atransferrinemia

Abbreviations: HJV, hemojuvelin; HAMP, hepcidin; TfR2, transferrin receptor 2.

clinicians should not wait for typical symptoms or findings of HH to appear before considering the diagnosis. However, once the diagnosis of HH is considered, either by an evaluation of abnormal screening iron studies, in the context of family studies, in a patient with an abnormal genetic test, or in the evaluation of a patient with any of the typical symptoms or clinical findings, definitive diagnosis is relatively straightforward. Transferrin saturation (serum iron divided by total iron-binding capacity [TIBC] or transferrin, times 100%) and ferritin levels should be obtained. Both of these will be elevated in a symptomatic patient. It must be remembered that ferritin is an acute-phase reactant and can be elevated in a number of other inflammatory disorders, such as rheumatoid arthritis, or in various neoplastic diseases, such as lymphoma or other cancers. Also, serum ferritin is elevated in a majority of patients with NASH, in the absence of iron overload.

At present, if patients have an elevated transferrin saturation or ferritin level, genetic testing should be performed; if they are a C282Y homozygote or a compound heterozygote (C282Y/H63D), the diagnosis is confirmed. If the ferritin is >1000 μg/L, the patient should be considered for liver biopsy because there is an increased frequency of advanced fibrosis in these individuals. If liver biopsy is performed, iron deposition is found in a periportal distribution with a periportal to pericentral gradient; iron is found predominantly in parenchymal cells, and Kupffer cells are spared.

TREATMENT Hereditary Hemochromatosis

Treatment of HH is relatively straightforward with weekly phlebotomy aimed to reduce iron stores, recognizing that each unit of blood contains 200 to 250 mg of iron. If patients are diagnosed and treated before the development of hepatic fibrosis, all complications of the disease can be avoided. Maintenance phlebotomy is required in most patients and usually can be achieved with 1 unit of blood removed every 2–3 months. Family studies should be performed with transferrin saturation, ferritin, and genetic testing offered to all first-degree relatives.

Wilson's disease

Wilson's disease is an inherited disorder of copper homeostasis first described in 1912. The Wilson's disease gene was discovered in 1993, with the identification of *ATP7B*. This P-type ATPase is involved in copper transport and is necessary for the export of copper from the hepatocyte. Thus, in patients with mutations in *ATP7B*, copper is retained in the liver, leading to increased copper storage and ultimately liver disease as a result.

The clinical presentation of Wilson's disease is variable and includes chronic hepatitis, hepatic steatosis, and cirrhosis in adolescents and young adults. Neurologic manifestations indicate that liver disease is present and include speech disorders and various movement disorders. Diagnosis includes the demonstration of a reduced ceruloplasmin level, increased urinary excretion of copper, the presence of Kayser-Fleischer rings in the corneas of the eyes, and an elevated hepatic copper level, in the appropriate clinical setting. The genetic diagnosis of Wilson's disease is difficult because >200 mutations in *ATP7B* have been described with different degrees of frequency and penetration in certain populations.

TREATMENT Wilson's Disease

Treatment consists of copper-chelating medications such as D-penicillamine and trientine. A role for zinc acetate has also been established. Medical treatment is lifelong, and severe relapses leading to liver failure and death can occur with cessation of therapy. Liver transplantation is curative with respect to the underlying metabolic defect and restores the normal phenotype with respect to copper homeostasis.

α₁ Antitrypsin deficiency

Alpha-1-antitrypsin (AAT) deficiency was first described in the late 1960s in patients with severe pulmonary disease. AAT is a 52-kD glycoprotein produced in hepatocytes, phagocytes, and epithelial cells in the lungs, which inhibits serine proteases, primarily neutrophil elastase. In AAT deficiency, increased amounts of neutrophil elastase can result in progressive lung injury from degradation of elastin leading to premature emphysema. In the 1970s, AAT deficiency was discovered as a cause of neonatal liver disease, so-called "neonatal hepatitis." It is now known to be a cause of liver disease in infancy, early childhood, adolescence, and adults.

In AAT deficiency, variants in the proteinase inhibitor (Pi) gene located on chromosome 14, alters AAT structure interfering with hepatocellular export. Aggregated, deformed polymers of AAT accumulate in the hepatocyte endoplasmic reticulum. There are over 75 different AAT variants. Conventional nomenclature identifies normal variants as PiMM; these individuals have normal blood levels of AAT. The most common abnormal variants are called S and Z. Individuals homozygous for the Z mutation (PiZZ) have low levels of AAT (about 15% of normal), and these patients are susceptible to liver and/or lung disease, yet only a proportion (about 25%) of PiZZ patients develop disease manifestations. Null variants have undetectable levels of AAT and are susceptible to premature lung disease.

AAT deficiency has been identified in all populations; however, the disorder is most common in patients of Northern European and Iberian descent. The disorder affects about 1 in 1500 to 2000 individuals in North America. The natural history of AAT deficiency is quite variable because many individuals with the PiZZ variant never develop disease, whereas others can develop childhood cirrhosis leading to liver transplantation.

In adults, the diagnosis often comes in the course of evaluation of patients with abnormal liver test abnormalities or in a work-up for cirrhosis. A hint to diagnosis may be coexistent lung disease at a relatively young age or a family history of liver and/or lung disease. Patients may have symptoms of pulmonary disease with cough and dyspnea. Liver disease may be asymptomatic other than fatigue, or patients may present with complications of decompensated liver disease.

Diagnosis of AAT deficiency is confirmed by blood tests showing reduced levels of serum AAT, accompanied by Pi determinations. Most patients with liver disease have either PiZZ or PiSZ; occasionally, patients with PiMZ have reduced levels of AAT, but they usually do not have a low enough level to cause disease. Liver biopsy is often performed to determine stage of hepatic fibrosis and shows characteristic PAS-positive, diastase-resistant globules in the periphery of the hepatic lobule.

TREATMENT α₁ Antitrypsin Deficiency

Treatment of AAT deficiency is usually nonspecific and supportive. For patients with liver involvement, other sources of liver injury, such as alcohol, should be avoided. Evidence for other liver diseases (e.g., viral hepatitis B and C, hemochromatosis, NAFLD, etc.) should be sought and treated if possible. Smoking can worsen lung disease progression in AAT and should be discontinued. Patients with lung disease may be eligible to receive infusions of AAT, which has been shown to halt further damage to the lungs. If liver disease becomes decompensated, transplantation should be pursued and is curative. Following transplant, patients express the Pi phenotype of the donor. Finally, risk of hepatocellular carcinoma is significantly increased in patients with cirrhosis due to AAT deficiency.

Cystic fibrosis

CF should also be considered as an inherited form of chronic liver disease, although the principal manifestations of CF include chronic lung disease and pancreatic insufficiency. A small percentage of patients with CF who survive to adulthood have a form of biliary cirrhosis characterized by cholestatic liver enzyme abnormalities and the development of chronic liver disease. Ursodeoxycholic acid is occasionally helpful in improving liver test abnormalities and in reducing symptoms. The disease is slowly progressive.

METABOLIC LIVER DISEASES

Nonalcoholic fatty liver disease

NAFLD was first described in the 1950s when fatty liver was characterized in a group of obese patients. In 1980, Ludwig and colleagues at the Mayo Clinic described 20 obese, diabetic, nonalcoholic patients who had similar findings on liver biopsy to patients with alcoholic liver disease, and the term nonalcoholic steatohepatitis was introduced. The prevalence of NAFLD in the United States and Europe ranges from 14–20%. This increased prevalence relates directly to the obesity epidemic seen in these populations. In the United States, NASH is thought to occur in ~3% of the general population, with fibrosis due to NASH being seen in >40% of obese patients. The spectrum of NAFLD includes simple hepatic steatosis, which, over time, can progress to NASH, with the subsequent development of fibrosis and cirrhosis. Causes of macrovesicular steatosis are listed in Table 44-2. It is now known that many patients with hitherto identified "cryptogenic" cirrhosis in fact have liver disease on the basis of NASH, with the resolution of the steatosis once patients become catabolic due to cirrhosis.

Most patients who come to medical attention with NAFLD are identified as a result of incidentally discovered elevated liver enzymes (ALT, AST). When patients are symptomatic, symptoms include fatigue or a vague right upper quadrant discomfort. ALT is

TABLE 44-2

CAUSES OF MACROVESICULAR STEATOSIS
Insulin resistance, hyperinsulinemia
Centripetal obesity
Type 2 diabetes
Medications
Glucocorticoids
Estrogens
Tamoxifen
Amiodarone
Nutritional
Starvation
Protein deficiency (kwashiorkor)
Choline deficiency
Liver disease
Wilson's disease
Chronic hepatitis C—genotype 3
Indian childhood cirrhosis
Jejunoileal bypass

generally higher than AST, and aminotransferases are only mildly (1.5–2 times the upper limit of normal) elevated. Recent studies have shown that many patients can have advanced fibrosis with NASH and even cirrhosis due to NASH with normal liver enzymes, indicating that the prevalence of the disease is likely to be even greater than was previously suspected. NASH is frequently seen in conjunction with other components of the metabolic syndrome (hypertension, diabetes mellitus, elevated lipids, and obesity), with NAFLD being considered the hepatic manifestation of this syndrome (Chap. 60). Insulin resistance is the underlying link between these various disorders and numerous studies have shown that virtually all patients with NASH have insulin resistance. Abnormal ferritin values are seen in ~50% of patients with NASH, and an elevated ferritin level may be a marker of insulin resistance in NASH.

The diagnosis of NAFLD requires a careful history to determine the amount of alcohol used. Most investigators in the field of fatty liver disease require that <20 g/d of alcohol be consumed to exclude alcoholic liver disease. Laboratory testing for other liver diseases such as hepatitis B and C, iron studies, ceruloplasmin, α_1 antitrypsin levels, and autoimmune serologies should also be determined. Imaging studies can show characteristic features of a fatty liver, but the ultimate diagnosis of either hepatic steatosis or NASH requires liver biopsy. Liver biopsy shows characteristic macrovesicular steatosis with occasional microvesicular fat being identified. A mixed inflammatory infiltrate is found in a lobular distribution. The histologic features of NASH are very similar to those seen in alcoholic liver disease; Mallory's hyaline can be seen in both disorders, although the number of hepatocytes containing Mallory's hyaline and the size of the deposits are frequently greater in alcoholic liver disease than in NASH. The fibrosis that occurs in NASH has a characteristic perivenular and perisinusoidal distribution. Most cross-sectional studies show that up to 30–40% of NASH patients can develop advanced fibrosis, with cirrhosis being identified in 10–15% of individuals in series. Increasingly, patients are being identified with cryptogenic cirrhosis who have most likely had NASH for decades. These patients can develop liver failure and require liver transplantation, and some patients can progress to the development of hepatocellular cancer. Often, when cirrhotic, these patients will not have steatosis on biopsy, but following transplant, NAFLD will frequently recur.

TREATMENT   Nonalcoholic Fatty Liver Disease

The mainstay of treatment of fatty liver disease is weight loss and exercise, which is often difficult to achieve in this population. As an aid to weight loss, orlistat, which is

a reversible inhibitor of gastric and pancreatic lipase, has been shown to result in a small decrease in body weight and is usually fairly well tolerated. This medication is now available over-the-counter. Bariatric surgery has been used and shows striking success, but is obviously a fairly drastic maneuver for induction of weight loss. Recent studies have focused on the presence of insulin resistance at the center of the pathophysiologic mechanisms of NAFLD. The thiazolidinedione medications are PPAR gamma inhibitors, which improve insulin sensitivity within the adipocyte and skeletal muscle by upregulating specific protein kinases involved in decreasing fatty acid synthesis. Two drugs—pioglitizone and rosiglitizone—are currently available and are being evaluated as potential therapeutic options in the treatment of NASH. Antioxidants have also been used, and a recent large multicenter study has shown benefit from vitamin E supplementation. Treatment of hyperlipidemia with statin-type agents has shown improvement in liver enzymes, but they have not been assessed for effects on histology. Ursodeoxycholic acid has been used and improves liver enzymes in patients with many liver diseases, but it has not been definitively helpful for fatty liver disease. At present, efforts should be directed to encouraging patients with NAFLD to lose weight and exercise.

Lipid storage diseases

There are a number of rare lipid storage diseases that involve the liver, including the inherited disorders of Gaucher's and Niemann-Pick disease. Other rare disorders include abetalipoproteinemia, Tangier disease, Fabray's disease, and types I and V hyperlipoproteinemia. Hepatomegaly is present due to increased fat deposition and increased glycogen found in the liver.

Porphyrias

The porphyrias are a group of metabolic disorders in which there are defects in the biosynthesis of heme necessary for incorporation into numerous hemoproteins such as hemoglobin, myoglobin, catalase, and the cytochromes. Porphyrias can present as either acute or chronic diseases, with the acute disorder causing recurring bouts of abdominal pain, and the chronic disorders characterized by painful skin lesions. Porphyria cutanea tarda (PCT) is the most commonly encountered porphyria. Patients present with characteristic vesicular lesions on sun-exposed areas of the skin, principally the dorsum of the hands, the tips of the ears, or the cheeks. About 40% of patients with PCT have mutations in the gene for hemochromatosis (HFE), and ~50% have hepatitis C; thus, iron studies and HFE mutation analysis as well as hepatitis C testing should be considered in all patients who present with PCT. PCT is also associated with excess alcohol use and some medications, most notably estrogens.

TREATMENT Porphyrias

The mainstay of treatment of PCT is iron reduction by therapeutic phlebotomy, which is successful in reversing the skin lesions in the majority of patients. If hepatitis C is present, this should be treated as well. Acute intermittent porphyria presents with abdominal pain, with the diagnosis made by avoidance of certain precipitating factors such as starvation or certain diets. Intravenous heme as hematin has been used for treatment.

INFILTRATIVE DISORDERS

Amyloidosis

Amyloidosis is a metabolic storage disease that results from deposition of insoluble proteins that are aberrantly folded and assembled and then deposited in a variety of tissues. Amyloidosis is divided into two types, primary and secondary, based on the broad concepts of association with myeloma (primary) or chronic inflammatory illnesses (secondary). The disease is generally considered rare, although, in certain disease states or in certain populations, it can be more common. For example, when associated with familial Mediterranean fever, it is seen in high frequency in Sephardic Jews and Armenians living in Armenia and less frequently in Ashkenazi Jews, Turks, and Arabs. Amyloidosis frequently affects patients suffering from tuberculosis and leprosy and can be seen in upwards of 10–15% of patients with ankylosing spondylitis, rheumatoid arthritis, or Crohn's disease. In one surgical pathology series, amyloid was found in <1% of cases. The liver is commonly involved in cases of systemic amyloidosis, but it is frequently inapparent clinically and only documented at autopsy. Pathologic findings in the liver include positive staining with the Congo red histochemical stain where there is an apple-green birefringence noted under polarizing light.

Granulomas

Granulomas are frequently found in the liver when patients are being evaluated for cholestatic liver enzyme abnormalities. Granulomas can be seen in primary biliary cirrhosis, but there are other characteristic clinical (e.g., pruritus, fatigue) and laboratory findings (cholestatic liver tests, antimitochondrial antibody) that allow for a definitive diagnosis of that disorder. Granulomatous infiltration can also be seen as the principal hepatic manifestation of sarcoidosis, and this is the most common presentation of hepatic granulomas. The vast majority of these patients do not require any specific treatment other than what would normally be used for treatment of their sarcoidosis. A small subset, however, can develop a particularly bothersome desmoplastic reaction with a significant increase in fibrosis, which can progress to cirrhosis and liver failure. These patients may require treatment with immunosuppressive therapy and may require liver transplantation. In patients who have granulomas in the liver not associated with sarcoidosis, treatment is rarely needed.

Diagnosis requires liver biopsy, and it is important to establish a diagnosis so that a cause for the elevated liver enzymes is carefully identified. Some medications can cause granulomatous infiltration of the liver, the most notable of which is allopurinol.

Lymphoma

Involvement of the liver with lymphoma can sometimes be with bulky mass lesions but can also be as a difficult-to-diagnose infiltrative disorder that does not show any characteristic findings on abdominal imaging studies. Patients may present with severe liver disease, jaundice, hypoalbuminemia, mild to moderately elevated aminotransferases, and an elevated alkaline phosphatase.

A liver biopsy is required for diagnosis and should be considered when routine blood testing does not lead to a diagnosis of the liver dysfunction.

CHAPTER 45

DISEASES OF THE GALLBLADDER AND BILE DUCTS

Norton J. Greenberger ■ Gustav Paumgartner

PHYSIOLOGY OF BILE PRODUCTION AND FLOW

BILE SECRETION AND COMPOSITION

Bile formed in the hepatic lobules is secreted into a complex network of canaliculi, small bile ductules, and larger bile ducts that run with lymphatics and branches of the portal vein and hepatic artery in portal tracts situated between hepatic lobules. These interlobular bile ducts coalesce to form larger septal bile ducts that join to form the right and left hepatic ducts, which in turn, unite to form the common hepatic duct. The common hepatic duct is joined by the cystic duct of the gallbladder to form the common bile duct (CBD), which enters the duodenum (often after joining the main pancreatic duct) through the ampulla of Vater.

Hepatic bile is an isotonic fluid with an electrolyte composition resembling blood plasma. The electrolyte composition of gallbladder bile differs from that of hepatic bile because most of the inorganic anions, chloride and bicarbonate, have been removed by reabsorption across the gallbladder epithelium. As a result of water reabsorption, total solute concentration of bile increases from 3–4 g/dL in hepatic bile to 10–15 g/dL in gallbladder bile.

Major solute components of bile by moles percent include bile acids (80%), lecithin and traces of other phospholipids (16%), and unesterified cholesterol (4.0%). In the lithogenic state, the cholesterol value can be as high as 8–10%. Other constituents include conjugated bilirubin; proteins (all immunoglobulins, albumin, metabolites of hormones, and other proteins metabolized in the liver); electrolytes; mucus; and, often, drugs and their metabolites.

The total daily basal secretion of hepatic bile is ~500–600 mL. Many substances taken up or synthesized by the hepatocyte are secreted into the bile canaliculi. The canalicular membrane forms microvilli and is associated with microfilaments of actin, microtubules, and other contractile elements. Prior to their secretion into the bile, many substances are taken up into the hepatocyte, while others, such as phospholipids, a portion of primary bile acids, and some cholesterol are synthesized de novo in the hepatocyte. Three mechanisms are important in regulating bile flow: (1) active transport of bile acids from hepatocytes into the bile canaliculi, (2) active transport of other organic anions, and (3) cholangiocellular secretion. The last is a secretin-mediated and cyclic AMP–dependent mechanism that results in the secretion of a sodium- and bicarbonate-rich fluid into the bile ducts.

Active vectorial secretion of biliary constituents from the portal blood into the bile canaliculi is driven by a set of polarized transport systems at the basolateral (sinusoidal) and the canalicular apical plasma membrane domains of the hepatocyte. Two sinusoidal bile salt uptake systems have been cloned in humans, the Na^+/taurocholate cotransporter (NTCP, SLC10A1) and the organic anion–transporting proteins (OATPs), which also transport a large variety of non-bile salt organic anions. Several ATP-dependent canalicular transport systems, "export pumps," (ATP-binding cassette transport proteins, also known as ABC transporters) have been identified, the most important of which are: the bile salt export pump (BSEP, ABCB11); the anionic conjugate export pump (MRP2, ABCC2), which mediates the canalicular excretion of various amphiphilic conjugates formed by phase II conjugation (e.g., bilirubin mono- and diglucuronides and drugs); the multidrug export pump (MDR1, ABCB1) for hydrophobic cationic compounds; and the phospholipid export pump (MDR3, ABCB4). Two hemitransporters ABCG5/G8, functioning as a couple, constitute the canalicular cholesterol and phytosterol transporter. F1C1 (ATP8B1) is an aminophospholipid transferase ("flippase") essential for maintaining the lipid asymmetry of the canalicular membrane. The canalicular membrane also contains ATP-independent transport systems such as the Cl/HCO$_3$ anion exchanger isoform 2 (AE2, SLC4A2) for canalicular bicarbonate secretion. For most of these transporters, genetic defects have been identified that are associated with various forms of cholestasis or defects of biliary excretion. F1C1 is defective in progressive familial intrahepatic cholestasis type 1 (PFIC1) and benign recurrent intrahepatic cholestasis type 1 (BRIC1) and results in ablation of all other ATP-dependent transporter functions. BSEP is defective in PFIC2 and BRIC2. Mutations of MRP2 (ABCC2) cause the Dubin-Johnson syndrome, an inherited form of conjugated hyperbilirubinemia (Chap. 37). A defective MDR3 (ABCB4) results in PFIC3. ABCG5/G8, the canalicular half transporters for cholesterol and other neutral sterols, are defective in sitosterolemia. The cystic fibrosis transmembrane regulator (CFTR, ABCC7) located on bile duct epithelial cells but not on canalicular membranes is defective in cystic fibrosis, which is associated with impaired cholangiocellular pH regulation during ductular bile formation and chronic cholestatic liver disease, occasionally resulting in biliary cirrhosis.

THE BILE ACIDS

The primary bile acids, cholic acid and chenodeoxycholic acid (CDCA), are synthesized from cholesterol in the liver, conjugated with glycine or taurine, and secreted into the bile. Secondary bile acids, including deoxycholate and lithocholate, are formed in the colon as bacterial metabolites of the primary bile acids. However, lithocholic acid is much less efficiently absorbed from the colon than deoxycholic acid. Another secondary bile acid, found in low concentration, is ursodeoxycholic acid (UDCA), a stereoisomer of CDCA. In healthy subjects, the ratio of glycine to taurine conjugates in bile is ~3:1.

Bile acids are detergent-like molecules that in aqueous solutions and above a critical concentration of about 2 mM form molecular aggregates called *micelles*. Cholesterol alone is sparingly soluble in aqueous environments, and its solubility in bile depends on both the total lipid concentration and the relative molar percentages of bile acids and lecithin. Normal ratios of these constituents favor the formation of solubilizing *mixed micelles*, while abnormal ratios promote the precipitation of cholesterol crystals in bile via an intermediate liquid crystal phase.

In addition to facilitating the biliary excretion of cholesterol, bile acids facilitate the normal intestinal absorption of dietary fats, mainly cholesterol and fat-soluble vitamins, via a micellar transport mechanism

(Chap. 15). Bile acids also serve as a major physiologic driving force for hepatic bile flow and aid in water and electrolyte transport in the small bowel and colon.

ENTEROHEPATIC CIRCULATION

Bile acids are efficiently conserved under normal conditions. Unconjugated, and to a lesser degree also conjugated, bile acids are absorbed by *passive diffusion* along the entire gut. Quantitatively much more important for bile salt recirculation, however, is the *active transport* mechanism for conjugated bile acids in the distal ileum (Chap. 15). The reabsorbed bile acids enter the portal bloodstream and are taken up rapidly by hepatocytes, reconjugated, and resecreted into bile (enterohepatic circulation).

The normal bile acid pool size is approximately 2–4 g. During digestion of a meal, the bile acid pool undergoes at least one or more enterohepatic cycles, depending on the size and composition of the meal. Normally, the bile acid pool circulates ~5–10 times daily. Intestinal absorption of the pool is about 95% efficient; therefore, fecal loss of bile acids is in the range of 0.2–0.4 g/d. In the steady state, this fecal loss is compensated by an equal daily synthesis of bile acids by the liver, and, thus, the size of the bile acid pool is maintained. Bile acids returning to the liver suppress de novo hepatic synthesis of primary bile acids from cholesterol by inhibiting the rate-limiting enzyme cholesterol 7-hydroxylase. While the loss of bile salts in stool is usually matched by increased hepatic synthesis, the maximum rate of synthesis is ~5 g/d, which may be insufficient to replete the bile acid pool size when there is pronounced impairment of intestinal bile salt reabsorption.

The expression of ABC transporters in the enterohepatic circulation and of the rate-limiting enzymes of bile acid and cholesterol synthesis are regulated in a coordinated fashion by nuclear receptors, which are ligand-activated transcription factors. The hepatic bile salt export pump (BSEP, ABCB11) is upregulated by the farnesoid X receptor (FXR), a bile acid sensor that also represses bile acid synthesis. The expression of the cholesterol transporter, ABCG5/G8, is upregulated by the liver X receptor (LXR), which is an oxysterol sensor.

GALLBLADDER AND SPHINCTERIC FUNCTIONS

In the fasting state, the sphincter of Oddi offers a high-pressure zone of resistance to bile flow from the CBD into the duodenum. This tonic contraction serves to (1) prevent reflux of duodenal contents into the pancreatic and bile ducts and (2) promote filling of the gallbladder. The major factor controlling the evacuation of the gallbladder is the peptide hormone cholecystokinin

(CCK), which is released from the duodenal mucosa in response to the ingestion of fats and amino acids. CCK produces (1) powerful contraction of the gallbladder, (2) decreased resistance of the sphincter of Oddi, and (3) enhanced flow of biliary contents into the duodenum.

Hepatic bile is "concentrated" within the gallbladder by energy-dependent transmucosal absorption of water and electrolytes. Almost the entire bile acid pool may be sequestered in the gallbladder following an overnight fast for delivery into the duodenum with the first meal of the day. The normal capacity of the gallbladder is ~30 mL of bile.

DISEASES OF THE GALLBLADDER

CONGENITAL ANOMALIES

Anomalies of the biliary tract are not uncommon and include abnormalities in number, size, and shape (e.g., agenesis of the gallbladder, duplications, rudimentary or oversized "giant" gallbladders, and diverticula). *Phrygian cap* is a clinically innocuous entity in which a partial or complete septum (or fold) separates the fundus from the body. Anomalies of position or suspension are not uncommon and include left-sided gallbladder, intrahepatic gallbladder, retrodisplacement of the gallbladder, and "floating" gallbladder. The latter condition predisposes to acute torsion, volvulus, or herniation of the gallbladder.

GALLSTONES

Epidemiology and pathogenesis

Gallstones are quite prevalent in most Western countries. In the United States, the third National Health and Nutrition Examination Survey (NHANES III) has revealed an overall prevalence of gallstones of 7.9% in men and 16.6% in women. The prevalence was high in Mexican Americans (8.9% in men, 26.7% in women), intermediate for non-Hispanic whites (8.6% in men, 16.6% in women), and low for African Americans (5.3% in men, 13.9% in women).

Gallstones are formed because of abnormal bile composition. They are divided into two major types: cholesterol stones account for more than 80% of the total, with pigment stones comprising less than 20%. Cholesterol gallstones usually contain >50% cholesterol monohydrate plus an admixture of calcium salts, bile pigments, and proteins. Pigment stones are composed primarily of calcium bilirubinate; they contain <20% cholesterol and are classified into "black" and "brown" types, the latter forming secondary to chronic biliary infection.

▬▬ Cholesterol stones and biliary sludge

Cholesterol is essentially water insoluble and requires aqueous dispersion into either micelles or vesicles, both of which require the presence of a second lipid to solubilize the cholesterol. Cholesterol and phospholipids are secreted into bile as unilamellar bilayered vesicles, which are converted into mixed micelles consisting of bile acids, phospholipids, and cholesterol by the action of bile acids. If there is an excess of cholesterol in relation to phospholipids and bile acids, unstable, cholesterol-rich vesicles remain, which aggregate into large multilamellar vesicles from which cholesterol crystals precipitate (**Fig. 45-1**).

There are several important mechanisms in the formation of lithogenic (stone-forming) bile. The most important is increased biliary secretion of cholesterol. This may occur in association with obesity, the metabolic syndrome, high-caloric and cholesterol-rich diets, or drugs (e.g., clofibrate) and may result from increased

FIGURE 45-1

Scheme showing pathogenesis of cholesterol gallstone formation. Conditions or factors that increase the ratio of cholesterol to bile acids and phospholipids (lecithin) favor gallstone formation. ABCB4, ATP-binding cassette transporter; ABCG5/8, ATP-binding cassette (ABC) transporter G5/G8; CYP7A1, cytochrome P450 7A1; MDR3, multidrug resistance protein 3, also called phospholipid export pump.

activity of hydroxymethylglutaryl-coenzyme A (HMG-CoA) reductase, the rate-limiting enzyme of hepatic cholesterol synthesis, and increased hepatic uptake of cholesterol from blood. In patients with gallstones, dietary cholesterol *increases* biliary cholesterol secretion. This does not occur in non–gallstone patients on high-cholesterol diets. In addition to environmental factors such as high-caloric and cholesterol-rich diets, genetic factors play an important role in gallstone disease. A large study of symptomatic gallstones in Swedish twins provided strong evidence for a role of genetic factors in gallstone pathogenesis. Genetic factors accounted for 25%, shared environmental factors for 13%, and individual environmental factors for 62% of the phenotypic variation among monozygotic twins. A single nucleotide polymorphism of the gene encoding the hepatic cholesterol transporter ABCG5/G8 has been found in 21% of patients with gallstones, but only in 9% of the general population. It is thought to cause a gain of function of the cholesterol transporter and to contribute to cholesterol hypersecretion. A high prevalence of gallstones is found among first-degree relatives of gallstone carriers and in certain ethnic populations such as American Indians as well as Chilean Indians and Chilean Hispanics. A common genetic trait has been identified for some of these populations by mitochondrial DNA analysis. In some patients, impaired hepatic conversion of cholesterol to bile acids may also occur, resulting in an increase of the lithogenic cholesterol/bile acid ratio. Although most cholesterol stones have a polygenic basis, there are rare monogenic (mendelian) causes. Recently, a mutation in the *CYP7A1* gene has been described that results in a deficiency of the enzyme cholesterol 7-hydroxylase, which catalyzes the initial step in cholesterol catabolism and bile acid synthesis. The homozygous state is associated with hypercholesterolemia and gallstones. Because the phenotype is expressed in the heterozygote state, mutations in the *CYP7A1* gene may contribute to the susceptibility to cholesterol gallstone disease in the population. Mutations in the *MDR3* (ABCB4) gene, which encodes the phospholipid export pump in the canalicular membrane of the hepatocyte, may cause defective phospholipid secretion into bile, resulting in cholesterol supersaturation of bile and formation of cholesterol gallstones in the gallbladder and in the bile ducts. Thus, an excess of biliary cholesterol in relation to bile acids and phospholipids is primarily due to hypersecretion of cholesterol, but hyposecretion of bile acids or phospholipids may contribute. An additional disturbance of bile acid metabolism that is likely to contribute to supersaturation of bile with cholesterol is enhanced conversion of cholic acid to deoxycholic acid, with replacement of the cholic acid pool by an expanded deoxycholic acid pool. It may result from enhanced dehydroxylation of cholic acid and increased absorption of newly formed deoxycholic acid.

An increased deoxycholate secretion is associated with hypersecretion of cholesterol into bile.

While supersaturation of bile with cholesterol is an important prerequisite for gallstone formation, it is generally not sufficient by itself to produce cholesterol precipitation in vivo. Most individuals with supersaturated bile do not develop stones because the time required for cholesterol crystals to nucleate and grow is longer than the time bile spends in the gallbladder.

An important mechanism is *nucleation* of cholesterol monohydrate crystals, which is greatly accelerated in human lithogenic bile. Accelerated nucleation of cholesterol monohydrate in bile may be due to either an *excess of pronucleating factors* or a *deficiency of antinucleating factors*. Mucin and certain non-mucin glycoproteins, principally immunoglobulins, appear to be pronucleating factors, while apolipoproteins A-I and A-II and other glycoproteins appear to be antinucleating factors. Cholesterol monohydrate crystal nucleation and crystal growth probably occur within the mucin gel layer. Vesicle fusion leads to liquid crystals, which, in turn, nucleate into solid cholesterol monohydrate crystals. Continued growth of the crystals occurs by direct nucleation of cholesterol molecules from supersaturated unilamellar or multilamellar biliary vesicles.

A third important mechanism in cholesterol gallstone formation is *gallbladder hypomotility*. If the gallbladder emptied all supersaturated or crystal-containing bile completely, stones would not be able to grow. A high percentage of patients with gallstones exhibit abnormalities of gallbladder emptying. Ultrasonographic studies show that gallstone patients display an increased gallbladder volume during fasting and also after a test meal (residual volume) and that fractional emptying after gallbladder stimulation is decreased.

Biliary sludge is a thick, mucous material that, upon microscopic examination, reveals lecithin-cholesterol liquid crystals, cholesterol monohydrate crystals, calcium bilirubinate, and mucin gels. Biliary sludge typically forms a crescent-like layer in the most dependent portion of the gallbladder and is recognized by characteristic echoes on ultrasonography (discussed later). The presence of biliary sludge implies two abnormalities: (1) the normal balance between gallbladder mucin secretion and elimination has become deranged and (2) nucleation of biliary solutes has occurred. That biliary sludge may be a precursor form of gallstone disease is evident from several observations. In one study, 96 patients with gallbladder sludge were followed prospectively by serial ultrasound studies. In 18%, biliary sludge disappeared and did not recur for at least 2 years. In 60%, biliary sludge disappeared and reappeared; in 14%, gallstones (8% asymptomatic, 6% symptomatic) developed; and in 6%, severe biliary pain with or without acute pancreatitis occurred. In 12 patients, cholecystectomies were performed, 6 for gallstone-associated biliary pain and 3 in symptomatic patients with sludge but without gallstones who had prior attacks of pancreatitis; the latter did not recur after cholecystectomy. It should be emphasized that biliary sludge can develop with disorders that cause gallbladder hypomotility; i.e., surgery, burns, total parenteral nutrition, pregnancy, and oral contraceptives—all of which are associated with gallstone formation. However, the presence of biliary sludge implies supersaturation of bile with either cholesterol or calcium bilirubinate.

Two other conditions are associated with cholesterol-stone or biliary-sludge formation: pregnancy and rapid weight reduction through a very low-calorie diet. There appear to be two key changes during pregnancy that contribute to a "cholelithogenic state": (1) a marked increase in cholesterol saturation of bile during the third trimester and (2) sluggish gallbladder contraction in response to a standard meal, resulting in impaired gallbladder emptying. That these changes are related to pregnancy per se is supported by several studies that show reversal of these abnormalities quite rapidly after delivery. During pregnancy, gallbladder sludge develops in 20–30% of women and gallstones in 5–12%. Although biliary sludge is a common finding during pregnancy, it is usually asymptomatic and often resolves spontaneously after delivery. Gallstones, which are less common than sludge and frequently associated with biliary colic, may also disappear after delivery because of spontaneous dissolution related to bile becoming unsaturated with cholesterol postpartum.

Approximately 10–20% of persons with rapid weight reduction achieved through very low calorie dieting develop gallstones. In a study involving 600 patients who completed a 16-week, 520-kcal/d diet, UDCA in a dosage of 600 mg/d proved highly effective in preventing gallstone formation; gallstones developed in only 3% of UDCA recipients, compared to 28% of placebo-treated patients.

To summarize, cholesterol gallstone disease occurs because of several defects, which include (1) bile supersaturation with cholesterol, (2) nucleation of cholesterol monohydrate with subsequent crystal retention and stone growth, and (3) abnormal gallbladder motor function with delayed emptying and stasis. Other important factors known to predispose to cholesterol-stone formation are summarized in **Table 45-1**.

Pigment stones

Black pigment stones are composed of either pure calcium bilirubinate or polymer-like complexes with calcium and mucin glycoproteins. They are more common in patients who have chronic hemolytic states (with increased conjugated bilirubin in bile), liver cirrhosis, Gilbert's syndrome, or cystic fibrosis. Gallbladder stones in patients with ileal diseases, ileal resection, or ileal bypass generally are also black pigment

TABLE 45-1

PREDISPOSING FACTORS FOR CHOLESTEROL AND PIGMENT GALLSTONE FORMATION

Cholesterol Stones

1. Demographic/genetic factors: Prevalence highest in North American Indians, Chilean Indians, and Chilean Hispanics, greater in Northern Europe and North America than in Asia, lowest in Japan; familial disposition; hereditary aspects
2. Obesity, metabolic syndrome: Normal bile acid pool and secretion but increased biliary secretion of cholesterol
3. Weight loss: Mobilization of tissue cholesterol leads to increased biliary cholesterol secretion while enterohepatic circulation of bile acids is decreased
4. Female sex hormones
   a. Estrogens stimulate hepatic lipoprotein receptors, increase uptake of dietary cholesterol, and increase biliary cholesterol secretion
   b. Natural estrogens, other estrogens, and oral contraceptives lead to decreased bile salt secretion and decreased conversion of cholesterol to cholesteryl esters
5. Increasing age: Increased biliary secretion of cholesterol, decreased size of bile acid pool, decreased secretion of bile salts
6. Gallbladder hypomotility leading to stasis and formation of sludge
   a. Prolonged parenteral nutrition
   b. Fasting
   c. Pregnancy
   d. Drugs such as octreotide
7. Clofibrate therapy: Increased biliary secretion of cholesterol
8. Decreased bile acid secretion
   a. Primary biliary cirrhosis
   b. Genetic defect of the *CYP7A1* gene
9. Decreased phospholipid secretion: Genetic defect of the *MDR3* gene
10. Miscellaneous
   a. High-calorie, high-fat diet
   b. Spinal cord injury

Pigment Stones

1. Demographic/genetic factors: Asia, rural setting
2. Chronic hemolysis
3. Alcoholic cirrhosis
4. Pernicious anemia
5. Cystic fibrosis
6. Chronic biliary tract infection, parasite infections
7. Increasing age
8. Ileal disease, ileal resection or bypass

stones. Enterohepatic recycling of bilirubin in ileal disease states contributes to their pathogenesis. Brown pigment stones are composed of calcium salts of unconjugated bilirubin with varying amounts of cholesterol and protein. They are caused by the presence of increased amounts of unconjugated, insoluble bilirubin in bile that precipitates to form stones. Deconjugation of an excess of soluble bilirubin mono- and diglucuronides may be mediated by endogenous β-glucuronidase but may also occur by spontaneous hydrolysis. Sometimes, the enzyme is also produced when bile is chronically infected by bacteria, and such stones are brown. Pigment stone formation is especially prominent in Asians and is often associated with infections in the gallbladder and biliary tree (Table 45-1).

Diagnosis

Procedures of potential use in the diagnosis of cholelithiasis and other diseases of the gallbladder are detailed in **Table 45-2**. Ultrasonography of the gallbladder is very accurate in the identification of cholelithiasis and has replaced oral cholecystography (**Fig. 45-2***A*). Stones as small as 1.5 mm in diameter may be confidently identified provided that firm criteria are used (e.g., acoustic "shadowing" of opacities that are within the gallbladder lumen and that change with the patient's position [by gravity]). In major medical centers, the false-negative and false-positive rates for ultrasound in gallstone patients are ~2–4%. Biliary sludge is material of low echogenic activity that typically forms a layer in the most dependent position of the gallbladder. This layer shifts with postural changes but fails to produce acoustic shadowing; these two characteristics distinguish sludges from gallstones. Ultrasound can also be used to assess the emptying function of the gallbladder.

The plain abdominal film may detect gallstones containing sufficient calcium to be radiopaque (10–15% of cholesterol and ~50% of pigment stones). Plain radiography may also be of use in the diagnosis of emphysematous cholecystitis, porcelain gallbladder, limey bile, and gallstone ileus.

Oral cholecystography (OCG) has historically been a useful procedure for the diagnosis of gallstones but has been replaced by ultrasound and is regarded as obsolete. It may be used to assess the patency of the cystic duct and gallbladder emptying function. Further, OCG can also delineate the size and number of gallstones and determine whether they are calcified.

Radiopharmaceuticals such as ^{99m}Tc-labeled *N*-substituted iminodiacetic acids (HIDA, DIDA, DISIDA, etc.) are rapidly extracted from the blood and are excreted into the biliary tree in high concentration even in the presence of mild to moderate serum bilirubin elevations. Failure to image the gallbladder in the presence of biliary ductal visualization may indicate cystic duct obstruction, acute or chronic cholecystitis, or surgical absence of the organ. Such scans have some application in the diagnosis of acute cholecystitis.

TABLE 45-2

DIAGNOSTIC EVALUATION OF THE GALLBLADDER

DIAGNOSTIC ADVANTAGES	DIAGNOSTIC LIMITATIONS	COMMENT
Gallbladder Ultrasound		
Rapid Accurate identification of gallstones (>95%) Simultaneous scanning of GB, liver, bile ducts, pancreas "Real-time" scanning allows assessment of GB volume, contractility Not limited by jaundice, pregnancy May detect very small stones	Bowel gas Massive obesity Ascites	Procedure of choice for detection of stones
Plain Abdominal X-Ray		
Low cost Readily available	Relatively low yield ? Contraindicated in pregnancy	Pathognomonic findings in: calcified gallstones Limey bile, porcelain GB Emphysematous cholecystitis Gallstone ileus
Radioisotope Scans (HIDA, DIDA, etc.)		
Accurate identification of cystic duct obstruction Simultaneous assessment of bile ducts	? Contraindicated in pregnancy Serum bilirubin >103–205 μmol/L (6–12 mg/dL) Cholecystogram of low resolution	Indicated for confirmation of suspected acute cholecystitis; less sensitive and less specific in chronic cholecystitis; useful in diagnosis of acalculous cholecystopathy, especially if given with CCK to assess gallbladder emptying

Abbreviations: CCK, cholecystokinin; GB, gallbladder.

FIGURE 45-2

Examples of ultrasound and radiologic studies of the biliary tract. A. An ultrasound study showing a distended gallbladder containing a single large stone (*arrow*), which casts an acoustic shadow. **B.** Endoscopic retrograde cholangiopancreatogram (ERCP) showing normal biliary tract anatomy. In addition to the endoscope and large vertical gallbladder filled with contrast dye, the common hepatic duct (CHD), common bile duct (CBD), and pancreatic duct (PD) are shown. The arrow points to the ampulla of Vater. **C.** Endoscopic retrograde cholangiogram (ERC) showing choledocholithiasis. The biliary tract is dilatated and contains multiple radiolucent calculi. **D.** ERCP showing sclerosing cholangitis. The common bile duct shows areas that are strictured and narrowed.

Symptoms of gallstone disease

Gallstones usually produce symptoms by causing inflammation or obstruction following their migration into the cystic duct or CBD. The most specific and characteristic symptom of gallstone disease is biliary colic that is a constant and often long-lasting pain (discussed later). Obstruction of the cystic duct or CBD by a stone produces increased intraluminal pressure and distention of the viscus that cannot be relieved by repetitive biliary contractions. The resultant visceral pain is characteristically a severe, steady ache or fullness in the epigastrium or right upper quadrant (RUQ) of the abdomen with frequent radiation to the interscapular area, right scapula, or shoulder.

Biliary colic begins quite suddenly and may persist with severe intensity for 15 min to 5 h, subsiding gradually or rapidly. It is steady rather than intermittent as would be suggested by the word *colic*, which must be regarded as a misnomer, although it is in widespread use. An episode of biliary pain persisting beyond 5 h should raise the suspicion of acute cholecystitis (discussed later). Nausea and vomiting frequently accompany episodes of biliary pain. An elevated level of serum bilirubin and/or alkaline phosphatase suggests a common duct stone. Fever or chills (rigors) with biliary pain usually imply a complication, i.e., cholecystitis, pancreatitis, or cholangitis. Complaints of vague epigastric fullness, dyspepsia, eructation, or flatulence, especially following a fatty meal, should not be confused with biliary pain. Such symptoms are frequently elicited from patients with or without gallstone disease but are not specific for biliary calculi. Biliary colic may be precipitated by eating a fatty meal, by consumption of a large meal following a period of prolonged fasting, or by eating a normal meal; it is frequently nocturnal, occurring within a few hours of retiring.

Natural history

Gallstone disease discovered in an asymptomatic patient or in a patient whose symptoms are not referable to cholelithiasis is a common clinical problem. The natural history of "silent," or asymptomatic, gallstones has occasioned much debate. A study of predominantly male silent gallstone patients suggests that the cumulative risk for the development of symptoms or complications is relatively low—10% at 5 years, 15% at 10 years, and 18% at 15 years. Patients remaining asymptomatic for 15 years were found to be unlikely to develop symptoms during further follow-up, and most patients who did develop complications from their gallstones experienced *prior* warning symptoms. Similar conclusions apply to diabetic patients with silent gallstones. Decision analysis has suggested that (1) the cumulative risk of death due to gallstone disease while on expectant management is small, and (2) prophylactic cholecystectomy is not warranted.

Complications requiring cholecystectomy are much more common in gallstone patients who have developed symptoms of biliary pain. Patients found to have gallstones at a young age are more likely to develop symptoms from cholelithiasis than are patients >60 years at the time of initial diagnosis. Patients with diabetes mellitus and gallstones may be somewhat more susceptible to septic complications, but the magnitude of risk of septic biliary complications in diabetic patients is incompletely defined.

TREATMENT Gallstones

SURGICAL THERAPY In asymptomatic gallstone patients, the risk of developing symptoms or complications requiring surgery is quite small (in the range of 1–2% per year). Thus, a recommendation for cholecystectomy in a patient with gallstones should probably be based on assessment of three factors: (1) the presence of symptoms that are frequent enough or severe enough to interfere with the patient's general routine; (2) the presence of a prior complication of gallstone disease, i.e., history of acute cholecystitis, pancreatitis, gallstone fistula, etc.; or (3) the presence of an underlying condition predisposing the patient to increased risk of gallstone complications (e.g., calcified or porcelain gallbladder and/or a previous attack of acute cholecystitis regardless of current symptomatic status). Patients with very large gallstones (>3 cm in diameter) and patients having gallstones in a congenitally anomalous gallbladder might also be considered for prophylactic cholecystectomy. Although young age is a worrisome factor in asymptomatic gallstone patients, few authorities would now recommend routine cholecystectomy in all young patients with silent stones. Laparoscopic cholecystectomy is a minimal-access approach for the removal of the gallbladder together with its stones. Its advantages include a markedly shortened hospital stay, minimal disability, as well as decreased cost, and it is the procedure of choice for most patients referred for elective cholecystectomy.

From several studies involving >4000 patients undergoing laparoscopic cholecystectomy, the following key points emerge: (1) complications develop in ~4% of patients, (2) conversion to laparotomy occurs in 5%, (3) the death rate is remarkably low (i.e., <0.1%), and (4) bile duct injuries are unusual (i.e., 0.2–0.5%) but more frequent than with open cholecystectomy. These data indicate why laparoscopic cholecystectomy has become the "gold standard" for treating symptomatic cholelithiasis.

MEDICAL THERAPY—GALLSTONE DISSOLUTION Ursodeoxycholic acid (UDCA) decreases cholesterol saturation of bile and also appears to produce a lamellar liquid crystalline phase in bile that allows a dispersion of cholesterol from stones by physical-chemical means. UDCA may also retard cholesterol crystal nucleation. In carefully selected patients with a functioning gallbladder and with radiolucent stones <10 mm in diameter, complete dissolution can be achieved in ~50% of patients within 6 months to 2 years. For good results within a reasonable time period, this therapy should be limited to radiolucent stones smaller than 5 mm in diameter. The dose of UDCA should be 10–15 mg/kg per day. Stones larger than 15 mm in size rarely dissolve. Pigment stones are not responsive to UDCA therapy. The highest success rate (i.e., >70%) occurs in patients with small (<5 mm) floating radiolucent gallstones. Probably ≤10% of patients with *symptomatic* cholelithiasis are candidates for such treatment. However, in addition to the vexing problem of recurrent stones (30–50% over 3–5 years of follow-up), there is also the factor of taking an expensive drug for up to 2 years. The advantages and success of laparoscopic cholecystectomy have largely reduced the role of gallstone dissolution to patients who wish to avoid or are not candidates for elective cholecystectomy. However, patients with cholesterol gallstone disease who develop recurrent choledocholithiasis after cholecystectomy should be on long-term treatment with ursodeoxycholic acid.

ACUTE AND CHRONIC CHOLECYSTITIS
Acute cholecystitis

Acute inflammation of the gallbladder wall usually follows obstruction of the cystic duct by a stone. Inflammatory response can be evoked by three factors: (1) *mechanical inflammation* produced by increased intraluminal pressure and distention with resulting ischemia of the gallbladder mucosa and wall, (2) *chemical inflammation* caused by the release of lysolecithin (due to the action of phospholipase on lecithin in bile) and other local tissue factors, and (3) *bacterial inflammation*, which may play a role in 50–85% of patients with acute cholecystitis. The organisms most frequently isolated by culture of gallbladder bile in these patients include *Escherichia coli*, *Klebsiella* spp., *Streptococcus* spp., and *Clostridium* spp.

Acute cholecystitis often begins as an attack of biliary pain that progressively worsens. Approximately 60–70% of patients report having experienced prior attacks that resolved spontaneously. As the episode progresses, however, the pain of acute cholecystitis becomes more generalized in the right upper abdomen. As with biliary colic, the pain of cholecystitis may radiate to the interscapular area, right scapula, or shoulder. Peritoneal signs of inflammation such as increased pain with jarring or on deep respiration may be apparent. The patient is anorectic and often nauseated. Vomiting is relatively common and may produce symptoms and signs of vascular and extracellular volume depletion. Jaundice is unusual early in the course of acute cholecystitis but may occur when edematous inflammatory changes involve the bile ducts and surrounding lymph nodes.

A low-grade fever is characteristically present, but shaking chills or rigors are not uncommon. The RUQ of the abdomen is almost invariably tender to palpation. An enlarged, tense gallbladder is palpable in 25–50% of patients. Deep inspiration or cough during subcostal palpation of the RUQ usually produces increased pain and inspiratory arrest (Murphy's sign). Localized rebound tenderness in the RUQ is common, as are abdominal distention and hypoactive bowel sounds from paralytic ileus, but generalized peritoneal signs and abdominal rigidity are usually lacking, in the absence of perforation.

The diagnosis of acute cholecystitis is usually made on the basis of a characteristic history and physical examination. The triad of sudden onset of RUQ tenderness, fever, and leukocytosis is highly suggestive. Typically, leukocytosis in the range of 10,000–15,000 cells per microliter with a left shift on differential count is found. The serum bilirubin is mildly elevated (<85.5 μmol/L [5 mg/dL]) in fewer than half of patients, while about one-fourth have modest elevations in serum aminotransferases (usually less than a fivefold elevation). Ultrasound will demonstrate calculi in 90–95% of cases and is useful for detection of signs of gallbladder inflammation including thickening of the wall, pericholecystic fluid, and dilation of the bile duct. The radionuclide (e.g., HIDA) biliary scan may be confirmatory if bile duct imaging is seen without visualization of the gallbladder.

Approximately 75% of patients treated medically have remission of acute symptoms within 2–7 days following hospitalization. In 25%, however, a complication of acute cholecystitis will occur despite conservative treatment (discussed later). In this setting, prompt surgical intervention is required. Of the 75% of patients with acute cholecystitis who undergo remission of symptoms, ~25% will experience a recurrence of cholecystitis within 1 year, and 60% will have at least one recurrent bout within 6 years. In view of the natural history of the disease, acute cholecystitis is best treated by early surgery whenever possible.

Mirizzi's syndrome is a rare complication in which a gallstone becomes impacted in the cystic duct or neck of the gallbladder causing compression of the CBD, resulting in CBD obstruction and jaundice. Ultrasound shows gallstone(s) lying outside the hepatic duct. Endoscopic retrograde cholangiopancreatography (ERCP) (Fig. 45-2B) or percutaneous transhepatic cholangiography (PTC) or magnetic resonance cholangiopancreatography (MRCP) will usually demonstrate the characteristic extrinsic compression of the CBD. Surgery consists of removing the cystic duct, diseased gallbladder, and the impacted stone. The preoperative diagnosis of Mirizzi's syndrome is important to avoid CBD injury.

Acalculous cholecystitis

In 5–10% of patients with acute cholecystitis, calculi obstructing the cystic duct are not found at surgery. In >50% of such cases, an underlying explanation for acalculous inflammation is not found. An increased risk for the development of acalculous cholecystitis is especially associated with serious trauma or burns, with the postpartum period following prolonged labor, and with orthopedic and other nonbiliary major surgical operations in the postoperative period. It may possibly complicate periods of prolonged parenteral hyperalimentation. For some of these cases, biliary sludge in the cystic duct may be responsible. Other precipitating factors include vasculitis, obstructing adenocarcinoma of the gallbladder, diabetes mellitus, torsion of the gallbladder, "unusual" bacterial infections of the gallbladder (e.g., *Leptospira*, *Streptococcus*, *Salmonella*, or *Vibrio cholerae*), and parasitic infestation of the gallbladder. Acalculous cholecystitis may also be seen with a variety of other systemic disease processes (sarcoidosis, cardiovascular disease, tuberculosis, syphilis, actinomycosis, etc.).

Although the clinical manifestations of acalculous cholecystitis are indistinguishable from those of calculous cholecystitis, the setting of acute gallbladder inflammation complicating severe underlying illness is characteristic of acalculous disease. Ultrasound, CT, or radionuclide examinations demonstrating a large, tense, static gallbladder without stones and with evidence of poor emptying over a prolonged period may be diagnostically useful in some cases. The complication rate for acalculous cholecystitis exceeds that for calculous cholecystitis. Successful management of acute acalculous cholecystitis appears to depend primarily on early diagnosis and surgical intervention, with meticulous attention to postoperative care.

Acalculous cholecystopathy

Disordered motility of the gallbladder can produce recurrent biliary pain in patients without gallstones. Infusion of an octapeptide of CCK can be used to measure the gallbladder ejection fraction during cholescintigraphy. The surgical findings have included abnormalities such as chronic cholecystitis, gallbladder muscle hypertrophy, and/or a markedly narrowed cystic duct. Some of these patients may well have had antecedent gallbladder disease. The following criteria can be used to identify patients with acalculous cholecystopathy: (1) recurrent episodes of typical RUQ pain characteristic of biliary tract pain, (2) abnormal CCK cholescintigraphy demonstrating a gallbladder ejection fraction of <40%, and (3) infusion of CCK reproduces the patient's pain. An additional clue would be the identification of a large gallbladder on ultrasound examination. Finally, it should be noted that sphincter of Oddi dysfunction can also give rise to recurrent RUQ pain and CCK-scintigraphic abnormalities.

Emphysematous cholecystitis

So-called emphysematous cholecystitis is thought to begin with acute cholecystitis (calculous or acalculous) followed by ischemia or gangrene of the gallbladder wall and infection by gas-producing organisms. Bacteria most frequently cultured in this setting include anaerobes, such as *C. welchii* or *C. perfringens*, and aerobes, such as *E. coli*. This condition occurs most frequently in elderly men and in patients with diabetes mellitus. The clinical manifestations are essentially indistinguishable from those of nongaseous cholecystitis. The diagnosis is usually made on plain abdominal film by finding gas within the gallbladder lumen, dissecting within the gallbladder wall to form a gaseous ring, or in the pericholecystic tissues. The morbidity and mortality rates with emphysematous cholecystitis are considerable. Prompt surgical intervention coupled with appropriate antibiotics is mandatory.

Chronic cholecystitis

Chronic inflammation of the gallbladder wall is almost always associated with the presence of gallstones and is thought to result from repeated bouts of subacute or acute cholecystitis or from persistent mechanical irritation of the gallbladder wall by gallstones. The presence of bacteria in the bile occurs in >25% of patients with chronic cholecystitis. The presence of infected bile in a patient with *chronic* cholecystitis undergoing elective cholecystectomy probably adds little to the operative risk. Chronic cholecystitis may be asymptomatic for years, may progress to symptomatic gallbladder disease or to acute cholecystitis, or may present with complications (see next section).

Complications of cholecystitis

Empyema and hydrops

Empyema of the gallbladder usually results from progression of acute cholecystitis with persistent cystic duct obstruction to superinfection of the stagnant bile with a pus-forming bacterial organism. The clinical picture resembles that of cholangitis with high fever; severe RUQ pain; marked leukocytosis; and often, prostration. Empyema of the gallbladder carries a high risk of gram-negative sepsis and/or perforation. Emergency surgical intervention with proper antibiotic coverage is required as soon as the diagnosis is suspected.

Hydrops or mucocele of the gallbladder may also result from prolonged obstruction of the cystic duct, usually by a large solitary calculus. In this instance, the obstructed gallbladder lumen is progressively distended, over a period of time, by mucus (mucocele) or by a clear transudate (hydrops) produced by mucosal epithelial cells. A visible, easily palpable, nontender mass sometimes extending from the RUQ into the right iliac fossa may be found on physical examination. The patient with hydrops of the gallbladder frequently remains asymptomatic, although chronic RUQ pain may also occur. Cholecystectomy is indicated, because empyema, perforation, or gangrene may complicate the condition.

Gangrene and perforation

Gangrene of the gallbladder results from ischemia of the wall and patchy or complete tissue necrosis. Underlying conditions often include marked distention of the gallbladder, vasculitis, diabetes mellitus, empyema, or torsion resulting in arterial occlusion. Gangrene usually predisposes to perforation of the gallbladder, but perforation may also occur in chronic cholecystitis without premonitory warning symptoms. *Localized perforations* are usually contained by the omentum or by adhesions produced by recurrent inflammation of the gallbladder. Bacterial superinfection of the walled-off gallbladder contents results in abscess formation. Most patients are best treated with cholecystectomy, but some seriously ill patients may be managed with cholecystostomy and drainage of the abscess. *Free perforation* is less common but is associated with a mortality rate of ~30%. Such patients may experience a sudden transient relief of RUQ pain as the distended gallbladder decompresses; this is followed by signs of generalized peritonitis.

Fistula formation and gallstone ileus

Fistulization into an adjacent organ adherent to the gallbladder wall may result from inflammation and adhesion formation. Fistulas into the duodenum are most common, followed in frequency by those involving the hepatic flexure of the colon, stomach or jejunum, abdominal wall, and renal pelvis. Clinically "silent" biliary-enteric fistulas occurring as a complication of acute cholecystitis have been found in up to 5% of patients undergoing cholecystectomy. Asymptomatic cholecystoenteric fistulas may sometimes be diagnosed by finding gas in the biliary tree on plain abdominal films. Barium contrast studies or endoscopy of the upper gastrointestinal tract or colon may demonstrate the fistula. Treatment in the symptomatic patient usually consists of cholecystectomy, CBD exploration, and closure of the fistulous tract.

Gallstone ileus refers to mechanical intestinal obstruction resulting from the passage of a large gallstone into the bowel lumen. The stone customarily enters the duodenum through a cholecystoenteric fistula at that level. The site of obstruction by the impacted gallstone is usually at the ileocecal valve, provided that the more proximal small bowel is of normal caliber. The majority of patients do not give a history of either prior biliary tract symptoms or complaints suggestive of acute cholecystitis or fistulization. Large stones, >2.5 cm in diameter, are thought to predispose to fistula formation by gradual erosion through the gallbladder fundus. Diagnostic confirmation may occasionally be found on the plain abdominal film (e.g., small-intestinal obstruction with gas in the biliary tree and a calcified, ectopic gallstone) or following an upper gastrointestinal series (cholecystoduodenal fistula with small-bowel obstruction at the ileocecal valve). Laparotomy with stone extraction (or propulsion into the colon) remains the procedure of choice to relieve obstruction. Evacuation of large stones within the gallbladder should also be performed. In general, the gallbladder and its attachment to the intestines should be left alone.

Limey (milk of calcium) bile and porcelain gallbladder

Calcium salts in the lumen of the gallbladder in sufficient concentration may produce calcium precipitation and diffuse, hazy opacification of bile or a layering effect on plain abdominal roentgenography. This so-called limey bile, or milk of calcium bile, is usually clinically innocuous, but cholecystectomy is recommended, especially when it occurs in a hydropic gallbladder. In the entity called *porcelain gallbladder*, calcium salt deposition within the wall of a chronically inflamed gallbladder may be detected on the plain abdominal film. Cholecystectomy is advised in all patients with porcelain gallbladder because in a high percentage of cases this finding appears to be associated with the development of carcinoma of the gallbladder.

TREATMENT Acute Cholecystitis

MEDICAL THERAPY Although surgical intervention remains the mainstay of therapy for acute cholecystitis and its complications, a period of in-hospital stabilization may be required before cholecystectomy. Oral intake is eliminated, nasogastric suction may be indicated, and extracellular volume depletion and electrolyte abnormalities are repaired. Meperidine or nonsteroidal anti-inflammatory drugs (NSAIDs) are usually employed for analgesia because they may produce less spasm of the sphincter of Oddi than drugs such as morphine. Intravenous antibiotic therapy is usually indicated in patients with severe acute cholecystitis, even though bacterial superinfection of bile may not have occurred in the early stages of the inflammatory process. Antibiotic therapy is guided by the most common organisms likely to be present, which are *E. coli*, *Klebsiella* spp., and *Streptococcus* spp. Effective antibiotics include ureidopenicillins such as piperacillin or mezlocillin, ampicillin sulbactam, ciprofloxacin, moxifloxacin, and third-generation cephalosporins. Anaerobic coverage by a drug such as metronidazole should be added if gangrenous or emphysematous cholecystitis is

suspected. Imipenem/meropenem represent potent parenteral antibiotics that cover the whole spectrum of bacteria causing ascending cholangitis. They should, however, be reserved for the most severe, life-threatening infections when other regimens have failed. Postoperative complications of wound infection, abscess formation, and sepsis are reduced in antibiotic-treated patients.

SURGICAL THERAPY The optimal timing of surgical intervention in patients with acute cholecystitis depends on stabilization of the patient. The clear trend is toward earlier surgery, and this is due in part to requirements for shorter hospital stays. Urgent (emergency) cholecystectomy or cholecystostomy is probably appropriate in most patients in whom a complication of acute cholecystitis such as empyema, emphysematous cholecystitis, or perforation is suspected or confirmed. Patients with uncomplicated acute cholecystitis should undergo early elective laparoscopic cholecystectomy, ideally within 72 h after diagnosis. The complication rate is not increased in patients undergoing early as opposed to delayed (>6 weeks after diagnosis) cholecystectomy. Delayed surgical intervention is probably best reserved for (1) patients in whom the overall medical condition imposes an unacceptable risk for early surgery and (2) patients in whom the diagnosis of acute cholecystitis is in doubt. Early cholecystectomy (within 72 h) is the treatment of choice for most patients with acute cholecystitis. Mortality figures for emergency cholecystectomy in most centers approach 3%, while the mortality risk for early elective cholecystectomy is ~0.5% in patients under age 60. Of course, the operative risks increase with age-related diseases of other organ systems and with the presence of long- or short-term complications of gallbladder disease. Seriously ill or debilitated patients with cholecystitis may be managed with cholecystostomy and tube drainage of the gallbladder. Elective cholecystectomy may then be done at a later date.

Postcholecystectomy complications

Early complications following cholecystectomy include atelectasis and other pulmonary disorders, abscess formation (often subphrenic), external or internal hemorrhage, biliary-enteric fistula, and bile leaks. Jaundice may indicate absorption of bile from an intraabdominal collection following a biliary leak or mechanical obstruction of the CBD by retained calculi, intraductal blood clots, or extrinsic compression.

Overall, cholecystectomy is a very successful operation that provides total or near-total relief of preoperative symptoms in 75–90% of patients. The most common cause of persistent postcholecystectomy symptoms is an overlooked symptomatic nonbiliary disorder (e.g., reflux esophagitis, peptic ulceration, pancreatitis, or—most often—irritable bowel syndrome). In a small percentage of patients, however, a disorder of the extrahepatic bile ducts may result in persistent symptomatology. These so-called postcholecystectomy syndromes may be due to (1) biliary strictures, (2) retained biliary calculi, (3) cystic duct stump syndrome, (4) stenosis or dyskinesia of the sphincter of Oddi, or (5) bile salt–induced diarrhea or gastritis.

Cystic duct stump syndrome

In the absence of cholangiographically demonstrable retained stones, symptoms resembling biliary pain or cholecystitis in the postcholecystectomy patient have frequently been attributed to disease in a long (>1 cm) cystic duct remnant (cystic duct stump syndrome). Careful analysis, however, reveals that postcholecystectomy complaints are attributable to other causes in almost all patients in whom the symptom complex was originally thought to result from the existence of a long cystic duct stump. Accordingly, considerable care should be taken to investigate the possible role of other factors in the production of postcholecystectomy symptoms before attributing them to cystic duct stump syndrome.

Papillary dysfunction, papillary stenosis, spasm of the sphincter of Oddi, and biliary dyskinesia

Symptoms of biliary colic accompanied by signs of recurrent, intermittent biliary obstruction may be produced by papillary stenosis, papillary dysfunction, spasm of the sphincter of Oddi, and biliary dyskinesia. Papillary stenosis is thought to result from acute or chronic inflammation of the papilla of Vater or from glandular hyperplasia of the papillary segment. Five criteria have been used to define papillary stenosis: (1) upper abdominal pain, usually RUQ or epigastric; (2) abnormal liver tests; (3) dilatation of the common bile duct upon ERCP examination; (4) delayed (>45 min) drainage of contrast material from the duct; and (5) increased basal pressure of the sphincter of Oddi, a finding that may be of only minor significance. An alternative to ERCP is magnetic resonance cholangiography (MRC) if ERCP and/or biliary manometry are either unavailable or not feasible. In patients with papillary stenosis, quantitative hepatobiliary scintigraphy has revealed delayed transit from the common bile duct to the bowel, ductal dilatation, and abnormal time-activity dynamics. This technique can also be used before and after sphincterotomy to document improvement in biliary emptying. Treatment consists of endoscopic or surgical sphincteroplasty to ensure wide patency of the distal portions of both the bile and pancreatic ducts. The greater the number of the preceding criteria present, the greater the likelihood that a patient does have a degree of papillary stenosis sufficient to justify correction. The factors usually considered as indications for sphincterotomy include (1) prolonged duration of symptoms, (2) lack of response to symptomatic treatment, (3) presence of severe disability, and (4) the patient's choice of sphincterotomy over surgery (given a clear understanding on his or her part of the risks involved in both procedures).

Criteria for diagnosing dyskinesia of the sphincter of Oddi are even more controversial than those for papillary stenosis. Proposed mechanisms include spasm of the sphincter, denervation sensitivity resulting in hypertonicity, and abnormalities of the sequencing or frequency rates of sphincteric-contraction waves. When thorough evaluation has failed to demonstrate another cause for the pain, and when cholangiographic and manometric criteria suggest a diagnosis of biliary dyskinesia, medical treatment with nitrites or anticholinergics to attempt pharmacologic relaxation of the sphincter has been proposed. Endoscopic biliary sphincterotomy (EBS) or surgical sphincteroplasty may be indicated in patients who fail to respond to a 2- to 3-month trial of medical therapy, especially if basal sphincter of Oddi pressures are elevated. EBS has become the procedure of choice for removing bile duct stones and for other biliary and pancreatic problems.

Bile salt–induced diarrhea and gastritis

Postcholecystectomy patients may develop symptoms of dyspepsia, which have been attributed to duodenogastric reflux of bile. However, firm data linking these symptoms to bile gastritis after surgical removal of the gallbladder are lacking. Cholecystectomy induces persistent changes in gut transit, and these changes effect a noticeable modification of bowel habits. Cholecystectomy shortens gut transit time by accelerating passage of the fecal bolus through the colon with marked acceleration in the right colon, thus causing an increase in colonic bile acid output and a shift in bile acid composition toward the more diarrheagenic secondary bile acids. Diarrhea that is severe enough, i.e., three or more watery movements per day, can be classified as postcholecystectomy diarrhea, and this occurs in 5–10% of patients undergoing elective cholecystectomy. Treatment with bile acid–sequestering agents such as cholestyramine or colestipol is often effective in ameliorating troublesome diarrhea.

THE HYPERPLASTIC CHOLECYSTOSES

The term *hyperplastic cholecystoses* is used to denote a group of disorders of the gallbladder characterized by excessive proliferation of normal tissue components.

Adenomyomatosis is characterized by a benign proliferation of gallbladder surface epithelium with glandlike formations, extramural sinuses, transverse strictures, and/or fundal nodule ("adenoma" or "adenomyoma") formation.

Cholesterolosis is characterized by abnormal deposition of lipid, especially cholesteryl esters within macrophages in the lamina propria of the gallbladder wall. In its diffuse form ("strawberry gallbladder"), the gallbladder mucosa is brick red and speckled with bright yellow flecks of lipid. The localized form shows solitary or multiple "cholesterol polyps" studding the gallbladder wall. Cholesterol stones of the gallbladder are found in nearly half the cases. Cholecystectomy is indicated in both adenomyomatosis and cholesterolosis when symptomatic or when cholelithiasis is present.

The prevalence of gallbladder polyps in the adult population is ~5%, with a marked male predominance. Few significant changes have been found over a 5-year period in asymptomatic patients with gallbladder polyps <10 mm in diameter. Cholecystectomy is recommended in symptomatic patients, as well as in asymptomatic patients >50 years of age, or in those whose polyps are >10 mm in diameter or associated with gallstones or polyp growth on serial ultrasonography.

DISEASES OF THE BILE DUCTS

CONGENITAL ANOMALIES

Biliary atresia and hypoplasia

Atretic and hypoplastic lesions of the extrahepatic and large intrahepatic bile ducts are the most common biliary anomalies of clinical relevance encountered in infancy. The clinical picture is one of severe obstructive jaundice during the first month of life, with pale stools. When biliary atresia is suspected on the basis of clinical, laboratory, and imaging findings the diagnosis is confirmed by surgical exploration and operative cholangiography. Approximately 10% of cases of biliary atresia are treatable with roux-en-Y choledochojejunostomy, with the Kasai procedure (hepatic portoenterostomy) being attempted in the remainder in an effort to restore some bile flow. Most patients, even those having successful biliary-enteric anastomoses, eventually develop chronic cholangitis, extensive hepatic fibrosis, and portal hypertension.

Choledochal cysts

Cystic dilatation may involve the free portion of the CBD, i.e., choledochal cyst, or may present as diverticulum formation in the intraduodenal segment. In the latter situation, chronic reflux of pancreatic juice into the biliary tree can produce inflammation and stenosis of the extrahepatic bile ducts leading to cholangitis or biliary obstruction. Because the process may be gradual, ~50% of patients present with onset of symptoms after age 10. The diagnosis may be made by ultrasound, abdominal CT, MRC, or cholangiography. Only one-third of patients show the classic triad of abdominal pain, jaundice, and an abdominal mass. Ultrasonographic detection of a cyst separate from the gallbladder should suggest the diagnosis of choledochal cyst, which can be confirmed by demonstrating the entrance of extrahepatic bile ducts into the cyst. Surgical treatment involves excision of the "cyst" and biliary-enteric anastomosis. Patients with choledochal cysts are at increased risk for the subsequent development of cholangiocarcinoma.

Congenital biliary ectasia

Dilatation of intrahepatic bile ducts may involve either the major intrahepatic radicles (Caroli's disease), the inter- and intralobular ducts (congenital hepatic fibrosis), or both. In Caroli's disease, clinical manifestations include recurrent cholangitis, abscess formation in and around the affected ducts, and, often, gallstone formation within portions of ectatic intrahepatic biliary radicles. Ultrasound, MRC, and CT are of great diagnostic value in demonstrating cystic dilatation of the intrahepatic bile ducts. Treatment with ongoing antibiotic therapy is usually undertaken in an effort to limit the frequency and severity of recurrent bouts of cholangitis. Progression to secondary biliary cirrhosis with portal hypertension, extrahepatic biliary obstruction, cholangiocarcinoma, or recurrent episodes of sepsis with hepatic abscess formation is common.

CHOLEDOCHOLITHIASIS

Pathophysiology and clinical manifestations

Passage of gallstones into the CBD occurs in ~10–15% of patients with cholelithiasis. The incidence of common duct stones increases with increasing age of the patient, so that up to 25% of elderly patients may have calculi in the common duct at the time of cholecystectomy. Undetected duct stones are left behind in ~1–5% of cholecystectomy patients. The overwhelming majority of bile duct stones are cholesterol stones formed in the gallbladder, which then migrate into the extrahepatic biliary tree through the cystic duct. Primary calculi arising de novo in the ducts are usually pigment stones developing in patients with (1) hepatobiliary parasitism or chronic, recurrent cholangitis; (2) congenital anomalies of the bile ducts (especially Caroli's disease); (3) dilated, sclerosed, or strictured ducts; or (4) an *MDR3* (ABCB4) gene defect leading to impaired biliary phospholipids secretion (low phospholipid–associated cholelithiasis). Common duct stones may remain asymptomatic for years, may pass spontaneously into the duodenum, or (most often) may present with biliary colic or a complication.

Complications

Cholangitis

Cholangitis may be acute or chronic, and symptoms result from inflammation, which usually is caused by at least partial obstruction to the flow of bile. Bacteria are present on bile culture in ~75% of patients with acute cholangitis early in the symptomatic course. The characteristic presentation of acute cholangitis involves biliary pain, jaundice, and spiking fevers with chills (Charcot's triad). Blood cultures are frequently positive, and leukocytosis is typical. *Nonsuppurative acute cholangitis* is most common and may respond relatively rapidly to supportive measures and to treatment with antibiotics. In *suppurative acute cholangitis*, however, the presence of pus under pressure in a completely obstructed ductal system leads to symptoms of severe toxicity—mental confusion, bacteremia, and septic shock. Response to antibiotics alone in this setting is relatively poor, multiple hepatic abscesses are often present, and the mortality rate approaches 100% unless prompt endoscopic or surgical relief of the obstruction and drainage of infected bile are carried out. Endoscopic management of bacterial cholangitis is as effective as surgical intervention. ERCP with endoscopic sphincterotomy is safe and the preferred initial procedure for both establishing a definitive diagnosis and providing effective therapy.

Obstructive jaundice

Gradual obstruction of the CBD over a period of weeks or months usually leads to initial manifestations of jaundice or pruritus without associated symptoms of biliary colic or cholangitis. Painless jaundice may occur in patients with choledocholithiasis, but is much more characteristic of biliary obstruction secondary to malignancy of the head of the pancreas, bile ducts, or ampulla of Vater.

In patients whose obstruction is secondary to choledocholithiasis, associated chronic calculous cholecystitis is very common, and the gallbladder in this setting may be relatively indistensible. The absence of a palpable gallbladder in most patients with biliary obstruction from duct stones is the basis for Courvoisier's law, i.e., that the presence of a palpably enlarged gallbladder suggests that the biliary obstruction is secondary to an underlying malignancy rather than to calculous disease. Biliary obstruction causes progressive dilatation of the intrahepatic bile ducts as intrabiliary pressures rise. Hepatic bile flow is suppressed, and reabsorption and regurgitation of conjugated bilirubin into the bloodstream lead to jaundice accompanied by dark urine (bilirubinuria) and light-colored (acholic) stools.

CBD stones should be suspected in any patient with cholecystitis whose serum bilirubin level is >85.5 μmol/L (5 mg/dL). The maximum bilirubin level is seldom >256.5 μmol/L (15.0 mg/dL) in patients with choledocholithiasis unless concomitant hepatic disease or another factor leading to marked hyperbilirubinemia exists. Serum bilirubin levels ≥342.0 μmol/L (20 mg/dL) should suggest the possibility of neoplastic obstruction. The serum alkaline phosphatase level is almost always elevated in biliary obstruction. A rise in alkaline phosphatase often precedes clinical jaundice and may be the only abnormality in routine liver function tests. There may be a two- to tenfold elevation of serum aminotransferases, especially in association with acute obstruction. Following relief of the obstructing process, serum aminotransferase elevations usually return rapidly to normal, while the serum bilirubin level may take 1–2 weeks to return to normal. The alkaline phosphatase level usually falls slowly, lagging behind the decrease in serum bilirubin.

Pancreatitis

The most common associated entity discovered in patients with nonalcoholic acute pancreatitis is biliary tract disease. Biochemical evidence of pancreatic inflammation complicates acute cholecystitis in 15% of cases and choledocholithiasis in >30%, and the common factor appears to be the passage of gallstones through the common duct. Coexisting pancreatitis should be suspected in patients with symptoms of cholecystitis who develop (1) back pain or pain to the left of the abdominal midline, (2) prolonged vomiting with paralytic ileus, or (3) a pleural effusion, especially on the left side. Surgical treatment of gallstone disease is usually associated with resolution of the pancreatitis.

Secondary biliary cirrhosis

Secondary biliary cirrhosis may complicate prolonged or intermittent duct obstruction with or without recurrent cholangitis. Although this complication may be seen in patients with choledocholithiasis, it is more common in cases of prolonged obstruction from stricture or neoplasm. Once established, secondary biliary cirrhosis may be progressive even after correction of the obstructing process, and increasingly severe hepatic cirrhosis may lead to portal hypertension or to hepatic failure and death. Prolonged biliary obstruction may also be associated with clinically relevant deficiencies of the fat-soluble vitamins A, D, E, and K.

Diagnosis and treatment

The diagnosis of choledocholithiasis is usually made by cholangiography (Table 45-3), either preoperatively by endoscopic retrograde cholangiogram (ERC) (Fig. 45-2C) or MRCP or intraoperatively at the time of cholecystectomy. As many as 15% of patients undergoing cholecystectomy will prove to have CBD stones. When CBD stones are suspected prior to laparoscopic cholecystectomy, preoperative ERCP with endoscopic papillotomy and stone extraction is the preferred approach.

TABLE 45-3

DIAGNOSTIC EVALUATION OF THE BILE DUCTS

DIAGNOSTIC ADVANTAGES	DIAGNOSTIC LIMITATIONS	CONTRAINDICATIONS	COMPLICATIONS	COMMENT
Hepatobiliary Ultrasound				
Rapid Simultaneous scanning of GB, liver, bile ducts, pancreas Accurate identification of dilated bile ducts Not limited by jaundice, pregnancy Guidance for fine-needle biopsy	Bowel gas Massive obesity Ascites Barium Partial bile duct obstruction Poor visualization of distal CBD	None	None	Initial procedure of choice in investigating possible biliary tract obstruction
Computed Tomography				
Simultaneous scanning of GB, liver, bile ducts, pancreas Accurate identification of dilated bile ducts, masses Not limited by jaundice, gas, obesity, ascites High-resolution image Guidance for fine-needle biopsy	Extreme cachexia Movement artifact Ileus Partial bile duct obstruction	Pregnancy	Reaction to iodinated contrast, if used	Indicated for evaluation of hepatic or pancreatic masses Procedure of choice in investigating possible biliary obstruction if diagnostic limitations prevent HBUS
Magnetic Resonance Cholangiopancreatography				
Useful modality for visualizing pancreatic and biliary ducts Has excellent sensitivity for bile duct dilatation, biliary stricture, and intraductal abnormalities Can identify pancreatic duct dilatation or stricture, pancreatic duct stenosis, and pancreas divisum	Cannot offer therapeutic intervention High cost	Claustrophobia Certain metals (iron)	None	
Endoscopic Retrograde Cholangiopancreatography				
Simultaneous pancreatography Best visualization of distal biliary tract Bile or pancreatic cytology Endoscopic sphincterotomy and stone removal Biliary manometry	Gastroduodenal obstruction ? Roux-en-Y biliary-enteric anastomosis	Pregnancy ? Acute pancreatitis ? Severe cardiopulmonary disease	Pancreatitis Cholangitis, sepsis Infected pancreatic pseudocyst Perforation (rare) Hypoxemia, aspiration	Cholangiogram of choice in: Absence of dilated ducts ? Pancreatic, ampullary or gastroduodenal disease Prior biliary surgery Endoscopic sphincterotomy a treatment possibility
Percutaneous Transhepatic Cholangiogram				
Extremely successful when bile ducts dilated Best visualization of proximal biliary tract Bile cytology/culture Percutaneous transhepatic drainage	Nondilated or sclerosed ducts	Pregnancy Uncorrectable coagulopathy Massive ascites ? Hepatic abscess	Bleeding Hemobilia Bile peritonitis Bacteremia, sepsis	Indicated when ERCP is contraindicated or failed
Endoscopic Ultrasound				
Most sensitive method to detect ampullary stones				

Abbreviations: CBD, common bile duct; ERCP, endoscopic retrograde cholangiopancreatography; GB, gallbladder; HBUS, hepatobiliary ultrasound.

It not only provides stone clearance but also defines the anatomy of the biliary tree in relationship to the cystic duct. CBD stones should be suspected in gallstone patients who have any of the following risk factors: (1) a history of jaundice or pancreatitis, (2) abnormal tests of liver function, and (3) ultrasonographic or MRCP evidence of a dilated CBD or stones in the duct. Alternatively, if intraoperative cholangiography reveals retained stones, postoperative ERCP can be carried out. The need for preoperative ERCP is expected to decrease further as laparoscopic techniques for bile duct exploration improve.

The widespread use of laparoscopic cholecystectomy and ERCP has decreased the incidence of complicated biliary tract disease and the need for choledocholithotomy and T-tube drainage of the bile ducts. EBS followed by spontaneous passage or stone extraction is the treatment of choice in the management of patients with common duct stones, especially in elderly or poor-risk patients.

TRAUMA, STRICTURES, AND HEMOBILIA

Most benign strictures of the extrahepatic bile ducts result from surgical trauma and occur in about 1 in 500 cholecystectomies. Strictures may present with bile leak or abscess formation in the immediate postoperative period or with biliary obstruction or cholangitis as long as 2 years or more following the inciting trauma. The diagnosis is established by percutaneous or endoscopic cholangiography. Endoscopic brushing of biliary strictures may be helpful in establishing the nature of the lesion and is more accurate than bile cytology alone. When positive exfoliative cytology is obtained, the diagnosis of a neoplastic stricture is established. This procedure is especially important in patients with primary sclerosing cholangitis (PSC) who are predisposed to the development of cholangiocarcinomas. Successful operative correction of non-PSC bile duct strictures by a skillful surgeon with duct-to-bowel anastomosis is usually possible, although mortality rates from surgical complications, recurrent cholangitis, or secondary biliary cirrhosis are high.

Hemobilia may follow traumatic or operative injury to the liver or bile ducts, intraductal rupture of a hepatic abscess or aneurysm of the hepatic artery, biliary or hepatic tumor hemorrhage, or mechanical complications of choledocholithiasis or hepatobiliary parasitism. Diagnostic procedures such as liver biopsy, PTC, and transhepatic biliary drainage catheter placement may also be complicated by hemobilia. Patients often present with a classic triad of biliary pain, obstructive jaundice, and melena or occult blood in the stools. The diagnosis is sometimes made by cholangiographic evidence of blood clot in the biliary tree, but selective angiographic verification may be required. Although minor episodes of hemobilia may resolve without operative intervention, surgical ligation of the bleeding vessel is frequently required.

EXTRINSIC COMPRESSION OF THE BILE DUCTS

Partial or complete biliary obstruction may be produced by extrinsic compression of the ducts. The most common cause of this form of obstructive jaundice is carcinoma of the head of the pancreas. Biliary obstruction may also occur as a complication of either acute or chronic pancreatitis or involvement of lymph nodes in the porta hepatis by lymphoma or metastatic carcinoma. The latter should be distinguished from cholestasis resulting from massive replacement of the liver by tumor.

HEPATOBILIARY PARASITISM

Infestation of the biliary tract by adult helminths or their ova may produce a chronic, recurrent pyogenic cholangitis with or without multiple hepatic abscesses, ductal stones, or biliary obstruction. This condition is relatively rare but does occur in inhabitants of southern China and elsewhere in Southeast Asia. The organisms most commonly involved are trematodes or flukes, including *Clonorchis sinensis*, *Opisthorchis viverrini* or *O. felineus*, and *Fasciola hepatica*. The biliary tract also may be involved by intraductal migration of adult *Ascaris lumbricoides* from the duodenum or by intrabiliary rupture of hydatid cysts of the liver produced by *Echinococcus* spp. The diagnosis is made by cholangiography and the presence of characteristic ova on stool examination. When obstruction is present, the treatment of choice is laparotomy under antibiotic coverage, with common duct exploration and a biliary drainage procedure.

SCLEROSING CHOLANGITIS

Primary or idiopathic sclerosing cholangitis is characterized by a progressive, inflammatory, sclerosing, and obliterative process affecting the extrahepatic and/or the intrahepatic bile ducts. The disorder occurs up to 75% in association with inflammatory bowel disease, especially ulcerative colitis. It may also be associated with autoimmune pancreatitis; multifocal fibrosclerosis syndromes such as retroperitoneal, mediastinal, and/or periureteral fibrosis; Riedel's struma; or pseudotumor of the orbit.

Immunoglobulin (IgG4)–associated cholangitis is a recently described biliary disease of unknown etiology that presents with biochemical and cholangiographic features indistinguishable from PSC, is often associated with autoimmune pancreatitis and other fibrosing conditions, and is characterized by elevated serum IgG4 and infiltration of IgG4-positive plasma cells in bile ducts and liver tissue. In contrast to PSC, it is not associated with inflammatory bowel disease and should be suspected if associated with increased serum IgG4 and unexplained pancreatic disease. Glucocorticoids are regarded as the initial treatment of choice. Relapse is common after steroid withdrawal especially with proximal strictures. Long-term treatment with glucocorticoids and/or azathioprine may be needed after relapse or for inadequate response (Chap. 48).

Patients with primary sclerosing cholangitis often present with signs and symptoms of chronic or intermittent biliary obstruction: RUQ abdominal pain, pruritus, jaundice, or acute cholangitis. Late in the course, complete biliary obstruction, secondary biliary cirrhosis, hepatic failure, or portal hypertension with bleeding varices may occur. The diagnosis is usually established by finding multifocal, diffusely distributed strictures with intervening segments of normal or dilated ducts, producing a beaded appearance on cholangiography (Fig. 45-2D). The cholangiographic techniques of choice in suspected cases are MRCP and ERCP. When a diagnosis of sclerosing cholangitis has been established, a search for associated diseases, especially for chronic inflammatory bowel disease, should be carried out.

A recent study describes the natural history and outcome for 305 patients of Swedish descent with primary sclerosing cholangitis; 134 (44%) of the patients were asymptomatic at the time of diagnosis and, not surprisingly, had a significantly higher survival rate. The independent predictors of a bad prognosis were age, serum bilirubin concentration, and liver histologic changes. Cholangiocarcinoma was found in 24 patients (8%). Inflammatory bowel disease was closely associated with primary sclerosing cholangitis and had a prevalence of 81% in this study population.

Small duct PSC is defined by the presence of chronic cholestasis and hepatic histology consistent with PSC but with normal findings on cholangiography. Small duct PSC is found in ~5% of patients with PSC and may represent an earlier stage of PSC associated with a significantly better long-term prognosis. However, such patients may progress to classic PSC and/or end-stage liver disease with consequent necessity of liver transplantation.

In patients with AIDS, cholangiopancreatography may demonstrate a broad range of biliary tract changes as well as pancreatic duct obstruction and occasionally pancreatitis. Further, biliary tract lesions in AIDS include infection and cholangiopancreatographic changes similar to those of PSC. Changes noted include: (1) diffuse involvement of intrahepatic bile ducts alone, (2) involvement of both intra- and extrahepatic bile ducts, (3) ampullary stenosis, (4) stricture of the intrapancreatic portion of the common bile duct, and (5) pancreatic duct involvement. Associated infectious organisms include *Cryptosporidium*, *Mycobacterium avium-intracellulare*, cytomegalovirus, *Microsporidia*, and *Isospora*. In addition, acalculous cholecystitis occurs in up to 10% of patients. ERCP sphincterotomy, while not without risk, provides significant pain reduction in patients with AIDS-associated papillary stenosis. Secondary sclerosing cholangitis may occur as a long-term complication of choledocholithiasis, cholangiocarcinoma, operative or traumatic biliary injury, or contiguous inflammatory processes.

TREATMENT   Sclerosing Cholangitis

Therapy with cholestyramine may help control symptoms of pruritus, and antibiotics are useful when cholangitis complicates the clinical picture. Vitamin D and calcium supplementation may help prevent the loss of bone mass frequently seen in patients with chronic cholestasis. Glucocorticoids, methotrexate, and cyclosporine have not been shown to be efficacious in PSC. UDCA in high dosage (20 mg/kg) improves serum liver tests, but an effect on survival has not been documented. In cases where high-grade biliary obstruction (dominant strictures) has occurred, balloon dilatation or stenting may be appropriate. Only rarely is surgical intervention indicated. Efforts at biliary-enteric anastomosis or stent placement may, however, be complicated by recurrent cholangitis and further progression of the stenosing process. The prognosis is unfavorable, with a median survival of 9 to 12 years following the diagnosis, regardless of therapy. Four variables (age, serum bilirubin level, histologic stage, and splenomegaly) predict survival in patients with PSC and serve as the basis for a risk score. PSC is one of the most common indications for liver transplantation.

SECTION VII

LIVER TRANSPLANTATION

CHAPTER 46

LIVER TRANSPLANTATION

Jules L. Dienstag ■ Raymond T. Chung

Liver transplantation—the replacement of the native, diseased liver by a normal organ (allograft)—has matured from an experimental procedure reserved for desperately ill patients to an accepted, lifesaving operation applied more optimally in the natural history of end-stage liver disease. The preferred and technically most advanced approach is *orthotopic transplantation*, in which the native organ is removed and the donor organ is inserted in the same anatomic location. Pioneered in the 1960s by Thomas Starzl at the University of Colorado and, later, at the University of Pittsburgh and by Roy Calne in Cambridge, England, liver transplantation is now performed routinely worldwide. Success measured as 1-year survival has improved from ~30% in the 1970s to ~90% today. These improved prospects for prolonged survival, dating back to the early 1980s, resulted from refinements in operative technique, improvements in organ procurement and preservation, advances in immunosuppressive therapy, and, perhaps most influentially, more enlightened patient selection and timing. Despite the perioperative morbidity and mortality, the technical and management challenges of the procedure, and its costs, liver transplantation has become the approach of choice for selected patients whose chronic or acute liver disease is progressive, life-threatening, and unresponsive to medical therapy. Based on the current level of success, the number of liver transplants has continued to grow each year; in 2009, 6320 patients received liver allografts in the United States. Still, the demand for new livers continues to outpace availability; as of mid-2010, 16,785 patients in the United States were on a waiting list for a donor liver. In response to this drastic shortage of donor organs, many transplantation centers supplement cadaver-organ liver transplantation with living-donor transplantation.

INDICATIONS

Potential candidates for liver transplantation are children and adults who, in the absence of contraindications (discussed later), suffer from severe, irreversible liver disease for which alternative medical or surgical treatments have been exhausted or are unavailable. *Timing of the operation is of critical importance.* Indeed, improved timing and better patient selection are felt to have contributed more to the increased success of liver transplantation in the 1980s and beyond than all the impressive technical and immunologic advances combined. Although the disease should be advanced, and although opportunities for spontaneous or medically induced stabilization or recovery should be allowed, the procedure should be done sufficiently early to give the surgical procedure a fair chance for success. Ideally, transplantation should be considered in patients with end-stage liver disease who are experiencing or have experienced a life-threatening complication of hepatic decompensation or whose quality of life has deteriorated to unacceptable levels. Although patients with well-compensated cirrhosis can survive for many years, many patients with quasi-stable chronic liver disease have much more advanced disease than may be apparent. As discussed later, the better the status of the patient prior to transplantation, the higher will be the anticipated success rate of transplantation. The decision about *when* to transplant is complex and requires the combined judgment of an experienced team of hepatologists, transplant surgeons, anesthesiologists, and specialists in support services, not to mention the well-informed consent of the patient and the patient's family.

TRANSPLANTATION IN CHILDREN

Indications for transplantation in children are listed in **Table 46-1**. The most common is *biliary atresia*.

TABLE 46-1

INDICATIONS FOR LIVER TRANSPLANTATION

CHILDREN	ADULTS
Biliary atresia	Primary biliary cirrhosis
Neonatal hepatitis	Secondary biliary cirrhosis
Congenital hepatic fibrosis	Primary sclerosing cholangitis
Alagille's syndrome[a]	Autoimmune hepatitis
Byler's disease[b]	Caroli's disease[c]
α_1-Antitrypsin deficiency	Cryptogenic cirrhosis
Inherited disorders of metabolism	Chronic hepatitis with cirrhosis
Wilson's disease	Hepatic vein thrombosis
Tyrosinemia	Fulminant hepatitis
Glycogen storage diseases	Alcoholic cirrhosis
Lysosomal storage diseases	Chronic viral hepatitis
Protoporphyria	Primary hepatocellular malignancies
Crigler-Najjar disease type I	Hepatic adenomas
Familial hypercholesterolemia	Nonalcoholic steatohepatitis
Primary hyperoxaluria type I	Familial amyloid polyneuropathy
Hemophilia	

[a]Arteriohepatic dysplasia, with paucity of bile ducts, and congenital malformations, including pulmonary stenosis.
[b]Intrahepatic cholestasis, progressive liver failure, mental and growth retardation.
[c]Multiple cystic dilatations of the intrahepatic biliary tree.

Inherited or genetic disorders of metabolism associated with liver failure constitute another major indication for transplantation in children and adolescents. In Crigler-Najjar disease type I and in certain hereditary disorders of the urea cycle and of amino acid or lactate-pyruvate metabolism, transplantation may be the only way to prevent impending deterioration of central nervous system function, despite the fact that the native liver is structurally normal. Combined heart and liver transplantation has yielded dramatic improvement in cardiac function and in cholesterol levels in children with homozygous familial hypercholesterolemia; combined liver and kidney transplantation has been successful in patients with primary hyperoxaluria type I. In hemophiliacs with transfusion-associated hepatitis and liver failure, liver transplantation has been associated with recovery of normal Factor VIII synthesis.

TRANSPLANTATION IN ADULTS

Liver transplantation is indicated for end-stage *cirrhosis* of all causes (Table 46-1). In *sclerosing cholangitis* and *Caroli's disease* (multiple cystic dilatations of the intrahepatic biliary tree), recurrent infections and sepsis associated with inflammatory and fibrotic obstruction of the biliary tree may be an indication for transplantation. Because prior biliary surgery complicates and is a relative contraindication for liver transplantation, surgical diversion of the biliary tree has been all but abandoned for patients with sclerosing cholangitis. In patients who undergo transplantation for *hepatic vein thrombosis (Budd-Chiari syndrome)*, postoperative anticoagulation is essential; underlying myeloproliferative disorders may have to be treated but are not a contraindication to liver transplantation. If a donor organ can be located quickly, before life-threatening complications—including cerebral edema—set in, patients with acute liver failure are candidates for liver transplantation. Routine candidates for liver transplantation are patients with *alcoholic cirrhosis*, *chronic viral hepatitis*, and *primary hepatocellular malignancies*. Although all three of these categories are considered to be high risk, liver transplantation can be offered to carefully selected patients. Currently, chronic hepatitis C and alcoholic liver disease are the most common indications for liver transplantation, accounting for over 40% of all adult candidates who undergo the procedure. Patients with alcoholic cirrhosis can be considered as candidates for transplantation if they meet strict criteria for abstinence and reform; however, these criteria still do not prevent recidivism in up to a quarter of cases. Patients with chronic hepatitis C have early allograft and patient survival comparable to those of other subsets of patients after transplantation; however, reinfection in the donor organ is universal, recurrent hepatitis C is insidiously progressive, the impact of antiviral therapy is limited, allograft cirrhosis develops in 20–30% at 5 years, and cirrhosis and late organ failure are being recognized with increasing frequency beyond 5 years. In patients with chronic hepatitis B, in the absence of measures to prevent recurrent hepatitis B, survival after transplantation is reduced by approximately 10–20%; however, prophylactic use of hepatitis B immune globulin (HBIg) during and after transplantation increases the success of transplantation to a level comparable to that seen in patients with nonviral causes of liver decompensation. Specific oral antiviral drugs (e.g., lamivudine, adefovir, entecavir, and tenofovir disoproxil fumarate) (Chap. 40) can be used both for prophylaxis against and for treatment of recurrent hepatitis B, facilitating further the management of patients undergoing liver transplantation for end-stage hepatitis B; most transplantation centers rely on a combination of HBIg and antiviral drugs to manage patients with hepatitis B. Issues of disease recurrence are discussed in more detail later. Patients with nonmetastatic primary hepatobiliary tumors—primary hepatocellular carcinoma (HCC), cholangiocarcinoma, hepatoblastoma, angiosarcoma, epithelioid hemangioendothelioma, and multiple or massive hepatic adenomata—have undergone liver transplantation; however, for some hepatobiliary malignancies, overall survival is significantly lower than that for other categories of liver disease. Most transplantation centers have reported 5-year recurrence-free survival rates in patients with unresectable HCC for single tumors <5 cm in diameter or for three or fewer lesions all <3 cm comparable to those seen in patients undergoing transplantation for nonmalignant indications. Consequently, liver transplantation is currently restricted to patients whose hepatic malignancies meet these criteria. Expanded criteria for patients with HCC are being evaluated. Because the likelihood of recurrent cholangiocarcinoma is very high, only highly selected patients with limited disease are being evaluated for transplantation after intensive chemotherapy and radiation.

CONTRAINDICATIONS

Absolute contraindications for transplantation include life-threatening systemic diseases, uncontrolled extrahepatic bacterial or fungal infections, preexisting advanced cardiovascular or pulmonary disease, multiple uncorrectable life-threatening congenital anomalies, metastatic malignancy, and active drug or alcohol abuse (Table 46-2). Because carefully selected patients in their sixties and even seventies have undergone transplantation successfully, advanced age per se is no longer considered an absolute contraindication; however, in older patients a more thorough preoperative evaluation should be undertaken to exclude ischemic cardiac disease and other comorbid conditions. Advanced age (>70 years), however, should be considered a *relative contraindication*—that is, a factor to be taken into account with other relative contraindications. Other relative contraindications include portal vein thrombosis, HIV infection, preexisting renal disease not associated with liver disease (which may prompt consideration of combined liver and kidney transplantation), intrahepatic or biliary sepsis, severe hypoxemia (Po2 <50 mmHg) resulting from right-to-left intrapulmonary shunts, portopulmonary hypertension with high mean pulmonary artery pressures (>35 mmHg), previous extensive hepatobiliary surgery, any uncontrolled serious psychiatric disorder, and lack of sufficient social supports. Any one of these relative contraindications is insufficient in and of itself to preclude transplantation. For example, the problem of portal vein thrombosis can be overcome by constructing a graft from the donor liver portal vein to the recipient's superior mesenteric vein. Now that highly active antiretroviral therapy has dramatically improved the survival of persons with HIV infection, and because end-stage liver disease caused by chronic hepatitis C and B has emerged as a serious source of morbidity and mortality in the HIV-infected population, liver transplantation has now been

TABLE 46-2

CONTRAINDICATIONS TO LIVER TRANSPLANTATION

ABSOLUTE	RELATIVE
Uncontrolled extrahepatobiliary infection	Age <70
Active, untreated sepsis	Prior extensive hepatobiliary surgery
Uncorrectable, life-limiting congenital anomalies	Portal vein thrombosis
Active substance or alcohol abuse	Renal failure not attributable to liver disease
Advanced cardiopulmonary disease	Previous extrahepatic malignancy (not including nonmelanoma skin cancer)
Extrahepatobiliary malignancy (not including nonmelanoma skin cancer)	Severe obesity
Metastatic malignancy to the liver	Severe malnutrition/wasting
Cholangiocarcinoma	Medical noncompliance
AIDS	HIV seropositivity with failure to control HIV viremia or CD4 <100/μL
Life-threatening systemic diseases	Intrahepatic sepsis
	Severe hypoxemia secondary to right-to-left intrapulmonary shunts (Po2 <50 mmHg)
	Severe pulmonary hypertension (mean pulmonary artery pressure >35 mmHg)
	Uncontrolled psychiatric disorder

performed successfully in selected HIV-positive persons who have excellent control of HIV infection. Selected patients with CD4+ T cell counts >100/μL and with pharmacologic suppression of HIV viremia have undergone transplantation for end-stage liver disease. HIV-infected persons who have received liver allografts for end-stage liver disease resulting from chronic hepatitis B have experienced survival rates compared to those of HIV-negative persons undergoing transplantation for the same indication. In contrast, recurrent hepatitis C virus (HCV) in the allograft has limited long-term success in persons with HCV-related end-stage liver disease.

TECHNICAL CONSIDERATIONS

CADAVER DONOR SELECTION

Cadaver donor livers for transplantation are procured primarily from victims of head trauma. Organs from brain-dead donors up to age 60 are acceptable if the following criteria are met: hemodynamic stability, adequate oxygenation, absence of bacterial or fungal infection, absence of abdominal trauma, absence of hepatic dysfunction, and serologic exclusion of hepatitis B (HBV) and C viruses and HIV. Occasionally, organs from donors with hepatitis B and C are used (e.g., for recipients with prior hepatitis B and C, respectively). Organs from donors with antibodies to hepatitis B core antigen (anti-HBc) can also be used when the need is especially urgent, and recipients of these organs are treated prophylactically with HBIg and other antiviral drugs. Cardiovascular and respiratory functions are maintained artificially until the liver can be removed. Transplantation of organs procured from deceased donors who have succumbed to cardiac death can be performed successfully under selected circumstances, when ischemic time is minimized and liver histology preserved. Compatibility in ABO blood group and organ size between donor and recipient are important considerations in donor selection; however, ABO-incompatible, split liver, or reduced-donor-organ transplants can be performed in emergencies or marked donor scarcity. Tissue typing for human leukocyte antigen (HLA) matching is not required, and preformed cytotoxic HLA antibodies do not preclude liver transplantation. Following perfusion with cold electrolyte solution, the donor liver is removed and packed in ice. The use of University of Wisconsin (UW) solution, rich in lactobionate and raffinose, has permitted the extension of cold ischemic time up to 20 h; however, 12 h may be a more reasonable limit. Improved techniques for harvesting multiple organs from the same donor have increased the availability of donor livers, but the availability of donor livers is far outstripped by the demand. Currently in the United States, all donor livers are distributed through a nationwide organ-sharing network (United Network for Organ Sharing [UNOS]) designed to allocate available organs based on regional considerations and recipient acuity. Recipients who have the highest disease severity generally have the highest priority, but allocation strategies that balance highest urgency against best outcomes continue to evolve to distribute cadaver organs most effectively. Allocation based on the Child-Turcotte-Pugh (CTP) score, which uses five clinical variables (encephalopathy stage, ascites, bilirubin, albumin, and prothrombin time) and waiting time, has been replaced by allocation based on urgency alone, calculated by the Model for End-Stage Liver Disease (MELD) score. The MELD score is based on a mathematical model that includes bilirubin, creatinine, and prothrombin time expressed as international normalized ratio (INR) (Table 46-3). Neither waiting time (except as a tie breaker between two potential recipients with the same MELD scores) nor posttransplantation outcome is taken into account, but the MELD score has been shown to reduce waiting list

TABLE 46-3

UNITED NETWORK FOR ORGAN SHARING (UNOS) LIVER TRANSPLANTATION WAITING LIST CRITERIA

Status 1	Fulminant hepatic failure (including primary graft nonfunction and hepatic artery thrombosis within 7 days after transplantation as well as acute decompensated Wilson's disease)[a]

The Model for End-Stage Liver Disease (MELD) score, on a continuous scale,[b] determines allocation of the remainder of donor organs. This model is based on the following calculation:

$3.78 \times \log_e$ bilirubin (mg/100 mL) + $11.2 \times \log_e$ International normalized ratio (INR) + $9.57 \times \log_e$ creatinine (mg/100 mL) + 6.43 ($\times 0$ for alcoholic and cholestatic liver disease, $\times 1$ for all other types of liver disease).[c,d,e]

Online calculators to determine MELD scores are available, such as the following: *http://optn.transplant.hrsa.gov/resources/professionalresources.asp?index=9.*

[a]For children <18 years of age, status 1 includes acute or chronic liver failure plus hospitalization in an intensive care unit or inborn errors of metabolism. Status 1 is retained for those persons with fulminant hepatic failure and supersedes the MELD score.
[b]The MELD scale is continuous, with 34 levels ranging between 6 and 40. Donor organs usually do not become available unless the MELD score exceeds 20.
[c]Patients with stage T2 hepatocellular carcinoma receive 22 disease-specific points. An α-fetoprotein level = 500 ng/mL is considered as stage I hepatocellular carcinoma even without evidence for a tumor on imaging.
[d]Creatinine is included because renal function is a validated predictor of survival in patients with liver disease. For adults undergoing dialysis twice a week, the creatinine in the equation is set to 4 mg/100 mL.
[e]For children <18 years of age, the Pediatric End-Stage Liver Disease (PELD) scale is used. This scale is based on albumin, bilirubin, INR, growth failure, and age. Status 1 is retained.

mortality, to reduce waiting time prior to transplantation, to be the best predictor of pretransplantation mortality, to satisfy the prevailing view that medical need should be the decisive determinant, and to eliminate both the subjectivity inherent in the CTP scoring system (presence and degree of ascites and hepatic encephalopathy) and the differences in waiting times among different regions of the country. Recent data indicate that liver recipients with MELD scores <15 experienced higher posttransplantation mortality rates than similarly classified patients who remained on the wait list. This observation has led to the modification of UNOS policy to allocate donor organs to candidates with MELD scores exceeding 15 within the local or regional procurement organization before offering the organ to local patients whose scores are <15. In addition, serum sodium, another important predictor of survival in liver transplantation candidates, is taken into consideration in allocating donor livers.

The highest priority (status 1) continues to be reserved for patients with fulminant hepatic failure or primary graft nonfunction. Because candidates for liver transplantation who have HCC may not be sufficiently decompensated to compete for donor organs based on urgency criteria alone, and because protracted waiting for cadaver donor organs often results in tumor growth beyond acceptable limits for transplantation, such patients are assigned disease-specific MELD points (Table 46-3).

LIVING DONOR TRANSPLANTATION

Occasionally, especially for liver transplantation in children, one cadaver organ can be split between two recipients (one adult and one child). A more viable alternative, transplantation of the right lobe of the liver from a healthy adult donor into an adult recipient, has gained increased popularity. Living donor transplantation of the left lobe (left lateral segment), introduced in the early 1990s to alleviate the extreme shortage of donor organs for small children, accounts currently for approximately one-third of all liver transplantation procedures in children. Driven by the shortage of cadaver organs, living donor transplantation involving the more sizable right lobe is being considered with increasing frequency in adults; however, living donor liver transplantation cannot be expected to solve the donor organ shortage; 219 such procedures were done in 2009, representing only about 4% of all liver transplant operations done in the United States.

Living donor transplantation can reduce waiting time and cold-ischemia time; is done under elective, rather than emergency, circumstances; and may be lifesaving in recipients who cannot afford to wait for a cadaver donor. The downside, of course, is the risk to the healthy donor (a mean of 10 weeks of medical disability; biliary complications in ~5%; postoperative complications such as wound infection, small-bowel obstruction, and incisional hernias in 9–19%; and even, in 0.2–0.4%, death) as well as the increased frequency of biliary (15–32%) and vascular (10%) complications in the recipient. Potential donors must participate voluntarily without coercion, and transplantation teams should go to great lengths to exclude subtle coercive or inappropriate psychological factors as well as outline carefully to both donor and recipient the potential benefits and risks of the procedure. Donors for the procedure should be 18–60 years old; have a compatible blood type with the recipient; have no chronic medical problems or history of major abdominal surgery; be related genetically or emotionally to the recipient; and pass an exhaustive series of clinical, biochemical, and serologic evaluations to unearth disqualifying medical disorders. The recipient should meet the same UNOS criteria for liver transplantation as recipients of a cadaver donor allograft.

Comprehensive outcome data on adult-to-adult living donor liver transplantation are being collected (*www.nih-a2all.org*).

SURGICAL TECHNIQUE

Removal of the recipient's native liver is technically difficult, particularly in the presence of portal hypertension with its associated collateral circulation and extensive varices and especially in the presence of scarring from previous abdominal operations. The combination of portal hypertension and coagulopathy (elevated prothrombin time and thrombocytopenia) may translate into large blood product transfusion requirements. After the portal vein and infrahepatic and suprahepatic inferior vena cavae are dissected, the hepatic artery and common bile duct are dissected. Then the native liver is removed and the donor organ inserted. During the anhepatic phase, coagulopathy, hypoglycemia, hypocalcemia, and hypothermia are encountered and must be managed by the anesthesiology team. Caval, portal vein, hepatic artery, and bile duct anastomoses are performed in succession, the last by end-to-end suturing of the donor and recipient common bile ducts or by choledochojejunostomy to a Roux-en-Y loop if the recipient common bile duct cannot be used for reconstruction (e.g., in sclerosing cholangitis). A typical transplant operation lasts 8 h, with a range of 6–18 h. Because of excessive bleeding, large volumes of blood, blood products, and volume expanders may be required during surgery; however, blood requirements have fallen sharply with improvements in surgical technique and experience.

As noted earlier, emerging alternatives to orthotopic liver transplantation include split-liver grafts, in which one donor organ is divided and inserted into two recipients; and living donor procedures, in which part of the left (for children), the left (for children or small adults), or the right (for adults) lobe of the liver is harvested from a living donor for transplantation into the recipient. In the adult procedure, once the right lobe is removed from the donor, the donor right hepatic vein is anastomosed to the recipient right hepatic vein remnant, followed by donor-to-recipient anastomoses of the portal vein and then the hepatic artery. Finally, the biliary anastomosis is performed, duct-to-duct if practical or via Roux-en-Y anastomosis. Heterotopic liver transplantation, in which the donor liver is inserted without removal of the native liver, has met with very limited success and acceptance, except in a very small number of centers. In attempts to support desperately ill patients until a suitable donor organ can be identified, several transplantation centers are studying extracorporeal perfusion with bioartificial liver cartridges constructed from hepatocytes bound to hollow fiber systems and used as temporary hepatic-assist devices, but their efficacy remains to be established. Areas of research with the potential to overcome the shortage of donor organs include hepatocyte transplantation and xenotransplantation with genetically modified organs of nonhuman origin (e.g., swine).

POSTOPERATIVE COURSE AND MANAGEMENT

IMMUNOSUPPRESSIVE THERAPY

The introduction in 1980 of cyclosporine as an immunosuppressive agent contributed substantially to the improvement in survival after liver transplantation. Cyclosporine, a calcineurin inhibitor (CNI), blocks early activation of T cells and is specific for T cell functions that result from the interaction of the T cell with its receptor and that involve the calcium-dependent signal transduction pathway. As a result, the activity of cyclosporine leads to inhibition of lymphokine gene activation, blocking interleukins 2, 3, and 4, tumor necrosis factor α, and other lymphokines. Cyclosporine also inhibits B cell functions. This process occurs without affecting rapidly dividing cells in the bone marrow, which may account for the reduced frequency of posttransplantation systemic infections. The most common and important side effect of cyclosporine therapy is nephrotoxicity. Cyclosporine causes dose-dependent renal tubular injury and direct renal artery vasospasm. Following renal function is therefore important in monitoring cyclosporine therapy, perhaps even a more reliable indicator than blood levels of the drug. Nephrotoxicity is reversible and can be managed by dose reduction. Other adverse effects of cyclosporine therapy include hypertension, hyperkalemia, tremor, hirsutism, glucose intolerance, and gingival hyperplasia.

Tacrolimus, a macrolide lactone antibiotic isolated from a Japanese soil fungus, *Streptomyces tsukubaensis*, has the same mechanism of action as cyclosporine but is 10–100 times more potent. Initially applied as "rescue" therapy for patients in whom rejection occurred despite the use of cyclosporine, tacrolimus was shown to be associated with a reduced frequency of acute, refractory, and chronic rejection. Although patient and graft survival are the same with these two drugs, the advantage of tacrolimus in minimizing episodes of rejection, reducing the need for additional glucocorticoid doses, and reducing the likelihood of bacterial and cytomegalovirus (CMV) infection has simplified the management of patients undergoing liver transplantation. In addition, the oral absorption of tacrolimus is more predictable than that of cyclosporine, especially during the early postoperative period when T-tube drainage interferes with the enterohepatic circulation of cyclosporine. As a result, in most transplantation centers tacrolimus has now supplanted cyclosporine for primary immunosuppression, and many centers rely on oral rather than IV administration from the outset. For transplantation centers that prefer cyclosporine, a better-absorbed microemulsion preparation is now available.

Although more potent than cyclosporine, tacrolimus is also more toxic and more likely to be discontinued for adverse events. The toxicity of tacrolimus is similar to that of cyclosporine; nephrotoxicity and neurotoxicity are the most commonly encountered adverse effects, and neurotoxicity (tremor, seizures, hallucinations, psychoses, coma) is more likely and more severe in tacrolimus-treated patients. Both drugs can cause diabetes mellitus, but tacrolimus does not cause hirsutism or gingival hyperplasia. Because of overlapping toxicity between cyclosporine and tacrolimus, especially nephrotoxicity, and because tacrolimus reduces cyclosporine clearance, these two drugs should not be used together. Because 99% of tacrolimus is metabolized by the liver, hepatic dysfunction reduces its clearance; in primary graft nonfunction (when, for technical reasons or because of ischemic damage prior to its insertion, the allograft is defective and does not function normally from the outset), tacrolimus doses have to be reduced substantially, especially in children. Both cyclosporine and tacrolimus are metabolized by the cytochrome P450 IIIA system, and, therefore, drugs that induce cytochrome P450 (e.g., phenytoin, phenobarbital, carbamazepine, rifampin) reduce available levels of cyclosporine and tacrolimus; drugs that inhibit cytochrome P450 (e.g., erythromycin, fluconazole, ketoconazole, clotrimazole, itraconazole, verapamil, diltiazem, nicardipine, cimetidine, danazol, metoclopramide, bromocriptine, and the HIV protease inhibitor ritonavir) increase cyclosporine and tacrolimus blood levels. Indeed, itraconazole is used occasionally to help boost tacrolimus levels. Like azathioprine, cyclosporine and tacrolimus appear to be associated with a risk of lymphoproliferative malignancies (discussed later), which may occur earlier after cyclosporine or tacrolimus than after azathioprine therapy. Because of these side effects, combinations of cyclosporine or tacrolimus with prednisone and an antimetabolite (azathioprine or mycophenolic acid, discussed later)—all at reduced doses—are preferable regimens for immunosuppressive therapy.

Mycophenolic acid, a nonnucleoside purine metabolism inhibitor derived as a fermentation product from several *Penicillium* species, is another immunosuppressive drug being used increasingly for patients undergoing liver transplantation. Mycophenolate has been shown to be better than azathioprine, when used with other standard immunosuppressive drugs, in preventing rejection after renal transplantation and has been adopted widely as well for use in liver transplantation. The most common adverse effects of mycophenolate are bone marrow suppression and gastrointestinal complaints.

In patients with pretransplantation renal dysfunction or renal deterioration that occurs intraoperatively or immediately postoperatively, tacrolimus or cyclosporine therapy may not be practical; under these circumstances, induction or maintenance of immunosuppression with antithymocyte globulin (ATG, thymoglobulin) or monoclonal antibodies to T cells, OKT3, may be appropriate. Therapy with these agents has been especially effective in reversing acute rejection in the posttransplant period and is the standard treatment for acute rejection that fails to respond to methylprednisolone boluses. Available data support the use of thymoglobulin induction to delay CNI use and its attendant nephrotoxicity. IV infusions of thymoglobulin may be complicated by fever and chills, which can be ameliorated by premedication with antipyretics and a low dose of glucocorticoids. Infusions of OKT3 may be complicated by fever, chills, and diarrhea, or by pulmonary edema, which can be fatal. Because OKT3 is such a potent immunosuppressive agent, its use is also more likely to be complicated by opportunistic infection or lymphoproliferative disorders; therefore, because of the availability of alternative immunosuppressive drugs, OKT3 is used less often nowadays.

Rapamycin, an inhibitor of later events in T cell activation, is approved for use in kidney transplantation but is not approved for use in liver transplant recipients because of the reported association with an increased frequency of hepatic artery thrombosis in the first month posttransplantation. In patients with CNI-related nephrotoxicity, conversion to rapamycin has been demonstrated to be effective in preventing rejection with accompanying improvements in renal function. Because of its profound antiproliferative effects, rapamycin has also been suggested to be a useful immunosuppressive agent in patients with a prior or current history of malignancy, such as HCC. Side effects include hyperlipidemia, peripheral edema, oral ulcers, and interstitial pneumonitis.

The most important principle of immunosuppression is that the ideal approach strikes a balance between immunosuppression and immunologic competence. In general, given sufficient immunosuppression, acute liver allograft rejection is nearly always reversible. On one hand, incompletely treated acute rejection predisposes to the development of chronic rejection, which can threaten graft survival. On the other hand, if the cumulative dose of immunosuppressive therapy is too large, the patient may succumb to opportunistic infection. In hepatitis C, pulse glucocorticoids or OKT3 use accelerate recurrent allograft hepatitis. Further complicating matters, acute rejection can be difficult to distinguish histologically from recurrent hepatitis C. Therefore, immunosuppressive drugs must be used judiciously,

with strict attention to the infectious consequences of such therapy and careful confirmation of the diagnosis of acute rejection. In this vein, efforts have been made to minimize the use of glucocorticoids, a mainstay of immunosuppressive regimens, and steroid-free immunosuppression can be achieved in some instances. Patients who undergo liver transplantation for autoimmune diseases such as primary biliary cirrhosis, autoimmune hepatitis, and primary sclerosing cholangitis are less likely to achieve freedom from glucocorticoids.

POSTOPERATIVE COMPLICATIONS

Complications of liver transplantation can be divided into nonhepatic and hepatic categories (Tables 46-4 and 46-5). In addition, both immediate postoperative and late complications are encountered. As a rule, patients who undergo liver transplantation have been chronically ill for protracted periods and may be

TABLE 46-4

NONHEPATIC COMPLICATIONS OF LIVER TRANSPLANTATION	
Fluid overload	
Cardiovascular instability	Arrhythmias
	Congestive heart failure
	Cardiomyopathy
Pulmonary compromise	Pneumonia
	Pulmonary capillary vascular permeability
	Fluid overload
Renal dysfunction	Prerenal azotemia
	Hypoperfusion injury (acute tubular necrosis)
	Drug nephrotoxicity
	↓ Renal blood flow secondary to ↑ intraabdominal pressure
Hematologic	Anemia 2° to gastrointestinal and/or intraabdominal bleeding
	Hemolytic anemia, aplastic anemia
	Thrombocytopenia
Infection	Bacterial: early, common postoperative infections
	Fungal/parasitic: late, opportunistic infections
	Viral: late, opportunistic infections, recurrent hepatitis
Neuropsychiatric	Seizures
	Metabolic encephalopathy
	Depression
	Difficult psychosocial adjustment
Diseases of donor	Infectious
	Malignant
Malignancy	B cell lymphoma (posttransplantation lymphoproliferative disorders)
	De novo neoplasms (particularly squamous cell skin carcinoma)

TABLE 46-5

HEPATIC COMPLICATIONS OF LIVER TRANSPLANTATION

Hepatic Dysfunction Common after Major Surgery

Prehepatic	Pigment load
	Hemolysis
	Blood collections (hematomas, abdominal collections)
Intrahepatic	
Early	Hepatotoxic drugs and anesthesia
	Hypoperfusion (hypotension, shock, sepsis)
	Benign postoperative cholestasis
Late	Transfusion-associated hepatitis
	Exacerbation of primary hepatic disease
Posthepatic	Biliary obstruction
	↓ Renal clearance of conjugated bilirubin (renal dysfunction)

Hepatic Dysfunction Unique to Liver Transplantation

Primary graft nonfunction	
Vascular compromise	Portal vein obstruction
	Hepatic artery thrombosis
	Anastomotic leak with intraabdominal bleeding
Bile duct disorder	Stenosis, obstruction, leak
Rejection	
Recurrent primary hepatic disease	

malnourished and wasted. The impact of such chronic illness and the multisystem failure that accompanies liver failure continue to require attention in the postoperative period. Because of the massive fluid losses and fluid shifts that occur during the operation, patients may remain fluid-overloaded during the immediate postoperative period, straining cardiovascular reserve; this effect can be amplified in the face of transient renal dysfunction and pulmonary capillary vascular permeability. Continuous monitoring of cardiovascular and pulmonary function, measures to maintain the integrity of the intravascular compartment and to treat extravascular volume overload, and scrupulous attention to potential sources and sites of infection are of paramount importance. Cardiovascular instability may also result from the electrolyte imbalance that may accompany reperfusion of the donor liver as well as from restoration of systemic vascular resistance following implantation. Pulmonary function may be compromised further by paralysis of the right hemidiaphragm associated with phrenic nerve injury. The hyperdynamic state with increased cardiac output that is characteristic of patients with liver failure reverses rapidly after successful liver transplantation.

Other immediate management issues include renal dysfunction. Prerenal azotemia, acute kidney injury associated with hypoperfusion (acute tubular necrosis), and renal toxicity caused by antibiotics, tacrolimus, or cyclosporine are encountered frequently in the postoperative period, sometimes necessitating dialysis. Hemolytic uremic syndrome can be associated with cyclosporine, tacrolimus, or OKT3. Occasionally, postoperative intraperitoneal bleeding may be sufficient to increase intraabdominal pressure, which, in turn, may reduce renal blood flow; this effect is rapidly reversible when abdominal distention is relieved by exploratory laparotomy to identify and ligate the bleeding site and to remove intraperitoneal clot.

Anemia may also result from acute upper gastrointestinal bleeding or from transient hemolytic anemia, which may be autoimmune, especially when blood group O livers are transplanted into blood group A or B recipients. This autoimmune hemolytic anemia is mediated by donor intrahepatic lymphocytes that recognize red blood cell A or B antigens on recipient erythrocytes. Transient in nature, this process resolves once the donor liver is repopulated by recipient bone marrow–derived lymphocytes; the hemolysis can be treated by transfusing blood group O red blood cells and/or by administering higher doses of glucocorticoids. Transient thrombocytopenia is also commonly encountered. Aplastic anemia, a late occurrence, is rare but has been reported in almost 30% of patients who underwent liver transplantation for acute, severe hepatitis of unknown cause.

Bacterial, fungal, or viral infections are common and may be life-threatening postoperatively. Early after transplant surgery, common postoperative infections predominate—pneumonia, wound infections, infected intraabdominal collections, urinary tract infections, and IV line infections—rather than opportunistic infections; these infections may involve the biliary tree and liver as well. Beyond the first postoperative month, the toll of immunosuppression becomes evident, and opportunistic infections—CMV, herpes viruses, fungal infections (*Aspergillus*, *Candida*, cryptococcal disease), mycobacterial infections, parasitic infections (*Pneumocystis*, *Toxoplasma*), bacterial infections (*Nocardia*, *Legionella*, and *Listeria*)—predominate. Rarely, early infections represent those transmitted with the donor liver, either infections present in the donor or infections acquired during procurement processing. De novo viral hepatitis infections acquired from the donor organ or, almost unheard of nowadays, from transfused blood products occur after typical incubation periods for these agents (well beyond the first month). Obviously, infections in an immunosuppressed host demand early recognition and prompt management; prophylactic antibiotic therapy is administered routinely in the immediate postoperative period. Use of sulfamethoxazole with trimethoprim reduces the incidence of postoperative *Pneumocystis carinii* pneumonia. Antiviral prophylaxis for CMV with ganciclovir should be administered in patients at high risk (e.g., when a CMV-seropositive donor organ is implanted into a CMV-seronegative recipient).

Neuropsychiatric complications include seizures (commonly associated with cyclosporine and tacrolimus toxicity), metabolic encephalopathy, depression, and difficult psychosocial adjustment. Rarely, diseases are transmitted by the allograft from the donor to the recipient. In addition to viral and bacterial infections, malignancies of donor origin have occurred. Posttransplantation lymphoproliferative disorders, especially B cell lymphoma, are a recognized complication associated with immunosuppressive drugs such as azathioprine, tacrolimus, and cyclosporine (discussed earlier). Epstein-Barr virus has been shown to play a contributory role in some of these tumors, which may regress when immunosuppressive therapy is reduced. De novo neoplasms appear at increased frequency after liver transplantation, particularly squamous cell carcinomas of the skin. Routine screening should be performed.

Long-term complications after liver transplantation attributable primarily to immunosuppressive medications include diabetes mellitus (associated with glucocorticoids) as well as hypertension, hyperlipidemia, and chronic renal insufficiency (associated with cyclosporine and tacrolimus). Monitoring and treating these disorders is a routine component of posttransplantation care; in some cases, they respond to changes in immunosuppressive regimen, while in others, specific treatment of the disorder is introduced.

HEPATIC COMPLICATIONS

Hepatic dysfunction after liver transplantation is similar to the hepatic complications encountered after major abdominal and cardiothoracic surgery; however, in addition, hepatic complications include primary graft failure, vascular compromise, failure or stricture of the biliary anastomoses, and rejection. As in nontransplant surgery, postoperative jaundice may result from prehepatic, intrahepatic, and posthepatic sources. *Prehepatic* sources represent the massive hemoglobin pigment load from transfusions, hemolysis, hematomas, ecchymoses, and other collections of blood. *Early intrahepatic* liver injury includes effects of hepatotoxic drugs and anesthesia; hypoperfusion injury associated with hypotension, sepsis, and shock; and benign postoperative cholestasis. *Late intrahepatic* sources of liver injury include posttransfusion hepatitis and exacerbation of primary disease. *Posthepatic* sources of hepatic dysfunction include biliary obstruction and reduced renal clearance of conjugated bilirubin. Hepatic complications unique to liver transplantation include primary graft failure associated with ischemic injury to the organ during harvesting; vascular compromise associated with thrombosis or stenosis of the portal vein or hepatic artery anastomoses; vascular

anastomotic leak; stenosis, obstruction, or leakage of the anastomosed common bile duct; recurrence of primary hepatic disorder (discussed later); and rejection.

TRANSPLANT REJECTION

Despite the use of immunosuppressive drugs, rejection of the transplanted liver still occurs in a proportion of patients, beginning 1–2 weeks after surgery. Clinical signs suggesting rejection are fever, right upper quadrant pain, and reduced bile pigment and volume. Leukocytosis may occur, but the most reliable indicators are increases in serum bilirubin and aminotransferase levels. Because these tests lack specificity, distinguishing among rejection, biliary obstruction, primary graft nonfunction, vascular compromise, viral hepatitis, CMV infection, drug hepatotoxicity, and recurrent primary disease may be difficult. Radiographic visualization of the biliary tree and/or percutaneous liver biopsy often help to establish the correct diagnosis. Morphologic features of acute rejection include a mixed portal cellular infiltrate, bile duct injury, and/or endothelial inflammation ("endothelialitis"); some of these findings are reminiscent of graft-versus-host disease, primary biliary cirrhosis, or recurrent allograft hepatitis C. As soon as transplant rejection is suspected, treatment consists of IV methylprednisolone in repeated boluses; if this fails to abort rejection, many centers use thymoglobulin or OKT3. Caution should be exercised when managing acute rejection with pulse glucocorticoids or OKT3 in patients with HCV infection, because of the high risk of triggering recurrent allograft hepatitis C.

Chronic rejection is a relatively rare outcome that can follow repeated bouts of acute rejection or that occurs unrelated to preceding rejection episodes. Morphologically, chronic rejection is characterized by progressive cholestasis, focal parenchymal necrosis, mononuclear infiltration, vascular lesions (intimal fibrosis, subintimal foam cells, fibrinoid necrosis), and fibrosis. This process may be reflected as ductopenia—the vanishing bile duct syndrome. Reversibility of chronic rejection is limited; in patients with therapy-resistant chronic rejection, retransplantation has yielded encouraging results.

OUTCOME

SURVIVAL

The survival rate for patients undergoing liver transplantation has improved steadily since 1983. One-year survival rates have increased from ~70% in the early 1980s to 85–90% from 2003 to 2009. Currently the 5-year survival rate exceeds 60%. An important observation is the relationship between clinical status before transplantation and outcome. For patients who undergo liver transplantation when their level of compensation is high (e.g., still working or only partially disabled), a 1-year survival rate of >85% is common. For those whose level of decompensation mandates continuous in-hospital care prior to transplantation, the 1-year survival rate is about 70%, while for those who are so decompensated that they require life support in an intensive care unit, the 1-year survival rate is ~50%. Since UNOS's adoption in 2002 of the MELD system for organ allocation, posttransplantation survival has been found to be affected adversely for candidates with MELD scores >25, considered high disease severity. Thus, irrespective of allocation scheme, high disease severity pretransplantation corresponds to diminished posttransplantation survival. Another important distinction in survival has been drawn between high- and low-risk patient categories. For patients who do not fit any "high-risk" designations, 1-year and 5-year survival rates of 85 and 80%, respectively, have been recorded. In contrast, among patients in high-risk categories—cancer, fulminant hepatitis, age >65, concurrent renal failure, respirator dependence, portal vein thrombosis, and history of a portacaval shunt or multiple right upper quadrant operations—survival statistics fall into the range of 60% at 1 year and 35% at 5 years. Survival after retransplantation for primary graft nonfunction is ~50%. Causes of failure of liver transplantation vary with time. Failures within the first 3 months result primarily from technical complications, postoperative infections, and hemorrhage. Transplant failures after the first 3 months are more likely to result from infection, rejection, or recurrent disease (such as malignancy or viral hepatitis).

RECURRENCE OF PRIMARY DISEASE

Features of autoimmune hepatitis, primary sclerosing cholangitis, and primary biliary cirrhosis overlap with those of rejection or posttransplantation bile duct injury. Whether autoimmune hepatitis and sclerosing choangitis recur after liver transplantation is controversial; data supporting recurrent autoimmune hepatitis (in up to one-third of patients in some series) are more convincing than those supporting recurrent sclerosing cholangitis. Similarly, reports of recurrent primary biliary cirrhosis after liver transplantation have appeared; however, the histologic features of primary biliary cirrhosis and chronic rejection are virtually indistinguishable and occur as frequently in patients with primary biliary cirrhosis as in patients undergoing transplantation for other reasons. The presence of a florid inflammatory bile duct lesion is highly suggestive of the recurrence of primary biliary cirrhosis, but even this lesion can be observed in acute rejection. Hereditary disorders such as Wilson's disease and α_1-antitrypsin deficiency have not recurred after liver transplantation; however, recurrence of disordered iron metabolism has been observed in some patients with hemochromatosis. Hepatic vein thrombosis (Budd-Chiari syndrome) may recur; this can be minimized by treating underlying myeloproliferative disorders and by anticoagulation. Because cholangiocarcinoma recurs almost invariably, few centers now offer transplantation to such patients; however, a few highly selected patients with operatively confirmed stage I or II cholangiocarcinoma who undergo liver transplantation combined with neoadjuvant chemoradiation may experience excellent outcomes. In patients with intrahepatic hepatocellular carcinoma who meet criteria for transplantation, 1- and 5-year survivals are similar to those observed in patients undergoing liver transplantation for nonmalignant disease. Finally, metabolic disorders such as nonalcoholic steatohepatitis recur frequently, especially if the underlying metabolic predisposition is not altered. The metabolic syndrome occurs commonly after liver transplantation as a result of recurrent nonalcoholic fatty liver, immunosuppressive medications, and/or, in patients with hepatitis C related to the impact of HCV infection on insulin resistance, diabetes, and fatty liver.

Hepatitis A can recur after transplantation for fulminant hepatitis A, but such acute reinfection has no serious clinical sequelae. In fulminant hepatitis B, recurrence is not the rule; however, in the absence of any prophylactic measures, hepatitis B usually recurs after transplantation for end-stage chronic hepatitis B. Before the introduction of prophylactic antiviral therapy, immunosuppressive therapy sufficient to prevent allograft rejection led inevitably to marked increases in hepatitis B viremia, regardless of pretransplantation levels. Overall graft and patient survival were poor, and some patients experienced a rapid recapitulation of severe injury—severe chronic hepatitis or even fulminant hepatitis—after transplantation. Also recognized in the era before availability of antiviral regimens was *fibrosing cholestatic hepatitis*, rapidly progressive liver injury associated with marked hyperbilirubinemia, substantial prolongation of the prothrombin time (both out of proportion to relatively modest elevations of aminotransferase activity), and rapidly progressive liver failure. This lesion has been suggested to represent a "choking off" of the hepatocyte by an overwhelming density of HBV proteins. Complications such as sepsis and pancreatitis were also observed more frequently in patients undergoing liver transplantation for hepatitis B prior to the introduction of antiviral therapy. The introduction of long-term prophylaxis with HBIg revolutionized liver transplantation for chronic hepatitis B. Preoperative hepatitis B vaccination, preoperative or postoperative interferon (IFN) therapy, or short-term (≤2 months) HBIg prophylaxis has not been shown to be effective, but a retrospective analysis of data from several hundred European patients followed for

3 years after transplantation has shown that long-term (≥6 months) prophylaxis with HBIg is associated with a lowering of the risk of HBV reinfection from ~75% to 35% and a reduction in mortality from ~50% to 20%.

As a result of long-term HBIg use following liver transplantation for chronic hepatitis B, similar improvements in outcome have been observed in the United States, with 1-year survival rates between 75% and 90%. Currently, with HBIg prophylaxis, the outcome of liver transplantation for chronic hepatitis B is indistinguishable from that for chronic liver disease unassociated with chronic hepatitis B; essentially, medical concerns regarding liver transplantation for chronic hepatitis B have been eliminated. Passive immunoprophylaxis with HBIg is begun during the anhepatic stage of surgery, repeated daily for the first 6 postoperative days, then continued with infusions that are given either at regular intervals of 4–6 weeks or, alternatively, when anti-hepatitis B surface (HBs) levels fall below a threshold of 100 mIU/mL. The current approach in most centers is to continue HBIg indefinitely, which can add approximately $20,000 per year to the cost of care; some centers are evaluating regimens that shift to less frequent administration or to IM administration in the late post-transplantation period or, in low-risk patients, maintenance with antiviral therapy (discussed later) alone. Still, "breakthrough" HBV infection occasionally occurs.

Further improving the outcome of liver transplantation for chronic hepatitis B is the current availability of such antiviral drugs as lamivudine, adefovir, entecavir, and tenofovir disoproxil fumarate (Chap. 40). When these drugs are administered to patients with decompensated liver disease, a proportion improve sufficiently to postpone imminent liver transplantation. In addition, lamivudine can be used to prevent recurrence of HBV infection when administered *prior* to transplantation; to treat hepatitis B that recurs *after* transplantation, including in patients who break through HBIg prophylaxis; and to reverse the course of otherwise fatal fibrosing cholestatic hepatitis. Clinical trials have shown that lamivudine antiviral therapy reduces the level of HBV replication substantially, sometimes even resulting in clearance of hepatitis B surface antigen (HBsAg); reduces alanine aminotransferase (ALT) levels; and improves histologic features of necrosis and inflammation. Long-term use of lamivudine is safe and effective, but after several months a proportion of patients become resistant to lamivudine, resulting from YMDD (tyrosine-methionine-aspartate-aspartate) mutations in the HBV polymerase motif (Chap. 40). In approximately one-half of such resistant patients, hepatic deterioration may ensue. Fortunately, adefovir or tenofovir disoproxil fumarate are available as well and can be used to treat lamivudine-associated YMDD variants, effectively "rescuing" patients experiencing hepatic decompensation

after lamivudine breakthrough. Currently, most liver transplantation centers combine HBIg plus lamivudine, adefovir, entecavir, or tenofovir disoproxil fumarate. Clinical trials are underway to define the optimal application of these antiviral agents in the management of patients undergoing liver transplantation for chronic hepatitis B; conceivably, in the future, combinations of oral antiviral drugs may supplant HBIg.

Prophylactic approaches applied to patients undergoing liver transplantation for chronic hepatitis B are being used as well for patients without hepatitis B who receive organs from donors with anti-hepatitis B core (HBc). Patients who undergo liver transplantation for chronic hepatitis B plus D are less likely to experience recurrent liver injury than patients undergoing liver transplantation for hepatitis B alone; still, such co-infected patients would also be offered standard posttransplantation prophylactic therapy for hepatitis B.

Accounting for up to 40% of all liver transplantation procedures, the most common indication for liver transplantation is end-stage liver disease resulting from chronic hepatitis C. Recurrence of HCV infection after liver transplantation can be documented in almost every patient. The clinical consequences of recurrent hepatitis C are limited during the first 5 years after transplantation. Nonetheless, despite the relative clinical benignity of recurrent hepatitis C in the early years after liver transplantation, and despite the negligible impact on patient survival during these early years, histologic studies have documented the presence of moderate to severe chronic hepatitis in more than one-half of all patients and bridging fibrosis or cirrhosis in ~10%. Moreover, progression to cirrhosis within 5 years is even more common, occurring in up to two-thirds of patients if moderate hepatitis is detected in a 1-year biopsy. Not surprisingly, then, for patients undergoing transplantation for hepatitis C, allograft and patient survival are diminished substantially between 5 and 10 years after transplantation. In a proportion of patients, even during the early posttransplantation period, recurrent hepatitis C may be sufficiently severe biochemically and histologically to merit antiviral therapy. Treatment with pegylated interferon (IFN) can *suppress* HCV-associated liver injury but rarely leads to *sustained* benefit. Sustained virologic responses are the exception, and reduced tolerability is often dose-limiting. Preemptive combination antiviral therapy with pegylated IFN and the nucleoside analogue ribavirin immediately after transplantation does not appear to provide any advantage over therapy introduced after clinical hepatitis has occurred. Similarly, although IFN-based antiviral therapy is not recommended for patients with decompensated liver disease, some centers have experimented with pretransplantation antiviral therapy in an attempt to eradicate HCV replication prior to transplantation;

preliminary results are promising, but IFN treatment of patients with end-stage liver disease can lead to worsening of hepatic decompensation, and HCV infection has recurred after transplantation in some of these recipients. Trials of hepatitis C immune globulin preparations to prevent recurrent hepatitis C after liver transplantation have not been successful.

A small number succumb to early HCV-associated liver injury, and a syndrome reminiscent of fibrosing cholestatic hepatitis (discussed earlier) has been observed rarely. Because patients with more episodes of rejection receive more immunosuppressive therapy, and because immunosuppressive therapy enhances HCV replication, patients with severe or multiple episodes of rejection are more likely to experience early recurrence of hepatitis C after transplantation. Both high viral levels and older donor age have been linked to recurrent HCV-induced liver disease and to earlier disease recurrence after transplantation.

Patients who undergo liver transplantation for end-stage alcoholic cirrhosis are at risk of resorting to drinking again after transplantation, a potential source of recurrent alcoholic liver injury. Currently, alcoholic liver disease is one of the more common indications for liver transplantation, accounting for 20–25% of all liver transplantation procedures, and most transplantation centers screen candidates carefully for predictors of continued abstinence. Recidivism is more likely in patients whose sobriety prior to transplantation was <6 months. For abstinent patients with alcoholic cirrhosis, liver transplantation can be undertaken successfully, with outcomes comparable to those for other categories of patients with chronic liver disease, when coordinated by a team approach that includes substance abuse counseling.

POSTTRANSPLANTATION QUALITY OF LIFE

Full rehabilitation is achieved in the majority of patients who survive the early postoperative months and escape chronic rejection or unmanageable infection. Psychosocial maladjustment interferes with medical compliance in a small number of patients, but most manage to adhere to immunosuppressive regimens, which must be continued indefinitely. In one study, 85% of patients who survived their transplant operations returned to gainful activities. In fact, some women have conceived and carried pregnancies to term after transplantation without demonstrable injury to their infants.

CHAPTER 47

APPROACH TO THE PATIENT WITH PANCREATIC DISEASE

Norton J. Greenberger ■ **Darwin L. Conwell** ■ **Peter A. Banks**

GENERAL CONSIDERATIONS

As emphasized in Chap. 48, the etiologies as well as the clinical manifestations of pancreatitis are quite varied. Although it is well-appreciated that pancreatitis is frequently secondary to biliary tract disease and alcohol abuse, it can also be caused by drugs, trauma, and viral infections and is associated with metabolic and connective tissue disorders. In ~30% of patients with acute pancreatitis and 25–40% of patients with chronic pancreatitis, the etiology initially can be obscure.

Although good data exist concerning the incidence of acute pancreatitis (about 5–35/100,000 new cases per year worldwide, with a mortality rate of about 3%), the number of patients who suffer with acute pancreatitis is largely increasing and is now estimated to be 70 hospitalizations/100,000 persons annually, resulting in >200,000 new cases of acute pancreatitis per year in the United States. Only one prospective study on the incidence of chronic pancreatitis is available; it showed an incidence of 8.2 new cases per 100,000 per year and a prevalence of 26.4 cases per 100,000. These numbers probably underestimate considerably the true incidence and prevalence, because non alcohol–induced pancreatitis has been largely ignored. At autopsy, the prevalence of chronic pancreatitis ranges from 0.04 to 5%. The relative inaccessibility of the pancreas to direct examination and the nonspecificity of the abdominal pain associated with pancreatitis make the diagnosis of pancreatitis difficult and usually dependent on elevation of blood amylase and/or lipase levels. Many patients with chronic pancreatitis do not have elevated blood amylase or lipase levels. Some patients with chronic pancreatitis develop signs and symptoms of pancreatic exocrine insufficiency, and, thus, objective evidence for pancreatic disease can be demonstrated. However, there is a very large reservoir of pancreatic exocrine function.

More than 90% of the pancreas must be damaged before maldigestion of fat and protein is manifested. Noninvasive, indirect tests of pancreatic exocrine function (fecal elastase) are much more likely to give abnormal results in patients with obvious pancreatic disease (i.e., pancreatic calcification, steatorrhea, or diabetes mellitus, than in patients with occult disease). Thus, the number of patients who have subclinical exocrine dysfunction (<90% loss of function) is unknown.

TESTS USEFUL IN THE DIAGNOSIS OF PANCREATIC DISEASE

Several tests have proved of value in the evaluation of pancreatic disease. Examples of specific tests and their usefulness in the diagnosis of acute and chronic pancreatitis are summarized in Table 47-1 and Fig. 47-1. At some institutions, pancreatic-function tests are available and performed if the diagnosis of pancreatic disease remains a possibility after noninvasive tests (ultrasound, CT, magnetic resonance cholangiopancreatography [MRCP]) or invasive tests (endoscopic retrograde cholangiopancreatography [ERCP], endoscopic ultrasonography [EUS]) have given normal or inconclusive results. In this regard, tests employing *direct* stimulation of the pancreas are the most sensitive.

Pancreatic enzymes in body fluids

The serum amylase and lipase levels are widely used as screening tests for acute pancreatitis in the patient with acute abdominal pain or back pain. Values greater than three times the upper limit of normal virtually clinch the diagnosis if gut perforation or infarction is excluded. In acute pancreatitis, the serum amylase and lipase are usually elevated within 24 h of onset and remain so for 3–7 days. Levels usually

TABLE 47-1

TESTS USEFUL IN THE DIAGNOSIS OF ACUTE AND CHRONIC PANCREATITIS AND PANCREATIC TUMORS

TEST	PRINCIPLE	COMMENT
Pancreatic Enzymes in Body Fluids		
Amylase		
1. Serum	Pancreatic inflammation leads to increased enzyme levels	Simple; 20–40% false negatives and positives; reliable if test results are three times the upper limit of normal
2. Urine	Renal clearance of amylase is increased in acute pancreatitis	Infrequently used
3. Ascitic fluid	Disruption of gland or main pancreatic duct leads to increased amylase concentration	Can help establish diagnosis of acute pancreatitis; false positives occur with intestinal obstruction and perforated ulcer
4. Pleural fluid	Exudative pleural effusion with pancreatitis	False positives occur with carcinoma of the lung and esophageal perforation
Serum lipase	Pancreatic inflammation leads to increased enzyme levels	New methods have greatly simplified determination; positive in 70–85% of cases
Studies Pertaining to Pancreatic Structure		
Radiologic and radionuclide tests		
1. Plain film of the abdomen	Can be abnormal in acute and chronic pancreatitis	Simple; normal in >50% of cases of both acute and chronic pancreatitis
2. Upper GI x-rays		Now obsolete
3. Ultrasonography (US)	Can provide information on edema, inflammation, calcification, pseudocysts, and mass lesions	Simple, noninvasive; sequential studies quite feasible; useful in diagnosis of pseudocyst limited by interference by bowel gas
4. CT scan	Permits detailed visualization of pancreas and surrounding structures, pancreatic fluid collection, pseudocyst, degree of necrosis	Useful in the diagnosis of pancreatic calcification, dilated pancreatic ducts, and pancreatic tumors; may not be able to distinguish between inflammatory and neoplastic mass lesions
5. Endoscopic retrograde cholangiopancreatography (ERCP)	Cannulation of pancreatic and common bile duct permits visualization of pancreatic-biliary ductal system	Can provide diagnostic data in 60–85% of cases; differentiation of chronic pancreatitis from pancreatic carcinoma may be difficult; now considered primarily a therapeutic procedure
6. Endoscopic ultrasonography (EUS)	High-frequency transducer employed with EUS can produce very high-resolution images and depict changes in the pancreatic duct and parenchyma with great detail	Can be used to assess chronic pancreatitis and pancreatic carcinoma
7. Magnetic resonance cholangiopancreatography	Three-dimensional rendering has been used to produce very good images of the pancreatic duct by a noninvasive technique	Has largely replaced ERCP as a diagnostic test
Pancreatic biopsy with US or CT guidance	Percutaneous aspiration biopsy with skinny needle and localization of lesion by US	High diagnostic yield; laparotomy avoided; can be done with EUS; requires special technical skills
Tests of Exocrine Pancreatic Function		
Direct stimulation of the pancreas with analysis of duodenal contents		
1. Secretin-pancreozymin (CCK) test	Secretin leads to increased output of pancreatic juice and HCO_3^-; CCK leads to increased output of pancreatic enzymes; pancreatic secretory response is related to the functional mass of pancreatic tissue	Sensitive enough to detect occult disease; involves duodenal intubation and fluoroscopy; poorly defined normal enzyme response; overlap in chronic pancreatitis; large secretory reserve capacity of the pancreas, currently done at only a few medical centers

(continued)

CHAPTER 47 Approach to the Patient with Pancreatic Disease

TABLE 47-1

TESTS USEFUL IN THE DIAGNOSIS OF ACUTE AND CHRONIC PANCREATITIS AND PANCREATIC TUMORS (*CONTINUED*)

TEST	PRINCIPLE	COMMENT
2. Endoscopic secretin—CCK test	Replaces need for tube placement duodenum	Sensitive enough to detect occult disease; avoids intubation and fluoroscopy; requires sedation
Measurement of intraluminal digestion products		
1. Microscopic examination of stool for undigested meat fibers and fat	Lack of proteolytic and lipolytic enzymes causes decreased digestion of meat fibers and triglycerides	Simple, reliable; not sensitive enough to detect milder cases of pancreatic insufficiency
2. Quantitative stool fat determination	Lack of lipolytic enzymes brings about impaired fat digestion	Reliable, reference standard for defining severity of malabsorption; does not distinguish between maldigestion and malabsorption
3. Fecal nitrogen	Lack of proteolytic enzymes leads to impaired protein digestion, resulting in an increase in stool nitrogen	Does not distinguish between maldigestion and malabsorption; low sensitivity
Measurement of pancreatic enzymes in feces		
1. Elastase	Pancreatic secretion of proteolytic enzymes; not degraded in intestine	Good sensitivity if stools not liquid

Abbreviation: CCK, cholecystokinin.

return to normal within 7 days unless there is pancreatic ductal disruption, ductal obstruction, or pseudocyst formation. Approximately 85% of patients with acute pancreatitis have a threefold or greater elevated serum amylase and lipase levels. The values may be normal if (1) there is a delay (of 2–5 days) before blood samples are obtained, (2) the underlying disorder is chronic pancreatitis rather than acute pancreatitis, or (3) hypertriglyceridemia is present. Patients with hypertriglyceridemia and proven pancreatitis have been found to have spuriously low levels of amylase and perhaps lipase activity. In the absence of objective evidence of pancreatitis by abdominal ultrasound, CT scan, MRCP, or EUS, mild to moderate elevations of amylase, and/or lipase are not helpful in making a diagnosis of chronic pancreatitis.

The serum amylase can be elevated in other conditions (Table 47-2), in part because the enzyme is found in many organs. In addition to the pancreas and salivary glands, small quantities of amylase are found in the tissues of the fallopian tubes, lung, thyroid, and tonsils and can be produced by various tumors (carcinomas of the lung, esophagus, breast, and ovary). Urinary amylase measurements, including the amylase/creatinine clearance ratio, are no more sensitive or specific than blood amylase levels and are rarely employed. Isoamylase determinations do not accurately distinguish elevated blood amylase levels due to bona fide pancreatitis from elevated blood amylase levels due to

a nonpancreatic source of amylase, especially when the blood amylase level is only moderately elevated.

Elevation of ascitic fluid amylase occurs in acute pancreatitis as well as in (1) pancreatogenous ascites due to disruption of the main pancreatic duct or a leaking pseudocyst and (2) other abdominal disorders that simulate pancreatitis (e.g., intestinal obstruction, intestinal infarction, or perforated peptic ulcer). Elevation of pleural fluid amylase can occur in acute pancreatitis, chronic pancreatitis, carcinoma of the lung, and esophageal perforation.

Lipase may now be the single best enzyme to measure for the diagnosis of acute pancreatitis. Improvements in substrates and technology offer clinicians improved options, especially when a turbidimetric assay is used. The newer lipase assays have colipase as a cofactor and are fully automated.

No single blood test is reliable for the diagnosis of acute pancreatitis in patients with renal failure. Determining whether a patient with renal failure and abdominal pain has pancreatitis remains a difficult clinical problem. One study found that serum amylase levels were elevated in patients with renal dysfunction only when creatinine clearance was <0.8 mL/s (<50 mL/min). In such patients, the serum amylase level was invariably <8.3 μkat/L (<500 IU/L) in the absence of objective evidence of acute pancreatitis. In that study, serum lipase and trypsin levels paralleled serum amylase values. With these limitations in mind,

FIGURE 47-1

A step-wise diagnostic approach to the patient with suspected chronic pancreatitis (CP). Endoscopic ultrasonography (EUS) and magnetic resonance cholangiopancreatography (sMRCP/MRCP) are appropriate diagnostic alternatives to endoscopic retrograde cholangiopancreatography (ERCP).

the recommended screening tests for acute pancreatitis are *serum lipase* and *serum amylase levels*. Serum lipase and amylase values greater than three times normal are highly specific.

Studies pertaining to pancreatic structure

Radiologic tests

Plain films of the abdomen, which once provided useful information in patients with acute and chronic pancreatitis, have been superceded by other detailed imaging procedures (US, EUS, CT, MRCP).

Ultrasonography can provide important information in patients with acute pancreatitis, chronic pancreatitis, pseudocysts, and pancreatic carcinoma. Echographic appearances can indicate the presence of edema, inflammation, and calcification (not obvious on plain films of the abdomen), as well as pseudocysts, mass lesions, and gallstones. In acute pancreatitis, the pancreas is characteristically enlarged. In pancreatic pseudocyst, the usual appearance is primarily that of smooth, round fluid collection. Pancreatic carcinoma distorts the usual landmarks, and mass lesions >3.0 cm are usually detected as localized, solid lesions. Ultrasound is often the initial investigation for most patients with suspected pancreatic disease. However, obesity and excess small- and large-bowel gas can interfere with pancreatic imaging by ultrasound studies.

TABLE 47-2

CAUSES OF HYPERAMYLASEMIA AND HYPERAMYLASURIA

Pancreatic Disease

I. Pancreatitis
  A. Acute
  B. Chronic: ductal
    obstruction
  C. Complications of
    pancreatitis
    1. Pancreatic pseudocyst
    2. Pancreatogenous
      ascites
    3. Pancreatic abscess
    4. Pancreatic necrosis
	II. Pancreatic
	    trauma
	III. Pancreatic
	    carcinoma

Nonpancreatic Disorders

I. Renal insufficiency
II. Salivary gland lesions
  A. Mumps
  B. Calculus
  C. Irradiation sialadenitis
  D. Maxillofacial surgery
III. "Tumor" hyperamylasemia
  A. Carcinoma of the lung
  B. Carcinoma of the
    esophagus
  C. Breast carcinoma,
    ovarian carcinoma
	IV. Macroamylasemia
	V. Burns
	VI. Diabetic
	    ketoacidosis
	VII. Pregnancy
	VIII. Renal
	    transplantation
	IX. Cerebral trauma
	X. Drugs: morphine

Other Abdominal Disorders

I. Biliary tract disease: cholecystitis, choledocholithiasis
II. Intraabdominal disease
  A. Perforated or penetrating peptic ulcer
  B. Intestinal obstruction or infarction
  C. Ruptured ectopic pregnancy
  D. Peritonitis
  E. Aortic aneurysm
  F. Chronic liver disease
  G. Postoperative hyperamylasemia

CT is the best imaging study for initial evaluation of a suspected pancreatic disorder and for the complications of acute and chronic pancreatitis. It is especially useful in the detection of pancreatic and peripancreatic acute fluid collections, fluid-containing lesions such as pseudocysts, walled-off necrosis, calcium deposits (see Chap. 48, Figs. 48-1, 48-2, and 48-4), and pancreatic neoplasms. Most lesions are characterized by (1) enlargement of the pancreatic outline, (2) distortion of the pancreatic contour, and/or (3) a fluid filling that has a different attenuation coefficient than normal pancreas. Oral, water-soluble contrast agents are used to opacify the stomach and duodenum during CT scans; this strategy permits more precise delineation of various organs as well as mass lesions. Dynamic CT (using rapid IV administration of

contrast) is useful in estimating the extent of pancreatic necrosis and in predicting morbidity and mortality. Spiral (helical) CT provides clear images much more rapidly and essentially negates artifact caused by patient movement.

EUS produces high-resolution images of the pancreatic parenchyma and pancreatic duct with a transducer fixed to an endoscope that can be directed onto the surface of the pancreas through the stomach or duodenum. EUS and MRCP have largely replaced ERCP for diagnostic purposes in many centers. EUS allows one to obtain information about the pancreatic duct as well as the parenchyma and has few procedure-related complications associated with it, in contrast to the 5–20% of post-ERCP pancreatitis observed. EUS is also helpful in detecting common bile duct stones. Pancreatic masses can be biopsied via EUS and one can deliver nerve-blocking agents through EUS fine-needle injection. Criteria for abnormalities on EUS in severe chronic pancreatic disease have been developed. Currently, chronic pancreatitis is considered diagnosed by EUS if five or more criteria listed in Table 47-3 are present. Recent studies comparing EUS and ERCP to the secretin test in patients with unexplained abdominal pain suspected of having chronic pancreatitis show equivalent diagnostic accuracy in detecting early changes of chronic pancreatitis. The exact role of EUS versus CT, ERCP, or function testing in the early diagnosis of chronic pancreatitis has yet to be clearly defined.

MRCP/MRI is now being used to view the bile ducts, pancreatic duct, and the pancreas parenchyma. Non breath–holding and three-dimensional turbo spin-echo techniques are being used to produce superb MRCP images. The main pancreatic duct and common bile duct can be seen well, but there is still a question as to whether changes can be detected consistently in the secondary ducts. The secondary ducts are not visualized in a normal pancreas. MRCP may be particularly useful to evaluate the pancreatic duct in high-risk patients such as the elderly because this is a noninvasive procedure. Secretin enhanced MRCP is currently under investigation but is emerging as a method to better evaluate ductal changes.

TABLE 47-3

ENDOSCOPIC ULTRASONOGRAPHIC CRITERIA FOR CHRONIC PANCREATITIS

DUCTAL	PARENCHYMAL
Stones	Echogenic strands
Echogenic ductal walls	Echogenic foci
Irregular ductal walls	Calcifications
Stricture	Lobular contour
Visible side branches	Cyst
Ductular dilatation	

Both EUS and MRCP have largely replaced diagnostic ERCP in most patients. As these techniques become more refined, they may well be the diagnostic tests of choice to evaluate the pancreatic duct. ERCP is still needed for treatment of bile duct and pancreatic duct lesions. ERCP is primarily of therapeutic value after CT, EUS, or MRCP have detected abnormalities requiring invasive endoscopic treatment. ERCP can also be helpful at clarification of equivocal findings discovered with other imaging techniques (see Chap. 48, Figs. 48-1*C*, 48-3*D*, and 48-4*B*). Pancreatic carcinoma is characterized by stenosis or obstruction of either the pancreatic duct or the common bile duct; both ductal systems are often abnormal. In chronic pancreatitis, ERCP abnormalities include (1) luminal narrowing; (2) irregularities in the ductal system with stenosis, dilation, sacculation, and ectasia; and (3) blockage of the pancreatic duct by calcium deposits. The presence of ductal stenosis and irregularity can make it difficult to distinguish chronic pancreatitis from carcinoma. It is important to be aware that ERCP changes interpreted as indicating chronic pancreatitis actually may be due to the effects of aging on the pancreatic duct or to the fact that the procedure was performed within several weeks of an attack of acute pancreatitis. Although aging may cause impressive ductal alterations, it does not affect the results of pancreatic function tests (i.e., the secretin test). Elevated serum amylase levels after ERCP have been reported in 25–75% of patients, and clinical pancreatitis in 5–20% of patients. There are no satisfactory means to pharmacologically prevent ERCP-induced pancreatitis, despite many agents such as octreotide and nitroglycerin having been suggested and evaluated. The best way to prevent ERCP-induced pancreatitis is to not perform this procedure for diagnostic purposes in high-risk patients, especially in women with acute relapsing pancreatitis in whom there is no evidence of biliary obstruction and patients with unexplained abdominal pain but no other abnormalities. If no lesion is found in the biliary and/or pancreatic ducts in a patient with repeated attacks of acute pancreatitis, manometric studies of the sphincter of Oddi may be indicated. Such studies, however, do increase the risk of post-ERCP/manometry acute pancreatitis. Such pancreatitis appears to be more common in patients with a nondilated pancreatic duct.

▮ Pancreatic biopsy with radiologic guidance
Percutaneous aspiration biopsy or a trucut biopsy of a pancreatic mass often distinguishes a pancreatic inflammatory mass from a pancreatic neoplasm.

TESTS OF EXOCRINE PANCREATIC FUNCTION

Pancreatic function tests (Table 47-1) can be divided into the following:

1. *Direct stimulation of the pancreas* by IV infusion of secretin or secretin plus cholecystokinin (CCK) followed by collection and measurement of duodenal contents
2. Study of *intraluminal digestion products*, such as undigested meat fibers, stool fat, and fecal nitrogen
3. *Measurement of fecal pancreatic enzymes* such as elastase

The secretin test, used to detect diffuse pancreatic disease, is based on the physiologic principle that the pancreatic secretory response is directly related to the functional mass of pancreatic tissue. In the standard assay, secretin is given IV in a dose of 0.2 μg/kg of synthetic human secretin as a bolus. Normal values for the standard secretin test are (1) volume output >2 mL/kg per hour, (2) bicarbonate (HCO_3^-) concentration >80 mmol/L, and (3) HCO_3^- output >10 mmol/L in 1 h. The most reproducible measurement, giving the highest level of discrimination between normal subjects and patients with chronic pancreatic exocrine insufficiency, appears to be the maximal bicarbonate concentration.

There may be a dissociation between the results of the secretin test and other tests of absorptive function. For example, patients with chronic pancreatitis often have abnormally low outputs of HCO_3^- after secretin but have normal fecal fat excretion. Thus the secretin test measures the secretory capacity of ductular epithelium, while fecal fat excretion indirectly reflects intraluminal lipolytic activity. Steatorrhea does not occur until intraluminal levels of lipase are markedly reduced, underscoring the fact that only small amounts of enzymes are necessary for intraluminal digestive activities. It must be noted that, an abnormal secretin test result suggests only that chronic pancreatic damage is present.

Measurement of *intraluminal digestion products* (i.e., undigested muscle fibers, stool fat, and fecal nitrogen) is discussed in Chap. 15. The amount of human elastase in stool reflects the pancreatic output of this proteolytic enzyme. Decreased elastase activity in stool is an excellent test to detect severe pancreatic exocrine insufficiency in patients with chronic pancreatitis and cystic fibrosis provided that the stool specimen is solid.

Tests useful in the diagnosis of exocrine pancreatic insufficiency and the differential diagnosis of malabsorption are also discussed in Chaps. 15 and 48.

CHAPTER 48

ACUTE AND CHRONIC PANCREATITIS

Norton J. Greenberger ■ Darwin L. Conwell
Bechien U. Wu ■ Peter A. Banks

BIOCHEMISTRY AND PHYSIOLOGY OF PANCREATIC EXOCRINE SECRETION

GENERAL CONSIDERATIONS

The pancreas secretes 1500–3000 mL of isosmotic alkaline (pH >8) fluid per day containing about 20 enzymes. The pancreatic secretions provide the enzymes needed to effect the major digestive activity of the gastrointestinal tract and provide an optimal pH for the function of these enzymes.

REGULATION OF PANCREATIC SECRETION

The exocrine pancreas is influenced by intimately interacting hormonal and neural systems. *Gastric acid* is the stimulus for the release of secretin from the duodenum, which stimulates the secretion of water and electrolytes from pancreatic ductal cells. Release of cholecystokinin (CCK) from the duodenum and proximal jejunum is largely triggered by long-chain fatty acids, certain essential amino acids (tryptophan, phenylalanine, valine, methionine), and gastric acid itself. CCK evokes an enzyme-rich secretion from acinar cells in the pancreas. The *parasympathetic nervous system* (via the vagus nerve) exerts significant control over pancreatic secretion. Secretion evoked by secretin and CCK depends on permissive roles of vagal afferent and efferent pathways. This is particularly true for enzyme secretion, whereas water and bicarbonate secretions are heavily dependent on the hormonal effects of secretin and to a lesser extent CCK. Also, vagal stimulation effects the release of vasoactive intestinal peptide (VIP), a secretin agonist.

Pancreatic exocrine secretion is influenced by inhibitory neuropeptides such as somatostatin, pancreatic polypeptide, peptide YY, neuropeptide Y, enkephalin, pancreastatin, calcitonin gene–related peptides, glucagon, and galanin. Although pancreatic polypeptide and peptide YY may act primarily on nerves outside the pancreas, somatostatin acts at multiple sites. Nitric oxide (NO) is also an important neurotransmitter. The mechanism of action of these various factors has not been fully defined.

WATER AND ELECTROLYTE SECRETION

Bicarbonate is the ion of primary physiologic importance within pancreatic secretion. The ductal cells secrete bicarbonate predominantly derived from plasma (93%) more than from intracellular metabolism (7%). Bicarbonate enters through the sodium bicarbonate cotransporter with depolarization caused by chloride efflux through the cystic fibrosis transmembrane conductance regulator (CFTR). Secretin and VIP, both of which increase intracellular cyclic AMP, act on the ductal cells opening the CFTR in promoting secretion. CCK, acting as a neuromodulator, markedly potentiates the stimulatory effects of secretin. Acetylcholine also plays an important role in ductal cell secretion. Bicarbonate helps neutralize gastric acid and creates the appropriate pH for the activity of pancreatic enzymes and bile salts.

ENZYME SECRETION

The acinar cell is highly compartmentalized and is concerned with the secretion of pancreatic enzymes. Proteins synthesized by the rough endoplasmic reticulum are processed in the Golgi and then targeted to the appropriate site, whether that be zymogen granules, lysosomes, or other cell compartments. The pancreas secretes amylolytic, lipolytic, and proteolytic enzymes. *Amylolytic enzymes* such as amylase, hydrolyze starch to oligosaccharides and to the disaccharide maltose. The *lipolytic enzymes* include lipase, phospholipase A_2, and cholesterol esterase. Bile salts inhibit lipase in isolation, but colipase, another constituent of pancreatic secretion, binds to lipase and prevents this inhibition. Bile salts activate phospholipase A and cholesterol esterase. *Proteolytic enzymes* include endopeptidases (trypsin, chymotrypsin), which act on internal peptide bonds of proteins and polypeptides; exopeptidases (carboxypeptidases, aminopeptidases), which act on the free carboxyl- and amino-terminal ends of peptides, respectively; and elastase. The proteolytic enzymes are secreted as inactive precursors and packaged as zymogens. Ribonucleases (deoxyribonucleases, ribonuclease) are also secreted. *Enterokinase*, an enzyme found in the duodenal mucosa, cleaves the lysine-isoleucine bond of trypsinogen to form trypsin. Trypsin then activates the other proteolytic zymogens and phospholipase A_2 in a cascade phenomenon. All pancreatic enzymes have pH optima in the alkaline range. The nervous system initiates pancreatic enzyme secretion. The neurologic stimulation is cholinergic, involving extrinsic innervation by the vagus nerve and subsequent innervation by intrapancreatic cholinergic nerves. The stimulatory neurotransmitters are acetylcholine and gastrin-releasing peptides. These neurotransmitters activate calcium-dependent second messenger systems, resulting in the release of zymogen granules. VIP is present in intrapancreatic nerves and potentiates the effect of acetylcholine. In contrast to other species, there are no CCK receptors on acinar cells in humans. CCK in physiologic concentrations stimulates pancreatic secretion by stimulating afferent vagal and intrapancreatic nerves.

AUTOPROTECTION OF THE PANCREAS

Autodigestion of the pancreas is prevented by the packaging of pancreatic proteases in precursor form and by the synthesis of protease inhibitor (i.e., pancreatic secretory trypsin inhibitor [PSTI] or SPINK1), which can bind and inactivate about 20% of trypsin activity. Mesotrypsin, chymotrypsin c, and enzyme y can also lyse and inactivate trypsin. These protease inhibitors are found in the acinar cell, the pancreatic secretions, and the α_1- and α_2-globulin fractions of plasma. In addition, low calcium concentration within the cytosol of acinar cells in the normal pancreas promotes the destruction of spontaneously activated trypsin. Loss of any of these protective mechanisms leads to zymogen activation, autodigestion, and acute pancreatitis.

EXOCRINE-ENDOCRINE RELATIONSHIPS

Insulin appears to be needed locally for secretin and CCK to promote exocrine secretion; thus, it acts in a permissive role for these two hormones.

ENTEROPANCREATIC AXIS AND FEEDBACK INHIBITION

Pancreatic enzyme secretion is controlled, at least in part, by a negative feedback mechanism induced by the presence of active serine proteases in the duodenum. To illustrate, perfusion of the duodenal lumen with phenylalanine causes a prompt result in increased plasma CCK levels as well as increased secretion of chymotrypsin and other pancreatic enzymes. However, simultaneous perfusion with trypsin blunts both responses. Conversely, perfusion of the duodenal lumen with protease inhibitors actually leads to enzyme hypersecretion. The available evidence supports the concept that the duodenum contains a peptide called *CCK-releasing factor* (CCK-RF) that is involved in stimulating CCK release. It appears that serine proteases inhibit pancreatic secretion by inactivating a CCK-releasing peptide in the lumen of the small intestine. Thus, the integrative result of both bicarbonate and enzyme secretion depends on a feedback process for both bicarbonate and pancreatic enzymes. Acidification of the duodenum releases secretin, which stimulates vagal and other neural pathways to activate pancreatic duct cells, which secrete bicarbonate. This bicarbonate then neutralizes the duodenal acid, and the feedback loop is completed. Dietary proteins bind proteases, thereby leading to an increase in free CCK-RF. CCK is then released into the blood in physiologic concentrations, acting primarily through the neural pathways (vagal-vagal). This leads to acetylcholine-mediated pancreatic enzyme secretion. Proteases continue to be secreted from the pancreas until the protein within the duodenum is digested. At this point, pancreatic protease secretion is reduced to basic levels, thus completing this step in the feedback process.

ACUTE PANCREATITIS

GENERAL CONSIDERATIONS

Pancreatic inflammatory disease may be classified as (1) acute pancreatitis or (2) chronic pancreatitis. The pathologic spectrum of acute pancreatitis varies from *interstitial pancreatitis*, which is usually a mild and self-limited disorder, to *necrotizing pancreatitis*, in which the extent of pancreatic necrosis may correlate with the severity of the attack and its systemic manifestations.

The incidence of pancreatitis varies in different countries and depends on cause (e.g., alcohol, gallstones, metabolic factors, and drugs [Table 48-1]). The estimated incidence in the United States is increasing and is now estimated to be 70 hospitalizations/100,000 persons annually, thus resulting in >200,000 new cases of acute pancreatitis per year.

TABLE 48-1

CAUSES OF ACUTE PANCREATITIS

Common Causes

Gallstones (including microlithiasis)
Alcohol (acute and chronic alcoholism)
Hypertriglyceridemia
Endoscopic retrograde cholangiopancreatography (ERCP), especially after biliary manometry
Trauma (especially blunt abdominal trauma)
Postoperative (abdominal and nonabdominal operations)
Drugs (azathioprine, 6-mercaptopurine, sulfonamides, estrogens, tetracycline, valproic acid, anti-HIV medications)
Sphincter of Oddi dysfunction

Uncommon Causes

Vascular causes and vasculitis (ischemic-hypoperfusion states after cardiac surgery)
Connective tissue disorders and thrombotic thrombocytopenic purpura (TTP)
Cancer of the pancreas
Hypercalcemia
Periampullary diverticulum
Pancreas divisum
Hereditary pancreatitis
Cystic fibrosis
Renal failure

Rare Causes

Infections (mumps, coxsackievirus, cytomegalovirus, echovirus, parasites)
Autoimmune (e.g., Sjögren's syndrome)

Causes to Consider in Patients with Recurrent Bouts of Acute Pancreatitis without an Obvious Etiology

Occult disease of the biliary tree or pancreatic ducts, especially microlithiasis, sludge
Drugs
Hypertriglyceridemia
Pancreas divisum
Pancreatic cancer
Sphincter of Oddi dysfunction
Cystic fibrosis
Idiopathic

ETIOLOGY AND PATHOGENESIS

There are many causes of acute pancreatitis (Table 48-1), but the mechanisms by which these conditions trigger pancreatic inflammation have not been fully elucidated. Gallstones continue to be the leading cause of acute pancreatitis in most series (30–60%). The risk of acute pancreatitis in patients with at least one gallstone <5 mm in diameter is fourfold greater than that in patients with larger stones. Alcohol is the second most common cause, responsible for 15–30% of

cases in the United States. The incidence of pancreatitis in alcoholics is surprisingly low (5/100,000), indicating that in addition to the amount of alcohol ingested unknown factors affect a person's susceptibility to pancreatic injury. The mechanism of injury is incompletely understood. Acute pancreatitis occurs in 5–20% of patients following endoscopic retrograde cholangiopancreatography (ERCP). Despite extensive research into the medical and endoscopic prevention of post-ERCP pancreatitis, there has been little decline in incidence. Use of prophylactic pancreatic duct stent after retrograde pancreatogram or pancreatic sphincterotomy has shown promise in reducing pancreatitis but requires further prospective evaluation. Risk factors for post-ERCP pancreatitis include minor papilla sphincterotomy, sphincter of Oddi dysfunction, prior history of post-ERCP pancreatitis, age <60 years, >2 contrast injections into the pancreatic duct, and endoscopic trainee involvement. Hypertriglyceridemia is the cause of acute pancreatitis in 1.3–3.8% of cases; serum triglyceride levels are usually >11.3 mmol/L (>1000 mg/dL). Most patients with hypertriglyceridemia, when subsequently examined, show evidence of an underlying derangement in lipid metabolism, probably unrelated to pancreatitis. Such patients are prone to recurrent episodes of pancreatitis. Any factor (e.g., drugs or alcohol) that causes an abrupt increase in serum triglycerides to levels >11 mmol/L (1000 mg/dL) can precipitate a bout of acute pancreatitis. Finally, patients with a deficiency of apolipoprotein CII have an increased incidence of pancreatitis; apolipoprotein CII activates lipoprotein lipase, which is important in clearing chylomicrons from the bloodstream. Patients with diabetes mellitus who have developed ketoacidosis and patients who are on certain medications such as oral contraceptives may also develop high triglyceride levels. Approximately 2–5% of cases of acute pancreatitis are drug related. Drugs cause pancreatitis either by a hypersensitivity reaction or by the generation of a toxic metabolite, although in some cases it is not clear which of these mechanisms is operative (Table 48-1).

Autodigestion is a currently accepted pathogenic theory; according to it, pancreatitis results when proteolytic enzymes (e.g., trypsinogen, chymotrypsinogen, proelastase, and lipolytic enzymes such as phospholipase A_2) are activated in the pancreas rather than in the intestinal lumen. A number of factors (e.g., endotoxins, exotoxins, viral infections, ischemia, anoxia, lysosomal calcium, and direct trauma) are believed to facilitate activation of trypsin. Activated proteolytic enzymes, especially trypsin, not only digest pancreatic and peripancreatic tissues but also can activate other enzymes, such as elastase and phospholipase A_2. Spontaneous activation of trypsin also can occur.

ACTIVATION OF PANCREATIC ENZYMES IN THE PATHOGENESIS OF ACUTE PANCREATITIS

Several recent studies have suggested that pancreatitis is a disease that evolves in three phases. The initial phase is characterized by intrapancreatic digestive enzyme activation and acinar cell injury. Trypsin activation appears to be mediated by lysosomal hydrolases such as cathepsin B that become colocalized with digestive enzymes in intracellular organelles; it is currently believed that acinar cell injury is the consequence of trypsin activation. The second phase of pancreatitis involves the activation, chemoattraction, and sequestration of leukocytes and macrophages in the pancreas, resulting in an enhanced intrapancreatic inflammatory reaction. Neutrophil depletion induced by prior administration of an antineutrophil serum has been shown to reduce the severity of experimentally induced pancreatitis. There is also evidence to support the concept that neutrophil sequestration can activate trypsinogen. Thus, intrapancreatic acinar cell activation of trypsinogen could be a two-step process (i.e., an early neutrophil-independent and a later neutrophil-dependent phase). The third phase of pancreatitis is due to the effects of activated proteolytic enzymes and cytokines, released by the inflamed pancreas, on distant organs. Activated proteolytic enzymes, especially trypsin, not only digest pancreatic and peripancreatic tissues but also activate other enzymes such as elastase and phospholipase A_2. The active enzymes and cytokines then digest cellular membranes and cause proteolysis, edema, interstitial hemorrhage, vascular damage, coagulation necrosis, fat necrosis, and parenchymal cell necrosis. Cellular injury and death result in the liberation of bradykinin peptides, vasoactive substances, and histamine that can produce vasodilation, increased vascular permeability, and edema with profound effects on many organs, most notably the lung. The systemic inflammatory response syndrome (SIRS) and acute respiratory distress syndrome (ARDS) as well as multiorgan failure may occur as a result of this cascade of local as well as distant effects.

There appear to be a number of genetic factors that can increase the susceptibility and/or modify the severity of pancreatic injury in acute pancreatitis. Four susceptibility genes have been identified: (1) cationic trypsinogen mutations (PRSS1m, R122Hm, and N291), (2) pancreatic secretory trypsin inhibitor (SPINK1), (3) CFTR, and (4) monocyte chemotactic protein (MCP-1). Experimental and clinical data indicate that MCP-1 may be an important inflammatory mediator in the early pathologic process of acute pancreatitis, a determinant of the severity of the inflammatory response, and a promoter of organ failure.

APPROACH TO THE PATIENT | **Abdominal Pain**

Abdominal pain is the major symptom of acute pancreatitis. Pain may vary from a mild and tolerable discomfort and more commonly to severe, constant, and incapacitating distress. Characteristically, the pain, which is steady and boring in character, is located in the epigastrium and periumbilical region and often radiates to the back as well as to the chest, flanks, and lower abdomen. The pain is frequently more intense when the patient is supine, and patients may obtain some relief by sitting with the trunk flexed and knees drawn up. Nausea, vomiting, and abdominal distention due to gastric and intestinal hypomotility and chemical peritonitis are also frequent complaints.

Physical examination frequently reveals a distressed and anxious patient. Low-grade fever, tachycardia, and hypotension are fairly common. Shock is not unusual and may result from (1) hypovolemia secondary to exudation of blood and plasma proteins into the retroperitoneal space and a "retroperitoneal burn" due to activated proteolytic enzymes; (2) increased formation and release of kinin peptides, which cause vasodilation and increased vascular permeability; and (3) systemic effects of proteolytic and lipolytic enzymes released into the circulation. Jaundice occurs infrequently; when present, it usually is due to edema of the head of the pancreas with compression of the intrapancreatic portion of the common bile duct. Erythematous skin nodules due to subcutaneous fat necrosis may occur. In 10–20% of patients, there are pulmonary findings, including basilar rales, atelectasis, and pleural effusion, the latter most frequently left sided. Abdominal tenderness and muscle rigidity are present to a variable degree, but, compared with the intense pain, these signs may be unimpressive. Bowel sounds are usually diminished or absent. An enlarged pancreas with walled off necrosis or a pseudocyst may be palpable in the upper abdomen later in the disease course (i.e., 4 to 6 weeks). A faint blue discoloration around the umbilicus (Cullen's sign) may occur as the result of hemoperitoneum, and a blue-red-purple or green-brown discoloration of the flanks (Turner's sign) reflects tissue catabolism of hemoglobin. The latter two findings, which are uncommon, indicate the presence of a severe necrotizing pancreatitis.

LABORATORY DATA

The diagnosis of acute pancreatitis is usually established by the detection of an increased level of serum amylase and lipase. Values threefold or more above normal virtually clinch the diagnosis if gut perforation, ischemia, and infarction are excluded. However, there appears to be no definite correlation between the severity of pancreatitis and the degree of serum lipase and amylase

TABLE 48-2

SEVERE ACUTE PANCREATITIS

Risk Factors for Severity

- Age >60 years
- Obesity, BMI >30
- Comorbid disease

Markers of Severity within 24 h

- SIRS (temperature >38° or <36°C [>100.4° or 96.8°F], pulse >90, tachypnea >24, ↑ WBC >12,000)
- Hemoconcentration (Hct >44%)
- BISAP
  - (B) Blood urea nitrogen (BUN) >22 mg%
  - (I) Impaired mental status
  - (S) SIRS: 2/4 present
  - (A) Age >60 years
  - (P) Pleural effusion
- Organ Failure
  - Cardiovascular: systolic BP <90 mmHg, heart rate >130
  - Pulmonary: Pao$_2$ <60 mmHg
  - Renal serum creatinine >2.0 mg

Markers of Severity during Hospitalization

- Persistent organ failure
- Pancreatic necrosis
- Hospital-acquired infection

Abbreviation: BISAP, Bedside Index of Severity in Acute Pancreatitis.

elevations. After 3 to 7 days, even with continuing evidence of pancreatitis, total serum amylase values tend to return toward normal. However, pancreatic isoamylase and lipase levels may remain elevated for 7 to 14 days. It will be recalled that amylase elevations in serum and urine occur in many conditions other than pancreatitis (see Chap. 47, Table 47-2). Importantly, patients with *acidemia* (arterial pH ≤7.32) may have spurious elevations in serum amylase. In one study, 12 of 33 patients with acidemia had elevated serum amylase, but only 1 had an elevated lipase value; in 9, salivary-type amylase was the predominant serum isoamylase. This finding explains why patients with diabetic ketoacidosis may have marked elevations in serum amylase without any other evidence of acute pancreatitis. Serum lipase activity increases in parallel with amylase activity. A three-fold elevated serum lipase value is usually diagnostic of acute pancreatitis; these tests are especially helpful in patients with nonpancreatic causes of hyperamylasemia (see Chap. 47, Table 47-2).

Leukocytosis (15,000–20,000 leukocytes per μL) occurs frequently. Patients with more severe disease may show hemoconcentration with hematocrit values >44% and/or azotemia with a blood urea nitrogen (BUN) level >22 mg/dL because of loss of plasma into the retroperitoneal space and peritoneal cavity. Hemoconcentration may be the harbinger of more severe disease (i.e., pancreatic necrosis), while azotemia is a significant risk factor for mortality. *Hyperglycemia* is common and is due to multiple factors, including decreased insulin release, increased glucagon release, and an increased output of adrenal glucocorticoids and catecholamines. *Hypocalcemia* occurs in ~25% of patients, and its pathogenesis is incompletely understood. Although earlier studies suggested that the response of the parathyroid gland to a decrease in serum calcium is impaired, subsequent observations have failed to confirm this phenomenon. Intraperitoneal saponification of calcium by fatty acids in areas of fat necrosis occurs occasionally, with large amounts (up to 6.0 g) dissolved or suspended in ascitic fluid. Such "soap formation" may also be significant in patients with pancreatitis, mild hypocalcemia, and little or no obvious ascites. *Hyperbilirubinemia* (serum bilirubin >68 μmol/L [>4.0 mg/dL]) occurs in ~10% of patients. However, jaundice is transient, and serum bilirubin levels return to normal in four to seven days. Serum alkaline phosphatase and aspartate aminotransferase levels are also transiently elevated and they parallel serum bilirubin values and may point to gallbladder-related disease. Markedly elevated serum lactic dehydrogenase levels (>8.5 μmol/L [>500 U/dL]) suggest a poor prognosis. *Hypertriglyceridemia* occurs in 5–10% of patients, and serum amylase levels in these individuals are often spuriously normal (Chap. 47). Approximately 5–10% of patients have *hypoxemia* (arterial PO$_2$ ≤ 60 mmHg), which may herald the onset of ARDS. Finally, the electrocardiogram is occasionally abnormal in acute pancreatitis with ST-segment and T-wave abnormalities simulating myocardial ischemia.

A CT scan can confirm the clinical impression of acute pancreatitis even with less than a threefold increase in serum amylase and lipase levels. Importantly, CT can be helpful in indicating the severity of acute pancreatitis and the risk of morbidity and mortality and in evaluating the complications of acute pancreatitis (Table 48-3). However, a CT scan obtained within the first several days of symptom onset may underestimate the extent of tissue injury. What may appear to be intestinal pancreatitis on initial CT scan may evolve to pancreatic necrosis on repeat CT scan 3 to 5 days later (Fig. 48-1). Sonography is useful in acute pancreatitis to evaluate the gallbladder if gallstone disease is suspected. Radiologic studies useful in the diagnosis of acute pancreatitis are discussed in Chap. 47, and listed in Table 47-1, and depicted in Figs. 48-1 to 48-3.

DIAGNOSIS

Any severe acute pain in the abdomen or back should suggest the possibility acute pancreatitis. The diagnosis is usually entertained when a patient with a possible predisposition to pancreatitis presents with severe and

TABLE 48-3

CT FINDINGS AND GRADING OF ACUTE PANCREATITIS (CT SEVERITY INDEX [CTSI])

GRADE	FINDINGS	SCORE
A	Normal pancreas: normal size, sharply defined, smooth contour, homogeneous enhancement, retroperitoneal peripancreatic fat without enhancement	0
B	Focal or diffuse enlargement of the pancreas, contour may show irregularity, enhancement may be inhomogeneous but there is no peripancreatic inflammation	1
C	Peripancreatic inflammation with intrinsic pancreatic abnormalities	2
D	Intrapancreatic or extrapancreatic fluid collections	3
E	Two or more large collections or gas in the pancreas or retroperitoneum	4

Necrosis score based on contrast-enhanced CT

Necrosis, %	Score
0	0
<33	2
33–50	4
≥50	6

Note: CT severity index equals unenhanced CT score plus necrosis score: maximum = 10; ≥6 = severe disease.
Source: Modified from EJ Balthazar et al: Radiology 1990;174:331.

constant abdominal pain, frequently associated with nausea, emesis, fever, tachycardia, and abnormal findings on abdominal examination. Laboratory studies may reveal leukocytosis, hypocalcemia, and hyperglycemia. The diagnosis of acute pancreatitis requires two of the following: typical abdominal pain, threefold or greater elevation in serum amylase and/or lipase level, and/or confirmatory findings on cross-sectional abdominal imaging. Although not required for diagnosis, markers of severity include hemoconcentration (hematocrit >44%), azotemia (BUN >22 mg/dL), and signs of organ failure (Table 48-2).

The *differential diagnosis* should include the following disorders: (1) perforated viscus, especially peptic ulcer; (2) acute cholecystitis and biliary colic; (3) acute intestinal obstruction; (4) mesenteric vascular occlusion; (5) renal colic; (6) myocardial infarction; (7) dissecting aortic aneurysm; (8) connective tissue disorders with vasculitis; (9) pneumonia; and (10) diabetic ketoacidosis. A penetrating duodenal ulcer can usually be identified by imaging studies or endoscopy. A perforated duodenal ulcer is readily diagnosed by the presence of free intraperitoneal air on abdominal imaging. It may be difficult to differentiate acute cholecystitis from acute pancreatitis, since an elevated serum amylase may be found in both disorders. Pain of biliary tract origin is more right sided or epigastric than periumbilical and can be more severe; ileus is usually absent. Sonography is helpful in establishing the diagnosis of cholelithiasis and cholecystitis. Intestinal obstruction due to mechanical factors can be differentiated from pancreatitis by the history of crescendo-decrescendo

CHAPTER 48   Acute and Chronic Pancreatitis

A   **B**   **C**

FIGURE 48-1

Acute pancreatitis: CT evolution. *A.* Contrast-enhanced CT scan of the abdomen performed on admission for a patient with clinical and biochemical parameters suggestive of acute pancreatitis. Note the abnormal enhancement of the pancreatic parenchyma (*arrow*) suggestive of interstitial pancreatitis. ***B.*** Contrast-enhanced CT scan of the abdomen performed on the same patient 6 days later for persistent fever and systemic inflammatory response syndrome. The pancreas now demonstrates significant areas of nonenhancement consistent with development of necrosis, particularly in the body and neck region (*arrow*). Note that an early CT scan obtained within the first 48 hours of hospitalization may underestimate or miss necrosis. ***C.*** Contrast-enhanced CT scan of the abdomen performed on the same patient 2 months after the initial episode of acute pancreatitis. CT now demonstrates evidence of a fluid collection consistent with walled-off pancreatic necrosis (*arrow*). (*Courtesy of Dr. KJ Mortele, Brigham and Women's Hospital; with permission.*)

A   *B*

C   *D*

FIGURE 48-2

A. Acute necrotizing pancreatitis: CT scan. Contrast-enhanced CT scan showing acute pancreatitis with necrosis. *Arrow* shows partially enhancing body/tail of pancreas surrounded by fluid with decreased enhancement in the neck/body of the pancreas. **B.** Acute fluid collection: CT scan. Contrast-enhanced CT scan showing fluid collection in the retroperitoneum (*arrow*) compressing the air-filled stomach arising from the pancreas in a patient with asparaginase-induced acute necrotizing pancreatitis. **C.** Walled-off pancreatic necrosis: CT scan. CT scan showing marked walled-off

necrosis of the pancreas and peripancreatic area (*arrow*) in a patient with necrotizing pancreatitis. Addendum: In past years, both of these CT findings (Figs. 48-2*B* and 48-2*C*) would have been misinterpreted as pseudocysts. **D.** Spiral CT showing a pseudocyst (*small arrow*) with a pseudoaneurysm (*light area in pseudocyst*). Note the demonstration of the main pancreatic duct (*big arrow*), even though this duct is minimally dilated by ERCP. (*A, B, C, courtesy of Dr. KJ Mortele, Brigham and Women's Hospital; D, courtesy of Dr. PR Ros, Brigham and Women's Hospital; with permission.*)

A   *B*   *C*

FIGURE 48-3

A. Pancreaticopleural fistula: pancreatic duct leak on ERCP. Pancreatic duct leak demonstrated (*arrow*) at the time of retrograde pancreatogram in a patient with acute exacerbation of alcohol-induced acute or chronic pancreatitis. **B.** Pancreaticopleural fistula: CT scan. Contrast-enhanced CT scan (coronal view) with *arrows* showing fistula tract from

pancreatic duct disruption in the pancreatic pleural fistula. **C.** Pancreaticopleural fistula: Chest x-ray. Large pleural effusion in the left hemithorax from a disrupted pancreatic duct. Analysis of pleural fluid revealed elevated amylase concentration. (*Courtesy of Dr. KJ Mortele, Brigham and Women's Hospital; with permission.*)

pain, findings on abdominal examination, and CT of the abdomen showing changes characteristic of mechanical obstruction. Acute mesenteric vascular occlusion is usually suspected in elderly debilitated patients with brisk leukocytosis, abdominal distention, and bloody diarrhea, confirmed by CT or MR angiography. Systemic lupus erythematosus and polyarteritis nodosa may be confused with pancreatitis, especially since pancreatitis may develop as a complication of these diseases. Diabetic ketoacidosis is often accompanied by abdominal pain and elevated total serum amylase levels, thus closely mimicking acute pancreatitis. However, the serum lipase level is not elevated in diabetic ketoacidosis.

COURSE OF THE DISEASE AND COMPLICATIONS

The initial assessment of severity in acute pancreatitis is critical for the appropriate triage and management of patients. The basis for the classification, severity, and complications of acute pancreatitis was initially established at the International Symposium held in Atlanta in 1992. While the definitions have come under greater scrutiny in recent years, it still serves as the common language for clinical care and research in acute pancreatitis. The criteria for severity in acute pancreatitis was defined as organ failure of at least one organ system (defined as a systolic blood pressure <90 mmHg, PaO_2 ≤60 mmHg, creatinine >2.0 mg/dL after rehydration, and gastrointestinal bleeding >500 mL/24 h) and the presence of a local complication such as necrosis, pseudocyst, and abscess.

Early predictors of severity at 48 h included ≥3 Ranson's signs and APACHE II score ≥8. Traditional severity indices such as APACHE II and Ranson's criteria have not been clinically useful since they are cumbersome, require collection of a large amount of clinical and laboratory data over time, and do not have acceptable positive and negative predictive value for severe acute pancreatitis. A recent simplified scoring system for the early prediction of mortality was developed from a large cohort of patients with acute pancreatitis. This scoring system, referred to as the Bedside Index of Severity in Acute Pancreatitis (BISAP), incorporates five clinical and laboratory parameters obtained within the first 24 h of hospitalization: (Table 48-2) (*B*UN >25, *I*mpaired mental status, *S*IRS, *A*ge >60 years, *P*leural effusion on radiography). Presence of three or more of these factors was associated with substantially increased risk for in-hospital mortality among patients with acute pancreatitis.

Apart from the severity indices, there are additional factors that can be used to assess severity in acute pancreatitis. They are best separated into risk factors for severity and markers of severity within 24 h of admission and during hospitalization. Risk factors for severe acute pancreatitis on admission include older age (>60 years), obesity (BMI ≥30), and comorbid disease. There is also evidence to support initial episode and alcohol use as additional risk factors for severity. At admission and during the first 24 h, markers of severity in acute pancreatitis include scoring systems such as BISAP score and APACHE II, SIRS, azotemia, hemoconcentration, and organ failure. During hospitalization, markers of severity include persistent organ failure lasting more than 48 h and pancreatic necrosis.

The course of acute pancreatitis is defined by two phases. In the first phase, which lasts 1 to 2 weeks, severity is defined by clinical parameters rather than morphologic findings. The most important clinical parameter is persistent organ failure (i.e., lasting longer than 48 h), which is the usual cause of death. Severity in the second phase is defined by both clinical parameters and morphologic criteria. The important clinical parameter of severity, as in the first phase, is persistent organ failure. The morphologic criteria of greatest interest is the development of necrotizing pancreatitis, especially when it prolongs hospitalization and/or it requires active intervention such as operative, endoscopic, or percutaneous therapy or requires supportive measures such as renal dialysis, ventilator support, or need for nasoenteric feeding.

The importance of the recognition of interstitial versus necrotizing acute pancreatitis has lead to the development of a CT severity index (Table 48-3) as another measure of severity that is best evaluated 3 to 5 days into hospitalization because it may not be possible to distinguish interstitial from necrotizing pancreatitis on contrast-enhanced CT scan on the day of admission. CT identification of local complications, particularly necrosis, is critical because patients with infected and sterile necrosis are at greatest risk of mortality (Figs. 48-1, 48-2). The median prevalence of organ failure is 54% in necrotizing pancreatitis. The prevalence of organ failure is perhaps slightly higher in infected versus sterile necrosis. With single organ system failure, the mortality is 3–10% but increases to 47% with multisystem organ failure. These data serve to highlight that a patient found to have pancreatic necrosis with multisystem organ failure is the most likely to die.

However, it should be noted that necrotizing pancreatitis is uncommon (10% of all patients with acute pancreatitis), and the far greater proportion of patients presenting in clinical practice have interstitial pancreatitis, which also is associated with organ failure in 10% and death in 3% of cases. This roughly translates to similar absolute mortality figures in the interstitial and necrotizing pancreatitis populations since interstitial disease is far more prevalent.

Mild acute pancreatitis

The majority of patients with mild acute pancreatitis and either no organ failure or only transient organ failure will respond to simple supportive care measures that form the hallmark of treatment in acute pancreatitis: bowel rest, intravenous hydration with crystalloid, and analgesia. Oral intake can be resumed once the patient is essentially pain free in the absence of parenteral analgesia, has no nausea or vomiting, normal bowel sounds, and is hungry. Typically, a clear or full liquid diet has been recommended for the initial meal, but a low-fat solid diet is a reasonable choice following recovery from mild acute pancreatitis. Patients with gallstone pancreatitis are at increased risk of recurrence. Therefore, following recovery from mild pancreatitis, consideration should be given to performing a laparoscopic cholecystectomy during the same admission. An alternative for patients who are not surgical candidates would be to perform an endoscopic biliary sphincterotomy.

Severe acute pancreatitis (See Figs. 48-1, 48-2)

Patients with predictive markers of severity on admission such as obesity or hemoconcentration are also managed with supportive measures outlined earlier. It is recommended that vigorous fluid resuscitation take place. Measurement of hematocrit and BUN every 12 h is recommended to ensure adequacy of fluid resuscitation. A decrease in hematocrit and BUN during the first 12 to 24 h is strong evidence that sufficient fluids are being administered. If the hematocrit remains elevated or increases further (particularly among those whose hematocrit on admission are >44), fluid resuscitation is inadequate.

Patients with persistent organ failure that does not respond to increased fluids (to counteract hypotension and increased serum creatinine) and/or nasal oxygen to overcome hypoxemia as well as those patients with labored respirations that may herald respiratory failure should be transferred to an intensive care unit for aggressive hydration and close monitoring for the possible need of intubation with mechanical ventilation, hemodialysis, and support of blood pressure.

TREATMENT   Acute Pancreatitis

In most patients (85–90%) with acute pancreatitis, the disease is self-limited and subsides spontaneously, usually within 3 to 7 days after treatment is instituted. Conventional measures include (1) analgesics for pain, (2) IV fluids and colloids to maintain normal intravascular volume, and (3) no oral alimentation.

Once it is clear that a patient will not be able to tolerate oral feeding (a determination that can usually be made within 48–72 h), enteral nutrition should be considered (rather than total parenteral nutrition [TPN])

since it maintains gut barrier integrity, thereby preventing bacterial translocation, is less expensive, and has fewer complications than TPN. The route through which enteral feeding is administered is under debate. Nasogastric access is easier to establish and may be as safe as nasojejunal enteral nutrition. However, enteral nutrition that bypasses the stomach and duodenum stimulates pancreatic secretions less and this rationale theoretically supports the use of the nasojejunal route. It has not been demonstrated whether either route is superior in altering morbidity and mortality. When patients with necrotizing pancreatitis begin oral intake of food, consideration should also be given to the addition of pancreatic enzyme supplementation and proton pump inhibitor therapy to assist with fat digestion and reduce gastric acid.

ROLE OF ANTIBIOTICS There is currently no role for prophylactic antibiotics in either interstitial or necrotizing pancreatitis. Although several early studies suggested a role for prophylactic antibiotics in patients with necrotizing pancreatitis, two recent double-blind, randomized controlled trials failed to demonstrate a reduction in pancreatic infection with use of antibiotic prophylaxis. However, it should also be noted that the overall rate of infected necrosis has been in decline over the past 10–15 years and currently is found in 20% of patients with necrotizing pancreatitis. It is reasonable to start antibiotics in a patient who appears septic while awaiting the results of cultures. If cultures are negative, the antibiotics should be discontinued to minimize the risk of developing fungal superinfection.

Percutaneous aspiration of necrosis with Gram stain and culture should generally not be performed until at least 7–10 days after establishing a diagnosis of necrotizing pancreatitis and only if there are ongoing signs of possible pancreatic infection such as sustained leukocytosis, fever, or organ failure. Once a diagnosis of infected necrosis is established, appropriate antibiotics should be instituted and surgical debridement should be undertaken. There exist minimally invasive alternative therapies such as endoscopic, percutaneous catheter, and retroperitoneal techniques for necrosectomy. However, there are currently no randomized studies supporting the use of one over another modality. For patients with sterile necrosis, medical management is usually maintained indefinitely unless patients develop serious complications such as compartment syndrome, intestinal perforation, pseudoaneurysms not responding to embolization, or inability to resume oral intake after 4 to 6 weeks of treatment (Fig. 48-2).

There are several clearly defined roles for ERCP in acute pancreatitis. Urgent ERCP (within 24 h) is indicated in patients who have severe acute biliary pancreatitis with organ failure and/or cholangitis. Elective ERCP with sphincterotomy can be considered in patients with persistent or incipient biliary obstruction, those deemed to be poor candidates for cholecystectomy, and for those in whom there is strong suspicion for bile duct stones after cholecystectomy. ERCP with stent placement is also indicated for pancreatic ductal disruptions that occur as part of the inflammatory process and result in peripancreatic fluid collections (Fig. 48-3A).

Several drugs have been evaluated by prospective controlled trials and found ineffective in the treatment of acute pancreatitis. The list, by no means complete, includes glucagon, H_2 blockers, protease inhibitors such as aprotinin, glucocorticoids, calcitonin, nonsteroidal anti-inflammatory drugs (NSAIDs), and lexipafant, a platelet-activating factor inhibitor. A recent meta-analysis of somatostatin, octreotide, and the antiprotease gabexate mesylate in the therapy of acute pancreatitis suggested (1) a reduced mortality rate but no change in complications with octreotide and (2) no effect on the mortality rate but reduced pancreatic damage with gabexate.

A dynamic contrast-enhanced CT (CECT) scan performed 3 to 5 days after hospitalization provides valuable information on the severity and prognosis of acute pancreatitis (Fig. 48-1). In particular, a CECT scan allows estimation of the presence and extent of pancreatic necrosis. Recent studies suggest that the likelihood of prolonged pancreatitis or a serious complication is negligible when the CT severity index is 1 or 2 and low with scores of 3–6. However, patients with scores of 7–10 had a 92% morbidity rate and a 17% mortality rate (Table 48-3). A few retrospective studies have raised concern that the use of IV contrast early in the course of acute pancreatitis might intensify pancreatic necrosis. However, since prospective human studies are not available, it is recommended that a CECT scan be obtained only after vigorous initial fluid resuscitation.

Elevation of serum amylase/lipase or persistent inflammatory changes seen on CT scans should not discourage feeding a hungry asymptomatic patient. In this regard, persistence of inflammatory changes on CT scans or persistent elevations in serum amylase/lipase may not resolve for weeks to months. The patient with unremitting severe necrotizing pancreatitis requires vigorous fluid resuscitation and close attention to complications such as cardiovascular collapse, respiratory insufficiency, and pancreatic infection. A useful indicator of severe/complicated forms of acute pancreatitis is the persistence of the systemic SIRS beyond 48 h. SIRS was defined in 1992 in a joint conference of the American College of Chest Physicians and Society of Critical Care Medicine as a standardized clinical syndrome to indicate the presence of systemic inflammation irrespective of etiology. Several studies have linked persistent SIRS with an increased risk of organ failure and death in acute pancreatitis. Complications from acute pancreatitis should be managed by a combination of radiologic and surgical means (discussed later). Although sterile necrosis is most often managed conservatively, surgical pancreatic debridement (necrosectomy) should be considered for definitive management of infected necrosis. Such decisions are influenced by response to antibiotic treatment. Multiple operations may be required. A recent study compared the step-up approach, i.e., percutaneous or endoscopic transgastric drainage with open necrosectomy for necrotizing pancreatitis. One third of the patients successfully treated with the step-up approach did not require major abdominal surgery. Enteral-feeding with a nasojejunal tube has been demonstrated to have fewer infectious complications than with total parenteral nutrition (TPN) and is the preferred method of nutritional support. In addition to nutritional support, enteral feeding helps to maintain integrity of the intestinal tract during severe acute pancreatitis.

Patients with severe gallstone-induced pancreatitis, complicated by cholangitis, may improve dramatically if papillotomy is carried out within the first 36–72 h of the attack. Studies indicate that only those patients with gallstone pancreatitis who are in the very severe group should be considered for urgent ERCP. Finally, the treatment for patients with hypertriglyceridemia-associated pancreatitis includes (1) weight loss to ideal weight, (2) a lipid-restricted diet, (3) exercise, (4) avoidance of alcohol and of drugs that can elevate serum triglycerides (i.e., estrogens, vitamin A, thiazides, and propranolol), and (5) control of diabetes.

Recurrent pancreatitis

Approximately 25% of patients who have had an attack of acute pancreatitis have a recurrence. The two most common etiologic factors are alcohol and cholelithiasis. In patients with recurrent pancreatitis without an obvious cause the differential diagnosis should encompass occult biliary tract disease including microlithiasis, hypertriglyceridemia, drugs, pancreatic cancer, sphincter of Oddi dysfunction, pancreas divisum, cystic fibrosis, and pancreatic cancer (Table 48-1). In one series of 31 patients diagnosed initially as having idiopathic or recurrent acute pancreatitis, 23 were found to have occult gallstone disease. Thus, approximately two-thirds of patients with recurrent acute pancreatitis without an obvious cause actually have occult gallstone disease due to microlithiasis. Genetic defects as in hereditary pancreatitis can result in recurrent pancreatitis. Other diseases of the biliary tree and pancreatic ducts that can cause acute pancreatitis include choledochocele; ampullary tumors; pancreas divisum; and pancreatic duct stones, stricture, and tumor. Approximately 2–4% of patients with pancreatic carcinoma present with acute pancreatitis.

INFECTED PANCREATIC NECROSIS AND PSEUDOCYST

Pancreatic necrosis does not usually become secondarily infected until at least 7–10 days after the onset of acute pancreatitis. Approximately one-half of cases of infected necrosis can be diagnosed between the 7th and 21st day, the remainder after 21 days. The diagnosis of pancreatic infection can be accomplished by CT-guided needle aspiration with Gram stain and culture. The organisms are most frequently gram-negative bacteria of intestinal origin. Clinical clues that should alert the clinician to the possibility of infected necrosis are persistent fever, leukocytosis, and organ failure in a patient with necrotizing pancreatitis. Some reports suggest that patients who have more than 50% pancreatic necrosis are more likely to have infected pancreatic necrosis than those who have lesser amounts of necrosis. Choices of treatment in infected pancreatic necrosis include surgical debridement; endoscopic debridement, if the pancreatic necrosis has been circumscribed into the entity termed *walled-off necrosis* that affects the posterior wall of the stomach; and, on occasion, radiologic catheter drainage with irrigation in an effort to eliminate at least some infected semisolid material as well as the infected liquid material. Radiologic approach is usually suggested to treat a patient who is too ill to undergo surgical debridement.

Walled-off necrosis

In necrotizing pancreatitis, there is invariably an intense inflammatory response involving the fat around the pancreas. This inflammatory process frequently results in peripancreatic necrosis. Eventually, after 3 to 6 weeks, there is coalescence of the pancreatic necrosis and peripancreatic fat necrosis into a structure that is encapsulated by fibrous tissue. The name that was originally used to describe this entity was "organized necrosis." New terminology now refers to it as "walled-off necrosis."

The walled-off necrosis contains semisolid necrotic tissue together with a considerable amount of dark fluid representing liquefaction of devitalized pancreatic and peripancreatic tissue as well as some blood.

Walled-off necrosis and a pancreatic pseudocyst may look very similar on first inspection of a contrast-enhanced CT scan. Both show a low attenuation nonenhancing round structure enclosed by a capsule containing fibrous tissue that enhances due to small blood vessels within the capsule. On closer inspection, a distinction can be made. In walled-off necrosis,

serial images clearly show that a portion of the pancreas as well as variable amounts of peripancreatic tissue are necrotic. In interstitial pancreatitis, the pancreas enhances normally in response to intravenous contrast, thereby confirming that the process is interstitial pancreatitis. The encapsulated structure is readily seen to be adjacent to the pancreas.

Pseudocysts

Pseudocysts of the pancreas are extrapancreatic collections of pancreatic fluid containing pancreatic enzymes and a small amount of debris. In contrast to true cysts, pseudocysts do not have an epithelial lining. The walls consist of necrotic tissue, granulation tissue, and fibrous tissue.

A pseudocyst should be distinguished from a postnecrotic fluid collection that contains heterogeneous material including residual necrotic debris. Disruption of the pancreatic ductal system is common. However, the subsequent course of this disruption varies widely, ranging from spontaneous healing to continuous leakage of pancreatic juice, which results in tense ascites. Pseudocysts are preceded by pancreatitis in 90% of cases and by trauma in 10%. Approximately 85% are located in the body or tail of the pancreas and 15% in the head. Some patients have two or more pseudocysts. Abdominal pain, with or without radiation to the back, is the usual presenting complaint. A palpable, tender mass may be found in the middle or left upper abdomen.

On imaging studies, 75% of pseudocysts can be seen to displace some portion of the gastrointestinal tract. Sonography, however, is reliable in detecting pseudocysts. Sonography also permits differentiation between an edematous, inflamed pancreas, which can give rise to a palpable mass, and an actual pseudocyst. Furthermore, serial ultrasound studies will indicate whether a pseudocyst has resolved. CT or MRI complements ultrasonography in the diagnosis of pancreatic pseudocyst, especially when the pseudocyst is infected as suggested by the rare finding of gas within the fluid collection.

In earlier studies with sonography, lesions thought to be pseudocysts were seen to resolve in 25–40% of patients. However, it is now recognized that it is important to distinguish between walled-off necrosis and pseudocysts that typically develop later in the course of acute pancreatitis. Pseudocysts that are >5 cm in diameter may persist for >6 weeks. Recent natural history studies have suggested that noninterventional, expectant management is the best course in selected patients with minimal symptoms and no evidence of active alcohol use in whom the pseudocyst appears mature by radiography and does not resemble a cystic neoplasm. A significant number of these pseudocysts resolve spontaneously in >6 weeks after their formation.

Also, these studies demonstrate that large pseudocyst size is not an absolute indication for interventional therapy and that many peripancreatic fluid collections detected on CT in cases of acute pancreatitis resolve spontaneously. A pseudocyst that does not resolve spontaneously can occasionally lead to serious complications, such as (1) pain caused by expansion of the lesion and pressure on other viscera, (2) rupture, (3) hemorrhage, and (4) abscess. Rupture of a pancreatic pseudocyst is a particularly serious complication. In this case, shock almost always supervenes, and mortality rates range from 14% if the rupture is not associated with hemorrhage to >60% if hemorrhage has occurred. Rupture and hemorrhage are the prime causes of death from pancreatic pseudocyst. A triad of findings—an increase in the size of the mass, a localized bruit over the mass, and a sudden decrease in hemoglobin level and hematocrit without obvious external blood loss—should alert one to the possibility of hemorrhage from a pseudocyst. Thus, in patients who are stable and free of complications and in whom serial ultrasound studies show that the pseudocyst is shrinking, conservative therapy is indicated. Conversely, if the pseudocyst is expanding and is complicated by severe pain, hemorrhage, or abscess, the patient should be operated on. Chronic pseudocysts can be treated safely and drainage can be accomplished by endoscopic, radiologic, or surgical means.

Pseudoaneurysms develop in up to 10% of patients with acute pancreatitis at sites reflecting the distribution of pseudocysts and fluid collections (Fig. 48-2D). The splenic artery is most frequently involved, followed by the inferior and superior pancreatic duodenal arteries. This diagnosis should be suspected in patients with pancreatitis who develop upper gastrointestinal bleeding without an obvious cause or in whom thin-cut CT scanning reveals a contrast-enhanced lesion within or adjacent to a suspected pseudocyst. CT angiography can identify the lesion, which can then be treated with angiographic embolization.

The local and systemic complications of acute pancreatitis are summarized in Table 48-4. Systemic complications include pulmonary, cardiovascular, hematologic, renal, metabolic, and central nervous system (CNS) abnormalities. *Purtscher's retinopathy*, a relatively unusual complication, is manifested by a sudden and severe loss of vision in a patient with acute pancreatitis. It is characterized by a peculiar funduscopic appearance with cotton-wool spots and hemorrhages confined to an area limited by the optic disc and macula; it is believed to be due to occlusion of the posterior retinal artery with aggregated granulocytes.

Pancreatitis in patients with AIDS

The incidence of acute pancreatitis is increased in patients with AIDS for two reasons: (1) the high

TABLE 48-4

COMPLICATIONS OF ACUTE PANCREATITIS

Local

Necrosis	Pancreatic ascites
Sterile	Disruption of main
Infected	pancreatic duct
Walled-off necrosis	Leaking pseudocyst
Pancreatic fluid collections	Involvement of
Pancreatic abscess	contiguous organs by
Pancreatic pseudocyst	necrotizing pancreatitis
Pain	Massive intraperitoneal
Rupture	hemorrhage
Hemorrhage	Thrombosis of blood
Infection	vessels (splenic vein,
Obstruction of	portal vein)
gastrointestinal	Bowel infarction
tract (stomach,	Obstructive jaundice
duodenum, colon)	

Systemic

Pulmonary	Renal
Pleural effusion	Oliguria
Atelectasis	Azotemia
Mediastinal abscess	Renal artery and/or renal
Pneumonitis	vein thrombosis
Acute respiratory	Acute tubular necrosis
distress syndrome	Metabolic
Cardiovascular	Hyperglycemia
Hypotension	Hypertriglyceridemia
Hypovolemia	Hypocalcemia
Sudden death	Encephalopathy
Nonspecific ST-T	Sudden blindness
changes in	(Purtscher's retinopathy)
electrocardiogram	Central nervous system
simulating myocardial	Psychosis
infarction	Fat emboli
Pericardial effusion	Fat necrosis
Hematologic	Subcutaneous tissues
Disseminated	(erythematous nodules)
intravascular	Bone
coagulation	Miscellaneous
Gastrointestinal	(mediastinum, pleura,
hemorrhage	nervous system)
Peptic ulcer disease	
Erosive gastritis	
Hemorrhagic pancreatic	
necrosis with erosion	
into major blood	
vessels	
Portal vein thrombosis,	
variceal hemorrhage	

incidence of infections involving the pancreas such as infections with cytomegalovirus, *Cryptosporidium*, and the *Mycobacterium avium* complex; and (2) the frequent use by patients with AIDS of medications such as didanosine, pentamidine, trimethoprim-sulfamethoxazole, and protease inhibitors.

PANCREATIC ASCITES AND PANCREATIC PLEURAL EFFUSIONS

Pancreatic ascites or pancreatic pleural effusion are initially identified based on CT or MRI imaging and are usually due to disruption of the main pancreatic duct, often by an internal fistula between the duct and the peritoneal cavity or a leaking pseudocyst (Fig. 48-3A). This diagnosis is suggested in a patient with a history of acute pancreatitis in whom the ascites or pleural fluid has both increased levels of albumin [>30 g/L (>3 g/dL)] and a markedly elevated level of amylase. An ERCP or magnetic resonance cholangiopancreatography (MRCP) confirms the clinical suspicion and radiologic findings and often demonstrates passage of contrast material from a disrupted major pancreatic duct or a pseudocyst into the peritoneal cavity. The differential diagnosis of pancreatic ascites should include intraperitoneal carcinomatosis, tuberculous peritonitis, constrictive pericarditis, and Budd–Chiari syndrome.

TREATMENT Pancreatic Ascites and Pancreatic Pleural Effusions

If the pancreatic duct disruption is posterior, an internal fistula may develop between the pancreatic duct and the pleural space, producing a pleural effusion (pancreaticopleural fistula) that is usually left-sided and often massive (Fig. 48-3). If the pancreatic duct disruption is anterior, amylase- and lipase-rich peritoneal fluid accumulate (pancreatic ascites). A leaking, disrupted pancreatic duct is best treated by ERCP and "bridging" stent placement and infrequently requires thoracentesis or chest tube drainage.

Treatment may also require enteral or parenteral alimentation to improve nutrition. If ascites or pleural fluid persists after 2 to 3 weeks of medical management, and the disruption is unable to be stented, the patient should be considered for surgical intervention after retrograde pancreatography to define the anatomy of the disrupted duct.

CHRONIC PANCREATITIS AND PANCREATIC EXOCRINE INSUFFICIENCY

PATHOPHYSIOLOGY

Chronic pancreatitis is a disease process characterized by irreversible damage to the pancreas as distinct from the reversible changes noted in acute pancreatitis. The condition is best defined by the presence of histologic abnormalities, including chronic inflammation,

TABLE 48-5

CHRONIC PANCREATITIS AND PANCREATIC EXOCRINE INSUFFICIENCY: TIGAR-O CLASSIFICATION SYSTEM

Toxic-metabolic
  Alcoholic
  Tobacco smoking
  Hypercalcemia
  Hyperlipidemia
  Chronic renal failure
  Medications—
    phenacetin abuse
  Toxins—organotin
    compounds
    (e.g., DBTC)
Idiopathic
  Early onset
  Late onset
  Tropical
Genetic
  Hereditary pancreatitis
  Cationic trypsinogen
  PRSS₁
  PRSS₂
  CFTR mutations
  SPINK1 mutations

Autoimmune
  Isolated autoimmune chronic pancreatitis
  Autoimmune chronic pancreatitis associated with Sjögren's syndrome
  Inflammatory bowel disease
  Primary biliary cirrhosis
Recurrent and Severe Acute Pancreatitis
  Postnecrotic (severe acute pancreatitis)
  Recurrent acute pancreatitis
  Vascular diseases/ischemia
  Postirradiation
Obstructive
  Pancreas divisum
  Sphincter of Oddi disorders (controversial)
  Duct obstruction (e.g., tumor)
  Preampullary duodenal wall cysts
  Posttraumatic pancreatic duct scars

Abbreviations: DBTC, dibutylin dichloride; TIGAR-O, toxic-metabolic, idiopathic, genetic, autoimmune, recurrent and severe acute pancreatitis, obstructive.

fibrosis, and progressive destruction of both exocrine and eventually endocrine tissue. A number of etiologies may result in chronic pancreatitis, and may result in the cardinal complications of chronic pancreatitis such as abdominal pain, steatorrhea, weight loss, and diabetes mellitus (Table 48-5).

The events that initiate the inflammatory process in the pancreas are incompletely understood. Current experimental and clinical observations have shown that alcohol has a direct toxic effect on the pancreas. While patients with alcohol-induced pancreatitis generally consume large amounts of alcohol, some consume as little as ≤50 g/d. Prolonged consumption of socially acceptable amounts of alcohol is compatible with the development of chronic pancreatitis. Findings of extensive pancreatic fibrosis in patients who died during their first attack of clinical acute alcohol-induced pancreatitis support the concept that such patients already had chronic pancreatitis.

There is a strong association of smoking and chronic pancreatitis. Cigarette smoke leads to an increased susceptibility to pancreatic self-digestion and predisposes to dysregulation of duct cell CFTR function. It has become increasingly apparent that smoking is an independent, dose-dependent risk factor for chronic pancreatitis and recurrent acute pancreatitis. Smoking is clearly associated with progression of disease in late-onset idiopathic chronic pancreatitis and with increased disease severity in alcohol-induced chronic pancreatitis.

Recent characterization of pancreatic stellate cells (PSC) has added insight to the underlying cellular responses behind development of chronic pancreatitis. Specifically, PSCs are believed to play a role in maintaining normal pancreatic architecture that can shift toward fibrogenesis in the case of chronic pancreatitis. The sentinel acute pancreatitis event (SAPE) hypothesis uniformly describes the events in the pathogenesis of chronic pancreatitis. It is believed that alcohol or additional stimuli lead to matrix metalloproteinase–mediated destruction of normal collagen in pancreatic parenchyma, which later allows for pancreatic remodeling. Proinflammatory cytokines, tumor necrosis factor α (TNF-α), interleukin 1 (IL-1), and interleukin 6 (IL-6) as well as oxidant complexes are able to induce PSC activity with subsequent new collagen synthesis. In addition to being stimulated by cytokines, oxidants, or growth factors, PSCs also possess transforming growth factor β (TGF-β)–mediated self-activating autocrine pathways that may explain disease progression in chronic pancreatitis even after removal of noxious stimuli.

ETIOLOGIC CONSIDERATIONS

Among adults in the United States, alcoholism is the most common cause of clinically apparent chronic pancreatitis, while cystic fibrosis is the most frequent cause in children. In up to 25% of adults in the United States with chronic pancreatitis, the cause is not known. That is, they are labeled as *idiopathic chronic pancreatitis*. Recent investigations have indicated that up to 15% of patients with idiopathic pancreatitis may have pancreatitis due to genetic defects (Table 48-5).

Whitcomb and associates studied several large families with hereditary chronic pancreatitis and were able to identify a genetic defect that affects the gene encoding for trypsinogen. Several additional defects of this gene have also been described. The defect prevents the destruction of trypsinogen and allows it to be resistant to the effect of trypsin inhibitor, become spontaneously activated, and to remain activated. It is hypothesized that this continual activation of digestive enzymes within the gland leads to acute injury and, finally, chronic pancreatitis. This group of investigators has also reported that another form of hereditary chronic pancreatitis tends to present later in life, has a female predominance, and frequently leads to chronic pancreatitis.

Several other groups of investigators have documented mutations of CFTR. This gene functions as a cyclic AMP–regulated chloride channel. In patients with cystic fibrosis, the high concentration of macromolecules can block the pancreatic ducts. It must be appreciated, however, that there is a great deal of heterogeneity in relationship to the CFTR gene defect. More than 1000 putative mutations of the CFTR gene have been identified. Attempts to elucidate the relationship between the genotype and pancreatic manifestations have been hampered by the number of mutations. The ability to detect CFTR mutations has led to the recognition that the clinical spectrum of the disease is broader than previously thought. Two recent studies have clarified the association between mutations of the CFTR gene and another monosymptomatic form of cystic fibrosis (i.e., chronic pancreatitis). It is estimated that in patients with idiopathic pancreatitis, the frequency of a single CFTR mutation is 11 times the expected frequency and the frequency of two mutant alleles is 80 times the expected frequency. In these studies, the patients were adults when the diagnosis of pancreatitis was made; none had any clinical evidence of pulmonary disease, and sweat test results were not diagnostic of cystic fibrosis. The prevalence of such mutations is unclear, and further studies are certainly needed. In addition, the therapeutic and prognostic implication of these findings with respect to managing pancreatitis remains to be determined. Long-term follow-up of affected patients is needed. CFTR mutations are common in the general population. It is unclear whether the CFTR mutation alone can lead to pancreatitis as an autosomal recessive disease. A recent study evaluated 39 patients with idiopathic chronic pancreatitis to assess the risk associated with these mutations. Patients with two CFTR mutations (compound heterozygotes) demonstrated CFTR function at a level between that seen in typical cystic fibrosis and cystic fibrosis carriers and had a fortyfold increased risk of pancreatitis. The presence of an N34S SPINK1 mutation increased the risk twentyfold. A combination of two CFTR mutations and an N34S SPINK1 mutation increased the risk of pancreatitis 900-fold. Table 48-5 lists recognized causes of chronic pancreatitis and pancreatic exocrine insufficiency.

AUTOIMMUNE PANCREATITIS (TABLE 48-6)

Autoimmune pancreatitis (AIP) is an uncommon disorder of presumed autoimmune causation with characteristic laboratory, histologic, and morphologic findings. AIP has been described as a primary pancreatic disorder; however, it is also associated with other clinical features such as parotid enlargement, submandibular adenopathy, thyroiditis, pericarditis, orbital mass lesions, and retroperitoneal fibrosis as part of a broader entity identified as IgG related disease. Mild symptoms, usually abdominal pain, are present but attacks of acute pancreatitis are unusual. Furthermore, AIP is not a common cause of idiopathic

TABLE 48-6

CLINICAL FEATURES OF AUTOIMMUNE PANCREATITIS (AIP)

- Mild symptoms usually abdominal pain, but without frequent attacks of pancreatitis, which are unusual
- Presentation with obstructive jaundice
- Diffuse swelling and enlargement of the pancreas, especially the head, the latter mimicking carcinoma of the pancreas
- Diffuse irregular narrowing of the pancreatic duct in ERCP
- Increased levels of serum gamma globulins especially IgG4
- Presence of other autoantibodies (ANA), rheumatoid factor (RF)
- Can occur with other autoimmune diseases: Sjögren's syndrome, primary sclerosing cholangitis, ulcerative colitis, rheumatoid arthritis
- Extra pancreatic bile duct changes such as stricture of the common bile duct and intrahepatic ducts
- Absence of pancreatic calcifications or cysts
- Pancreatic biopsies reveal extensive fibrosis and lymphoplasmacytic infiltration
- Glucocorticoids are effective in alleviating symptoms, decreasing size of the pancreas, and reversing histopathologic changes
- Two-thirds of patients present with either obstructive jaundice or a "mass" in the head of the pancreas mimicking carcinoma

recurrent pancreatitis. In the United States, 50–75% of patients with AIP present with obstructive jaundice.

Weight loss and new onset of diabetes may also occur. An obstructive pattern on liver tests is common (i.e., disproportionately elevated serum alkaline phosphatase and minimally elevated serum aminotransferases). Elevated serum levels of immunoglobulin G4 (IgG4) provide a marker for the disease, particularly in Western populations. Serum IgG4 normally accounts for only 5–6% of the total IgG4 in healthy patients but is elevated at least twofold higher than 135 mg/dL in those with AIP. CT scans reveal abnormalities in the majority of patients and include diffuse enlargement, focal enlargement, and a distinct enlargement at the head of the pancreas. ERCP or MRCP reveals strictures in the bile duct in more than one-third of patients with AIP; these may be common bile duct strictures, intrahepatic bile duct strictures, or proximal bile duct strictures, with accompanying narrowing of the pancreatic bile duct. This has been termed autoimmune cholangitis. Characteristic histologic findings include extensive lymphoplasmacytic infiltrates with dense fibrosis around pancreatic ducts, as well as a lymphoplasmacytic infiltration, resulting in an obliterative phlebitis.

The Mayo Clinic criteria indicate that AIP can be diagnosed with at least one of three abnormalities: (1) diagnostic histology; (2) characteristic findings on

CT and pancreatography combined with elevated IgG4 levels; and (3) response to glucocorticoid therapy, with improvement in pancreatic and extrapancreatic manifestations.

Glucocorticoids have shown efficacy in alleviating symptoms, decreasing the size of the pancreas, and reversing histopathologic features in patients with AIP. Patients may respond dramatically to glucocorticoid therapy within a 2- to 4-week period. Prednisone is usually administered at an initial dose of 40 mg/d for 4 weeks followed by a taper of the daily dosage by 5 mg/week based on monitoring of clinical parameters. Relief of symptoms, serial changes in abdominal imaging of the pancreas and bile ducts, decreased serum γ-globulin and IgG4 levels, and improvements in liver tests are parameters to follow. A poor response to glucocorticoids over a 2- to 4-week period should raise suspicion of pancreatic cancer or other forms of chronic pancreatitis. In most reports, 50–70% of patients responded to glucocorticoids, but about 25% required a second course of treatment while a smaller number required maintenance treatment with prednisone at a dosage of 5–10 mg/d. Patients with bile duct strictures are less likely to have a sustained response to glucocorticoids and may require immunosuppressive therapy with azathioprine or 6-mercaptopurine.

Clinical features of chronic pancreatitis

Patients with chronic pancreatitis seek medical attention predominantly because of two symptoms: abdominal pain or maldigestion and weight loss. The abdominal pain may be quite variable in location, severity, and frequency. The pain can be constant or intermittent with frequent pain-free intervals. Eating may exacerbate the pain, leading to a fear of eating with consequent weight loss. The spectrum of abdominal pain ranges from mild to quite severe, with narcotic dependence as a frequent consequence. Maldigestion is manifested as chronic diarrhea, steatorrhea, weight loss, and fatigue. Patients with chronic abdominal pain may or may not progress to maldigestion, and ~20% of patients will present with symptoms of maldigestion without a history of abdominal pain. Patients with chronic pancreatitis have significant morbidity and mortality and utilize appreciable amounts of societal resources. Despite the steatorrhea, clinically apparent deficiencies of fat-soluble vitamins are surprisingly uncommon. Physical findings in these patients are usually unimpressive so that there is a disparity between the severity of abdominal pain and the physical signs that usually consist of some mild tenderness.

In contrast to acute pancreatitis, the serum amylase and lipase levels are usually not strikingly elevated in chronic pancreatitis. Elevation of serum bilirubin and alkaline phosphatase may indicate cholestasis secondary to common bile duct stricture caused by chronic inflammation. Many patients have impaired glucose tolerance with elevated fasting blood glucose levels. The diagnostic test with the best sensitivity and specificity is the hormone stimulation test utilizing secretin. It becomes abnormal when ≥60% of the pancreatic exocrine function has been lost. This usually correlates well with the onset of chronic abdominal pain. In earlier studies, approximately 40% of patients with chronic pancreatitis had cobalamin (vitamin B_{12}) malabsorption. This can be corrected by the administration of oral pancreatic enzymes. The fecal elastase-1 and small bowel biopsy are useful in the evaluation of patients with suspected pancreatic steatorrhea. The fecal elastase level will be abnormal and small bowel histology will be normal in such patients. A decrease of fecal elastase level to <100 μg per gram of stool strongly suggests severe pancreatic exocrine insufficiency.

Utilizing radiographic techniques (Fig. 48-4), it can be shown that diffuse calcifications noted on plain film of the abdomen usually indicate significant damage to the pancreas. While alcohol is by far the most common cause of pancreatic calcification such calcification may also be noted in hereditary pancreatitis, posttraumatic pancreatitis, hypercalcemic pancreatitis, islet cell tumors, idiopathic chronic pancreatitis, and tropical pancreatitis. Abdominal ultrasonography, CT scanning, and MRCP greatly aid in the diagnosis of pancreatic disease (Fig. 48-4). In addition to excluding a pseudocyst and pancreatic cancer, CT may show calcification, dilated ducts, or an atrophic pancreas. MRCP provides a direct view of the pancreatic duct and is now the diagnostic procedure of choice. The role of endoscopic ultrasonography (EUS) in diagnosing early chronic pancreatitis is still being defined. A total of nine endosonographic features have been described in chronic pancreatitis. The presence of five or more features is considered diagnostic of chronic pancreatitis. EUS complements pancreatic function tests, and a combination of a hormone-stimulation function test and EUS is a modality to evaluate the pancreatic duct morphology, parenchymal architecture, and secretory function for the presence or extent of chronic pancreatitis (Chap. 47). Whether EUS alone can detect early, noncalcific chronic pancreatitis with the same degree of accuracy as the hormone-stimulation test is controversial. Data comparing these modalities head-to-head have indicated that EUS is not a sensitive enough test for detecting early chronic pancreatitis (Chap. 47) and may show positive features in patients who have dyspepsia or even in normal controls. However, recent data suggest that EUS can be combined with endoscopic pancreatic function testing (EUS-ePFT) during a single endoscopy to screen for chronic pancreatitis in patients with chronic abdominal pain.

FIGURE 48-4
A. Chronic pancreatitis and pancreatic calculi: CT scan. In this contrast-enhanced CT scan of the abdomen, there is evidence of an atrophic pancreas with multiple calcifications and stones in the parenchyma and dilated pancreatic duct (*arrow*). **B.** In this contrast-enhanced CT scan of the abdomen, there is evidence of an atrophic pancreas with multiple calcifications (*arrows*). Note the markedly dilated pancreatic duct seen in this section through the body and tail (*open arrows*). **C.** Chronic pancreatitis on MRCP: dilated duct with filling defects. Gadolinium-enhanced MRI/MRCP reveals a dilated pancreatic duct (*arrow*) in chronic pancreatitis with multiple filling defects suggestive of pancreatic duct calculi. (*A, C, courtesy of Dr. KJ Mortele, Brigham and Women's Hospital; with permission.*)

CHAPTER 48 Acute and Chronic Pancreatitis

512

TABLE 48-7

COMPLICATIONS OF CHRONIC PANCREATITIS	
Narcotic addiction	Gastrointestinal bleeding
Impaired glucose tolerance	Jaundice
Gastroparesis	Cholangitis and/or biliary
Cobalamin malabsorption	cirrhosis
Nondiabetic retinopathy	Subcutaneous fat necrosis
Effusions with high amylase	Bone pain
content	Pancreatic cancer

Complications of chronic pancreatitis

The complications of chronic pancreatitis are protean and are listed in Table 48-7. Although most patients have impaired glucose tolerance, diabetic ketoacidosis and coma are uncommon. Likewise, end-organ damage (retinopathy, neuropathy, nephropathy) is also uncommon. A nondiabetic retinopathy may be due to either vitamin A and/or zinc deficiency. Gastrointestinal bleeding may occur from peptic ulceration, gastritis, a pseudocyst eroding into the duodenum, or ruptured varices secondary to splenic vein thrombosis due to chronic inflammation of the tail of the pancreas. Jaundice, cholestasis, and biliary cirrhosis may occur from the chronic inflammatory reaction around the intrapancreatic portion of the common bile duct. Twenty years after the diagnosis of calcific chronic pancreatitis, the cumulative risk of pancreatic carcinoma is 4%. Patients with hereditary pancreatitis are at a tenfold higher risk for pancreatic cancer.

TREATMENT Chronic Pancreatitis

The treatment of steatorrhea with pancreatic enzymes is straightforward even though complete correction of steatorrhea is unusual. Enzyme therapy usually brings diarrhea under control and restores absorption of fat to an acceptable level and effects weight gain. Thus, pancreatic enzymes have been the cornerstone of pancreatic therapy. In treating steatorrhea, it is important to use a potent pancreatic formulation that will deliver sufficient lipase into the duodenum to correct maldigestion and decrease steatorrhea (Table 48-8). In an attempt to standardize the enzyme activity, potency and bioavailability, the Food and Drug Administration (FDA) required that all pancreas enzyme drugs in the United States obtain a New Drug Application (NDA) by April 2008. Table 48-8 lists frequently utilized formulations but availability will be based on compliance with the FDA mandate. Recent data suggests that dosages up to 80,000–100,000 units of lipase per meal may be necessary to normalize nutritional parameters in malnourished chronic pancreatitis patients.

The management of pain in patients with chronic pancreatitis is problematic.

Recent meta-analyses have shown no consistent benefit of enzyme therapy at reducing pain in chronic pancreatitis. In some patients with idiopathic chronic pancreatitis, conventional nonenteric coated enzyme preparations containing high concentrations of serine proteases may relieve mild abdominal pain or discomfort. The pain relief experienced by these patients actually may be due to improvements in the dyspepsia from maldigestion. Table 48-8 lists the frequently utilized pancreatic enzyme preparations in the United States.

Oxidative stress has also been implicated in the pathophysiology of the pain of chronic pancreatitis. A recent randomized prospective study from India showed antioxidant therapy to be beneficial at reducing pain in mild chronic pancreatitis. Gastroparesis is also quite common in patients with chronic pancreatitis. It is important to recognize this because treatment with enzymes may fail simply because gastroparesis is preventing the appropriate delivery of enzymes into the upper intestine where the enzymes can then act via a feedback inhibition process. In patients with painful chronic pancreatitis, it is important to evaluate gastric emptying and, if gastric emptying is impaired, to effect proper emptying with prokinetic agents. In this setting, enzyme therapy is more apt to be successful.

Endoscopic treatment of chronic pancreatitis pain may involve sphincterotomy, stenting, stone extraction, and drainage of a pancreatic pseudocyst. Therapy directed to the pancreatic duct would seem to be most appropriate in the setting of a dominant stricture, if a ductal stone has led to obstruction. The use of endoscopic stenting for patients with chronic pain, but without a dominant stricture, has not been subjected to any controlled trials. It is now appreciated that significant complications can occur from stenting (i.e., bleeding, cholangitis, stent migration, and stent clogging). All of these may lead to pancreatitis. Importantly, damage to the pancreatic duct and the pancreatic parenchyma can occur following stenting. In patients with large-duct disease usually from alcohol-induced chronic pancreatitis, ductal decompression has been the therapy of choice. Among such patients, 80% seem to obtain immediate relief; however, at the end of three years, one-half the patients have recurrence of pain. Two randomized prospective trials comparing endoscopic to surgical therapy for chronic pancreatitis demonstrated that surgical therapy was superior to endoscopy at decreasing pain and improving quality of life in selected patients with dilated ducts and abdominal pain. This would suggest that chronic pancreatitis patients with dilated ducts and pain should be considered for surgical intervention. The role of preoperative stenting prior to surgery as a predictor of response has yet to be proven.

A Whipple procedure as well as total pancreatectomy and autologous islet cell transplantation have been

TABLE 48-8

FREQUENTLY UTILIZED PANCREATIC ENZYME PREPARATIONS

ENZYME PREPARATIONS	MANUFACTURER, LOCATION	LIPASE[a]	PROTEASE[a]	AMYLASE[a]
Enteric Coated (EC)				
Ultrase	Axcan Pharma, Birmingham, AL			
[EC microspheres in capsules]				
Ultrase		4500	25,000	20,000
Ultrase 12		12,000	39,000	39,000
Ultrase 18		18,000	58,500	58,500
Ultrase 20		20,000	65,000	65,000
Creon	Solvay Pharmaceuticals, Marietta, GA			
[delayed-release capsules containing EC spheres]				
Creon 6		6000	19,000	30,000
Creon 12		12,000	38,000	60,000
Creon 24		24,000	76,000	120,000
Pancrease	Ortho-McNeil Pharmaceuticals, Riritan, NJ			
[EC microtablets in capsule]				
Pancrease MT 4		4000	12,000	12,000
Pancrease MT 10		10,000	30,000	30,000
Pancrease MT 16		16,000	48,000	48,000
Pancrease MT 20		20,000	44,000	56,000
Pancreacarb	Digestive Care, Inc., Bethlehem, PA			
(EC microspheres [buffered] in delayed-release capsule)				
Pancreacarb MS-8		8000	45,000	40,000
Nonenteric Coated				
Viokase	Axcan Scandipharm, Birmingham, AL			
(pancrelipase, USP) Tablets, Powder				
Viokase 8		8000	30,000	30,000
Viokase 16		16,000	60,000	60,000
Viokase Powder: Lactose, sodium chloride, each 0.7 g (1/4 teaspoonful)		16,800	70,000	70,000
Ku-zyme/Kutrase	UCB Inc., Rochester, NY			
Ku-zyme		1200	15,000	15,000
Kutrase		1200	30,000	30,000

[a]United States Pharmacopeia (USP) units per tablet or capsule

Note: FDA has mandated all enzyme manufacturers to submit new drug applications (NDAs) for all pancreatic extract drug products after reviewing data that showed substantial variations among currently marketed products. Numerous manufacturers have investigations underway to seek FDA approval for the treatment of exocrine pancreatic insufficiency (EPI) due to cystic fibrosis (CF) or other conditions under the new guidelines for this class of drugs (www.fda.gov).

used in selected patients with chronic pancreatitis and abdominal pain refractory to conventional therapy. The patients who have benefited the most from total pancreatectomy have chronic pancreatitis without prior pancreatic surgery or evidence of islet cell insufficiency. The role of this procedure remains to be fully defined but may be an option in lieu of ductal decompression surgery or pancreatic resection in patients with intractable, painful small-duct disease, particularly as the

standard surgical procedures tend to decrease islet cell yield. Celiac plexus block has not been demonstrated to provide long-lasting pain relief.

HEREDITARY PANCREATITIS

Hereditary pancreatitis is a rare disease that is similar to chronic pancreatitis except for an early age of onset and evidence of hereditary factors (involving an autosomal dominant gene with incomplete penetrance). A genomewide search using genetic linkage analysis identified the hereditary pancreatitis gene on chromosome 7. Mutations in ion codons 29 (exon 2) and 122 (exon 3) of the cationic trypsinogen gene cause autosomal dominant forms of hereditary pancreatitis. The codon 122 mutations lead to a substitution of the corresponding arginine with another amino acid, usually histidine. This substitution, when it occurs, eliminates a fail-safe trypsin self-destruction site necessary to eliminate trypsin that is prematurely activated within the acinar cell. These patients have recurring attacks of severe abdominal pain that may last from a few days to a few weeks. The serum amylase and lipase levels may be elevated during acute attacks but are usually normal. Patients frequently develop pancreatic calcification, diabetes mellitus, and steatorrhea; in addition, they have an increased incidence of pancreatic carcinoma, with the cumulative incidence being as high as 40% by age 70 years. A recent natural history study of hereditary pancreatitis in more than 200 patients from France reported that abdominal pain started in childhood at age 10 years, steatorrhea developed at age 29 years, diabetes at age 38 years, and pancreatic carcinoma at age 55 years. Such patients often require surgical ductal decompression for pain relief. Abdominal complaints in relatives of patients with hereditary pancreatitis should raise the question of pancreatic disease.

Pancreatic secretory trypsin inhibitor (PSTI) gene mutations

PSTI, or SPINK1, is a 56-amino-acid peptide that specifically inhibits trypsin by physically blocking its active site. SPINK1 acts as the first line of defense against prematurely activated trypsinogen in the acinar cell. Recently, it has been shown that the frequency of SPINK1 mutations in patients with idiopathic chronic pancreatitis is markedly increased, suggesting that these mutations may be associated with pancreatitis.

PANCREATIC ENDOCRINE TUMORS

Pancreatic endocrine tumors are discussed in Chap. 52.

OTHER CONDITIONS

ANNULAR PANCREAS

When the ventral pancreatic anlage fails to migrate correctly to make contact with the dorsal anlage, the result may be a ring of pancreatic tissue encircling the duodenum. Such an annular pancreas may cause intestinal obstruction in the neonate or the adult. Symptoms of postprandial fullness, epigastric pain, nausea, and vomiting may be present for years before the diagnosis is entertained. The radiographic findings are symmetric dilation of the proximal duodenum with bulging of the recesses on either side of the annular band, effacement but not destruction of the duodenal mucosa, accentuation of the findings in the right anterior oblique position, and lack of change on repeated examinations. The differential diagnosis should include duodenal webs, tumors of the pancreas or duodenum, postbulbar peptic ulcer, regional enteritis, and adhesions. Patients with annular pancreas have an increased incidence of pancreatitis and peptic ulcer. Because of these and other potential complications, the treatment is surgical even if the condition has been present for years. Retrocolic duodenojejunostomy is the procedure of choice, although some surgeons advocate Billroth II gastrectomy, gastroenterostomy, and vagotomy.

PANCREAS DIVISUM

Pancreas divisum occurs when the embryologic ventral and dorsal pancreatic anlagen fail to fuse, so that pancreatic drainage is accomplished mainly through the accessory papilla. Pancreas divisum is the most common congenital anatomic variant of the human pancreas. Current evidence indicates that this anomaly does not predispose to the development of pancreatitis in the great majority of patients who harbor it. However, the combination of pancreas divisum and a small accessory orifice could result in dorsal duct obstruction. The challenge is to identify this subset of patients with dorsal duct pathology. Cannulation of the dorsal duct by ERCP is not as easily done as is cannulation of the ventral duct. Patients with pancreatitis and pancreas divisum demonstrated by MRCP or ERCP should be treated with conservative measures. In many of these patients, pancreatitis is idiopathic and unrelated to the pancreas divisum. Endoscopic or surgical intervention is indicated only if pancreatitis recurs and no other cause can be found. If marked dilation of the dorsal duct can be demonstrated, surgical ductal decompression should be performed. It should be stressed that the ERCP appearance of pancreas divisum (i.e., a small-caliber ventral duct with an arborizing pattern) may be mistaken as representing an obstructed main pancreatic duct secondary to a mass lesion.

MACROAMYLASEMIA

In macroamylasemia, amylase circulates in the blood in a polymer form too large to be easily excreted by the kidney. Patients with this condition demonstrate an elevated serum amylase value, a low urinary amylase value, and a C_{am}/C_{cr} ratio of <1%. The presence of macroamylase can be documented by chromatography of the serum. The prevalence of macroamylasemia is 1.5% of the nonalcoholic general adult hospital population. Usually macroamylasemia is an incidental finding and is not related to disease of the pancreas or other organs.

Macrolipasemia has now been documented in a few patients with cirrhosis or non–Hodgkin's lymphoma. In these patients, the pancreas appeared normal on ultrasound and CT examination. Lipase was shown to be complexed with immunoglobulin A. Thus, the possibility of *both* macroamylasemia and macrolipasemia should be considered in patients with elevated blood levels of these enzymes.

ACKNOWLEDGMENTS

This chapter represents a revised version of the chapter by Dr. Norton J. Greenberger and Dr. Phillip P. Toskes that was in the previous editions of Harrison's Principles of Internal Medicine.

SECTION IX

NEOPLASTIC DISEASES OF THE GASTROINTESTINAL SYSTEM

CHAPTER 49
GASTROINTESTINAL TRACT CANCER

Robert J. Mayer

The gastrointestinal tract is the second most common noncutaneous site for cancer and the second major cause of cancer-related mortality in the United States.

ESOPHAGEAL CANCER

INCIDENCE AND ETIOLOGY

Cancer of the esophagus is a relatively uncommon but extremely lethal malignancy. The diagnosis was made in 16,640 Americans in 2010 and led to 14,500 deaths. Worldwide, the incidence, of esophageal cancer varies strikingly. It occurs frequently within a geographic region extending from the southern shore of the Caspian Sea on the west to northern China on the east and encompassing parts of Iran, Central Asia, Afghanistan, Siberia, and Mongolia. Familial increased risk has been seen in regions with high incidence, though gene associations are not yet defined. High-incidence "pockets" of the disease are also present in such disparate locations as Finland, Iceland, Curaçao, southeastern Africa, and northwestern France. In North America and western Europe, the disease is more common in blacks than whites and in males than females; it appears most often after age 50 and seems to be associated with a lower socioeconomic status.

A variety of causative factors have been implicated in the development of the disease (Table 49-1). In the United States, esophageal cancer cases are either squamous cell carcinomas or adenocarcinomas. The etiology of squamous cell esophageal cancer is related to excess alcohol consumption and/or cigarette smoking. The relative risk increases with the amount of tobacco smoked or alcohol consumed, with these factors acting synergistically. The consumption of whiskey is linked to a higher incidence than the consumption of wine or beer. Squamous cell esophageal carcinoma has also been associated with the ingestion of nitrites, smoked opiates, and fungal toxins in pickled vegetables, as well as mucosal damage caused by such physical insults as long-term exposure to extremely hot tea, the ingestion of lye, radiation-induced strictures, and chronic achalasia. The presence of an esophageal web in association with glossitis and iron deficiency (i.e., Plummer-Vinson or Paterson-Kelly syndrome) and congenital hyperkeratosis and pitting of the palms and soles (i.e., tylosis palmaris et plantaris) have each been linked with squamous cell esophageal cancer, as have dietary deficiencies of molybdenum, zinc, selenium, and vitamin A. Bisphosphonates may increase the risk in patients with Barrett's esophagus. Patients with head and neck cancer are at increased risk of squamous cell cancer of the esophagus.

TABLE 49-1

SOME ETIOLOGIC FACTORS BELIEVED TO BE ASSOCIATED WITH ESOPHAGEAL CANCER
Excess alcohol consumption
Cigarette smoking
Other ingested carcinogens
Nitrates (converted to nitrites)
Smoked opiates
Fungal toxins in pickled vegetables
Mucosal damage from physical agents
Hot tea
Lye ingestion
Radiation-induced strictures
Chronic achalasia
Host susceptibility
Esophageal web with glossitis and iron deficiency (i.e., Plummer-Vinson or Paterson-Kelly syndrome)
Congenital hyperkeratosis and pitting of the palms and soles (i.e., tylosis palmaris et plantaris)
? Dietary deficiencies of selenium, molybdenum, zinc, and vitamin A
? Celiac sprue
Chronic gastric reflux (i.e., Barrett's esophagus) for adenocarcinoma

For unclear reasons, the incidence of squamous cell esophageal cancer has decreased somewhat in both the black and white population in the United States over the past 30 years, while the rate of adenocarcinoma has risen dramatically, particularly in white males (M:F 6:1). Adenocarcinomas arise in the distal esophagus in the presence of chronic gastric reflux and gastric metaplasia of the epithelium (Barrett's esophagus), which is more common in obese persons. Adenocarcinomas arise within dysplastic columnar epithelium in the distal esophagus. Even before frank neoplasia is detectable, aneuploidy and p53 mutations are found in the dysplastic epithelium. These adenocarcinomas behave clinically like gastric adenocarcinoma and now account for >70% of esophageal cancers.

CLINICAL FEATURES

About 10% of esophageal cancers occur in the upper third of the esophagus (cervical esophagus), 35% in the middle third, and 55% in the lower third. Squamous cell carcinomas and adenocarcinomas cannot be distinguished radiographically or endoscopically.

Progressive dysphagia and weight loss of short duration are the initial symptoms in the vast majority of patients. Dysphagia initially occurs with solid foods and gradually progresses to include semisolids and liquids. By the time these symptoms develop, the disease is usually incurable, since difficulty in swallowing does not occur until >60% of the esophageal circumference is infiltrated with cancer. Dysphagia may be associated with pain on swallowing (odynophagia), pain radiating to the chest and/or back, regurgitation or vomiting, and aspiration pneumonia. The disease most commonly spreads to adjacent and supraclavicular lymph nodes, liver, lungs, pleura, and bone. Tracheoesophageal fistulas may develop as the disease advances, leading to severe suffering. As with other squamous cell carcinomas, hypercalcemia may occur in the absence of osseous metastases, probably from parathormone-related peptide secreted by tumor cells.

DIAGNOSIS

Attempts at endoscopic and cytologic screening for carcinoma in patients with Barrett's esophagus, while effective as a means of detecting high-grade dysplasia, have not yet been shown to improve the prognosis in individuals found to have a carcinoma. Routine contrast radiographs effectively identify esophageal lesions large enough to cause symptoms. In contrast to benign esophageal leiomyomas, which result in esophageal narrowing with preservation of a normal mucosal pattern, esophageal carcinomas show ragged, ulcerating changes in the mucosa in association with deeper infiltration,

producing a picture resembling achalasia. Smaller, potentially resectable tumors are often poorly visualized despite technically adequate esophagograms. Because of this, esophagoscopy should be performed in all patients suspected of having an esophageal abnormality, to visualize the tumor and to obtain histopathologic confirmation of the diagnosis. Because the population of persons at risk for squamous cell carcinoma of the esophagus (i.e., smokers and drinkers) also has a high rate of cancers of the lung and the head and neck region, endoscopic inspection of the larynx, trachea, and bronchi should also be done. A thorough examination of the fundus of the stomach (by retroflexing the endoscope) is imperative as well. Endoscopic biopsies of esophageal tumors fail to recover malignant tissue in one-third of cases because the biopsy forceps cannot penetrate deeply enough through normal mucosa pushed in front of the carcinoma. Taking multiple biopsies increases the yield. Cytologic examination of tumor brushings complements standard biopsies and should be performed routinely. The extent of tumor spread to the mediastinum and para-aortic lymph nodes should be assessed by CT scans of the chest and abdomen and by endoscopic ultrasound. Positron emission tomography scanning provides a useful assessment of resectability, offering accurate information regarding spread to mediastinal lymph nodes. Most patients have advanced disease at presentation.

TREATMENT   Esophageal Cancer

The prognosis for patients with esophageal carcinoma is poor. Fewer than 5% of patients survive 5 years after the diagnosis; thus, management focuses on symptom control. Surgical resection of all gross tumor (i.e., total resection) is feasible in only 45% of cases, with residual tumor cells frequently present at the resection margins. Such esophagectomies have been associated with a postoperative mortality rate of approximately 5% due to anastomotic fistulas, subphrenic abscesses, and respiratory complications. About 20% of patients who survive a total resection live 5 years. The efficacy of primary radiation therapy (5500–6000 cGy) for squamous cell carcinomas is similar to that of radical surgery, sparing patients perioperative morbidity but often resulting in less satisfactory palliation of obstructive symptoms. The evaluation of chemotherapeutic agents in patients with esophageal carcinoma has been hampered by ambiguity in the definition of "response" and the debilitated physical condition of many treated individuals. Nonetheless, significant reductions in the size of measurable tumor masses have been reported in 15–25% of patients given single-agent treatment and in 30–60% of patients treated with drug combinations that include cisplatin. Combination chemotherapy and radiation therapy as the initial therapeutic approach, either alone or followed by an attempt at operative resection, seems to be beneficial. When administered along with radiation therapy, chemotherapy produces a better survival outcome than radiation therapy alone. The use of preoperative chemotherapy and radiation therapy followed by esophageal resection appears to prolong survival as compared with controls in small, randomized trials, and some reports suggest that no additional benefit accrues when surgery is added if significant shrinkage of tumor has been achieved by the chemoradiation combination.

For the incurable, surgically unresectable patient with esophageal cancer, dysphagia, malnutrition, and the management of tracheoesophageal fistulas are major issues. Approaches to palliation include repeated endoscopic dilatation, the surgical placement of a gastrostomy or jejunostomy for hydration and feeding, and endoscopic placement of an expansive metal stent to bypass the tumor. Endoscopic fulguration of the obstructing tumor with lasers is the most promising of these techniques.

TUMORS OF THE STOMACH

GASTRIC ADENOCARCINOMA

Incidence and epidemiology

For unclear reasons, the incidence and mortality rates for gastric cancer have decreased markedly worldwide during the past 75 years. The mortality rate from gastric cancer in the United States has dropped in men from 28 to 5.8 per 100,000 persons, while in women the rate has decreased from 27 to 2.8 per 100,000. Nonetheless, 21,000 new cases of stomach cancer were diagnosed in the United States, and 10,570 Americans died of the disease in 2010. Gastric cancer incidence has decreased worldwide but remains high in Japan, China, Chile, and Ireland.

The risk of gastric cancer is greater among lower socioeconomic classes. Migrants from high- to low-incidence nations maintain their susceptibility to gastric cancer, while the risk for their offspring approximates that of the new homeland. These findings suggest that an environmental exposure, probably beginning early in life, is related to the development of gastric cancer, with dietary carcinogens considered the most likely factor(s).

Pathology

About 85% of stomach cancers are adenocarcinomas, with 15% due to lymphomas and gastrointestinal stromal tumors (GIST) and leiomyosarcomas. Gastric adenocarcinomas may be subdivided into two categories:

a *diffuse type*, in which cell cohesion is absent, so that individual cells infiltrate and thicken the stomach wall without forming a discrete mass; and an *intestinal type*, characterized by cohesive neoplastic cells that form glandlike tubular structures. The diffuse carcinomas occur more often in younger patients, develop throughout the stomach (including the cardia), result in a loss of distensibility of the gastric wall (so-called linitis plastica, or "leather bottle" appearance), and carry a poorer prognosis. Diffuse cancers have defective intercellular adhesion, mainly as a consequence of loss of expression of E-cadherin. Intestinal-type lesions are frequently ulcerative, more commonly appear in the antrum and lesser curvature of the stomach, and are often preceded by a prolonged precancerous process, often initiated by *Helicobacter pylori* infection. While the incidence of diffuse carcinomas is similar in most populations, the intestinal type tends to predominate in the high-risk geographic regions and is less likely to be found in areas where the frequency of gastric cancer is declining. Thus, different etiologic factor(s) are likely involved in these two subtypes. In the United States, ~30% of gastric cancers originate in the distal stomach, ~20% arise in the midportion of the stomach, and ~37% originate in the proximal third of the stomach. The remaining 13% involve the entire stomach.

Etiology

The long-term ingestion of high concentrations of nitrates in dried, smoked, and salted foods appears to be associated with a higher risk. The nitrates are thought to be converted to carcinogenic nitrites by bacteria (Table 49-2). Such bacteria may be introduced exogenously through the ingestion of partially decayed foods,

TABLE 49-2

NITRATE-CONVERTING BACTERIA AS A FACTOR IN THE CAUSATION OF GASTRIC CARCINOMA[a]

Exogenous sources of nitrate-converting bacteria:
  Bacterially contaminated food (common in lower socioeconomic classes, who have a higher incidence of the disease; diminished by improved food preservation and refrigeration)
  ? *Helicobacter pylori* infection
Endogenous factors favoring growth of nitrate-converting bacteria in the stomach:
  Decreased gastric acidity
  Prior gastric surgery (antrectomy) (15- to 20-year latency period)
  Atrophic gastritis and/or pernicious anemia
  ? Prolonged exposure to histamine H_2-receptor antagonists

[a]Hypothesis: Dietary nitrates are converted to carcinogenic nitrites by bacteria.

which are consumed in abundance worldwide by the lower socioeconomic classes. Bacteria such as *H. pylori* may also contribute to this effect by causing chronic gastritis, loss of gastric acidity, and bacterial growth in the stomach. The effect of *H. pylori* eradication on the subsequent risk for gastric cancer in high-incidence areas is under investigation. Loss of acidity may occur when acid-producing cells of the gastric antrum have been removed surgically to control benign peptic ulcer disease or when achlorhydria, atrophic gastritis, and even pernicious anemia develop in the elderly. Serial endoscopic examinations of the stomach in patients with atrophic gastritis have documented replacement of the usual gastric mucosa by intestinal-type cells. This process of intestinal metaplasia may lead to cellular atypia and eventual neoplasia. Since the declining incidence of gastric cancer in the United States primarily reflects a decline in distal, ulcerating, intestinal-type lesions, it is conceivable that better food preservation and the availability of refrigeration to all socioeconomic classes have decreased the dietary ingestion of exogenous bacteria. *H. pylori* has not been associated with the diffuse, more proximal form of gastric carcinoma.

Several additional etiologic factors have been associated with gastric carcinoma. Gastric ulcers and adenomatous polyps have occasionally been linked, but data on a cause-and-effect relationship are unconvincing. The inadequate clinical distinction between benign gastric ulcers and small ulcerating carcinomas may, in part, account for this presumed association. The presence of extreme hypertrophy of gastric rugal folds (i.e., Ménétrier's disease), giving the impression of polypoid lesions, has been associated with a striking frequency of malignant transformation; such hypertrophy, however, does not represent the presence of true adenomatous polyps. Individuals with blood group A have a higher incidence of gastric cancer than persons with blood group O; this observation may be related to differences in the mucous secretion, leading to altered mucosal protection from carcinogens. A germ-line mutation in the E-cadherin gene (*CDH1*), inherited in an autosomal dominant pattern and coding for a cell adhesion protein, has been linked to a high incidence of occult diffuse-type gastric cancers in young asymptomatic carriers. Duodenal ulcers are not associated with gastric cancer.

In keeping with the stepwise model of carcinogenesis, K-ras mutations appear to be early events in intestinal-type gastric cancer. C-met expression is amplified in about 1 in 5 cases and correlates with advanced stage. About half of intestinal-type tumors have mutations in tumor suppressor genes such as *TP53*, *TP73*, *APC* (adenomatous polyposis coli), *TFF* (trefoid factor family), *DCC* (deleted in colon cancer), and *FHIT* (fragile histidine triad). Cyclin E overexpression is associated with progression from dysplasia. Epigenetic changes (especially increased methylation) has been correlated with higher risk of invasive disease. Beta-catenin has been found in the nucleus of tumor cells at the leading edge of invasion.

Clinical features

Gastric cancers, when superficial and surgically curable, usually produce no symptoms. As the tumor becomes more extensive, patients may complain of an insidious upper abdominal discomfort varying in intensity from a vague, postprandial fullness to a severe, steady pain. Anorexia, often with slight nausea, is very common but is not the usual presenting complaint. Weight loss may eventually be observed, and nausea and vomiting are particularly prominent with tumors of the pylorus; dysphagia and early satiety may be the major symptoms caused by diffuse lesions originating in the cardia. There are no early physical signs. A palpable abdominal mass indicates long-standing growth and predicts regional extension.

Gastric carcinomas spread by direct extension through the gastric wall to the perigastric tissues, occasionally adhering to adjacent organs such as the pancreas, colon, or liver. The disease also spreads via lymphatics or by seeding of peritoneal surfaces. Metastases to intraabdominal and supraclavicular lymph nodes occur frequently, as do metastatic nodules to the ovary (Krukenberg's tumor), periumbilical region ("Sister Mary Joseph node"), or peritoneal cul-de-sac (Blumer's shelf palpable on rectal or vaginal examination); malignant ascites may also develop. The liver is the most common site for hematogenous spread of tumor.

The presence of iron-deficiency anemia in men and of occult blood in the stool in both sexes mandates a search for an occult gastrointestinal tract lesion. A careful assessment is of particular importance in patients with atrophic gastritis or pernicious anemia. Unusual clinical features associated with gastric adenocarcinomas include migratory thrombophlebitis, microangiopathic hemolytic anemia, diffuse seborrheic keratoses (so-called Leser-Trélat sign), and acanthosis nigricans.

Diagnosis

A double-contrast radiographic examination is the simplest diagnostic procedure for the evaluation of a patient with epigastric complaints. The use of double-contrast techniques helps to detect small lesions by improving mucosal detail. The stomach should be distended at some time during every radiographic examination, since decreased distensibility may be the only indication of a diffuse infiltrative carcinoma. Although gastric ulcers can be detected fairly early, distinguishing benign from malignant lesions radiographically is difficult. The anatomic location of an ulcer is not in itself an indication of the presence or absence of a cancer.

TABLE 49-3

STAGING SYSTEM FOR GASTRIC CARCINOMA

STAGE	TNM	FEATURES	NO. OF CASES, %	5-YEAR SURVIVAL, %
			DATA FROM ACS	
0	T$_{is}$N0M0	Node negative; limited to mucosa	1	90
IA	T1N0M0	Node negative; invasion of lamina propria or submucosa	7	59
IB	T2N0M0 T1N1M0	Node negative; invasion of muscularis propria	10	44
II	T1N2M0 T2N1M0	Node positive; invasion beyond mucosa but within wall	17	29
	T3N0M0	or Node negative; extension through wall		
IIIA	T2N2M0 T3N1-2M0	Node positive; invasion of muscularis propria or through wall	21	15
IIIB	T4N0-1M0	Node negative; adherence to surrounding tissue	14	9
IIIC	T4N2-3M0 T3N3M0	>3 nodes positive; invasion of serosa or adjacent structures 7 or more positive nodes; penetrates wall without invading serosa or adjacent structures		
IV	T4N2M0	Node positive; adherence to surrounding tissue or	30	3
	T1-4N0-2M1	Distant metastases		

Abbreviation: ACS, American Cancer Society; TNM, tumor, node, metastasis.

Gastric ulcers that appear benign by radiography present special problems. Some physicians believe that gastroscopy is not mandatory if the radiographic features are typically benign, if complete healing can be visualized by x-ray within 6 weeks, and if a follow-up contrast radiograph obtained several months later shows a normal appearance. However, we recommend gastroscopic biopsy and brush cytology for all patients with a gastric ulcer in order to exclude a malignancy. Malignant gastric ulcers must be recognized before they penetrate into surrounding tissues, because the rate of cure of early lesions limited to the mucosa or submucosa is >80%. Since gastric carcinomas are difficult to distinguish clinically or radiographically from gastric lymphomas, endoscopic biopsies should be made as deeply as possible, due to the submucosal location of lymphoid tumors.

The staging system for gastric carcinoma is shown in Table 49–3.

TREATMENT ▸ Gastric Adenocarcinoma

Complete surgical removal of the tumor with resection of adjacent lymph nodes offers the only chance for cure. However, this is possible in less than a third of patients. A subtotal gastrectomy is the treatment of choice for patients with distal carcinomas, while total or near-total gastrectomies are required for more proximal tumors. The inclusion of extended lymph node dissection in these procedures appears to confer an added risk for complications without enhancing survival. The prognosis following complete surgical resection depends on the degree of tumor penetration into the stomach wall and is adversely influenced by regional lymph node involvement, vascular invasion, and abnormal DNA content (i.e., aneuploidy), characteristics found in the vast majority of American patients. As a result, the probability of survival after 5 years for the 25–30% of patients able to undergo complete resection is ~20% for distal tumors and <10% for proximal tumors, with recurrences continuing for at least 8 years after surgery. In the absence of ascites or extensive hepatic or peritoneal metastases, even patients whose disease is believed to be incurable by surgery should be offered resection of the primary lesion. Reduction of tumor bulk is the best form of palliation and may enhance the probability of benefit from subsequent therapy.

Gastric adenocarcinoma is a relatively radioresistant tumor, and adequate control of the primary tumor requires doses of external beam irradiation that exceed the tolerance of surrounding structures, such as bowel mucosa and spinal cord. As a result, the major role of radiation therapy in patients has been palliation of pain. Radiation therapy alone after a complete resection does not prolong survival. In the setting of surgically unresectable disease limited to the epigastrium, patients treated with 3500–4000 cGy did not live longer than similar patients not receiving radiotherapy; however, survival was prolonged slightly when 5-fluorouracil (5-FU) plus leucovorin was given in combination with radiation therapy (3-year survival 50% vs 41% for radiation therapy alone). In this clinical setting, the 5-FU may be functioning as a radiosensitizer.

The administration of combinations of cytotoxic drugs to patients with advanced gastric carcinoma has been associated with partial responses in 30–50% of cases; responders appear to benefit from treatment. Such drug combinations have generally included cisplatin combined with epirubicin or docetaxel and infusional 5-FU, or with irinotecan. Despite this encouraging response rate, complete remissions are uncommon, the partial responses are transient, and the overall influence of multidrug therapy on survival has been unclear. The use of adjuvant chemotherapy alone following the complete resection of a gastric cancer has only minimally improved survival. However, combination chemotherapy administered before and after surgery (*perioperative treatment*) as well as postoperative chemotherapy combined with radiation therapy reduces the recurrence rate and prolongs survival.

PRIMARY GASTRIC LYMPHOMA

Primary lymphoma of the stomach is relatively uncommon, accounting for <15% of gastric malignancies and ~2% of all lymphomas. The stomach is, however, the most frequent extranodal site for lymphoma, and gastric lymphoma has increased in frequency during the past 30 years. The disease is difficult to distinguish clinically from gastric adenocarcinoma; both tumors are most often detected during the sixth decade of life; present with epigastric pain, early satiety, and generalized fatigue; and are usually characterized by ulcerations with a ragged, thickened mucosal pattern demonstrated by contrast radiographs. The diagnosis of lymphoma of the stomach may occasionally be made through cytologic brushings of the gastric mucosa but usually requires a biopsy at gastroscopy or laparotomy. Failure of gastroscopic biopsies to detect lymphoma in a given case should not be interpreted as being conclusive, since superficial biopsies may miss the deeper lymphoid infiltrate. The macroscopic pathology of gastric lymphoma may also mimic adenocarcinoma, consisting of either a bulky ulcerated lesion localized in the corpus or antrum or a diffuse process spreading throughout the entire gastric submucosa and even extending into the duodenum. Microscopically, the vast majority of gastric lymphoid tumors are non-Hodgkin's lymphomas of B cell origin; Hodgkin's disease involving the stomach is extremely uncommon. Histologically, these tumors may range from well-differentiated, superficial processes (mucosa-associated lymphoid tissue [MALT]) to high-grade, large-cell lymphomas. Like gastric adenocarcinoma, infection with *H. pylori* increases the risk for gastric lymphoma in general and MALT lymphomas in particular. Gastric lymphomas spread initially to regional lymph nodes (often to Waldeyer's ring) and may then disseminate. Gastric lymphomas are staged like other lymphomas.

| TREATMENT | Primary Gastric Lymphoma |

Primary gastric lymphoma is a far more treatable disease than adenocarcinoma of the stomach, a fact that underscores the need for making the correct diagnosis. Antibiotic treatment to eradicate *H. pylori* infection has led to regression of about 75% of gastric MALT lymphomas and should be considered before surgery, radiation therapy, or chemotherapy are undertaken in patients having such tumors. A lack of response to such antimicrobial treatment has been linked to a specific chromosomal abnormality, i.e., t(11;18). Responding patients should undergo periodic endoscopic surveillance because it remains unclear whether the neoplastic clone is eliminated or merely suppressed, although the response to antimicrobial treatment is quite durable. Subtotal gastrectomy, usually followed by combination chemotherapy, has led to 5-year survival rates of 40–60% in patients with localized high-grade lymphomas. The need for a major surgical procedure has been questioned, particularly in patients with preoperative radiographic evidence of nodal involvement, for whom chemotherapy (CHOP [cyclophosphamide, doxorubicin, vincristine, and prednisone]) plus rituximab is effective therapy. A role for radiation therapy is not defined because most recurrences develop at distant sites.

GASTRIC (NONLYMPHOID) SARCOMA

Leiomyosarcomas and GISTs make up 1–3% of gastric neoplasms. They most frequently involve the anterior and posterior walls of the gastric fundus and often ulcerate and bleed. Even those lesions that appear benign on histologic examination may behave in a malignant fashion. These tumors rarely invade adjacent viscera and characteristically do not metastasize to lymph nodes, but they may spread to the liver and lungs. The treatment of choice is surgical resection. Combination chemotherapy should be reserved for patients with metastatic disease. All such tumors should be analyzed for a mutation in the c-*kit* receptor. GISTs are unresponsive to conventional chemotherapy; yet ~50% of patients experience objective response and prolonged survival when treated with imatinib mesylate (Gleevec) (400–800 mg PO daily), a selective inhibitor of the c-*kit* tyrosine kinase. Many patients with GIST whose tumors have become refractory to imatinib subsequently benefit from sunitinib (Sutent), another inhibitor of the c-*kit* tyrosine kinase.

COLORECTAL CANCER

INCIDENCE

Cancer of the large bowel is second only to lung cancer as a cause of cancer death in the United States: 142,570 new cases occurred in 2010, and 51,370 deaths were due to colorectal cancer. The incidence rate has decreased significantly during the past 20 years, likely due to enhanced and more compliantly followed screening practices. Similarly, mortality rates in the United States have decreased by approximately 25%, resulting largely from improved treatment and earlier detection.

POLYPS AND MOLECULAR PATHOGENESIS

Most colorectal cancers, regardless of etiology, arise from adenomatous polyps. A polyp is a grossly visible protrusion from the mucosal surface and may be classified pathologically as a nonneoplastic hamartoma (*juvenile polyp*), a hyperplastic mucosal proliferation (*hyperplastic polyp*), or an adenomatous polyp. Only adenomas are clearly premalignant, and only a minority of such lesions becomes cancer. Adenomatous polyps may be found in the colons of ~30% of middle-aged and ~50% of elderly people; however, <1% of polyps ever become malignant. Most polyps produce no symptoms and remain clinically undetected. Occult blood in the stool is found in <5% of patients with polyps.

A number of molecular changes are noted in adenomatous polyps, dysplastic lesions, and polyps containing microscopic foci of tumor cells (carcinoma in situ), which are thought to reflect a multistep process in the evolution of normal colonic mucosa to life-threatening invasive carcinoma. These developmental steps toward carcinogenesis include, but are not restricted to, point mutations in the K-*ras* protooncogene; hypomethylation of DNA, leading to gene activation; loss of DNA (*allelic loss*) at the site of a tumor-suppressor gene (the adenomatous polyposis coli [*APC*] gene) on the long arm of chromosome 5 (5q21); allelic loss at the site of a tumor-suppressor gene located on chromosome 18q (the deleted in colorectal cancer [*DCC*] gene); and allelic loss at chromosome 17p, associated with mutations in the p53 tumor-suppressor gene. Thus, the altered proliferative pattern of the colonic mucosa,

which results in progression to a polyp and then to carcinoma, may involve the mutational activation of an oncogene followed by and coupled with the loss of genes that normally suppress tumorigenesis. It remains uncertain whether the genetic aberrations always occur in a defined order. Based on this model, however, cancer is believed to develop only in those polyps in which most (if not all) of these mutational events take place.

Clinically, the probability of an adenomatous polyp becoming a cancer depends on the gross appearance of the lesion, its histologic features, and its size. Adenomatous polyps may be pedunculated (stalked) or sessile (flat-based). Cancers develop more frequently in sessile polyps. Histologically, adenomatous polyps may be tubular, villous (i.e., papillary), or tubulovillous. Villous adenomas, most of which are sessile, become malignant more than three times as often as tubular adenomas. The likelihood that any polypoid lesion in the large bowel contains invasive cancer is related to the size of the polyp, being negligible (<2%) in lesions <1.5 cm, intermediate (2–10%) in lesions 1.5–2.5 cm, and substantial (10%) in lesions >2.5 cm in size.

Following the detection of an adenomatous polyp, the entire large bowel should be visualized endoscopically or radiographically, since synchronous lesions are noted in about one-third of cases. Colonoscopy should then be repeated periodically, even in the absence of a previously documented malignancy, since such patients have a 30–50% probability of developing another adenoma and are at a higher-than-average risk for developing a colorectal carcinoma. Adenomatous polyps are thought to require >5 years of growth before becoming clinically significant; colonoscopy need not be carried out more frequently than every 3 years.

ETIOLOGY AND RISK FACTORS

Risk factors for the development of colorectal cancer are listed in **Table 49-4**.

TABLE 49-4

RISK FACTORS FOR THE DEVELOPMENT OF COLORECTAL CANCER

Diet: Animal fat
Hereditary syndromes (autosomal dominant inheritance)
  Polyposis coli
  Nonpolyposis syndrome (Lynch syndrome)
Inflammatory bowel disease
Streptococcus bovis bacteremia
Ureterosigmoidostomy
? Tobacco use

Diet

The etiology for most cases of large-bowel cancer appears to be related to environmental factors. The disease occurs more often in upper socioeconomic populations who live in urban areas. Mortality from colorectal cancer is directly correlated with per capita consumption of calories, meat protein, and dietary fat and oil as well as elevations in the serum cholesterol concentration and mortality from coronary artery disease. Geographic variations in incidence are unrelated to genetic differences, since migrant groups tend to assume the large-bowel cancer incidence rates of their adopted countries. Furthermore, population groups such as Mormons and Seventh Day Adventists, whose lifestyle and dietary habits differ somewhat from those of their neighbors, have significantly lower-than-expected incidence and mortality rates for colorectal cancer. Colorectal cancer has increased in Japan since that nation has adopted a more "Western" diet. At least three hypotheses have been proposed to explain the relationship to diet, none of which is fully satisfactory.

▮ Animal fats

One hypothesis is that the ingestion of animal fats found in red meats and processed meat leads to an increased proportion of anaerobes in the gut microflora, resulting in the conversion of normal bile acids into carcinogens. This provocative hypothesis is supported by several reports of increased amounts of fecal anaerobes in the stools of patients with colorectal cancer. Diets high in animal (but not vegetable) fats are also associated with high serum cholesterol, which is also associated

with enhanced risk for the development of colorectal adenomas and carcinomas.

▮ Insulin resistance

The large number of calories in Western diets coupled with physical inactivity has been associated with a higher prevalence of obesity. Obese persons develop insulin resistance with increased circulating levels of insulin, leading to higher circulating concentrations of insulin-like growth factor type I (IGF-I). This growth factor appears to stimulate proliferation of the intestinal mucosa.

▮ Fiber

Contrary to prior beliefs, the results of randomized trials and case-controlled studies have failed to show any value for dietary fiber or diets high in fruits and vegetables in preventing the recurrence of colorectal adenomas or the development of colorectal cancer. The weight of epidemiologic evidence, however, implicates diet as being the major etiologic factor for colorectal cancer, particularly diets high in animal fat and in calories.

HEREDITARY FACTORS AND SYNDROMES

Up to 25% of patients with colorectal cancer have a family history of the disease, suggesting a hereditary predisposition. Inherited large-bowel cancers can be divided into two main groups: the well-studied but uncommon polyposis syndromes and the more common nonpolyposis syndromes (Table 49-5).

TABLE 49-5

HEREDITABLE (AUTOSOMAL DOMINANT) GASTROINTESTINAL POLYPOSIS SYNDROMES

SYNDROME	DISTRIBUTION OF POLYPS	HISTOLOGIC TYPE	MALIGNANT POTENTIAL	ASSOCIATED LESIONS
Familial adenomatous polyposis	Large intestine	Adenoma	Common	None
Gardner's syndrome	Large and small intestines	Adenoma	Common	Osteomas, fibromas, lipomas, epidermoid cysts, ampullary cancers, congenital hypertrophy of retinal pigment epithelium
Turcot's syndrome	Large intestine	Adenoma	Common	Brain tumors
Nonpolyposis syndrome (Lynch syndrome)	Large intestine (often proximal)	Adenoma	Common	Endometrial and ovarian tumors
Peutz-Jeghers syndrome	Small and large intestines, stomach	Hamartoma	Rare	Mucocutaneous pigmentation; tumors of the ovary, breast, pancreas, endometrium
Juvenile polyposis	Large and small intestines, stomach	Hamartoma, rarely progressing to adenoma	Rare	Various congenital abnormalities

Polyposis coli

Polyposis coli (familial polyposis of the colon) is a rare condition characterized by the appearance of thousands of adenomatous polyps throughout the large bowel. It is transmitted as an autosomal dominant trait; the occasional patient with no family history probably developed the condition due to a spontaneous mutation. Polyposis coli is associated with a deletion in the long arm of chromosome 5 (including the *APC* [adenomatous polyposis coli] gene) in both neoplastic (somatic mutation) and normal (germ-line mutation) cells. The loss of this genetic material (i.e., allelic loss) results in the absence of tumor-suppressor genes whose protein products would normally inhibit neoplastic growth. The presence of soft tissue and bony tumors, congenital hypertrophy of the retinal pigment epithelium, mesenteric desmoid tumors, and ampullary cancers in addition to the colonic polyps characterizes a subset of polyposis coli known as *Gardner's syndrome*. The appearance of malignant tumors of the central nervous system accompanying polyposis coli defines *Turcot's syndrome*. The colonic polyps in all these conditions are rarely present before puberty but are generally evident in affected individuals by age 25. If the polyposis is not treated surgically, colorectal cancer will develop in almost all patients before age 40. Polyposis coli results from a defect in the colonic mucosa, leading to an abnormal proliferative pattern and impaired DNA repair mechanisms. Once the multiple polyps are detected, patients should undergo a total colectomy. Medical therapy with nonsteroidal anti-inflammatory drugs (NSAIDs) such as sulindac and cyclooxygenase-2 inhibitors such as celecoxib can decrease the number and size of polyps in patients with polyposis coli; however, this effect on polyps is only temporary, and NSAIDs are not proven to reduce the risk of cancer. Colectomy remains the primary therapy/prevention. The offspring of patients with polyposis coli, who often are prepubertal when the diagnosis is made in the parent, have a 50% risk for developing this premalignant disorder and should be carefully screened by annual flexible sigmoidoscopy until age 35. Proctosigmoidoscopy is a sufficient screening procedure because polyps tend to be evenly distributed from cecum to anus, making more-invasive and expensive techniques such as colonoscopy or barium enema unnecessary. Testing for occult blood in the stool is an inadequate screening maneuver. An alternative method for identifying carriers is testing DNA from peripheral blood mononuclear cells for the presence of a mutated *APC* gene. The detection of such a germ-line mutation can lead to a definitive diagnosis before the development of polyps.

Hereditary nonpolyposis colon cancer

Hereditary nonpolyposis colon cancer (HNPCC), also known as *Lynch syndrome*, is another autosomal dominant trait. It is characterized by the presence of three or more relatives with histologically documented colorectal cancer, one of whom is a first-degree relative of the other two; one or more cases of colorectal cancer diagnosed before age 50 in the family; and colorectal cancer involving at least two generations. In contrast to polyposis coli, HNPCC is associated with an unusually high frequency of cancer arising in the proximal large bowel. The median age for the appearance of an adenocarcinoma is <50 years, 10–15 years younger than the median age for the general population. Despite having a poorly differentiated histologic appearance, the proximal colon tumors in HNPCC have a better prognosis than sporadic tumors from patients of similar age. Families with HNPCC often include individuals with multiple primary cancers; the association of colorectal cancer with either ovarian or endometrial carcinomas is especially strong in women. It has been recommended that members of such families undergo biennial colonoscopy beginning at age 25 years, with intermittent pelvic ultrasonography and endometrial biopsy for afflicted women; such a screening strategy has not yet been validated. HNPCC is associated with germ-line mutations of several genes, particularly *hMSH2* on chromosome 2 and *hMLH1* on chromosome 3. These mutations lead to errors in DNA replication and are thought to result in DNA instability because of defective repair of DNA mismatches resulting in abnormal cell growth and tumor development. Testing tumor cells through molecular analysis of DNA or immunohistochemical staining of paraffin-fixed tissue for "microsatellite instability" (sequence changes reflecting defective mismatch repair) in patients younger than age 50 with colorectal cancer and a positive family history for colorectal or endometrial cancer may identify probands with HNPCC.

INFLAMMATORY BOWEL DISEASE

(Chap. 17) Large-bowel cancer is increased in incidence in patients with long-standing inflammatory bowel disease (IBD). Cancers develop more commonly in patients with ulcerative colitis than in those with granulomatous colitis, but this impression may result in part from the occasional difficulty of differentiating these two conditions. The risk of colorectal cancer in a patient with IBD is relatively small during the initial 10 years of the disease, but then it appears to increase at a rate of ~0.5–1% per year. Cancer may develop in 8–30% of patients after 25 years. The risk is higher in younger patients with pancolitis.

Cancer surveillance in patients with IBD is unsatisfactory. Symptoms such as bloody diarrhea, abdominal cramping, and obstruction, which may signal the appearance of a tumor, are similar to the complaints caused by a flare-up of the underlying disease. In patients with a history of IBD lasting ≥15 years who continue to experience exacerbations, the surgical removal of the colon can significantly reduce the risk for cancer and also eliminate the target organ for the underlying chronic gastrointestinal disorder. The value of such surveillance techniques as colonoscopy with mucosal biopsies and brushings for less-symptomatic individuals with chronic IBD is uncertain. The lack of uniformity regarding the pathologic criteria that characterize dysplasia and the absence of data that such surveillance reduces the development of lethal cancers have made this costly practice an area of controversy.

OTHER HIGH-RISK CONDITIONS

Streptococcus bovis *bacteremia*

For unknown reasons, individuals who develop endocarditis or septicemia from this fecal bacterium have a high incidence of occult colorectal tumors and, possibly, upper gastrointestinal cancers as well. Endoscopic or radiographic screening appears advisable.

Tobacco use

Cigarette smoking is linked to the development of colorectal adenomas, particularly after >35 years of tobacco use. No biologic explanation for this association has yet been proposed.

PRIMARY PREVENTION

Several orally administered compounds have been assessed as possible inhibitors of colon cancer. The most effective class of chemopreventive agents is aspirin and other NSAIDs, which are thought to suppress cell proliferation by inhibiting prostaglandin synthesis. Regular aspirin use reduces the risk of colon adenomas and carcinomas as well as death from large-bowel cancer; such use also appears to diminish the likelihood for developing additional premalignant adenomas following treatment for a prior colon carcinoma. This effect of aspirin on colon carcinogenesis increases with the duration and dosage of drug use. Oral folic acid supplements and oral calcium supplements reduce the risk of adenomatous polyps and colorectal cancers in case-controlled studies. The value of vitamin D as a form of chemoprevention is under study. Antioxidant vitamins such as ascorbic acid, tocopherols, and β-carotene are ineffective at reducing the incidence of subsequent adenomas in patients who have undergone the removal of a colon adenoma. Estrogen-replacement therapy has been associated with a reduction in the risk of colorectal cancer in women, conceivably by an effect on bile acid synthesis and composition or by decreasing synthesis of IGF-I. The otherwise unexplained reduction in colorectal cancer mortality rate in women may be a result of the widespread use of estrogen replacement in postmenopausal individuals.

SCREENING

The rationale for colorectal cancer screening programs is that earlier detection of localized, superficial cancers in asymptomatic individuals will increase the surgical cure rate. Such screening programs are important for individuals having a family history of the disease in first-degree relatives. The relative risk for developing colorectal cancer increases to 1.75 in such individuals and may be even higher if the relative was afflicted before age 60. The prior use of proctosigmoidoscopy as a screening tool was based on the observation that 60% of early lesions are located in the rectosigmoid. For unexplained reasons, however, the proportion of large-bowel cancers arising in the rectum has been decreasing during the past several decades, with a corresponding increase in the proportion of cancers in the more proximal descending colon. As such, the potential for rigid proctosigmoidoscopy to detect a sufficient number of occult neoplasms to make the procedure cost-effective has been questioned. Flexible, fiberoptic sigmoidoscopes permit trained operators to visualize the colon for up to 60 cm, which enhances the capability for cancer detection. However, this technique still leaves the proximal half of the large bowel unscreened.

Most programs directed at the early detection of colorectal cancers have focused on digital rectal examinations and fecal occult blood testing. The digital examination should be part of any routine physical evaluation in adults older than age 40 years, serving as a screening test for prostate cancer in men, a component of the pelvic examination in women, and an inexpensive maneuver for the detection of masses in the rectum. The development of the Hemoccult test has greatly facilitated the detection of occult fecal blood. Unfortunately, even when performed optimally, the Hemoccult test has major limitations as a screening technique. About 50% of patients with documented colorectal cancers have a negative fecal Hemoccult test, consistent with the intermittent bleeding pattern of these tumors. When random cohorts of asymptomatic persons have been tested, 2–4% have Hemoccult-positive stools. Colorectal cancers have been found in <10% of these "test-positive" cases, with benign polyps being detected in an additional 20–30%. Thus, a colorectal neoplasm will not be found in most asymptomatic individuals with occult blood in their stool. Nonetheless, persons found to have Hemoccult-positive stool routinely undergo further medical evaluation, including sigmoidoscopy, barium enema, and/or colonoscopy—procedures that are not only uncomfortable and expensive but also associated with a small risk for significant complications. The added cost of these studies would appear justifiable if the small number of patients found to have occult neoplasms because of Hemoccult screening could be shown to have an improved prognosis and prolonged survival. Prospectively controlled trials showed a statistically significant reduction in mortality rate from colorectal cancer for individuals undergoing annual screening. However, this benefit only emerged after >13 years of follow-up and was extremely expensive to achieve, since all positive tests (most of which were false-positive) were followed by colonoscopy. Moreover, these colonoscopic examinations quite likely provided the opportunity for cancer prevention through the removal of potentially premalignant adenomatous polyps since the eventual development of cancer was reduced by 20% in the cohort undergoing annual screening.

Screening techniques for large-bowel cancer in asymptomatic persons remain unsatisfactory. Compliance with any screening strategy within the general population is poor. At present, the American Cancer Society suggests fecal Hemoccult screening annually and flexible sigmoidoscopy every 5 years beginning at age 50 for asymptomatic individuals having no colorectal cancer risk factors. The American Cancer Society has also endorsed a "total colon examination" (i.e., colonoscopy or double-contrast barium enema) every 10 years as an alternative to Hemoccult testing with periodic flexible sigmoidoscopy. Colonoscopy has been shown to be superior to double-contrast barium enema and also to have a higher sensitivity for detecting villous or dysplastic adenomas or cancers than the strategy employing occult fecal blood testing and flexible sigmoidoscopy. Whether colonoscopy performed every 10 years beginning after age 50 will prove to be cost-effective and whether it may be supplanted as a screening maneuver by sophisticated radiographic techniques ("virtual colonoscopy") remains unclear. More effective techniques for screening are needed, perhaps taking advantage of the molecular changes that have been described in these tumors. Analysis of fecal DNA for multiple mutations associated with colorectal cancer is being tested.

CLINICAL FEATURES

Presenting symptoms

Symptoms vary with the anatomic location of the tumor. Since stool is relatively liquid as it passes through the ileocecal valve into the right colon, cancers arising in the cecum and ascending colon may become quite large without resulting in any obstructive symptoms or noticeable alterations in bowel habits. Lesions of the right colon commonly ulcerate, leading to chronic, insidious blood loss without a change in the appearance of the stool. Consequently, patients with tumors of the ascending colon often present with symptoms such as

FIGURE 49-1
Double-contrast air-barium enema revealing a sessile tumor of the cecum in a patient with iron-deficiency anemia and guaiac-positive stool. The lesion at surgery was a stage II adenocarcinoma.

fatigue, palpitations, and even angina pectoris and are found to have a hypochromic, microcytic anemia indicative of iron deficiency. Since the cancer may bleed intermittently, a random fecal occult blood test may be negative. As a result, the unexplained presence of iron-deficiency anemia in any adult (with the possible exception of a premenopausal, multiparous woman) mandates a thorough endoscopic and/or radiographic visualization of the entire large bowel **(Fig. 49-1)**.

Since stool becomes more formed as it passes into the transverse and descending colon, tumors arising there tend to impede the passage of stool, resulting in the development of abdominal cramping, occasional obstruction, and even perforation. Radiographs of the abdomen often reveal characteristic annular, constricting lesions ("apple-core" or "napkin-ring") **(Fig. 49-2)**.

Cancers arising in the rectosigmoid are often associated with hematochezia, tenesmus, and narrowing of the caliber of stool; anemia is an infrequent finding. While these symptoms may lead patients and their physicians to suspect the presence of hemorrhoids, the development of rectal bleeding and/or altered bowel habits demands a prompt digital rectal examination and proctosigmoidoscopy.

Staging, prognostic factors, and patterns of spread

The prognosis for individuals having colorectal cancer is related to the depth of tumor penetration into the bowel wall and the presence of both regional lymph

FIGURE 49-2

Annular, constricting adenocarcinoma of the descending colon. This radiographic appearance is referred to as an "apple-core" lesion and is always highly suggestive of malignancy.

node involvement and distant metastases. These variables are incorporated into the staging system introduced by Dukes and applied to a TNM classification method, in which T represents the depth of tumor penetration, N the presence of lymph node involvement, and M the presence or absence of distant metastases (Fig. 49-3). Superficial lesions that do not involve regional lymph nodes and do not penetrate through the submucosa (T1) or the muscularis (T2) are designated as *stage I* (T1–2N0M0) disease; tumors that penetrate through the muscularis but have not spread to lymph nodes are *stage II* disease (T3N0M0); regional lymph node involvement defines *stage III* (TXN$_1$M$_0$) disease; and metastatic spread to sites such as liver, lung, or bone indicates *stage IV* (TXNXM$_1$) disease. Unless gross evidence of metastatic disease is present, disease stage cannot be determined accurately before surgical resection and pathologic analysis of the operative specimens. It is not clear whether the detection of nodal metastases by special immunohistochemical molecular techniques has the same prognostic implications as disease detected by routine light microscopy.

Most recurrences after a surgical resection of a large-bowel cancer occur within the first 4 years, making 5-year survival a fairly reliable indicator of cure. The likelihood for 5-year survival in patients with colorectal cancer is stage-related (Fig. 49-3). That likelihood has improved during the past several decades when similar surgical stages have been compared. The most plausible explanation for this improvement is more thorough intraoperative and pathologic staging. In particular, more exacting attention to pathologic detail has revealed that the prognosis following the resection of a colorectal cancer is not related merely to the presence or absence of regional lymph node involvement. Prognosis may be more precisely gauged by the number of involved lymph nodes (one to three lymph nodes versus four or more lymph nodes) and the number of nodes

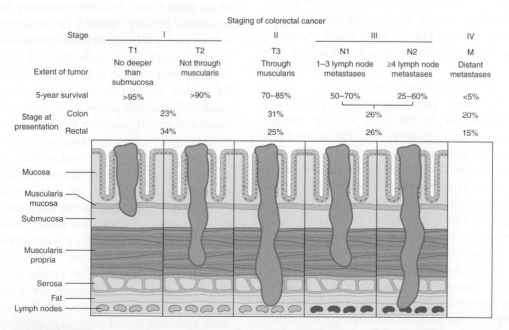

Staging of colorectal cancer

	Stage	I		II	III		IV
		T1	T2	T3	N1	N2	M
Extent of tumor		No deeper than submucosa	Not through muscularis	Through muscularis	1–3 lymph node metastases	≥4 lymph node metastases	Distant metastases
5-year survival		>95%	>90%	70–85%	50–70%	25–60%	<5%
Stage at presentation	Colon	23%		31%	26%		20%
	Rectal	34%		25%	26%		15%

Mucosa
Muscularis mucosa
Submucosa
Muscularis propria
Serosa
Fat
Lymph nodes

FIGURE 49-3

Staging and prognosis for patients with colorectal cancer.

TABLE 49-6

PREDICTORS OF POOR OUTCOME FOLLOWING TOTAL SURGICAL RESECTION OF COLORECTAL CANCER

Tumor spread to regional lymph nodes
Number of regional lymph nodes involved
Tumor penetration through the bowel wall
Poorly differentiated histology
Perforation
Tumor adherence to adjacent organs
Venous invasion
Preoperative elevation of CEA titer (>5 ng/mL)
Aneuploidy
Specific chromosomal deletion (e.g., allelic loss on chromosome 18q)

Abbreviation: CEA, carcinoembryonic antigen.

examined. A minimum of 12 sampled lymph nodes is thought necessary to accurately define tumor stage, and the more nodes examined the better. Other predictors of a poor prognosis after a total surgical resection include tumor penetration through the bowel wall into pericolic fat, poorly differentiated histology, perforation and/or tumor adherence to adjacent organs (increasing the risk for an anatomically adjacent recurrence), and venous invasion by tumor **(Table 49-6)**. Regardless of the clinicopathologic stage, a preoperative elevation of the plasma carcinoembryonic antigen (CEA) level predicts eventual tumor recurrence. The presence of aneuploidy and specific chromosomal deletions, such as allelic loss in chromosome 18q (involving the *DCC* gene) in tumor cells, appears to predict a higher risk for metastatic spread, particularly in patients with stage II (T3N0M0) disease. Conversely, the detection of microsatellite instability in tumor tissue indicates a more favorable outcome. In contrast to most other cancers, the prognosis in colorectal cancer is not influenced by the size of the primary lesion when adjusted for nodal involvement and histologic differentiation.

Cancers of the large bowel generally spread to regional lymph nodes or to the liver via the portal venous circulation. The liver represents the most frequent visceral site of metastasis; it is the initial site of distant spread in one-third of recurring colorectal cancers and is involved in more than two-thirds of such patients at the time of death. In general, colorectal cancer rarely spreads to the lungs, supraclavicular lymph nodes, bone, or brain without prior spread to the liver. A major exception to this rule occurs in patients having primary tumors in the distal rectum, from which tumor cells may spread through the paravertebral venous plexus, escaping the portal venous system and thereby reaching the lungs or supraclavicular lymph nodes without hepatic involvement. The median survival after the detection of distant metastases has ranged in the

past from 6–9 months (hepatomegaly, abnormal liver chemistries) to 24–30 months (small liver nodule initially identified by elevated CEA level and subsequent CT scan), but effective systemic therapy is improving the prognosis.

Efforts to use gene expression profiles to identify patients at risk of recurrence or those particularly likely to benefit from adjuvant therapy have not yet yielded practice changing results. Despite a burgeoning literature examining a host of prognostic factors, pathologic stage at diagnosis is the best predictor of long-term prognosis. Patients with lymphovascular invasion and high preoperative CEA levels are likely to have a more aggressive clinical course.

TREATMENT Colorectal Cancer

Total resection of tumor is the optimal treatment when a malignant lesion is detected in the large bowel. An evaluation for the presence of metastatic disease, including a thorough physical examination, chest radiograph, biochemical assessment of liver function, and measurement of the plasma CEA level, should be performed before surgery. When possible, a colonoscopy of the entire large bowel should be performed to identify synchronous neoplasms and/or polyps. The detection of metastases should not preclude surgery in patients with tumor-related symptoms such as gastrointestinal bleeding or obstruction, but it often prompts the use of a less radical operative procedure. At the time of laparotomy, the entire peritoneal cavity should be examined, with thorough inspection of the liver, pelvis, and hemidiaphragm and careful palpation of the full length of the large bowel. Following recovery from a complete resection, patients should be observed carefully for 5 years by semiannual physical examinations and yearly blood chemistry measurements. If a complete colonoscopy was not performed preoperatively, it should be carried out within the first several postoperative months. Some authorities favor measuring plasma CEA levels at 3-month intervals because of the sensitivity of this test as a marker for otherwise undetectable tumor recurrence. Subsequent endoscopic or radiographic surveillance of the large bowel, probably at triennial intervals, is indicated, since patients who have been cured of one colorectal cancer have a 3–5% probability of developing an additional bowel cancer during their lifetime and a >15% risk for the development of adenomatous polyps. Anastomotic ("suture-line") recurrences are infrequent in colorectal cancer patients, provided the surgical resection margins are adequate and free of tumor. The value of periodic CT scans of the abdomen, assessing for an early, asymptomatic indication of tumor recurrence, is an area of uncertainty, with some experts recommending the test be performed annually for the first 3 postoperative years.

Radiation therapy to the pelvis is recommended for patients with rectal cancer because it reduces the 20–25% probability of regional recurrences following complete surgical resection of stage II or III tumors, especially if they have penetrated through the serosa. This alarmingly high rate of local disease recurrence is believed to be due to the fact that the contained anatomic space within the pelvis limits the extent of the resection and because the rich lymphatic network of the pelvic side wall immediately adjacent to the rectum facilitates the early spread of malignant cells into surgically inaccessible tissue. The use of sharp rather than blunt dissection of rectal cancers (*total mesorectal excision*) appears to reduce the likelihood of local disease recurrence to ~10%. Radiation therapy, either pre- or postoperatively, reduces the likelihood of pelvic recurrences but does not appear to prolong survival. Combining postoperative radiation therapy with 5-fluorouracil-based chemotherapy lowers local recurrence rates and improves overall survival. Preoperative radiotherapy is indicated for patients with large, potentially unresectable rectal cancers; such lesions may shrink enough to permit subsequent surgical removal. Radiation therapy is not effective in the primary treatment of colon cancer.

Systemic therapy for patients with colorectal cancer has become more effective. 5-FU remains the backbone of treatment for this disease. Partial responses are obtained in 15–20% of patients. The probability of tumor response appears to be somewhat greater for patients with liver metastases when chemotherapy is infused directly into the hepatic artery, but intraarterial treatment is costly and toxic and does not appear to appreciably prolong survival. The concomitant administration of folinic acid (leucovorin) improves the efficacy of 5-FU in patients with advanced colorectal cancer, presumably by enhancing the binding of 5-FU to its target enzyme, thymidylate synthase. A threefold improvement in the partial response rate is noted when folinic acid is combined with 5-FU; however, the effect on survival is marginal, and the optimal dose schedule remains to be defined. 5-FU is generally administered intravenously but may also be given orally in the form of capecitabine (Xeloda) with seemingly similar efficacy.

Irinotecan (CPT-11), a topoisomerase 1 inhibitor, prolongs survival when compared to supportive care in patients whose disease has progressed on 5-FU. Furthermore, the addition of irinotecan to 5-FU and leucovorin (LV) improves response rates and survival of patients with metastatic disease. The *FOLFIRI regimen* is as follows: irinotecan, 180 mg/m^2 as a 90-min infusion on day 1; LV, 400 mg/m^2 as a 2-h infusion during irinotecan administration; immediately followed by 5-FU bolus,

400 mg/m^2, and 46-h continuous infusion of 2.4–3 g/m^2 every 2 weeks. Diarrhea is the major side effect from irinotecan. Oxaliplatin, a platinum analogue, also improves the response rate when added to 5-FU and LV as initial treatment of patients with metastatic disease. The *FOLFOX regimen* is the following: 2-h infusion of LV (400 mg/m^2 per day) followed by a 5-FU bolus (400 mg/m^2 per day) and 22-h infusion (1200 mg/m^2) every 2 weeks, together with oxaliplatin, 85 mg/m^2 as a 2-h infusion on day 1. Oxaliplatin frequently causes a dose-dependent sensory neuropathy that often resolves following the cessation of therapy. FOLFIRI and FOLFOX are equal in efficacy. In metastatic disease, these regimens may produce median survivals of 2 years.

Monoclonal antibodies are also effective in patients with advanced colorectal cancer. Cetuximab (Erbitux) and panitumumab (Vectibix) are directed against the epidermal growth factor receptor (EGFR), a transmembrane glycoprotein involved in signaling pathways affecting growth and proliferation of tumor cells. Both cetuximab and panitumumab, when given alone, have been shown to benefit a small proportion of previously treated patients, and cetuximab appears to have therapeutic synergy with such chemotherapeutic agents as irinotecan, even in patients previously resistant to this drug; this suggests that cetuximab can reverse cellular resistance to cytotoxic chemotherapy. The antibodies are not effective in the subset of colon tumors that contain mutated *K-ras*. The use of both cetuximab and panitumumab can lead to an acne-like rash, with the development and severity of the rash being correlated with the likelihood of antitumor efficacy. Inhibitors of the EGFR tyrosine kinase such as erlotinib (Tarceva) do not appear to be effective in colorectal cancer.

Bevacizumab (Avastin) is a monoclonal antibody directed against the vascular endothelial growth factor (VEGF) and is thought to act as an anti-angiogenesis agent. The addition of bevacizumab to irinotecan-containing combinations and to FOLFOX initially appeared to improve the outcome observed with chemotherapy alone, but subsequent studies have been less convincing. The use of bevacizumab can lead to hypertension, proteinuria, and an increased likelihood of thromboembolic events.

Patients with solitary hepatic metastases without clinical or radiographic evidence of additional tumor involvement should be considered for partial liver resection, because such procedures are associated with 5-year survival rates of 25–30% when performed on selected individuals by experienced surgeons.

The administration of 5-FU and LV for 6 months after resection of tumor in patients with stage III disease leads to a 40% decrease in recurrence rates and 30% improvement in survival. The likelihood of recurrence has been further reduced when oxaliplatin has been combined with 5-FU and LV (e.g., FOLFOX); unexpectedly, the addition of irinotecan to 5-FU and LV as well as the addition of either bevacizumab or cetuximab to FOLFOX did not enhance outcome. Patients with stage II tumors do not appear to benefit applicably from adjuvant therapy with the use of such treatment generally restricted to those patients having biologic characteristics (e.g., perforated tumors, Ty lesions, lymphovascular invasion) that place them at higher than usual risk for recurrence. In rectal cancer, the delivery of preoperative or postoperative combined modality therapy (5-FU plus radiation therapy) reduces the risk of recurrence and increases the chance of cure for patients with stages II and III tumors, with the preoperative approach being better tolerated. The 5-FU acts as a radiosensitizer when delivered together with radiation therapy. Life-extending adjuvant therapy is used in only about half of patients older than age 65 years. This age bias is completely inappropriate as the benefits and likely the tolerance of adjuvant therapy in patients aged 65+ years appear similar to those seen in younger individuals.

TUMORS OF THE SMALL INTESTINE

Small-bowel tumors comprise <3% of gastrointestinal neoplasms. Because of their rarity, a correct diagnosis is often delayed. Abdominal symptoms are usually vague and poorly defined, and conventional radiographic studies of the upper and lower intestinal tract often appear normal. Small-bowel tumors should be considered in the differential diagnosis in the following situations: (1) recurrent, unexplained episodes of crampy abdominal pain; (2) intermittent bouts of intestinal obstruction, especially in the absence of IBD or prior abdominal surgery; (3) intussusception in the adult; and (4) evidence of chronic intestinal bleeding in the presence of negative conventional contrast radiographs. A careful small-bowel barium study is the diagnostic procedure of choice; the diagnostic accuracy may be improved by infusing barium through a nasogastric tube placed into the duodenum (enteroclysis).

BENIGN TUMORS

The histology of benign small-bowel tumors is difficult to predict on clinical and radiologic grounds alone. The symptomatology of benign tumors is not distinctive, with pain, obstruction, and hemorrhage being the most frequent symptoms. These tumors are usually discovered during the fifth and sixth decades of life, more often in the distal rather than the proximal small intestine. The most common benign tumors are adenomas, leiomyomas, lipomas, and angiomas.

Adenomas

These tumors include those of the islet cells and Brunner's glands as well as polypoid adenomas. *Islet cell adenomas* are occasionally located outside the pancreas; the associated syndromes are discussed in Chap. 52. *Brunner's gland adenomas* are not truly neoplastic but represent a hypertrophy or hyperplasia of submucosal duodenal glands. These appear as small nodules in the duodenal mucosa that secrete a highly viscous alkaline mucus. Most often, this is an incidental radiographic finding not associated with any specific clinical disorder.

Polypoid adenomas

About 25% of benign small-bowel tumors are polypoid adenomas (Table 49-5). They may present as single polypoid lesions or, less commonly, as papillary villous adenomas. As in the colon, the sessile or papillary form of the tumor is sometimes associated with a coexisting carcinoma. Occasionally, patients with Gardner's syndrome develop premalignant adenomas in the small bowel; such lesions are generally in the duodenum. Multiple polypoid tumors may occur throughout the small bowel (and occasionally the stomach and colorectum) in the Peutz-Jeghers syndrome. The polyps are usually hamartomas (juvenile polyps) having a low potential for malignant degeneration. Mucocutaneous melanin deposits as well as tumors of the ovary, breast, pancreas, and endometrium are also associated with this autosomal dominant condition.

Leiomyomas

These neoplasms arise from smooth-muscle components of the intestine and are usually intramural, affecting the overlying mucosa. Ulceration of the mucosa may cause gastrointestinal hemorrhage of varying severity. Cramping or intermittent abdominal pain is frequently encountered.

Lipomas

These tumors occur with greatest frequency in the distal ileum and at the ileocecal valve. They have a characteristic radiolucent appearance and are usually intramural and asymptomatic, but on occasion cause bleeding.

Angiomas

While not true neoplasms, these lesions are important because they frequently cause intestinal bleeding. They may take the form of telangiectasia or hemangiomas. Multiple intestinal telangiectasias occur in a nonhereditary form confined to the gastrointestinal tract or as part of the hereditary Osler-Rendu-Weber syndrome. Vascular tumors may also take the form of isolated hemangiomas, most commonly in the jejunum. Angiography, especially during bleeding, is the best procedure for evaluating these lesions.

MALIGNANT TUMORS

While rare, small-bowel malignancies occur in patients with long-standing regional enteritis and celiac sprue as well as in individuals with AIDS. Malignant tumors of the small bowel are frequently associated with fever, weight loss, anorexia, bleeding, and a palpable abdominal mass. After ampullary carcinomas (many of which arise from biliary or pancreatic ducts), the most frequently occurring small-bowel malignancies are adenocarcinomas, lymphomas, carcinoid tumors, and leiomyosarcomas.

Adenocarcinomas

The most common primary cancers of the small bowel are adenocarcinomas, accounting for ~50% of malignant tumors. These cancers occur most often in the distal duodenum and proximal jejunum, where they tend to ulcerate and cause hemorrhage or obstruction. Radiologically, they may be confused with chronic duodenal ulcer disease or with Crohn's disease if the patient has long-standing regional enteritis. The diagnosis is best made by endoscopy and biopsy under direct vision. Surgical resection is the treatment of choice.

Lymphomas

Lymphoma in the small bowel may be primary or secondary. A diagnosis of a primary intestinal lymphoma requires histologic confirmation in a clinical setting in which palpable adenopathy and hepatosplenomegaly are absent and no evidence of lymphoma is seen on chest radiograph, CT scan, or peripheral blood smear or on bone marrow aspiration and biopsy. Symptoms referable to the small bowel are present, usually accompanied by an anatomically discernible lesion. Secondary lymphoma of the small bowel consists of involvement of the intestine by a lymphoid malignancy extending from involved retroperitoneal or mesenteric lymph nodes.

Primary intestinal lymphoma accounts for ~20% of malignancies of the small bowel. These neoplasms are non-Hodgkin's lymphomas; they usually have a diffuse, large-cell histology and are of T cell origin. Intestinal lymphoma involves the ileum, jejunum, and duodenum, in decreasing frequency—a pattern that mirrors the relative amount of normal lymphoid cells in these anatomic areas. The risk of small-bowel lymphoma is increased in patients with a prior history of malabsorptive conditions (e.g., celiac sprue), regional enteritis, and depressed immune function due to congenital immunodeficiency syndromes, prior organ transplantation, autoimmune disorders, or AIDS.

The development of localized or nodular masses that narrow the lumen results in periumbilical pain (made worse by eating) as well as weight loss, vomiting, and occasional intestinal obstruction. The diagnosis of small-bowel lymphoma may be suspected from the appearance on contrast radiographs of patterns such as infiltration and thickening of mucosal folds, mucosal nodules, areas of irregular ulceration, or stasis of contrast material. The diagnosis can be confirmed by surgical exploration and resection of involved segments. Intestinal lymphoma can occasionally be diagnosed by peroral intestinal mucosal biopsy, but since the disease mainly involves the lamina propria, full-thickness surgical biopsies are usually required.

Resection of the tumor constitutes the initial treatment modality. While postoperative radiation therapy has been given to some patients following a total resection, most authorities favor short-term (three cycles) systemic treatment with combination chemotherapy. The frequent presence of widespread intraabdominal disease at the time of diagnosis and the occasional multicentricity of the tumor often make a total resection impossible. The probability of sustained remission or cure is ~75% in patients with localized disease but is ~25% in individuals with unresectable lymphoma. In patients whose tumors are not resected, chemotherapy may lead to bowel perforation.

A unique form of small-bowel lymphoma, diffusely involving the entire intestine, was first described in oriental Jews and Arabs and is referred to as *immunoproliferative small intestinal disease* (IPSID), *Mediterranean lymphoma*, or α *heavy chain disease*. This is a B cell tumor. The typical presentation includes chronic diarrhea and steatorrhea associated with vomiting and abdominal cramps; clubbing of the digits may be observed. A curious feature in many patients with IPSID is the presence in the blood and intestinal secretions of an abnormal IgA that contains a shortened α heavy chain and is devoid of light chains. It is suspected that the abnormal α chains are produced by plasma cells infiltrating the small bowel. The clinical course of patients with IPSID is generally one of exacerbations and remissions, with death frequently resulting from either progressive malnutrition and wasting or the development of an aggressive lymphoma. The use of oral antibiotics such as tetracycline appears to be beneficial in the early phases of the disorder, suggesting a possible infectious etiology. Combination chemotherapy has been administered during later stages of the disease, with variable results. Results are better when antibiotics and chemotherapy are combined.

Carcinoid tumors

Carcinoid tumors arise from argentaffin cells of the crypts of Lieberkühn and are found from the distal duodenum to the ascending colon, areas embryologically derived from the midgut. More than 50% of intestinal carcinoids are found in the distal ileum, with most congregating close to the ileocecal valve. Most intestinal carcinoids are asymptomatic and of low malignant potential, but invasion and metastases may occur, leading to the carcinoid syndrome (Chap. 52).

Leiomyosarcomas

Leiomyosarcomas often are >5 cm in diameter and may be palpable on abdominal examination. Bleeding, obstruction, and perforation are common. Such tumors should be analyzed for the expression of mutant c-*kit* receptor (defining GIST), and in the presence of metastatic disease, justifying treatment with imatinib mesylate (Gleevec) or, in imatinib-refractory patients, sunitinib (Sutent).

CANCERS OF THE ANUS

Cancers of the anus account for 1–2% of the malignant tumors of the large bowel. Most such lesions arise in the anal canal, the anatomic area extending from the anorectal ring to a zone approximately halfway between the pectinate (or dentate) line and the anal verge. Carcinomas arising proximal to the pectinate line (i.e., in the transitional zone between the glandular mucosa of the rectum and the squamous epithelium of the distal anus) are known as *basaloid*, *cuboidal*, or *cloacogenic* tumors; about one-third of anal cancers have this histologic pattern. Malignancies arising distal to the pectinate line have squamous histology, ulcerate more frequently, and constitute ~55% of anal cancers. The prognosis for

patients with basaloid and squamous cell cancers of the anus is identical when corrected for tumor size and the presence or absence of nodal spread.

The development of anal cancer is associated with infection by human papillomavirus, the same organism etiologically linked to cervical cancer. The virus is sexually transmitted. The infection may lead to anal warts (condyloma acuminata), which may progress to anal intraepithelial neoplasia and on to squamous cell carcinoma. The risk for anal cancer is increased among homosexual males, presumably related to anal intercourse. Anal cancer risk is increased in both men and women with AIDS, possibly because their immunosuppressed state permits more severe papillomavirus infection. Anal cancers occur most commonly in middle-aged persons and are more frequent in women than men. At diagnosis, patients may experience bleeding, pain, sensation of a perianal mass, and pruritus.

Radical surgery (abdominal-perineal resection with lymph node sampling and a permanent colostomy) was once the treatment of choice for this tumor type. The 5-year survival rate after such a procedure was 55–70% in the absence of spread to regional lymph nodes and <20% if nodal involvement was present. An alternative therapeutic approach combining external beam radiation therapy with concomitant chemotherapy has resulted in biopsy-proven disappearance of all tumor in >80% of patients whose initial lesion was <3 cm in size. Tumor recurrences develop in <10% of these patients, meaning that ~70% of patients with anal cancers can be cured with nonoperative treatment. Surgery should be reserved for the minority of individuals who are found to have residual tumor after being managed initially with radiation therapy combined with chemotherapy.

CHAPTER 50

TUMORS OF THE LIVER AND BILIARY TREE

Brian I. Carr

HEPATOCELLULAR CARCINOMA

INCIDENCE

Hepatocellular carcinoma (HCC) is one of the most common malignancies worldwide. The annual global incidence is approximately 1 million cases, with a male to female ratio of approximately 4:1 (1:1 without cirrhosis to 9:1 in many high-incidence countries). The incidence rate equals the death rate. In the United States, approximately 22,000 new cases are diagnosed annually, with 18,000 deaths. The death rates in males in low-incidence countries such as the United States are 1.9 per 100,000 per year; in intermediate areas such as Austria and South Africa, they range from 5.1–20; and in high-incidence areas such as in the Orient (China and Korea) as high as 23.1–150 per 100,000 per year (Table 50-1). The incidence of HCC in the United States is approximately 3 per 100,000 persons, with significant gender, ethnic, and geographic variations. These numbers are rapidly increasing and may be an underestimate. Approximately 4 million chronic hepatitis C virus (HCV) carriers are in the United States alone. Approximately 10% of them or 400,000 are likely to develop cirrhosis. Approximately 5% or 20,000 of these may develop HCC annually. Add to this the two other common predisposing factors—hepatitis B virus (HBV) and chronic alcohol consumption—and 60,000 new HCC cases annually seem possible. Future advances in HCC survival will likely depend in part on immunization strategies for HBV (and HCV) and earlier diagnosis by screening of patients at risk of HCC development.

Current directions

With the U.S. HCV epidemic, HCC is increasing in most states, and obesity-associated liver disease (nonalcoholic steatohepatitis [NASH]) is increasingly recognized as a cause.

EPIDEMIOLOGY

There are two general types of epidemiologic studies of HCC—those of country-based incidence rates (Table 50-1) and those of migrants. Endemic hot spots occur in areas of China and sub-Saharan Africa, which are associated both with high endemic hepatitis B carrier rates as well as mycotoxin contamination of foodstuffs (aflatoxin B_1), stored grains, drinking water, and soil. Environmental factors are important, for example, Japanese in Japan have a higher

TABLE 50-1

AGE-ADJUSTED INCIDENCE RATES FOR HEPATOCELLULAR CARCINOMA

| COUNTRY | PERSONS PER 100,000 PER YEAR | |
	MALE	FEMALE
Argentina	6.0	2.5
Brazil, Recife	9.2	8.3
Brazil, Sao Paulo	3.8	2.6
Mozambique	112.9	30.8
South Africa, Cape: Black	26.3	8.4
South Africa, Cape: White	1.2	0.6
Senegal	25.6	9.0
Nigeria	15.4	3.2
Gambia	33.1	12.6
Burma	25.5	8.8
Japan	7.2	2.2
Korea	13.8	3.2
China, Shanghai	34.4	11.6
India, Bombay	4.9	2.5
India, Madras	2.1	0.7
Great Britain	1.6	0.8
France	6.9	1.2
Italy, Varese	7.1	2.7
Norway	1.8	1.1
Spain, Navarra	7.9	4.7

incidence than those living in Hawaii, who in turn have a higher incidence than those living in California.

ETIOLOGIC FACTORS

Chemical carcinogens

Causative agents for HCC have been studied along two general lines. First are agents identified as carcinogenic in experimental animals (particularly rodents) that are thought to be present in the human environment **(Table 50-2)**. Second is the association of HCC with various other clinical conditions. Probably the best-studied and most potent ubiquitous natural chemical carcinogen is a product of the *Aspergillus* fungus, called aflatoxin B_1. This mold and aflatoxin product can be found in a variety of stored grains in hot, humid places, where peanuts and rice are stored in unrefrigerated conditions. Aflatoxin contamination of foodstuffs correlates well with incidence rates in Africa and to some extent in China. In endemic areas of China, even farm animals such as ducks have HCC. The most potent carcinogens appear to be natural products of plants, fungi, and bacteria, such as bush trees containing pyrrolizidine alkaloids as well as tannic acid and safrole. Pollutants such as pesticides and insecticides are known rodent carcinogens.

Hepatitis

Both case-control and cohort studies have shown a strong association between chronic hepatitis B carrier rates and increased incidence of HCC. In Taiwanese male postal carriers who were hepatitis B surface antigen (HBsAg)-positive, a 98-fold greater risk for HCC was found compared to HBsAg-negative individuals. The incidence of HCC in Alaskan natives is markedly increased related to a high prevalence of HBV infection. HBV-based HCC may involve rounds of hepatic destruction with subsequent proliferation and not

TABLE 50-2

FACTORS ASSOCIATED WITH AN INCREASED RISK OF DEVELOPING HCC	
COMMON	**UNUSUAL**
Cirrhosis from any cause	Primary biliary cirrhosis
Hepatitis B or C chronic infection	Hemochromatosis
Ethanol chronic consumption	α_1-Antitrypsin deficiency
NASH/NAFL	Glycogen storage diseases
Aflatoxin B_1 or other mycotoxins	Citrullinemia
	Porphyria cutanea tarda
	Hereditary tyrosinemia
	Wilson's disease

Abbreviations: NAFL, nonalcoholic fatty liver; NASH, nonalcoholic steatohepatitis.

necessarily frank cirrhosis. The increase in Japanese HCC incidence rates in the last three decades is thought to be from hepatitis C. A large-scale World Health Organization (WHO)-sponsored intervention study is currently underway in Asia involving HBV vaccination of the newborn. HCC in African blacks is not associated with severe cirrhosis but is poorly differentiated and very aggressive. Despite uniform HBV carrier rates among the South African Bantu, there is a ninefold difference in HCC incidence between Mozambicans living along the coast and inland. These differences are attributed to the additional exposure to dietary aflatoxin B_1 and other carcinogenic mycotoxins. A typical interval between HCV-associated transfusion and subsequent HCC is approximately 30 years. HCV-associated HCC patients tend to have more frequent and advanced cirrhosis, but in HBV-associated HCC, only half the patients have cirrhosis; the remainder having chronic active hepatitis (Chap. 40).

Other etiologic conditions

The 75–85% association of HCC with underlying cirrhosis has long been recognized, more typically with macronodular cirrhosis in Southeast Asia, but also with micronodular cirrhosis (alcohol) in Europe and the United States (Chap. 42). It is still not clear whether cirrhosis itself is a predisposing factor to the development of HCC or whether the underlying causes of the cirrhosis are actually the carcinogenic factors. However, ~20% of U.S. patients with HCC do not have underlying cirrhosis. Several underlying conditions are associated with an increased risk for cirrhosis-associated HCC (Table 50-2), including hepatitis, alcohol, autoimmune chronic active hepatitis, cryptogenic cirrhosis, and NASH. A less common association is with primary biliary cirrhosis and several metabolic diseases including hemochromatosis, Wilson's disease, α_1-antitrypsin deficiency, tyrosinemia, porphyria cutanea tarda, glycogenesis types 1 and 3, citrullinemia. and orotic aciduria. The etiology of HCC in those 20% of patients who have no cirrhosis is currently unclear, and their HCC natural history is not well-defined.

Current directions

Many patients have multiple etiologies, and the interactions of either hepatitis or alcohol and smoking, or with aflatoxins, are just beginning to be explored.

CLINICAL FEATURES

Symptoms

These include abdominal pain, weight loss, weakness, abdominal fullness and swelling, jaundice, and nausea **(Table 50-3)**. Presenting signs

TABLE 50-3

HEPATOCELLULAR CARCINOMA CLINICAL PRESENTATION (N = 547)

SYMPTOM	PATIENT # (%)
No symptom	129(24)
Abdominal pain	219(40)
Other (workup of anemia and various diseases)	64(12)
Routine physical exam finding, elevated LFTs	129(24)
Weight loss	112(20)
Appetite loss	59 (11)
Weakness/malaise	83(15)
Jaundice	30(5)
Routine CT scan screening of known cirrhosis	92(17)
Cirrhosis symptoms (ankle swelling, abdominal bloating, increased girth, pruritus, GI bleed)	98(18)
Diarrhea	7 (1)
Tumor rupture	1

Patient Characteristics

Mean age (yr)	56 ± 13
Male:Female	3:1
Ethnicity	
White	72 %
Middle Eastern	10 %
Asian	13 %
African American	5 %
Cirrhosis	81 %
No cirrhosis	19 %

Tumor Characteristics

Hepatic tumor numbers	
1	20 %
2	25 %
3 or more	65 %
Portal vein invasion	75 %
Unilobar	25 %
Bilobar	75 %

Abbreviations: GI, gastrointestinal; LFT, liver function test.

and symptoms differ somewhat between high- and low-incidence areas. In high-risk areas, especially in South African blacks, the most common symptom is abdominal pain; by contrast, only 40–50% of Chinese and Japanese patients present with abdominal pain. Abdominal swelling may occur as a consequence of ascites due to the underlying chronic liver disease or may be due to a rapidly expanding tumor. Occasionally, central necrosis or acute hemorrhage into the peritoneal cavity leads to death. In countries with an active surveillance program, HCC tends to be identified at an earlier stage, when symptoms may be due only to the underlying disease. Jaundice is usually due to obstruction of the intrahepatic ducts from underlying liver disease. Hematemesis may occur due to esophageal varices from the underlying portal hypertension. Bone pain is

seen in 3–12% of patients, but necropsies show pathologic bone metastases in ~20% of patients. However, 25% of patients may be asymptomatic.

Physical signs

Hepatomegaly is the most common physical sign, occurring in 50–90% of the patients. Abdominal bruits are noted in 6–25%, and ascites occurs in 30–60% of patients. Ascites should be examined by cytology. Splenomegaly is mainly due to portal hypertension. Weight loss and muscle wasting are common, particularly with rapidly growing or large tumors. Fever is found in 10–50% of patients, from unclear cause. The signs of chronic liver disease may often be present, including jaundice, dilated abdominal veins, palmar erythema, gynecomastia, testicular atrophy, and peripheral edema. Budd-Chiari syndrome can occur due to HCC invasion of the hepatic veins, with tense ascites and a large tender liver (Chap. 42).

Paraneoplastic syndromes

Most paraneoplastic syndromes in HCC are biochemical abnormalities without associated clinical consequences. They include hypoglycemia (also caused by end-stage liver failure), erythrocytosis, hypercalcemia, hypercholesterolemia, dysfibrinogenemia, carcinoid syndrome, increased thyroxin-binding globulin, changes in secondary sex characteristics (gynecomastia, testicular atrophy, and precocious puberty), and porphyria cutanea tarda. Mild hypoglycemia occurs in rapidly growing HCC as part of terminal illness, and profound hypoglycemia may occur, although the cause is unclear. Erythrocytosis occurs in 3–12% of patients and hypercholesterolemia in 10–40%. A high percent of patients have thrombocytopenia or leukopenia, resulting from portal hypertension, and not from cancer infiltration of bone marrow, as in other tumor types.

STAGING

Multiple clinical staging systems for HCC have been described. A widely used one has been the American Joint Commission for Cancer (AJCC)/tumor-node-metastasis (TNM) classification. However, the Cancer of the Liver Italian Program (CLIP) system is now popular as it takes the cirrhosis into account, based on the Okuda system (Table 50-4). Other staging systems have been proposed, and a consensus is needed. They are all based on combining the prognostic features of liver damage with those of tumor aggressiveness and include systems from Spain (Barcelona Clinic Liver Cancer [BCLC]), Japan, Hong Kong, and others (Chinese University Prognostic Index [CUPI], Japan Integrated Staging [JIS], and SLiDe, which stands for S,

TABLE 50-4

CLIP AND OKUDA STAGING SYSTEMS FOR HEPATOCELLULAR CARCINOMA

CLIP Classification

	POINTS		
VARIABLES	**0**	**1**	**2**
i. Tumor number	Single	Multiple	–
Hepatic replacement by tumor (%)	<50	<50	<50
ii. Child-Pugh score	A	B	C
iii. α Fetoprotein level (ng/mL)	<400	≥400	–
iv. Portal vein thrombosis (CT)	No	Yes	–

CLIP stages (score = sum of points): CLIP 0, 0 points; CLIP 1, 1 point; CLIP 2, 2 points; CLIP 3, 3 points.

Okuda Classification

TUMOR EXTENT[a]		ASCITES		ALBUMIN (g/L)		BILIRUBIN (mg/dL)	
≥50%	<50	+	(–)	≤3	>3	≥3	<3
(+)	(–)	(+)	(–)	(+)	(–)	(+)	(–)

Okuda stages: stage 1, all (–); stage 2, 1 or 2 (+); stage 3, 3 or 4 (+)

Abbreviation: CLIP, Cancer of the Liver Italian Program.
[a]Extent of liver occupied by tumor.

---

stage; Li, liver damage; De, des-γ-carboxy prothrombin). The best prognosis is for stage I, solitary tumors of less than 2-cm diameter without vascular invasion. Adverse prognostic features include ascites, jaundice, vascular invasion, and elevated α-fetoproteins (AFPs). Vascular invasion in particular has profound effects on prognosis and may be microscopic or macroscopic (visible on CT scans). Most large tumors have microscopic vascular invasion, so full staging can usually be made only after surgical resection. Stage III disease contains a mixture of lymph node–positive and –negative tumors. Stage III patients with positive lymph node disease have a poor prognosis, and few patients survive 1 year. The prognosis of stage IV is poor after either resection or transplantation and 1–year survival is rare. A working staging system based entirely on clinical grounds that incorporates the contribution of the underlying liver disease was originally developed by Okuda et al. (Table 50-4). Patients with Okuda stage III have a dire prognosis because they usually cannot be curatively resected, and the condition of their liver typically precludes chemotherapy.

New directions

Consensus is needed on staging. These systems will soon be upended by proteomics.

Hepatocellular Carcinoma

HISTORY AND PHYSICAL The history is important in evaluating putative predisposing factors, including a history of hepatitis or jaundice, blood transfusion, or use of intravenous drugs. A family history of HCC or hepatitis should be sought and a detailed social history taken to include job descriptions for industrial exposure to possible carcinogenic drugs as well as contraceptive hormones. Physical examination should include assessing stigmata of underlying liver disease such as jaundice, ascites, peripheral edema, spider nevi, palmar erythema, and weight loss. Evaluation of the abdomen for hepatic size, masses or ascites, hepatic nodularity and tenderness, and splenomegaly is needed, as is assessment of overall performance status and psychosocial evaluation.

SEROLOGIC ASSAYS AFP is a serum tumor marker for HCC; however, it is only increased in approximately one-half of U.S. patients. The lens culinaris agglutinin-reactive fraction of AFP (AFP-L3) assay is thought to be more specific. The other widely used assay is that for des-γ-carboxy prothrombin (DCP), a protein induced by vitamin K absence (PIVKA-2). This protein is increased in as many as 80% of HCC patients but may also be elevated in patients with vitamin K deficiency; it is always elevated after Coumadin use. It may predict for portal vein invasion. Both AFP-L3 and DCP are FDA-approved. Many other assays have been developed, such as glypican-3, but none have greater aggregate sensitivity and specificity. In a patient presenting with either a new hepatic mass or other indications of recent hepatic decompensation, carcinoembryonic antigen (CEA), vitamin B_{12}, AFP, ferritin, PIVKA-2, and anti-mitochondrial Ab should be measured, and standard liver function tests should be performed, including prothrombin time (PT), partial thromboplastin time (PTT), albumin, transaminases, γ-glutamyl transpeptidase, and alkaline phosphatase. Decreases in platelet count and white blood cell count may reflect portal hypertension and associated hypersplenism. Hepatitis A, B, and C serology should be measured. If HBV or HCV serology is positive, quantitative measurements of HBV DNA or HCV RNA are needed.

New Directions Newer biomarkers are being evaluated, especially tissue- and serum-based genomics profiling.

RADIOLOGY An ultrasound examination of the liver is an excellent screening tool. The two characteristic vascular abnormalities are hypervascularity of the tumor mass (neovascularization or abnormal tumor-feeding arterial vessels) and thrombosis by tumor invasion of otherwise normal portal veins. To determine tumor size and extent and the presence of portal vein invasion accurately, a helical/triphasic CT scan of the abdomen and pelvis, with fast-contrast bolus technique should be performed to detect the vascular lesions typical of HCC. Portal vein invasion is normally detected as an obstruction and expansion of the vessel. A chest CT is used to exclude metastases. MRI can also provide detailed information, especially with the newer contrast agents. Ethiodol (Lipiodol) is an ethiodized oil emulsion retained by liver tumors that can be delivered by hepatic artery injection (5–15 mL) for CT imaging 1 week later. For small tumors, Ethiodol injection is very helpful before biopsy because the histologic presence of the dye constitutes proof that the needle biopsied the mass under suspicion. A prospective comparison of triphasic CT, gadolinium-enhanced MRI, ultrasound, and fluorodeoxyglucose positron emission tomography (FDG-PET) showed similar results for CT, MRI, and ultrasound; PET imaging was unsuccessful.

New Directions The altered tumor vascularity that is a consequence of molecularly targeted therapies is the basis for newer imaging techniques including contrast-enhanced ultrasound (CEUS) and dynamic MRI.

PATHOLOGIC DIAGNOSIS Histologic proof of the presence of HCC is obtained through a core liver biopsy of the liver mass under ultrasound guidance, as well as random biopsy of the underlying liver. Bleeding risk is increased compared to other cancers because (1) the tumors are hypervascular, and (2) patients often have thrombocytopenia and decreased liver-dependent clotting factors. Bleeding risk is further increased in the presence of ascites. Tracking of tumor has an uncommon problem. Fine-needle aspirates can provide sufficient material for diagnosis of cancer, but core biopsies are preferred. Tissue architecture allows the distinction between HCC and adenocarcinoma. Laparoscopic approaches can also be used. For patients suspected of having portal vein involvement, a core biopsy of the portal vein may be performed safely. If positive, this is regarded as an exclusion criterion for transplantation for HCC.

New Directions Immunohistochemistry has become mainstream. Prognostic subgroupings are being defined based on growth signaling pathway proteins and genotyping strategies. Furthermore, molecular profiling of the underlying liver has provided evidence for a "field-effect" of cirrhosis in generating recurrent or new HCCs after primary resection.

SCREENING HIGH-RISK POPULATIONS

Screening has not been shown to save lives. Prospective studies in high-risk populations showed that ultrasound was more sensitive than AFP elevations. An Italian study in patients with cirrhosis identified a yearly HCC incidence of 3% but showed no increase in the rate of detection of potentially curable tumors with aggressive screening. Prevention strategies including universal vaccination against hepatitis are more likely to be effective than screening efforts. Despite absence of formal guidelines, most practitioners obtain 6-monthly AFP and CT (or ultrasound) when following high-risk patients (HBV carriers, HCV cirrhosis, family history of HCC).

Current directions

Cost-benefit analysis is not yet convincing, even though screening is intuitively sound. However, studies from areas of high HBV carrier rates have shown a survival benefit for screening as a result of earlier stage at diagnosis. Gamma-glutamyl transpeptidase appears useful for detecting small tumors.

TREATMENT Hepatocellular Carcinoma

Most HCC patients have two liver diseases, cirrhosis and HCC, each of which is an independent cause of death. The presence of cirrhosis usually places constraints on resection surgery, ablative therapies, and chemotherapy. Thus patient assessment and treatment planning has to take the severity of the nonmalignant liver disease into account. The clinical management choices for HCC can be complex (Fig. 50-1, Tables 50-5 and 50-6). The natural history of HCC is highly variable. Patients presenting with advanced tumors (vascular invasion, symptoms, extrahepatic spread) have a median survival of ~4 months, with or without treatment. Treatment results from the literature are difficult to interpret. Survival is not always a measure of the efficacy of therapy because of the adverse effects on survival of the underlying liver disease. A multidisciplinary team, including a hepatologist, interventional radiologist, surgical oncologist, transplant surgeon, and medical oncologist, is important for the comprehensive management of HCC patients.

STAGES I AND II HCC Early-stage tumors are successfully treated using various techniques, including surgical resection, local ablation (thermal or radiofrequency [RFA]), and local injection therapies (Table 50-6). Because the majority of patients with HCC suffer from a field defect in the cirrhotic liver, they are at risk for subsequent multiple primary liver tumors. Many will also have significant underlying liver disease and may not tolerate major surgical loss of hepatic parenchyma, and they may be eligible for orthotopic liver transplant (OLTX). Living related donor transplants have increased in popularity resulting in absence of waiting for a transplant. An important principle in treating early-stage

HEPATOCELLULAR CARCINOMA TREATMENT ALGORITHM

FIGURE 50-1

Hepatocellular carcinoma treatment algorithm. Treatment approach to patients with hepatocellular carcinoma. The initial clinical evaluation is aimed at assessing the extent of the tumor and the underlying functional compromise of the liver by cirrhosis. Patients are classified as having resectable disease, unresectable disease, or as transplantation candidates. LN, lymph node; OLTX, orthotopic liver transplantation; PEI, percutaneous ethanol injection; RFA, radiofrequency ablation; TACE, transarterial chemoembolization; UNOS, United Network for Organ Sharing. Child's A/B/C refers to the Child-Pugh classification of liver failure.

TABLE 50-5

TREATMENT OPTIONS FOR HEPATOCELLULAR CARCINOMA
Surgery
Resection
Liver transplantation
Local Ablative Therapies
Cryosurgery
Radiofrequency ablation (RFA)
Percutaneous ethanol injection (PEI)
Regional Therapies: Hepatic Artery Transcatheter Treatments
Transarterial chemotherapy
Transarterial embolization
Transarterial chemoembolization
Transarterial drug-eluting beads
Transarterial radiotherapies:
^{90}Yttrium microspheres
^{131}Iodine - Ethiodol
Conformal External-Beam Radiation
Systemic therapies
Molecularly targeted therapies (sorafenib, etc.)
Chemotherapy
Immunotherapy
Hormonal therapy + growth control
Supportive Therapies

HCC is to use liver-sparing treatments and to focus on treatment of both the tumor and the cirrhosis.

Surgical Excision The risk of major hepatectomy is high (5–10% mortality rate) due to the underlying liver disease and the potential for liver failure, but acceptable in selected cases. Preoperative portal vein occlusion can sometimes be performed to cause atrophy of the HCC-involved lobe and compensatory hypertrophy of the noninvolved liver, permitting safer resection. Intraoperative ultrasound (US) is useful for planning the surgical approach. The US can image the proximity of major vascular structures that may be encountered during the dissection. In cirrhotic patients, any major liver surgery can result in liver failure. The Child-Pugh classification of liver failure is still a reliable prognosticator for tolerance of hepatic surgery and only Child A patients should be considered for surgical resection. Child B and C patients with stages I and II HCC should be referred for OLTX if appropriate, as well as patients with ascites or a recent history of variceal bleeding. Although open surgical excision is the most reliable, the patient may be better served with a laparoscopic approach to resection, using RFA or percutaneous ethanol injection (PEI). No adequate comparisons of these different techniques have been undertaken and the choice of treatment is usually based on physician skill.

TABLE 50-6

SOME RANDOMIZED CLINICAL TRIALS INVOLVING TRANSHEPATIC ARTERY CHEMOEMBOLIZATION (TACE) FOR HEPATOCELLULAR CARCINOMA

AUTHOR	YEAR	AGENTS 1	AGENTS 2	SURVIVAL EFFECT
Kawaii	1992	Doxorubicin + Embo	Embo	No
Chang	1994	Cisplatin + Embo	Embo	No
Hatanaka	1995	Cisplatin, Doxorubicin + Embo	Same + Lipiodol	No
Uchino	1993	Cisplatin, Doxorubicin + oral FU	Same + Tamoxifen	No
Lin	1988	Embo	Embo + IV FU	No
Yoshikawa	1994	Epirubicin + Ethiodol	Epirubicin	No
Pelletier	1990	Doxorubicin + Gelfoam	None	No
Trinchet	1995	Cisplatin + Gelfoam	None	No
Bruix	1998	Coils and Gelfoam	None	No
Pelletier	1998	Cisplatin + Ethiodol	None	No
Trinchet	1995	Cisplatin + Gelfoam	None	No
Lo	2002	Cisplatin + Ethiodol	None	Yes
Llovet	2002	Doxorubicin + Ethiodol	None	Yes

Abbreviations: Embo, embolization; FU, 5-fluorouracil.

Local Ablation Strategies Radiofrequency ablation (RFA) uses heat to ablate tumors. The maximum size of the probe arrays allows for a 7-cm zone of necrosis, which would be adequate for a 3- to 4-cm tumor. The heat reliably kills cells within the zone of necrosis. Treatment of tumors close to the main portal pedicles can lead to bile duct injury and obstruction. This limits the location of tumors that are anatomically suited for this technique. RFA can be performed percutaneously with CT or ultrasound guidance, or at the time of laparoscopy with ultrasound guidance.

Local Injection Therapy Numerous agents have been used for local injection into tumors, most commonly, ethanol (PEI). The relatively soft HCC within the hard background cirrhotic liver allows for injection of large volumes of ethanol into the tumor without diffusion into the hepatic parenchyma or leakage out of the liver. PEI causes direct destruction of cancer cells, but it is not selective for cancer and will destroy normal cells in the vicinity. However, it usually requires multiple injections (average three), in contrast to one for RFA. The maximum size of tumor reliably treated is 3 cm, even with multiple injections.

Current Directions Resection and RFA each obtain similar results.

Liver Transplantation (OLTX) A viable option for stages I and II tumors in the setting of cirrhosis is OLTX, with survival approaching that for noncancer cases. OLTX for patients with a single lesion ≤5 cm or three or fewer nodules, each ≤3 cm (Milan criteria), resulted in excellent tumor-free survival (≥70% at 5 years). For advanced HCC, OLTX has been abandoned

due to high tumor recurrence rates. Priority scoring for OLTX previously led to HCC patients waiting too long for their OLTX, resulting in some tumors becoming too advanced during the patient's wait for a donated liver. A variety of therapies were used as a "bridge" to OLTX, including RFA, polyethylenimine, and transcatheter arterial chemoembolization (TACE). It seems clear that these pretransplant treatments allow patients to remain on the waiting list longer, giving them greater opportunities to be transplanted. What remains unclear, however, is whether this translates into prolonged survival after transplant. Further, it is not known whether patients who have had their tumor(s) treated preoperatively follow the recurrence pattern predicted by their tumor status at the time of transplant (i.e., post–local ablative therapy), or if they follow the course set by their tumor parameters present before such treatment. The United Network for Organ Sharing (UNOS) point system for priority scoring of OLTX recipients now includes additional points for patients with HCC. The success of living related donor liver transplantation programs has also led to patients receiving transplantation earlier for HCC and often with greater than minimal tumors.

Current Directions Expanded criteria for larger HCCs beyond the Milan criteria (one lesion <5 cm or three lesions, each <3 cm) are being increasingly accepted by various UNOS areas for OLTX with satisfactory longer-term survival. Furthermore, downstaging HCCs by medical therapy (TACE) is increasingly recognized as acceptable treatment before OLTX.

Adjuvant Therapy The role of adjuvant chemotherapy for patients after resection or OLTX remains unclear. Both adjuvant and neoadjuvant approaches have been studied, but no clear advantage in disease-free or overall survival has been found. However, a meta-analysis of several trials revealed a significant improvement in disease-free and overall survival. Although analysis of postoperative adjuvant systemic chemotherapy trials demonstrated no disease-free or overall survival advantage, single studies of TACE and neoadjuvant ^{131}I-Ethiodol showed enhanced survival post-resection.

Current Directions A large adjuvant trial examining resection with or without sorafenib (discussed later) is in progress.

STAGES III AND IV HCC Fewer surgical options exist for stage III tumors involving major vascular structures. In patients without cirrhosis, a major hepatectomy is feasible, although prognosis is poor. Patients with Child's A cirrhosis may be resected, but a lobectomy is associated with significant morbidity and mortality rates, and long-term prognosis is poor. Nevertheless, a small percentage of patients will achieve long-term survival, justifying an attempt at resection when feasible. Because of the advanced nature of these tumors, even successful resection can be followed by rapid recurrence. These patients are not considered candidates for transplantation because of the high tumor recurrence rates, unless their tumors can first be downstaged with neoadjuvant therapy. Decreasing the size of the primary tumor allows for less surgery, and the delay in surgery allows for extrahepatic disease to manifest on imaging studies and avoid unhelpful OLTX. The prognosis is poor for stage IV tumors, and no surgical treatment is recommended.

Systemic Chemotherapy A large number of controlled and uncontrolled clinical studies have been performed with most of the major classes of cancer chemotherapy. No single agent or combination of agents given systemically reproducibly leads to even a 25% response rate or has any effect on survival.

Regional Chemotherapy In contrast to the dismal results of systemic chemotherapy, a variety of agents given via the hepatic artery have activity for HCC confined to the liver (Table 50-6). Two randomized controlled trials have shown a survival advantage for TACE in a selected subset of patients. One used doxorubicin and the other used cisplatin. Despite the fact that increased hepatic extraction of chemotherapy has been shown for very few drugs, some drugs such as cisplatin, doxorubicin, mitomycin C, and possibly neocarzinostatin, produce substantial objective responses when administered regionally. Few data are available on continuous hepatic arterial infusion for HCC, although

pilot studies with cisplatin have shown encouraging responses. Because the reports have not usually stratified responses or survival based on TNM staging, it is difficult to know long-term prognosis in relation to tumor extent. Most of the studies on regional hepatic arterial chemotherapy also use an embolizing agent such as Ethiodol, gelatin sponge particles (Gelfoam), starch (Spherex), or microspheres. Two products are composed of microspheres of defined size ranges—Embospheres (Biospheres) and Contour SE—using particles of 40–120, 100–300, 300–500, and 500–1000 μm in size. The optimal diameter of the particles for TACE has yet to be defined. Consistently higher objective response rates are reported for arterial administration of drugs together with some form of hepatic artery occlusion compared with any form of systemic chemotherapy to date. The widespread use of some form of embolization in addition to chemotherapy has added to its toxicities. These include a frequent, but transient fever, abdominal pain, and anorexia (all in >60% of patients). In addition, >20% of patients have increased ascites or transient elevation of transaminases. Cystic artery spasm and cholecystitis are also not uncommon. However, higher responses have also been obtained. The hepatic toxicities associated with embolization may be ameliorated by the use of degradable starch microspheres, with 50–60% response rates. Two randomized studies of TACE vs. placebo showed a survival advantage for treatment (Table 50-6). In addition, it is not clear that formal oncologic CT response criteria are adequate for HCC. A loss of vascularity on CT without size change may be an index of loss of viability and thus of response to TACE. A major problem that TACE trials have had in showing a survival advantage is that many HCC patients die of their underlying cirrhosis, not the tumor. However, improving quality of life is a legitimate goal of regional therapy.

New Therapies The major finding has been a survival advantage for oral sorafenib (Nexavar) vs. placebo controls in two randomized trials, leading to its approval by the FDA. However, tumor responses were negligible, and the survival in the treatment arm in Asians was below the placebo arm in the Western trial (Table 50-7). Furthermore, prolonged survival has been reported in phase II trials using newer agents, such as bevacizumab plus erlotinib. Several forms of *radiation therapy* have been used in the treatment of HCC, including external beam radiation and conformal radiation therapy. Radiation hepatitis remains a dose-limiting problem. The pure beta emitter [90]Yttrium attached to either glass or resin microspheres has been assessed in phase II trials of HCC and has encouraging survival effects with minimal toxicities. Randomized trials have yet to be performed. Vitamin K has been assessed in clinical trials at high

TABLE 50-7

TARGETED THERAPIES IN HCC: TRIALS

PHASE III	TARGET	SURVIVAL (mo)
Sorafenib vs placebo	Raf, VEGFR, PDGFR	10.7 vs. 7.9
Sorafenib vs placebo (Asians)	Raf, WGFR, PDGFR	6.5 vs. 4.2
Phase II		
Sorafenib		9
Sorafenib (Asians)		5
Sunitinib		9.8, 8 (2 trials)
Bevacizumab	VEGF	12.4
Bevacizumab plus erlotinib	VEGF plus EGFR	15.6
Bevacizumab plus capecitabine		8
Erlotinib	EGFR	13, 10.7 (2 trials)
Linifanib	VEGFR, PDGF	9.7
Brivanib	VEGFR, FGFR	10

Abbreviations: EGFR, epidermal growth factor receptor; FGFR, fibroblast growth factor receptor; PDGF, platelet-derived growth factor; PDGFR, platelet-derived growth factor receptor; Raf, rapidly accelerated fibrosarcoma; VEGF, vascular endothelial growth factor; VEGFR, vascular endothelial growth factor receptor.

dosage for its HCC-inhibitory actions. This idea is based on the characteristic biochemical defect in HCC of elevated plasma levels of immature prothrombin (DCP or PIVKA-2), due to a defect in the activity of prothrombin carboxylase, a vitamin K-dependent enzyme. Two vitamin K randomized controlled trials from Japan show decreased tumor occurrence.

Current Directions A number of new treatments are being evaluated for HCC (Table 50-8). These include the biologicals, such as Raf kinase and vascular endothelial growth factor (VEGF) inhibitors; ^{90}Yttrium looks promising without chemotherapy toxicities, and vitamin K_2 appears to prevent recurrences post-resection. The bottleneck of liver donors for OLTX is at last widening with increasing use of living donors, and criteria for OLTX for larger HCCs are slowly expanding. Patient participation in clinical trials assessing new therapies is encouraged (*www.clinicaltrials.gov*).

SUMMARY (TABLE 50-5)

The most common modes of patient presentation

1. A patient with known history of hepatitis, jaundice, or cirrhosis, with an abnormality on US or CT scan, or rising AFP or DCP (PIVKA-2)
2. A patient with an abnormal liver function test as part of a routine examination

TABLE 50-8

SOME NOVEL MEDICAL TREATMENTS FOR HEPATOCELLULAR CARCINOMA

EGF receptor antagonists: erlotinib, gefitinib, lapatinib, cetuximab, brivanib
Multikinase antagonists: sorafenib, sunitinib
VEGF antagonist: bevacizumab
VEGFR antagonist: ABT-869 (linifanib)
mTOR antagonists: sirolimus, temsirolimus, everolimus
Proteasome inhibitors: bortezomib
Vitamin K
^{131}I – Ethiodol (lipiodol)
^{131}I – Ferritin
^{90}Yttrium microspheres (TheraSphere, SIR-spheres)
^{166}Holmium, ^{188}Rhenium
Three-dimensional conformal radiation
Proton beam high-dose radiotherapy
Gamma knife, CyberKnife
New targets: inhibitors of cyclin dependent kinases (Cdk) and caspases

Abbreviations: EGF, epidermal growth factor; VEGF, vascular endothelial growth factor; VEGFR vascular endothelial growth factor receptor.

3. Radiologic workup for liver transplant for cirrhosis
4. Symptoms of HCC including cachexia, abdominal pain, or fever

History and physical examination

1. Clinical jaundice, asthenia, itching (scratches), tremors, or disorientation
2. Hepatomegaly, splenomegaly, ascites, peripheral edema, skin signs of liver failure

Clinical evaluation

1. Blood tests: full blood count (splenomegaly), liver function tests, ammonia levels, electrolytes, AFP and DCP (PIVKA-2), Ca^{2+} and Mg^{2+}; hepatitis B, C, and D serology (and quantitative HBV DNA or HCV RNA, if either is positive); neurotensin (specific for fibrolamellar HCC)
2. Triphasic dynamic helical (spiral) CT scan of liver (if inadequate, then follow with an MRI); chest CT scan; upper and lower gastrointestinal endoscopy (for varices, bleeding, ulcers); and brain scan (only if symptoms suggest)
3. Core biopsy: of the tumor and separate biopsy of the underlying liver

Therapy (Tables 50-5 and 50-6)

1. HCC <2 cm: RFA, PEI, or resection
2. HCC >2 cm, no vascular invasion: liver resection, RFA, or OLTX

3. Multiple unilobar tumors or tumor with vascular invasion: TACE or sorafenib
4. Bilobar tumors, no vascular invasion: TACE with OLTX for patients with tumor response
5. Extrahepatic HCC or elevated bilirubin: sorafenib or bevacizumab plus erlotinib (combination agent trials are in progress)

OTHER PRIMARY LIVER TUMORS

FIBROLAMELLAR HCC (FL-HCC)

This rarer variant of HCC has a quite different biology than adult-type HCC. None of the known HCC causative factors seem important here. It is typically a disease of younger adults, often teenagers and predominantly females. It is AFP-negative, but patients typically have elevated blood neurotensin levels, normal liver function tests, and no cirrhosis. Radiology is similar for HCC, except that characteristic adult-type portal vein invasion is less common. Although it is often multifocal in the liver, and therefore not resectable, metastases are common, especially to lungs and locoregional lymph nodes, but survival is often much better than with adult-type HCC. Resectable tumors are associated with 5-year survival ≥50%. Patients often present with a huge liver or unexplained weight loss, fever, or elevated liver function tests on routine evaluations. These huge masses suggest quite slow growth for many tumors. Surgical resection is the best management option, even for metastases, as these tumors respond much less well to chemotherapy than adult-type HCC. Although several series of OLTX for FL-HCC have been reported, the patients seem to die from tumor recurrences, with a 2- to 5-year lag compared with OLTX for adult-type HCC. Anecdotal responses to gemcitabine plus cisplatin-TACE are reported.

EPITHELIOID HEMANGIOENDOTHELIOMA (EHE)

This rare vascular tumor of adults is also usually multifocal and can also be associated with prolonged survival, even in the presence of metastases, which are commonly in the lung. There is usually no underlying cirrhosis. Histologically, these tumors are usually of borderline malignancy and express factor VIII, confirming their endothelial origin. OLTX may produce prolonged survival.

CHOLANGIOCARCINOMA (CCC)

CCC typically refers to mucin-producing adenocarcinomas (different from HCC) that arise from the bile ducts. They are grouped by their anatomic site of origin, as intrahepatic, hilar (central, ~65% of CCCs), and peripheral (or distal, ~30% of CCCs). They arise on the basis of cirrhosis less frequently than HCC, excepting primary biliary cirrhosis. Nodular tumors arising at the bifurcation of the common bile duct are called *Klatskin* tumors and are often associated with a collapsed gallbladder, a finding that mandates visualization of the entire biliary tree. The approach to management of central and peripheral CCC is quite different. Incidence is increasing. Although most CCCs have no obvious cause, a number of predisposing factors have been identified. Predisposing diseases include primary sclerosing cholangitis (10–20% of primary sclerosing cholangitis [PSC] patients), an autoimmune disease, and liver fluke in Asians, especially *Opisthorchis viverrini* and *Clonorchis sinensis*. CCC seems also to be associated with any cause of chronic biliary inflammation and injury, with alcoholic liver disease, choledocholithiasis, choledochal cysts (10%), and Caroli's disease (a rare inherited form of bile duct ectasia). CCC most typically presents as painless jaundice, often with pruritus or weight loss. Diagnosis is made by biopsy, percutaneously for peripheral liver lesions, or more commonly via endoscopic retrograde cholangiopancreatography (ERCP) under direct vision for central lesions. The tumors often stain positively for cytokeratins 7, 8, and 19 and negatively for cytokeratin 20. However, histology alone cannot usually distinguish CCC from metastases from colon or pancreas primary tumors. Serologic tumor markers appear to be nonspecific, but CEA, CA 19–9, and CA-125 are often elevated in CCC patients and are useful for following response to therapy. Radiologic evaluation typically starts with ultrasound, which is very useful in visualizing dilated bile ducts, and then proceeds with either MRI or magnetic resonance cholangiopancreatography (MRCP) or helical CT scans. Invasive cholangiopancreatography (ERCP) is then needed to define the biliary tree and obtain a biopsy or is needed therapeutically to decompress an obstructed biliary tree with internal stent placement. If that fails, then percutaneous biliary drainage will be needed, with the biliary drainage flowing into an external bag. Central tumors often invade the porta hepatis, and locoregional lymph node involvement by tumor is frequent.

TREATMENT   Cholangiocarcinoma

Hilar CCC is resectable in ~30% of patients and usually involves bile duct resection and lymphadenectomy. Typical survival is approximately 24 months, with recurrences being mainly in the operative bed but with ~30% in the lungs and liver. Distal CCC, which involves the main ducts, is normally treated by resection of the extrahepatic bile ducts, often with pancreaticoduodenectomy.

Survival is similar. Due to the high rates of locoregional recurrences or positive surgical margins, many patients receive postoperative adjuvant radiotherapy. Its effect on survival has not been assessed. Intraluminal brachyradiotherapy has also shown some promise. However, photodynamic therapy enhanced survival in one study. In this technique, sodium porfimer is injected intravenously and then subjected to intraluminal red light laser photoactivation. OLTX has been assessed for treatment of unresectable CCC. Five-year survival was ~20%, so enthusiasm waned. However, neoadjuvant radiotherapy with sensitizing chemotherapy has shown better survival rates for CCC treated by OLTX and is currently used by UNOS for perihilar CCC, size <3 cm with neither intrahepatic or extrahepatic metastases. Multiple chemotherapeutic agents have been assessed for activity and survival in unresectable CCC. Most have been inactive. However, both systemic and hepatic arterial gemcitabine have shown promising results. The combination of cisplatin plus gemcitabine has produced a survival advantage compared with gemcitabine alone and is considered standard therapy for unresectable CCC.

GALLBLADDER CANCER (GB Ca)

GB Ca has an even worse prognosis than CCC, and with typical survival ~6 months or less. Women are affected much more commonly than men (4:1), unlike HCC or CCC, and GB Ca occurs more frequently than CCC. Most patients have a history of antecedent gallstones, but very few patients with gallstones develop GB Ca (~0.2%). It presents similarly to CCC and is often diagnosed unexpectedly during gallstone or cholecystitis surgery. Presentation is typically that of chronic cholecystitis, chronic right upper quadrant pain and weight loss. Useful but nonspecific serum markers include CEA and CA 19-9. CT scans or MRCP typically reveal a gallbladder mass. The mainstay of treatment is surgical, either simple or radical cholecystectomy for stages I or II disease, respectively. Survival rates are near 100% at 5 years for stage I, and range from 60–90% at 5 years for stage II. More advanced GB Ca has worse survival, and many patients are unresectable. Adjuvant radiotherapy, used in the presence of local lymph node disease, has not been shown to enhance survival. Chemotherapy is not useful in advanced or metastatic GB Ca.

CARCINOMA OF THE AMPULLA OF VATER

This tumor arises within 2 cm of the distal end of the common bile duct and is mainly (90%) an adenocarcinoma. Locoregional lymph nodes are commonly involved (50%), and the liver is the most frequent site for metastases. The most common clinical presentation is jaundice, and many patients also have pruritus, weight loss, and epigastric pain. Initial evaluation is performed with an abdominal ultrasound to assess vascular involvement, biliary dilation, and liver lesions. This is followed by a CT scan, or MRI and especially MRCP. The most effective therapy is resection by pylorus-sparing pancreaticoduodenectomy, an aggressive procedure resulting in better survival rates than with local resection. Survival rates are ~25% at 5 years in operable patients with involved lymph nodes and ~50% in patients without involved nodes. Unlike CCC, approximately 80% of patients are thought to be resectable at diagnosis. Adjuvant chemotherapy or radiotherapy has not been shown to enhance survival. For metastatic tumors, chemotherapy is currently experimental.

TUMORS METASTATIC TO THE LIVER

These are predominantly from colon, pancreas, and breast primary tumors but can originate from any organ primary. Ocular melanomas are prone to liver metastasis. Tumor spread to the liver normally carries a poor prognosis for that tumor type. Colorectal and breast hepatic metastases were previously treated with continuous hepatic arterial infusion chemotherapy. However, more effective systemic drugs for each of these two cancers, especially the addition of oxaliplatin to colorectal cancer regimens, have reduced the use of hepatic artery infusion therapy. In a large randomized study of systemic versus infusional plus systemic chemotherapy for resected colorectal metastases to the liver, the patients receiving infusional therapy had no survival advantage, mainly due to extrahepatic tumor spread. [90]Yttrium resin beads are approved in the United States for treatment of colorectal hepatic metastases. The role of this modality, either alone or in combination with chemotherapy, is being evaluated in many centers. Palliation my be obtained from chemoembolization, PEI, or RFA.

BENIGN LIVER TUMORS

Three common benign tumors occur and all are found predominantly in women. They are *hemangiomas, adenomas,* and *focal nodular hyperplasia* (FNH). FNH is typically benign, and usually no treatment is needed. Hemangiomas are the most common and are entirely benign. Treatment is unnecessary unless their expansion causes symptoms. Adenomas are associated with contraceptive hormone use. They can cause pain and can bleed or rupture, causing acute problems. Their main interest for the physician is a low potential for malignant change and a 30% risk of bleeding. For this reason, considerable effort has gone into differentiating these three entities radiologically. On discovery of a liver mass, patients are usually advised to stop taking sex steroids, as adenoma regression may then occasionally occur. Adenomas can often be large masses ranging from 8–15 cm. Due to their size and definite, but low, malignant potential and potential for bleeding, adenomas are typically resected. The most useful diagnostic differentiating tool is a triphasic CT scan performed with HCC fast bolus protocol for arterial-phase imaging, together with subsequent delayed venous-phase imaging. Adenomas usually do not appear on the basis

of cirrhosis, although both adenomas and HCCs are intensely vascular on the CT arterial phase and both can exhibit hemorrhage (40% of adenomas). However, adenomas have smooth, well-defined edges, and enhance homogeneously, especially in the portal venous phase on delayed images, when HCCs no longer enhance. FNHs exhibit a characteristic central scar that is hypovascular on the arterial-phase and hypervascular on the delayed-phase CT images. MRI is even more sensitive in depicting the characteristic central scar of FNH.

CHAPTER 51

PANCREATIC CANCER

Irene Chong ■ David Cunningham

Pancreatic cancer is the fourth leading cause of cancer death in the United States and is associated with a poor prognosis. Endocrine tumors affecting the pancreas are discussed in Chap. 52. Infiltrating ductal adenocarcinomas, the subject of this chapter, account for the vast majority of cases and arise most frequently in the head of pancreas. At the time of diagnosis 85–90% of patients have inoperable or metastatic disease, which is reflected in the 5-year survival rate of only 5% for all stages combined. An improved 5-year survival of up to 20% may be achieved when the tumor is detected at an early stage and when complete surgical resection is accomplished.

EPIDEMIOLOGY

Pancreatic cancer represents 3% of all newly diagnosed malignancies in the United States. The most common age group at diagnosis is 60–79 years for both sexes. Pancreatic cancer will be diagnosed in approximately 43,140 patients and account for 36,800 deaths in 2010. Over the past 30 years, 5-year survival rates have not improved substantially.

RISK FACTORS

Cigarette smoking may be the cause of up to 20–25% of all pancreatic cancers and is the most common environmental risk factor for this disease. Other risk factors are not well established due to inconsistent results from epidemiological studies, but include chronic pancreatitis and diabetes. It is difficult to evaluate whether these conditions are causally related, or develop as a consequence of cancer. Alcohol does not appear to be a risk factor unless excess consumption gives rise to chronic pancreatitis.

GENETIC CONSIDERATIONS

Pancreatic cancer is associated with a number of well-defined molecular hallmarks. The most frequent genetic aberrations comprise *KRAS* mutations, mostly affecting codon 12, which are observed in 60–75% of pancreatic cancers. The tumor-suppressor genes *p16, p53,* and *SMAD4* are frequently inactivated; the *p16* gene locus on chromosome 9p21 is deleted in up to 95% of tumors, the *p53* gene is inactivated by mutation or deleted in 50–70% of tumors, and the *SMAD4* gene is deleted in 55% of pancreatic tumors. Furthermore, *SMAD4* gene inactivation is associated with poorer survival in patients with surgically resected pancreatic adenocarcinoma.

IGF-1R and focal adhesion kinase (*FAK*) interact to promote cell proliferation and survival, and their simultaneous inhibition synergistically inhibits pancreatic cell growth. Overexpression and/or aberrant activation of *c-Src* is frequently observed, which results in cell adhesion, enhanced migration, invasion, and cell proliferation. Survivin is overexpressed in more than 80% of pancreatic tumors, which results in resistance to apoptosis, and genomic sequencing has identified *PALB2* as a susceptibility gene for pancreatic cancer.

Up to 16% of pancreatic cancers are thought to be inherited. This occurs in three separate clinical settings: (1) familial multi-organ cancer syndromes, (2) genetically driven chronic diseases, and (3) familial pancreatic cancer with as yet unidentified genetic abnormalities, which comprise the largest proportion of inherited pancreatic cancer. The familial multi-organ cancer syndromes consist of Peutz-Jeghers syndrome, familial atypical multiple mole melanoma (FAMMM), familial breast-ovarian cancer associated with germ-line mutations in *BRCA1* and *BRCA2*, hereditary nonpolyposis colorectal cancer (HNPCC), familial adenomatous polyposis (FAP), and Li-Fraumeni syndrome. Peutz-Jeghers, associated with mutations in the *STK11* gene, carries the highest lifetime risk of pancreatic cancer with a relative risk of approximately 132-fold above that of the general population. Genetically driven chronic causes of pancreatic cancer include hereditary pancreatitis, cystic fibrosis, and ataxia telangiectasia. The absolute number of affected first-degree relatives is also correlated with increased cancer risk, and patients with at least two first-degree relatives with pancreatic cancer should be considered to have familial pancreatic cancer until proven otherwise.

SCREENING AND EARLY DETECTION

Screening is not routinely recommended as putative tumor markers such as Ca 19-9 and CEA have insufficient sensitivity, and computed tomography (CT) has inadequate resolution to detect pancreatic dysplasia. Endoscopic ultrasound (EUS) is a more promising screening tool, and preclinical efforts are focused on identifying biomarkers that may detect pancreatic cancer at an early stage. Consensus practice recommendations based largely on expert opinion have chosen a threshold of >tenfold increased risk for developing pancreatic cancer to select individuals who may benefit from screening. This includes family members with ≥3 first-degree relatives with pancreatic cancer, and patients with FAMMM, Peutz-Jeghers syndrome, or hereditary pancreatitis.

CLINICAL FEATURES

CLINICAL PRESENTATION

Obstructive jaundice occurs frequently when the cancer is located in the head of pancreas. This may be accompanied by symptoms of abdominal discomfort, pruritus, lethargy, and weight loss. Less common presenting features include epigastric pain, backache, new-onset diabetes mellitus, and acute pancreatitis caused by pressure effects on the pancreatic duct. Nausea and vomiting, resulting from gastroduodenal obstruction, may also be a symptom of this disease.

PHYSICAL SIGNS

Patients can present with jaundice and cachexia, and scratch marks may be present. Of patients with operable tumors 25% have a palpable gallbladder (Courvoisier's sign). Physical signs related to the development of distant metastases include hepatomegaly, ascites, left supraclavicular lymphadenopathy (Virchow's node), and periumbilical lymphadenopathy (Sister Mary Joseph's nodes).

DIAGNOSIS

DIAGNOSTIC IMAGING

Patients who present with clinical features suggestive of pancreatic cancer undergo imaging to confirm the

FIGURE 51-1
Coronal CT showing pancreatic cancer and dilated intrahepatic and pancreatic ducts (*arrows*).

presence of a tumor, and to establish whether the mass is likely to be inflammatory or malignant in nature. Other imaging objectives include the local and distant staging of the tumor, which will determine resectability and provide prognostic information. Dual phase, contrast-enhanced spiral CT is the imaging modality of choice **(Fig. 51-1)**. It provides accurate visualization of surrounding viscera, vessels, and lymph nodes, thus determining tumor resectability. Intestinal infiltration, and liver and lung metastases are also reliably depicted on CT. There is no advantage of magnetic resonance imaging (MRI) over CT in predicting tumor resectability, but selected cases may benefit from MRI to characterize the nature of small indeterminate liver lesions and to evaluate the cause of biliary dilatation when no obvious mass is seen on CT. Endoscopic retrograde cholangiopancreatography (ERCP) is useful for revealing small pancreatic lesions, identifying stricture or obstruction in pancreatic or common bile ducts, and facilitating stent placement **(Fig. 51-2)**. Magnetic resonance

FIGURE 51-2
ERCP showing contrast in dilated pancreatic duct (*arrows*).

cholangiopancreatography (MRCP) is a noninvasive method for accurately depicting the level and degree of bile and pancreatic duct dilatation. EUS is highly sensitive in detecting lesions less than 3 cm in size, and is useful as a local staging tool for assessing vascular invasion and lymph node involvement. Fluorodeoxyglucose positron emission tomography (FDG-PET) should be considered before surgery or radical chemoradiotherapy (CRT), as it is superior to conventional imaging in detecting distant metastases.

TISSUE DIAGNOSIS AND CYTOLOGY

Preoperative confirmation of malignancy is not always necessary in patients with radiological appearances consistent with operable pancreatic cancer. However, EUS-guided fine-needle aspiration is the technique of choice when there is any doubt, and also for use in patients who require neoadjuvant treatment. It has an accuracy of approximately 90% and has a smaller risk of intraperitoneal dissemination compared with the percutaneous route. Percutaneous biopsy of the pancreatic primary or liver metastases is only acceptable in patients with inoperable or metastatic disease. ERCP is a useful method for obtaining ductal brushings, but the diagnostic value of pancreatic juice sampling is only in the order of 25–30%.

SERUM MARKERS

Tumor-associated carbohydrate antigen 19-9 (CA 19-9) is elevated in approximately 70–80% of patients with pancreatic carcinoma, but is not recommended as a routine diagnostic or screening test as its sensitivity and specificity are inadequate for accurate diagnosis. Preoperative CA 19-9 levels correlate with tumor stage, and postresection CA 19-9 level has prognostic value. It is an indicator of asymptomatic recurrence in patients with completely resected tumors and is used as a biomarker of response in patients with advanced disease undergoing chemotherapy. A number of studies have established a high pretreatment CA 19-9 level as an independent prognostic factor.

STAGING

The American Joint Committee on Cancer (AJCC) tumor–node–metastasis (TNM) staging of pancreatic cancer takes into account the location and size of the tumor, the involvement of lymph nodes, and distant metastasis. This information is then combined to assign a stage (Fig. 51-3). From a practical standpoint, patients are grouped according to whether the cancer is resectable, locally advanced (unresectable, but without distant spread), or metastatic.

TREATMENT ▶ Pancreatic Cancer

RESECTABLE DISEASE Approximately 10% of patients present with localized nonmetastatic disease that is potentially suitable for surgical resection. Approximately 30% of patients have R1 resection (microscopic residual disease) following surgery. Those who undergo R0 resection (no microscopic or macroscopic residual tumor), and who receive adjuvant treatment have the best chance of cure, with an estimated median survival of 20–23 months and a 5-year survival of approximately 20%. Outcomes are more favorable in patients with small (<3 cm), well-differentiated tumors, and lymph node-negative disease.

Patients should have surgery in dedicated pancreatic centers that have lower postoperative morbidity and mortality rates. The standard surgical procedure for patients with tumors of the pancreatic head or uncinate process is a pylorus-preserving pancreaticoduodenectomy (modified Whipple's procedure). The procedure of choice for tumors of the pancreatic body and tail is a distal pancreatectomy, which routinely includes splenectomy.

Postoperative treatment, either chemotherapy or CRT, improves long-term outcomes in this group of patients. Adjuvant chemotherapy, comprising six cycles of fluorouracil (5FU) and folinic acid (FA) or gemcitabine, is common practice in Europe based on data from three randomized controlled trials (Table 51-1): Results from the European Study Group for Pancreatic Cancer 1 trial (ESPAC-1) revealed a median survival improvement from 14.7 months with surgery alone to 20.1 months with surgery plus adjuvant 5FU/FA, and patients did not benefit from CRT in this study. The Charité Onkologie trial (CONKO 001) found that the use of gemcitabine after complete resection significantly delayed the development of recurrent disease compared with surgery alone. The ESPAC-3 trial, which investigated the benefit of adjuvant 5FU/FA versus gemcitabine, revealed no survival difference between the two drugs. However, the safety profile of adjuvant gemcitabine, with respect to the incidence of stomatitis and diarrhea, was superior to 5FU/FA.

A different treatment strategy using adjuvant 5FU based CRT following gemcitabine as advocated by the Radiation Therapy Oncology Group (RTOG) 97-04 trial is preferred in the United States. This approach may be most beneficial in patients with bulky tumors involving the pancreatic head and in patients with R1 resection.

INOPERABLE LOCALLY ADVANCED DISEASE Approximately 30% of patients present with locally advanced unresectable but nonmetastatic pancreatic carcinoma. The median survival with gemcitabine is 9 months, and patients who respond to or achieve

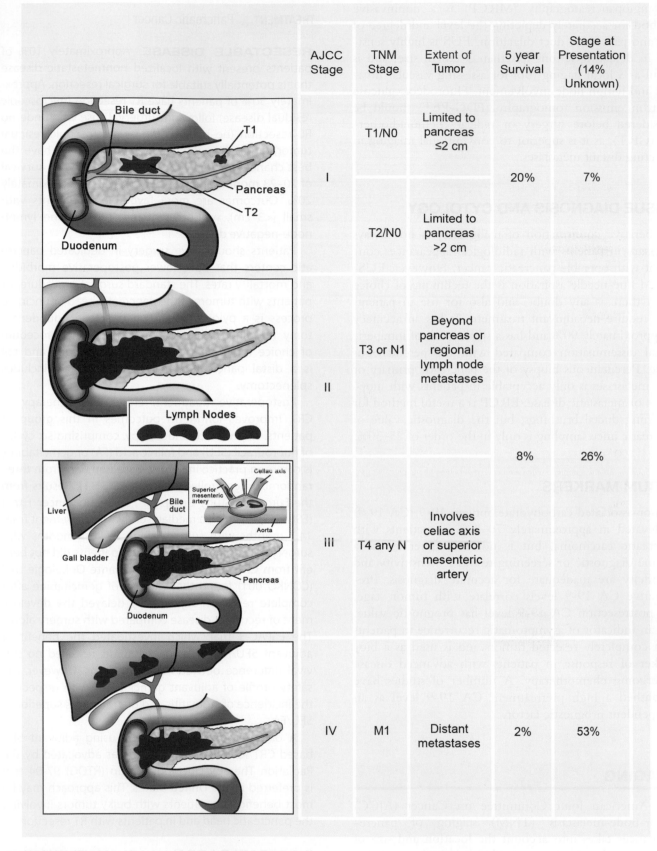

AJCC Stage	TNM Stage	Extent of Tumor	5 year Survival	Stage at Presentation (14% Unknown)
I	T1/N0	Limited to pancreas ≤2 cm	20%	7%
	T2/N0	Limited to pancreas >2 cm		
II	T3 or N1	Beyond pancreas or regional lymph node metastases	8%	26%
III	T4 any N	Involves celiac axis or superior mesenteric artery		
IV	M1	Distant metastases	2%	53%

FIGURE 51-3

Staging of pancreatic cancer, and survival according to stage. (*Illustration by Stephen Millward.*)

TABLE 51-1

PHASE III STUDIES OF ADJUVANT CHEMOTHERAPY IN RESECTED PANCREATIC CANCER

STUDY	COMPARATOR ARM	PATIENT NUMBER	SURVIVAL	
			PFS/DFS (MONTHS)	MEDIAN SURVIVAL (MONTHS)
ESPAC 1 Neoptolemos et al. (2004)	Chemotherapy (Folinic acid + bolus 5FU) vs No chemotherapy	550	PFS 15.3 vs 9.4. ($p = 0.02$)	20.1 vs 14.7 (HR 0.71, 95% CI 0.55 to 0.92, $p = 0.009$)
CONKO 001 Oettle et al. (2007)	Gemcitabine vs Observation	368	Median DFS 13.4 vs 6.9 ($p < 0.001$)	22.1 vs 20.2 ($p = 0.06$)
ESPAC 3 Neoptolemos et al. (2010)	5FU/LV vs Gemcitabine	1088		23 vs 23.6 (HR 0.94, 95% CI 0.81 to 1.08, $p = 0.39$)

Abbreviations: CI, confidence interval; CONKO, Charite ONKOlogie; DFS, disease-free survival; ESPAC, European Study Group for Pancreatic Cancer; 5FU, fluorouracil; HR, hazard ratio; LV, leucovorin; PFS, progression-free survival.

TABLE 51-2

SELECTED PHASE III STUDIES EVALUATING CHEMOTHERAPY TREATMENT IN ADVANCED PANCREATIC CANCER

STUDY	COMPARATOR ARM	PATIENT NUMBER	SURVIVAL	
			PFS (MONTHS)	MEDIAN SURVIVAL (MONTHS)
Moore M et al. (2007)	Gemcitabine vs Gemcitabine + erlotinib	569	3.55 vs 3.75 (HR 0.77, 95% CI 0.64 to 0.92, $p = 0.004$)	5.91 vs 6.24 (HR 0.82, 95% CI 0.69 to 0.99, $p = 0.038$)
GEM-CAP Cunningham et al. (2009)	Gemcitabine vs Gemcitabine + capecitabine (GEM-CAP)	533	3.8 vs 5.3 (HR 0.78, 95% CI 0.66 to 0.93, $p = 0.004$)	6.2 vs 7.1 (HR 0.86, 95% CI 0.72 to 1.02, $p = 0.08$)
GEM-CAP meta-analysis Cunningham et al. (2009)	Gemcitabine vs GEM-CAP	935		Overall survival in favor of GEM-CAP (HR 0.86, 95% CI 0.75 to 0.98, $p = 0.02$)

stable disease after 3–6 months of gemcitabine may derive benefit from consolidation radiotherapy.

METASTATIC DISEASE Approximately 60% of patients with pancreatic cancer present with metastatic disease. Patients with poor performance status do not benefit from chemotherapy. Gemcitabine is the standard treatment with a median survival of 6 months and a 1-year survival rate of only 20%. The toxicities associated with gemcitabine need to be weighed against the potential benefits of treatment.

Adding other drugs to gemcitabine to improve outcome has been generally unsuccessful with the exception of erlotinib, an oral HER1/EGFR tyrosine kinase inhibitor. The combination of erlotinib with gemcitabine resulted in an improved 1-year survival compared with gemcitabine alone (23% versus 17%, $p = 0.023$) (Table 51-2). Capecitabine, an oral fluoropyrimidine, has been combined with gemcitabine (GEM-CAP) in a phase III trial that showed an improvement in response rate and progression-free survival over single-agent gemcitabine, but no survival benefit. However, pooling of two other randomized controlled trials with this trial in a meta-analysis resulted in a survival advantage with GEM-CAP.

A trial in good performance status patients with metastatic pancreatic cancer showed improved survival with the combination of 5FU/FA, irinotecan and oxaliplatin (FOLFIRINOX) compared with gemcitabine, but with increased toxicity. Nab-paclitaxel (Abraxane), an albumin bound nano-particle formulation of paclitaxel, given with gemcitabine also shows promising activity.

FUTURE DIRECTIONS

The early detection and future treatment of pancreatic cancer relies on an improved understanding of molecular pathways involved in the development of this disease. This will ultimately lead to the discovery of novel agents, and the identification of patient groups who are likely to benefit most from targeted therapy.

CHAPTER 52

ENDOCRINE TUMORS OF THE GASTROINTESTINAL TRACT AND PANCREAS

Robert T. Jensen

GENERAL FEATURES OF GASTROINTESTINAL (GI) NEUROENDOCRINE TUMORS

Gastrointestinal neuroendocrine tumors (NETs) are tumors derived from the diffuse neuroendocrine system of the GI tract; that system is composed of amine- and acid-producing cells with different hormonal profiles, depending on the site of origin. The tumors historically are divided into carcinoid tumors and pancreatic endocrine tumors (PETs), although recent pathologic classifications have proposed that they all be classified as gastrointestinal NETs. In this chapter the term *carcinoid tumor* is retained because it is widely used. These tumors originally were classified as APUDomas (for *amine precursor uptake and decarboxylation*), as were pheochromocytomas, melanomas, and medullary thyroid carcinomas, because they share certain cytochemical features as well as various pathologic, biologic, and molecular features **(Table 52-1)**. It was originally proposed that APUDomas had a similar embryonic origin from neural crest cells, but it is now known the peptide-secreting cells are not of neuroectodermal origin. Nevertheless, the concept of APUDomas is useful because the tumors from the cells have important similarities as well as some differences (Table 52-1). In this section, the areas of similarity between PETs and carcinoids will be discussed together and areas in which there are important differences will be discussed separately.

CLASSIFICATION/PATHOLOGY/TUMOR BIOLOGY OF NETS

NETs generally are composed of monotonous sheets of small round cells with uniform nuclei, and mitoses are uncommon. They can be identified tentatively on routine histology; however, these tumors are now recognized principally by their histologic staining patterns due to shared cellular proteins. Historically, silver staining was used, and tumors were classified as showing an argentaffin reaction if they took up and reduced silver or as being argyrophilic if they did not reduce it. More recently immunocytochemical localization of chromogranins (A, B, C), neuron-specific enolase, and synaptophysin, which are all neuroendocrine cell markers, is used (Table 52-1). Chromogranin A is currently the most widely used.

Ultrastructurally, these tumors possess electron-dense neurosecretory granules and frequently contain small clear vesicles that correspond to synaptic vesicles of neurons. NETs synthesize numerous peptides, growth factors, and bioactive amines that may be ectopically secreted, giving rise to a specific clinical syndrome **(Table 52-2)**. The diagnosis of the specific syndrome requires the clinical features of the disease (Table 52-2) and cannot be made from the immunocytochemistry results alone. The presence or absence of a specific clinical syndrome also cannot be predicted from the immunocytochemistry alone (Table 52-1). Furthermore, pathologists cannot distinguish between benign and malignant NETs unless metastases or invasion is present.

Carcinoid tumors frequently are classified according to their anatomic area of origin (i.e., foregut, midgut, hindgut) because tumors with similar areas of origin share functional manifestations, histochemistry, and secretory products **(Table 52-3)**. Foregut tumors generally have a low serotonin (5-HT) content; are argentaffin-negative but argyrophilic; occasionally secrete adrenocorticotropic hormone (ACTH) or 5-hydroxytryptophan (5-HTP), causing an atypical carcinoid syndrome **(Fig. 52-1)**; are often multihormonal; and may metastasize to bone. They uncommonly produce a clinical syndrome due to the secreted products.

TABLE 52-1

GENERAL CHARACTERISTICS OF GASTROINTESTINAL NEUROENDOCRINE TUMORS (CARCINOIDS, PANCREATIC ENDOCRINE TUMORS [PETS])

A. Share general neuroendocrine cell markers (identification used for diagnosis)
   1. Chromogranins (A, B, C) are acidic monomeric soluble proteins found in the large secretory granules. Chromogranin A is the most widely used.
   2. Neuron-specific enolase (NSE) is the γ-γ dimer of the enzyme enolase and is a cytosolic marker of neuroendocrine differentiation.
   3. Synaptophysin is an integral membrane glycoprotein of 38,000 molecular weight found in small vesicles of neurons and neuroendocrine tumors.

B. Pathologic similarities
   1. All are APUDomas showing amine precursor uptake and decarboxylation.
   2. Ultrastructurally they have dense-core secretory granules (>80 nm).
   3. Histologically, generally appear similar with few mitoses and uniform nuclei.
   4. Frequently synthesize multiple peptides/amines, which can be detected immunocytochemically but may not be secreted.
   5. Presence or absence of clinical syndrome or type cannot be predicted by immunocytochemical studies.
   6. Histologic classifications increasingly predictive of biologic behavior. Only invasion or metastases establish malignancy.

C. Similarities of biologic behavior
   1. Generally slow growing, but a proportion are aggressive.
   2. Secrete biologically active peptides/amines, which can cause clinical symptoms.
   3. Generally have high densities of somatostatin receptors, which are used for both localization and treatment.

D. Similarities/differences in molecular abnormalities
   1. Similarities
      a. Uncommon—alterations in common oncogenes (*ras, jun, fos,* etc).
      b. Uncommon—alterations in common tumor-suppressor genes (p53, retinoblastoma).
      c. Alterations at MEN 1 locus (11q13) and p16^{INK4a} (9p21) occur in a proportion (10–45%).
      d. Methylation of various genes occurs in 40–87% (ras-associated domain family I, p14, p16, O^6 methyl guanosine methyltransferases, retinoic acid receptor β)
   2. Differences
      a. PETs—loss of 1p (21%), 3p (8–47%), 3q (8–41%), 11q (21–62%), 6q (18–68%). Gains at 17q (10–55%), 7q (16–68%), 4q (33%).
      b. Carcinoids—loss of 18q (38–67%) >18p (33–43%) >9p, 16q21(21–23%). Gains at 17q, 19p (57%), 4q (33%), 14q (20%).

Abbreviation: MEN 1, multiple endocrine neoplasia type 1.

Midgut carcinoids are argentaffin–positive, have a high serotonin content, most frequently cause the typical carcinoid syndrome when they metastasize (Table 52-3, Fig. 52-1), release serotonin and tachykinins (substance P, neuropeptide K, substance K), rarely secrete 5-HTP or ACTH, and less commonly metastasize to bone. Hindgut carcinoids (rectum, transverse and descending colon) are argentaffin–negative, are often argyrophilic, rarely contain serotonin or cause the carcinoid syndrome (Fig. 52-1, Table 52-3), rarely secrete 5-HTP or ACTH, contain numerous peptides, and may metastasize to bone.

Pancreatic endocrine tumors can be classified into nine well-established specific functional syndromes (Table 52-2), five possible specific functional syndromes (PETs secreting calcitonin, renin, luteinizing hormone, erythropoietin, or insulin-like growth factor II) (Table 52-2), and nonfunctional PETs (pancreatic polypeptide-secreting tumors; PPomas). Other functional hormonal syndromes due to nonpancreatic tumors

(usually intraabdominal in location) have been described only rarely and are not included in Table 52-2. They include secretion of glucagon-like peptide-2 (GLP-2) that causes intestinal villus hypertrophy (enteroglucagonomas), secretion of GLP-1 that causes hypoglycemia and delayed transit, and intestinal and ovarian tumors secreting peptide tyrosine tyrosine (PYY) that result in altered motility and constipation. Each of the functional syndromes listed in Table 52-2 is associated with symptoms due to the specific hormone released. In contrast, nonfunctional PETs release no products that cause a specific clinical syndrome. "Nonfunctional" is a misnomer in the strict sense because those tumors frequently ectopically secrete a number of peptides (pancreatic polypeptide [PP], chromogranin A, ghrelin, neurotensin, α subunits of human chorionic gonadotropin, neuron-specific enolase); however, they cause no specific clinical syndrome. The symptoms caused by nonfunctional PETs are entirely due to the tumor per se.

TABLE 52-2

GASTROINTESTINAL NEUROENDOCRINE TUMOR SYNDROME

NAME	BIOLOGICALLY ACTIVE PEPTIDE(S) SECRETED	INCIDENCE (NEW CASES/10⁶ POPULATION/ YEAR)	TUMOR LOCATION	MALIGNANT, %	ASSOCIATED WITH MEN 1, %	MAIN SYMPTOMS/ SIGNS
I. Established Specific Functional Syndrome						
A. Carcinoid tumor						
Carcinoid syndrome	Serotonin, possibly tachykinins, motilin, prostaglandins	0.5–2	Midgut (75–87%) Foregut (2–33%) Hindgut (1–8%) Unknown (2–15%)	95–100	Rare	Diarrhea (32–84%) Flushing (63–75%) Pain (10–34%) Asthma (4–18%) Heart disease (11–41%)
B. Pancreatic endocrine tumor						
Zollinger-Ellison syndrome	Gastrin	0.5–1.5	Duodenum (70%) Pancreas (25%) Other sites (5%)	60–90	20–25	Pain (79–100%) Diarrhea (30–75%) Esophageal symptoms (31–56%)
Insulinoma	Insulin	1–2	Pancreas (>99%)	<10	4–5	Hypoglycemic symptoms (100%)
VIPoma (Verner-Morrison syndrome, pancreatic cholera, WDHA)	Vasoactive intestinal peptide	0.05–0.2	Pancreas (90%, adult) Other (10%, neural, adrenal, periganglionic)	40–70	6	Diarrhea (90–100%) Hypokalemia (80–100%) Dehydration (83%)
Glucagonoma	Glucagon	0.01–0.1	Pancreas (100%)	50–80	1–20	Rash (67–90%) Glucose intolerance (38–87%) Weight loss (66–96%)
Somatostatinoma	Somatostatin	Rare	Pancreas (55%) Duodenum/ jejunum (44%)	>70	45	Diabetes mellitus (63–90%) Cholelithiases (65–90%) Diarrhea (35–90%)
GRFoma	Growth hormone–releasing hormone	Unknown	Pancreas (30%) Lung (54%) Jejunum (7%) Other (13%)	>60	16	Acromegaly (100%)
ACTHoma	ACTH	Rare	Pancreas (4–16% all ectopic Cushing's)	>95	Rare	Cushing's syndrome (100%)
PET causing carcinoid syndrome	Serotonin, ?tachykinins	Rare (43 cases)	Pancreas (<1% all carcinoids)	60–88	Rare	Same as carcinoid syndrome above
PET causing hypercalcemia	PTHrP Others unknown	Rare	Pancreas (rare cause of hypercalcemia)	84	Rare	Abdominal pain due to hepatic metastases
II. Possible Specific Functional Syndrome						
PET secreting calcitonin	Calcitonin	Rare	Pancreas (rare cause of hyper-calcitonemia)	>80	16	Diarrhea (50%)
PET secreting renin	Renin	Rare	Pancreas	Unknown	No	Hypertension

(continued)

TABLE 52-2

GASTROINTESTINAL NEUROENDOCRINE TUMOR SYNDROME (*CONTINUED*)

NAME	BIOLOGICALLY ACTIVE PEPTIDE(S) SECRETED	INCIDENCE (NEW CASES/10⁶ POPULATION/ YEAR)	TUMOR LOCATION	MALIGNANT, %	ASSOCIATED WITH MEN 1, %	MAIN SYMPTOMS/ SIGNS
PET secreting luteinizing hormone	Luteinizing hormone	Rare	Pancreas	Unknown	No	Anovulation, virilization (female); reduced libido (male)
PET secreting erythropoietin	Erythropoietin	Rare	Pancreas	100	No	Polycythemia
PET secreting IF-II	Insulin-like growth growth factor II	Rare	Pancreas	Unknown	No	Hypoglycemia
III. No Functional Syndrome						
PPoma/ nonfunctional	None	1–2	Pancreas (100%)	>60	18–44	Weight loss (30–90%) Abdominal mass (10–30%) Pain (30–95%)

Abbreviations: ACTH, adrenocorticotropic hormone; GRFoma, growth hormone-releasing factor secreting pancreatic endocrine tumor; IF-II, insulin-like growth factor 2; MEN, multiple endocrine neoplasia; PET, pancreatic endocrine tumor; PPoma, tumor secreting pancreatic polypeptide; PTHrP, parathyroid hormone–related peptide; VIPoma, tumor secreting vasoactive intestinal peptide; WDHA, *watery diarrhea, hypokalemia, and achlorhydria* syndrome.

Carcinoid tumors can occur in almost any GI tissue (Table 52-3); however, at present most (70%) have their origin in one of three sites: bronchus, jejunoileum, or colon/rectum. In the past, carcinoid tumors most frequently were reported in the appendix (i.e., 40%); however, the bronchus/lung, rectum, and small intestine are now the most common sites. Overall, the GI tract is the most common site for these tumors, accounting for 64%, with the respiratory tract a distant second at 28%. Both race and sex can affect the frequency as well as the distribution of carcinoid tumors. African Americans have a high incidence of carcinoids, and rectal carcinoids are the most common. Females have a lower incidence of small-intestinal and pancreatic carcinoids.

The term *pancreatic endocrine tumor*, although widely used and therefore retained here, is also a misnomer, strictly speaking, because these tumors can occur either almost entirely in the pancreas (insulinomas, glucagonomas, nonfunctional PETs, PETs causing hypercalcemia) or at both pancreatic and extrapancreatic sites (gastrinomas, VIPomas [vasoactive intestinal peptide], somatostatinomas, GRFomas [growth hormone–releasing factor]). PETs are also called islet cell tumors; however, the use of this term is discouraged because it is not established that they originate from the islets and many can occur at extrapancreatic sites.

A number of new classification systems have been proposed for both carcinoids and PETs. In the World Health Organization (WHO) classification it has been proposed that these tumors all be classified as GI neuroendocrine tumors (including carcinoids and PETs), which divides them into three general categories: (1a) well-differentiated NETs, (1b) well-differentiated neuroendocrine carcinomas that have low-grade malignancy, and (2) poorly differentiated neuroendocrine carcinomas that are usually small cell neuroendocrine carcinomas of high-grade malignancy. The term *carcinoid* is synonymous with *well-differentiated NETs* (1a). This classification is further divided on the basis of tumor location and biology. In addition, for the first time a standard TNM (tumor, node, metastasis) classification and grading system has been proposed for GI neuroendocrine tumors. The new WHO classification and the TNM classification and grading system were proposed to facilitate the comparison and evaluation of clinical, pathologic, and prognostic features and results of treatment in GI NETs from different studies. These classification systems may provide important prognostic information that can guide treatment (**Table 52-4**).

The exact incidence of carcinoid tumors or PETs varies according to whether only symptomatic tumors or all tumors are considered. The incidence of clinically significant carcinoids is 7–13 cases/million population per year, whereas any malignant carcinoids at autopsy are reported in 21–84 cases/million population per year. The incidence of GI NETs is approximately 25–50 cases

TABLE 52-3

CARCINOID TUMOR LOCATION, FREQUENCY OF METASTASES, AND ASSOCIATION WITH THE CARCINOID SYNDROME

	LOCATION (% OF TOTAL)	INCIDENCE OF METASTASES	INCIDENCE OF CARCINOID SYNDROME
Foregut			
Esophagus	<0.1	—	—
Stomach	4.6	10	9.5
Duodenum	2.0	—	3.4
Pancreas	0.7	71.9	20
Gallbladder	0.3	17.8	5
Bronchus, lung, trachea	27.9	5.7	13
Midgut			
Jejunum	1.8	{58.4	9
Ileum	14.9		9
Meckel's diverticulum	0.5	—	13
Appendix	4.8	38.8	<1
Colon	8.6	51	5
Liver	0.4	32.	—
Ovary	1.0	2 32	50
Testis	<0.1	—	50
Hindgut			
Rectum	13.6	3.9	—

Source: Location is from the PAN-SEER data (1973–1999), and incidence of metastases from the SEER data (1992–1999), reported by IM Modlin et al: Cancer 97:934, 2003. Incidence of carcinoid syndrome is from 4349 cases studied from 1950–1971, reported by JD Godwin: Cancer 36:560, 1975.

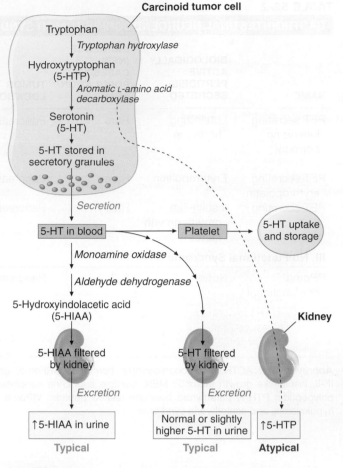

FIGURE 52-1
Synthesis, secretion, and metabolism of serotonin (5-HT) in patients with typical and atypical carcinoid syndromes. 5-HIAA, 5-hydroxyindolacetic acid.

per million in the United States, which makes them less common than adenocarcinomas of the GI tract. However, their incidence has increased sixfold in the last 30 years. Clinically significant PETs have a prevalence of 10 cases/million population, with insulinomas, gastrinomas, and nonfunctional PETs having an incidence of 0.5–2 cases/million population per year (Table 52-2). VIPomas are two to eight times less common, glucagonomas are 17 to 30 times less common, and somatostatinomas are the least common. In autopsy studies 0.5–1.5% of all cases have a PET; however, in less than 1 in 1000 cases was a functional tumor thought to occur.

Both carcinoid tumors and PETs commonly show malignant behavior (Tables 52-2 and 52-3). With PETs, except for insulinomas in which <10% are malignant, 50–100% in different series are malignant. With carcinoid tumors the percentage showing malignant behavior varies in different locations. For the three most common sites of occurrence, the incidence of metastases varies greatly from jejunoileum (58%) > lung/bronchus (6%) > rectum (4%) (Table 52-3). With both carcinoid

tumors and PETs, a number of factors, summarized in Table 52-4, are important prognostic factors in determining survival and the aggressiveness of the tumor. Patients with PETs (excluding insulinomas) generally have a poorer prognosis than do patients with GI NETs (carcinoids). The presence of liver metastases is the single most important prognostic factor in single and multivariate analyses for both carcinoid tumors and PETs. Particularly important in the development of liver metastases is the size of the primary tumor. For example, with small-intestinal carcinoids, which are the most common cause of the carcinoid syndrome due to metastatic disease in the liver (Table 52-2), metastases occur in 15–25% if the tumor diameter is <1 cm, 58–80% if it is 1–2 cm in diameter, and >75% if it is >2 cm in diameter. Similar data exist for gastrinomas and other PETs in which the size of the primary tumor is an independent predictor of the development of liver metastases. The presence of lymph node metastases; the depth of invasion; the rapid rate of growth; various histologic features (differentiation, mitotic rates, growth indices, vessel density, vascular endothelial growth factor [VEGF], and CD10

TABLE 52-4

PROGNOSTIC FACTORS IN NEUROENDOCRINE TUMORS

I. Both carcinoid tumors and PETs
- Presence of liver metastases ($p < .001$)
- Extent of liver metastases ($p < .001$)
- Presence of lymph node metastases ($p < .001$)
- Depth of invasion ($p < .001$)
- Rapid rate of tumor growth
- Elevated serum alkaline phosphatase levels ($p = .003$)
- Primary tumor site ($p < .001$)
- Primary tumor size ($p < .005$)
- Various histologic features
  - Tumor differentiation ($p < .001$)
  - High growth indices (high K_{i-67} index, PCNA expression)
  - High mitotic counts ($p < .001$)
  - Necrosis present
  - Presence of cytokeratin 19 ($p < .02$)
  - Vascular or perineural invasion
  - Vessel density (low microvessel density, increased lymphatic density)
  - High CD10 metalloproteinase expression (in series with all grades of NETs)
  - Flow cytometric features (i.e., aneuploidy)
  - High VEGF expression (in low-grade or well-differentiated NETs only)
- WHO, TNM, and grading classification
- Presence of a pancreatic NET rather than GI NET associated with poorer prognosis ($p = .0001$)
- Older age ($p < .01$)

II. Carcinoid tumors
- Presence of carcinoid syndrome
- Laboratory results (urinary 5-HIAA levels [$p < .01$], plasma neuropeptide K [$p < .05$], serum chromogranin A [$p < .01$])
- Presence of a second malignancy
- Male sex ($p < .001$)
- Mode of discovery (incidental > symptomatic)
- Molecular findings (TGF-α expression [$p < .05$], chr 16q LOH or gain chr 4p [$p < .05$])
- WHO, TNM, and grading classification
- Molecular findings (gain in chr 14, loss of 3p13 [ileal carcinoid], upregulation of Hoxc6)

III. PETs
- Ha-*ras* oncogene or p53 overexpression
- Female gender
- MEN 1 syndrome absent
- Presence of nonfunctional tumor (some studies, not all)
- WHO, TNM, and grading classification
- Laboratory findings (increased chromogranin A in some studies; gastrinomas—increased gastrin level)
- Molecular findings: increased HER2/*neu* expression ($p = .032$), chr 1q, 3p, 3q, or 6q LOH ($p = .0004$), EGF receptor overexpression ($p = .034$), gains in chr 7q, 17q, 17p, 20q; alterations in the VHL gene (deletion, methylation)

Abbreviations: 5-HIAA, 5-hydroxyindoleacetic acid; chr, chromosome; EGF, epidermal growth factor; Ki-67, proliferation-associated nuclear antigen recognized by Ki-67 monoclonal antibody; LOH, loss of heterozygosity; MEN, multiple endocrine neoplasia; NET, neuroendocrine tumors; PCNA, proliferating cell nuclear antigen; PET, pancreatic endocrine tumor; TGF-α, transforming growth factor α; TNM, tumor, node, metastasis; VEGF, vascular endothelial growth factor; WHO, World Health Organization.

metalloproteinase expression); necrosis; presence of cyto-keratin; elevated serum alkaline phosphatase levels; older age; advanced stages in WHO, TNM, or grading classification systems; and flow cytometric results such as the presence of aneuploidy are all important prognostic factors for the development of metastatic disease (Table 52-4). For patients with carcinoid tumors, additional associations with a worse prognosis include the development of the carcinoid syndrome (especially the development of carcinoid heart disease), male sex, the presence of a symptomatic tumor or greater increases in a number of tumor markers (5-hydroxyindolacetic acid [5-HIAA], neuropeptide K, chromogranin A), and the presence of various molecular features. With PETs or gastrinomas, which have been the best studied PET long-term, a worse prognosis is associated with female sex, overexpression of the Ha-*ras* oncogene or p53, the absence of multiple endocrine neoplasia type 1 (MEN 1), higher levels of various tumor markers (i.e., chromogranin A, gastrin), and various molecular features (Table 52-4).

A number of diseases due to various genetic disorders are associated with an increased incidence of neuroendocrine tumors **(Table 52-5)**. Each one is caused by a loss of a possible tumor-suppressor gene. The most

important is MEN 1, which is an autosomal dominant disorder due to a defect in a 10-exon gene on 11q13, which encodes for a 610-amino-acid nuclear protein, menin. Patients with MEN 1 develop hyperparathyroidism due to parathyroid hyperplasia in 95–100% of cases, PETs in 80–100%, pituitary adenomas in 54–80%, adrenal adenomas in 27–36%, bronchial carcinoids in 8%, thymic carcinoids in 8%, gastric carcinoids in 13–30% of patients with Zollinger-Ellison syndrome, skin tumors (angiofibromas [88%], collagenomas [72%]), central nervous system (CNS) tumors (meningiomas [<8%]), and smooth-muscle tumors (leiomyomas, leiomyosarcomas [1–7%]). Among patients with MEN 1, 80–100% develop nonfunctional PETs (most are microscopic with 0–13% large/symptomatic), functional PETs occur in 20–80% in different series with a mean of 54% developing Zollinger-Ellison syndrome, 18% insulinomas, 3% glucagonomas, 3% VIPomas, and <1% GRFomas or somatostatinomas. MEN 1 is present in 20–25% of all patients with Zollinger-Ellison syndrome, 4% of patients with insulinomas, and a low percentage (<5%) of patients with the other PETs.

Three phacomatoses associated with neuroendocrine tumors are von Hippel–Lindau disease (VHL),

TABLE 52-5

GENETIC SYNDROMES ASSOCIATED WITH AN INCREASED INCIDENCE OF NEUROENDOCRINE TUMORS (NETS) (CARCINOIDS OR PANCREATIC ENDOCRINE TUMORS [PETS])

SYNDROME	LOCATION OF GENE MUTATION AND GENE PRODUCT	NETS SEEN/FREQUENCY
Multiple endocrine neoplasia type 1 (MEN 1)	11q13 (encodes 610-amino-acid protein, menin)	80–100% develop PETs (microscopic), 20–80% (clinical): (nonfunctional > gastrinoma > insulinoma) Carcinoids: gastric (13–30%), bronchial/thymic (8%)
von Hippel–Lindau disease	3q25 (encodes 213-amino-acid protein)	12–17% develop PETs (almost always nonfunctional)
von Recklinghausen's disease (neurofibromatosis 1 [NF-1])	17q11.2 (encodes 2485-amino-acid protein, neurofibromin)	0–10% develop PETs, primarily duodenal somatostatinomas (usually nonfunctional) Rarely insulinoma, gastrinoma
Tuberous sclerosis	9q34 (TSCI) (encodes 1164-amino-acid protein, hamartin) 16p13 (TSC2) (encodes 1807-amino-acid protein, tuberin)	Uncommonly develop PETs (nonfunctional and functional [insulinoma, gastrinoma])

von Recklinghausen's disease (neurofibromatosis type 1 [NF-1]), and tuberous sclerosis (Bourneville's disease) (Table 52-5). VHL is an autosomal dominant disorder due to defects on chromosome 3p25, which encodes for a 213-amino-acid protein that interacts with the elongin family of proteins as a transcriptional regulator. In addition to cerebellar hemangioblastomas, renal cancer, and pheochromocytomas, 10–17% develop a PET. Most are nonfunctional, although insulinomas and VIPomas have been reported. Patients with NF-1 (von Recklinghausen's disease) have defects in a gene on chromosome 17q11.2 that encodes for a 2845-amino-acid protein, neurofibromin, which functions in normal cells as a suppressor of the ras signaling cascade. Up to 10% of these patients develop an upper GI carcinoid tumor, characteristically in the periampullary region (54%). Many are classified as somatostatinomas because they contain somatostatin immunocytochemically; however, they uncommonly secrete somatostatin and rarely produce a clinical somatostatinoma syndrome. NF-1 has rarely been associated with insulinomas and Zollinger-Ellison syndrome. NF-1 accounts for 48% of all duodenal somatostatinomas and 23% of all ampullary carcinoid tumors. Tuberous sclerosis is caused by mutations that alter either the 1164-amino-acid protein hamartin (TSC1) or the 1807-amino-acid protein tuberin (TSC2). Both hamartin and tuberin interact in a pathway related to phosphatidylinositol 3-kinases and mTor signaling cascades. A few cases including nonfunctional and functional PETs (insulinomas and gastrinomas) have been reported in these patients (Table 52-5).

In contrast to most common nonendocrine tumors, such as carcinoma of the breast, colon, lung, or stomach, in neither PETs nor carcinoid tumors have alterations in common oncogenes (*ras, myc, fos, src, jun*) or common tumor-suppressor genes (p53, retinoblastoma susceptibility gene) been found to be generally important in their molecular pathogenesis (Table 52-1). Alterations that may be important in their pathogenesis include changes in the *MEN 1* gene, p16/MTS1 tumor-suppressor gene, and *DPC 4/Smad 4 gene*; amplification of the HER-2/*neu* protooncogene; alterations in transcription factors (Hoxc6 [GI carcinoids]), growth factors, and their receptor expression; methylation of a number of genes that probably results in their inactivation; and deletions of unknown tumor-suppressor genes as well as gains in other unknown genes (Table 52-1). Comparative genomic hybridization, genome-wide allelotyping studies, and genome-wide single-nucleotide polymorphism analyses have shown that chromosomal losses and gains are common in PETs and carcinoids, but they differ between these two NETs and some have prognostic significance (Table 52-4). Mutations in the *MEN 1* gene are probably particularly important. There is loss of heterozygosity at the MEN 1 locus on chromosome 11q13 in 93% of sporadic PETs (i.e., in patients without MEN 1) and in 26–75% of sporadic carcinoid tumors. Mutations in the *MEN 1* gene are reported in 31–34% of sporadic gastrinomas. The presence of a number of these molecular alterations (PET or carcinoid) correlates with tumor growth, tumor size, and disease extent or invasiveness and may have prognostic significance.

CARCINOID TUMORS AND CARCINOID SYNDROME

CHARACTERISTICS OF THE MOST COMMON GI CARCINOID TUMORS

Appendiceal carcinoids

Appendiceal carcinoids occur in 1 in every 200–300 appendectomies, usually in the appendiceal tip. Most (i.e., >90%) are <1 cm in diameter without metastases in older studies, but more recently 2–35% have had metastases (Table 52-3). In the SEER data of 1570 appendiceal carcinoids, 62% were localized, 27% had regional metastases, and 8% had distant metastases. Approximately 50% between 1 and 2 cm metastasized to lymph nodes. Their percentage of the total number of carcinoids decreased from 43.9% (1950–1969) to 2.4% (1992–1999).

Small-intestinal carcinoids

Small-intestinal carcinoids account for approximately one-third of all small-bowel tumors in various surgical series. These are frequently multiple; 70–80% are present in the ileum, and 70% within 6 cm (24 in.) of the ileocecal valve. Forty percent are <1 cm in diameter, 32% are 1–2 cm, and 29% are >2 cm. Between 35 and 70% are associated with metastases (Table 52-3). They characteristically cause a marked fibrotic reaction, which can lead to intestinal obstruction. Distant metastases occur to liver in 36–60%, to bone in 3%, and to lung in 4%. As discussed previously, tumor size is an important variable in the frequency of metastases. However, even a proportion of small carcinoid tumors of the small intestine (<1 cm) have metastases in 15–25% of cases, whereas the proportion increases to 58–100% for tumors 1–2 cm in diameter. Carcinoids also occur in the duodenum, with 31% having metastases. No duodenal tumor <1 cm in two series metastasized, whereas 33% of those >2 cm had metastases. Small-intestinal carcinoids are the most common cause (60–87%) of the carcinoid syndrome and are discussed in a later section (Table 52-6).

Rectal carcinoids

Rectal carcinoids represent 1–2% of all rectal tumors. They are found in approximately 1 in every 2500 proctoscopies. Nearly all occur between 4 and 13 cm above the dentate line. Most are small, with 66–80% being <1 cm in diameter, and rarely metastasize (5%). Tumors between 1 and 2 cm can metastasize in 5–30%, and those >2 cm, which are uncommon, in >70%.

Bronchial carcinoids

Bronchial carcinoids account for 1–2% of primary lung tumors. The frequency of bronchial carcinoids has increased more than fivefold over the last 30 years. A number of different classifications of bronchial carcinoid tumors have been proposed. In some studies, lung NETs are classified into four categories: typical carcinoid (also called bronchial carcinoid tumor, Kulchitsky cell carcinoma I [KCC-I]), atypical carcinoid (also called well-differentiated neuroendocrine carcinoma

TABLE 52-6

CLINICAL CHARACTERISTICS IN PATIENTS WITH CARCINOID SYNDROME

	AT PRESENTATION	DURING COURSE OF DISEASE
Symptoms/signs		
Diarrhea	32–73%	68–84%
Flushing	23–65%	63–74%
Pain	10%	34%
Asthma/wheezing	4–8%	3–18%
Pellagra	2%	5%
None	12%	22%
Carcinoid heart disease present	11%	14–41%
Demographics		
Male	46–59%	46–61%
Age		
Mean	57 yrs	52–54 yrs
Range	25–79 yrs	9–91 yrs
Tumor location		
Foregut	5–9%	2–33%
Midgut	78–87%	60–87%
Hindgut	1–5%	1–8%
Unknown	2–11%	2–15%

[KC-II]), intermediate small cell neuroendocrine carcinoma, and small cell neuroendocarcinoma (KC-III). Another proposed classification includes three categories of lung NETs: benign or low-grade malignant (typical carcinoid), low-grade malignant (atypical carcinoid), and high-grade malignant (poorly differentiated carcinoma of the large cell or small cell type). The WHO classification includes four general categories: typical carcinoid, atypical carcinoid, large cell neuroendocrine carcinoma, and small cell carcinoma. These different categories of lung NETs have different prognoses, varying from excellent for typical carcinoid to poor for small cell neuroendocrine carcinomas. The occurrence of large cell and small cell lung carcinoids, but not typical or atypical lung carcinoids, is related to tobacco use.

Gastric carcinoids

Gastric carcinoids account for 3 of every 1000 gastric neoplasms. Three different subtypes of gastric carcinoids are proposed to occur. Each originates from gastric enterochromaffin-like cells (ECL cells), one of the six types of gastric neuroendocrine cells, in the gastric mucosa. Two subtypes are associated with hypergastrinemic states, either chronic atrophic gastritis (type I) (80% of all gastric carcinoids) or Zollinger-Ellison syndrome, which is almost always a part of the MEN 1 syndrome (type II) (6% of all cases). These tumors generally pursue a benign course, with type I uncommonly

(<10%) associated with metastases, whereas type II tumors are slightly more aggressive with 10–30% associated with metastases. They are usually multiple and small and infiltrate only to the submucosa. The third subtype of gastric carcinoid (type III) (sporadic) occurs without hypergastrinemia (14–25% of all gastric carcinoids) and has an aggressive course, with 54–66% developing metastases. Sporadic carcinoids are usually single, large tumors; 50% have atypical histology, and they can be a cause of the carcinoid syndrome. Gastric carcinoids as a percentage of all carcinoids are increasing in frequency (1.96% [1969–1971], 3.6% [1973–1991], 5.8% [1991–1999]).

CARCINOID TUMORS WITHOUT THE CARCINOID SYNDROME

The age of patients at diagnosis ranges from 10 to 93 years, with a mean age of 63 years for the small intestine and 66 years for the rectum. The presentation is diverse and is related to the site of origin and the extent of malignant spread. In the appendix, carcinoid tumors usually are found incidentally during surgery for suspected appendicitis. Small-intestinal carcinoids in the jejunoileum present with periodic abdominal pain (51%), intestinal obstruction with ileus/invagination (31%), an abdominal tumor (17%), or GI bleeding (11%). Because of the vagueness of the symptoms, the diagnosis usually is delayed approximately 2 years from onset of the symptoms, with a range up to 20 years. Duodenal, gastric, and rectal carcinoids are most frequently found by chance at endoscopy. The most common symptoms of rectal carcinoids are melena/bleeding (39%), constipation (17%), and diarrhea (12%). Bronchial carcinoids frequently are discovered as a lesion on a chest radiograph, and 31% of the patients are asymptomatic. Thymic carcinoids present as anterior mediastinal masses, usually on chest radiograph or CT scan. Ovarian and testicular carcinoids usually present as masses discovered on physical examination or ultrasound. Metastatic carcinoid tumor in the liver frequently presents as hepatomegaly in a patient who may have minimal symptoms and nearly normal liver function test results.

CARCINOID TUMORS WITH SYSTEMIC SYMPTOMS DUE TO SECRETED PRODUCTS

Carcinoid tumors immunocytochemically can contain numerous GI peptides: gastrin, insulin, somatostatin, motilin, neurotensin, tachykinins (substance K, substance P, neuropeptide K), glucagon, gastrin-releasing peptide, vasoactive intestinal peptide (VIP), pancreatic polypeptide (PP), ghrelin, other biologically active peptides

(ACTH, calcitonin, growth hormone), prostaglandins, and bioactive amines (serotonin). These substances may or may not be released in sufficient amounts to cause symptoms. In various studies of patients with carcinoid tumors, elevated serum levels of PP were found in 43%, motilin in 14%, gastrin in 15%, and VIP in 6%. Foregut carcinoids are more likely to produce various GI peptides than are midgut carcinoids. Ectopic ACTH production causing Cushing's syndrome is seen increasingly with foregut carcinoids (respiratory tract primarily) and in some series has been the most common cause of the ectopic ACTH syndrome, accounting for 64% of all cases. Acromegaly due to growth hormone–releasing factor release occurs with foregut carcinoids, as does the somatostatinoma syndrome, but rarely occurs with duodenal carcinoids. The most common systemic syndrome with carcinoid tumors is the carcinoid syndrome, which is discussed in detail in the next section.

CARCINOID SYNDROME

Clinical features

The cardinal features from a number of series at presentation as well as during the disease course are shown in Table 52-6. Flushing and diarrhea are the two most common symptoms, occurring in up to 73% initially and in up to 89% during the course of the disease. The characteristic flush is of sudden onset; it is a deep red or violaceous erythema of the upper body, especially the neck and face, often associated with a feeling of warmth and occasionally associated with pruritus, lacrimation, diarrhea, or facial edema. Flushes may be precipitated by stress; alcohol; exercise; certain foods, such as cheese; or certain agents, such as catecholamines, pentagastrin, and serotonin reuptake inhibitors. Flushing episodes may be brief, lasting 2 to 5 min, especially initially, or may last hours, especially later in the disease course. Flushing usually is associated with metastatic midgut carcinoids but can also occur with foregut carcinoids. With bronchial carcinoids the flushes frequently are prolonged for hours to days, reddish in color, and associated with salivation, lacrimation, diaphoresis, diarrhea, and hypotension. The flush associated with gastric carcinoids can also be reddish in color, but with a patchy distribution over the face and neck, although the classic flush seen with midgut carcinoids can also be seen with gastric carcinoids. It may be provoked by food and have accompanying pruritus.

Diarrhea is present in 32–73% initially and 68–84% at some time in the disease course. Diarrhea usually occurs with flushing (85% of cases). The diarrhea usually is described as watery, with 60% of patients having <1 L/d of diarrhea. Steatorrhea is present in 67%, and in 46% it is greater than 15 g/d (normal <7 g).

Abdominal pain may be present with the diarrhea or independently in 10–34% of cases.

Cardiac manifestations occur in 11–20% initially of patients with carcinoid syndrome and in 17–56% (mean 40%) at some time in the disease course. The cardiac disease is due to the formation of fibrotic plaques (composed of smooth-muscle cells, myofibroblasts, and elastic tissue) involving the endocardium, primarily on the right side, although lesions on the left side also occur occasionally, especially if a patent foramen ovale exists. The dense fibrous deposits are most commonly on the ventricular aspect of the tricuspid valve and less commonly on the pulmonary valve cusps. They can result in constriction of the valves, and pulmonic stenosis is usually predominant, whereas the tricuspid valve is often fixed open, resulting in regurgitation predominating. Overall, in patients with carcinoid heart disease, 97% have tricuspid insufficiency, 59% tricuspid stenosis, 50% pulmonary insufficiency, 25% pulmonary stenosis, and 11% (0–25%) left-side lesions. Up to 80% of patients with cardiac lesions develop heart failure. Lesions on the left side are much less extensive, occur in 30% at autopsy, and most frequently affect the mitral valve.

Other clinical manifestations include wheezing or asthma-like symptoms (8–18%) and pellagra-like skin lesions (2–25%). A variety of noncardiac problems due to increased fibrous tissue have been reported, including retroperitoneal fibrosis causing urethral obstruction, Peyronie's disease of the penis, intraabdominal fibrosis, and occlusion of the mesenteric arteries or veins.

Pathobiology

Carcinoid syndrome occurred in 8% of 8876 patients with carcinoid tumors, with a rate of 1.4–18.4% in different studies. It occurs only when sufficient concentrations of products secreted by the tumor reach the systemic circulation. In 91% of cases this occurs after distant metastases to the liver. Rarely, primary gut carcinoids with nodal metastases with extensive retroperitoneal invasion, pancreatic carcinoids with retroperitoneal lymph nodes, or carcinoids of the lung or ovary with direct access to the systemic circulation can cause the carcinoid syndrome without hepatic metastases. All carcinoid tumors do not have the same propensity to metastasize and cause the carcinoid syndrome (Table 52-3). Midgut carcinoids account for 60–67% of cases of carcinoid syndrome, foregut tumors for 2–33%, hindgut for 1–8%, and an unknown primary location for 2–15%.

One of the main secretory products of carcinoid tumors involved in the carcinoid syndrome is serotonin (5-hydroxytryptamine [5-HT]) (Fig. 52-1), which is synthesized from tryptophan. Up to 50% of dietary tryptophan can be used in this synthetic pathway by tumor cells, and this can result in inadequate supplies for conversion to niacin; hence, some patients (2.5%) develop pellagra-like lesions. Serotonin has numerous biologic effects, including stimulating intestinal secretion with inhibition of absorption, stimulating increases in intestinal motility, and stimulating fibrogenesis. In various studies 56–88% of all carcinoid tumors were associated with serotonin overproduction; however, 12–26% of the patients did not have the carcinoid syndrome. In one study platelet serotonin was elevated in 96% of patients with midgut carcinoids, 43% with foregut tumors, and 0% with hindgut tumors. In 90–100% of patients with the carcinoid syndrome there is evidence of serotonin overproduction. Serotonin is thought to be predominantly responsible for the diarrhea because of its effects on gut motility and intestinal secretion, primarily through $5\text{-}HT_3$ and, to a lesser degree, $5\text{-}HT_4$ receptors. Serotonin receptor antagonists (especially $5\text{-}HT_3$ antagonists) relieve the diarrhea in many, but not all, patients. Additional studies suggest that prostaglandin E_2 (PGE_2) and tachykinins may be important mediators of the diarrhea in some patients. In one study, plasma tachykinin levels correlated with symptoms of both flushing and diarrhea. Serotonin does not appear to be involved in the flushing because serotonin receptor antagonists do not relieve flushing. In patients with gastric carcinoids the characteristic red, patchy pruritic flush probably is due to histamine release because H_1- and H_2-receptor antagonists can prevent it. Numerous studies have shown that tachykinins are stored in carcinoid tumors and released during flushing. However, some studies have demonstrated that octreotide can relieve the flushing induced by pentagastrin in these patients without altering the stimulated increase in plasma substance P, suggesting that other mediators must be involved in the flushing. A correlation between plasma tachykinin levels, but not substance P levels, and flushing has been reported. Both histamine and serotonin may be responsible for the wheezing as well as the fibrotic reactions involving the heart, causing Peyronie's disease and intraabdominal fibrosis. The exact mechanism of the heart disease has remained unclear, although increasing evidence supports a central role for serotonin. The valvular heart disease caused by the appetite-suppressant drug dexfenfluramine is histologically indistinguishable from that observed in carcinoid disease. Furthermore, ergot-containing dopamine receptor agonists used for Parkinson's disease (pergolide, cabergoline) cause valvular heart disease that closely resembles that seen in the carcinoid syndrome. Metabolites of fenfluramine, as well as the dopamine receptor agonists, have high affinity for serotonin receptor subtype $5\text{-}HT_{2B}$ receptors, whose activation is known to cause fibroblast mitogenesis. Serotonin receptor subtypes $5\text{-}HT_{1B,1D,2A,2B}$ normally are expressed in human heart valve interstitial cells. High levels of

5-HT_{2B} receptors are known to occur in heart valves and occur in cardiac fibroblasts and cardiomyocytes. Studies of cultured interstitial cells from human cardiac valves have demonstrated that these valvulopathic drugs induce mitogenesis by activating 5-HT_{2B} receptors and stimulating upregulation of transforming growth factor β and collagen biosynthesis. These observations support the conclusion that serotonin overproduction by carcinoid tumors is important in mediating the valvular changes, possibly by activating 5-HT_{2B} receptors in the endocardium. Both the magnitude of serotonin overproduction and prior chemotherapy are important predictors of progression of the heart disease. Atrial natriuretic peptide (ANP) overproduction also has been reported in patients with cardiac disease, but its role in the pathogenesis is unknown. However, high plasma levels of ANP have a worse prognosis. Plasma connective tissue growth factor levels are elevated in many fibrotic conditions; elevated levels occur in patients with carcinoid heart disease and correlate with the presence of right-ventricular dysfunction and the extent of valvular regurgitation in patients with carcinoid tumors.

Patients may develop either a typical or, rarely, an atypical carcinoid syndrome. In patients with the typical form, which characteristically is caused by a midgut carcinoid tumor, the conversion of tryptophan to 5-HTP is the rate-limiting step (Fig. 52-1). Once 5-HTP is formed, it is rapidly converted to 5-HT and stored in secretory granules of the tumor or in platelets. A small amount remains in plasma and is converted to 5-HIAA, which appears in large amounts in the urine. These patients have an expanded serotonin pool size, increased blood and platelet serotonin, and increased urinary 5-hydroxyindolacetic acid (5-HIAA). Some carcinoid tumors cause an atypical carcinoid syndrome that is thought to be due to a deficiency in the enzyme dopa decarboxylase; thus, 5-HTP cannot be converted to 5-HT (serotonin), and 5-HTP is secreted into the bloodstream (Fig. 52-1). In these patients, plasma serotonin levels are normal but urinary levels may be increased because some 5-HTP is converted to 5-HT in the kidney. Characteristically, urinary 5-HTP and 5-HT are increased, but urinary 5-HIAA levels are only slightly elevated. Foregut carcinoids are the most likely to cause an atypical carcinoid syndrome.

One of the most immediate life-threatening complications of the carcinoid syndrome is the development of a carcinoid crisis. This is more common in patients who have intense symptoms or have greatly increased urinary 5-HIAA levels (i.e., >200 mg/d). The crises may occur spontaneously or be provoked by stress, anesthesia, chemotherapy, or a biopsy. Patients develop intense flushing, diarrhea, abdominal pain, cardiac abnormalities including tachycardia, hypertension, or hypotension. If not adequately treated, this can be a terminal event.

DIAGNOSIS OF THE CARCINOID SYNDROME AND CARCINOID TUMORS

The diagnosis of carcinoid syndrome relies on measurement of urinary or plasma serotonin or its metabolites in the urine. The measurement of 5-HIAA is used most frequently. False-positive elevations may occur if the patient is eating serotonin-rich foods such as bananas, pineapples, walnuts, pecans, avocados, or hickory nuts or is taking certain medications (cough syrup containing guaifenesin, acetaminophen, salicylates, serotonin reuptake inhibitors, or L-dopa). The normal range in daily urinary 5-HIAA excretion is 2–8 mg/d. Serotonin overproduction was noted in 92% of patients with carcinoid syndrome in one study, and in another study, 5-HIAA had 73% sensitivity and 100% specificity for carcinoid syndrome.

Most physicians use only the urinary 5-HIAA excretion rate; however, plasma and platelet serotonin levels, if available, may provide additional information. Platelet serotonin levels are more sensitive than urinary 5-HIAA but are not generally available. Because patients with foregut carcinoids may produce an atypical carcinoid syndrome, if this syndrome is suspected and the urinary 5-HIAA is minimally elevated or normal, other urinary metabolites of tryptophan, such as 5-HTP and 5-HT, should be measured (Fig. 52-1).

Flushing occurs in a number of other diseases, including systemic mastocytosis, chronic myeloid leukemia with increased histamine release, menopause, reactions to alcohol or glutamate, side effects of chlorpropamide, calcium channel blockers, and nicotinic acid. None of these conditions cause increased urinary 5-HIAA.

The diagnosis of carcinoid tumor can be suggested by the carcinoid syndrome, recurrent abdominal symptoms in a healthy-appearing individual, or the discovery of hepatomegaly or hepatic metastases associated with minimal symptoms. Ileal carcinoids, which make up 25% of all clinically detected carcinoids, should be suspected in patients with bowel obstruction, abdominal pain, flushing, or diarrhea.

Serum chromogranin A levels are elevated in 56–100% of patients with carcinoid tumors, and the level correlates with tumor bulk. Serum chromogranin A levels are not specific for carcinoid tumors because they are also elevated in patients with PETs and other neuroendocrine tumors. Plasma neuron-specific enolase levels are also used as a marker of carcinoid tumors but are less sensitive than chromogranin A, being increased in only 17–47% of patients.

TREATMENT	Carcinoid Syndrome and Nonmetastatic Carcinoid Tumors

CARCINOID SYNDROME Treatment includes avoiding conditions that precipitate flushing, dietary supplementation with nicotinamide, treatment of heart failure with diuretics, treatment of wheezing with oral bronchodilators, and control of the diarrhea with anti-diarrheal agents such as loperamide and diphenoxylate. If patients still have symptoms, serotonin receptor antagonists or somatostatin analogues (Fig. 52-2) are the drugs of choice.

There are 14 subclasses of serotonin receptors, and antagonists for many are not available. The 5-HT$_1$ and 5-HT$_2$ receptor antagonists methylsergide, cyproheptadine, and ketanserin have all been used to control

FIGURE 52-2

Structure of somatostatin and synthetic analogues used for diagnostic or therapeutic indications.

the diarrhea but usually do not decrease flushing. The use of methylsergide is limited because it can cause or enhance retroperitoneal fibrosis. Ketanserin diminishes diarrhea in 30–100% of patients. 5-HT$_3$ receptor antagonists (ondansetron, tropisetron, alosetron) can control diarrhea and nausea in up to 100% of patients and occasionally ameliorate the flushing. A combination of histamine H$_1$- and H$_2$-receptor antagonists (i.e., diphenhydramine and cimetidine or ranitidine) may control flushing in patients with foregut carcinoids.

Synthetic analogues of somatostatin (octreotide, lanreotide) are now the most widely used agents to control the symptoms of patients with carcinoid syndrome (Fig. 52-2). These drugs are effective at relieving symptoms and decreasing urinary 5-HIAA levels in patients with this syndrome. Octreotide-LAR and lanreotide-SR/autogel (Somatuline) control symptoms in 74% and 68%, respectively, of patients with carcinoid syndrome and show a biochemical response in 51% and 39%. Patients with mild to moderate symptoms usually are treated initially with octreotide 100 µg SC every 8 h and begun on long-acting monthly depot forms (octreotide-LAR or lanreotide-autogel). Forty percent of patients escape control after a median time of 4 months, and the depot dosage may have to be increased as well as supplemented with the shorter-acting formulation, SC octreotide.

Carcinoid heart disease is associated with a decreased mean survival (3.8 years), and therefore it should be sought for and carefully assessed in all patients with carcinoid syndrome. Transthoracic echocardiography remains a key element in establishing the diagnosis of carcinoid heart disease and determining the extent and type of cardiac abnormalities. Treatment with diuretics and somatostatin analogues can reduce the negative hemodynamic effects and secondary heart failure. It remains unclear whether long-term treatment with these drugs will decrease the progression of carcinoid heart disease. Balloon valvuloplasty for stenotic valves or cardiac valve surgery may be required.

In patients with carcinoid crises, somatostatin analogues are effective at both treating the condition and preventing their development during known precipitating events such as surgery, anesthesia, chemotherapy, and stress. It is recommended that octreotide 150–250 µg SC every 6 to 8 h be used 24–48 h before anesthesia and then continued throughout the procedure.

Currently, sustained-release preparations of both octreotide (octreotide-LAR [long-acting release], 10, 20, 30 mg) and lanreotide (lanreotide-PR [prolonged release, lanreotide-autogel], 60, 90, 120 mg) are available and widely used because their use greatly facilitates long-term treatment. Octreotide-LAR (30 mg/month) gives a plasma level ≥1 ng/mL for 25 days, whereas this requires three to six injections a day of the non-sustained-release form. Lanreotide autogel (Somatuline) is given every 4–6 weeks.

Short-term side effects occur in up to one-half of patients. Pain at the injection site and side effects related to the GI tract (59% discomfort, 15% nausea, diarrhea) are the most common. They are usually short-lived and do not interrupt treatment. Important long-term side effects include gallstone formation, steatorrhea, and deterioration in glucose tolerance. The overall incidence of gallstones/biliary sludge in one study was 52%, with 7% having symptomatic disease that required surgical treatment.

Interferon α is reported to be effective in controlling symptoms of the carcinoid syndrome either alone or combined with hepatic artery embolization. With interferon α alone the response rate is 42%, and with interferon α with hepatic artery embolization, diarrhea was controlled for 1 year in 43% and flushing was controlled in 86%.

Hepatic artery embolization alone or with chemotherapy (chemoembolization) has been used to control the symptoms of carcinoid syndrome. Embolization alone is reported to control symptoms in up to 76% of patients, and chemoembolization (5-fluorouracil, doxorubicin, cisplatin, mitomycin) in 60–75% of patients. Hepatic artery embolization can have major side effects, including nausea, vomiting, pain, and fever. In two studies 5–7% of patients died from complications of hepatic artery occlusion.

Other drugs have been used successfully in small numbers of patients to control the symptoms of carcinoid syndrome. Parachlorophenylanine can inhibit tryptophan hydroxylase and therefore the conversion of tryptophan to 5-HTP. However, its severe side effects, including psychiatric disturbances, make it intolerable for long-term use. α-Methyldopa inhibits the conversion of 5-HTP to 5-HT, but its effects are only partial.

Peptide radioreceptor therapy (using radiotherapy with radiolabeled somatostatin analogues), the use of radiolabeled microspheres, and other methods for treatment of advanced metastatic disease may facilitate control of the carcinoid syndrome and are discussed in a later section dealing with treatment of advanced disease.

CARCINOID TUMORS (NONMETASTATIC)

Surgery is the only potentially curative therapy. Because with most carcinoids the probability of metastatic disease increases with increasing size, the extent of surgical resection is determined accordingly. With appendiceal carcinoids <1 cm, simple appendectomy was curative in 103 patients followed for up to 35 years. With rectal carcinoids <1 cm, local resection is curative. With small-intestinal carcinoids <1 cm, there is not complete agreement. Because 15–69% of small-intestinal carcinoids this size have metastases in different studies, some

recommend a wide resection with en bloc resection of the adjacent lymph-bearing mesentery. If the carcinoid tumor is >2 cm for rectal, appendiceal, or small-intestinal carcinomas, a full cancer operation should be done. This includes a right hemicolectomy for appendiceal carcinoid, an abdominoperineal resection or low anterior resection for rectal carcinoids, and an en bloc resection of adjacent lymph nodes for small-intestinal carcinoids. For carcinoids 1–2 cm in diameter for appendiceal tumors, a simple appendectomy is proposed by some, whereas others favor a formal right hemicolectomy. For rectal carcinoids 1–2 cm, it is recommended that a wide local full-thickness excision be performed.

With type I or II gastric carcinoids, which are usually <1 cm, endoscopic removal is recommended. In type I or II gastric carcinoids, if the tumor is >2 cm or if there is local invasion, some recommend total gastrectomy, whereas others recommend antrectomy in type I to reduce the hypergastrinemia, which led to regression of the carcinoids in a number of studies. For types I and II gastric carcinoids of 1–2 cm, there is no agreement, with some recommending endoscopic treatment followed by chronic somatostatin treatment and careful follow-up and others recommending surgical treatment. With type III gastric carcinoids >2 cm, excision and regional lymph node clearance are recommended. Most tumors <1 cm are treated endoscopically.

Resection of isolated or limited hepatic metastases may be beneficial and will be discussed in a later section on treatment of advanced disease.

PANCREATIC ENDOCRINE TUMORS

Functional PETs usually present clinically with symptoms due to the hormone-excess state. Only late in the course of the disease does the tumor per se cause prominent symptoms such as abdominal pain. In contrast, all the symptoms due to nonfunctional PETs are due to the tumor per se. The overall result of this is that some functional PETs may present with severe symptoms with a small or undetectable primary tumor, whereas nonfunctional tumors usually present late in the disease course with large tumors, which are frequently metastatic. The mean delay between onset of continuous symptoms and diagnosis of a functional PET syndrome is 4–7 years. Therefore, the diagnoses frequently are missed for extended periods.

TREATMENT   Pancreatic Endocrine Tumor

Treatment of PETs requires two different strategies. First, treatment must be directed at the hormone-excess state such as the gastric acid hypersecretion in gastrinomas or the hypoglycemia in insulinomas. Ectopic hormone secretion usually causes the presenting symptoms and can cause life-threatening complications. Second, with all the tumors except insulinomas, >50% are malignant (Table 52-2); therefore, treatment must also be directed against the tumor per se. Because in many patients these tumors are not surgically curable due to the presence of advanced disease at diagnosis, surgical resection for cure, which addresses both treatment aspects, is often not possible.

GASTRINOMA (ZOLLINGER-ELLISON SYNDROME) (ZES)

A gastrinoma is a neuroendocrine tumor that secretes gastrin; the resultant hypergastrinemia causes gastric acid hypersecretion (Zollinger-Ellison syndrome). The chronic hypergastrinemia results in marked gastric acid hypersecretion and growth of the gastric mucosa with increased numbers of parietal cells and proliferation of gastric ECL cells. The gastric acid hypersecretion characteristically causes peptic ulcer disease, often refractory and severe, as well as diarrhea. The most common presenting symptoms are abdominal pain (70–100%), diarrhea (37–73%), and gastroesophageal reflux disease (GERD) (30–35%); 10–20% have diarrhea only. Although peptic ulcers may occur in unusual locations, most patients have a typical duodenal ulcer. Important observations that should suggest this diagnosis include peptic ulcer disease (PUD); with diarrhea; PUD in an unusual location or with multiple ulcers; PUD refractory to treatment or persistent; PUD associated with prominent gastric folds; PUD associated with findings suggestive of MEN 1 (endocrinopathy, family history of ulcer or endocrinopathy, nephrolithiases); and PUD without *Helicobacter pylori* present. *H. pylori* is present in >90% of idiopathic peptic ulcers but is present in <50% of patients with gastrinomas. Chronic unexplained diarrhea also should suggest gastrinoma.

Approximately 20–25% of patients with ZES have MEN 1, and in most cases hyperparathyroidism is present before the gastrinoma. These patients are treated differently from those without MEN 1; therefore, MEN 1 should be sought in all patients by family history and by measuring plasma ionized calcium and prolactin levels and plasma hormone levels (parathormone, growth hormone).

Most gastrinomas (50–70%) are present in the duodenum, followed by the pancreas (20–40%) and other intraabdominal sites (mesentery, lymph nodes, biliary tract, liver, stomach, ovary). Rarely, the tumor may involve extraabdominal sites. In MEN 1 the gastrinomas are also usually in the duodenum (70–90%), followed by the pancreas (10–30%), and are almost always

multiple. About 60–90% of gastrinomas are malignant (Table 52-2) with metastatic spread to lymph nodes and liver. Distant metastases to bone occur in 12–30% of patients with liver metastases.

Diagnosis

The diagnosis of ZES requires the demonstration of inappropriate fasting hypergastrinemia, usually by demonstrating hypergastrinemia occurring with an increased basal gastric acid output (BAO) (hyperchlorhydria). More than 98% of patients with gastrinomas have fasting hypergastrinemia, although in 40–60% the level may be elevated less than tenfold. Therefore, when the diagnosis is suspected, a fasting gastrin should be determined first. It is important to remember that potent gastric acid suppressant drugs such as proton pump inhibitors (omeprazole, esomeprazole, pantoprazole, lansoprazole, rabeprazole) can suppress acid secretion sufficiently to cause hypergastrinemia; because of their prolonged duration of action, these drugs have to be discontinued for a week before the gastrin determination. Withdrawal of proton pump inhibitors (PPIs) should be performed carefully and is best done in consultation with GI units with experience in this area. The widespread use of PPIs can confound the diagnosis of ZES by raising a false-positive diagnosis by causing hypergastrinemia in a patient being treated with idiopathic peptic disease (without ZES) and lead to a false-negative diagnosis because at routine doses used to treat patients with idiopathic peptic disease, PPIs control symptoms in most ZES patients and thus mask the diagnosis. If ZES is suspected and the gastrin level is elevated, it is important to show that it is increased when gastric pH is ≤2.0 because physiologically hypergastrinemia secondary to achlorhydria (atrophic gastritis, pernicious anemia) is one of the most common causes of hypergastrinemia. Nearly all gastrinoma patients have a fasting pH ≤2 when off antisecretory drugs. If the fasting gastrin is >1000 pg/mL (increased tenfold) and the pH is ≤2.0, which occurs in 40–60% of patients with gastrinoma, the diagnosis of ZES is established after the possibility of retained antrum syndrome has been ruled out by history. In patients with hypergastrinemia with fasting gastrins <1000 pg/mL and gastric pH ≤2.0, other conditions, such as *H. pylori* infections, antral G-cell hyperplasia/hyperfunction, gastric outlet obstruction, and, rarely, renal failure, can masquerade as ZES. To establish the diagnosis in this group, a determination of BAO and a secretin provocative test should be done. In patients with ZES without previous gastric acid–reducing surgery, the BAO is usually (>90%) elevated (i.e., >15 meq/h). The secretin provocative test is usually positive, with the criterion of a >120-pg/mL increase over the basal level having the highest sensitivity (94%) and specificity (100%).

TREATMENT   Gastrinomas

Gastric acid hypersecretion in patients with gastrinomas can be controlled in almost every case by oral gastric antisecretory drugs. Because of their long duration of action and potency, which allows dosing once or twice a day, the PPIs (H^+,K^+-ATPase inhibitors) are the drugs of choice. Histamine H_2-receptor antagonists are also effective, although more frequent dosing (q 4–8 h) and high doses are required. In patients with MEN 1 with hyperparathyroidism, correction of the hyperparathyroidism increases the sensitivity to gastric antisecretory drugs and decreases the basal acid output. Long-term treatment with PPIs (>15 years) has proved to be safe and effective, without development of tachyphylaxis. Although patients with ZES, especially those with MEN 1, more frequently develop gastric carcinoids, no data suggest that the long-term use of PPIs increases this risk in these patients. With long-term PPI use in ZES patients, vitamin B_{12} deficiency can develop; thus, vitamin B_{12} levels should be assessed during follow-up.

With the increased ability to control acid hypersecretion, more than 50% of patients who are not cured (>60% of patients) will die from tumor-related causes. At presentation, careful imaging studies are essential to localize the extent of the tumor. A third of patients present with hepatic metastases, and in <15% of those patients the disease is limited, so that surgical resection may be possible. Surgical short-term cure is possible in 60% of all patients without MEN 1 or liver metastases (40% of all patients) and in 30% of patients long-term. In patients with MEN 1, long-term surgical cure is rare because the tumors are multiple, frequently with lymph node metastases. Therefore, all patients with gastrinomas without MEN 1 or a medical condition that limits life expectancy should undergo surgery by a surgeon experienced in the treatment of these disorders.

INSULINOMAS

An insulinoma is an endocrine tumor of the pancreas that is thought to be derived from beta cells that ectopically secrete insulin, which results in hypoglycemia. The average age of occurrence is 40–50 years old. The most common clinical symptoms are due to the effect of the hypoglycemia on the CNS (neuroglycemic symptoms) and include confusion, headache, disorientation, visual difficulties, irrational behavior, and even coma. Also, most patients have symptoms due to excess catecholamine release secondary to the hypoglycemia, including sweating, tremor, and palpitations. Characteristically, these attacks are associated with fasting.

Insulinomas are generally small (>90% <2 cm) and usually not multiple (90%); only 5–15% are malignant, and they almost invariably occur only in the pancreas, distributed equally in the pancreatic head, body, and tail.

Insulinomas should be suspected in all patients with hypoglycemia, especially when there is a history suggesting that attacks are provoked by fasting, or with a family history of MEN 1. Insulin is synthesized as proinsulin, which consists of a 21-amino-acid α chain and a 30-amino-acid β chain connected by a 33-amino-acid connecting peptide (C peptide). In insulinomas, in addition to elevated plasma insulin levels, elevated plasma proinsulin levels are found, and C-peptide levels can be elevated.

Diagnosis

The diagnosis of insulinoma requires the demonstration of an elevated plasma insulin level at the time of hypoglycemia. A number of other conditions may cause fasting hypoglycemia, such as the inadvertent or surreptitious use of insulin or oral hypoglycemic agents, severe liver disease, alcoholism, poor nutrition, and other extrapancreatic tumors. Furthermore, postprandial hypoglycemia can be caused by a number of conditions that confuse the diagnosis of insulinoma. Particularly important here is the increased occurrence of hypoglycemia after gastric bypass surgery for obesity, which is now widely performed. The most reliable test to diagnose insulinoma is a fast up to 72 h with serum glucose, C-peptide, proinsulin, and insulin measurements every 4–8 h. If at any point the patient becomes symptomatic or glucose levels are persistently below <2.2 mmol/L (40 mg/dL), the test should be terminated and repeat samples for the above studies should be obtained before glucose is given. Some 70–80% of patients will develop hypoglycemia during the first 24 h, and 98% by 48 h. In nonobese normal subjects, serum insulin levels should decrease to <43 pmol/L (<6 μU/mL) when blood glucose decreases to <2.2 mmol/L (<40 mg/dL) and the ratio of insulin to glucose is <0.3 (in mg/dL). In addition to having an insulin level >6 μU/mL when blood glucose is <40 mg/dL, some investigators also require an elevated C-peptide and serum proinsulin level, an insulin/glucose ratio >0.3, and a decreased plasma β-hydroxybutyrate level for the diagnosis of insulinomas. Surreptitious use of insulin or hypoglycemic agents may be difficult to distinguish from insulinomas. The combination of proinsulin levels (normal in exogenous insulin/hypoglycemic agent users), C-peptide levels (low in exogenous insulin users), antibodies to insulin (positive in exogenous insulin users), and measurement of sulfonylurea levels in serum or plasma will allow the correct diagnosis to be made. The diagnosis of insulinoma has been complicated by the introduction of specific insulin assays that do not also interact with proinsulin, as do many of the older radioimmunoassays (RIAs), and therefore give lower plasma insulin levels. The increased use of these specific insulin assays has resulted in increased numbers of patients with insulinomas having lower plasma insulin values than the 6 μU/mL levels proposed to be characteristic of insulinomas by RIA. In these patients the assessment of proinsulin and C-peptide levels at the time of hypoglycemia is particularly helpful for establishing the correct diagnosis. An elevated proinsulin level when the fasting glucose level is <45 mg/dL is sensitive and specific.

TREATMENT Insulinomas

Only 5–15% of insulinomas are malignant; therefore, after appropriate imaging (discussed later), surgery should be performed. In different studies, 75–100% of patients are cured by surgery. Before surgery, the hypoglycemia can be controlled by frequent small meals and the use of diazoxide (150–800 mg/d). Diazoxide is a benzothiadiazide whose hyperglycemic effect is attributed to inhibition of insulin release. Its side effects are sodium retention and GI symptoms such as nausea. Approximately 50–60% of patients respond to diazoxide. Other agents effective in some patients to control the hypoglycemia include verapamil and diphenylhydantoin. Long-acting somatostatin analogues such as octreotide and lanreotide are acutely effective in 40% of patients. However, octreotide must be used with care because it inhibits growth hormone secretion and can alter plasma glucagon levels; therefore, in some patients it can worsen the hypoglycemia.

For the 5–15% of patients with malignant insulinomas, these drugs or somatostatin analogues are used initially. In a small number of patients with insulinomas, some with malignant tumors, mammalian target of rapamycin (mTor) inhibitors (everolimus, rapamycin) are reported to control the hypoglycemia. If they are not effective, various antitumor treatments such as hepatic arterial embolization, chemoembolization, chemotherapy, and peptide receptor radiotherapy have been used (discussed later).

Insulinomas, which are usually benign (>90%) and intrapancreatic in location, are increasingly resected using a laparoscopic approach, which has lower morbidity rates. This approach requires that the insulinoma be localized on preoperative imaging studies.

GLUCAGONOMAS

A glucagonoma is an endocrine tumor of the pancreas that secretes excessive amounts of glucagon, which causes a distinct syndrome characterized by dermatitis, glucose intolerance or diabetes, and weight loss. Glucagonomas principally occur between 45 and 70 years of age. The tumor is clinically heralded by a characteristic dermatitis (migratory necrolytic erythema) (67–90%), accompanied by glucose intolerance (40–90%), weight loss (66–96%), anemia (33–85%), diarrhea (15–29%), and thromboembolism (11–24%).

The characteristic rash usually starts as an annular erythema at intertriginous and periorificial sites, especially in the groin or buttock. It subsequently becomes raised, and bullae form; when the bullae rupture, eroded areas form. The lesions can wax and wane. The development of a similar rash in patients receiving glucagon therapy suggests that the rash is a direct effect of the hyperglucagonemia. A characteristic laboratory finding is hypoaminoacidemia, which occurs in 26–100% of patients.

Glucagonomas are generally large tumors at diagnosis (5–10 cm). Some 50–80% occur in the pancreatic tail. From 50 to 82% have evidence of metastatic spread at presentation, usually to the liver. Glucagonomas are rarely extrapancreatic and usually occur singly.

Diagnosis

The diagnosis is confirmed by demonstrating an increased plasma glucagon level. Characteristically, plasma glucagon levels exceed 1000 pg/mL (normal is <150 pg/mL) in 90%; 7% are between 500 and 1000 pg/mL, and 3% are <500 pg/mL. A trend toward lower levels at diagnosis has been noted in the last decade. A plasma glucagon level >1000 pg/mL is considered diagnostic of glucagonoma. Other diseases causing increased plasma glucagon levels include renal insufficiency, acute pancreatitis, hypercorticism, hepatic insufficiency, severe stress, and prolonged fasting or familial hyperglucagonemia, as well as danazol treatment. With the exception of cirrhosis, these disorders do not increase plasma glucagon >500 pg/mL.

Necrolytic migratory erythema is not pathognomonic for glucagonoma and occurs in myeloproliferative disorders, hepatitis B infection, malnutrition, short-bowel syndrome, inflammatory bowel disease, and malabsorption disorders.

TREATMENT Glucagonomas

In 50–80% of patients, hepatic metastases are present, and so curative surgical resection is not possible. Surgical debulking in patients with advanced disease or other antitumor treatments may be beneficial (discussed later). Long-acting somatostatin analogues such as octreotide and lanreotide improve the skin rash in 75% of patients and may improve the weight loss, pain, and diarrhea but usually do not improve the glucose intolerance.

SOMATOSTATINOMA SYNDROME

The somatostatinoma syndrome is due to an NET that secretes excessive amounts of somatostatin, which causes a distinct syndrome characterized by diabetes mellitus, gallbladder disease, diarrhea, and steatorrhea. There is no general distinction in the literature between a tumor that contains somatostatin-like immunoreactivity (somatostatinoma) and does (11–45%) or does not (55–90%) produce a clinical syndrome (somatostatinoma syndrome) by secreting somatostatin. In a review of 173 cases of somatostatinomas, only 11% were associated with the somatostatinoma syndrome. The mean age is 51 years. Somatostatinomas occur primarily in the pancreas and small intestine, and the frequency of the symptoms and occurrence of the somatostatinoma syndrome differ in each. Each of the usual symptoms is more common in pancreatic than in intestinal somatostatinomas: diabetes mellitus (95% vs. 21%), gallbladder disease (94% vs. 43%), diarrhea (92% vs. 38%), steatorrhea (83% vs. 12%), hypochlorhydria (86% vs. 12%), and weight loss (90% vs. 69%). The somatostatinoma syndrome occurs in 30–90% of pancreatic and 0–5% of small-intestinal somatostatinomas. In various series 43% of all duodenal NETs contain somatostatin; however, the somatostatinoma syndrome is rarely present (<2%). Somatostatinomas occur in the pancreas in 56–74% of cases, with the primary location being the pancreatic head. The tumors are usually solitary (90%) and large (mean size 4.5 cm). Liver metastases are common, being present in 69–84% of patients. Somatostatinomas are rare in patients with MEN 1, occurring in only 0.65%.

Somatostatin is a tetradecapeptide that is widely distributed in the CNS and GI tract, where it functions as a neurotransmitter or has paracrine and autocrine actions. It is a potent inhibitor of many processes, including release of almost all hormones, acid secretion, intestinal and pancreatic secretion, and intestinal absorption. Most of the clinical manifestations are directly related to these inhibitory actions.

Diagnosis

In most cases somatostatinomas have been found by accident either at the time of cholecystectomy or during endoscopy. The presence of psammoma bodies in a duodenal tumor should particularly raise suspicion. Duodenal somatostatin-containing tumors are increasingly associated with von Recklinghausen's disease. Most of these tumors (>98%) do not cause the somatostatinoma syndrome. The diagnosis of the somatostatinoma syndrome requires the demonstration of elevated plasma somatostatin levels.

TREATMENT   Somatostatinomas

Pancreatic tumors are frequently (70–92%) metastatic at presentation, whereas 30–69% of small-intestinal somatostatinomas have metastases. Surgery is the treatment of choice for those without widespread hepatic metastases. Symptoms in patients with the somatostatinoma syndrome are also improved by octreotide treatment.

VIPOMAS

VIPomas are endocrine tumors that secrete excessive amounts of vasoactive intestinal peptide, which causes a distinct syndrome characterized by large-volume diarrhea, hypokalemia, and dehydration. This syndrome also is called Verner-Morrison syndrome, pancreatic cholera, and WDHA syndrome for *w*atery *d*iarrhea, *h*ypokalemia, and *a*chlorhydria, which some patients develop. The mean age of patients with this syndrome is 49 years; however, it can occur in children, and when it does, it is usually caused by a ganglioneuroma or ganglioneuroblastoma.

The principal symptoms are large-volume diarrhea (100%) severe enough to cause hypokalemia (80–100%), dehydration (83%), hypochlorhydria (54–76%), and flushing (20%). The diarrhea is secretory in nature, persisting during fasting, and is almost always >1 L/d and in 70% is >3 L/d. In a number of studies, the diarrhea was intermittent initially in up to half the patients. Most patients do not have accompanying steatorrhea (16%), and the increased stool volume is due to increased excretion of sodium and potassium, which, with the anions, accounts for the osmolality of the stool. Patients frequently have hyperglycemia (25–50%) and hypercalcemia (25–50%).

VIP is a 28-amino-acid peptide that is an important neurotransmitter, ubiquitously present in the CNS and GI tract. Its known actions include stimulation of small-intestinal chloride secretion as well as effects on smooth muscle contractility, inhibition of acid secretion, and vasodilatory effects, which explain most features of the clinical syndrome.

In adults 80–90% of VIPomas are pancreatic in location, with the rest due to VIP-secreting pheochromocytomas, intestinal carcinoids, and rarely ganglioneuromas. These tumors are usually solitary, 50–75% are in the pancreatic tail, and 37–68% have hepatic metastases at diagnosis. In children <10 years old, the syndrome is usually due to ganglioneuromas or ganglioblastomas and is less often malignant (10%).

Diagnosis

The diagnosis requires the demonstration of an elevated plasma VIP level and the presence of large-volume diarrhea. A stool volume <700 mL/d is proposed to exclude the diagnosis of VIPoma. When the patient fasts, a number of diseases can be excluded that can cause marked diarrhea. Other diseases that can produce a secretory large-volume diarrhea include gastrinomas, chronic laxative abuse, carcinoid syndrome, systemic mastocytosis, rarely medullary thyroid cancer, diabetic diarrhea, sprue, and AIDS. Among these conditions, only VIPomas caused a marked increase in plasma VIP. Chronic surreptitious use of laxatives/diuretics can be particularly difficult to detect clinically. Hence, in a patient with unexplained chronic diarrhea, screens for laxatives should be performed; they will detect many, but not all, laxative abusers.

TREATMENT Vasoactive Intestinal Peptidomas

The most important initial treatment in these patients is to correct their dehydration, hypokalemia, and electrolyte losses with fluid and electrolyte replacement. These patients may require 5 L/d of fluid and >350 meq/d of potassium. Because 37–68% of adults with VIPomas have metastatic disease in the liver at presentation, a significant number of patients cannot be cured surgically. In these patients long-acting somatostatin analogues such as octreotide and lanreotide are the drugs of choice.

Octreotide/lanreotide will control the diarrhea short- and long-term in 75–100% of patients. In nonresponsive patients the combination of glucocorticoids and octreotide/lanreotide has proved helpful in a small number of patients. Other drugs reported to be helpful in small numbers of patients include prednisone (60–100 mg/d), clonidine, indomethacin, phenothiazines, loperamide, lidamidine, lithium, propranolol, and metoclopramide. Treatment of advanced disease with embolization, chemoembolization, chemotherapy, radiotherapy, radiofrequency ablation, and peptide receptor radiotherapy may be helpful (discussed later).

NONFUNCTIONAL PANCREATIC ENDOCRINE TUMORS (NF-PETs)

NF-PETs are endocrine tumors that originate in the pancreas and secrete no products, or their products do not cause a specific clinical syndrome. The symptoms are due entirely to the tumor per se. NF-PETs secrete chromogranin A (90–100%), chromogranin B (90–100%), PP (58%), α-HCG (human chorionic gonadotropin) (40%), and β-HCG (20%). Because the symptoms are due to the tumor mass, patients with NF-PETs usually present late in the disease course with invasive tumors and hepatic metastases (64–92%) and the tumors are usually large (72% >5 cm). NF-PETs are usually solitary except in patients with MEN 1, in which case they are multiple. They occur primarily in the pancreatic head. Even though these tumors do not cause a functional syndrome, immunocytochemical studies show that they synthesize numerous peptides and cannot be distinguished from functional tumors by immunocytochemistry. In MEN 1, 80–100% of patients have

microscopic NF-PETs, but they become large or symptomatic in only a minority (0–13%) of cases. In VHL 12–17% develop NF-PETs, and in 4% they are ≥3 cm in diameter.

The most common symptoms are abdominal pain (30–80%), jaundice (20–35%), and weight loss, fatigue, or bleeding; 10–30% are found incidentally. The average time from the beginning of symptoms to diagnosis is 5 years.

Diagnosis

The diagnosis is established by histologic confirmation in a patient without either the clinical symptoms or the elevated plasma hormone levels of one of the established syndromes. The principal difficulty in diagnosis is to distinguish an NF-PET from a nonendocrine pancreatic tumor, which is more common. Even though chromogranin A levels are elevated in almost every patient, this is not specific for this disease as it can be found in functional PETs, carcinoids, and other neuroendocrine disorders. Plasma pancreatic polypeptide is increased in 22–71% of patients and should strongly suggest the diagnosis in a patient with a pancreatic mass because it is usually normal in patients with pancreatic adenocarcinomas. Elevated plasma PP is not diagnostic of this tumor because it is elevated in a number of other conditions, such as chronic renal failure, old age, inflammatory conditions, and diabetes. A positive somatostatin receptor scan in a patient with a pancreatic mass should suggest the presence of PET/NF-PET rather than a nonendocrine tumor.

TREATMENT Nonfunctional Pancreatic Endocrine Tumors

Overall survival in patients with sporadic NF-PET is 30–63% at 5 years, with a median survival of 6 years. Unfortunately, surgical curative resection can be considered only in a minority of these patients because 64–92% present with metastatic disease. Treatment needs to be directed against the tumor per se using the various modalities discussed later for advanced disease. The treatment of NF-PETs in either MEN 1 patients or patients with VHL is controversial. Most recommend surgical resection for any tumor >2–3 cm in diameter; however, there is no consensus on smaller NF-PETs, with most recommending careful surveillance of these patients.

GRFOMAS

GRFomas are endocrine tumors that secrete excessive amounts of growth hormone–releasing factor (GRF) that cause acromegaly. GRF is a 44-amino-acid peptide, and 25–44% of PETs have GRF immunoreactivity, although it is uncommonly secreted. GRFomas are lung tumors in 47–54% of cases, PETs in 29–30%, and small-intestinal carcinoids in 8–10%; up to 12% occur at other sites. Patients have a mean age of 38 years, and the symptoms usually are due to either acromegaly or the tumor per se. The acromegaly caused by GRFomas is indistinguishable from classic acromegaly. The pancreatic tumors are usually large (>6 cm), and liver metastases are present in 39%. They should be suspected in any patient with acromegaly and an abdominal tumor, a patient with MEN 1 with acromegaly, or a patient without a pituitary adenoma with acromegaly or associated with hyperprolactinemia, which occurs in 70% of GRFomas. GRFomas are an uncommon cause of acromegaly. GRFomas occur in <1% of MEN 1 patients. The diagnosis is established by performing plasma assays for GRF and growth hormone. Most GRFomas have a plasma GRF level >300 pg/mL (normal <5 pg/mL men, <10 pg/mL women). Patients with GRFomas also have increased plasma levels of insulin-like growth factor type I (IGF-I) levels similar to those in classic acromegaly. Surgery is the treatment of choice if diffuse metastases are not present. Long-acting somatostatin analogues such as octreotide and lanreotide are the agents of choice, with 75–100% of patients responding.

OTHER RARE PANCREATIC ENDOCRINE TUMOR SYNDROMES

Cushing's syndrome (ACTHoma) due to a PET occurs in 4–16% of all ectopic Cushing's syndrome cases. It occurs in 5% of cases of sporadic gastrinomas, almost invariably in patients with hepatic metastases, and is an independent poor prognostic factor. Paraneoplastic hypercalcemia due to PETs releasing parathyroid hormone–related peptide (PTHrP), a PTH-like material, or unknown factor, is rarely reported. The tumors are usually large, and liver metastases are usually present. Most (88%) appear to be due to release of PTHrP. PETs occasionally can cause the carcinoid syndrome. PETs secreting calcitonin have been proposed as a specific clinical syndrome. One-half of the patients have diarrhea, which disappears with resection of the tumor. The proposal that this could be a discrete syndrome is supported by the finding that 25–42% of patients with medullary thyroid cancer with hypercalcitonemia develop diarrhea, probably secondary to a motility disorder. This is classified in Table 52-2 as a possible specific disorder because so few cases have been described. Similarly classified with only a few cases described are a renin-producing PET in a patient presenting with hypertension; PETs secreting luteinizing hormone, resulting in masculinization or decreased libido; a PET-secreting erythropoietin resulting in polycythemia; and

PETs secreting insulin-like growth factor II causing hypoglycemia (Table 52-2). Ghrelin is a 28-amino-acid peptide with a number of metabolic functions. Even though it is detectable immunohistochemically in most PETs, no specific syndrome is associated with release of ghrelin by the PET.

TUMOR LOCALIZATION

Localization of the primary tumor and knowledge of the extent of the disease are essential to the proper management of all carcinoids and PETs. Without proper localization studies it is not possible to determine whether the patient is a candidate for curative resection or cytoreductive surgery or requires antitumor treatment or to predict the patient's prognosis reliably.

Numerous tumor localization methods are used in both types of NETs, including conventional imaging studies (computed tomographic scanning, magnetic resonance imaging, transabdominal ultrasound, selective angiography), somatostatin receptor scintigraphy (SRS), and positron emission tomographic scanning. In PETs, endoscopic ultrasound (EUS) and functional localization by measuring venous hormonal gradients are also reported to be useful. Bronchial carcinoids are usually detected by standard chest radiography and assessed by CT. Rectal, duodenal, colonic, and gastric carcinoids are usually detected by GI endoscopy.

PETs, as well as carcinoid tumors, frequently overexpress high-affinity somatostatin receptors in both their primary tumors and their metastases. Of the five types of somatostatin receptors (sst_{1-5}), radiolabeled octreotide binds with high affinity to sst_2 and sst_5, has a lower affinity for sst_3, and has a very low affinity for sst_1 and sst_4. Between 90 and 100% of carcinoid tumors and PETs possess sst_2, and many also have the other four sst subtypes. Interaction with these receptors can be used to localize NETs by using [^{111}In-DTPA-D-Phe^1] octreotide and radionuclide scanning (SRS) as well as for treatment of the hormone-excess state with octreotide or lanreotide, as discussed earlier. Because of its sensitivity and ability to localize tumor throughout the body, SRS is the initial imaging modality of choice for localizing both the primary and metastatic NETs. SRS localizes tumor in 73–89% of patients with carcinoids and in 56–100% of patients with PETs, except insulinomas. Insulinomas are usually small and have low densities of sst receptors, resulting in SRS being positive in only 12–50% of patients with insulinomas. **Figure 52-3** shows an example of the increased sensitivity of SRS in a patient with a carcinoid tumor. The CT scan showed a single liver metastasis, whereas the SRS demonstrated three metastases in the liver in multiple locations. Occasional false-positive responses with SRS can occur (12% in one study) because numerous other normal tissues

CT Scan

FIGURE 52-3

Ability of CT scanning (*top*) or somatostatin receptor scintigraphy (SRS) (*bottom*) to localize metastatic carcinoid in the liver.

as well as diseases can have high densities of sst receptors, including granulomas (sarcoid, tuberculosis, etc.), thyroid diseases (goiter, thyroiditis), and activated lymphocytes (lymphomas, wound infections). For PETs in the pancreas, EUS is highly sensitive, localizing 77–100% of insulinomas, which occur almost exclusively within the pancreas. Endoscopic ultrasound is less sensitive for extrapancreatic tumors. It is increasingly used in patients with MEN 1 and to a lesser extent VHL to detect small PETs not seen with other modalities or for serial PET assessments to determine size changes or rapid growth in patients in whom surgery is deferred. EUS with cytologic evaluation also is used frequently to distinguish an NF-PET from a pancreatic adenocarcinoma or another nonendocrine pancreatic tumor.

Insulinomas overexpress receptors for GLP-1; a radiolabeled GLP-1 analogue can detect occult insulinomas not localized by other imaging modalities. Functional localization by measuring hormonal gradients is now uncommonly used with gastrinomas (after

intraarterial secretin injections) but is still frequently used in insulinoma patients in whom other imaging studies are negative (assessing hepatic vein insulin concentrations post-intraarterial calcium injections). The intraarterial calcium test may also allow differentiation of the cause of the hypoglycemia and indicate whether it is due to an insulinoma or a nesidioblastosis. The latter entity is becoming increasingly important because hypoglycemia after gastric bypass surgery for obesity is increasing in frequency, and it is primarily due to nesidioblastosis, although it can occasionally be due to an insulinoma.

If liver metastases are identified by SRS, to plan the proper treatment either a CT or an MRI is recommended to assess the size and exact location of the metastases because SRS does not provide information on tumor size. Functional localization measuring hormone gradients after intraarterial calcium injections in insulinomas (insulin) or gastrin gradients after secretin injections in gastrinoma is a sensitive method, being positive in 80–100% of patients. However, this method provides only regional localization and therefore is reserved for cases in which the other imaging modalities are negative.

Two newer imaging modalities (positron emission tomography and use of hybrid scanners such as CT and SRS) may have increased sensitivity. Positron emission tomographic scanning with ^{18}F-fluoro-DOPA in patients with carcinoids or with ^{11}C-5-HTP or ^{68}gallium-labeled somatostatin analogues in patients with PETs or carcinoids has greater sensitivity than conventional imaging studies or SRS and probably will be used increasingly in the future. Positron emission tomographic scanning for GI NETs is not currently approved in the United States.

TREATMENT | **Advanced Disease (Diffuse Metastatic Disease)**

The single most important prognostic factor for survival is the presence of liver metastases (Fig. 52-4). For patients with foregut carcinoids without hepatic metastases, the 5-year survival in one study was 95%, and with distant metastases, it was 20% (Fig. 52-4, bottom). With gastrinomas the 5-year survival without liver metastases is 98%; with limited metastases in one hepatic lobe, it is 78%; and with diffuse metastases, 16% (Fig. 52-4, top). In a large study of 156 patients (67 PETs, rest carcinoids) the overall 5-year survival rate was 77%; it was 96% without liver metastases, 73% with liver metastases, and 50% with distant disease. Therefore, treatment for advanced metastatic disease is an important challenge. A number of different modalities are reported to be effective, including cytoreductive

FIGURE 52-4

Effect of the presence and extent of liver metastases on survival in patients with gastrinomas **(A)** or carcinoid tumors **(B)**. ZES, Zollinger-Ellison syndrome. (*Top panel is drawn from data from 199 patients with gastrinomas modified from F Yu et al: J Clin Oncol 17:615, 1999. Bottom panel is drawn from data from 71 patients with foregut carcinoid tumors from EW McDermott et al: Br J Surg 81:1007, 1994.*)

surgery (surgically or by radio frequency ablation [RFA]), treatment with chemotherapy, somatostatin analogues, interferon α, hepatic embolization alone or with chemotherapy (chemoembolization), radiotherapy with radiolabeled beads/microspheres, peptide radio-receptor therapy, and liver transplantation.

SPECIFIC ANTITUMOR TREATMENTS Cytoreductive surgery, unfortunately, is possible in only 9–22% of patients who present with limited hepatic metastases. Although no randomized studies have proved that it extends life, results from a number of studies suggest that it probably increases survival; therefore, it is recommended, if possible. Radio frequency thermal ablation can be applied to GI NET liver metastases if they are limited in number (usually <5) and size (usually <3.5 cm in diameter). Response rates

are >80%, the morbidity rate is low, and this procedure may be particularly helpful in patients with functional PETs that are difficult to control medically.

Chemotherapy for metastatic carcinoid tumors has generally been disappointing, with response rates of 0–40% with various two- and three-drug combinations. Chemotherapy for PETs has been more successful, with tumor shrinkage reported in 30–70% of patients. The current regimen of choice is streptozotocin and doxorubicin. In poorly differentiated PETs, chemotherapy with cisplatin, etoposide, or their derivatives is the recommended treatment, with response rates of 40–70%; however, responses are generally short-lived. Some newer combinations of chemotherapeutic agents show promise in small numbers of patients, including temozolomide (TMZ) alone, especially in PETs, which frequently have O^6-methylguanine DNA methyltransferase deficiency, which increases their TMZ sensitivity (34% response rate), and TMZ plus capecitabine (response rate 59–71%, retrospective studies).

Long-acting somatostatin analogues such as octreotide, lanreotide, and interferon α rarely decrease tumor size (i.e., 0–17%); however, these drugs have tumoristatic effects, stopping additional growth in 26–95% of patients with NETs. A randomized, double-blind study in patients with metastatic midgut carcinoids demonstrated a marked lengthening of time to progression (14.3 vs. 6 months, $p = .000072$) from the use of octreotide-LAR. This improvement was seen in patients with limited liver involvement. Whether this change will result in extended survival has not been proved. Somatostatin analogues can induce apoptosis in carcinoid tumors, and interferon α can decrease Bcl-2 protein expression, which probably contributes to its antiproliferative effects.

Hepatic embolization and chemoembolization (with dacarbazine, cisplatin, doxorubicin, 5-fluorouracil, or streptozotocin) have been reported to decrease tumor bulk and help control the symptoms of the hormone-excess state. These modalities generally are reserved for liver-directed therapy in cases in which treatment with somatostatin analogues, interferon (carcinoids), or chemotherapy (PETs) fails. Embolization, when combined with treatment with octreotide and interferon α, significantly reduces tumor progression ($p = .008$) compared with treatment with embolization and octreotide alone in patients with advanced midgut carcinoids.

Radiotherapy with radiolabeled somatostatin analogues that are internalized by the tumors is being investigated. Three different radionuclides are being used. High doses of [^{111}In-DTPA-D-Phe^1]octreotide, which emits γ-rays, internal conversion, and Auger electrons; yttrium-90, which emits high-energy β-particles coupled by a DOTA chelating group to octreotide or octreotate; and [177]lutetium-coupled analogues, which emit both, are all in clinical studies. [111]Indium-, [90]yttrium-, and [177]lutetium-labeled compounds caused tumor stabilization in 41–81%, 44–88%, and 23–40%, respectively, and a decrease in tumor size in 8–30%, 6–37%, and 38%, respectively, of patients with advanced metastatic NETs. Use of ^{177}Lu-labeled analogues to treat 504 patients with malignant NETs produced a reduction of tumor size of >50% in 30% of patients (2% complete) and tumor stabilization in 51%. An effect on survival has not been established. These results suggest that this novel therapy may be helpful, especially in patients with widespread metastatic disease.

Selective internal radiation therapy (SIRT) using [90]yttrium glass or resin microspheres is being evaluated in patients with unresectable NET liver metastases. The treatment requires careful evaluation for vascular shunting before treatment and generally is reserved for patients without extrahepatic metastatic disease and with adequate hepatic reserve. The ^{90}Y-microspheres are delivered to the liver by intraarterial injection from percutaneous placed catheters. In four studies involving metastatic NETs, the response rate varied from 50–61% (partial or complete), tumor stabilization occurred in 22–41%, and overall survival varied from 25–70 months. In the largest study (148 patients), no radiation-induced liver failure occurred and the most common side effect was fatigue (6.5%).

The use of liver transplantation has been abandoned for treatment of most metastatic tumors to the liver. However, for metastatic NETs, it is still a consideration. In a review of 103 cases of malignant NETs (48 PETs, 43 carcinoids) the 2- and 5-year survival rates were 60% and 47%, respectively. However, recurrence-free survival was low (<24%). For younger patients with metastatic NETs limited to the liver, liver transplantation may be justified.

Newer approaches show some promise in the treatment of advanced GI NETs. They include the use of growth factor inhibitors or inhibitors of their receptors (using tyrosine kinase inhibitors, monoclonal antibodies), inhibitors of mTor signaling (everolimus, temsirolimus), angiogenesis inhibitors, and VEGF or vascular endothelial growth factor receptor (VEGFR) tyrosine kinase inhibitors. A number of these agents, particularly sunitinib (tyrosine kinase inhibitor), various mTor inhibitors, and bevacizumub (monoclonal antibody against VEGF), show impressive activity. Additional value may result from selected combinations of agents.

SECTION X

NUTRITION

CHAPTER 53

NUTRIENT REQUIREMENTS AND DIETARY ASSESSMENT

Johanna Dwyer

Nutrients are substances that are not synthesized in sufficient amounts in the body and therefore must be supplied by the diet. Nutrient requirements for groups of healthy persons have been determined experimentally. For good health, we require energy-providing nutrients (protein, fat, and carbohydrate), vitamins, minerals, and water. Human requirements for organic nutrients include 9 essential amino acids, several fatty acids, glucose, 4 fat-soluble vitamins, 10 water-soluble vitamins, dietary fiber, and choline. Several inorganic substances, including 4 minerals, 7 trace minerals, 3 electrolytes, and the ultra trace elements, must also be supplied by diet.

The required amounts of the essential nutrients differ by age and physiologic state. Conditionally essential nutrients are not required in the diet but must be supplied to individuals who do not synthesize them in adequate amounts, such as those with genetic defects, those having pathologic states with nutritional implications, and developmentally immature infants. Many other organic and inorganic compounds present in foods have health effects. For example, lead and pesticide residues may have toxic effects.

ESSENTIAL NUTRIENT REQUIREMENTS

ENERGY

For weight to remain stable, energy intake must match energy output. The major components of energy output are resting energy expenditure (REE) and physical activity; minor sources include the energy cost of metabolizing food (thermic effect of food or specific dynamic action) and shivering thermogenesis (e.g., cold-induced thermogenesis). The average energy intake is about 2600 kcal/d for American men and about 1900 kcal/d for American women, though these estimates vary with body size and activity level. Formulas for estimating

REE are useful for assessing the energy needs of an individual whose weight is stable. Thus, for males, REE = 900 + 10m, and for females, REE = 700 + 7m, where m is mass in kilograms. The calculated REE is then adjusted for physical activity level by multiplying by 1.2 for sedentary, 1.4 for moderately active, or 1.8 for very active individuals. The final figure provides an estimate of total caloric needs in a state of energy balance. For further discussion of energy balance in health and disease, see Chap. 55.

PROTEIN

Dietary protein consists of both essential and nonessential amino acids that are required for protein synthesis. The nine essential amino acids are histidine, isoleucine, leucine, lysine, methionine/cystine, phenylalanine/tyrosine, threonine, tryptophan, and valine. Certain amino acids, such as alanine, can also be used for energy and gluconeogenesis. When energy intake is inadequate, protein intake must be increased, because ingested amino acids are diverted into pathways of glucose synthesis and oxidation. In extreme energy deprivation, protein–calorie malnutrition may ensue (Chap. 55).

For adults, the recommended dietary allowance (RDA) for protein is about 0.6 g/kg desirable body mass per day, assuming that energy needs are met and that the protein is of relatively high biologic value. Current recommendations for a healthy diet call for at least 10 to 14% of calories from protein. Most American diets provide at least those amounts. Biologic value tends to be highest for animal proteins, followed by proteins from legumes (beans), cereals (rice, wheat, corn), and roots. Combinations of plant proteins that complement one another in biologic value, or combinations of animal and plant proteins, can increase biologic value and lower total protein requirements.

Protein needs increase during growth, pregnancy, lactation, and rehabilitation after injury or malnutrition. Tolerance to dietary protein is decreased in renal insufficiency (causing uremia) and in liver failure. Normal protein intake can precipitate encephalopathy in patients with cirrhosis of the liver.

FAT AND CARBOHYDRATE

Fats are a concentrated source of energy and constitute, on average, 34% of calories in U.S. diets. However, for optimal health, fat intake should total no more than 30% of calories. Saturated fat and trans-fat should be limited to <10% of calories, and polyunsaturated fats to <10% of calories, with monounsaturated fats comprising the remainder of fat intake. At least 45–55% of total calories should be derived from carbohydrates. The brain requires about 100 g/d of glucose for fuel; other tissues use about 50 g/d. Some tissues (e.g., brain and red blood cells) rely on glucose supplied either exogenously or from muscle proteolysis. Over time, adaptations in carbohydrate needs are possible during hypocaloric states.

WATER

For adults, 1 to 1.5 mL water per kcal of energy expenditure is sufficient under usual conditions to allow for normal variations in physical activity, sweating, and solute load of the diet. Water losses include 50 to 100 mL/d in the feces; 500 to 1000 mL/d by evaporation or exhalation; and, depending on the renal solute load, ≥1000 mL/d in the urine. If external losses increase, intakes must increase accordingly to avoid underhydration. Fever increases water losses by approximately 200 mL/d per °C; diarrheal losses vary, but may be as great as 5 L/d in severe diarrhea. Heavy sweating and vomiting also increase water losses. When renal function is normal and solute intakes are adequate, the kidneys can adjust to increased water intake by excreting up to 18 L/d of excess water. However, obligatory urine outputs can compromise hydration status when there is inadequate intake or when losses increase in disease or kidney damage.

Infants have high requirements for water because of their large ratio of surface area to volume, the limited capacity of the immature kidney to handle high renal solute loads, and their inability to communicate their thirst. Increased water needs during pregnancy are about 30 mL/d. During lactation, milk production increases water requirements so that approximately 1000 mL/d of additional water is needed, or 1 mL for each mL of milk produced. Special attention must be paid to the water needs of the elderly, who have reduced total body water and blunted thirst sensation, and are more likely to be taking medications such as diuretics.

OTHER NUTRIENTS

See Chap. 54 for detailed descriptions of vitamins and trace minerals.

DIETARY REFERENCE INTAKES AND RECOMMENDED DIETARY ALLOWANCES

Fortunately, human life and well-being can be maintained within a fairly wide range for most nutrients. However, the capacity for adaptation is not infinite—too much, as well as too little, intake of a nutrient could have adverse effects or alter the health benefits conferred by another nutrient. Therefore, benchmark recommendations regarding nutrient intakes have been developed to guide clinical practice. These quantitative estimates of nutrient intakes are collectively referred to as the *dietary reference intakes* (DRIs). The DRIs supplant the *recommended daily allowances* (RDAs), the single reference values used in the United States until the early 1990s. DRIs include the *estimated average requirement* (EAR) for nutrients as well as other reference values used for dietary planning for individuals: the RDA, the *adequate intake* (AI), and the tolerable *upper level* (UL). The DRI also include acceptable macronutrient distribution ranges (AMDR) for protein, fat, and carbohydrate. The current DRIs for vitamins and elements are provided in **Tables 53-1** and **53-2**, respectively.

ESTIMATED AVERAGE REQUIREMENT

When florid manifestations of the classic dietary deficiency diseases such as rickets (deficiency of vitamin D and calcium), scurvy (deficiency of vitamin C), xerophthalmia (deficiency of vitamin A), and protein-calorie malnutrition were common, nutrient adequacy was inferred from the absence of their clinical signs. Later, biochemical and other changes were found to be evident long before the clinical deficiency became apparent. Consequently, criteria of adequacy are now based on biologic markers when they are available. Current efforts focus on the amount of a nutrient that reduces the risk of chronic degenerative diseases. Priority is given to sensitive biochemical, physiologic, or behavioral tests that reflect early changes in regulatory processes; maintenance of body stores of nutrients; or, if available, the amount of a nutrient that minimizes risk of chronic degenerative disease.

The EAR is the amount of a nutrient estimated to be adequate for half of the healthy individuals of a specific age and sex. The types of evidence and criteria used to establish nutrient requirements vary by nutrient, age, and physiologic group. The EAR is not an effective estimate of nutrient adequacy in individuals because it

DIETARY REFERENCE INTAKES: RECOMMENDED INTAKES FOR INDIVIDUALS—VITAMINS

| LIFE-STAGE GROUP | VITAMIN, µg/d | | | | | THIAMINE, mg/d | RIBOFLAVIN, mg/d | NIACIN, mg/d[e] | VITAMIN B6, mg/d | FOLATE, µg/d[f] | VITAMIN B12, µg/d | PANTOTHENIC ACID, mg/d | BIOTIN, µg/d | CHOLINE, mg/d[g] |
	A[a]	C	D[b,c]	E[d]	K									
Infants														
0–6 mo	400	40	5	4	2.0	0.2	0.3	2	0.1	65	0.4	1.7	5	125
7–12 mo	500	50	5	5	2.5	0.3	0.4	4	0.3	80	0.5	1.8	6	150
Children														
1–3 y	300	15	5	6	30	0.5	0.5	6	0.5	150	0.9	2	8	200
4–8 y	400	25	5	7	55	0.6	0.6	8	0.6	200	1.2	3	12	250
Males														
9–13 y	600	45	5	11	60	0.9	0.9	12	1.0	300	1.8	4	20	375
14–18 y	900	75	5	15	75	1.2	1.3	16	1.3	400	2.4	5	25	550
19–30 y	900	90	5	15	120	1.2	1.3	16	1.3	400	2.4	5	30	550
31–50 y	900	90	5	15	120	1.2	1.3	16	1.3	400	2.4	5	30	550
51–70 y	900	90	10	15	120	1.2	1.3	16	1.7	400	2.4[h]	5	30	550
>70 y	900	90	15	15	120	1.2	1.3	16	1.7	400	2.4[h]	5	30	550
Females														
9–13 y	600	45	5	11	60	0.9	0.9	12	1.0	300	1.8	4	20	375
14–18 y	700	65	5	15	75	1.0	1.0	14	1.2	400[i]	2.4	5	25	400
19–30 y	700	75	5	15	90	1.1	1.1	14	1.3	400[i]	2.4	5	30	425
31–50 y	700	75	5	15	90	1.1	1.1	14	1.3	400[i]	2.4	5	30	425
51–70 y	700	75	10	15	90	1.1	1.1	14	1.5	400	2.4[h]	5	30	425
>70 y	700	75	15	15	90	1.1	1.1	14	1.5	400	2.4[h]	5	30	425
Pregnancy														
≤18 y	750	80	5	15	75	1.4	1.4	18	1.6	600[j]	2.6	6	30	450
19–30 y	770	85	5	15	90	1.4	1.4	18	1.9	600[j]	2.6	6	30	450
31–50 y	770	85	5	15	90	1.4	1.4	18	1.9	600[j]	2.6	6	30	450

Lactation													
≤18 y	**1200**	**115**	5	19	**75**	**1.4**	**1.6**	**17**	**2.0**	**500**	**2.8**	7	35	550
19–30 y	**1300**	**120**	5	19	**90**	**1.4**	**1.6**	**17**	**2.0**	**500**	**2.8**	7	35	550
31–50 y	**1300**	**120**	5	19	**90**	**1.4**	**1.6**	**17**	**2.0**	**500**	**2.8**	7	35	550

Note: This table presents recommended dietary allowances (RDAs) in **bold type** and adequate intakes (AIs) in ordinary type. RDAs and AIs may both be used as goals for individual intake. RDAs are set to meet the needs of almost all individuals (97–98%) in a group. For healthy breastfed infants, the AI is the mean intake. The AI for other life stage and gender groups is believed to cover needs of all individuals in the group, but lack of data or uncertainty in the data prevent being able to specify with confidence the percentage of individuals covered by this intake.

[a]As retinol activity equivalents (RAEs). 1 RAE = 1 μg retinol, 12 μg β-carotene, 24 μg α-carotene, or 24 μg β-cryptoxanthin. To calculate RAEs from retinol equivalents (REs) of provitamin A carotenoids in foods, divide the REs by 2. For preformed vitamin A in foods or supplements and for provitamin A carotenoids in supplements, 1 RE = 1 RAE.

[b]As calciferol. 1 μg calciferol = 40 IU vitamin D.

[c]In the absence of adequate exposure to sunlight.

[d]As α-tocopherol. α-Tocopherol includes *RRR*-α-tocopherol, the only form of α-tocopherol that occurs naturally in foods, and the *2R*-stereoisomeric forms of α-tocopherol (*RRR*-, *RSR*-, *RSR*-, *RRS*-, and *RSS*-α-tocopherol) that occur in fortified foods and supplements. It does not include the 2S-stereoisomeric forms of α-tocopherol (*SRR*-, *SSR*-, *SRS*-, and *SSS*-α-tocopherol), also found in fortified foods and supplements.

[e]As niacin equivalents (NE). 1 mg of niacin = 60 mg of tryptophan; 0–6 months = preformed niacin (not NE).

[f]As dietary folate equivalents (DFEs). 1 DFE = 1 μg food folate = 0.6 μg of folic acid from fortified food or as a supplement consumed with food = 0.5 μg of a supplement taken on an empty stomach.

[g]Although AIs have been set for choline, there are few data to assess whether a dietary supply of choline is needed at all stages of the life cycle, and it may be that the choline requirement can be met by endogenous synthesis at some of these stages.

[h]Because 10 to 30% of older people may malabsorb food-bound B₁₂, it is advisable for those >50 years to meet their RDA mainly by consuming foods fortified with B₁₂ or a supplement containing B₁₂.

[i]In view of evidence linking inadequate folate intake with neural tube defects in the fetus, it is recommended that all women capable of becoming pregnant consume 400 μg from supplements or fortified foods in addition to intake of food folate from a varied diet.

[j]It is assumed that women will continue consuming 400 μg from supplements or fortified food until their pregnancy is confirmed and they enter prenatal care, which ordinarily occurs after the end of the periconceptional period—the critical time for formation of the neural tube.

Source: Food and Nutrition Board, Institute of Medicine—National Academy of Sciences Dietary Reference Intakes, 2000, 2002, reprinted with permission. Courtesy of the National Academy Press, Washington, DC. *http://www.nap.edu.*

TABLE 53-2

DIETARY REFERENCE INTAKES: RECOMMENDED INTAKES FOR INDIVIDUALS—ELEMENTS

LIFE-STAGE GROUP	CALCIUM, mg/d	CHROMIUM, µg/d	COPPER, µg/d	FLUORIDE, mg/d	IODINE, µg/d	IRON, mg/d	MAGNESIUM, mg/d	MANGANESE, mg/d	MOLYBDENUM, µg/d	PHOSPHORUS, mg/d	SELENIUM, µg/d	ZINC, mg/d
Infants												
0–6 mo	210	0.2	200	0.01	110	0.27	30	0.003	2	100	15	2
7–12 mo	270	5.5	220	0.5	130	11	75	0.6	3	275	20	3
Children												
1–3 y	500	11	340	0.7	90	7	80	1.2	17	460	20	3
4–8 y	800	15	440	1	90	10	130	1.5	22	500	30	5
Males												
9–13 y	1300	25	700	2	120	8	240	1.9	34	1250	40	8
14–18 y	1300	35	890	3	150	11	410	2.2	43	1250	55	11
19–30 y	1000	35	900	4	150	8	400	2.3	45	700	55	11
31–50 y	1000	35	900	4	150	8	420	2.3	45	700	55	11
51–70 y	1200	30	900	4	150	8	420	2.3	45	700	55	11
>70 y	1200	30	900	4	150	8	420	2.3	45	700	55	11
Females												
9–13 y	1300	21	700	2	120	8	240	1.6	34	1250	40	8
14–18 y	1300	24	890	3	150	15	360	1.6	43	1250	55	9
19–30 y	1000	25	900	3	150	18	310	1.8	45	700	55	8
31–50 y	1000	25	900	3	150	18	320	1.8	45	700	55	8
51–70 y	1200	20	900	3	150	8	320	1.8	45	700	55	8
>70 y	1200	20	900	3	150	8	320	1.8	45	700	55	8
Pregnancy												
≤18 y	1300	29	1000	3	220	27	400	2.0	50	1250	60	12
19–30 y	1000	30	1000	3	220	27	350	2.0	50	700	60	11
31–50 y	1000	30	1000	3	220	27	360	2.0	50	700	60	11
Lactation												
≤18 y	1300	44	1300	3	290	10	360	2.6	50	1250	70	13
19–30 y	1000	45	1300	3	290	9	310	2.6	50	700	70	12
31–50 y	1000	45	1300	3	290	9	320	2.6	50	700	70	12

Note: This table presents recommended dietary allowances (RDAs) in **bold type** and adequate intakes (AIs) in ordinary type. RDAs and AIs may both be used as goals for individual intake. RDAs are set to meet the needs of almost all individuals (97–98%) in a group. For healthy breastfed infants, the AI is the mean intake. The AI for other life stage and gender groups is believed to cover needs of all individuals in the group, but lack of data or uncertainty in the data prevent being able to specify with confidence the percentage of individuals covered by this intake.

Source: Food and Nutrition Board, Institute of Medicine—National Academy of Sciences Dietary Reference Intakes, 2000, 2002, reprinted with permission. Courtesy of the National Academy Press, Washington, DC. *http://www.nap.edu.*

is a median requirement for a group; 50% of individuals in a group fall below the requirement and 50% fall above it. Thus, a person with a usual intake at the EAR has a 50% risk of an inadequate intake. For these reasons, other standards, described later, are more useful for clinical purposes.

RECOMMENDED DIETARY ALLOWANCES

The RDA is the average daily dietary intake level that meets the nutrient requirements of nearly all healthy persons of a specific sex, age, life stage, or physiologic condition (such as pregnancy or lactation). The RDA is the nutrient-intake goal for planning diets of individuals.

The RDA is defined statistically as two standard deviations (SD) above the EAR to ensure that the needs of any given individual are met. Recommendations for individuals of a given age, sex, and weight are easily obtained from a Web-based calculator at *http://fnic.nal.usda.gov/interactiveDRI/*. This online tool allows health professionals to calculate daily nutrient recommendations for dietary planning based on the DRIs for individuals.

The RDAs are used to formulate food guides such as the U.S. Department of Agriculture (USDA) Food Guide Pyramid for individuals, to create food-exchange lists for therapeutic diet planning, and as a standard for describing the nutritional content of processed foods and nutrient-containing dietary supplements. The nutrient content in a food is stated by weight or as a percent of the daily value (DV), a variant of the RDA used in food labeling on the nutrition facts panel that, for an adult, represents the highest RDA for an adult consuming 2000 kcal/d.

The risk of dietary inadequacy increases as intake falls below the RDA. However, the RDA is an overly generous criterion for evaluating nutrient adequacy. For example, by definition the RDA exceeds the actual requirements of all but about 2 to 3% of the population. Therefore, many people whose intake falls below the RDA may still be getting enough of the nutrient.

ADEQUATE INTAKE

It is not possible to set an RDA for some nutrients that do not have an established EAR. In this circumstance, the AI is based on observed, or experimentally determined, approximations of nutrient intakes in healthy people. In the DRIs, AIs rather than RDAs are proposed for infants up to age 1 year, as well as for calcium, chromium, vitamin D, fluoride, manganese, pantothenic acid, biotin, and choline for persons of all ages. Vitamin D and calcium are currently being reevaluated, and more precise values may be available in the near future.

TOLERABLE UPPER LEVELS OF NUTRIENT INTAKE

Excessive nutrient intake can disturb body functions and cause acute, progressive, or permanent disabilities. The tolerable UL is the highest level of chronic nutrient intake (usually daily) that is unlikely to pose a risk of adverse health effects for most of the population. Data on the adverse effects of large amounts of many nutrients are unavailable or too limited to establish a UL. Therefore, the lack of a UL does *not* mean that the risk of adverse effects from high intake is nonexistent. Healthy individuals derive no established benefit from consuming nutrient levels above the RDA or AI. Nutrients in commonly eaten foods rarely exceed the UL. However, highly fortified foods and dietary supplements provide more concentrated amounts of nutrients per serving and, thus, pose a potential risk of toxicity. Nutrient supplements are labeled with supplement facts that express the amount of nutrient in absolute units or as the percent of the DV provided per recommended serving size. Total nutrient consumption, including foods; supplements; and over-the-counter medications, such as antacids, should not exceed RDA levels.

ACCEPTABLE MACRONUTRIENT DISTRIBUTION RANGES

The AMDR is a range of energy providing intakes that the Food and Nutrition Board considers to be healthful for macronutrients. These ranges are 10–35% calories for protein, 20–35% calories for fat, and 45–65% of calories for carbohydrate. Alcohol, which also provides energy, is not a nutrient and recommendations, therefore, are not provided for it.

FACTORS ALTERING NUTRIENT NEEDS

The DRIs are affected by age, sex, rate of growth, pregnancy, lactation, physical activity, concomitant diseases, drugs, and dietary composition. If requirements for nutrient sufficiency are close to levels indicating excess, dietary planning is difficult.

PHYSIOLOGIC FACTORS

Growth, strenuous physical activity, pregnancy, and lactation increase needs for energy and several essential nutrients. Energy needs rise during pregnancy due to the demands of fetal growth and during lactation because of the increased energy required for milk production. Energy needs decrease with loss of lean body mass, the major determinant of REE. Because both health and physical activity tend to decline with age, energy needs of older persons, especially those over 70, tend to be less than those of younger persons.

DIETARY COMPOSITION

Dietary composition affects the biologic availability and use of nutrients. For example, the absorption of iron may be impaired by high amounts of calcium or lead; also, non-heme iron uptake may be impaired by the lack of ascorbic acid and amino acids in the meal. Protein use by the body may be decreased when essential amino acids are not present in sufficient amounts. Animal foods, such as milk, eggs, and meat, have high biologic values with most of the needed amino acids present in adequate amounts. Plant proteins in corn (maize), soy, and wheat have lower biologic values and must be combined with other plant or animal proteins to achieve optimal use by the body.

ROUTE OF ADMINISTRATION

The RDAs apply only to oral intakes. When nutrients are administered parenterally, similar values can sometimes be used for amino acids, carbohydrates, fats, sodium, chloride, potassium, and most of the vitamins, because their intestinal absorption is nearly 100%. However, the oral bioavailability of most mineral elements may be only half that obtained by parenteral administration. For some nutrients that are not readily stored in the body or cannot be stored in large amounts, timing of administration may also be important. For example, amino acids cannot be used for protein synthesis if they are not supplied together; instead, they will be used for energy production.

DISEASE

Specific dietary deficiency diseases include: protein-calorie malnutrition; iron, iodine, and vitamin A deficiency; megaloblastic anemia due to vitamin B_{12} or folic acid deficiency; vitamin D–deficiency rickets and osteomalacia; and scurvy, beriberi, and pellagra (Chaps. 54 and 55). Each deficiency disease is characterized by imbalances at the cellular level between the supply of nutrients or energy and the body's nutritional needs for growth, maintenance, and other functions. Imbalances and excess in nutrient intakes are recognized as risk factors for certain chronic degenerative diseases, such as saturated fat and cholesterol in coronary artery disease; sodium in hypertension; obesity in hormone–dependent endometrial and breast cancers; and ethanol in alcoholism. Because the etiology and pathogenesis of these disorders are multifactorial, diet is only one of many risk factors. Osteoporosis, for example, is associated with calcium deficiency, as well as risk factors related to environment (e.g., smoking, sedentary lifestyle), physiology (e.g., estrogen

deficiency), genetic determinants (e.g., defects in collagen metabolism), and drug use (chronic steroids).

DIETARY ASSESSMENT

In clinical situations, nutritional assessment is an iterative process that involves: (1) screening for malnutrition, (2) assessing the diet and other data to establish either the absence or presence of malnutrition and its possible causes, (3) planning and implementing the most appropriate nutritional therapy, and (4) reassessing intakes to make sure that they were consumed. Some disease states affect the bioavailability, requirement, use, or excretion of specific nutrients. In these circumstances, specific measurements of various nutrients or their biomarkers may be required to ensure adequate replacement.

Most health care facilities have nutrition-screening processes in place for identifying possible malnutrition after hospital admission. Nutritional screening is required by the Joint Commission on Accreditation of Healthcare Organizations (JCAHO), but there are no universally recognized or validated standards. The factors that are usually assessed include: abnormal weight for height or body mass index (e.g., BMI <19 or >25); reported weight change (involuntary loss or gain of >5 kg in the past 6 months) (Chap. 10); diagnoses with known nutritional implications (metabolic disease, any disease affecting the gastrointestinal tract, alcoholism, and others); present therapeutic dietary prescription; chronic poor appetite; presence of chewing and swallowing problems or major food intolerances; need for assistance with preparing or shopping for food, eating, or other aspects of self-care; and social isolation. Reassessment of nutrition status should occur periodically in hospitalized patients—at least once every week.

A more complete dietary assessment is indicated for patients who exhibit a high risk of or frank malnutrition on nutrition screening. The type of assessment varies based on the clinical setting, severity of the patient's illness, and stability of his or her condition.

ACUTE CARE SETTINGS

In acute care settings, anorexia, various diseases, test procedures, and medications can compromise dietary intake. Under such circumstances, the goal is to identify and avoid inadequate intake and assure appropriate alimentation. Dietary assessment focuses on what patients are currently eating, whether or not they are able and willing to eat, and whether or not they experience any problems with eating. Dietary intake assessment is based on information from observed intakes; medical record; history; clinical examination; and anthropometric, biochemical, and functional status. The objective is to gather enough information to establish the likelihood of malnutrition due to poor dietary intake or other causes to assess whether nutritional therapy is indicated (Chap. 56).

Simple observations may suffice to suggest inadequate oral intake. These include dietitians' and nurses' notes, the amount of food eaten on trays, frequent tests and procedures that are likely to cause meals to be skipped, nutritionally inadequate diet orders such as clear liquids or full liquids for more than a few days, fever, gastrointestinal distress, vomiting, diarrhea, a comatose state, and diseases or treatments that involve any part of the alimentary tract. Acutely ill patients with diet-related diseases such as diabetes need assessment because an inappropriate diet may exacerbate these conditions and adversely affect other therapies. Abnormal biochemical values (serum albumin levels <35 g/L [<3.5 mg/dL]; serum cholesterol levels <3.9 mmol/L [<150 mg/dL]) are nonspecific but may also indicate a need for further nutritional assessment.

Most therapeutic diets offered in hospitals are calculated to meet individual nutrient requirements and the RDA *if they are eaten.* Exceptions include clear liquids, some full-liquid diets, and test diets (such as preparation for gastrointestinal procedures), which are inadequate for several nutrients and should not be used, if possible, for more than 24 h. As much as half of the food served to hospitalized patients is not eaten, and so it cannot be assumed that the intakes of hospitalized patients are adequate. Dietary assessment should compare how much and what food the patient has consumed with the diet that has been provided. Major deviations in intakes of energy, protein, fluids, or other nutrients of special concern for the patient's illness should be noted and corrected.

Nutritional monitoring is especially important for patients who are very ill and who have extended lengths of stay. Patients who are fed by special enteral and parenteral routes also require special nutritional assessment and monitoring by physicians and/or dietitians with certification in nutrition support (Chap. 56).

AMBULATORY SETTINGS

The aim of dietary assessment in the outpatient setting is to determine whether or not the patient's usual diet is a health risk in itself or if it contributes to existing chronic disease-related problems. Dietary assessment also provides the basis for planning a diet that fulfills therapeutic goals while ensuring patient adherence. The outpatient dietary assessment should review the adequacy of present and usual food intakes, including vitamin and mineral supplements, medications, and alcohol, because all of these may affect the patient's nutritional status. The assessment should focus on the dietary constituents that are most likely to be involved or compromised by a specific diagnosis, as well as any co morbidities that are present. More than one day's intake should be reviewed to provide a better representation of the usual diet.

There are many ways to assess the adequacy of the patient's habitual diet. These include a food guide, a food-exchange list, a diet history, or a food-frequency questionnaire. A commonly used food guide for healthy persons is the USDA's food pyramid, which is useful as a basis for identifying inadequate intakes of essential nutrients, as well as likely excesses in fat, saturated fat, sodium, sugar, and alcohol (Table 53-3). The Web version of the guide provides a calculator that tailors the number of servings

TABLE 53-3

MY PYRAMID: THE USDA FOOD GUIDE PYRAMID FOR HEALTHY PERSONS

SERVINGS AND EXAMPLES OF STANDARD PORTION SIZES	LOWER: 1600 kcal	MODERATE: 2200 kcal	HIGHER: 2800 kcal
Fruits, cups	1.5	2	2.5
Vegetables, cups	2	3	3.5
Grains, oz eq (1 slice bread, 1 cup ready to eat cereal, 0.5 cup cooked rice, pasta, cooked cereal)	5	7	10
Meat and beans, oz eq (1 oz lean meat, poultry, or fish; 1 egg, 1 Tbsp. peanut butter, 0.25 cup cooked dry beans, or 0.5 oz nuts or seeds)	5	6	7
Milk, cups (1 cup milk or yogurt, 1.5 oz natural or 2 oz processed cheese)	3	3	3
Oils, tsp	5	6	8
Discretionary calorie allowance, kcal (remaining calories after accounting for all of the above)	132	290	426

Abbreviation: oz eq, ounce equivalent.
Source: Data from United States Department of Agriculture. *http://www.MyPyramid.gov.*

suggested for healthy patients of different weights, sexes, ages, and life-cycle stages: *http://www.mypyramidtracker.gov/planner/launchpage.aspx*. Patients who follow ethnic or unusual dietary patterns may need extra instruction on how foods should be categorized, as well as the appropriate portion sizes that constitute a serving. The process of reviewing the guide with patients helps them transition to healthier dietary patterns and identifies food groups eaten in excess of recommendations or in insufficient quantities. For those on therapeutic diets, assessment against food-exchange lists may be useful. These include, for example, the American Diabetes Association food-exchange lists for diabetes or the American Dietetic Association food-exchange lists for renal disease.

NUTRITIONAL STATUS ASSESSMENT

Full nutritional status assessment is reserved for seriously ill patients and those at very high nutritional risk when the cause of malnutrition is still uncertain after initial clinical evaluation and dietary assessment. It involves multiple dimensions, including documentation of dietary intake, anthropometric measurements, biochemical measurements of blood and urine, clinical examination, health history, and functional status. Therapeutic dietary prescriptions and menu plans for most diseases are available from most hospitals and from the American Dietetic Association. For further discussion of nutritional assessment, see Chap. 55.

GLOBAL CONSIDERATIONS

The DRI such as the EAR, UL, and energy needs are estimates of physiologic requirements based on experimental evidence. Assuming appropriate adjustments are made for age, sex, body size, and physical activity level, they should be applicable to individuals in most parts of the world. However, the AI are based on customary and adequate intakes in U.S. and Canadian populations, which appear to be compatible with good health, rather than being based on a large body of direct experimental evidence. Similarly, the AMDR represent expert opinion of approximate intakes of energy providing nutrients that are healthful in these North American populations. As such, they should be used with caution in other settings. Nutrient-based standards like the DRI have also been developed by the World Health Organization/Food and Agricultural Organization of the United Nations (WHO/FAO) and are available at their Web site: *http://www.who.int/nutrition/topics/nutrecomm/en/index.html*. The different standards have many similarities in their basic concepts, definitions, and nutrient-recommendation levels, but there are some differences from the DRI, due to the functional criteria chosen, environmental differences, the timeliness of the evidence reviewed, and expert judgment.

CHAPTER 54

VITAMIN AND TRACE MINERAL DEFICIENCY AND EXCESS

Robert M. Russell ■ Paolo M. Suter

Vitamins and trace minerals are required constituents of the human diet since they are inadequately synthesized or not synthesized in the human body. Only small amounts of these substances are needed to carry out essential biochemical reactions (e.g., by acting as coenzymes or prosthetic groups). Overt vitamin or trace mineral deficiencies are rare in Western countries due to a plentiful, varied, and inexpensive food supply; however, multiple nutrient deficiencies may appear together in persons who are chronically ill or alcoholic. After gastric bypass surgery, patients are at high risk for multiple nutrient deficiencies. Moreover, subclinical vitamin and trace mineral deficiencies, as diagnosed by laboratory testing, are quite common in the normal population, especially in the geriatric age group.

 Victims of famine, emergency-affected and displaced populations, and refugees are at increased risk for protein-energy malnutrition and classic micronutrient deficiencies (vitamin A, iron, iodine) as well as for thiamine (beriberi), riboflavin, vitamin C (scurvy), and niacin (pellagra) overt deficiencies.

Body stores of vitamins and minerals vary tremendously. For example, vitamin B_{12} and vitamin A stores are large, and an adult may not become deficient for 1 or more years after being on a deficient diet. However, folate and thiamine may become depleted within weeks among those eating a deficient diet. Therapeutic modalities can deplete essential nutrients from the body; for example, hemodialysis removes water-soluble vitamins, which must be replaced by supplementation.

There are several roles for vitamins and trace minerals in diseases: (1) deficiencies of vitamins and minerals may be caused by disease states such as malabsorption; (2) both deficiency and excess of vitamins and minerals can cause disease in and of themselves (e.g., vitamin A intoxication and liver disease); and (3) vitamins and minerals in high doses may be used as drugs (e.g., niacin for

hypercholesterolemia). The hematologic-related vitamins and minerals either are not considered or are considered only briefly in this chapter, as are the bone-related vitamins and minerals (vitamin D, calcium, phosphorus, since they are covered elsewhere (Tables 54-1 and 54-2 and Fig. 54-1).

VITAMINS

THIAMINE (VITAMIN B₁)

Thiamine was the first B vitamin to be identified and therefore is referred to as vitamin B_1. Thiamine functions in the decarboxylation of α-ketoacids, such as pyruvate α-ketoglutarate, and branched-chain amino acids and thus is essential for energy generation. In addition, thiamine pyrophosphate acts as a coenzyme for a transketolase reaction that mediates the conversion of hexose and pentose phosphates. It has been postulated that thiamine plays a role in peripheral nerve conduction, although the exact chemical reactions underlying this function are not known.

Food sources

The median intake of thiamine in the United States from food alone is 2 mg/d. Primary food sources for thiamine include yeast, organ meat, pork, legumes, beef, whole grains, and nuts. Milled rice and grains contain little thiamine, if any. Thiamine deficiency is therefore more common in cultures that rely heavily on a rice-based diet. Tea, coffee (regular and decaffeinated), raw fish, and shellfish contain thiaminases, which can destroy the vitamin. Thus, drinking large amounts of tea or coffee can theoretically lower thiamine body stores.

TABLE 54-1

PRINCIPAL CLINICAL FINDINGS OF VITAMIN MALNUTRITION

NUTRIENT	CLINICAL FINDING	DIETARY LEVEL PER DAY ASSOCIATED WITH OVERT DEFICIENCY IN ADULTS	CONTRIBUTING FACTORS TO DEFICIENCY
Thiamine	Beriberi: neuropathy, muscle weakness and wasting, cardiomegaly, edema, ophthalmoplegia, confabulation	<0.3 mg/1000 kcal	Alcoholism, chronic diuretic use, hyperemesis
Riboflavin	Magenta tongue, angular stomatitis, seborrhea, cheilosis	<0.6 mg	—
Niacin	Pellagra: pigmented rash of sun-exposed areas, bright red tongue, diarrhea, apathy, memory loss, disorientation	<9.0 niacin equivalents	Alcoholism, vitamin B_6 deficiency, riboflavin deficiency, tryptophan deficiency
Vitamin B_6	Seborrhea, glossitis, convulsions, neuropathy, depression, confusion, microcytic anemia	<0.2 mg	Alcoholism, isoniazid
Folate	Megaloblastic anemia, atrophic glossitis, depression, ↑ homocysteine	<100 µg/d	Alcoholism, sulfasalazine, pyrimethamine, triamterene
Vitamin B_{12}	Megaloblastic anemia, loss of vibratory and position sense, abnormal gait, dementia, impotence, loss of bladder and bowel control, ↑ homocysteine, ↑ methylmalonic acid	<1.0 µg/d	Gastric atrophy (pernicious anemia), terminal ileal disease, strict vegetarianism, acid-reducing drugs (e.g., H_2 blockers)
Vitamin C	Scurvy: petechiae, ecchymosis, coiled hairs, inflamed and bleeding gums, joint effusion, poor wound healing, fatigue	<10 mg/d	Smoking, alcoholism
Vitamin A	Xerophthalmia, night blindness, Bitot's spots, follicular hyperkeratosis, impaired embryonic development, immune dysfunction	<300 µg/d	Fat malabsorption, infection, measles, alcoholism, protein-energy malnutrition
Vitamin D	Rickets: skeletal deformation, rachitic rosary, bowed legs; osteomalacia	<2.0 µg/d	Aging, lack of sunlight exposure, fat malabsorption, deeply pigmented skin
Vitamin E	Peripheral neuropathy, spinocerebellar ataxia, skeletal muscle atrophy, retinopathy	Not described unless underlying contributing factor is present	Occurs only with fat malabsorption or genetic abnormalities of vitamin E metabolism/transport
Vitamin K	Elevated prothrombin time, bleeding	<10 µg/d	Fat malabsorption, liver disease, antibiotic use

Deficiency

Most dietary deficiency of thiamine worldwide is the result of poor dietary intake. In Western countries, the primary causes of thiamine deficiency are alcoholism and chronic illnesses such as cancer. Alcohol interferes directly with the absorption of thiamine and with the synthesis of thiamine pyrophosphate. Thiamine should always be replenished when a patient with alcoholism is being refed, as carbohydrate repletion without adequate thiamine can precipitate acute thiamine deficiency with lactic acidosis. Other at-risk populations are women with prolonged hyperemesis gravidarum

and anorexia, patients with overall poor nutritional status on parenteral glucose, patients after bariatric bypass surgery, and patients on chronic diuretic therapy due to increased urinary thiamine losses. Maternal thiamine deficiency can lead to infantile beriberi in breast-fed children. Thiamine deficiency should be considered in the setting of motor vehicle accidents associated with head injury.

Thiamine deficiency in its early stage induces anorexia and nonspecific symptoms (e.g., irritability, decrease in short-term memory). Prolonged thiamine deficiency causes beriberi, which is classically categorized as wet or dry, although there is considerable overlap. In either

TABLE 54-2

DEFICIENCIES AND TOXICITIES OF METALS

ELEMENT	DEFICIENCY	TOXICITY	TOLERABLE UPPER (DIETARY) INTAKE LEVEL
Boron	No biologic function determined	Developmental defects, male sterility, testicular atrophy	20 mg/d (extrapolated from animal data)
Calcium	Reduced bone mass, osteoporosis	Renal insufficiency (milk-alkali syndrome), nephrolithiasis, impaired iron absorption	2500 mg/d (milk-alkali)
Copper	Anemia, growth retardation, defective keratinization and pigmentation of hair, hypothermia, degenerative changes in aortic elastin, osteopenia, mental deterioration	Nausea, vomiting, diarrhea, hepatic failure, tremor, mental deterioration, hemolytic anemia, renal dysfunction	10 mg/d (liver toxicity)
Chromium	Impaired glucose tolerance	Occupational: renal failure, dermatitis, pulmonary cancer	ND
Fluoride	↑ Dental caries	Dental and skeletal fluorosis, osteosclerosis	10 mg/d (fluorosis)
Iodine	Thyroid enlargement, ↓ T_4, cretinism	Thyroid dysfunction, acne-like eruptions	1100 µg/d (thyroid dysfunction)
Iron	Muscle abnormalities, koilonychia, pica, anemia, ↓ work performance, impaired cognitive development, premature labor, ↑ perinatal maternal mortality	Gastrointestinal effects (nausea, vomiting, diarrhea, constipation), iron overload with organ damage, acute systemic toxicity	45 mg/d of elemental iron (GI side effects)
Manganese	Impaired growth and skeletal development, reproduction, lipid and carbohydrate metabolism; upper body rash	General: neurotoxicity, Parkinson-like symptoms; occupational: encephalitis-like syndrome, Parkinson-like syndrome, psychosis, pneumoconiosis	11 mg/d (neurotoxicity)
Molybdenum	Severe neurologic abnormalities	Reproductive and fetal abnormalities	2 mg/d extrapolated from animal data
Selenium	Cardiomyopathy, heart failure, striated muscle degeneration	General: alopecia, nausea, vomiting, abnormal nails, emotional lability, peripheral neuropathy, lassitude, garlic odor to breath, dermatitis; occupational: lung and nasal carcinomas, liver necrosis, pulmonary inflammation	400 µg/d (hair, nail changes)
Phosphorus	Rickets (osteomalacia), proximal muscle weakness, rhabdomyolysis, paresthesia, ataxia, seizure, confusion, heart failure, hemolysis, acidosis	Hyperphosphatemia	4000 mg/d
Zinc	Growth retardation, ↓ taste and smell, alopecia, dermatitis, diarrhea, immune dysfunction, failure to thrive, gonadal atrophy, congenital malformations	General: reduced copper absorption, gastritis, sweating, fever, nausea, vomiting; occupational: respiratory distress, pulmonary fibrosis	40 mg/d (impaired copper metabolism)

Abbreviations: GI, gastrointestinal; ND, not determined.

form of beriberi, patients may complain of pain and paresthesia. *Wet beriberi* presents primarily with cardiovascular symptoms, due to impaired myocardial energy metabolism and dysautonomia, and can occur after 3 months of a thiamine-deficient diet. Patients present with an enlarged heart, tachycardia, high-output congestive heart failure, peripheral edema, and peripheral neuritis. Patients with *dry beriberi* present with a symmetric peripheral neuropathy of the motor and sensory systems with diminished reflexes. The neuropathy affects the legs most markedly, and these patients have difficulty rising from a squatting position.

Alcoholic patients with chronic thiamine deficiency also may have central nervous system (CNS) manifestations

Vitamin	Active derivative or cofactor form	Principal function
Thiamine (B₁)	Thiamine pyrophosphate	Coenzyme for cleavage of carbon-carbon bonds; amino acid and carbohydrate metabolism
Riboflavin (B₂)	Flavin mononucleotide (FMN) and flavin adenine dinucleotide (FAD)	Cofactor for oxidation, reduction reactions, and covalently attached prosthetic groups for some enzymes
Niacin	Nicotinamide adenine dinucleotide phosphate (NADP) and nicotinamide adenine dinucleotide (NAD)	Coenzymes for oxidation and reduction reactions
Vitamin B₆	Pyridoxal phosphate	Cofactor for enzymes of amino acid metabolism
Folate	Polyglutamate forms of (5, 6, 7, 8) tetrahydrofolate with carbon unit attachments	Coenzyme for one carbon transfer in nucleic acid and amino acid metabolism
Vitamin B₁₂	Methylcobalamine Adenosylcobalamin	Coenzyme for methionine synthase and L-methylmalonyl-CoA mutase

FIGURE 54-1
The structures and principal functions of vitamins associated with human disorders.

Vitamin	Active derivative or cofactor form	Principal function
Vitamin C $O=C-C=C-C-C-CH_2OH$ $\quad\ OH\ OH\quad OH$	Ascorbic acid and dehydroascorbic acid	Participation as a redox ion in many biologic oxidation and hydrogen transfer reactions
Vitamin A (β-Carotene) CH_2OH (Retinol)	Retinol, retinaldehyde, and retinoic acid	Formation of rhodopsin (vision) and glycoproteins (epithelial cell function); also regulates gene transcription
Vitamin D OH CH_2 $HO \quad OH$	1,25-Dihydroxyvitamin D	Maintenance of blood calcium and phosphorus levels; antiproliferative hormone
Vitamin E CH_3 $HO \quad CH_2[CH_2-CH_2-CH-CH_2]_3H$	Tocopherols and tocotrienols	Antioxidants
Vitamin K O R O	Vitamin K hydroquinone	Cofactor for posttranslation carboxylation of many proteins including essential clotting factors

FIGURE 54-1
(*Continued*)

known as *Wernicke's encephalopathy*, consisting of horizontal nystagmus, ophthalmoplegia (due to weakness of one or more extraocular muscles), cerebellar ataxia, and mental impairment. When there is an additional loss of memory and a confabulatory psychosis, the syndrome is known as *Wernicke-Korsakoff syndrome*. Despite the typical clinical picture and history, Wernicke-Korsakoff syndrome is underdiagnosed.

The laboratory diagnosis of thiamine deficiency usually is made by a functional enzymatic assay of transketolase activity measured before and after the addition of thiamine pyrophosphate. A >25% stimulation by the addition of thiamine pyrophosphate (an activity coefficient of 1.25) is interpreted as abnormal. Thiamine or the phosphorylated esters of thiamine in serum or blood also can be measured by high-performance liquid chromatography (HPLC) to detect deficiency.

TREATMENT Thiamine Deficiency

In acute thiamine deficiency with either cardiovascular or neurologic signs, 100 mg/d of thiamine should be given parenterally for 7 days, followed by 10 mg/d orally until there is complete recovery. Cardiovascular and ophthalmoplegic improvement occurs within 24 h. Other manifestations gradually clear, although psychosis in Wernicke-Korsakoff syndrome may be permanent or persist for several months.

Toxicity

Although anaphylaxis has been reported after high doses of thiamine, no adverse effects have been recorded from either food or supplements at high doses. Thiamine supplements may be bought over the counter in doses of up to 50 mg/d.

RIBOFLAVIN (VITAMIN B$_2$)

Riboflavin is important for the metabolism of fat, carbohydrate, and protein, reflecting its role as a respiratory coenzyme and an electron donor. Enzymes that contain flavin adenine dinucleotide (FAD) or flavin mononucleotide (FMN) as prosthetic groups are known as *flavoenzymes* (e.g., succinic acid dehydrogenase, monoamine oxidase, glutathione reductase). FAD is a cofactor for methyltetrahydrofolate reductase and therefore modulates homocysteine metabolism. The vitamin also plays a role in drug and steroid metabolism, including detoxification reactions.

Although much is known about the chemical and enzymatic reactions of riboflavin, the clinical manifestations of riboflavin deficiency are nonspecific and are similar to those of other deficiences of B vitamins. Riboflavin deficiency is manifested principally by lesions of the mucocutaneous surfaces of the mouth and skin (Table 54-1). In addition to the mucocutaneous lesions, corneal vascularization, anemia, and personality changes have been described with riboflavin deficiency.

Deficiency and excess

Riboflavin deficiency almost always is due to dietary deficiency. Milk, other dairy products, and enriched breads and cereals are the most important dietary sources of riboflavin in the United States, although lean meat, fish, eggs, broccoli, and legumes are also good sources. Riboflavin is extremely sensitive to light, and milk should be stored in containers that protect against photodegradation. Laboratory diagnosis of riboflavin deficiency can be made by measurement of red blood cell or urinary riboflavin concentrations or by measurement of erythrocyte glutathione reductase activity, with and without added FAD. Because the capacity of the gastrointestinal tract to absorb riboflavin is limited (~20 mg if given in one oral dose), riboflavin toxicity has not been described.

NIACIN (VITAMIN B$_3$)

The term *niacin* refers to nicotinic acid and nicotinamide and their biologically active derivatives. Nicotinic acid and nicotinamide serve as precursors of two coenzymes, nicotinamide adenine dinucleotide (NAD) and NAD phosphate (NADP), which are important in numerous oxidation and reduction reactions in the body. In addition, NAD and NADP are active in adenine diphosphate–ribose transfer reactions involved in DNA repair and calcium mobilization.

Metabolism and requirements

Nicotinic acid and nicotinamide are absorbed well from the stomach and small intestine. Niacin bioavailability is high from beans, milk, meat, and eggs; bioavailability from cereal grains is lower. Since flour is enriched with the "free" niacin (i.e., non-coenzyme form), bioavailability is excellent. Median intakes of niacin in the United States considerably exceed the recommended dietary allowance (RDA).

The amino acid tryptophan can be converted to niacin with an efficiency of 60:1 by weight. Thus, the RDA for niacin is expressed in niacin equivalents. A lower conversion of tryptophan to niacin occurs in vitamin B$_6$ and/or riboflavin deficiencies and in the presence of isoniazid. The urinary excretion products of niacin include 2-pyridone and 2-methyl nicotinamide, measurements of which are used in the diagnosis of niacin deficiency.

Deficiency

Niacin deficiency causes *pellagra*, which is found mostly among people eating corn-based diets in parts of China, Africa, and India. Pellagra in North America is found mainly among alcoholics; in patients with congenital defects of intestinal and kidney absorption of tryptophan (Hartnup disease); and in patients with carcinoid syndrome (Chap. 52), in which there is increased conversion of tryptophan to serotonin. In the setting of famine or population displacement, the occurrence of pellagra results from the absolute lack of niacin but also from the deficiency of micronutrients required for the conversion of tryptophan to niacin (e.g., iron, riboflavin, and pyridoxine). The early symptoms of pellagra include loss of appetite, generalized weakness and irritability, abdominal pain, and vomiting. Bright red glossitis then ensues, followed by a characteristic skin rash that is pigmented and scaling, particularly in skin areas exposed to sunlight. This rash is known as *Casal's necklace* because it forms a ring around the neck; it is seen in advanced cases. Vaginitis and esophagitis also may occur. Diarrhea (in part due to proctitis and in part due to malabsorption), depression, seizures, and dementia are also part of the pellagra syndrome—the four *D*s: *d*ermatitis, *d*iarrhea, and *d*ementia leading to *d*eath.

TREATMENT   Pellagra

Treatment of pellagra consists of oral supplementation of 100–200 mg of nicotinamide or nicotinic acid three times daily for 5 days. High doses of nicotinic acid (2 g/d in a time-release form) are used for the treatment of elevated cholesterol and triglyceride levels and/or a low high-density lipoprotein (HDL) cholesterol level.

Toxicity

Prostaglandin-mediated flushing due to binding of the vitamin to a G protein–coupled receptor has been observed at daily doses as low as 50 mg of niacin when taken as a supplement or as therapy for dyslipidemia. There is no evidence of toxicity from niacin derived from food sources. Flushing always starts in the face and may be accompanied by skin dryness, itching, paresthesia, and headache. Pharmaceutical preparations of nicotinic acid combined with laropiprant, a selective prostaglandin D_2 receptor 1 antagonist, or premedication with aspirin may alleviate these symptoms. Flushing is subject to tachyphylaxis and often improves with time. Nausea, vomiting, and abdominal pain also occur at similar doses of niacin. Hepatic toxicity is the most serious toxic reaction caused by niacin and may present as jaundice with elevated aspartate aminotransferase (AST) and alanine aminotransferase (ALT) levels. A few cases of fulminant hepatitis requiring liver transplantation have been reported at doses of 3–9 g/d. Other toxic reactions include glucose intolerance, hyperuricemia, macular edema, and macular cysts. The combination of nicotinic acid preparations for dyslipidemia with 3-hydroxy-3-methylglutaryl coenzyme A (HMG-CoA) reductase inhibitors may increase the risk of rhabdomyolysis. The upper limit for daily niacin intake has been set at 35 mg. However, this upper limit does not pertain to the therapeutic use of niacin.

PYRIDOXINE (VITAMIN B₆)

Vitamin B_6 refers to a family of compounds that include pyridoxine, pyridoxal, pyridoxamine, and their 5′-phosphate derivatives. 5′-Pyridoxal phosphate (PLP) is a cofactor for more than 100 enzymes involved in amino acid metabolism. Vitamin B_6 also is involved in heme and neurotransmitter synthesis and in the metabolism of glycogen, lipids, steroids, sphingoid bases, and several vitamins, including the conversion of tryptophan to niacin.

Dietary sources

Plants contain vitamin B_6 in the form of pyridoxine, whereas animal tissues contain PLP and pyridoxamine phosphate. The vitamin B_6 contained in plants is less bioavailable than that in animal tissues. Rich food sources of vitamin B_6 include legumes, nuts, wheat bran, and meat, although it is present in all food groups.

Deficiency

Symptoms of vitamin B_6 deficiency include epithelial changes, as seen frequently with other B vitamin deficiencies. In addition, severe vitamin B_6 deficiency can lead to peripheral neuropathy, abnormal electroencephalograms, and personality changes that include depression and confusion. In infants, diarrhea, seizures, and anemia have been reported. Microcytic hypochromic anemia is due to diminished hemoglobin synthesis, since the first enzyme involved in heme biosynthesis (aminolevulinate synthase) requires PLP as a cofactor. In some case reports, platelet dysfunction has been reported. Since vitamin B_6 is necessary for the conversion of homocysteine to cystathionine, it is possible that chronic low-grade vitamin B_6 deficiency may result in hyperhomocysteinemia and increased risk of cardiovascular disease. Independent of homocysteine, low levels of circulating vitamin B_6 have been associated with inflammation and elevated levels of C-reactive protein.

Certain medications, such as isoniazid, L-dopa, penicillamine, and cycloserine, interact with PLP due to a reaction with carbonyl groups. Pyridoxine should be given concurrently with isoniazid to avoid neuropathy. The increased ratio of AST to ALT seen in alcoholic liver disease reflects the relative vitamin B_6 dependence of ALT. Vitamin B_6 dependency syndromes that require pharmacologic doses of vitamin B_6 are rare; they include cystathionine β-synthase deficiency, pyridoxine-responsive (primarily sideroblastic) anemias, and gyrate atrophy with chorioretinal degeneration due to decreased activity of the mitochondrial enzyme ornithine aminotransferase. In these situations, 100–200 mg/d of oral vitamin B_6 is required for treatment.

High doses of vitamin B_6 have been used to treat carpal tunnel syndrome, premenstrual syndrome, schizophrenia, autism, and diabetic neuropathy but have not been found to be effective.

The laboratory diagnosis of vitamin B_6 deficiency is generally made on the basis of low plasma PLP values (<20 nmol/L). Treatment of vitamin B_6 deficiency is done with 50 mg/d; higher doses of 100–200 mg/d are given if the deficiency is related to medication use. Vitamin B_6 should not be given with L-dopa, since the vitamin interferes with the action of this drug.

Toxicity

The safe upper limit for vitamin B_6 has been set at 100 mg/d, although no adverse effects have been associated with high intakes of vitamin B_6 from food sources only. When toxicity occurs, it causes a severe sensory neuropathy, leaving patients unable to walk. Some cases of photosensitivity and dermatitis have been reported.

FOLATE, VITAMIN B₁₂

Folates are related compounds that build on a backbone of pteroylglutamic acid. The biologically active form of folate is reduced (dihydro- and tetrahydrofolate) and contains a methyl group that it donates to uridylate to make thymidylate, the rate-limiting step in DNA synthesis. Folates are also involved in purine synthesis and methionine synthesis. Folate is also involved in the development of the nervous system. Folate deficiency during pregnancy can lead to spina bifida and other neural tube defects in the baby. However, the most common manifestation of folate deficiency is megaloblastic anemia due to the shortage of thymidylate. Folate deficiency is rare due to folate food supplementation. Folates are found in virtually every kind of food but even more is required in the setting of high red cell turnover such as hemolytic anemia or rapid growth such as pregnancy.

Vitamin B_{12} or cobalamin exists in a variety of forms that all have a cobalt atom within a corrin ring. The 2-deoxyadenosyl form is located in the mitochondria and is a coafactor for methylmalonyl coenzyme A mutase, which is involved in myelin synthesis and other reactions. Methylcobalamin is a cofactor for methionine synthase and participates in the reduction and methylation of folate to donate a methyl group for thymidylate synthesis. Vitamin B_{12} is found only in meat, fish, and dairy products, not plants. Its absorption is mediated by intrinsic factor produced by parietal cells in the stomach and the intrinsic factor-B_{12} complex is absorbed in the terminal ileum. Gastritis and acid blockers can inhibit intrinsic factor production. Diseases of the terminal ileum may also inhibit absorption. Because folate corrects the anemia of B_{12} deficiency, folate food supplementation has also reduced the detection of B_{12} deficiency from anemia symptoms. Accordingly, it is now more common to detect B_{12} deficiency in older patients with balance difficulties from posterior columns demyelination, B_{12} deficiency is also a reversible cause of dementia.

VITAMIN C

Both ascorbic acid and its oxidized product dehydroascorbic acid are biologically active. Actions of vitamin C include antioxidant activity, promotion of nonheme iron absorption, carnitine biosynthesis, the conversion of dopamine to norepinephrine, and the synthesis of many peptide hormones. Vitamin C is also important for connective tissue metabolism and cross-linking (proline hydroxylation), and it is a component of many drug-metabolizing enzyme systems, particularly the mixed-function oxidase systems.

Absorption and dietary sources

Almost complete absorption of vitamin C occurs if <100 mg is administered in a single dose; however, only 50% or less is absorbed at doses >1 g. Enhanced

degradation and fecal and urinary excretion of vitamin C occur at higher intake levels.

Good dietary sources of vitamin C include citrus fruits, green vegetables (especially broccoli), tomatoes, and potatoes. Consumption of five servings of fruits and vegetables a day provides vitamin C in excess of the RDA of 90 mg/d for males and 75 mg/d for females. In addition, approximately 40% of the U.S. population consumes vitamin C as a dietary supplement in which "natural forms" of the vitamin are no more bioavailable than synthetic forms. Smoking, hemodialysis, pregnancy, and stress (e.g., infection, trauma) appear to increase vitamin C requirements.

Deficiency

Vitamin C deficiency causes scurvy. In the United States, this is seen primarily among the poor and elderly, in alcoholics who consume <10 mg/d of vitamin C, and in individuals consuming macrobiotic diets. Vitamin C deficiency also can occur in young adults who eat severely unbalanced diets. In addition to generalized fatigue, symptoms of scurvy primarily reflect impaired formation of mature connective tissue and include bleeding into skin (petechiae, ecchymoses, perifollicular hemorrhages); inflamed and bleeding gums; and manifestations of bleeding into joints, the peritoneal cavity, the pericardium, and the adrenal glands. In children, vitamin C deficiency may cause impaired bone growth. Laboratory diagnosis of vitamin C deficiency is made on the basis of low plasma or leukocyte levels.

Administration of vitamin C (200 mg/d) improves the symptoms of scurvy within a matter of several days. High-dose vitamin C supplementation (e.g., 1–2 g/d) may slightly decrease the symptoms and duration of upper respiratory tract infections. Vitamin C supplementation has also been reported to be useful in Chédiak-Higashi syndrome and osteogenesis imperfecta. Diets high in vitamin C have been claimed to lower the incidence of certain cancers, particularly esophageal and gastric cancers. If proved, this effect may be due to the fact that vitamin C can prevent the conversion of nitrites and secondary amines to carcinogenic nitrosamines. However, an intervention study from China did not show vitamin C to be protective. Parenteral ascorbic acid has been suggested to have a potential therapeutic role in the treatment of advanced cancers.

Toxicity

Taking >2 g of vitamin C in a single dose may result in abdominal pain, diarrhea, and nausea. Since vitamin C may be metabolized to oxalate, it is feared that chronic high-dose vitamin C supplementation could result in an increased prevalence of kidney stones. However, this has not been borne out in several trials, except in patients with preexisting renal disease. Thus, it is reasonable to advise patients with a past history of kidney stones not to take large doses of vitamin C. There is also an unproven but possible risk that chronic high doses of vitamin C could promote iron overload in patients taking supplemental iron. High doses of vitamin C can induce hemolysis in patients with glucose-6-phosphate dehydrogenase deficiency, and doses >1 g/d can cause false-negative guaiac reactions as well as interfere with tests for urinary glucose. High doses may interfere with certain drugs (e.g., bortezomib in myeloma patients).

BIOTIN

Biotin is a water-soluble vitamin that plays a role in gene expression, gluconeogenesis, and fatty acid synthesis and serves as a CO_2 carrier on the surface of both cytosolic and mitochondrial carboxylase enzymes. The vitamin also functions in the catabolism of specific amino acids (e.g., leucine). Excellent food sources of biotin include organ meat such as liver or kidney, soy, beans, yeast, and egg yolks; however, egg white contains the protein avidin, which strongly binds the vitamin and reduces its bioavailability.

Biotin deficiency due to low dietary intake is rare; rather, deficiency is due to inborn errors of metabolism. Biotin deficiency has been induced by experimental feeding of egg white diets and in patients with short bowels who received biotin-free parenteral nutrition. In adults, biotin deficiency results in mental changes (depression, hallucinations), paresthesia, anorexia, and nausea. A scaling, seborrheic, and erythematous rash may occur around the eyes, nose, and mouth as well as on the extremities. In infants, biotin deficiency presents as hypotonia, lethargy, and apathy. In addition, infants may develop alopecia and a characteristic rash that includes the ears. The laboratory diagnosis of biotin deficiency can be established on the basis of a decreased urinary concentration or an increased urinary excretion of 3-hydroxyisovaleric acid after a leucine challenge. Treatment requires pharmacologic doses of biotin, using up to 10 mg/d. No toxicity is known.

PANTOTHENIC ACID (VITAMIN B₅)

Pantothenic acid is a component of coenzyme A and phosphopantetheine, which are involved in fatty acid metabolism and the synthesis of cholesterol, steroid hormones, and all compounds formed from isoprenoid units. In addition, pantothenic acid is involved in the acetylation of proteins. The vitamin is excreted in the urine, and the laboratory diagnosis of deficiency is made on the basis of low urinary vitamin levels.

The vitamin is ubiquitous in the food supply. Liver, yeast, egg yolks, whole grains, and vegetables are particularly good sources. Human pantothenic acid deficiency has been demonstrated only in experimental feeding of diets low in pantothenic acid or by giving a specific pantothenic acid antagonist. The symptoms of pantothenic acid deficiency are nonspecific and include gastrointestinal disturbance, depression, muscle cramps, paresthesia, ataxia, and hypoglycemia. Pantothenic acid deficiency is believed to have caused the burning feet syndrome seen in prisoners of war during World War II. No toxicity of this vitamin has been reported.

CHOLINE

Choline is a precursor for acetylcholine, phospholipids, and betaine. Choline is necessary for the structural integrity of cell membranes, cholinergic neurotransmission, lipid and cholesterol metabolism, methyl-group metabolism, and transmembrane signaling. Recently, a recommended adequate intake was set at 550 mg/d for adult males and 425 mg/d for adult females, although certain genetic polymorphisms can increase an individual's requirement. Choline is thought to be a "conditionally essential" nutrient in that de novo synthesis occurs in the liver and is less than the vitamin's utilization only under certain stress conditions (e.g., alcoholic liver disease). The dietary requirement of choline depends on the status of other methyl-group donors (folate, vitamin B_{12}, and methionine) and thus varies widely. Choline is widely distributed in food (e.g., egg yolk, wheat germ, organ meat, milk) in the form of lecithin (phosphatidylcholine). Choline deficiency has occurred in patients receiving parenteral nutrition devoid of choline. Deficiency results in fatty liver, elevated transaminase levels, and skeletal muscle damage with high creatine phosphokinase values. The diagnosis of choline deficiency is currently made on the basis of low plasma levels, although nonspecific conditions (e.g., heavy exercise) may suppress plasma levels.

Toxicity from choline results in hypotension, cholinergic sweating, diarrhea, salivation, and a fishy body odor. The upper limit for choline has been set at 3.5 g/d. Therapeutically, choline has been suggested for patients with dementia and patients at high risk of cardiovascular disease, due to its ability to lower cholesterol and homocysteine levels. However, such benefits have not been firmly documented. Choline- and betaine-restricted diets are of therapeutic value in trimethylaminuria (fish odor syndrome).

FLAVONOIDS

Flavonoids constitute a large family of polyphenols that contribute to the aroma, taste, and color of fruits and vegetables. Major groups of dietary flavonoids include anthocyanidins in berries; catechins in green tea and chocolate; flavonols (e.g., quercitin) in broccoli, kale, leeks, onion, and the skins of grapes and apples; and isoflavones (e.g., genistein) in legumes. Isoflavones have a low bioavailability and are partially metabolized by the intestinal flora. The dietary intake of flavonoids is estimated to be between 10 and 100 mg/d, although this is almost certainly an underestimate due to the lack of knowledge of their concentrations in many foods. Several flavonoids have been shown to have antioxidant activity and to affect cell signaling. From observational epidemiologic studies and limited clinical human and animal studies, flavonoids have been postulated to play a role in the prevention of several chronic diseases, including neurodegenerative disease, diabetes, and osteoporosis. The ultimate importance and usefulness of their compounds against human disease have not been demonstrated.

VITAMIN A

Vitamin A, in the strictest sense, refers to retinol. However, the oxidized metabolites, retinaldehyde and retinoic acid, are also biologically active compounds. The term *retinoids* includes all molecules (including synthetic molecules) that are chemically related to retinol. Retinaldehyde (11-*cis*) is the essential form of vitamin A that is required for normal vision, whereas retinoic acid is necessary for normal morphogenesis, growth, and cell differentiation. Retinoic acid does not function in vision and, in contrast to retinol, is not involved in reproduction. Vitamin A also plays a role in iron utilization, humoral immunity, T cell–mediated immunity, natural killer cell activity, and phagocytosis. Vitamin A is commercially available in esterified forms (e.g., acetate, palmitate) since it is more stable as an ester.

There are more than 600 carotenoids in nature, and approximately 50 of them can be metabolized to vitamin A. β-Carotene is the most prevalent carotenoid in the food supply that has provitamin A activity. In humans, significant fractions of carotenoids are absorbed intact and are stored in liver and fat. It is now estimated that 12 μg or more (range, 4–27 μg) of dietary all-trans β-carotene is equivalent to 1 μg of retinol activity, whereas 24 μg or more of other dietary provitamin A carotenoids (e.g., cryptoxanthin, α-carotene) is equivalent to 1 μg of retinol activity. The vitamin A equivalency for a β-carotene supplement in an oily solution is 2:1.

Metabolism

The liver contains approximately 90% of the vitamin A reserves and secretes vitamin A in the form of retinol, which is bound to retinol-binding protein. Once this has occurred, the retinol-binding protein complex interacts with a second protein, transthyretin. This trimolecular complex functions to prevent vitamin A from being filtered by the kidney glomerulus to protect the body against the toxicity of retinol and to allow retinol to be taken up by specific cell-surface receptors that recognize retinol-binding protein. A certain amount of vitamin A enters peripheral cells even if it is not bound to retinol-binding protein. After retinol is internalized by the cell, it becomes bound to a series of cellular retinol-binding proteins, which function as sequestering and transporting agents as well as co-ligands for enzymatic reactions. Certain cells also contain retinoic acid–binding proteins, which have sequestering functions but also shuttle retinoic acid to the nucleus and enable its metabolism.

Retinoic acid is a ligand for certain nuclear receptors that act as transcription factors. Two families of receptors (RAR and RXR receptors) are active in retinoid-mediated gene transcription. Retinoid receptors regulate transcription by binding as dimeric complexes to specific DNA sites, the retinoic acid response elements, in target genes. The receptors can either stimulate or repress gene expression in response to their ligands. RAR binds all-*trans* retinoic acid and 9-*cis*-retinoic acid, whereas RXR binds only 9-*cis*-retinoic acid.

The retinoid receptors play an important role in controlling cell proliferation and differentiation. Retinoic acid is useful in the treatment of promyelocytic leukemia and also is used in the treatment of cystic acne because it inhibits keratinization, decreases sebum secretion, and possibly alters the inflammatory reaction. RXRs dimerize with other nuclear receptors to function as coregulators of genes responsive to retinoids, thyroid hormone, and calcitriol. RXR agonists induce insulin sensitivity experimentally, perhaps because RXR is a cofactor for the peroxisome-proliferator-activated receptors (PPARs), which are targets for thiazolidinedione drugs such as rosiglitazone and troglitazone.

Dietary sources

The retinol activity equivalent (RAE) is used to express the vitamin A value of food. One RAE is defined as 1 μg of retinol (0.003491 mmol), 12 μg of β-carotene, and 24 μg of other provitamin A carotenoids. In older literature, vitamin A often was expressed in international units (IU), with 1 μg of retinol being equal to 3.33 IU of retinol and 20 IU of β-carotene, but these units are no longer in scientific use.

Liver, fish, and eggs are excellent food sources for preformed vitamin A; vegetable sources of provitamin A carotenoids include dark green and deeply colored fruits and vegetables. Moderate cooking of vegetables enhances carotenoid release for uptake in the gut. Carotenoid absorption is also aided by some fat in a meal. Infants are particularly susceptible to vitamin A deficiency because neither breast nor cow's milk supplies enough vitamin A to prevent deficiency. In developing countries, chronic dietary deficiency is the main cause of vitamin A deficiency and is exacerbated by infection. In early childhood, low vitamin A status results from inadequate intakes of animal food sources and edible oils, both of which are expensive, coupled with seasonal unavailability of vegetables and fruits and lack of marketed fortified food products. Concurrent zinc deficiency can interfere with the mobilization of vitamin A from liver stores. Alcohol interferes with the conversion of retinol to retinaldehyde in the eye by competing for alcohol (retinol) dehydrogenase. Drugs that interfere with the absorption of vitamin A include mineral oil, neomycin, and cholestyramine.

Deficiency

Vitamin A deficiency is endemic in areas where diets are chronically poor, especially in southern Asia, sub-Saharan Africa, some parts of Latin America, and the western Pacific, including parts of China. Vitamin A status is usually assessed by measuring serum retinol (normal range, 1.05–3.50 μmol/L [30–100 μg/dL]) or blood spot retinol or by tests of dark adaptation. There are stable isotopic or invasive liver biopsy methods to estimate total body stores of vitamin A. Based on deficient serum retinol (<0.70 μmol/L [20 μg/dL]), there are >90 million preschool-age children with vitamin A deficiency, among whom >4 million have an ocular manifestation of deficiency termed *xerophthalmia*. This condition includes milder stages of night blindness and conjunctival xerosis (dryness) with Bitot's spots (white patches of keratinized epithelium appearing on the sclera) as well as rare, potentially blinding corneal ulceration and necrosis. Keratomalacia (softening of the cornea) leads to corneal scarring that blinds at least a quarter of a million children each year and is associated with a fatality rate of 4–25%. However, vitamin A deficiency at any stage poses an increased risk of mortality from diarrhea, dysentery, measles, malaria, and respiratory disease. Vitamin A deficiency can compromise barrier and innate and acquired immune defenses to infection. Vitamin A supplementation can markedly reduce risk of child mortality (23–34%, on average) in areas where deficiency is widely prevalent. About 10% of pregnant women in undernourished settings also develop night blindness, assessed by history, during the latter half of pregnancy, and this moderate vitamin A deficiency is associated with an increased risk of maternal infection and mortality rate.

TREATMENT   Vitamin A Deficiency

Any stage of xerophthalmia should be treated with 60 mg of vitamin A in oily solution, usually contained in a soft-gel capsule. The same dose is repeated 1 and 14 days later. Doses should be reduced by half for patients 6–11 months of age. Mothers with night blindness or Bitot's spots should be given vitamin A orally, either 3 mg daily or 7.5 mg twice a week for 3 months. These regimens are efficacious, and they are less expensive and more widely available than injectable water-miscible vitamin A. A common approach to prevention is to supplement young children in high-risk areas with 60 mg every 4–6 months, with a half dose given to infants 6–11 months of age.

Uncomplicated vitamin A deficiency rarely occurs in industrialized countries. One high-risk group, extremely low-birth-weight infants (<1000 g), is likely to be vitamin A–deficient and should be supplemented with 1500 μg (or RAE) of vitamin A three times a week for 4 weeks. Severe measles in any society can lead to secondary vitamin A deficiency. Children hospitalized with measles should receive two 60-mg doses of vitamin A on 2 consecutive days. Vitamin A deficiency most often occurs in patients with malabsorptive diseases (e.g., celiac sprue, short-bowel syndrome) who have abnormal dark adaptation or symptoms of night blindness without other ocular changes. Typically, such patients are treated for 1 month with 15 mg/d of a water-miscible preparation of vitamin A. This is followed by a lower maintenance dose, with the exact amount determined by monitoring serum retinol.

There are no specific deficiency signs or symptoms that result from carotenoid deficiency. It was postulated that β-carotene would be an effective chemopreventive agent for cancer because numerous epidemiologic studies had shown that diets high in β-carotene were associated with lower incidences of cancers of the respiratory and digestive systems. However, intervention studies in smokers found that treatment with high doses of β-carotene actually resulted in more lung cancers than did treatment with placebo. Non–provitamin A carotenoids such as lutein and zeaxanthin have been suggested to protect against macular degeneration, and large-scale intervention studies have been undertaken to test this hypothesis. The non–provitamin A carotenoid lycopene has been proposed to protect against prostate cancer. However, the effectiveness of these agents has not been proved by intervention studies, and the mechanisms underlying these purported biologic actions are unknown.

Selective plant breeding techniques that lead to a higher provitamin A content of staple foods may improve vitamin A malnutrition in low-income countries. Moreover, a recently developed genetically modified food (Golden Rice) showed an improved β-carotene to vitamin A conversion ratio of ~3:1.

Toxicity

Acute toxicity of vitamin A was first noted in Arctic explorers who ate polar bear liver and has also been seen after administration of 150 mg in adults or 100 mg in children. Acute toxicity is manifested by increased intracranial pressure, vertigo, diplopia, bulging fontanels in children, seizures, and exfoliative dermatitis; it may result in death. In children being treated for vitamin A deficiency according to the protocols outlined earlier, transient bulging of fontanels occurs in 2% of infants, and transient nausea, vomiting, and headache occur in 5% of preschoolers. Chronic vitamin A intoxication is largely a concern in industrialized countries and has been seen in normal adults who ingest 15 mg/d and children who ingest 6 mg/d of vitamin A over a period of several months. Manifestations include dry skin, cheilosis, glossitis, vomiting, alopecia, bone demineralization and pain, hypercalcemia, lymph node enlargement, hyperlipidemia, amenorrhea, and features of pseudotumor cerebri with increased intracranial pressure and papilledema. Liver fibrosis with portal hypertension and bone demineralization may result from chronic vitamin A intoxication. When vitamin A is provided in excess to pregnant women, congenital malformations have included spontaneous abortions, craniofacial abnormalities, and valvular heart disease. In pregnancy, the daily dose of vitamin A should not exceed 3 mg. Commercially available retinoid derivatives are also toxic, including 13-*cis*-retinoic acid, which has been associated with birth defects. As a result, contraception should be continued for a least 1 year and possibly longer in women who have taken 13-*cis*-retinoic acid.

In malnourished children, vitamin A supplements (100,000–200,000 IU) as a function of age in several rounds over 2 years are considered to amplify nonspecific effects of vaccines. However, for unclear reasons, there may be a negative effect on mortality rates in incompletely vaccinated girls.

High doses of carotenoids do not result in toxic symptoms but should be avoided in smokers due to an increased risk of lung cancer. Very high doses of β-carotene (~200 mg/d) have been used to treat or prevent the skin rashes of erythropoietic protoporphyria. Carotenemia, which is characterized by a yellowing of the skin (creases of the palms and soles) but not the sclerae, may be present after ingestion of >30 mg of β-carotene daily. Hypothyroid patients are particularly susceptible to the development of carotenemia due to impaired breakdown of carotene to vitamin A. Reduction of carotenes from the diet results in the disappearance of skin yellowing and carotenemia over a period of 30–60 days.

VITAMIN D

The biologic effects of vitamin D are mediated by vitamin D receptors, which are found in most tissues, thus potentially expanding vitamin D actions on nearly all cell systems and organs (e.g., immune cells, brain, breast, colon, and prostate) as well as exerting classic endocrine effects on calcium metabolism and bone health. Vitamin D is thought to be important for maintaining normal function of many nonskeletal tissues such as muscle (including heart muscle), immune function, and inflammation as well as cell proliferation and differentiation. Studies have shown that it may be useful as adjunctive treatment for tuberculosis, psoriasis, and multiple sclerosis or for the prevention of certain cancers. Vitamin D insufficiency may increase the risk of type 1 diabetes mellitus, cardiovascular disease (insulin resistance, hypertension, or low-grade inflammation), or brain dysfunction (e.g., depression). However, the importance of the exact physiologic role of vitamin D in these nonskeletal diseases has not been clarified.

A major source of vitamin D is its synthesis in the skin upon ultraviolet B (UV-B) (wavelength, 290–315 nm) exposure. Except for fish, food (unless fortified) contains only limited amounts of vitamin D. Vitamin D_2 (ergocalciferol) is obtained from plant sources and is the chemical form found in some supplements.

Deficiency

Vitamin D status has been assessed by measuring serum 25-dihydroxyvitamin D (25[OH]$_2$ vitamin D) levels; however, there is no consensus on a uniform assay methodology or on optimal serum levels. The optimal level might, in fact, differ according to the targeted disease entity. Based on epidemiologic and experimental data, a 25(OH)$_2$ vitamin D level >20 ng/mL (≥50 nmol/L; to convert ng/mL to nmol/L, multiply by 2.496) is sufficient for good bone health. Some experts advocate higher serum levels (e.g., >30 ng/mL) for other desirable endpoints of vitamin D action.

Risk factors for vitamin D deficiency are old age, lack of sun exposure, dark skin (especially among those living in northern latitudes), fat malabsorption, and obesity. Rickets represents the classic disease of vitamin D deficiency. Signs of deficiency are muscle soreness, weakness, and bone pain. Some of these effects are independent of calcium intake.

The U.S. National Academy of Science recently concluded that the majority of North Americans are receiving adequate amounts of vitamin D (RDA = 15 μg/d or 600 IU/d; Chap. 53). However, for people older than 70 years, the RDA is set at 20 μg/d (800 IU/d). The consumption of fortified or enriched foods as well as suberythemal sun exposure should be encouraged for people at risk for vitamin D deficiency. If an adequate intake cannot be achieved, vitamin D supplements should be taken, especially during the winter months. Vitamin D deficiency can be treated by the oral administration of 50,000 IU/week for 6–8 weeks followed by a maintenance dose of 800 IU/d (100 μg/d) from food and supplements after achievement of normal plasma levels. The physiologic effects of vitamin D_2 and D_3 are identical when ingested over long periods.

Toxicity

The upper limit of intake has been set at 4000 IU/d. Contrary to earlier beliefs, acute vitamin D intoxication is rare and usually is caused by the uncontrolled and excessive ingestion of supplements or faulty food fortification practices. High plasma $1,25(OH)_2$ vitamin D and high plasma calcium levels are central features of toxicity. Stopping vitamin D and calcium supplements is mandatory, and treatment of hypercalcemia may be required.

VITAMIN E

Vitamin E is a collective name for all stereoisomers of tocopherols and tocotrienols, although only the *RR* tocopherols meet human requirements. Vitamin E acts as a chain-breaking antioxidant and is an efficient pyroxyl radical scavenger that protects low-density lipoproteins (LDLs) and polyunsaturated fats in membranes from oxidation. A network of other antioxidants (e.g., vitamin C, glutathione) and enzymes maintains vitamin E in a reduced state. Vitamin E also inhibits prostaglandin synthesis and the activities of protein kinase C and phospholipase A_2.

Absorption and metabolism

After absorption, vitamin E is taken up from chylomicrons by the liver, and a hepatic α-tocopherol transport protein mediates intracellular vitamin E transport and incorporation into very low density lipoprotein (VLDL). The transport protein has particular affinity for the RRR isomeric form of α-tocopherol; thus, this natural isomer has the most biologic activity.

Requirement

Vitamin E is widely distributed in the food supply and is particularly high in sunflower oil, safflower oil, and wheat germ oil; γ-tocotrienols are notably present in soybean and corn oils. Vitamin E is also found in meats, nuts, and cereal grains, and small amounts are present in fruits and vegetables. Vitamin E pills containing doses of 50–1000 mg are ingested by about 10% of the U.S. population. The RDA for vitamin E is 15 mg/d (34.9 μmol or 22.5 IU) for all adults. Diets high in polyunsaturated fats may necessitate a slightly higher intake of vitamin E.

Dietary deficiency of vitamin E does not exist. Vitamin E deficiency is seen in only severe and prolonged malabsorptive diseases, such as celiac disease, or after small-intestinal resection. Children with cystic fibrosis or prolonged cholestasis may develop vitamin E deficiency characterized by areflexia and hemolytic anemia. Children with abetalipoproteinemia cannot absorb or transport vitamin E and become deficient quite rapidly. A familial form of isolated vitamin E deficiency also exists; it is due to a defect in the α-tocopherol transport protein. Vitamin E deficiency causes axonal degeneration of the large myelinated axons and results in posterior column and spinocerebellar symptoms. Peripheral neuropathy is initially characterized by areflexia, with progression to an ataxic gait, and by decreased vibration and position sensations. Ophthalmoplegia, skeletal myopathy, and pigmented retinopathy may also be features of vitamin E deficiency. Either vitamin E or selenium deficiency in the host has been shown to increase certain viral mutations and, therefore, virulence. The laboratory diagnosis of vitamin E deficiency is made on the basis of low blood levels of α-tocopherol (<5 μg/mL, or <0.8 mg of α-tocopherol per gram of total lipids).

TREATMENT   Vitamin E Deficiency

Symptomatic vitamin E deficiency should be treated with 800–1200 mg of α-tocopherol per day. Patients with abetalipoproteinemia may need as much as 5000–7000 mg/d. Children with symptomatic vitamin E deficiency should be treated with 400 mg/d orally of water-miscible esters; alternatively, 2 mg/kg per d may be administered intramuscularly. Vitamin E in high doses may protect against oxygen-induced retrolental fibroplasia and bronchopulmonary dysplasia as well as intraventricular hemorrhage of prematurity. Vitamin E has been suggested to increase sexual performance, treat intermittent claudication, and slow the aging process, but evidence for these properties is lacking. When given in combination with other antioxidants, vitamin E may help prevent macular degeneration. High doses (60–800 mg/d) of vitamin E have been shown in controlled trials to improve parameters of immune function and reduce colds in nursing home residents, but intervention studies using vitamin E to prevent cardiovascular disease or cancer have not shown efficacy, and at doses >400 mg/d, vitamin E may even increase all-cause mortality rates.

Toxicity

All forms of vitamin E are absorbed and could contribute to toxicity. *High* doses of vitamin E (>800 mg/d) may reduce platelet aggregation and interfere with vitamin K metabolism and are therefore contraindicated in patients taking warfarin and antiplatelet agents (such as aspirin or clopidogrel). Nausea, flatulence, and diarrhea have been reported at doses >1 g/d.

VITAMIN K

There are two natural forms of vitamin K: vitamin K_1, also known as *phylloquinone*, from vegetable and animal sources, and vitamin K$_2$, or *menaquinone*, which is synthesized by bacterial flora and found in hepatic tissue. Phylloquinone can be converted to menaquinone in some organs.

Vitamin K is required for the posttranslational carboxylation of glutamic acid, which is necessary for calcium binding to γ-carboxylated proteins such as prothrombin (factor II); factors VII, IX, and X; protein C; protein S; and proteins found in bone (osteocalcin) and vascular smooth muscle (e.g., matrix Gla protein). However, the importance of vitamin K for bone mineralization and prevention of vascular calcification is not known. Warfarin-type drugs inhibit γ-carboxylation by preventing the conversion of vitamin K to its active hydroquinone form.

Dietary sources

Vitamin K is found in green leafy vegetables such as kale and spinach, and appreciable amounts are also present in margarine and liver. Vitamin K is present in vegetable oils; olive, canola, and soybean oils are particularly rich sources. The average daily intake by Americans is estimated to be approximately 100 μg/d.

Deficiency

The symptoms of vitamin K deficiency are due to hemorrhage, and newborns are particularly susceptible because of low fat stores, low breast milk levels of vitamin K, sterility of the infantile intestinal tract, liver immaturity, and poor placental transport. Intracranial bleeding, as well as gastrointestinal and skin bleeding, can occur in vitamin K–deficient infants 1–7 days after birth. Thus, vitamin K (1 mg IM) is given prophylactically at the time of delivery.

Vitamin K deficiency in adults may be seen in patients with chronic small-intestinal disease (e.g., celiac disease, Crohn's disease), in those with obstructed biliary tracts, or after small-bowel resection. Broad-spectrum antibiotic treatment can precipitate vitamin K deficiency by reducing gut bacteria, which synthesize menaquinones, and by inhibiting the metabolism of vitamin K. In patients with warfarin therapy, the antiobesity drug orlistat can lead to international normalized ratio (INR) changes due to vitamin K malabsorption. The diagnosis of vitamin K deficiency usually is made on the basis of an elevated prothrombin time or reduced clotting factors, although vitamin K may also be measured directly by HPLC. Vitamin K deficiency is treated by using a parenteral dose of 10 mg. For patients with chronic malabsorption, 1–2 mg/d of vitamin K should be given orally, or 1–2 mg/week can be taken parenterally. Patients with liver disease may have an elevated prothrombin time because of liver cell destruction as well as vitamin K deficiency. If an elevated prothrombin time does not improve on vitamin K therapy, it can be deduced that it is not the result of vitamin K deficiency.

Toxicity

Toxicity from dietary phylloquinones and menaquinones has not been described. High doses of vitamin K can impair the actions of oral anticoagulants.

MINERALS

Table 54-2.

ZINC

Zinc is an integral component of many metalloenzymes in the body; it is involved in the synthesis and stabilization of proteins, DNA, and RNA and plays a structural role in ribosomes and membranes. Zinc is necessary for the binding of steroid hormone receptors and several other transcription factors to DNA. Zinc is absolutely required for normal spermatogenesis, fetal growth, and embryonic development.

Absorption

The absorption of zinc from the diet is inhibited by dietary phytate, fiber, oxalate, iron, and copper, as well as by certain drugs, including penicillamine, sodium valproate, and ethambutol. Meat, shellfish, nuts, and legumes are good sources of bioavailable zinc, whereas zinc in grains and legumes is less available for absorption.

Deficiency

Mild zinc deficiency has been described in many diseases, including diabetes mellitus, HIV/AIDS, cirrhosis, alcoholism, inflammatory bowel disease, malabsorption syndromes, and sickle cell disease. In these diseases, mild chronic zinc deficiency can cause stunted growth in children, decreased taste sensation (hypogeusia), and impaired immune function. Severe chronic zinc deficiency has been described as a cause of hypogonadism and dwarfism in several Middle Eastern countries. In these children, hypopigmented hair is also part of the syndrome. Acrodermatitis enteropathica is a rare autosomal recessive disorder characterized by abnormalities in zinc absorption. Clinical manifestations include diarrhea, alopecia, muscle wasting, depression, irritability, and a rash involving the extremities, face, and perineum. The rash is characterized by vesicular and pustular crusting with scaling and erythema. Occasional patients with Wilson's disease have developed zinc deficiency as a consequence of penicillamine therapy.

The diagnosis of zinc deficiency is usually made by a serum zinc level <12 μmol/L (<70 μg/dL). Pregnancy and birth control pills may cause a slight depression in serum zinc levels, and hypoalbuminemia from any cause can result in hypozincemia. In acute stress situations, zinc may be redistributed from serum into tissues. Zinc deficiency may be treated with 60 mg elemental zinc, orally twice a day. Zinc gluconate lozenges (13 mg elemental zinc every 2 h while awake) have been reported to reduce the duration and symptoms of the common cold in adults, but studies are conflicting.

Zinc deficiency is prevalent in many developing countries and usually coexists with other micronutrient deficiencies (especially iron). Zinc (20 mg/d) may be an effective adjunctive therapeutic strategy for diarrheal disease and pneumonia in children.

Toxicity

Acute zinc toxicity after oral ingestion causes nausea, vomiting, and fever. Zinc fumes from welding may also be toxic and cause fever, respiratory distress, excessive salivation, sweating, and headache. Chronic large doses of zinc may depress immune function and cause hypochromic anemia as a result of copper deficiency. Intranasal zinc preparations should be avoided because they may lead to irreversible damage of nasal mucosa and anosmia.

COPPER

Copper is an integral part of numerous enzyme systemsz, including amine oxidases, ferroxidase (ceruloplasmin), cytochrome-*c* oxidase, superoxide dismutase, and dopamine hydroxylase. Copper is also a component of ferroprotein, a transport protein involved in the basolateral transfer of iron during absorption from the enterocyte. As such, copper plays a role in iron metabolism, melanin synthesis, energy production, neurotransmitter synthesis, and CNS function; the synthesis and cross-linking of elastin and collagen; and the scavenging of superoxide radicals. Dietary sources of copper include shellfish, liver, nuts, legumes, bran, and organ meats.

Deficiency

Dietary copper deficiency is relatively rare, although it has been described in premature infants who are fed milk diets and in infants with malabsorption (Table 54-2). Copper-deficiency anemia has been reported in patients with malabsorptive diseases and nephrotic syndrome and in patients treated for Wilson's disease with chronic high doses of oral zinc, which can interfere with copper absorption. Menkes' kinky hair syndrome is an X-linked metabolic disturbance of copper metabolism characterized by mental retardation, hypocupremia, and decreased circulating ceruloplasmin. It is caused by mutations in the copper-transporting *ATP7A* gene. Children with this disease often die within 5 years because of dissecting aneurysms or cardiac rupture. Aceruloplasminemia is

a rare autosomal recessive disease characterized by tissue iron overload, mental deterioration, microcytic anemia, and low serum iron and copper concentrations.

The diagnosis of copper deficiency is usually made on the basis of low serum levels of copper (<65 μg/dL) and low ceruloplasmin levels (<20 mg/dL). Serum levels of copper may be elevated in pregnancy or stress conditions since ceruloplasmin is an acute-phase reactant and 90% of circulating copper is bound to ceruloplasmin.

Toxicity

Copper toxicity is usually accidental (Table 54-2). In severe cases, kidney failure, liver failure, and coma may ensue. In Wilson's disease, mutations in the copper-transporting *ATP7B* gene lead to accumulation of copper in the liver and brain, with low blood levels due to decreased ceruloplasmin.

SELENIUM

Selenium, in the form of selenocysteine, is a component of the enzyme glutathione peroxidase, which serves to protect proteins, cell membranes, lipids, and nucleic acids from oxidant molecules. As such, selenium is being actively studied as a chemopreventive agent against certain cancers, such as prostate cancer. Selenocysteine is also found in the deiodinase enzymes, which mediate the deiodination of thyroxine to triiodothyronine. Rich dietary sources of selenium include seafood, muscle meat, and cereals, although the selenium content of cereal is determined by the soil concentration. Countries with low soil concentrations include parts of Scandinavia, China, and New Zealand. *Keshan disease* is an endemic cardiomyopathy found in children and young women residing in regions of China where dietary intake of selenium is low (<20 μg/d). Concomitant deficiencies of iodine and selenium may worsen the clinical manifestations of cretinism. Chronic ingestion of high amounts of selenium leads to selenosis, characterized by hair and nail brittleness and loss, garlic breath odor, skin rash, myopathy, irritability, and other abnormalities of the nervous system.

CHROMIUM

Chromium potentiates the action of insulin in patients with impaired glucose tolerance, presumably by increasing insulin receptor–mediated signaling, although its usefulness in treating type 2 diabetes is uncertain. In addition, improvement in blood lipid profiles has been reported in some patients. The usefulness of chromium supplements in muscle building has not been substantiated. Rich food sources of chromium include yeast, meat, and grain products. Chromium in the trivalent state is found in supplements and is largely nontoxic; however, chromium-6 is a product of stainless steel welding and is a known pulmonary carcinogen as well as a cause of liver, kidney, and CNS damage.

MAGNESIUM

Magnesium is the major intracellular divalent cation and is essential for normal neuromuscular activity. Magnesium is a cofactor for a wide range of biochemical process in the cell including enzymes, transporters, and nucleic acids. The serum concentration is generally 1.7-2.4 mg/dL (0.7-1 mmol/L or 1.4-2 mEq/L). Total body magnesium is about 25 grams about half of which is in bone. Vitamin D facilitates intestinal absorption. About 140-360 mg of magnesium are ingested in the normal diet each day and about 100 mg/d is absorbed and is matched by the levels of excretion.

Hypomagnesemia is generally a reflection of increased losses through nausea, vomiting, diarrhea, or increased renal excretion due to failure of reabsorption. Hypomagnesemic patients may have tetany, tremor, muscle weakness, ataxia, nystagmus, vertigo, seizures, apathy, depression, irritability, delirium, or psychosis. Cardiac arrhythmias may also occur. Hypocalcemia and hypokalemia may also be seen. Magnesium supplementation is usually corrective

Hypermagnesemia occurs mainly in the setting of renal failure or overingestion of magnesium-containing cathartics. Vasodilatation is the common result with hypotension refractory to pressors, nausea, lethargy, weakness, ileus, dilated pupils, and heart rhythm disturbances including heart block. Hydration and hemodialysis may be needed to bring magnesium levels down. Calcium administration may provide temporary relief of some symptoms.

FLUORIDE, MANGANESE, AND ULTRATRACE ELEMENTS

An essential function for fluoride in humans has not been described, although it is useful for the maintenance of structure in teeth and bone. Adult fluorosis results in mottled and pitted defects in tooth enamel as well as brittle bone (skeletal fluorosis).

Manganese and molybdenum deficiencies have been reported in patients with rare genetic abnormalities and in a few patients receiving prolonged total parenteral nutrition. Several manganese-specific enzymes have been identified (e.g., manganese superoxide dismutase). Deficiencies of manganese have been reported to result in bone demineralization, poor growth, ataxia, disturbances in carbohydrate and lipid metabolism, and convulsions.

Ultratrace elements are defined as those needed in amounts <1 mg/d. Essentiality has not been established for most ultratrace elements, although selenium, chromium, and iodine are clearly essential. *Molybdenum* is necessary for the activity of sulfite and xanthine oxidase, and molybdenum deficiency may result in skeletal and brain lesions.

CHAPTER 55

MALNUTRITION AND NUTRITIONAL ASSESSMENT

Douglas C. Heimburger

Malnutrition can arise from primary or secondary causes, with the former resulting from inadequate or poor-quality food intake and the latter from diseases that alter food intake or nutrient requirements, metabolism, or absorption. Primary malnutrition occurs mainly in developing countries and under conditions of political unrest, war, or famine. Secondary malnutrition, the main form encountered in industrialized countries, was largely unrecognized until the early 1970s, when it was appreciated that persons with adequate food supplies can become malnourished as a result of acute or chronic diseases that alter nutrient intake or metabolism, particularly diseases that cause acute or chronic inflammation. Various studies have shown that protein-energy malnutrition (PEM) affects one-third to one-half of patients on general medical and surgical wards in teaching hospitals. The consistent finding that nutritional status influences patient prognosis underscores the importance of preventing, detecting, and treating malnutrition.

PROTEIN-ENERGY MALNUTRITION

Definitions for forms of PEM are in flux. Traditionally, the two major types of PEM have been *marasmus* and *kwashiorkor*. These conditions are compared in **Table 55-1**. Marasmus has been considered the end result of a long-term deficit of dietary energy, whereas kwashiorkor has been understood to result from a protein-poor diet. Although the former concept remains essentially correct, evidence is accumulating that PEM syndromes are distinguished by two main features: dietary intake and underlying inflammatory processes. Energy-poor diets with minimal inflammation cause gradual erosion of body mass, resulting in classic marasmus. By contrast, inflammation from acute illnesses such as injury

or sepsis and chronic illnesses such as cancer, lung or heart disease, and HIV can erode lean body mass even in the presence of relatively sufficient dietary intake, leading to a kwashiorkor-like state. Quite often, inflammatory illnesses impair appetite and dietary intake, producing combinations of the two.

An international consensus committee has proposed the following revised definitions. *Starvation-related malnutrition* is suggested for instances of chronic starvation without inflammation, *chronic disease–related malnutrition* when inflammation is chronic and of mild to moderate degree, and *acute disease– or injury-related malnutrition* when inflammation is acute and of a severe degree. However, because distinguishing diagnostic criteria for these conditions have not been elaborated, this chapter outlines criteria that have served well and are embedded in the medical literature.

MARASMUS OR CACHEXIA

Marasmus is a state in which virtually all available body fat stores have been exhausted due to starvation. Cachexia is a state that involves substantial loss of lean body mass due to chronic systemic inflammation. Conditions that produce cachexia in high-income countries tend to be chronic and indolent, such as cancer and chronic pulmonary disease, whereas marasmus occurs in patients with anorexia nervosa. These conditions are relatively easy to detect because of the patient's starved appearance. The diagnosis is based on fat and muscle wastage resulting from prolonged calorie deficiency and/or inflammation. Diminished skinfold thickness reflects the loss of fat reserves; reduced arm muscle circumference with temporal and interosseous muscle wasting reflects the catabolism of protein throughout the body, including vital organs such as the heart, liver, and kidneys.

TABLE 55-1

COMPARISON OF MARASMUS/CACHEXIA AND KWASHIORKOR/PROTEIN-CALORIE MALNUTRITION		
	MARASMUS OR CACHEXIA	**KWASHIORKOR OR PROTEIN-CALORIE MALNUTRITION[a]**
Clinical setting	↓ Energy intake	↓ Protein intake during stress state
Time course to develop	Months or years	Weeks
Clinical features	Starved appearance Weight <80% standard for height Triceps skinfold <3 mm Midarm muscle circumference <15 cm	Well-nourished appearance Easy hair pluckability[b] Edema
Laboratory findings	Creatinine-height index <60% standard	Serum albumin <2.8 g/dL Total iron-binding capacity <200 μg/dL Lymphocytes <1500/μL Anergy
Clinical course	Reasonably preserved responsiveness to short-term stress	Infections Poor wound healing, decubitus ulcers, skin breakdown
Mortality	Low unless related to underlying disease	High
Diagnostic criteria	Triceps skinfold <3 mm Midarm muscle circumference <15 cm	Serum albumin <2.8 g/dL At least one of the following: Poor wound healing, decubitus ulcers, or skin breakdown Easy hair pluckability[b] Edema

[a]The findings used to diagnose kwashiorkor must be unexplained by other causes.
[b]Tested by *firmly* pulling a lock of hair from the top (not the sides or back), grasping with the thumb and forefinger. An average of three or more hairs removed easily and painlessly is considered abnormal hair pluckability.

Routine laboratory findings in cachexia/marasmus are relatively unremarkable. The creatinine–height index (24-h urinary creatinine excretion compared with normal values based on height) is low, reflecting the loss of muscle mass. Occasionally, the serum albumin level is reduced, but it stays above 2.8 g/dL in uncomplicated cases. Despite a morbid appearance, immunocompetence, wound healing, and the ability to handle short-term stress are reasonably well preserved in most patients.

Pure starvation-related malnutrition is a chronic, fairly well adapted form of starvation rather than an acute illness; it should be treated cautiously in an attempt to reverse the downward trend gradually. Although nutritional support is necessary, overly aggressive repletion can result in severe, even life-threatening metabolic imbalances such as hypophosphatemia and cardiorespiratory failure (refeeding syndrome). When possible, oral or enteral nutritional support is preferred; treatment started slowly allows readaptation of metabolic and intestinal functions (Chap. 56).

KWASHIORKOR OR PROTEIN-CALORIE MALNUTRITION (PCM)

By contrast, kwashiorkor or PCM in developed countries occurs mainly in connection with acute, life-threatening illnesses such as trauma and sepsis. The physiologic stress produced by these illnesses increases protein and energy requirements at a time when intake is often limited. A classic scenario for PCM is an acutely stressed patient who receives only 5% dextrose solutions for periods as brief as 2 weeks; this gives rise to the proposed term *acute disease– or injury-related malnutrition*. Although the etiologic mechanisms are not fully known, the protein-sparing response normally seen in starvation is blocked by the stressed state and by carbohydrate infusion.

In its early stages, the physical findings of kwashiorkor/PCM are few and subtle. Fat reserves and muscle mass are initially unaffected, giving the deceptive appearance of adequate nutrition. Signs that support the diagnosis of kwashiorkor/PCM include easy hair pluckability, edema, skin breakdown, and poor wound healing. The major sine qua non is severe reduction of levels of serum proteins such as albumin (<2.8 g/dL) and transferrin (<150 mg/dL) or iron-binding capacity (<200 μg/dL). Cellular immune function is depressed, reflected by lymphopenia (<1500 lymphocytes/μL in adults and older children) and lack of response to skin test antigens (anergy).

The prognosis of adult patients with full-blown kwashiorkor/PCM is not good even with aggressive nutritional support. Surgical wounds often dehisce (fail to heal), pressure sores develop, gastroparesis and diarrhea can occur with enteral feeding, the risk of gastrointestinal bleeding from stress ulcers is increased, host defenses are compromised, and death from overwhelming infection may occur despite antibiotic therapy. Unlike treatment in marasmus, aggressive nutritional support is indicated to restore better metabolic balance rapidly (Chap. 56). Although kwashiorkor in children is less foreboding, perhaps because a lesser degree of stress is required to precipitate the disorder, it is still a serious condition.

PHYSIOLOGIC CHARACTERISTICS OF HYPOMETABOLIC AND HYPERMETABOLIC STATES

The metabolic characteristics and nutritional needs of hypermetabolic patients who are stressed from injury, infection, or chronic inflammatory illness differ from those of hypometabolic patients who are unstressed but chronically starved. In both cases, nutritional support is important, but misjudgments in selecting the appropriate approach may have serious adverse consequences.

The hypometabolic patient is typified by the relatively less stressed but mildly catabolic and chronically starved individual who, with time, will develop cachexia/marasmus. The hypermetabolic patient stressed from injury or infection is catabolic (experiencing rapid breakdown of body mass) and is at high risk for developing PCM/kwashiorkor if nutritional needs are not met and/or the illness does not resolve quickly. As summarized in **Table 55-2**, the two states are distinguished by differing perturbations of metabolic rate, rates of protein breakdown (proteolysis), and rates of gluconeogenesis. These differences are mediated by proinflammatory cytokines and counterregulatory hormones—tumor necrosis factor, interleukins 1 and 6, C-reactive protein, catecholamines (epinephrine and norepinephrine), glucagon, and cortisol—that are relatively reduced in hypometabolic patients and increased in hypermetabolic patients. Although insulin levels are also elevated in stressed patients, insulin resistance in the target tissues blocks insulin-mediated anabolic effects.

METABOLIC RATE

In starvation and semistarvation, the resting metabolic rate falls between 10 and 30% as an adaptive response to energy restriction, slowing the rate of weight loss. By contrast, resting metabolic rate rises in the presence of physiologic stress in proportion to the degree of the insult. It may increase by about 10% after elective surgery, 20–30% after bone fractures, 30–60% with severe infections such as peritonitis or gram-negative septicemia, and as much as 110% after major burns.

TABLE 55-2

PHYSIOLOGIC CHARACTERISTICS OF HYPOMETABOLIC AND HYPERMETABOLIC STATES

PHYSIOLOGIC CHARACTERISTICS	HYPOMETABOLIC, NONSTRESSED PATIENT (MARASMIC)	HYPERMETABOLIC, STRESSED PATIENT (KWASHIORKOR RISK[a])
Cytokines, catecholamines, glucagon, cortisol, insulin	↓	↑
Metabolic rate, O_2 consumption	↓	↑
Proteolysis, gluconeogenesis	↓	↑
Ureagenesis, urea excretion	↓	↑
Fat catabolism, fatty acid utilization	Relative ↑	Absolute ↑
Adaptation to starvation	Normal	Abnormal

[a]These changes characterize the stressed, kwashiorkor-risk patient seen in developed countries; they differ in some respects from the characteristics of primary kwashiorkor seen in developing countries.

If the metabolic rate (energy requirement) is not matched by energy intake, weight loss results, slowly in hypometabolism and quickly in hypermetabolism. Losses of up to 10% of body mass are unlikely to be detrimental; however, losses greater than this in acutely ill hypermetabolic patients may be associated with rapid deterioration in body function.

PROTEIN CATABOLISM

The rate of endogenous protein breakdown (catabolism) to supply energy needs normally falls during uncomplicated energy deprivation. After about 10 days of total starvation, an unstressed individual loses about 12–18 g/d protein (equivalent to approximately 2 oz of muscle tissue or 2–3 g of nitrogen). By contrast, in injury and sepsis, protein breakdown accelerates in proportion to the degree of stress, reaching 30–60 g/d after elective surgery, 60–90 g/d with infection, 100–130 g/d with severe sepsis or skeletal trauma, and >175 g/d with major burns or head injuries. These losses are reflected by proportional increases in the excretion of urea nitrogen, the major by-product of protein breakdown.

GLUCONEOGENESIS

The major aim of protein catabolism during a state of starvation is to provide the glucogenic amino acids (especially alanine and glutamine) that serve as substrates for endogenous glucose production (gluconeogenesis) in the liver. In the hypometabolic/starved state, protein breakdown for gluconeogenesis is minimized, especially as ketones derived from fatty acids become the substrate preferred by certain tissues. In the hypermetabolic/stress state, gluconeogenesis increases dramatically and in proportion to the degree of the insult to increase the supply of glucose (the major fuel of reparation). Glucose is the only fuel that can be utilized by hypoxemic tissues (anaerobic glycolysis), white blood cells, and newly generated fibroblasts. Infusions of glucose partially offset a negative energy balance but do not significantly suppress the high rates of gluconeogenesis in catabolic patients. Hence, adequate supplies of protein are needed to replace the amino acids utilized for this metabolic response.

In summary, a hypometabolic patient is adapted to starvation and conserves body mass by reducing the metabolic rate and using fat as the primary fuel (rather than glucose and its precursor amino acids). A hypermetabolic patient also uses fat as a fuel but rapidly breaks down body protein to produce glucose, causing loss of muscle and organ tissue and endangering vital body functions.

MICRONUTRIENT MALNUTRITION

The same illnesses and reductions in nutrient intake that lead to PEM often produce deficiencies of vitamins and minerals as well (Chap. 54). Deficiencies of nutrients that are stored in small amounts (such as the water-soluble vitamins) are lost through external secretions, such as zinc in diarrhea fluid or burn exudate, and are probably more common than generally recognized.

Deficiencies of vitamin C, folic acid, and zinc are reasonably common in sick patients. Signs of scurvy such as corkscrew hairs on the lower extremities are found frequently in chronically ill and/or alcoholic patients. The diagnosis can be confirmed with plasma vitamin C levels. Folic acid intakes and blood levels are often less than optimal, even among healthy persons; when illness, alcoholism, poverty, or poor dentition is present, these deficiencies are common. Low blood zinc levels are prevalent in patients with malabsorption syndromes such as inflammatory bowel disease. Patients with zinc deficiency often exhibit poor wound healing, pressure ulcer formation, and impaired immunity. Thiamine deficiency is a common complication of alcoholism but may be prevented by therapeutic doses of thiamine in patients treated for alcohol abuse.

Patients with low plasma vitamin C levels usually respond to the doses in multivitamin preparations, but patients with deficiencies should be supplemented with 250–500 mg/d. Folic acid is absent from some oral multivitamin preparations; patients with deficiencies should be supplemented with about 1 mg/d. Patients with zinc deficiencies resulting from large external losses sometimes require oral supplementation with 220 mg of zinc sulfate one to three times daily. For these reasons, laboratory assessments of the micronutrient status of patients at high risk are desirable.

Hypophosphatemia develops in hospitalized patients with remarkable frequency and generally results from rapid intracellular shifts of phosphate in cachectic or alcoholic patients receiving intravenous glucose. The adverse clinical sequelae are numerous; some, such as acute cardiopulmonary failure, are collectively called refeeding syndrome and can be life-threatening.

GLOBAL CONSIDERATIONS

Many developing countries are still faced with high prevalences of the classic forms of PEM: marasmus and kwashiorkor. *Food insecurity*, which characterizes many poor countries, prevents consistent dietary sufficiency and/or quality and leads to endemic or cyclic malnutrition. Factors threatening food security include marked seasonal variations in agricultural productivity (rainy season–dry season cycles), periodic droughts, political unrest or injustice, and disease epidemics, especially HIV/AIDS. The coexistence of malnutrition and disease epidemics exacerbates the latter and increases complications and mortality rates, creating vicious cycles of malnutrition and disease.

As economic prosperity improves, developing countries have been observed to undergo an epidemiologic transition, a component of which has been termed the *nutrition transition*. As improved economic resources make greater dietary diversity possible, middle-income populations (e.g., southern Asia, China, and Latin America) typically begin to adopt lifestyle habits of industrialized nations, with increased consumption of energy and fat and decreased levels of physical activity. This leads to rising levels of obesity, metabolic syndrome, diabetes, cardiovascular disease, and cancer, sometimes coexisting in populations with persistent undernutrition.

Micronutrient deficiencies also remain prevalent in many countries of the world, impairing functional status and productivity and increasing mortality rates. Vitamin A deficiency affects perhaps 20% of the world's population, impairing vision and increasing morbidity and mortality rates from infections, for example, measles. Community vitamin A supplementation programs have significantly reduced measles mortality rates in vulnerable populations. Mild to moderate iron deficiency may be prevalent in up to 50% of the world, resulting from poor dietary diversity coupled with periodic blood loss and pregnancies. Iodine deficiency remains prevalent in about 35% of the world's population, causing goiter, hypothyroidism, and cretinism. Zinc deficiency is endemic in many populations, producing growth retardation, hypogonadism, and dermatoses, and impairing wound healing.

NUTRITIONAL ASSESSMENT

Because interactions between illness and nutrition are complex, many physical and laboratory findings reflect both underlying disease and nutritional status. Therefore, the nutritional evaluation of a patient requires an integration of the history, physical examination, anthropometrics, and laboratory studies. This approach helps both to detect nutritional problems and to prevent concluding that isolated findings indicate nutritional problems when they do not. For example, hypoalbuminemia caused by an underlying illness does not necessarily indicate malnutrition.

NUTRITIONAL HISTORY

A nutritional history is directed toward identifying underlying mechanisms that put patients at risk for nutritional depletion or excess. These mechanisms include inadequate intake, impaired absorption, decreased utilization, increased losses, and increased requirements of nutrients.

Individuals with the characteristics listed in Table 55-3 are at particular risk for nutritional deficiencies.

PHYSICAL EXAMINATION

Physical findings that suggest vitamin, mineral, and protein–energy deficiencies and excesses are outlined in Table 55-4. Most of the physical findings are not specific for individual nutrient deficiencies and must be integrated with the historic, anthropometric, and laboratory findings. For example, the finding of follicular hyperkeratosis on the back of the arms is a fairly

TABLE 55-3

THE HIGH-RISK PATIENT
Underweight (body mass index <18.5) and/or recent loss of ≥10% of usual body mass
Poor intake: anorexia, food avoidance (e.g., psychiatric condition), or NPO status for more than about 5 days
Protracted nutrient losses: malabsorption, enteric fistulas, draining abscesses or wounds, renal dialysis
Hypermetabolic states: sepsis, protracted fever, extensive trauma or burns
Alcohol abuse or use of drugs with antinutrient or catabolic properties: steroids, antimetabolites (e.g., methotrexate), immunosuppressants, antitumor agents
Impoverishment, isolation, advanced age

common, normal finding. However, if it is widespread in a person who consumes little fruit and vegetables and smokes regularly (increasing ascorbic acid requirements), vitamin C deficiency is likely. Similarly, easily pluckable hair may be a consequence of chemotherapy, but in a hospitalized patient who has poorly healing surgical wounds and hypoalbuminemia, it suggests PCM/ kwashiorkor.

ANTHROPOMETRICS

Anthropometric measurements provide information on body muscle mass and fat reserves. The most practical and commonly used measurements are body weight, height, triceps skinfold (TSF), and midarm muscle circumference (MAMC). Body weight is one of the most useful nutritional parameters to follow in patients who are acutely or chronically ill. Unintentional weight loss during illness often reflects loss of lean body mass (muscle and organ tissue), especially if it is rapid and is not caused by diuresis. This can be an ominous sign since it indicates use of vital body protein stores for metabolic fuel. The reference standard for normal body weight, body mass index (BMI: weight in kilograms divided by height, in meters, squared), is discussed in Chap. 58. BMIs <18.5 are considered underweight, 18.5–24.9 are normal, 25–29.9 are overweight, and ≥30 are obese.

Measurement of skinfold thickness is useful for estimating body fat stores, because about 50% of body fat is normally in the subcutaneous region. Skinfold thickness can also permit discrimination of fat mass from muscle mass. The TSF is a convenient site that is generally representative of the body's overall fat level. A thickness <3 mm suggests virtually complete exhaustion of fat stores. The MAMC can be used to estimate skeletal muscle mass, calculated as follows:

$$\text{MAMC (cm)} = \text{upper arm circumference (cm)} - [0.314 \times \text{TSF (mm)}]$$

LABORATORY STUDIES

A number of laboratory tests used routinely in clinical medicine can yield valuable information about a patient's nutritional status if a slightly different approach to their interpretation is used. For example, abnormally low serum albumin levels, total iron-binding capacity, and anergy may have a distinct explanation, but collectively they may represent kwashiorkor. In the clinical setting of a hypermetabolic, acutely ill patient who is edematous and has easily pluckable hair and inadequate protein intake, the diagnosis of PCM/kwashiorkor is clear-cut. Commonly used laboratory tests for assessing nutritional status are outlined in Table 55-5. The table also provides tips to avoid assigning nutritional significance to tests that may be abnormal for nonnutritional reasons.

TABLE 55-4

PHYSICAL FINDINGS OF NUTRITIONAL DEFICIENCIES

CLINICAL FINDINGS	POSSIBLE DEFICIENCY[a]	POSSIBLE EXCESS
Hair, Nails		
Corkscrew hairs and unemerged coiled hairs	Vitamin C	
Easily pluckable hair	Protein	
Flag sign (transverse depigmentation of hair)	Protein	
Sparse hair	Protein, biotin, zinc	Vitamin A
Transverse ridging of nails	Protein	
Skin		
Cellophane appearance	Protein	
Cracking (flaky paint or crazy pavement dermatosis)	Protein	
Follicular hyperkeratosis	Vitamins A, C	
Petechiae (especially perifollicular)	Vitamin C	
Purpura	Vitamins C, K	
Pigmentation, scaling of sun-exposed areas	Niacin	
Poor wound healing, decubitus ulcers	Protein, vitamin C, zinc	
Scaling	Vitamin A, essential fatty acids, biotin	Vitamin A
Yellow pigmentation sparing sclerae (benign)	Zinc (hyperpigmented)	Carotene
Eyes		
Night blindness	Vitamin A	
Papilledema		Vitamin A
Perioral		
Angular stomatitis	Riboflavin, pyridoxine, niacin	
Cheilosis (dry, cracking, ulcerated lips)	Riboflavin, pyridoxine, niacin	
Oral		
Atrophic lingual papillae (slick tongue)	Riboflavin, niacin, folate, vitamin B_{12}, protein, iron	
Glossitis (scarlet, raw tongue)	Riboflavin, niacin, pyridoxine, folate, vitamin B_{12}	
Hypogeusesthesia, hyposmia	Zinc	
Swollen, retracted, bleeding gums (if teeth present)	Vitamin C	
Bones, Joints		
Beading of ribs, epiphyseal swelling, bowlegs	Vitamin D	
Tenderness, subperiosteal hemorrhage in children	Vitamin C	
Neurologic		
Confabulation, disorientation	Thiamine (Korsakoff's psychosis)	
Drowsiness, lethargy, vomiting		Vitamin A
Dementia	Niacin, vitamin B_{12}, folate	
Headache		Vitamin A
Ophthalmoplegia	Thiamine, phosphorus	
Peripheral neuropathy (e.g., weakness, paresthesias, ataxia, footdrop, and decreased tendon reflexes, fine tactile sense, vibratory sense, and position sense)	Thiamine, pyridoxine, vitamin B_{12}	Pyridoxine
Tetany	Calcium, magnesium	
Other		
Edema	Protein, thiamine	
Heart failure	Thiamine ("wet" beriberi), phosphorus	
Hepatomegaly	Protein	Vitamin A
Parotid enlargement	Protein (consider also bulimia)	
Sudden heart failure, death	Vitamin C	

[a]In this table, "protein deficiency" is used to signify kwashiorkor/PCM.

TABLE 55-5

607

CHAPTER 55 Malnutrition and Nutritional Assessment

LABORATORY TESTS FOR NUTRITIONAL ASSESSMENT

TEST (NORMAL VALUES)	NUTRITIONAL USE	CAUSES OF NORMAL VALUE DESPITE MALNUTRITION	OTHER CAUSES OF ABNORMAL VALUE

Serum albumin (3.5–5.5 g/dL)	2.8–3.5: Compromised protein status
	 <2.8: Possible kwashiorkor
	 Increasing value reflects positive protein balance
		Dehydration
		
		 Infusion of albumin, fresh-frozen plasma, or whole blood
			Low
			 Common:
			   Infection and other stress, especially with poor protein intake
			   Burns, trauma
			   Congestive heart failure
			   Fluid overload
			   Severe liver disease
			 Uncommon:
			   Nephrotic syndrome
			   Zinc deficiency
			   Bacterial stasis/overgrowth of small intestine

Serum prealbumin, also called transthyretin (20–40 mg/dL; lower in prepubertal children)	10–15 mg/dL: Mild protein depletion 5–10 mg/dL: Moderate protein depletion <5 mg/dL: Severe protein depletion Increasing value reflects positive protein balance	Chronic renal failure	Similar to serum albumin
Serum total iron-binding capacity (TIBC) 240–450 µg/dL	<200: Compromised protein status, possible kwashiorkor Increasing value reflects positive protein balance More labile than albumin	Iron deficiency	**Low** Similar to serum albumin **High** Iron deficiency
Prothrombin time 12.0–15.5 s	Prolongation: vitamin K deficiency		**Prolonged** Anticoagulant therapy (warfarin) Severe liver disease
Serum creatinine 0.6–1.6 mg/dL	<0.6: Muscle wasting due to prolonged energy deficit Reflects muscle mass		**High** Despite muscle wasting: Renal failure Severe dehydration
24-h urinary creatinine 500–1200 mg/d (standardized for height and sex)	Low value: muscle wasting due to prolonged energy deficit	>24-h collection Decreasing serum creatinine	**Low** Incomplete urine collection Increasing serum creatinine Neuromuscular wasting
24-h urinary urea nitrogen (UUN) <5 g/d (depends on level of protein intake)	Determine level of catabolism (as long as protein intake is ≥10 g below calculated protein loss or <20 g total, but at least 100 g carbohydrate is provided) 5–10 g/d = mild catabolism or normal fed state 10–15 g/d = moderate catabolism >15 g/d = severe catabolism Estimate protein balance Protein balance = protein intake – protein loss where protein loss (protein catabolic rate) = [24-h UUN (g) + 4] × 6.25		

(continued)

TABLE 55-5

LABORATORY TESTS FOR NUTRITIONAL ASSESSMENT (*CONTINUED*)

TEST (NORMAL VALUES)	NUTRITIONAL USE	CAUSES OF NORMAL VALUE DESPITE MALNUTRITION	OTHER CAUSES OF ABNORMAL VALUE
	Adjustments required in burn patients and others with large nonurinary nitrogen losses and in patients with fluctuating BUN levels (e.g., renal failure)		
Blood urea nitrogen (BUN) 8–23 mg/dL	<8: Possibly inadequate protein intake 12–23: Possibly adequate protein intake >23: Possibly excessive protein intake If serum creatinine is normal, use BUN If serum creatinine is elevated, use BUN/creatinine ratio (normal range is essentially the same as for BUN)		**Low** Severe liver disease Anabolic state Syndrome of inappropriate antidiuretic hormone **High** Despite poor protein intake: Renal failure (use BUN/creatinine ratio) Congestive heart failure Gastrointestinal hemorrhage

Assessment of circulating (visceral) proteins

The serum proteins most commonly used to assess nutritional status include albumin, total iron-binding capacity (or transferrin), thyroxine-binding prealbumin (or transthyretin), and retinol-binding protein. Because they have differing synthesis rates and half-lives—the half-life of serum albumin is about 21 days, whereas those of prealbumin and retinol-binding protein are about 2 days and 12 h, respectively—some of these proteins reflect changes in nutritional status more quickly than do others. However, rapid fluctuations can also make shorter-half-life proteins less reliable.

Levels of circulating proteins are influenced by their rates of synthesis and catabolism, "third spacing" (loss into interstitial spaces), and, in some cases, external loss. Although an adequate intake of calories and protein is necessary to achieve optimal circulating protein levels, serum protein levels generally do not reflect protein intake. For example, a drop in the serum level of albumin or transferrin often accompanies significant physiologic stress (e.g., from infection or injury) and is not necessarily an indication of malnutrition or poor intake. A low serum albumin level in a burned patient with both hypermetabolism and increased dermal losses of protein may not indicate malnutrition. However, adequate nutritional support of the patient's calorie and protein needs is critical for returning circulating proteins to normal levels as stress resolves. Thus low values by themselves do not define malnutrition, but they often point to increased risk of malnutrition because of the hypermetabolic stress state. As long as significant

physiologic stress persists, serum protein levels remain low, even with aggressive nutritional support. However, if the levels do not rise after the underlying illness improves, the patient's protein and calorie needs should be reassessed to ensure that intake is sufficient.

Assessment of vitamin and mineral status

The use of laboratory tests to confirm suspected micronutrient deficiencies is desirable because the physical findings for those deficiencies are often equivocal or nonspecific. Low blood micronutrient levels can predate more serious clinical manifestations and also may indicate drug-nutrient interactions.

ESTIMATING ENERGY AND PROTEIN REQUIREMENTS

A patient's basal energy expenditures (BEE, measured in kilocalories per day) can be estimated from height, weight, age, and gender by using the Harris-Benedict equations:

$$\text{Men: BEE} = 66.47 + 13.75W + 5.00H - 6.76A$$
$$\text{Women: BEE} = 655.10 + 9.56W + 1.85H - 4.68A$$

where W is weight in kilograms; H is height in centimeters, and A is age in years. After these equations are solved, total energy requirements are estimated by multiplying BEE by a factor that accounts for the stress of illness. Multiplying by 1.1–1.4 yields a range 10–40% above basal that estimates the 24-h energy expenditure of the majority of patients. The lower value (1.1) is used for patients without evidence of significant physiologic stress; the higher value (1.4) is appropriate for patients with marked stress such as sepsis or trauma. The result is used as a 24-h energy goal for feeding.

When it is important to have a more accurate assessment of energy expenditure, it can be measured at the bedside by using indirect calorimetry. This technique is useful in patients who are believed to be hypermetabolic from sepsis or trauma and whose body weights cannot be obtained accurately. Indirect calorimetry can also be useful in patients who have difficulty weaning from a ventilator, as their energy needs should not be exceeded to avoid excessive CO_2 production. Patients at the extremes of weight (e.g., obese persons) and/or age are good candidates as well, because the Harris-Benedict equations were developed from measurements in adults with roughly normal body weights.

Because urea is a major by-product of protein catabolism, the amount of urea nitrogen excreted each day can be used to estimate the rate of protein catabolism and determine whether protein intake is adequate to offset it. Total protein loss and protein balance can be calculated from urinary urea nitrogen (UUN) as follows:

$$\text{Protein catabolic rate (g/d)} = [\text{24-h UUN (g)} + 4] \times 6.25 \text{ (g protein/g nitrogen)}$$

The value of 4 g added to the UUN represents a liberal estimate of the unmeasured nitrogen lost in the urine (e.g., creatinine and uric acid), sweat, hair, skin, and feces. When protein intake is low (e.g., less than about 20 g/d), the equation indicates both the patient's protein requirement and the severity of the catabolic state (Table 55-5). More substantial protein intakes can raise the UUN because some of the ingested (or infused) protein is catabolized and converted to UUN. Thus, at lower protein intakes the equation is useful for estimating *requirements*, and at higher protein intakes it is useful for assessing protein *balance*.

$$\text{Protein balance (g/d)} = \text{protein intake} - \text{protein catabolic rate}$$

CHAPTER 56

ENTERAL AND PARENTERAL NUTRITION THERAPY

Bruce R. Bistrian ■ David F. Driscoll

The ability to provide specialized nutritional support (SNS) represents a major advance in medical therapy. Nutritional support, via either enteral or parenteral routes, is used in two main settings: (1) to provide adequate nutritional intake during the recuperative phase of illness or injury, when the patient's ability to ingest or absorb nutrients is impaired, and (2) to support the patient during the systemic response to inflammation, injury, or infection during an extended critical illness. SNS is also used in patients with permanent loss of intestinal length or function. In addition, an increasing number of elderly patients living in nursing homes and chronic care facilities receive enteral feeding, usually as a consequence of inadequate nutritional intake.

Enteral refers to feeding via a tube placed into the gut to deliver liquid formulas containing all essential nutrients. *Parenteral* refers to the infusion of complete nutrient solutions into the bloodstream via a peripheral vein or, more commonly, by central venous access to meet nutritional needs. Enteral feeding is generally the preferred route because of benefits derived from maintaining the digestive, absorptive, and immunologic barrier functions of the gastrointestinal tract. Small-bore pliable tubes have largely replaced large-bore rubber tubes, making placement easier and more acceptable to patients. Infusion pumps have also improved the delivery of nutrient solutions.

For short-term use, enteral tubes can be placed via the nose into the stomach, duodenum, or jejunum. For long-term use, these sites can be accessed through the abdominal wall using endoscopic, radiologic, or surgical procedures. Intestinal tolerance of tube feeding may be limited during acute illness by gastric retention or diarrhea. Parenteral feeding has greater risk of infection, reflecting the need for venous access, and a greater propensity for inducing hyperglycemia. However, these risks can generally be managed successfully by SNS teams. For the postoperative patient with preexisting malnutrition, or in trauma patients who were previously well nourished, SNS is cost-effective. In the most critically ill patient in the intensive care unit, SNS can enhance survival. Although enteral nutrition (EN) can be provided by most health care teams caring for hospitalized patients, safe and effective parenteral nutrition (PN) usually requires specialized teams.

APPROACH TO THE PATIENT: Requirements for Specialized Nutritional Support

INDICATIONS FOR SPECIALIZED NUTRITIONAL SUPPORT Although at least 15–20% of patients in acute care hospitals have evidence of significant malnutrition, only a small fraction will benefit from SNS. For others, wasting is an inevitable component of a terminal disease and the course of the disease will not be altered by SNS. The decision to use SNS should be based on the likelihood that preventing protein-calorie malnutrition (PCM) will increase the likelihood of recovery, reduce infection rates, improve healing, or otherwise shorten the hospital stay. In the case of the elderly or chronically ill patient for whom full recovery is not anticipated, the decision to feed is usually based on whether SNS will extend the duration or quality of life. The decision-making process used to assess whether to use SNS is depicted in **Fig. 56-1**.

The first step in deciding to administer SNS is to consider the nutritional implications of the disease process. Is the condition or its treatment likely to impair food intake and absorption for a prolonged period of time? For example, a well-nourished individual can tolerate approximately 7 days of starvation while experiencing a systemic response to inflammation (SRI). The second step is to determine if the patient is already significantly

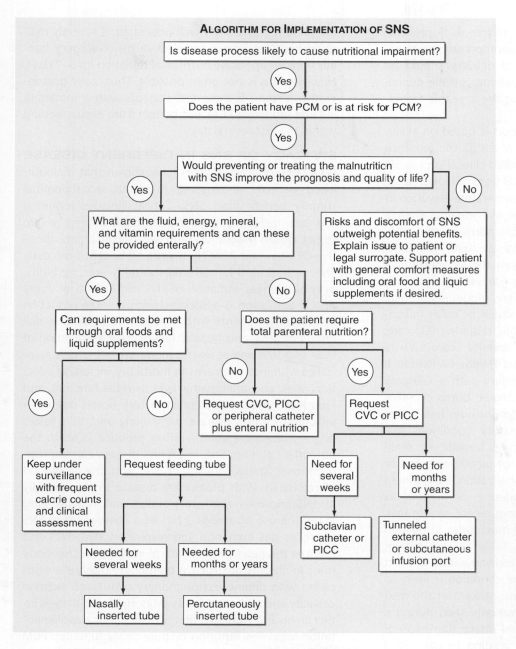

ALGORITHM FOR IMPLEMENTATION OF SNS

Is disease process likely to cause nutritional impairment?

Yes

Does the patient have PCM or is at risk for PCM?

Yes

Would preventing or treating the malnutrition with SNS improve the prognosis and quality of life?

Yes — No

What are the fluid, energy, mineral, and vitamin requirements and can these be provided enterally?

Risks and discomfort of SNS outweigh potential benefits. Explain issue to patient or legal surrogate. Support patient with general comfort measures including oral food and liquid supplements if desired.

Yes — No

Can requirements be met through oral foods and liquid supplements?

Does the patient require total parenteral nutrition?

No — Yes

Request CVC, PICC or peripheral catheter plus enteral nutrition

Request CVC or PICC

Yes — No

Keep under surveillance with frequent calorie counts and clinical assessment

Request feeding tube

Need for several weeks

Need for months or years

Subclavian catheter or PICC

Tunneled external catheter or subcutaneous infusion port

Needed for several weeks

Needed for months or years

Nasally inserted tube

Percutaneously inserted tube

FIGURE 56-1

Decision-making for the implementation of specialized nutrition support (SNS). CVC, central venous catheter; PICC, peripherally inserted central catheter. (*Adapted from chapter in Harrison's Principles of Internal Medicine, 16e, by Lyn Howard, MD.*)

malnourished to the degree that critical functions such as wound healing, immune responses, or ventilatory function are impaired (Chap. 55). An unintentional weight loss of >10% during the previous 6 months or a weight/height <90% of standard, when associated with physiologic impairment, represents significant PCM. Weight loss >20% of usual or <80% of standard reflects severe PCM. The presence or absence of SRI should be noted, since inflammation, injury, and infection increase the rate of lean tissue loss. SRI also has pathophysiologic effects that influence nutritional responses such as fluid retention and hyperglycemia, as well as impairment of anabolic responses to nutritional support.

Once it is determined that a patient is already or at risk of becoming malnourished, the next step is to decide whether SNS will impact positively on the patient's response to disease. In the end stages of many chronic illnesses with accompanying PCM, particularly those due to cancer or terminal neurologic disorders, nutrition may not reverse the PCM or improve quality of life. While the provision of food and water is part of basic medical care, nutrition delivered by tube or catheter, either enterally or parenterally, is associated with risk and discomfort. Thus, SNS should be recommended only when potential benefits exceed risks, and it should be undertaken with the consent of the patient. Like other life support measures, enteral or parenteral therapy is difficult to withdraw once started. Initiating nutrition support may be appropriate before a final prognosis can be determined, but this should not preclude its subsequent withdrawal. If preventing or treating PCM with SNS is appropriate, nutritional requirements and the method of delivery should be determined. The optimal route depends on the degree of gut function and somewhat on the available technical resources.

The timing of nutritional support is based on evaluation of the preexisting nutritional status, the presence and extent of SRI, and the anticipated clinical course. SRI is identified by the standard clinical signs of leukocytosis, tachycardia, tachypnea, and/or temperature elevation or depression. Although the degree of hypoalbuminemia provides an estimate of SRI severity, normal serum albumin levels will not be restored by adequate nutritional support until the SRI remits, even though nutritional benefits can be achieved by adequate feeding.

The SRI can be graded as severe, moderate, or mild. Examples of severe SRI include sepsis or other inflammatory conditions like pancreatitis requiring ICU care, multiple trauma with an Injury Severity Score >20–25 or Acute Physiology and Chronic Health Evaluation II (APACHE II) >25, closed head injury with a Glasgow Coma Scale <8, or major third-degree burns of >40% of body surface area. Moderate SRI includes less severe infections, injuries, or inflammatory conditions like pneumonia, major surgery, acute hepatic or renal insufficiency, and exacerbations of ulcerative colitis or regional enteritis requiring hospitalization. PCM should also be defined as severe, moderate, or minimal as assessed by weight/height, percent recent weight loss, and body mass index. The body mass index in relation to nutritional status is listed in Table 56-1. A patient with a severe SRI requires early feeding within the first several days of care because the condition is likely to produce inadequate spontaneous intake over the next 7 days. A moderate SRI, as commonly seen during a postoperative period without oral intake that exceeds 5 days, benefits from adequate feeding by day 5–7 if

the patient was initially well nourished. If severely malnourished, candidates for elective major surgery benefit from preoperative nutritional repletion for 5–7 days. However, this is not often possible. Thus, early postoperative feeding is indicated. Patients with a moderate SRI and moderate PCM also benefit from earlier feeding within the first several days.

EFFICACY OF SNS IN DIFFERENT DISEASE STATES Efficacy studies have shown that malnourished patients undergoing major thoracoabdominal surgery benefit from SNS. Critical illnesses requiring ICU care, including major burns, major trauma, severe sepsis, closed head injury, and severe pancreatitis (positive CT scan and APACHE II >10), all benefit from early SNS, as indicated by reduced mortality and morbidity. In critical illness, initiation of SNS within 24 h of injury or ICU admission is associated with a ~50% reduction in mortality. Patients with nitrogen accumulation disorders of renal and hepatic failure have a likelihood of PCM of >50% and at least a moderate SRI. SNS is associated with improvements in morbidity, including infection rates, encephalopathy, liver or renal function, and length of hospital stay. Inflammatory bowel disease—including Crohn's disease particularly and, to a lesser degree, ulcerative colitis—often produce PCM. In the outpatient setting, SNS in Crohn's disease can improve nutritional status, quality of life, and the likelihood of remission. With pulmonary disease in the critically ill, SNS improves ventilatory status, and in acute lung injury the use of omega-3 fats as a component of SNS improves gas exchange and respiratory dynamics and reduces the need for mechanical ventilation. Low body mass in chronic obstructive pulmonary disease is associated with diminished pulmonary status and exercise capacity and higher mortality rates. However, there is little convincing evidence that SNS as caloric supplementation improves nutrition or pulmonary function. PCM is also common in the course of cancer and HIV disease, although less so in the latter with the advent of highly active antiretroviral therapy. When PCM develops as a consequence of SRI in these conditions, there is limited likelihood of substantial efficacy or benefit from SNS. However, when PCM develops as a consequence of gastrointestinal dysfunction, SNS can be effective. Although no randomized trials have been performed for SNS provided for hyperemesis gravidarum, there is considerable clinical evidence that it improves pregnancy outcomes.

RISKS AND BENEFITS OF SPECIALIZED NUTRITION SUPPORT The risks are determined primarily by patient factors such as state of alertness, swallowing competence, the route of delivery, underlying conditions, and the experience of the supervising clinical team. The safest and least costly approach is to avoid SNS by close attention to oral food intake, by adding an oral

TABLE 56-1

BODY MASS INDEX (BMI) AND NUTRITIONAL STATUS

BMI	NUTRITIONAL STATUS
>30 kg/m^2	Obese
>25–30 kg/m^2	Overweight
20–25 kg/m^2	Normal
<18.5 kg/m^2	Moderate malnutrition
<16 kg/m^2	Severe malnutrition
<13 kg/m^2	Lethal in males
<11 kg/m^2	Lethal in females

Source: From D Driscoll, B Bistrian: Parenteral and enteral nutrition in the intensive care unit, in *Intensive Care Medicine*, R Irwin, J Rippe (eds). Lippincott Williams & Wilkins, Philadelphia, 2003.

liquid supplement, or in certain chronic conditions by using medications to stimulate appetite. Nutrient intake monitoring by frequent calorie counts or oral formula selection is best performed by a nutritionist.

Enteral tube feeding is often required in patients with anorexia, impaired swallowing, or bowel disease. The bowel and its associated digestive organs derive 70% of their required nutrients directly from food in the lumen. Arginine, glutamine, short-chain fatty acids, long-chain omega-3 fatty acids, and nucleotides available in some specialty enteral formulas are particularly important for maintaining immunity. Enteral feeding also supports gut function by stimulating splanchnic blood flow, neuronal activity, IgA antibody release, and secretion of gastrointestinal hormones that stimulate gut trophic activity. These factors support the gut as an immunologic barrier against enteric pathogens. For these reasons, some luminal nutrition should be provided, even when PN is required to provide most of the nutritional support. The combination of some enteral feeding either by mouth or by enteral tube with parenteral feeding often shortens the transition to full enteral feeding, which can generally be used when >50% of requirements can be met enterally. Substantial nutritional benefit can be achieved by providing ~50% of energy needs for periods of up to 10 days, if protein and other essential nutrient requirements are met. For longer periods of time, it may be preferable to provide 75–80% of energy needs, rather than full feeding, if this improves gastrointestinal tolerance, glycemic control, and avoidance of excess fluid administration.

In the past, bowel rest through PN was the cornerstone of treatment for many severe gastrointestinal disorders. However, the value of providing even minimal amounts of EN is now widely accepted. Protocols to facilitate more widespread use of EN include initiation within 24 h of ICU admission; aggressive use of the head-upright position; postpyloric and nasojejunal feeding tubes; prokinetic agents; more rapid increases in feeding rates; tolerance of higher gastric residuals; and nurse-administered algorithms for feeding progression. PN alone is generally necessary only for severe gut dysfunction due to prolonged ileus, obstruction, or severe hemorrhagic pancreatitis. In the critically ill, feeding adequately by PN beginning within the first 24 h of care improves mortality and is more effective than delayed EN. Early feeding of the critically ill in the ICU is associated with a 50% reduction in mortality, but there is also a 50% increase in infection risk. Much of the increase in morbidity related to PN and EN is due to hyperglycemia, which can be significantly reduced by intensive insulin therapy. The level of glycemia necessary to accomplish this goal, whether <110 mg/dL or only <150 mg/dL, is not yet defined. Surgical patients being adequately fed may benefit from the lower glucose range, but studies of intensive insulin therapy alone without full feeding have shown improved morbidity and mortality outcome with looser control of glucose <180 mg/dL.

Although PN was initially relatively expensive, its components are now often less expensive than specialty enteral formulas. Percutaneous placement of a central venous catheter into the subclavian or internal jugular vein with advancement into the superior vena cava can be accomplished at the bedside by trained personnel using sterile techniques. Peripherally inserted central catheters (PICCs) can also be placed within the lumen in the central vein, but this technique is usually more appropriate for non-ICU patients. Subclavian or internal jugular catheters carry a greater risk, including pneumothorax or serious vascular damage, but they are well tolerated and can be exchanged over a wire rather than requiring reinsertion when ruling out catheter infection. The peripherally inserted catheters are subject to position-related flow, and the catheter cannot be changed over a wire. Inserting a nasogastric tube is a bedside procedure, but many critically ill patients have impaired gastric emptying that increases the risk of aspiration pneumonia. This risk can be reduced by feeding directly into the jejunum beyond the ligament of Treitz. This usually requires fluoroscopic guidance or endoscopic placement. In patients who have planned laparotomies or other conditions likely to require a prolonged need for SNS, it is advantageous to place a jejunal feeding tube at the time of surgery.

Although most SNS is delivered in hospitals, some patients require it on a long-term basis. If they have a safe environment and a willingness to learn the self-care techniques, SNS can be administered at home. The clinical outcomes of patients with severe intestinal disorders treated with home PN or EN are summarized in Table 56-2. PN infused at home is usually cycled overnight to give greater daytime freedom. Other important considerations in determining the appropriateness of home PN or EN are that the patient's prognosis is longer than several months and that the therapy benefits quality of life. Recent advances in surgical techniques and immunosuppressive therapies have made intestinal transplantation a viable alternative for some patients who require life-long home parenteral nutrition. Although the quality of life can be improved with intestinal transplantation relative to home PN, long-term survival even in the most accomplished centers is still somewhat less with transplantation.

DISEASE-SPECIFIC NUTRITIONAL SUPPORT
SNS is basically a support therapy and is primary therapy only for the treatment or prevention of malnutrition. Certain conditions require modification of nutritional support because of organ or system impairment.

TABLE 56-2

SUMMARY OF OUTCOMES FOR PATIENTS ON HOME PARENTERAL AND ENTERAL NUTRITION (HPEN)

DIAGNOSIS	NUMBER IN GROUP	AGE IN YEARS	SURVIVAL[a] ON THERAPY, %	THERAPY STATUS, % AT 1 YEAR[b] FULL ORAL NUTRITION	CONTINUED ON HPEN RX	DIED	REHABILITATION[c] STATUS, % IN 1ST YEAR C	P	M	COMPLICATIONS[d] PER PATIENT-YEAR HPEN	NONHPEN
Home Parenteral Nutrition											
Crohn's disease	562	36	96	70	25	2	60	38	2	0.9	1.1
Ischemic bowel disease	331	49	87	27	48	19	53	41	6	1.4	1.1
Motility disorder	299	45	87	31	44	21	49	39	12	1.3	1.1
Congenital bowel defect	172	5	94	42	47	9	63	27	11	2.1	1.0
Hyperemesis gravidarum	112	28	100	100	0	0	83	16	1	1.5	3.5
Chronic pancreatitis	156	42	90	82	10	5	60	38	2	1.2	2.5
Radiation enteritis	145	58	87	28	49	22	42	49	9	0.8	1.1
Chronic adhesive obstructions	120	53	83	47	34	13	23	68	10	1.7	1.4
Cystic fibrosis	51	17	50	38	13	36	24	66	16	0.8	3.7
Cancer	2122	44	20	26	8	63	29	57	14	1.1	3.3
AIDS	280	33	10	13	6	73	8	63	29	1.6	3.3
Home Enteral Nutrition											
Neurologic disorders of swallowing	1134	65	55	19	25	48	5	24	71	0.3	0.9
Cancer	1644	61	30	30	6	59	21	59	21	0.4	2.7

[a]Survival rates on therapy are values at 1 year, calculated by the life table method. This will differ from the percentage listed as died under Therapy Status, since all patients with known endpoints are considered in this latter measure. The ratio of observed versus expected deaths is equivalent to a Standard Mortality Ratio.
[b]Not shown are those patients who were back in hospital or who had changed therapy type by 12 months.
[c]Rehabilitation is designated complete (C), partial (P), or minimal (M), relative to the patient's ability to sustain normal age-related activity.
[d]Complications refer only to those complications that resulted in rehospitalization.
Source: Derived from North American HPEN Registry. Adapted from chapter in *Harrison's Principles of Internal Medicine*, 16e, by Lyn Howard, MD.

For instance, in nitrogen accumulation disorders, protein intake may need to be reduced. However, in renal disease, except for brief periods of several days, protein intakes should approach requirement levels of at least 0.8 g/kg or higher up to 1.2 g/kg as long as the blood urea nitrogen does not exceed 100 mg/dL. If this is not possible, then dialysis or other renal replacement therapy should be considered to allow better feeding.

In hepatic failure, intakes of 1.2–1.4 g/kg up to the optimal 1.5 g/kg should be attempted, as long as encephalopathy due to protein intolerance is not encountered. In the presence of protein intolerance, formulas containing 33–50% branched-chain amino acids are available and should be provided at the 1.2–1.4-g/kg level. Cardiac patients, and many severely stressed patients, often benefit from fluid and sodium restriction to levels of 1000 mL of total parenteral nutrition (TPN) formula and 5–20 meq of sodium per day. In patients with severe chronic PCM characterized by severe weight loss and tissue wasting, TPN must be instituted gradually because of the profound antinatriuresis, antidiuresis, and intracellular accumulation of potassium, magnesium, and phosphorus that develop as a consequence of high insulin levels. This modification of TPN is usually accomplished by limiting fluid intakes initially to about 1000 mL containing modest carbohydrate content of 10–20% dextrose, low sodium, and ample potassium, magnesium, and phosphorus, with careful daily assessment of fluid and electrolyte status. Protein need not be restricted.

THE DESIGN OF INDIVIDUAL REGIMENS

FLUID REQUIREMENTS

The normal daily requirement for fluid is 30 mL/kg of body mass from all sources (IV infusions, per tube, or oral intake), plus any replacement of abnormal losses such as from an osmotic diuresis, nasogastric drainage, wound output, or diarrheal/ostomy losses. Electrolyte and mineral losses can be estimated or measured and also need to be replaced (Table 56-3). Fluid restriction may be necessary in patients with fluid overload, and fluid inputs can be limited to 1200 mL/d if urine is the only significant fluid output. When severe fluid overload is present, the optimal TPN solution for central venous administration is a concentrated 1-L solution of 7% crystalline amino acids (70 g) and 21% dextrose (210 g), which provides an amount of nitrogen and glucose that is optimally effective at protein-sparing.

Patients requiring PN or EN in the acute care setting generally have some element of associated hormonal adaptations to their underlying critical illness (e.g., increased secretion of antidiuretic hormone,

aldosterone, insulin, glucagon, or cortisol) that cause fluid retention and hyperglycemia. Weight gain in the critically ill, whether receiving SNS or not, is invariably the consequence of fluid retention, since lean tissue accretion, even with feeding, is minimal in the acute phase of illness. Because excess fluid removal can be difficult, limiting fluid intake to allow for balanced intake and output is more effective.

ENERGY REQUIREMENTS

Total energy expenditure comprises resting energy expenditure, activity energy expenditure, and the thermal effect of feeding (Chap. 55). Resting energy expenditure (two-thirds) includes the calories necessary for basal metabolism at bed rest. Activity energy expenditure represents one-fourth to one-third of the total, and the thermal effect of feeding is about 10% of the total energy expenditure. For normally nourished healthy individuals, the total energy expenditure is about 30–35 kcal/kg. Although critical illness increases resting energy expenditure, only in initially well-nourished individuals with the highest systemic inflammatory response, such as that from severe multiple trauma, burns, closed head injury, or sepsis, do total energy expenditures reach 40–45 kcal/kg. The chronically ill patient with lean tissue loss has reduced basal energy expenditure, as well as inactivity, which results in a total energy expenditure of about 20–25 kcal/kg. About 95% of such patients need <30 kcal/kg to achieve energy balance. Because providing about 50% of measured energy expenditure as SNS is at least equally efficacious for the first 10 days of critical illness, actual measurement of energy expenditure is not generally necessary in the early period of SNS. However, in patients who remain critically ill beyond several weeks, in the severely malnourished for whom estimates of energy expenditure are unreliable, or in those who are difficult to wean from ventilators, it is reasonable to actually measure energy expenditure and

TABLE 56-3

ENTERIC FLUID VOLUMES AND THEIR ELECTROLYTE CONTENT[a]

	L/d	Na	K	Cl	HCO₃	H
Oral intake	2–3					
Enteric secretions						
Saliva	1–2	15	30	15	50	—
Gastric juice	1.5–2	50–70	5–15	90–120	0	70–100
Bile	0.5–1.5	120–150	5–15	80–120	30–50	—
Pancreatic	0.5–1	100–140	10	70–100	60–110	—
Small intestine	1–2	80–140	10–20	80–120	20–40	—

[a]All in meq/L.

Source: Adapted from chapter in *Harrison's Principles of Internal Medicine*, 16e, by Lyn Howard, MD.

to aim for energy balance to 1.2 times measured expenditure with SNS.

Insulin resistance due to SRI is associated with increased gluconeogenesis and reduced peripheral glucose utilization, predisposing a patient to hyperglycemia. This is aggravated in patients receiving exogenous carbohydrate from SNS. Normalization of blood glucose levels by insulin infusion in critically ill patients receiving SNS reduces morbidity and mortality. In mild or moderately malnourished patients, a reasonable goal is to provide metabolic support to improve protein synthesis and maintain metabolic homeostasis. Hypocaloric nutrition providing only about 1000 kcal/d and 70 g protein for up to 10 days requires less fluid and reduces the likelihood of poor glycemic control. Energy content can be advanced to 20–25 kcal/kg with 1.5 g protein/kg as metabolic conditions permit and definitely during the second week of SNS. Patients with multiple trauma, closed head injury, and severe burns often have much higher energy expenditures, but there is little evidence that providing more than 30 kcal/kg has additional benefit, and it substantially increases the risks of hyperglycemia.

Generally, because glucose is an essential tissue fuel, glucose and amino acids are provided parenterally until the level of resting energy expenditure is reached. At this point, adding fat becomes beneficial, since more parenteral glucose stimulates de novo lipogenesis by the liver—an energy-inefficient process. Polyunsaturated long-chain triglycerides as soybean oil are the chief ingredient in most parenteral fat emulsions and the majority of the fat in enteral feeding formulas. These vegetable oil–based emulsions provide essential fatty acids. Enteral feeding formulas have fat content that ranges from 3% of calories up to as much as 50% of calories, while parenteral fat comes in separate containers as 10%, 20%, and 30% emulsions that can be infused separately or mixed by the pharmacy under controlled conditions as all-in-one or total nutrient admixture with glucose, amino acids, lipid, electrolytes, vitamins, and minerals. Although parenteral fat is required at only about 3% of energy requirements to meet essential fatty acid requirements, when provided as an all-in-one mixture of carbohydrate, fat, and protein, 2–3% fat in the TPN mixtures, representing about 20–30% of calories as fat, is provided to ensure emulsion stability. If given separately, parenteral fat should not be provided at rates exceeding 0.11 g/kg body mass per h or about 100 g over 12 h—equivalent to 1 L of 10% parenteral fat and 500 mL of 20% parenteral fat.

Medium-chain triglycerides, which contain saturated fatty acids with chain lengths of 6, 8, 10, or 12 carbons, are provided in a number of enteral feeding formulas because they are absorbed preferentially. Fish oil contains polyunsaturated fatty acids of the omega-3 family, which have been shown to improve immune function and reduce the inflammatory response.

Carbohydrates are provided as hydrous glucose providing 3.4 kcal/g in PN formulas. In enteral formulas, glucose is the carbohydrate source in so-called monomeric diets. These diets provide protein as amino acids and fat in minimal amounts (3%) to meet essential fatty acid requirements. Monomeric formulas are designed to optimize absorption in the seriously compromised gut. These formulas, like the immune-enhancing diets, are quite expensive. In polymeric diets, the carbohydrate source is usually an osmotically less active polysaccharide, protein is usually soy or casein protein, and fat is present in amounts from 25 to 50%. Such formulas are usually well tolerated by patients with normal intestinal length, and some are acceptable for oral consumption.

PROTEIN OR AMINO ACID REQUIREMENTS

Although the recommended dietary allowance for protein is 0.8 g/kg per d, maximal rates of repletion occur with 1.5 g/kg in the malnourished. In the severely catabolic patient, this higher level minimizes protein loss. In patients requiring SNS in the acute care setting, at least 1 g/kg is recommended, with greater amounts up to 1.5 g/kg as volume, renal, and hepatic tolerances allow. The standard parenteral and enteral formulas contain protein of high biologic value and meet the requirements for the eight essential amino acids when nitrogen needs are met. In protein-intolerant conditions such as renal and hepatic failure, modified amino acid formulas should be considered. In hepatic failure, higher branched-chain amino acid–enriched formulas appear to improve outcomes. Conditionally essential amino acids like arginine and glutamine may also have some benefit in supplemental amounts.

Protein (nitrogen) balance provides a measure of feeding efficacy of PN or EN. It is calculated as protein intake/6.25 because proteins are on average 16% nitrogen (N), minus the 24-h urine urea N (UUN) plus 4 g N, which reflects other N losses. In the critically ill, a mild negative balance of 2–4 g N/d is usually achievable with a similarly mild positive balance in the recuperating patient. Each g N represents approximately 30 g lean tissue.

MINERAL AND VITAMIN REQUIREMENTS

Parenteral electrolyte, vitamin, and trace mineral requirements are summarized in **Tables 56-4**, **56-5**, and **56-6**. Electrolyte modifications are necessary with substantial gastrointestinal losses from nasogastric drainage or intestinal losses from fistulas, diarrhea, or ostomy outputs. Such losses also imply extra calcium, magnesium, and zinc losses. Excessive urine or potassium losses with amphotericin, or magnesium losses with

TABLE 56-4

USUAL DAILY ELECTROLYTE ADDITIONS TO PARENTERAL NUTRITION

ELECTROLYTE	PARENTERAL EQUIVALENT OF RDA	USUAL INTAKE
Sodium		1–2 meq/kg + replacement, but can be as low as 5–40 meq/d
Potassium		40–100 meq/d + replacement of unusual losses
Chloride		As needed for acid-base balance, but usually 2:1 to 1:1 with acetate
Acetate		As needed for acid-base balance
Calcium	10 meq	10–20 meq/d
Magnesium	10 meq	8–16 meq/d
Phosphorus	30 mmol	20–40 mmol

cisplatin or in renal failure, necessitate adjustments in sodium, potassium, magnesium, phosphorus, and acid-base balance. Vitamin and trace element requirements are met by the daily provision of a complete parenteral vitamin supplement and trace elements for PN, and with the provision of adequate amounts of enteral feeding formulas that contain these micronutrients.

TABLE 56-5

PARENTERAL MULTIVITAMIN REQUIREMENTS FOR ADULTS

VITAMIN	RECENTLY REVISED VALUE
Vitamin A	3300 IU
Thiamin (B_1)	6 mg
Riboflavin (B_2)	3.6 mg
Niacin (B_3)	40 mg
Folic acid	600 µg
Pantothenic acid	15 mg
Pyridoxine (B_6)	6 mg
Cyanocobalamin (B_{12})	5 µg
Biotin	60 µg
Ascorbic acid (C)	200 mg
Vitamin D	200 IU
Vitamin E	10 IU
Vitamin K[a]	150 µg

[a]A product is available without vitamin K. Vitamin K supplementation is recommended at 2–4 mg/week in patients not receiving oral anticoagulation therapy if using this product.

TABLE 56-6

PARENTERAL TRACE METAL SUPPLEMENTATION FOR ADULTS[a]

TRACE MINERAL	INTAKE
Zinc	2.5–4 mg/d, an additional 10–15 mg/d per L of stool or ileostomy output
Copper	0.5–1.5 mg/d, possibility of retention in biliary tract obstruction
Manganese	0.1–0.3 mg/d, possibility of retention in biliary tract obstruction
Chromium	10–15 µg/d
Selenium	20–100 µg/d, necessary for long-term PN, optional for short-term TPN
Molybdenum	20–120 µg/d, necessary for long-term PN, optional for short-term PN
Iodine	75–150 µg/d, necessary for long-term PN, optional for short-term PN

[a]Commercial products are available with the first four, first five, and all seven of these metals in recommended amounts.
Abbreviations: PN, parenteral nutrition; TPN, total parenteral nutrition.

PARENTERAL NUTRITION

INFUSION TECHNIQUE AND PATIENT MONITORING

Parenteral feeding through a peripheral vein is limited by osmolality and volume constraints. Solutions that contain more than 3% amino acids and 5% glucose (290 kcal/L) are poorly tolerated peripherally. Parenteral fat (20%) can be given to increase the calories delivered. The total volume required to provide a marginal protein intake of 60 g and 1680 total kcal is 2.5 L. Moreover, the risk of significant morbidity and mortality from incompatibilities of calcium and phosphate salts is greatest in these low-osmolality, low-glucose regimens. Parenteral feeding via a peripheral vein is generally intended as a supplement to oral feeding and is not optimal for the critically ill. Peripheral parenteral nutrition may benefit from small amounts of heparin at 1000 U/L and co-infusion with parenteral fat to reduce osmolality, but volume constraints still limit the value of this therapy. PICCs can be used for the short term to provide concentrated glucose parenteral solutions of 20–25% dextrose and 4–7% amino acids, while avoiding some of the complications of catheter placement via a large central vein. With PICC lines, however, flow can be position-related, and the lines cannot be exchanged over a wire for infection monitoring. For these reasons, in the critically ill, centrally placed catheters are preferred. The subclavian approach is best tolerated by the patient and is the easiest to dress. The jugular approach is less likely to lead to a pneumothorax. The femoral approach is discouraged because of the greater risk of catheter infection. For long-term feeding in the home, tunneled catheters and implanted ports reduce infection risk and are more acceptable to patients. However, tunneled catheters require placement in the operating room.

Catheters are made of silastic, polyurethane, or polyvinyl chloride. Silastic catheters are less thrombogenic and are best for tunneled catheters. Polyurethane is best for temporary catheters. Dressing changes with dry gauze at regular intervals should be performed by nurses skilled in catheter care to avoid infection. Chlorhexidine solution is more effective than alcohol or iodine compounds. Appropriate monitoring for patients receiving PN is summarized in Table 56-7.

COMPLICATIONS

Mechanical

The insertion of a central venous catheter should be performed by trained and experienced personnel using aseptic techniques to limit the major common complications of pneumothorax and inadvertent arterial

TABLE 56-7

MONITORING THE PATIENT ON PARENTERAL NUTRITION

Clinical Data Monitored Daily

General sense of well-being

Strength as evidenced in getting out of bed, walking, resistance exercise as appropriate

Vital signs including temperature, blood pressure, pulse, and respiratory rate

Fluid balance: weight at least several times weekly, fluid intake (parenteral and enteral) vs. fluid output (urine, stool, gastric drainage, wound, ostomy)

Parenteral nutrition delivery equipment: tubing, pump, filter, catheter, dressing

Nutrient solution composition

Laboratory Daily

Finger-stick glucose	Three times daily until stable
Blood glucose, Na, K, Cl, HCO₃, BUN	Daily until stable and fully advanced, then twice weekly
Serum creatinine, albumin, PO₄, Ca, Mg, Hb/Hct, WBC	Baseline, then twice weekly
INR	Baseline, then weekly
Micronutrient tests	As indicated

Abbreviations: BUN, blood urea nitrogen; Hb, hemoglobin; Hct, hematocrit; INR, international normalized ratio; WBC, white blood cell count.
Source: Adapted from chapter in *Harrison's Principles of Internal Medicine,* 16e, by Lyn Howard, MD.

puncture or injury. Catheter position should be radiographically confirmed to be in the superior vena cava distal to the junction with the jugular or subclavian vein and not directly against the vessel wall. Thrombosis related to the catheter may occur at the site of entry into the vein and extend to encase the catheter. Catheter infection predisposes to thrombosis, as does the SRI. The addition of 6000 U of heparin in the daily parenteral formula in hospitalized patients with temporary catheters reduces the risk of fibrin sheath formation and catheter infection. Temporary catheters that develop a thrombus should be removed and, based on clinical findings, treated with anticoagulants. Thrombolytic therapy can be considered for patients with permanent catheters, depending on the ease of replacement and presence of alternate, reasonably acceptable venous access sites. Low-dose warfarin therapy of 1 mg/d reduces the risk of thrombosis in permanent catheters used for home PN, but full anticoagulation may be required in patients who have recurrent thrombosis related to permanent catheters. A recent U.S. Food and Drug Administration mandate to reformulate parenteral multivitamins to include vitamin K at a dose of 150 μg daily may affect the efficacy of low-dose warfarin therapy. There is a "no vitamin K" version available for patients receiving this therapy. Catheters can become mechanically occluded and may also become occluded by fibrin at the tip, or by fat, minerals, or drugs intraluminally. These occlusions can be managed with low-dose alteplase for fibrin, with indwelling 70% alcohol for fat, with 0.1 N hydrochloric acid for mineral precipitates, and with either 0.1 N hydrochloric acid or 0.1 N sodium hydroxide for drugs, depending on their pH.

Metabolic

The most common problems related to PN are fluid overload and hyperglycemia (Table 56-8). Hypertonic dextrose stimulates a much higher insulin level than meal feeding. Because insulin is a potent antinatriuretic and antidiuretic hormone, hyperinsulinemia leads to sodium and fluid retention. In the absence of gastrointestinal losses or renal dysfunction, net fluid retention is likely when total fluid intake exceeds 2000 mL/d. Close monitoring of body mass, as well as fluid intake and output, is necessary to prevent this complication. In the absence of significant renal impairment, the sodium content of the urine is likely to be <10 meq/L. Providing sodium in limited amounts of 40 meq/d and the use of both glucose and fat in the PN mixture to lower total glucose and sodium will help reduce fluid retention. The elevated insulin also increases the intracellular transport of potassium, magnesium, and phosphorus, which can precipitate a dangerous refeeding syndrome if the total glucose content of the PN solution is advanced too quickly in severely malnourished

TABLE 56-8

SELECTED METABOLIC DISTURBANCES AND THEIR CORRECTION

DISTURBANCE	CAUSE	CORRECTIVE ACTION WITH PN
Hyponatremia	Increased total body water or decreased total body sodium	Decrease free water or increase sodium
Hypernatremia	Occurs commonly with excessive isotonic or hypertonic fluid followed by diuretic administration with free water clearance; can also occur with dehydration and normal total body sodium	Increase free water to produce net positive fluid balance maintaining sodium and chloride balance
Hypokalemia	Inadequate intake relative to need Excessive diuresis, tubular dysfunction Magnesium deficiency Metabolic alkalosis Hyperinsulinemia	Use supplements Use supplements Increase PN magnesium Correct alkalosis Maintain constant PN, increase potassium
Hyperkalemia	Excessive provision Metabolic acidosis Renal deterioration	Reduce supplements Evaluate acidosis, treat with PN acetate salt and decrease potassium Evaluate patient and adjust PN as indicated
Hypocalcemia	Reciprocal response to phosphorus repletion Critical illness effect Severe malabsorption	Increase calcium Increase calcium Supplement calcium
Hypercalcemia	Excessive administration or pathologic (cancer, hyperparathyroidism)	Reduce or eliminate calcium
Hypomagnesemia	Increased requirements due to diuretic use, alcoholism, malabsorption, malnutrition Critical illness	Supplement magnesium Supplement magnesium
Hypophosphatemia	Inadequate intake relative to needs related to malnutrition, alcohol use Increased calcium intake	Supplement phosphorus Use supplements
Hyperphosphatemia	Excessive administration or worsening renal function	Reduce phosphorus
Azotemia	Excessive amino acid infusion or worsening renal function	Reduce amino acid level but consider renal replacement therapy if cannot provide 1 g protein per kg for prolonged periods

Abbreviation: PN, parenteral nutrition.

patients. It is generally best to start PN with <200 g glucose/d to assess glucose tolerance. Regular insulin can be added to the PN formula to establish glycemic control, and the insulin doses can be increased proportionately as the glucose is advanced. As a general rule, patients with insulin-dependent diabetes require about twice their usual home insulin doses when they are receiving TPN at 20–25 kcal/kg, largely as a consequence of parenteral glucose administration and some loss of insulin to the TPN container. As a rough estimate, the amount of insulin can be provided in a similar proportion to the amount of calories provided as TPN relative to full feeding, and the insulin can be placed in the TPN formula. Subcutaneous (SC) regular insulin can be provided to improve glucose control as assessed by measurements of blood glucose every 6 h. About two-thirds of the total 24-h amount can be added to the next day's order, with SC insulin supplements as needed. Advances in TPN concentration should be made when reasonable glucose control is established, and the insulin dose adjusted proportionately to the calories added as glucose and amino acids. These are general rules, and they are conservative. Given the adverse clinical impact of hyperglycemia, it may be necessary to use intensive insulin therapy as a separate infusion with a standard protocol to initially establish control. Once established, this insulin dose can be added to the PN formula. Acid-base imbalance is also common during PN therapy. Amino acid formulas are buffered, but critically ill patients are prone to metabolic acidosis, often due to renal tubular impairment. The use of sodium and potassium acetate salts in the PN formula may address this problem. Bicarbonate salts should not be used because they are incompatible with TPN formulations.

Nasogastric drainage produces a hypochloremic alkalosis that can be managed by attention to chloride balance. Occasionally, hydrochloric acid may be required for a more rapid response or when diuretic therapy limits the ability to provide substantial sodium chloride. Up to 100 meq/L and up to 150 meq of hydrochloric acid per day may be placed in a fat-free TPN formula.

Infectious

Infections of the central access catheter rarely occur in the first 72 h. Fever during this period is usually from infection elsewhere or another cause. Fever that develops during PN can be addressed by checking the catheter site and, if the site looks clean, exchanging the catheter over a wire with cultures taken through the catheter and at the catheter tip. If these cultures are negative, as they are most of the time, the new catheter can continue to be used. If a culture is positive for a relatively nonpathogenic bacteria like *Staphylococcus epidermidis*, consider a second exchange over a wire with repeat cultures or replace the catheter depending on the clinical circumstances. If cultures are positive for more pathogenic bacteria, or for fungi like *Candida albicans*, it is generally best to replace the catheter at a new site. Whether antibiotic treatment is required is a clinical decision, but *C. albicans* grown from the blood culture in a patient receiving PN should always be treated because the consequences of failure to treat can be dire.

Catheter infections can be minimized by dedicating the feeding catheter to TPN, without blood sampling or medication administration. Central catheter infections are a serious complication with an attributed mortality of 12–25%. Infections in central venous catheters dedicated to feeding should occur less frequently than 3 per 1000 catheter-days. Home TPN catheters that become infected may be treated through the catheter without removal of the catheter, particularly if the offending organism is *S. epidermidis*. Clearing of the biofilm and fibrin sheath by local treatment of the catheter with indwelling alteplase may increase the likelihood of eradication. Antibiotic lock therapy with high concentrations of antibiotic, with or without heparin in addition to systemic therapy, may improve efficacy. Sepsis with hypotension should precipitate catheter removal in either the temporary or permanent TPN setting.

ENTERAL NUTRITION

TUBE PLACEMENT AND PATIENT MONITORING

The types of enteral feeding tubes, methods of insertion, their clinical uses, and potential complications are outlined in Table 56-9. The different types of enteral

formulas are listed in Table 56-10. Patients receiving EN are at risk for many of the same metabolic complications as those who receive PN and should be monitored in the same manner. EN can be a source of similar problems, but not to the same degree, because the insulin response to EN is about half of that seen with PN. Enteral feeding formulas have fixed electrolyte compositions that are generally modest in sodium and somewhat higher in potassium content. Acid-base disturbances can be addressed to a more limited extent with EN. Acetate salts can be added to the formula to treat chronic metabolic acidosis. Calcium chloride can be added to treat mild chronic metabolic alkalosis. Medications and other additives to enteral feeding formulas can clog the tubes (e.g., calcium chloride may interact with casein-based formulas to produce insoluble calcium caseinate products) and may reduce the efficacy of some drugs (e.g., phenytoin). Since small-bore tubes are easily displaced, tube position should be checked at intervals by aspirating and measuring the pH of the gut fluid (<4 in the stomach, >6 in the jejunum).

COMPLICATIONS

Aspiration

The debilitated patient with poor gastric emptying and impairment of swallowing and cough is at risk for aspiration; this is particularly true for those who are mechanically ventilated. Tracheal suctioning induces coughing and gastric regurgitation, and cuffs on endotracheal or tracheostomy tubes seldom protect against aspiration. Preventive measures include elevating the head of the bed to 30 degrees, using nurse-directed algorithms for formula advancement, combining enteral with parenteral feeding, and using post–ligament of Treitz feeding. Tube feeding should not be discontinued for gastric residuals of <300 mL unless there are other signs of gastrointestinal intolerance such as nausea, vomiting, or abdominal distention. Continuous feeding using pumps is better tolerated intragastrically and is essential for feeding into the jejunum. For small-bowel feeding, residuals are not assessed but abdominal pain and distention should be monitored.

Diarrhea

Enteral feeding often leads to diarrhea, especially if bowel function is compromised by disease or drugs, particularly broad-spectrum antibiotics. Diarrhea may be controlled by the use of a continuous drip, with a fiber-containing formula, or by adding an antidiarrheal agent to the formula. However, *Clostridium difficile*, which is a common cause of diarrhea in patients being tube fed, should be ruled out before using antidiarrheal agents. H$_2$ blockers may also assist in reducing

TABLE 56-9

ENTERAL FEEDING TUBES

TYPE/INSERTION TECHNIQUE	CLINICAL USES	POTENTIAL COMPLICATIONS
Nasogastric Tube		
External measurement: nostril, ear, xiphisternum; tube stiffened by ice water or stylet; position verified by injecting air and auscultating, or by x-ray	Short-term clinical situation (weeks) or longer periods with intermittent insertion; bolus feeding simpler, but continuous drip with pump better tolerated	Aspiration; ulceration of nasal and esophageal tissues, leading to stricture
Nasoduodenal Tube		
External measurement: nostril, ear, anterior superior iliac spine; tube stiffened by stylet and passed through pylorus under fluoroscopy or with endoscopic loop	Short-term clinical situations where gastric emptying impaired or proximal leak suspected; requires continuous drip with pump	Spontaneous pulling back into stomach (position verified by aspirating content, pH >6); diarrhea common, fiber-containing formulas may help
Gastrostomy Tube		
Percutaneous placement endoscopically, radiologically, or surgically; after tract established, can be converted to a gastric "button"	Long-term clinical situations, swallowing disorders, or impaired small-bowel absorption requiring continuous drip	Aspiration; irritation around tube exit site; peritoneal leak; balloon migration and obstruction of pylorus
Jejunostomy Tube		
Percutaneous placement endoscopically or radiologically via pylorus or endoscopically or surgically directly into the jejunum	Long-term clinical situations where gastric emptying impaired; requires continuous drip with pump; direct endoscopic placement (PEJ) is the most comfortable for patient	Clogging or displacement of tube; jejunal fistula if large-bore tube used; diarrhea from dumping; irritation of surgical anchoring suture
Combined Gastrojejunostomy Tube		
Percutaneous placement endoscopically, radiologically, or surgically; intragastric arm for continuous or intermittent gastric suction; jejunal arm for enteral feeding	Used for patients with impaired gastric emptying and at high risk for aspiration or patients with acute pancreatitis or proximal leaks	Clogging: especially of small-bore jejunal tube

Note: All small tubes are at risk for clogging, especially if used for crushed medications. In long-term enteral patients, gastrostomy and jejunostomy tubes can be exchanged for a low-profile "button" once the tract is established. PEJ, percutaneous endoscopic jejunostomy.
Source: Adapted from chapter in *Harrison's Principles of Internal Medicine*, 16e, by Lyn Howard, MD.

TABLE 56-10

ENTERAL FORMULAS

COMPOSITION CHARACTERISTICS	CLINICAL INDICATIONS
Standard Enteral Formula	

1. Complete dietary products (+)[a]
   a. Caloric density 1 kcal/mL
   b. Protein ~14% cals, caseinates, soy, lactalbumin
   c. CHO ~60% cals, hydrolyzed corn starch, maltodextrin, sucrose
   d. Fat ~30% cals, corn, soy, safflower oils
   e. Recommended daily intake of all minerals and vitamins in >1500 kcal/d
   f. Osmolality (mosmol/kg): ~300
	Suitable for most patients requiring tube feeding; some can be used orally

Modified Enteral Formulas	
1. Caloric density 1.5–2 kcal/mL (+) 2. a. High protein ~20–25% protein (+) b. Hydrolyzed protein to small peptides (+)	Fluid-restricted patients Critically ill patients Impaired absorption

(continued)

TABLE 56-10

ENTERAL FORMULAS (*CONTINUED*)

COMPOSITION CHARACTERISTICS	CLINICAL INDICATIONS
Modified Enteral Formulas	
c. ↑ Arginine, glutamine, nucleotides, ω3 fat (+++)	Immune-enhancing diets
d. ↑ Branched-chain amino acids, ↓ aromatic amino acids (+++)	Liver failure patients intolerant of 0.8 g/kg protein
e. Low protein of high biologic value	Renal failure patient for brief periods if critically ill
3. a. Low-fat partial MCT substitution (+)	Fat malabsorption
b. ↑ Fat >40% cals (++)	Pulmonary failure with CO_2 retention on standard formula, limited utility
c. ↑ Fat from MUFA (++)	Improvement in glycemic index control in diabetes
d. ↑ Fat from ω3 and ↓ ω6 linoleic acid (+++)	Improved ventilation in ARDS
4. Fiber provided as soy polysaccharide (+)	Improved laxation

^aCost: +, inexpensive; ++, moderately expensive; +++, very expensive.
Abbreviations: ARDS, acute respiratory distress syndrome; CHO, carbohydrate; MCT, medium-chain triglyceride; MUFA, monounsaturated fatty acids; ω3 or ω6, polyunsaturated fat with first double bond at carbon 3 (fish oils) or carbon 6 (vegetable oils).
Source: Adapted from chapter in *Harrison's Principles of Internal Medicine*, 16e, by Lyn Howard, MD.

the net fluid presented to the colon. Diarrhea associated with enteral feeding does not necessarily imply inadequate absorption of nutrients other than water and electrolytes. Amino acids and glucose are particularly well absorbed in the upper small bowel except in the most diseased or shortest bowel. Since luminal nutrients exert trophic effects on the gut mucosa, it is often appropriate to persist with tube feeding, despite the diarrhea, even when this necessitates supplemental parenteral fluid support.

Global Considerations

In the United States the only parenteral lipid emulsion available is made with soybean oil, and it has been suggested that its constituent fatty acids may be immunosuppressive under certain circumstances. In Europe and Japan there are a number of other lipid emulsions available, including those containing fish oil only; mixtures of fish oil, medium-chain triglycerides, and long-chain triglycerides as olive oil and/or soybean oil; mixtures of medium-chain triglycerides and long-chain triglycerides as soybean oil; and long-chain triglyceride mixtures of olive oil and soybean oil, which may be more beneficial in terms of metabolism and hepatic and immune function. Furthermore, a glutamine-containing dipeptide for inclusion in TPN formulas is available in Europe and may be helpful in terms of immune function and resistance to infection.

ACKNOWLEDGMENT

The authors acknowledge the contributions of Lyn Howard, MD, the author in earlier editions of Harrison's Principles of Internal Medicine, to material in this chapter.

SECTION XI

OBESITY AND EATING DISORDERS

CHAPTER 57

BIOLOGY OF OBESITY

Jeffrey S. Flier ■ Eleftheria Maratos-Flier

In a world where food supplies are intermittent, the ability to store energy in excess of what is required for immediate use is essential for survival. Fat cells, residing within widely distributed adipose tissue depots, are adapted to store excess energy efficiently as triglyceride and, when needed, to release stored energy as free fatty acids for use at other sites. This physiologic system, orchestrated through endocrine and neural pathways, permits humans to survive starvation for as long as several months. However, in the presence of nutritional abundance and a sedentary lifestyle, and influenced importantly by genetic endowment, this system increases adipose energy stores and produces adverse health consequences.

DEFINITION AND MEASUREMENT

Obesity is a state of excess adipose tissue mass. Although often viewed as equivalent to increased body weight, this need not be the case—lean but very muscular individuals may be overweight by numerical standards without having increased adiposity. Body weights are distributed continuously in populations, so that choice of a medically meaningful distinction between lean and obese is somewhat arbitrary. Obesity is therefore more effectively defined by assessing its linkage to morbidity or mortality.

Although not a direct measure of adiposity, the most widely used method to gauge obesity is the *body mass index* (BMI), which is equal to weight/height^2 (in kg/m^2) (Fig. 57-1). Other approaches to quantifying obesity include anthropometry (skinfold thickness), densitometry (underwater weighing), CT or MRI, and electrical impedance. Using data from the Metropolitan Life Tables, BMIs for the midpoint of all heights and frames among both men and women range from 19 to 26 kg/m^2; at a similar BMI, women have more body fat than men. Based on data of substantial morbidity, a BMI of 30 is most commonly used as a threshold for obesity

in both men and women. Large-scale epidemiologic studies suggest that all-cause, metabolic, cancer, and cardiovascular morbidity begin to rise (albeit at a slow rate) when BMIs are ≥25, suggesting that the cutoff for obesity should be lowered. Most authorities use the term *overweight* (rather than obese) to describe individuals with BMIs between 25 and 30. A BMI between 25 and 30 should be viewed as medically significant and worthy of therapeutic intervention, especially in the presence of risk factors that are influenced by adiposity such as hypertension and glucose intolerance.

The distribution of adipose tissue in different anatomic depots also has substantial implications for morbidity. Specifically, intraabdominal and abdominal subcutaneous fat have more significance than subcutaneous fat present in the buttocks and lower extremities. This distinction is most easily made clinically by determining the waist-to-hip ratio, with a ratio >0.9 in women and >1.0 in men being abnormal. Many of the most important complications of obesity such as insulin resistance, diabetes, hypertension, hyperlipidemia, and hyperandrogenism in women, are linked more strongly to intraabdominal and/or upper body fat than to overall adiposity (Chap. 60). The mechanism underlying this association is unknown but may relate to the fact that intraabdominal adipocytes are more lipolytically active than those from other depots. Release of free fatty acids into the portal circulation has adverse metabolic actions, especially on the liver. Whether adipokines and cytokines secreted by visceral adipocytes play an additional role in systemic complications of obesity is an area of active investigation.

PREVALENCE

Data from the National Health and Nutrition Examination Surveys (NHANES) show that the percentage of the American adult population with obesity (BMI >30) has increased from 14.5% (between 1976

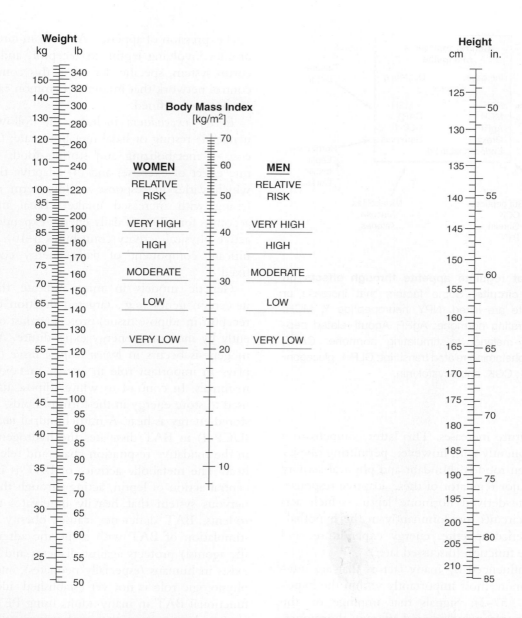

FIGURE 57-1

Nomogram for determining body mass index. To use this nomogram, place a ruler or other straight edge between the body weight (without clothes) in kilograms or pounds located on the left-hand line and the height (without shoes) in centimeters or inches located on the right-hand line. The body mass index is read from the middle of the scale and is in metric units. (*Copyright 1979, George A. Bray, MD; used with permission.*)

and 1980) to 33.9% (between 2007 and 2008). As many as 68% of U.S. adults aged ≥20 years were overweight (defined as BMI >25) between the years of 2007 and 2008. Extreme obesity (BMI ≥40) has also increased and affects 5.7% of the population. The increasing prevalence of medically significant obesity raises great concern. Obesity is more common among women and in the poor, and among blacks and Hispanics; the prevalence in children is also rising at a worrisome rate.

PHYSIOLOGIC REGULATION OF ENERGY BALANCE

Substantial evidence suggests that body weight is regulated by both endocrine and neural components that ultimately influence the effector arms of energy intake and expenditure. This complex regulatory system is necessary because even small imbalances between energy intake and expenditure will ultimately have large effects on body weight. For example, a 0.3% positive imbalance over 30 years would result in a 9-kg (20-lb) weight gain. This exquisite regulation of energy balance cannot be monitored easily by calorie-counting in relation to physical activity. Rather, body weight regulation or dysregulation depends on a complex interplay of hormonal and neural signals. Alterations in stable weight by forced overeeeding or food deprivation induce physiologic changes that resist these perturbations: with weight loss, appetite increases and energy expenditure falls; with overfeeding, appetite falls and

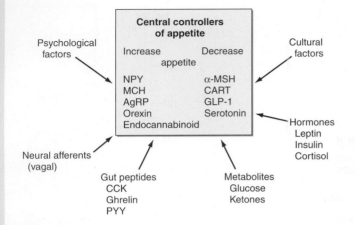

FIGURE 57-2

The factors that regulate appetite through effects on central neural circuits. Some factors that increase or decrease appetite are listed. NPY, neuropeptide Y; MCH, melanin-concentrating hormone; AgRP, Agouti-related peptide; α-MSH, α-melanocyte-stimulating hormone; CART, cocaine- and amphetamine-related transcript; GLP-1, glucagon-related peptide-1; CCK, cholecystokinin.

energy expenditure increases. This latter compensatory mechanism frequently fails, however, permitting obesity to develop when food is abundant and physical activity is limited. A major regulator of these adaptive responses is the adipocyte-derived hormone leptin, which acts through brain circuits (predominantly in the hypothalamus) to influence appetite, energy expenditure, and neuroendocrine function (discussed later).

Appetite is influenced by many factors that are integrated by the brain, most importantly within the hypothalamus **(Fig. 57-2)**. Signals that impinge on the hypothalamic center include neural afferents, hormones, and metabolites. Vagal inputs are particularly important, bringing information from viscera, such as gut distention. Hormonal signals include leptin, insulin, cortisol, and gut peptides. Among the latter is ghrelin, which is made in the stomach and stimulates feeding, and peptide YY (PYY) and cholecystokinin, which is made in the small intestine and signal to the brain through direct action on hypothalamic control centers and/or via the vagus nerve. Metabolites, including glucose, can influence appetite, as seen by the effect of hypoglycemia to induce hunger; however, glucose is not normally a major regulator of appetite. These diverse hormonal, metabolic, and neural signals act by influencing the expression and release of various hypothalamic peptides (e.g., neuropeptide Y [NPY], Agouti-related peptide [AgRP], α-melanocyte-stimulating hormone [α-MSH], and melanin-concentrating hormone [MCH]) that are integrated with serotonergic, catecholaminergic, endocannabinoid, and opioid signaling pathways (discussed later). Psychological and cultural factors also play a role in the final expression of appetite. Apart from rare genetic syndromes involving leptin, its receptor, and the melanocortin system, specific defects in this complex appetite control network that influence common cases of obesity are not well defined.

Energy expenditure includes the following components: (1) resting or basal metabolic rate; (2) the energy cost of metabolizing and storing food; (3) the thermic effect of exercise; and (4) adaptive thermogenesis, which varies in response to long-term caloric intake (rising with increased intake). Basal metabolic rate accounts for ~70% of daily energy expenditure, whereas active physical activity contributes 5–10%. Thus, a significant component of daily energy consumption is fixed.

Genetic models in mice indicate that mutations in certain genes (e.g., targeted deletion of the insulin receptor in adipose tissue) protect against obesity, apparently by increasing energy expenditure. Adaptive thermogenesis occurs in *brown adipose tissue* (BAT), which plays an important role in energy metabolism in many mammals. In contrast to white adipose tissue, which is used to store energy in the form of lipids, BAT expends stored energy as heat. A mitochondrial *uncoupling protein* (UCP-1) in BAT dissipates the hydrogen ion gradient in the oxidative respiration chain and releases energy as heat. The metabolic activity of BAT is increased by a central action of leptin, acting through the sympathetic nervous system that heavily innervates this tissue. In rodents, BAT deficiency causes obesity and diabetes; stimulation of BAT with a specific adrenergic agonist (β3 agonist) protects against diabetes and obesity. BAT exists in humans (especially neonates), and although its physiologic role is not yet established, identification of functional BAT in many adults using PET imaging has increased interest in the implications of the tissue for pathogenesis and therapy of obesity.

THE ADIPOCYTE AND ADIPOSE TISSUE

Adipose tissue is composed of the lipid-storing adipose cell and a stromal/vascular compartment in which cells including preadipocytes and macrophages reside. Adipose mass increases by enlargement of adipose cells through lipid deposition, as well as by an increase in the number of adipocytes. Obese adipose tissue is also characterized by increased numbers of infiltrating macrophages. The process by which adipose cells are derived from a mesenchymal preadipocyte involves an orchestrated series of differentiation steps mediated by a cascade of specific transcription factors. One of the key transcription factors is *peroxisome proliferator-activated receptor γ* (PPARγ), a nuclear receptor that binds the thiazolidinedione class of insulin-sensitizing drugs used in the treatment of type 2 diabetes.

FIGURE 57-3

Factors released by the adipocyte that can affect peripheral tissues. PAI, plasminogen activator inhibitor; TNF, tumor necrosis factor; RBP4, retinal binding protein 4.

Although the adipocyte has generally been regarded as a storage depot for fat, it is also an endocrine cell that releases numerous molecules in a regulated fashion (Fig. 57-3). These include the energy balance–regulating hormone leptin, cytokines such as tumor necrosis factor (TNF)-α and interleukin (IL)-6, complement factors such as factor D (also known as *adipsin*), prothrombotic agents such as plasminogen activator inhibitor I, and a component of the blood pressure–regulating system, angiotensinogen. Adiponectin, an abundant adipose-derived protein whose levels are reduced in obesity, enhances insulin sensitivity and lipid oxidation and it has vascular-protective effects, whereas resistin and RBP4, whose levels are increased in obesity, may induce insulin resistance. These factors, and others not yet identified, play a role in the physiology of lipid homeostasis, insulin sensitivity, blood pressure control, coagulation, and vascular health, and are likely to contribute to obesity-related pathologies.

ETIOLOGY OF OBESITY

Although the molecular pathways regulating energy balance are beginning to be illuminated, the causes of obesity remain elusive. In part, this reflects the fact that obesity is a heterogeneous group of disorders. At one level, the pathophysiology of obesity seems simple: a chronic excess of nutrient intake relative to the level of energy expenditure. However, due to the complexity of the neuroendocrine and metabolic systems that regulate energy intake, storage, and expenditure, it has been difficult to quantitate all the relevant parameters (e.g., food intake and energy expenditure) over time in human subjects.

Role of genes versus environment

Obesity is commonly seen in families, and the heritability of body weight is similar to that for height. Inheritance is usually not Mendelian, however, and it is difficult to distinguish the role of genes and environmental factors. Adoptees more closely resemble their biologic than adoptive parents with respect to obesity, providing strong

support for genetic influences. Likewise, identical twins have very similar BMIs whether reared together or apart, and their BMIs are much more strongly correlated than those of dizygotic twins. These genetic effects appear to relate to both energy intake and expenditure.

Whatever the role of genes, it is clear that the environment plays a key role in obesity, as evidenced by the fact that famine prevents obesity in even the most obesity-prone individual. In addition, the recent increase in the prevalence of obesity in the United States is far too rapid to be due to changes in the gene pool. Undoubtedly, genes influence the susceptibility to obesity in response to specific diets and availability of nutrition. Cultural factors are also important—these relate to both availability and composition of the diet and to changes in the level of physical activity. In industrial societies, obesity is more common among poor women, whereas in underdeveloped countries, wealthier women are more often obese. In children, obesity correlates to some degree with time spent watching television. Although the role of diet composition in obesity continues to generate controversy, it appears that high-fat diets may promote obesity when combined with diets rich in simple, rapidly absorbed carbohydrates.

Additional environmental factors may contribute to the increasing obesity prevalence. Both epidemiologic correlations and experimental data suggest that sleep deprivation leads to increased obesity. Changes in gut microbiome with capacity to alter energy balance are receiving experimental support from animal studies, and a possible role for obesigenic viral infections continues to receive sporadic attention.

Specific genetic syndromes

For many years, obesity in rodents has been known to be caused by a number of distinct mutations distributed through the genome. Most of these single-gene mutations cause both hyperphagia and diminished energy expenditure, suggesting a physiologic link between these two parameters of energy homeostasis. Identification of the *ob* gene mutation in genetically obese (ob/ob) mice represented a major breakthrough in the field. The ob/ob mouse develops severe obesity, insulin resistance, and hyperphagia, as well as efficient metabolism (e.g., it gets fat even when ingesting the same number of calories as lean litter mates). The product of the *ob* gene is the peptide leptin, a name derived from the Greek root *leptos*, meaning thin. Leptin is secreted by adipose cells and acts primarily through the hypothalamus. Its level of production provides an index of adipose energy stores (Fig. 57-4). High leptin levels decrease food intake and increase energy expenditure. Another mouse mutant, db/db, which is resistant to leptin, has a mutation in the leptin receptor and

Brain

Hypothalamus

→ Glucose and lipid metabolism

→ Hunger/satiety

→ Thermogenesis/autonomic system

→ Neuroendocrine function

Blood-brain barrier

Peripheral targets — Beta cells / Immune cells / Others

↑ Leptin — Fed state/obesity

↓ Leptin — Fasted state

Adipocyte

FIGURE 57-4

The physiologic system regulated by leptin. Rising or falling leptin levels act through the hypothalamus to influence appetite, energy expenditure, and neuroendocrine function and through peripheral sites to influence systems such as the immune system.

develops a similar syndrome. The *ob* gene is present in humans where it is also expressed in fat. Several families with morbid, early-onset obesity caused by inactivating mutations in either leptin or the leptin receptor have been described, thus demonstrating the biologic relevance of the leptin pathway in humans. Obesity in these individuals begins shortly after birth, is severe, and is accompanied by neuroendocrine abnormalities. The most prominent of these is hypogonadotropic hypogonadism, which is reversed by leptin replacement in the leptin-deficient subset. Central hypothyroidism and growth retardation are seen in the mouse model, but their occurrence in leptin-deficient humans is less clear. To date, there is no evidence that mutations in the leptin or leptin receptor genes play a prominent role in common forms of obesity.

Mutations in several other genes cause severe obesity in humans **(Table 57-1)**; each of these syndromes is rare. Mutations in the gene encoding proopiomelanocortin (POMC) cause severe obesity through failure to synthesize α-MSH, a key neuropeptide that inhibits appetite in the hypothalamus. The absence of POMC also causes secondary adrenal insufficiency due to absence of adrenocorticotropic hormone (ACTH), as well as pale skin and red hair due to absence of α-MSH. Proenzyme convertase 1 (PC-1) mutations are thought to cause obesity by preventing synthesis of α-MSH from its precursor peptide, POMC. α-MSH binds to the type 4 melanocortin receptor (MC4R), a key hypothalamic receptor that inhibits eating. Heterozygous loss-of-function mutations of this receptor account for as much as 5% of severe obesity. These five genetic defects define a pathway through which leptin (by stimulating POMC and increasing α-MSH) restricts food intake and limits weight **(Fig. 57-5)**. The results of genomewide association studies to identify genetic loci responsible for obesity in the general population have so far been disappointing. More than 10 replicated

TABLE 57-1

SOME OBESITY GENES IN HUMANS AND MICE

GENE	GENE PRODUCT	MECHANISM OF OBESITY	IN HUMAN	IN RODENT
Lep (ob)	Leptin, a fat-derived hormone	Mutation prevents leptin from delivering satiety signal; brain perceives starvation	Yes	Yes
LepR (db)	Leptin receptor	Same as above	Yes	Yes
POMC	Proopiomelanocortin, a precursor of several hormones and neuropeptides	Mutation prevents synthesis of melanocyte-stimulating hormone (MSH), a satiety signal	Yes	Yes
MC4R	Type 4 receptor for MSH	Mutation prevents reception of satiety signal from MSH	Yes	Yes
AgRP	Agouti-related peptide, a neuropeptide expressed in the hypothalamus	Overexpression inhibits signal through *MC4R*	No	Yes
PC-1	Prohormone convertase 1, a processing enzyme	Mutation prevents synthesis of neuropeptide, probably MSH	Yes	No
Fat	Carboxypeptidase E, a processing enzyme	Same as above	No	Yes
Tub	Tub, a hypothalamic protein of unknown function	Hypothalamic dysfunction	No	Yes
TrkB	TrkB, a neurotrophin receptor	Hyperphagia due to uncharacterized hypothalamic defect	Yes	Yes

FIGURE 57-5

A central pathway through which leptin acts to regulate appetite and body weight. Leptin signals through proopiomelanocortin (POMC) neurons in the hypothalamus to induce increased production of α-melanocyte-stimulating hormone (α-MSH), requiring the processing enzyme PC-1 (proenzyme convertase 1). α-MSH acts as an agonist on melanocortin-4 receptors to inhibit appetite, and the neuropeptide AgRp (Agouti-related peptide) acts as an antagonist of this receptor. Mutations that cause obesity in humans are indicated by the solid green arrows.

loci linked to obesity have been identified, but together they account for less than 3% of interindividual variation in BMI. The most replicated of these is a gene named FTO, which is of unknown function, but like many of the other recently described candidates, is expressed in the brain. Since the heritability of obesity is estimated to be 40–70%, it is likely that many more loci remain to be identified.

In addition to these human obesity genes, studies in rodents reveal several other molecular candidates for hypothalamic mediators of human obesity or leanness. The *tub* gene encodes a hypothalamic peptide of unknown function; mutation of this gene causes late-onset obesity. The *fat* gene encodes carboxypeptidase E, a peptide-processing enzyme; mutation of this gene is thought to cause obesity by disrupting production of one or more neuropeptides. AgRP is coexpressed with NPY in arcuate nucleus neurons. AgRP antagonizes α-MSH action at MC4 receptors, and its overexpression induces obesity. In contrast, a mouse deficient in the peptide MCH, whose administration causes feeding, is lean.

A number of complex human syndromes with defined inheritance are associated with obesity (Table 57-2). Although specific genes have limited definition at present, their identification will likely enhance our understanding of more common forms of human obesity. In the Prader-Willi syndrome, a multigenic neurodevelopmental disorder, obesity coexists with short stature, mental retardation, hypogonadotropic hypogonadism, hypotonia, small hands and feet, fish-shaped mouth, and hyperphagia. Most patients have a deletion in the 15q11-13 chromosomal region, and reduced expression of the signaling protein necdin may be an important cause of defective hypothalamic neural development in this disorder. Bardet-Biedl syndrome (BBS) is a genetically heterogeneous disorder characterized by obesity, mental retardation, retinitis pigmentosa, diabetes, renal and cardiac malformations, polydactyly, and hypogonadotropic hypogonadism. At least 12 genetic loci have been identified, and most of the encoded proteins form two multiprotein complexes that are involved in ciliary function and microtubule-based intracellular transport. Recent evidence suggests that mutations might disrupt leptin receptor trafficking in key hypothalamic neurons, causing leptin resistance.

Other specific syndromes associated with obesity

Cushing's syndrome

Although obese patients commonly have central obesity, hypertension, and glucose intolerance, they lack other specific stigmata of Cushing's syndrome. Nonetheless, a potential diagnosis of Cushing's syndrome is often entertained. Cortisol production and urinary metabolites (17OH steroids) may be increased in simple obesity. Unlike in Cushing's syndrome, however, cortisol levels in blood and urine in the basal state and in response to corticotropin-releasing hormone (CRH) or ACTH are normal; the overnight 1-mg dexamethasone suppression test is normal in 90%, with the remainder being normal on a standard 2-day low-dose dexamethasone suppression test. Obesity may be associated with excessive local reactivation of cortisol in fat by 11β-hydroxysteroid dehydrogenase 1, an enzyme that converts inactive cortisone to cortisol.

Hypothyroidism

The possibility of hypothyroidism should be considered, but it is an uncommon cause of obesity; hypothyroidism is easily ruled out by measuring thyroid-stimulating hormone (TSH). Much of the weight gain that occurs in hypothyroidism is due to myxedema.

Insulinoma

Patients with insulinoma often gain weight as a result of overeating to avoid hypoglycemic symptoms. The increased substrate plus high insulin levels promote energy storage in fat. This can be marked in some individuals but is modest in most.

Craniopharyngioma and other disorders involving the hypothalamus

Whether through tumors, trauma, or inflammation, hypothalamic dysfunction of systems controlling satiety, hunger, and energy expenditure can cause varying degrees of obesity. It is uncommon to identify a discrete anatomic basis for these disorders. Subtle

TABLE 57-2

A COMPARISON OF SYNDROMES OF OBESITY—HYPOGONADISM AND MENTAL RETARDATION

	SYNDROME				
FEATURE	**PRADER-WILLI**	**LAURENCE-MOON-BIEDL**	**AHLSTROM'S**	**COHEN'S**	**CARPENTER'S**
Inheritance	Sporadic; two-thirds have defect	Autosomal recessive	Autosomal recessive	Probably autosomal recessive	Autosomal recessive
Stature	Short	Normal; infrequently short	Normal; infrequently short	Short or tall	Normal
Obesity	Generalized Moderate to severe Onset 1–3 years	Generalized Early onset, 1–2 years	Truncal Early onset, 2–5 years	Truncal Mid-childhood, age 5	Truncal, gluteal
Craniofacies	Narrow bifrontal diameter Almond-shaped eyes Strabismus V-shaped mouth High-arched palate	Not distinctive	Not distinctive	High nasal bridge Arched palate Open mouth Short philtrum	Acrocephaly Flat nasal bridge High-arched palate
Limbs	Small hands and feet Hypotonia	Polydactyly	No abnormalities	Hypotonia Narrow hands and feet	Polydactyly Syndactyly Genu valgum
Reproductive status	1° Hypogonadism	1° Hypogonadism	Hypogonadism in males but not in females	Normal gonadal function or hypo-gonadotrophic hypogonadism	2° Hypogonadism
Other features	Enamel hypoplasia Hyperphagia Temper tantrums Nasal speech			Dysplastic ears Delayed puberty	
Mental retardation	Mild to moderate		Normal intelligence	Mild	Slight

hypothalamic dysfunction is probably a more common cause of obesity than can be documented using currently available imaging techniques. Growth hormone (GH), which exerts lipolytic activity, is diminished in obesity and is increased with weight loss. Despite low GH levels, insulin-like growth factor (IGF)-I (somatomedin) production is normal, suggesting that GH suppression is a compensatory response to increased nutritional supply.

Pathogenesis of common obesity

Obesity can result from increased energy intake, decreased energy expenditure, or a combination of the two. Thus, identifying the etiology of obesity should involve measurements of both parameters. However, it

is difficult to perform direct and accurate measurements of energy intake in free-living individuals; and the obese, in particular, often underreport intake. Measurements of chronic energy expenditure are possible using doubly labeled water or metabolic chamber/rooms. In subjects at stable weight and body composition, energy intake equals expenditure. Consequently, these techniques allow assessment of energy intake in free-living individuals. The level of energy expenditure differs in established obesity, during periods of weight gain or loss, and in the pre- or postobese state. Studies that fail to take note of this phenomenon are not easily interpreted.

There is continued interest in the concept of a body weight "set point." This idea is supported by physiologic mechanisms centered around a sensing system in adipose tissue that reflects fat stores and a receptor, or "adipostat," that is in the hypothalamic centers. When fat stores are depleted, the adipostat signal is low, and the hypothalamus responds by stimulating hunger and decreasing energy expenditure to conserve energy. Conversely, when fat stores are abundant, the signal is increased, and the hypothalamus responds by decreasing hunger and increasing energy expenditure. The recent discovery of the *ob* gene, and its product leptin, and the *db* gene, whose product is the leptin receptor, provides important elements of a molecular basis for this physiologic concept (discussed earlier).

What is the status of food intake in obesity? (Do the obese eat more than the lean?)

This question has stimulated much debate, due in part to the methodologic difficulties inherent in determining food intake. Many obese individuals believe that they eat small quantities of food, and this claim has often been supported by the results of food intake questionnaires. However, it is now established that average energy expenditure increases as individuals get more obese, due primarily to the fact that metabolically active lean tissue mass increases with obesity. Given the laws of thermodynamics, the obese person must therefore eat more than the average lean person to maintain their increased weight. It may be the case, however, that a subset of individuals who are predisposed to obesity have the capacity to become obese initially without an absolute increase in caloric consumption.

What is the state of energy expenditure in obesity?

The average total daily energy expenditure is higher in obese than lean individuals when measured at stable weight. However, energy expenditure falls as weight is lost, due in part to loss of lean body mass and to decreased sympathetic nerve activity. When reduced to near-normal weight and maintained there for awhile, (some) obese individuals have lower energy expenditure than (some) lean individuals. There is also a tendency for those who will develop obesity as infants or children to have lower resting energy expenditure rates than those who remain lean.

The physiologic basis for variable rates of energy expenditure (at a given body weight and level of energy intake) is essentially unknown. A mutation in the human β_3-adrenergic receptor may be associated with increased risk of obesity and/or insulin resistance in certain (but not all) populations.

One recently described component of thermogenesis, called *nonexercise activity thermogenesis* (NEAT), has been linked to obesity. It is the thermogenesis that accompanies physical activities other than volitional exercise such as the activities of daily living, fidgeting, spontaneous muscle contraction, and maintaining posture. NEAT accounts for about two-thirds of the increased daily energy expenditure induced by overfeeding. The wide variation in fat storage seen in overfed individuals is predicted by the degree to which NEAT is induced. The molecular basis for NEAT and its regulation is unknown.

Leptin in typical obesity

The vast majority of obese persons have increased leptin levels but do not have mutations of either leptin or its receptor. They appear, therefore, to have a form of functional "leptin resistance." Data suggesting that some individuals produce less leptin per unit fat mass than others or have a form of relative leptin deficiency that predisposes to obesity are at present contradictory and unsettled. The mechanism for leptin resistance, and whether it can be overcome by raising leptin levels or combining leptin with other treatments in a subset of obese individuals, is not yet established. Some data suggest that leptin may not effectively cross the blood-brain barrier as levels rise. It is also apparent from animal studies that leptin signaling inhibitors, such as SOCS3 and PTP1b, are involved in the leptin-resistant state.

PATHOLOGIC CONSEQUENCES OF OBESITY

(See also Chap. 58) Obesity has major adverse effects on health. Obesity is associated with an increase in mortality, with a 50–100% increased risk of death from all causes compared to normal-weight individuals, mostly due to cardiovascular causes. Obesity and overweight together are the second leading cause of preventable death in the United States, accounting for 300,000 deaths per year. Mortality rates rise as obesity increases, particularly when obesity is associated with increased intraabdominal fat (discussed earlier). Life expectancy of a moderately obese individual could be shortened by 2–5 years, and a 20- to 30-year-old male with a BMI >45 may lose 13 years of life. It is also apparent that the degree to which obesity affects particular organ systems is influenced by susceptibility genes that vary in the population.

Insulin resistance and type 2 diabetes mellitus

Hyperinsulinemia and insulin resistance are pervasive features of obesity, increasing with weight gain and diminishing with weight loss (Chap. 60). Insulin resistance is more strongly linked to intraabdominal fat than to fat in other depots. Molecular links between obesity and insulin resistance in fat, muscle, and liver have been sought for many years. Major factors include: (1) insulin itself, by inducing receptor downregulation; (2) free fatty acids that are increased and capable of impairing insulin action; (3) intracellular lipid accumulation; and (4) several circulating peptides produced by adipocytes, including the cytokines TNF-α and IL-6, RBP4, and the "adipokines" adiponectin and resistin that have altered expression in obese adipocytes, and can modify insulin action. Additional mechanisms are obesity-linked inflammation, including infiltration of macrophages into tissues including fat, and induction of the endoplasmic reticulum stress response, that can bring about resistance to insulin action in cells. Despite the prevalence of insulin resistance, most obese individuals do not develop diabetes, suggesting that diabetes requires an interaction between obesity-induced insulin resistance and other factors such as impaired insulin secretion. Obesity, however, is a major risk factor for diabetes, and as many as 80% of patients with type 2 diabetes mellitus are obese. Weight loss and exercise, even of modest degree, increase insulin sensitivity and often improve glucose control in diabetes.

Reproductive disorders

Disorders that affect the reproductive axis are associated with obesity in both men and women. Male hypogonadism is associated with increased adipose tissue, often distributed in a pattern more typical of females. In men whose weight is >160% ideal body weight (IBW), plasma testosterone and sex hormone–binding globulin (SHBG) are often reduced, and estrogen levels (derived from conversion of adrenal androgens in adipose tissue) are increased. Gynecomastia may be seen. However, masculinization, libido, potency, and spermatogenesis are preserved in most of these individuals. Free testosterone may be decreased in morbidly obese men whose weight is >200% IBW.

Obesity has long been associated with menstrual abnormalities in women, particularly in women with upper body obesity. Common findings are increased androgen production, decreased SHBG, and increased peripheral conversion of androgen to estrogen. Most obese women with oligomenorrhea have the polycystic ovarian syndrome (PCOS), with its associated anovulation and ovarian hyperandrogenism; 40% of women with PCOS are obese. Most nonobese women with PCOS are also insulin-resistant, suggesting that insulin resistance, hyperinsulinemia, or the combination of the two are causative or contribute to the ovarian pathophysiology in PCOS in both obese and lean individuals. In obese women with PCOS, weight loss or treatment with insulin-sensitizing drugs often restores normal menses. The increased conversion of androstenedione to estrogen, which occurs to a greater degree in women with lower body obesity, may contribute to the increased incidence of uterine cancer in postmenopausal women with obesity.

Cardiovascular disease

The Framingham Study revealed that obesity was an independent risk factor for the 26-year incidence of cardiovascular disease in men and women (including coronary disease, stroke, and congestive heart failure [CHF]). The waist-to-hip ratio may be the best predictor of these risks. When the additional effects of hypertension and glucose intolerance associated with obesity are included, the adverse impact of obesity is even more evident. The effect of obesity on cardiovascular mortality in women may be seen at BMIs as low as 25. Obesity, especially abdominal obesity, is associated with an atherogenic lipid profile; with increased low–density lipoprotein cholesterol, very low density lipoprotein, and triglyceride; and with decreased high-density lipoprotein cholesterol and decreased levels of the vascular protective adipokine adiponectin. Obesity is also associated with hypertension. Measurement of blood pressure in the obese requires use of a larger cuff size to avoid artifactual increases. Obesity-induced hypertension is associated with increased peripheral resistance and cardiac output, increased sympathetic nervous system tone, increased salt sensitivity, and insulin-mediated salt retention; it is often responsive to modest weight loss.

Pulmonary disease

Obesity may be associated with a number of pulmonary abnormalities. These include reduced chest wall compliance, increased work of breathing, increased minute ventilation due to increased metabolic rate, and decreased functional residual capacity and expiratory reserve volume. Severe obesity may be associated with obstructive sleep apnea and the "obesity hypoventilation syndrome" with attenuated hypoxic and hypercapnic ventilatory responses. Sleep apnea can be obstructive (most common), central, or mixed and is associated with hypertension. Weight loss (10–20 kg) can bring substantial improvement, as can major weight loss following gastric bypass or restrictive surgery. Continuous positive airway pressure has been used with some success.

Hepatobiliary disease

Obesity is frequently associated with the common disorder nonalcoholic fatty liver disease (NAFLD). This hepatic fatty infiltration of NAFLD can progress in a subset to inflammatory nonalcoholic steatohepatitis (NASH) and more rarely to cirrhosis and hepatocellular carcinoma. Steatosis has been noted to improve following weight loss, secondary to diet or bariatric surgery. The mechanism for the association remains unclear. Obesity is associated with enhanced biliary secretion of cholesterol, supersaturation of bile, and a higher incidence of gallstones, particularly cholesterol gallstones (Chap. 45). A person 50% above IBW has about a sixfold increased incidence of symptomatic gallstones. Paradoxically, fasting increases supersaturation of bile by decreasing the phospholipid component. Fasting-induced cholecystitis is a complication of extreme diets.

Cancer

Obesity in males is associated with higher mortality from cancer, including cancer of the esophagus, colon, rectum, pancreas, liver, and prostate; obesity in females is associated with higher mortality from cancer of the gallbladder, bile ducts, breasts, endometrium, cervix, and ovaries. Some of the latter may be due to increased rates of conversion of androstenedione to estrone in adipose tissue of obese individuals. Other possible

mechanistic links are other hormones whose levels are linked to nutritional state, including insulin, leptin, adiponectin, and IGF-I. It has been estimated that obesity accounts for 14% of cancer deaths in men and 20% in women in the United States.

Bone, joint, and cutaneous disease

Obesity is associated with an increased risk of osteoarthritis, no doubt partly due to the trauma of added weight bearing, but potentially linked as well to activation of inflammatory pathways that could promote synovial pathology. The prevalence of gout may also be increased. Among the skin problems associated with obesity is acanthosis nigricans, manifested by darkening and thickening of the skinfolds on the neck, elbows, and dorsal interphalangeal spaces. Acanthosis reflects the severity of underlying insulin resistance and diminishes with weight loss. Friability of skin may be increased, especially in skinfolds, enhancing the risk of fungal and yeast infections. Finally, venous stasis is increased in the obese.

CHAPTER 58

EVALUATION AND MANAGEMENT OF OBESITY

Robert F. Kushner

Over 66% of U.S. adults are categorized as overweight or obese, and the prevalence of obesity is increasing rapidly in most of the industrialized world. Children and adolescents also are becoming more obese, indicating that the current trends will accelerate over time. Obesity is associated with an increased risk of multiple health problems, including hypertension, type 2 diabetes, dyslipidemia, degenerative joint disease, and some malignancies. Thus, it is important for physicians to identify, evaluate, and treat patients for obesity and associated comorbid conditions.

EVALUATION

Physicians should screen all adult patients for obesity and offer intensive counseling and behavioral interventions to promote sustained weight loss. The five main steps in the evaluation of obesity, as described in the following sections, are (1) focused obesity-related history, (2) physical examination to determine the degree and type of obesity, (3) comorbid conditions, (4) fitness level, and (5) the patient's readiness to adopt lifestyle changes.

The obesity-focused history

Information from the history should address the following six questions:

- What factors contribute to the patient's obesity?
- How is the obesity affecting the patient's health?
- What is the patient's level of risk from obesity?
- What are the patient's goals and expectations?
- Is the patient motivated to begin a weight management program?
- What kind of help does the patient need?

Although the vast majority of cases of obesity can be attributed to behavioral features that affect diet and physical activity patterns, the history may suggest secondary causes that merit further evaluation. Disorders to consider include polycystic ovarian syndrome, hypothyroidism, Cushing's syndrome, and hypothalamic disease. Drug-induced weight gain also should be considered. Common causes include medications for diabetes (insulin, sulfonylureas, thiazolidinediones); steroid hormones; psychotropic agents; mood stabilizers (lithium); antidepressants (tricyclics, monoamine oxidase inhibitors, paroxetine, mirtazapine); and antiepileptic drugs (valproate, gabapentin, carbamazepine). Other medications, such as nonsteroidal anti-inflammatory drugs and calcium channel blockers, may cause peripheral edema but do not increase body fat.

The patient's current diet and physical activity patterns may reveal factors that contribute to the development of obesity in addition to identifying behaviors to target for treatment. This type of historic information is best obtained by using a questionnaire in combination with an interview.

BMI and waist circumference

Three key anthropometric measurements are important to evaluate the degree of obesity: weight, height, and waist circumference. The body mass index (BMI), calculated as weight (kg)/height (m)^2, or weight (lbs)/height (inches)^2 × 703, is used to classify weight status and risk of disease (Tables 58-1 and 58-2). BMI is used since it provides an estimate of body fat and is related to risk of disease. Lower BMI thresholds for overweight and obesity have been proposed for the Asia-Pacific region since this population appears to be at risk for glucose and lipid abnormalities at lower body weights.

Excess abdominal fat, assessed by measurement of waist circumference or waist-to-hip ratio, is independently associated with higher risk for diabetes mellitus and cardiovascular disease. Measurement of the waist circumference is a surrogate for visceral adipose tissue and should be performed in the horizontal plane above the iliac crest (Table 58-3).

TABLE 58-1
BODY MASS INDEX (BMI) TABLE

BMI	19	20	21	22	23	24	25	26	27	28	29	30	31	32	33	34	35
HEIGHT, INCHES								BODY WEIGHT, POUNDS									
58	91	96	100	105	110	115	119	124	129	134	138	143	148	153	158	162	167
59	94	99	104	109	114	119	124	128	133	138	143	148	153	158	163	168	173
60	97	102	107	112	118	123	128	133	138	143	148	153	158	163	168	174	179
61	100	106	111	116	122	127	132	137	143	148	153	158	164	169	174	180	185
62	104	109	115	120	126	131	136	142	147	153	158	164	169	175	180	186	191
63	107	113	118	124	130	135	141	146	152	158	163	169	175	180	186	191	197
64	110	116	122	128	134	140	145	151	157	163	169	174	180	186	192	197	204
65	114	120	126	132	138	144	150	156	162	168	174	180	186	192	198	204	210
66	118	124	130	136	142	148	155	161	167	173	179	186	192	198	204	210	216
67	121	127	134	140	146	153	159	166	172	178	185	191	198	204	211	217	223
68	125	131	138	144	151	158	164	171	177	184	190	197	203	210	216	223	230
69	128	135	142	149	155	162	169	176	182	189	196	203	209	216	223	230	236
70	132	139	146	153	160	167	174	181	188	195	202	209	216	222	229	236	243
71	136	143	150	157	165	172	179	186	193	200	208	215	222	229	236	243	250
72	140	147	154	162	169	177	184	191	199	206	213	221	228	235	242	250	258
73	144	151	159	166	174	182	189	197	204	212	219	227	235	242	250	257	265
74	148	155	163	171	179	186	194	202	210	218	225	233	241	249	256	264	272
75	152	160	168	176	184	192	200	208	216	224	232	240	248	256	264	272	279
76	156	164	172	180	189	197	205	213	221	230	238	246	254	263	271	279	287

BMI	36	37	38	39	40	41	42	43	44	45	46	47	48	49	50	51	52	53	54
58	172	177	181	186	191	196	201	205	210	215	220	224	229	234	239	244	248	253	258
59	178	183	188	193	198	203	208	212	217	222	227	232	237	242	247	252	257	262	267
60	184	189	194	199	204	209	215	220	225	230	235	240	245	250	255	261	266	271	276
61	190	195	201	206	211	217	222	227	232	238	243	248	254	259	264	269	275	280	285
62	196	202	207	213	218	224	229	235	240	246	251	256	262	267	273	278	284	289	295
63	203	208	214	220	225	231	237	242	248	254	259	265	270	278	282	287	293	299	304
64	209	215	221	227	232	238	244	250	256	262	267	273	279	285	291	296	302	308	314
65	216	222	228	234	240	246	252	258	264	270	276	282	288	294	300	306	312	318	324
66	223	229	235	241	247	253	260	266	272	278	284	291	297	303	309	315	322	328	334
67	230	236	242	249	255	261	268	274	280	287	293	299	306	312	319	325	331	338	344
68	236	243	249	256	262	269	276	282	289	295	302	308	315	322	328	335	341	348	354
69	243	250	257	263	270	277	284	291	297	304	311	318	324	331	338	345	351	358	365
70	250	257	264	271	278	285	292	299	306	313	320	327	334	341	348	355	362	369	376
71	257	265	272	279	286	293	301	308	315	322	329	338	343	351	358	365	372	379	386
72	265	272	279	287	294	302	309	316	324	331	338	346	353	361	368	375	383	390	397
73	272	280	288	295	302	310	318	325	333	340	348	355	363	371	378	386	393	401	408
74	280	287	295	303	311	319	326	334	342	350	358	365	373	381	389	396	404	412	420
75	287	295	303	311	319	327	335	343	351	359	367	375	383	391	399	407	415	423	431
76	295	304	312	320	328	336	344	353	361	369	377	385	394	402	410	418	426	435	443

Physical fitness

Several prospective studies have demonstrated that physical fitness, reported by questionnaire or measured by a maximal treadmill exercise test, is an important predictor of all-cause mortality rate independent of BMI and body composition. These observations highlight the importance of taking an exercise history during examination as well as emphasizing physical activity as a treatment approach.

Obesity-associated comorbid conditions

The evaluation of comorbid conditions should be based on presentation of symptoms, risk factors, and index of suspicion. All patients should have a fasting lipid panel (total, low-density lipoprotein [LDL], and high-density lipoprotein [HDL] cholesterol and triglyceride levels) and fasting blood glucose along with blood pressure determination. Symptoms and diseases that are directly or indirectly related to obesity are listed in Table 58-4.

TABLE 58-2

	BMI (kg/m²)	**OBESITY CLASS**	**RISK OF DISEASE**

CLASSIFICATION OF WEIGHT STATUS AND RISK OF DISEASE

	BMI (kg/m²)	OBESITY CLASS	RISK OF DISEASE
Underweight	<18.5		
Healthy weight	18.5–24.9		
Overweight	25.0–29.9		Increased
Obesity	30.0–34.9	I	High
Obesity	35.0–39.9	II	Very high
Extreme Obesity	≥40	III	Extremely high

Source: Adapted from National Institutes of Health, National Heart, Lung, and Blood Institute: *Clinical Guidelines on the Identification, Evaluation, and Treatment of Overweight and Obesity in Adults.* U.S. Department of Health and Human Services, Public Health Service, 1998.

Although individuals vary, the number and severity of organ-specific comorbid conditions usually rise with increasing levels of obesity. Patients at very high absolute risk include those with the following: established coronary heart disease; presence of other atherosclerotic diseases, such as peripheral arterial disease, abdominal aortic aneurysm, and symptomatic carotid artery disease; type 2 diabetes; and sleep apnea.

TABLE 58-3

ETHNIC-SPECIFIC VALUES FOR WAIST CIRCUMFERENCE

ETHNIC GROUP	WAIST CIRCUMFERENCE
Europeans	
Men	>94 cm (37 in)
Women	>80 cm (31.5 in)
South Asians and Chinese	
Men	>90 cm (35 in)
Women	>80 cm (31.5 in)
Japanese	
Men	>85 cm (33.5 in)
Women	>90 cm (35 in)
Ethnic South and Central Americans	Use south Asian recommendations until more specific data are available.
Sub-Saharan Africans	Use European data until more specific data are available.
Eastern Mediterranean and Middle East (Arab) populations	Use European data until more specific data are available.

Source: From KGMM Alberti et al for the IDF Epidemiology Task Force Consensus Group: Lancet 366:1059, 2005.

TABLE 58-4

OBESITY-RELATED ORGAN SYSTEMS REVIEW

Cardiovascular
- Hypertension
- Congestive heart failure
- Cor pulmonale
- Varicose veins
- Pulmonary embolism
- Coronary artery disease

Endocrine
- Metabolic syndrome
- Type 2 diabetes
- Dyslipidemia
- Polycystic ovarian syndrome

Musculoskeletal
- Hyperuricemia and gout
- Immobility
- Osteoarthritis (knees and hips)
- Low back pain
- Carpal tunnel syndrome

Psychological
- Depression/low self-esteem
- Body image disturbance
- Social stigmatization

Integument
- Striae distensae
- Stasis pigmentation of legs
- Lymphedema
- Cellulitis
- Intertrigo, carbuncles
- Acanthosis nigricans
- Acrochordon (skin tags)
- Hidradenitis suppurativa

Respiratory
- Dyspnea
- Obstructive sleep apnea
- Hypoventilation syndrome
- Pickwickian syndrome
- Asthma

Gastrointestinal
- Gastroesophageal reflux disease
- Nonalcoholic fatty liver disease
- Cholelithiasis
- Hernias
- Colon cancer

Genitourinary
- Urinary stress incontinence
- Obesity-related glomerulopathy
- Hypogonadism (male)
- Breast and uterine cancer
- Pregnancy complications

Neurologic
- Stroke
- Idiopathic intracranial hypertension
- Meralgia paresthetica
- Dementia

Assessing the patient's readiness to change

An attempt to initiate lifestyle changes when the patient is not ready usually leads to frustration and may hamper future weight-loss efforts. Assessment includes patient motivation and support, stressful life events, psychiatric status, time availability and constraints, and appropriateness of goals and expectations. Readiness can be viewed as the balance of two opposing forces: (1) motivation, or the patient's desire to change, and (2) resistance, or the patient's resistance to change.

A helpful method to begin a readiness assessment is to "anchor" the patient's interest and confidence to change on a numerical scale. With this technique, the patient is asked to rate his or her level of interest and confidence on a scale from 0 to 10, with 0 being not so important (or confident) and 10 being very important (or confident) to lose weight at this time. This exercise helps establish readiness to change and also serves as a basis for further dialogue.

TREATMENT Obesity

THE GOAL OF THERAPY The primary goal of treatment is to improve obesity-related comorbid conditions and reduce the risk of developing future comorbidities. Information obtained from the history,

physical examination, and diagnostic tests is used to determine risk and develop a treatment plan (Fig. 58-1). The decision of how aggressively to treat the patient and which modalities to use is determined by the patient's risk status, expectations, and available resources. Therapy for obesity always begins with lifestyle management and may include pharmacotherapy or surgery, depending on BMI risk category (Table 58-5). Setting an initial weight-loss goal of 10% over 6 months is a realistic target.

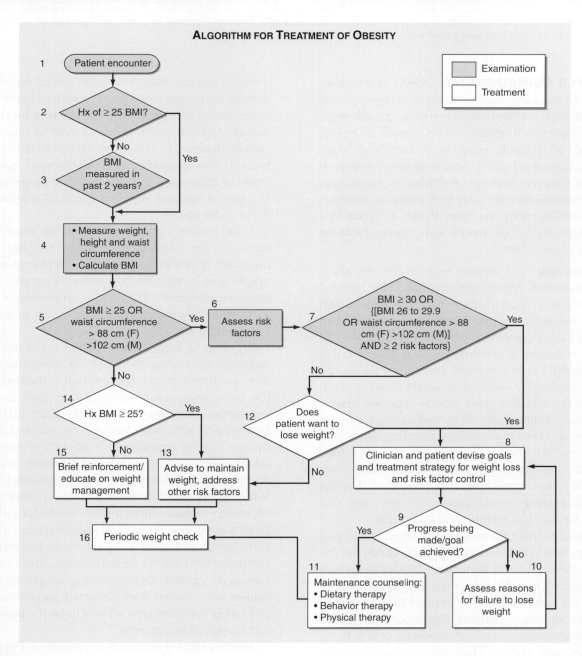

ALGORITHM FOR TREATMENT OF OBESITY

FIGURE 58-1

Treatment algorithm. This algorithm applies only to the assessment for overweight and obesity and subsequent decisions on that assessment. It does not reflect any initial overall assessment for other conditions that the physician may wish to perform. BMI, body mass index; Ht, height;

Hx, history; Wt, weight. (*From National, Heart, Lung, and Blood Institute: Clinical guidelines on the identification, evaluation, and treatment of overweight and obesity in adults: The evidence report. Washington, DC, U.S. Department of Health and Human Services, 1998.*)

TABLE 58-5

A GUIDE TO SELECTING TREATMENT

TREATMENT	BMI CATEGORY				
	25–26.9	27–29.9	30–35	35–39.9	≥40
Diet, exercise, behavior therapy	With comorbidities	With comorbidities	+	+	+
Pharmacotherapy		With comorbidities	+	+	+
Surgery				With comorbidities	+

Source: From National Heart, Lung, and Blood Institute, North American Association for the Study of Obesity: Practical guide: Identification, evaluation, and treatment of overweight and obesity in adults. Bethesda, MD, National Institutes of Health pub number 00-4084, Oct. 2000. Available online at www.nhlbi.nih.gov/guidelines/obesity/practgde.htm.

LIFESTYLE MANAGEMENT Obesity care involves attention to three essential elements of lifestyle: dietary habits, physical activity, and behavior modification. Because obesity is fundamentally a disease of energy imbalance, all patients must learn how and when energy is consumed (diet), how and when energy is expended (physical activity), and how to incorporate this information into their daily lives (behavior therapy). Lifestyle management has been shown to result in a modest (typically 3–5 kg) weight loss compared with no treatment or usual care.

Diet Therapy The primary focus of diet therapy is to reduce overall calorie consumption. The National Heart, Lung, and Blood Institute (NHLBI) guidelines recommend initiating treatment with a calorie deficit of 500–1000 kcal/d compared with the patient's habitual diet. This reduction is consistent with a goal of losing approximately 1–2 lb per week. This calorie deficit can be accomplished by suggesting substitutions or alternatives to the diet. Examples include choosing smaller portion sizes, eating more fruits and vegetables, consuming more whole-grain cereals, selecting leaner cuts of meat and skimmed dairy products, reducing fried foods and other added fats and oils, and drinking water instead of caloric beverages. It is important that the dietary counseling remain patient-centered and that the goals be practical, realistic, and achievable.

The macronutrient composition of the diet will vary with the patient's preference and medical condition. The 2005 U.S. Department of Agriculture Dietary Guidelines for Americans (Chap. 53), which focus on health promotion and risk reduction, can be applied to treatment of overweight or obese patients. The recommendations include maintaining a diet rich in whole grains, fruits, vegetables, and dietary fiber; consuming two servings (8 oz) of fish high in omega-3 fatty acids per week; decreasing sodium to <2300 mg/d; consuming 3 cups of milk (or equivalent low-fat or fat-free dairy products) per day; limiting cholesterol to <300 mg/d; and keeping total fat between 20 and 35% of daily calories and saturated fats to <10% of daily calories. Application of these

guidelines to specific calorie goals can be found on the website *www.mypyramid.gov*. The revised Dietary Reference Intakes for Macronutrients released by the Institute of Medicine recommends 45–65% of calories from carbohydrates, 20–35% from fat, and 10–35% from protein. The guidelines also recommend daily fiber intake of 38 g (men) and 25 g (women) for persons over 50 years of age and 30 g (men) and 21 g (women) for those under age 50.

Since portion control is one of the most difficult strategies for patients to manage, the use of pre-prepared products such as meal replacements is a simple and convenient suggestion. Examples include frozen entrees, canned beverages, and bars. Use of meal replacements in the diet has been shown to result in a 7–8% weight loss.

An ongoing area of investigation is the use of low-carbohydrate, high-protein diets for weight loss. These diets are based on the concept that carbohydrates are the primary cause of obesity and lead to insulin resistance. Most low-carbohydrate diets (e.g., South Beach, Zone, and Sugar Busters!) recommend a carbohydrate level of approximately 40–46% of energy. The Atkins diet contains 5–15% carbohydrate, depending on the phase of the diet. Low-carbohydrate, high-protein diets appear to be more effective in lowering BMI; improving coronary heart disease risk factors, including an increase in HDL cholesterol and a decrease in triglyceride levels; and controlling satiety in the short term compared with low-fat diets. However, after 12 months, there is no significance difference among diets. Multiple studies have shown that sustained adherence to the diet rather than diet type is likely to be the best predictor of weight-loss outcome.

Another dietary approach to consider is the concept of energy density, which refers to the number of calories (energy) a food contains per unit of weight. People tend to ingest a constant volume of food regardless of caloric or macronutrient content. Adding water or fiber to a food decreases its energy density by increasing weight without affecting caloric content.

Examples of foods with low-energy density include soups, fruits, vegetables, oatmeal, and lean meats. Dry foods and high-fat foods such as pretzels, cheese, egg yolks, potato chips, and red meat have a high-energy density. Diets containing low-energy dense foods have been shown to control hunger and result in decreased caloric intake and weight loss.

Occasionally, very low calorie diets (VLCDs) are prescribed as a form of aggressive dietary therapy. The primary purpose of a VLCD is to promote a rapid and significant (13–23 kg) short-term weight loss over a 3- to 6-month period. These propriety formulas typically supply ≤800 kcal, 50–80 g protein, and 100% of the recommended daily intake for vitamins and minerals. According to a review by the National Task Force on the Prevention and Treatment of Obesity, indications for initiating a VLCD include well-motivated individuals who are moderately to severely obese (BMI >30), have failed at more conservative approaches to weight loss, and have a medical condition that would be immediately improved with rapid weight loss. These conditions include poorly controlled type 2 diabetes, hypertriglyceridemia, obstructive sleep apnea, and symptomatic peripheral edema. The risk for gallstone formation increases exponentially at rates of weight loss >1.5 kg/week (3.3 lb/week). Prophylaxis against gallstone formation with ursodeoxycholic acid, 600 mg/d, is effective in reducing this risk. Because of the need for close metabolic monitoring, these diets usually are prescribed by physicians specializing in obesity care.

Physical Activity Therapy Although exercise alone is only moderately effective for weight loss, the combination of dietary modification and exercise is the most effective behavioral approach for the treatment of obesity. The most important role of exercise appears to be in the maintenance of the weight loss. The 2008 Physical Activity Guidelines for Americans recommends that adults should engage in 150 min a week of moderate-intensity or 75 min a week of vigorous-intensity aerobic physical activity performed in episodes of at least 10 min, preferably spread throughout the week. The guidelines can be found at *www.health.gov/paguidelines*. Focusing on simple ways to add physical activity into the normal daily routine through leisure activities, travel, and domestic work should be suggested. Examples include walking, using the stairs, doing home and yard work, and engaging in sport activities. Asking the patient to wear a pedometer to monitor total accumulation of steps as part of the activities of daily living is a useful strategy. Step counts are highly correlated with activity level. Studies have demonstrated that lifestyle activities are as effective as structured exercise programs for improving cardiorespiratory fitness and weight loss. A high amount of physical activity (more than 300 min of moderate-intensity activity a week) is often needed to lose weight and sustain weight loss. These exercise recommendations are daunting to most patients and need to be implemented gradually. Consultation with an exercise physiologist or personal trainer may be helpful.

Behavioral Therapy Cognitive behavioral therapy is used to help change and reinforce new dietary and physical activity behaviors. Strategies include self-monitoring techniques (e.g., journaling, weighing, and measuring food and activity); stress management; stimulus control (e.g., using smaller plates, not eating in front of the television or in the car); social support; problem solving; and cognitive restructuring to help patients develop more positive and realistic thoughts about themselves. When recommending any behavioral lifestyle change, have the patient identify what, when, where, and how the behavioral change will be performed. The patient should keep a record of the anticipated behavioral change so that progress can be reviewed at the next office visit. Because these techniques are time-consuming to implement, they are often provided by ancillary office staff such as a nurse clinician or registered dietitian.

PHARMACOTHERAPY Adjuvant pharmacologic treatments should be considered for patients with a BMI >30 kg/m^2 or a BMI >27 kg/m^2 for those who also have concomitant obesity-related diseases and for whom dietary and physical activity therapy has not been successful. When an antiobesity medication is prescribed, patients should be actively engaged in a lifestyle program that provides the strategies and skills needed to use the drug effectively since this support increases total weight loss.

There are several potential targets of pharmacologic therapy for obesity. The most thoroughly explored treatment is suppression of appetite via centrally active medications that alter monoamine neurotransmitters. A second strategy is to reduce the absorption of selective macronutrients from the gastrointestinal (GI) tract, such as fat.

Centrally Acting Anorexiant Medications Appetite-suppressing drugs, or anorexiants, affect satiety—the absence of hunger after eating—and hunger—a biologic sensation that initiates eating. By increasing satiety and decreasing hunger, these agents help patients reduce caloric intake without a sense of deprivation. The target site for the actions of anorexiants is the ventromedial and lateral hypothalamic regions in the central nervous system (Chap. 57). Their biologic effect on appetite regulation is produced by augmenting the neurotransmission of three monoamines: norepinephrine; serotonin (5-hydroxytryptamine

[5-HT]); and, to a lesser degree, dopamine. The classic sympathomimetic adrenergic agents (benzphetamine, phendimetrazine, diethylpropion, mazindol, and phentermine) function by stimulating norepinephrine release or by blocking its reuptake. In contrast, sibutramine (Meridia) functions as a serotonin and norepinephrine reuptake inhibitor. Unlike other previously used anorexiants, sibutramine is not pharmacologically related to amphetamine and has no addictive potential.

Sibutramine was the only available anorexiant approved by the U.S. Food and Drug Administration (FDA) for long-term use until it was voluntarily withdrawn from the U.S. market by the manufacturer in October 2010, due to an increased risk of nonfatal myocardial infarction and nonfatal stroke among individuals with preexisting cardiovascular disease.

Peripherally Acting Medications Orlistat (Xenical) is a synthetic hydrogenated derivative of a naturally occurring lipase inhibitor, lipostatin, produced by the mold *Streptomyces toxytricini*. Orlistat is a potent, slowly reversible inhibitor of pancreatic, gastric, and carboxylester lipases and phospholipase A_2, which are required for the hydrolysis of dietary fat into fatty acids and monoacylglycerols. The drug acts in the lumen of the stomach and small intestine by forming a covalent bond with the active site of these lipases. Taken at a therapeutic dose of 120 mg tid, orlistat blocks the digestion and absorption of about 30% of dietary fat. After discontinuation of the drug, fecal fat usually returns to normal concentrations within 48–72 h.

Multiple randomized, double-blind, placebo-controlled studies have shown that after 1 year, orlistat produces a weight loss of about 9–10%, compared with a 4–6% weight loss in the placebo-treated groups. Because orlistat is minimally (<1%) absorbed from the GI tract, it has no systemic side effects. Tolerability to the drug is related to the malabsorption of dietary fat and subsequent passage of fat in the feces. GI tract adverse effects are reported in at least 10% of orlistat-treated patients. These effects include flatus with discharge, fecal urgency, fatty/oily stool, and increased defecation. These side effects generally are experienced early, diminish as patients control their dietary fat intake, and infrequently cause patients to withdraw from clinical trials. Psyllium mucilloid is helpful in controlling the orlistat-induced GI side effects when taken concomitantly with the medication. Serum concentrations of the fat-soluble vitamins D and E and β-carotene may be reduced, and vitamin supplements are recommended to prevent potential deficiencies. Orlistat was approved for over-the-counter use in 2007.

The Endocannabinoid System Cannabinoid receptors and their endogenous ligands have been implicated in a variety of physiologic functions, including feeding, modulation of pain, emotional behavior, and peripheral lipid metabolism. Cannabis and its main ingredient, Δ^9-tetrahydrocannabinol (THC), is an exogenous cannabinoid compound. Two endocannabinoids have been identified: anandamide and 2-arachidonyl glyceride. Two cannabinoid receptors have been identified: CB_1 (abundant in the brain) and CB_2 (present in immune cells). The brain endocannabinoid system is thought to control food intake by reinforcing motivation to find and consume foods with high incentive value and to regulate actions of other mediators of appetite. The first selective cannabinoid CB_1 receptor antagonist, rimonabant, was discovered in 1994. The medication antagonizes the orexigenic effect of THC and suppresses appetite. Several large prospective, randomized controlled trials have demonstrated the effectiveness of rimonabant as a weight-loss agent with concomitant improvements in waist circumference and cardiovascular risk factors. However, increased risk of neurologic and psychiatric side effects—seizures, depression, anxiety, insomnia, aggressiveness, and suicidal thoughts among patients randomized to rimonabant—resulted in a ruling against approval of the drug by the FDA in June 2007. Although the drug was available in 56 countries around the world in 2008, approval was officially withdrawn by the European Medicines Agency (EMEA) in January 2009, stating that the benefits of rimonabant no longer outweighed its risks. Development of CB_1 antagonists that do not enter the brain and selectively target the peripheral endocannabinoid system is needed.

Antiobesity Drugs in Development An emerging theme in pharmacotherapy for obesity is to target several points in the regulatory pathways that control body weight. Several combination drug therapies have completed phase III trials and have been submitted to the FDA for approval. Bupropion and naltrexone (Contrave), a dopamine and norepinephrine reuptake inhibitor and an opioid receptor antagonist, respectively, are combined to dampen the motivation/reinforcement that food brings (dopamine effect) and the pleasure/palatability of eating (opioid effect). Another formulation of bupropion with zonisamide (Empatic) combines bupropion with an anticonvulsant that has serotonergic and dopaminergic activity. Lastly, a formulation of phentermine and topiramate (Qnexa) combines a catecholamine releaser and an anticonvulsant, respectively, that have independently been shown to result in weight loss. The mechanism responsible for topiramate's weight loss is uncertain but is thought to be mediated through its modulation of γ-aminobutyric acid (GABA) receptors, inhibition of carbonic anhydrase, and antagonism of glutamate to reduce food intake. In October 2010, the FDA rejected

Qnexa's initial application as a new drug, citing clinical concerns regarding the potential teratogenic risks of topiramate in women of childbearing age. An additional investigational drug, lorcaserin, a 5-HT$_2$C receptor agonist, has completed phase III trials as a single agent. The FDA rejected lorcaserin's initial application as a new drug, citing clinical concerns that the weight loss efficacy in overweight and obese individuals without type 2 diabetes is marginal and nonclinical concerns related to mammary adenocarcinomas in female rats.

SURGERY Bariatric surgery can be considered for patients with severe obesity (BMI ≥40 kg/m^2) or those with moderate obesity (BMI ≥35 kg/m^2) associated with a serious medical condition. Surgical weight loss functions by reducing caloric intake and, depending on the procedure, macronutrient absorption.

Weight-loss surgeries fall into one of two categories: restrictive and restrictive-malabsorptive (Fig. 58-2). Restrictive surgeries limit the amount of food the stomach can hold and slow the rate of gastric emptying. The vertical banded gastroplasty (VBG) is the prototype of this category but is currently performed on a very limited basis due to lack of effectiveness in long-term trials. Laparoscopic adjustable silicone gastric banding (LASGB) has replaced the VBG as the most commonly performed restrictive operation. The first banding device, the LAP-BAND, was approved for use in the United States in 2001, and the second, the REALIZE band, in 2007. In contrast to previous devices, the diameters of these bands are adjustable by way of their connection to a reservoir that is implanted under the skin. Injection or removal of saline into the reservoir tightens or loosens the band's internal diameter, thus changing the size of the gastric opening.

The three restrictive-malabsorptive bypass procedures combine the elements of gastric restriction and selective malabsorption. These procedures include Roux-en-Y gastric bypass (RYGB), biliopancreatic diversion (BPD), and biliopancreatic diversion with duodenal switch (BPDDS) (Fig. 58-2). RYGB is the most commonly performed and accepted bypass procedure. It may be performed with an open incision or laparoscopically.

Although no recent randomized controlled trials compare weight loss after surgical and nonsurgical interventions, data from meta-analyses and large databases, primarily obtained from observational studies, suggest that bariatric surgery is the most effective weight-loss therapy for those with clinically severe obesity. These procedures generally produce a 30–35% average total body weight loss that is maintained in nearly 60% of patients at 5 years. In general, mean weight loss is greater after the combined restrictive-malabsorptive procedures

FIGURE 58-2
Bariatric surgical procedures. Examples of operative interventions used for surgical manipulation of the gastrointestinal tract. **A.** Laparoscopic gastric band (LAGB). **B.** The Roux-en-Y gastric bypass. **C.** Biliopancreatic diversion with duodenal switch. **D.** Biliopancreatic diversion. (*From ML Kendrick, GF Dakin: Mayo Clin Proc 815:518, 2006; with permission.*)

than after the restrictive procedures. An abundance of data supports the positive impact of bariatric surgery on obesity-related morbid conditions, including diabetes mellitus, hypertension, obstructive sleep apnea, dyslipidemia, and nonalcoholic fatty liver disease. The rapid improvement seen in diabetes after restrictive-malabsorptive procedures is thought to be due to surgery-specific, weight-independent effects on glucose homeostasis brought about by alteration of gut hormones.

Surgical mortality rate from bariatric surgery is generally <1% but varies with the procedure, patient's age and comorbid conditions, and experience of the surgical team. The most common surgical complications include stomal stenosis or marginal ulcers (occurring in 5–15% of patients) that present as prolonged nausea and vomiting after eating or inability to advance the diet to solid foods. These complications typically are treated by endoscopic balloon dilatation and acid suppression therapy, respectively. For patients who undergo LASGB, there are no intestinal absorptive abnormalities other than mechanical reduction in gastric size and outflow. Therefore, selective deficiencies occur uncommonly unless eating habits become unbalanced. In contrast, the restrictive-malabsorptive procedures increase risk for micronutrient deficiencies of vitamin B_{12}, iron, folate, calcium, and vitamin D. Patients with restrictive-malabsorptive procedures require lifelong supplementation with these micronutrients.

CHAPTER 59

EATING DISORDERS

B. Timothy Walsh ■ Evelyn Attia

Anorexia nervosa and bulimia nervosa are characterized by severe disturbances of eating behavior. The salient feature of *anorexia nervosa* (AN) is a voluntary restriction of food intake relative to caloric requirements leading to an inappropriately low body weight. *Bulimia nervosa* (BN) is characterized by recurrent episodes of binge eating followed by abnormal compensatory behaviors, such as self-induced vomiting. AN and BN are distinct clinical syndromes but share common features. Both disorders occur primarily among previously healthy young women who become overly concerned with body shape and weight. Many patients with BN have past histories of AN, and many patients with AN engage in binge eating and purging behavior. In the current diagnostic system, the critical distinction between AN and BN depends on body weight: patients with AN are, by definition, significantly underweight, whereas patients with BN have body weights in the normal range or above. *Binge eating disorder* (BED) is a more recently described syndrome characterized by repeated episodes of binge eating, similar to those of BN, in the absence of inappropriate compensatory behavior.

ANOREXIA NERVOSA

EPIDEMIOLOGY

Among women, the lifetime prevalence of the full syndrome of AN is approximately 1%. AN is much less common in males. AN is more prevalent in cultures where food is plentiful and being thin is associated with attractiveness. Individuals who pursue interests that place a premium on thinness, such as ballet and modeling, are at greater risk. The incidence of AN has increased in recent decades.

ETIOLOGY

The etiology of AN is unknown but appears to involve a combination of psychological, biologic, and cultural risk factors. Some factors, such as sexual or physical abuse and a family history of mood disturbance, are best viewed as nonspecific risk factors that increase vulnerability to a range of psychiatric disorders, including AN.

Patients who develop AN are inclined to be more obsessional and perfectionist than their peers. The disorder often begins as a diet not distinguishable at the outset from those undertaken by many adolescents and young women. As weight loss progresses, the fear of gaining weight grows; dieting becomes stricter; and psychological, behavioral, and medical aberrations increase. Eating disorders, including AN, may develop among individuals with type 1 diabetes mellitus and are associated with poorer glycemic control and an increased frequency of complications.

Numerous physiologic disturbances, including abnormalities in a variety of neurotransmitter systems, have been described in AN (discussed later). It is difficult to distinguish neurochemical, metabolic, and hormonal changes that may have a role in the initiation or perpetuation of the syndrome from those that are secondary to the disorder. The resolution of most of these abnormalities with weight restoration argues against an etiologic role.

Genetic factors contribute to the risk of development of AN, as its incidence is greater in families with one affected member and the concordance in monozygotic twins is greater than in dizygotic twins. However, specific genes or risk factor loci have not been identified.

CLINICAL FEATURES

AN typically begins in mid to late adolescence, sometimes in association with a stressful life event such as leaving home for school (Table 59-1). The disorder

TABLE 59-1

COMMON CHARACTERISTICS OF ANOREXIA NERVOSA, BULIMIA NERVOSA, AND BINGE EATING DISORDER

	ANOREXIA NERVOSA[a]	BULIMIA NERVOSA	BINGE EATING DISORDER[b]
Clinical Characteristics			
Onset	Mid-adolescence	Late adolescence/early adulthood	Late adolescence/early adulthood
Female:male	10:1	10:1	2:1
Lifetime prevalence	1% of women	1–3% of women	4% of men and women
Weight	Markedly decreased	Usually normal	Usually obese
Menstruation	Absent	Usually normal	Usually normal
Binge eating	25–50%	Required for diagnosis	Required for diagnosis
Mortality	~5% per decade	Low	Low
Physical and Laboratory Findings[a]			
Skin/extremities	Lanugo Acrocyanosis Edema	Callus/abrasion on dorsum of hand	
Cardiovascular	Bradycardia Hypotension		
Gastrointestinal	Salivary gland enlargement Slow gastric emptying Constipation Elevated liver enzymes	Salivary gland enlargement Dental erosion	
Hematopoietic	Normochromic, normocytic anemia Leukopenia		
Fluid/Electrolyte	Increased BUN, creatinine Hypokalemia Hypophosphatemia, Hypomagnesemia	Hypokalemia Hypochloremia Alkalosis	
Endocrine	Hypoglycemia Low estrogen or testosterone Low LH and FSH Low-normal thyroxine Normal TSH Increased cortisol		
Bone	Osteopenia		

[a]Patients with anorexia nervosa who frequently induce purging may also exhibit the physical and laboratory findings associated with bulimia nervosa.
[b]Obese patients with binge eating disorder are at risk for complications of obesity.
Abbreviations: BUN, blood urea nitrogen; FSH, follicle-stimulating hormone; LH, luteinizing hormone; TSH, thyroid-stimulating hormone.

occasionally develops in early puberty, before menarche, but seldom begins after age 40. Despite being underweight, patients with AN are irrationally afraid of gaining weight. They also exhibit a distortion of body image; despite being emaciated, patients with AN may believe that their body as a whole, or some part of their body, is too fat. Further weight loss is viewed by the patient as a fulfilling accomplishment, whereas weight gain is seen as a personal failure. Patients with AN rarely complain of hunger or fatigue and often exercise extensively. Despite the denial of hunger, one-quarter to one-half of patients with AN engage in eating binges. Patients tend to become socially withdrawn and increasingly committed to work or study, dieting, and exercise. As weight loss progresses, thoughts of food dominate mental life and idiosyncratic rules develop around eating. Patients with AN may obsessively collect cookbooks and recipes and be drawn to food-related occupations.

Physical features

Patients with AN typically have few physical complaints but may note cold intolerance. Gastrointestinal motility is diminished, leading to reduced gastric emptying and constipation. Some women who develop AN after menarche report that their menses ceased before significant weight loss occurred. Weight and height should be measured to allow calculation of body mass index (BMI; kg/m^2). Vital signs may reveal bradycardia, hypotension, and mild hypothermia. Soft, downy hair growth (lanugo) sometimes occurs, as does alopecia. Salivary gland enlargement, which is associated with starvation as well as with binge eating and vomiting, may make the face appear surprisingly full in contrast to the marked general wasting. Acrocyanosis of the digits is common, and peripheral edema can be seen in the absence of hypoalbuminemia, particularly when the patient begins to regain weight. Consumption of large amounts of vegetables containing vitamin A can result in a yellow tint to the skin (*hypercarotenemia*), which is especially notable on the palms.

Laboratory abnormalities

Mild normochromic, normocytic anemia is frequent, as is mild to moderate leukopenia, with a disproportionate reduction of polymorphonuclear leukocytes. Dehydration may result in slightly increased levels of blood urea nitrogen and creatinine. Serum transaminase levels may increase, especially during the early phases of refeeding. The level of serum proteins is usually normal. Blood sugar is often low and serum cholesterol may be moderately elevated. Hypokalemia, often accompanied by alkalosis, suggests self-induced vomiting or use of diuretics. Hyponatremia is common and may result from excess fluid intake and disturbances in the secretion of antidiuretic hormone. Hypophosphatemia and hypomagnesemia may be present in severe AN, especially as part of a refeeding syndrome.

Endocrine abnormalities

The regulation of virtually every endocrine system is altered in AN, but the most striking changes occur in the reproductive system. Amenorrhea is hypothalamic in origin and reflects diminished production of gonadotropin-releasing hormone (GnRH). The resulting gonadotropin deficiency causes low plasma estrogen in women and reduced testosterone in men. The hypothalamic GnRH pulse generator is exquisitely sensitive, particularly in women, to body weight, stress, and exercise, each of which may contribute to *hypothalamic amenorrhea* in AN.

Serum leptin levels are markedly reduced in AN as a result of undernutrition and decreased body-fat mass. The reduction in leptin is the primary factor responsible for the disturbances of the hypothalamic-pituitary-gonadal axis, and an important mediator of the other neuroendocrine abnormalities characteristic of AN (Chap. 57).

Serum cortisol and 24-h urine-free cortisol levels are generally elevated but without characteristic clinical signs of cortisol excess. Thyroid function tests resemble the pattern seen in euthyroid sick syndrome. Thyroxine (T_4) and free T_4 levels are usually in the low-normal range, triiodothyronine (T_3) levels are reduced, and reverse T_3 (rT_3) is elevated. The level of thyroid-stimulating hormone (TSH) is normal or partially suppressed. Growth hormone is increased, but insulin-like growth factor I (IGF-I), which is produced mainly by the liver, is reduced, as in other conditions of starvation. Diminished bone density is routinely observed in AN and reflects the effects of multiple nutritional deficiencies, reduced gonadal steroids, increased cortisol, and reduced IGF-I. The degree of bone-density reduction is proportional to the length of the illness, and patients are at risk for the development of symptomatic fractures. The occurrence of AN during adolescence may lead to the premature cessation of linear bone growth and a failure to achieve expected adult height.

Cardiac abnormalities

Cardiac output is reduced, and congestive heart failure occurs rarely during rapid refeeding. The electrocardiogram usually shows sinus bradycardia, reduced QRS voltage, and nonspecific ST-T-wave abnormalities. Some patients develop a prolonged QT_c interval, which may predispose to serious arrhythmias, particularly when electrolyte abnormalities are present.

DIAGNOSIS

The diagnosis of AN is based on the presence of characteristic behavioral, psychological, and physical attributes (Table 59-2). Widely accepted diagnostic criteria are provided by the American Psychiatric Association's *Diagnostic and Statistical Manual of Mental Disorders* (DSM-IV). These criteria include maintenance of a less than minimally normal body weight for age and height. Weights less than 85% of that expected, roughly equivalent to a BMI of 18.5 kg/m^2, are commonly considered to meet this criterion, but a patient weighing somewhat more who meets all other diagnostic criteria would still merit the diagnosis of AN. The current diagnostic criteria require that women with AN not have spontaneous menses, patients who have other characteristics of AN but report menstrual activity probably merit the diagnosis.

The diagnosis of AN can usually be made confidently in a patient with a history of weight loss accomplished by restrictive dieting and excessive exercise

TABLE 59-2

DIAGNOSTIC FEATURES OF ANOREXIA NERVOSA

Refusal to maintain body weight at or above a minimally normal weight for age and height. (This includes a failure to achieve weight gain expected during a period of growth leading to an abnormally low body weight.)

Intense fear of weight gain or becoming fat.

Distortion of body image (e.g., feeling fat despite an objectively low weight or minimizing the seriousness of low weight).

Amenorrhea. (This criterion is met if menstrual periods occur only following hormone—e.g., estrogen—administration.)

accompanied by a marked reluctance to gain weight. Patients with AN often deny that they have a serious problem and may be brought to medical attention by concerned family or friends. Especially in atypical presentations, other causes of significant weight loss in previously healthy young people should be considered, including inflammatory bowel disease, gastric outlet obstruction, diabetes mellitus, CNS tumors, or neoplasm (Chap. 10).

PROGNOSIS

The course and outcome of AN are highly variable. One-quarter to one-half of patients eventually recover fully, with few psychological or physical sequelae. However, many patients have persistent difficulties with weight maintenance, depression, and eating disturbances, including BN. The development of obesity following AN is rare. The long-term mortality of AN is among the highest associated with any psychiatric disorder. Approximately 5% of patients die per decade of follow-up, primarily due to the physical effects of chronic starvation or by suicide.

Virtually all of the physiologic abnormalities associated with AN are observed in other forms of starvation and markedly improve or disappear with weight gain. A worrisome exception is the reduction in bone mass, which may not recover fully, particularly if AN occurs during adolescence when peak bone mass is normally achieved.

TREATMENT Anorexia Nervosa

Because of the profound physiologic and psychological effects of starvation, there is a broad consensus that weight restoration to at least 90% of predicted weight is the primary goal in the treatment of AN. Unfortunately, because most patients resist this goal, the management of AN is often accompanied by frustration for the patient, the family, and the physician. Patients typically

exaggerate their food intake and minimize their symptoms. Some patients resort to subterfuge to make their weights appear higher, for example, by water-loading before they are weighed. In attempting to engage the patient in treatment, it may be useful to elicit the patient's physical concerns (e.g., about osteoporosis, weakness, or fertility), and provide education about the importance of normalizing nutritional status in order to address those concerns. The physician should reassure the patient that weight gain will not be permitted to get out of control but simultaneously emphasize that weight restoration is medically and psychologically imperative.

The intensity of the initial treatment, including the need for hospitalization, is determined by the patient's current weight, the rapidity of recent weight loss, and the severity of medical and psychological complications (Fig. 59-1). Hospitalization should be strongly considered for patients weighing <75% of that expected age and height, even if the results of routine blood studies are within normal limits. Acute medical problems, such as severe electrolyte imbalances, should be identified and addressed. Nutritional restoration can almost

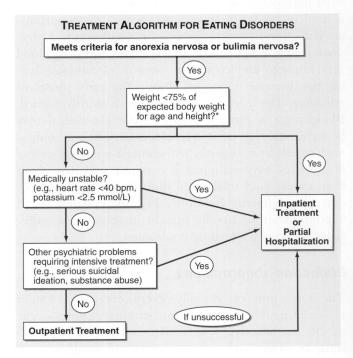

TREATMENT ALGORITHM FOR EATING DISORDERS

FIGURE 59-1

An algorithm for basic treatment decisions regarding patients with anorexia nervosa or bulimia nervosa. Based on the American Psychiatric Association practice guidelines for the treatment of patients with eating disorders. *Although outpatient management may be considered for patients with anorexia nervosa weighing more than 75% of expected, there should be a low threshold for using more intensive interventions if the weight loss has been rapid or if current weight is <80% of expected.

always be successfully accomplished by oral feeding, and parenteral methods are rarely required. For severely underweight patients, sufficient calories (approximately 1200–1800 kcal/d) should be provided initially in divided meals as food or liquid supplements to maintain weight and permit physiological stabilization. Calories can then be gradually increased to achieve a weight gain of 1–2 kg (2–4 lb) per week, typically requiring an intake of 3000–4000 kcal/d. Meals must be supervised, ideally by personnel who are firm regarding the necessity of food consumption, empathic regarding the challenges entailed, and reassuring about the patient's eventual recovery. Patients have great psychological difficulty complying with the need for increased caloric consumption, and the assistance of psychiatrists or psychologists experienced in the treatment of AN is usually necessary.

Less severely affected patients may be treated in a partial hospitalization program where medical and psychiatric supervision is available and several meals can be monitored each day. Outpatient treatment may suffice for mildly ill patients. Weight must be monitored at frequent intervals, and explicit goals agreed on for weight gain, with the understanding that more intensive treatment will be required if the level of care initially employed is not successful. For younger patients, the active involvement of the family in treatment is crucial regardless of treatment setting. Outpatient interventions that help parents refeed their child have been be quite successful at achieving weight restoration.

Psychiatric treatment focuses primarily on two issues. First, patients require much emotional support during the period of weight gain. They often intellectually agree with the need to gain weight, but strenuously resist increases in caloric intake, and often surreptitiously discard food that is provided. Second, patients must learn to base their self-esteem not on the achievement of an inappropriately low weight, but on the development of satisfying personal relationships and the attainment of reasonable academic and occupational goals. While this is often possible, some patients with AN develop other serious emotional and behavioral symptoms such as depression, self-mutilation, obsessive-compulsive behavior, and suicidal ideation. These symptoms may require additional therapeutic interventions, in the form of psychotherapy, medication, or hospitalization.

Medical complications occasionally occur during refeeding. Especially in the early stages of treatment, severely malnourished patients may develop a "refeeding syndrome" characterized by hypophosphatemia, hypomagnesemia, and cardiovascular instability. Acute gastric dilatation has been described when refeeding is rapid. As in other forms of malnutrition, fluid retention and peripheral edema may occur, but they generally do not require specific treatment in the absence of cardiac, renal, or hepatic dysfunction. Transient modest elevations in serum liver enzyme levels occasionally occur. Multivitamins should be given, and an adequate intake of vitamin D (400 IU/d) and calcium (1500 mg/d) should be provided.

No psychotropic medications are of established value in the treatment of AN, although there is recent preliminary evidence that the atypical antipsychotic medication olanzapine may assist some patients by increasing the rate of weight gain and decreasing obsessive thinking. Medications that may prolong the QT_c interval should be avoided. The alterations of cortisol and thyroid hormone metabolism do not require specific treatment and correct with weight gain. Estrogen treatment appears to offer no benefit to bone density in underweight patients, and the small benefit of bisphosphonate treatment appears to be outweighed by the potential risks of such agents in young women.

BULIMIA NERVOSA

EPIDEMIOLOGY

In women, the full syndrome of BN occurs with a lifetime prevalence of 1–3%. Variants of the disorder, such as occasional binge eating or purging, are much more common and occur in 5–10% of young women. The frequency of BN among men is less than one-tenth of that among women. The prevalence of BN increased dramatically in the early 1970s and 1980s but may have leveled off or declined somewhat in recent years.

ETIOLOGY

As with AN, the etiology of BN is likely to be multifactorial. Patients who develop BN describe a higher-than-expected prevalence of childhood and parental obesity, suggesting that a predisposition toward obesity may increase vulnerability to this eating disorder. The marked increase in the number of cases of BN during the past 30 years and the rarity of BN in underdeveloped countries imply that cultural factors are important.

CLINICAL FEATURES

The typical patient presenting for treatment of BN is a woman of normal weight in her mid-twenties who reports binge eating and purging 5–10 times a week for 5–10 years (Table 59-3). The disorder usually begins in late adolescence or early adulthood during or following a diet, often in association with depressed mood. The self-imposed caloric restriction leads to increased hunger and to overeating. In an attempt to

TABLE 59-3

DIAGNOSTIC FEATURES OF BULIMIA NERVOSA

Recurrent episodes of binge eating, which is characterized by the consumption of a large amount of food in a short period of time and a feeling that the eating is out of control.

Recurrent inappropriate behavior to compensate for the binge eating, such as self-induced vomiting.

The occurrence of both the binge eating and the inappropriate compensatory behavior at least twice weekly, on average, for 3 months.

Overconcern with body shape and weight.

Note: If the diagnostic criteria for anorexia nervosa are simultaneously met, only the diagnosis of anorexia nervosa is given.

avoid weight gain, the patient induces vomiting, takes laxatives or diuretics, or engages in some other form of compensatory behavior. During binges, patients with this disorder tend to consume large amounts of sweet foods with a high fat content, such as dessert items. The most frequent compensatory behaviors are self-induced vomiting and laxative abuse, but a wide variety of techniques have been described, including the omission of insulin injections by individuals with type 1 diabetes mellitus. Initially, patients may experience a sense of satisfaction that appealing food can be eaten without weight gain. However, as the disorder progresses, patients perceive diminished control overeating. Binges increase in size and frequency and are provoked by a variety of stimuli, such as transient depression, anxiety, or a sense that too much food has been consumed in a normal meal. Between binges, patients restrict caloric intake, which increases hunger and sets the stage for the next binge. Typically, patients with BN are ashamed of their behavior and endeavor to keep their disorder hidden from family and friends. Like patients with AN, those with BN place an unusual emphasis on weight and shape as a basis for their self-esteem. Many patients with BN have mild symptoms of depression. Some patients exhibit serious mood and behavioral disturbances, such as suicide attempts, sexual promiscuity, and drug and alcohol abuse. Although vomiting may be triggered initially by manual stimulation of the gag reflex, most patients with BN develop the ability to induce vomiting at will. Rarely, patients resort to the regular use of syrup of ipecac. Laxatives and diuretics are frequently taken in impressive quantities, such as 30 or 60 laxative pills on a single occasion. The resulting fluid loss produces dehydration and a feeling of emptiness but has little impact on caloric balance.

The physical abnormalities associated with BN primarily result from the purging behavior. Painless bilateral salivary gland hypertrophy (sialadenosis) may be noted. A scar or callus on the dorsum of the hand may develop due to repeated trauma from the teeth among patients who manually stimulate the gag reflex. Recurrent vomiting and the exposure of the lingual surfaces of the teeth to stomach acid lead to loss of dental enamel and eventually to chipping and erosion of the front teeth. Laboratory abnormalities are surprisingly infrequent, but hypokalemia, hypochloremia, and hyponatremia are observed occasionally. Repeated vomiting may lead to alkalosis, whereas repeated laxative abuse may produce a mild metabolic acidosis. Serum amylase may be slightly elevated due to an increase in the salivary isoenzyme.

Serious physical complications resulting from BN are rare. Oligomenorrhea and amenorrhea are more frequent than among women without eating disorders. Arrhythmias occasionally occur secondary to electrolyte disturbances. Tearing of the esophagus and rupture of the stomach have been reported and constitute life-threatening events. Some patients who chronically abuse laxatives or diuretics develop transient peripheral edema when this behavior ceases, presumably due to high levels of aldosterone secondary to persistent fluid and electrolyte depletion.

DIAGNOSIS

The critical diagnostic features of BN are repeated episodes of binge eating followed by inappropriate behaviors aimed at avoiding weight gain (Table 59-3). The diagnosis of BN requires a candid history from the patient detailing frequent, large eating binges followed by the purposeful use of inappropriate mechanisms to avoid weight gain. Most patients with BN who present for treatment are distressed by their inability to control their eating behavior and are able to provide such details if queried in a supportive and nonjudgmental fashion.

PROGNOSIS

The prognosis of BN is much more favorable than that of AN. Mortality is low, and full recovery occurs in approximately 50% of patients within 10 years. Approximately 25% of patients have persistent symptoms of BN over many years. Few patients progress from BN to AN.

TREATMENT Bulimia Nervosa

BN can usually be treated on an outpatient basis (Fig. 59-1). Cognitive behavioral therapy (CBT) is a short-term (4–6 months) psychological treatment that focuses on the intense concern with shape and weight, the persistent dieting, and the binge eating and purging that characterize this disorder. Patients are directed to monitor the circumstances, thoughts, and emotions associated with binge/purge episodes, to eat regularly, and to challenge their assumptions linking weight to self-esteem. CBT produces symptomatic remission in 25–50% of patients.

Numerous double-blind, placebo-controlled trials have documented that antidepressant medications are useful in the treatment of BN but are probably somewhat less effective than CBT. Although efficacy has been established for virtually all chemical classes of antidepressants, only the selective serotonin reuptake inhibitor fluoxetine (Prozac) has been approved for use in BN by the U.S. Food and Drug Administration. Antidepressant medications are helpful even for patients with BN who are not depressed, and the dose of fluoxetine recommended for BN (60 mg/d) is higher than that typically used to treat depression. These observations suggest that different mechanisms may underlie the utility of these medications in BN and in depression.

A subset of patients does not respond to CBT, antidepressant medication, or their combination. More intensive forms of treatment, including hospitalization, may be required.

BINGE EATING DISORDER

Binge eating disorder (BED) is characterized by frequent episodes of eating unusually large amounts of food accompanied by feeling loss of control. In contrast to those with BN, patients with BED do not frequently engage in appropriate behavior to compensate for binge eating. In addition, BED is commonly associated with obesity (Table 59-1). BED occurs more frequently than AN and BN in both clinical and community population samples, and males constitute a greater fraction of affected individuals. Compared with obese individuals without BED, those with BED have higher rates of anxiety, depression, and health care use. A range of psychological treatments, such as CBT and interpersonal therapy (IPT) and medications, including antidepressants and weight-loss agents, appear helpful in reducing binge eating. Surprisingly, cessation of binge eating is not routinely followed by loss of weight.

GLOBAL CONSIDERATIONS

Eating disorders are more common in cultures where food is available and thinness is idealized. Nevertheless, eating disorders have been reported across the world, including in many parts of Asia and Africa. Cultural variation may contribute to differing presentations of eating disorder symptoms. For example, in some cultural groups, the rationale for food refusal of low weight individuals who exhibit many symptoms of AN may not include the DSM IV criterion, "intense fear of gaining weight or becoming fat."

CHAPTER 60

THE METABOLIC SYNDROME

Robert H. Eckel

The metabolic syndrome (syndrome X, insulin resistance syndrome) consists of a constellation of metabolic abnormalities that confer increased risk of cardiovascular disease (CVD) and diabetes mellitus (DM). The criteria for the metabolic syndrome have evolved since the original definition by the World Health Organization in 1998, reflecting growing clinical evidence and analysis by a variety of consensus conferences and professional organizations. The major features of the metabolic syndrome include central obesity, hypertriglyceridemia, low high-density lipoprotein (HDL) cholesterol, hyperglycemia, and hypertension **(Table 60-1)**.

EPIDEMIOLOGY

The prevalence of metabolic syndrome varies around the world, in part reflecting the age and ethnicity of the populations studied and the diagnostic criteria applied. In general, the prevalence of metabolic syndrome increases with age. The highest recorded prevalence worldwide is in Native Americans, with nearly 60% of women ages 45–49 and 45% of men ages 45–49 meeting National Cholesterol Education Program and Adult Treatment Panel III (NCEP:ATPIII) criteria. In the United States, metabolic syndrome is less

TABLE 60-1

NCEP:ATPIII 2001 AND IDF CRITERIA FOR THE METABOLIC SYNDROME

NCEP:ATPIII 2001	IDF CRITERIA FOR CENTRAL ADIPOSITY[a]		
Three or more of the following: Central obesity: Waist circumference >102 cm (M), >88 cm (F) Hypertriglyceridemia: Triglycerides ≥150 mg/dL or specific medication Low HDL cholesterol: <40 mg/dL and <50 mg/dL, respectively, or specific medication Hypertension: Blood pressure ≥130 mm systolic or ≥85 mm diastolic or specific medication Fasting plasma glucose ≥100 mg/dL or specific medication or previously diagnosed type 2 diabetes	**WAIST CIRCUMFERENCE**		
	MEN	**WOMEN**	**ETHNICITY**
	≥94 cm	≥80 cm	Europid, Sub-Saharan African, Eastern and Middle Eastern
	≥90 cm	≥80 cm	South Asian, Chinese, and ethnic South and Central American
	≥85 cm	≥90 cm	Japanese

Two or more of the following:
Fasting triglycerides >150 mg/dL or specific medication
HDL cholesterol <40 mg/dL and <50 mg/dL for men and women, respectively, or specific medication
Blood pressure >130 mm systolic or >85 mm diastolic or previous diagnosis or specific medication
Fasting plasma glucose ≥100 mg/dL or previously diagnosed type 2 diabetes

[a]In this analysis, the following thresholds for waist circumference were used: white men, ≥94 cm; African-American men, ≥94 cm; Mexican-American men, ≥90 cm; white women, ≥80 cm; African-American women, ≥80 cm; Mexican-American women, ≥80 cm. For participants whose designation was "other race—including multiracial," thresholds that were once based on Europid cut points (≥94 cm for men and ≥80 cm for women) and once based on South Asian cut points (≥90 cm for men and ≥80 cm for women) were used. For participants who were considered "other Hispanic," the IDF thresholds for ethnic South and Central Americans were used.
Abbreviations: HDL, high-density lipoprotein; IDF, International Diabetes Foundation; NCEP:ATPIII, National Cholesterol Education Program, Adult Treatment Panel III.

FIGURE 60-1
Prevalence of the metabolic syndrome components, from NHANES III. NHANES, National Health and Nutrition Examination Survey; TG, triglyceride; HDL, high-density lipoprotein; BP, blood pressure. The prevalence of elevated glucose includes individuals with known diabetes mellitus. (*Created from data in ES Ford et al: Diabetes Care 27:2444, 2004.*)

common in African-American men and more common in Mexican-American women. Based on data from the National Health and Nutrition Examination Survey (NHANES) 1999–2000, the age-adjusted prevalence of the metabolic syndrome in United States adults who did not have diabetes is 28% for men and 30% for women. In France, a cohort 30 to 60 years old has shown a <10% prevalence for each sex, although 17.5% are affected in the age range 60–64. Greater industrialization worldwide is associated with rising rates of obesity, which is anticipated to increase prevalence of the metabolic syndrome dramatically, especially as the population ages. Moreover, the rising prevalence and severity of obesity in children is initiating features of the metabolic syndrome in a younger population.

The frequency distribution of the five components of the syndrome for the U.S. population (NHANES III) is summarized in **Fig. 60-1.** Increases in waist circumference predominate in women, whereas fasting triglycerides >150 mg/dL and hypertension are more likely in men.

RISK FACTORS
Overweight/obesity

Although the first description of the metabolic syndrome occurred in the early twentieth century, the worldwide overweight/obesity epidemic has been the driving force for more recent recognition of the syndrome. Central adiposity is a key feature of the syndrome, reflecting the fact that the syndrome's prevalence is driven by the strong relationship between waist circumference and increasing adiposity. However, despite the importance

of obesity, patients who are normal weight may also be insulin-resistant and have the syndrome.

Sedentary lifestyle

Physical inactivity is a predictor of CVD events and related mortality rate. Many components of the metabolic syndrome are associated with a sedentary lifestyle, including increased adipose tissue (predominantly central), reduced HDL cholesterol, and a trend toward increased triglycerides, high blood pressure, and increased glucose in the genetically susceptible. Compared with individuals who watched television or videos or used the computer <1 h daily, those who carried out those behaviors for >4 h daily had a twofold increased risk of the metabolic syndrome.

Aging

The metabolic syndrome affects 44% of the U.S. population older than age 50. A greater percentage of women over age 50 have the syndrome than men. The age dependency of the syndrome's prevalence is seen in most populations around the world.

Diabetes mellitus

DM is included in both the NCEP and International Diabetes Foundation (IDF) definitions of the metabolic syndrome. It is estimated that the great majority (~75%) of patients with type 2 diabetes or impaired glucose tolerance (IGT) have the metabolic syndrome. The presence of the metabolic syndrome in these populations relates to a higher prevalence of CVD compared with patients with type 2 diabetes or IGT without the syndrome.

Coronary heart disease

The approximate prevalence of the metabolic syndrome in patients with coronary heart disease (CHD) is 50%, with a prevalence of 37% in patients with premature coronary artery disease (age ≤45), particularly in women. With appropriate cardiac rehabilitation and changes in lifestyle (e.g., nutrition, physical activity, weight reduction, and, in some cases, pharmacologic agents), the prevalence of the syndrome can be reduced.

Lipodystrophy

Lipodystrophic disorders in general are associated with the metabolic syndrome. Both genetic (e.g., Berardinelli-Seip congenital lipodystrophy, Dunnigan familial partial lipodystrophy) and acquired (e.g., HIV-related lipodystrophy in patients treated with highly active antiretroviral therapy) forms of lipodystrophy may give rise to severe insulin resistance and many of the components of the metabolic syndrome.

ETIOLOGY

Insulin resistance

The most accepted and unifying hypothesis to describe the pathophysiology of the metabolic syndrome is insulin resistance, which is caused by an incompletely understood defect in insulin action. The onset of insulin resistance is heralded by postprandial hyperinsulinemia, followed by fasting hyperinsulinemia and, ultimately, hyperglycemia.

An early major contributor to the development of insulin resistance is an overabundance of circulating fatty acids (Fig. 60-2). Plasma albumin-bound free fatty acids (FFAs) are derived predominantly from adipose tissue triglyceride stores released by lipolytic enzymes lipase. Fatty acids are also derived from the lipolysis of triglyceride-rich lipoproteins in tissues by lipoprotein lipase (LPL). Insulin mediates both antilipolysis and the stimulation of LPL in adipose tissue. Of note, the inhibition of lipolysis in adipose tissue is the most sensitive pathway of insulin action. Thus, when insulin resistance develops, increased lipolysis produces more fatty acids, which further decrease the antilipolytic effect of insulin. Excessive fatty acids enhance substrate availability and create insulin resistance by modifying downstream signaling. Fatty acids impair insulin-mediated glucose uptake and accumulate as triglycerides in both skeletal and cardiac muscle, whereas increased glucose production and triglyceride accumulation are seen in liver.

The oxidative stress hypothesis provides a unifying theory for aging and the predisposition to the metabolic

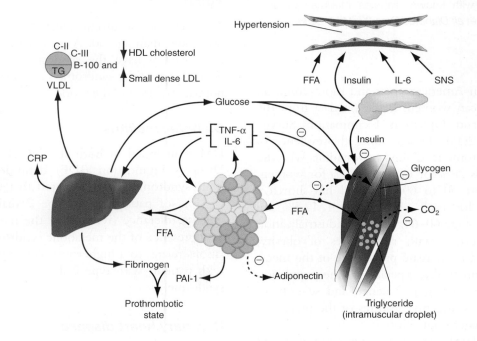

FIGURE 60-2

Pathophysiology of the metabolic syndrome. Free fatty acids (FFAs) are released in abundance from an expanded adipose tissue mass. In the liver, FFAs result in an increased production of glucose and triglycerides and secretion of very low density lipoproteins (VLDLs). Associated lipid/lipoprotein abnormalities include reductions in high-density lipoprotein (HDL) cholesterol and an increased density of low-density lipoproteins (LDLs). FFAs also reduce insulin sensitivity in muscle by inhibiting insulin-mediated glucose uptake. Associated defects include a reduction in glucose partitioning to glycogen and increased lipid accumulation in triglyceride (TG). Increases in circulating glucose, and to some extent FFA, increase pancreatic insulin secretion, resulting in hyperinsulinemia. Hyperinsulinemia may result in enhanced sodium reabsorption and increased sympathetic nervous system (SNS) activity and contribute to the hypertension, as might increased levels of circulating FFAs. The proinflammatory state is superimposed and contributory to the insulin resistance produced by excessive FFAs. The enhanced secretion of interleukin 6 (IL-6) and tumor necrosis factor α (TNF-α) produced by adipocytes and monocyte-derived macrophages results in more insulin resistance and lipolysis of adipose tissue triglyceride stores to circulating FFAs. IL-6 and other cytokines also enhance hepatic glucose production, VLDL production by the liver, and insulin resistance in muscle. Cytokines and FFAs also increase the hepatic production of fibrinogen and adipocyte production of plasminogen activator inhibitor 1 (PAI-1), resulting in a prothrombotic state. Higher levels of circulating cytokines also stimulate the hepatic production of C-reactive protein (CRP). Reduced production of the anti-inflammatory and insulin-sensitizing cytokine adiponectin is also associated with the metabolic syndrome. (*Reprinted from RH Eckel et al: Lancet 365:1415, 2005, with permission from Elsevier.*)

syndrome. In studies carried out in insulin-resistant subjects with obesity or type 2 diabetes, the offspring of patients with type 2 diabetes, and the elderly, a defect has been identified in mitochondrial oxidative phosphorylation, leading to the accumulation of triglycerides and related lipid molecules in muscle. The accumulation of lipids in muscle is associated with insulin resistance.

Increased waist circumference

Waist circumference is an important component of the most recent and frequently applied diagnostic criteria for the metabolic syndrome. However, measuring waist circumference does not reliably distinguish increases in subcutaneous adipose tissue vs. visceral fat; this distinction requires CT or MRI. With increases in visceral adipose tissue, adipose tissue-derived FFAs are directed to the liver. In contrast, increases in abdominal subcutaneous fat release lipolysis products into the systemic circulation and avoid more direct effects on hepatic metabolism. Relative increases in visceral versus subcutaneous adipose tissue with increasing waist circumference in Asians and Asian Indians may explain the greater prevalence of the syndrome in those populations compared with African-American men in whom subcutaneous fat predominates. It is also possible that visceral fat is a marker for, but not the source of, excess postprandial FFAs in obesity.

Dyslipidemia

In general, FFA flux to the liver is associated with increased production of apoB-containing, triglyceride-rich very low density lipoproteins (VLDLs). The effect of insulin on this process is complex, but *hypertriglyceridemia* is an excellent marker of the insulin-resistant condition.

The other major lipoprotein disturbance in the metabolic syndrome is a *reduction in HDL cholesterol*. This reduction is a consequence of changes in HDL composition and metabolism. In the presence of hypertriglyceridemia, a decrease in the cholesterol content of HDL is a consequence of reduced cholesteryl ester content of the lipoprotein core in combination with cholesteryl ester transfer protein–mediated alterations in triglyceride, making the particle small and dense. This change in lipoprotein composition also results in increased clearance of HDL from the circulation. The relationships of these changes in HDL to insulin resistance are probably indirect, occurring in concert with the changes in triglyceride-rich lipoprotein metabolism.

In addition to HDL, low-density lipoproteins (LDLs) are modified in composition. With fasting serum triglycerides >2.0 mM (~180 mg/dL), there is almost always a predominance of small dense LDLs. Small dense LDLs are thought to be more atherogenic. They may be toxic to the endothelium, and they are able to transit through the endothelial basement membrane and adhere to glycosaminoglycans. They also have increased susceptibility to oxidation and are selectively bound to scavenger receptors on monocyte-derived macrophages. Subjects with increased small dense LDL particles and hypertriglyceridemia also have increased cholesterol content of both VLDL1 and VLDL2 subfractions. This relatively cholesterol-rich VLDL particle may contribute to the atherogenic risk in patients with metabolic syndrome.

Glucose intolerance

The defects in insulin action lead to impaired suppression of glucose production by the liver and kidney and reduced glucose uptake and metabolism in insulin-sensitive tissues, i.e., muscle and adipose tissue. The relationship between impaired fasting glucose (IFG) or impaired glucose tolerance (IGT) and insulin resistance is well supported by human, nonhuman primate, and rodent studies. To compensate for defects in insulin action, insulin secretion and/or clearance must be modified to sustain euglycemia. Ultimately, this compensatory mechanism fails, usually because of defects in insulin secretion, resulting in progress from IFG and/or IGT to DM.

Hypertension

The relationship between insulin resistance and hypertension is well established. Paradoxically, under normal physiologic conditions, insulin is a vasodilator with secondary effects on sodium reabsorption in the kidney. However, in the setting of insulin resistance, the vasodilatory effect of insulin is lost but the renal effect on sodium reabsorption is preserved. Sodium reabsorption is increased in whites with the metabolic syndrome but not in Africans or Asians. Insulin also increases the activity of the sympathetic nervous system, an effect that also may be preserved in the setting of the insulin resistance. Finally, insulin resistance is characterized by pathway-specific impairment in phosphatidylinositol-3-kinase signaling. In the endothelium, this may cause an imbalance between the production of nitric oxide and the secretion of endothelin 1, leading to decreased blood flow. Although these mechanisms are provocative, when insulin action is assessed by levels of fasting insulin or by the Homeostasis Model Assessment (HOMA), insulin resistance contributes only modestly to the increased prevalence of hypertension in the metabolic syndrome.

Proinflammatory cytokines

The increases in proinflammatory cytokines, including interleukin (IL)-1, IL-6, IL-18, resistin, tumor necrosis factor (TNF) α, and C-reactive protein (CRP), reflect overproduction by the expanded adipose tissue mass (Fig. 60-2). Adipose tissue-derived macrophages may be the primary source of proinflammatory cytokines locally and in the systemic circulation. It remains unclear, however, how much of the insulin resistance is caused by the paracrine vs. endocrine effects of these cytokines.

Adiponectin

Adiponectin is an anti-inflammatory cytokine produced exclusively by adipocytes. Adiponectin enhances insulin sensitivity and inhibits many steps in the inflammatory process. In the liver, adiponectin inhibits the expression of gluconeogenic enzymes and the rate of glucose production. In muscle, adiponectin increases glucose transport and enhances fatty acid oxidation, partially due to activation of adenosine monophosphate (AMP) kinase. Adiponectin is reduced in the metabolic syndrome. The relative contribution of adiponectin deficiency versus overabundance of the proinflammatory cytokines is unclear.

CLINICAL FEATURES

Symptoms and signs

The metabolic syndrome is typically not associated with symptoms. On physical examination, waist circumference may be expanded and blood pressure elevated. The presence of one or either of these signs should alert the clinician to search for other biochemical abnormalities that may be associated with the metabolic syndrome. Less frequently, lipoatrophy or acanthosis nigricans is found on examination. Because these physical findings typically are associated with severe insulin resistance, other components of the metabolic syndrome should be expected.

Associated diseases

Cardiovascular disease

The relative risk for new-onset CVD in patients with the metabolic syndrome, in the absence of diabetes, averages between 1.5-fold and threefold. However, in an 8-year follow-up of middle-aged men and women in the Framingham Offspring Study (FOS), the population-attributable risk for patients with the metabolic syndrome to develop CVD was 34% in men and only 16% in women. In the same study, both the metabolic syndrome and diabetes predicted ischemic stroke, with greater risk for patients with the metabolic syndrome than for those with diabetes alone (19% vs. 7%), particularly in women (27% vs. 5%). Patients with metabolic syndrome are also at increased risk for peripheral vascular disease.

Type 2 diabetes

Overall, the risk for type 2 diabetes in patients with the metabolic syndrome is increased three- to fivefold. In the FOS's 8-year follow-up of middle-aged men and women, the population-attributable risk for developing type 2 diabetes was 62% in men and 47% in women.

Other associated conditions

In addition to the features specifically associated with metabolic syndrome, insulin resistance is accompanied by other metabolic alterations. Those alterations include increases in apoB and apoC-III, uric acid, prothrombotic factors (fibrinogen, plasminogen activator inhibitor 1), serum viscosity, asymmetric dimethylarginine, homocysteine, white blood cell count, proinflammatory cytokines, CRP, microalbuminuria, nonalcoholic fatty liver disease (NAFLD) and/or nonalcoholic steatohepatitis (NASH), polycystic ovarian disease (PCOS), and obstructive sleep apnea (OSA).

Nonalcoholic fatty liver disease

(See also Chap. 44) Fatty liver is relatively common. However, in NASH, both triglyceride accumulation and inflammation coexist. NASH is now present in 2–3% of the population in the United States and other Western countries. As the prevalence of overweight/obesity and the metabolic syndrome increases, NASH may become one of the more common causes of end-stage liver disease and hepatocellular carcinoma.

Hyperuricemia

Hyperuricemia reflects defects in insulin action on the renal tubular reabsorption of uric acid, whereas the increase in asymmetric dimethylarginine, an endogenous inhibitor of nitric oxide synthase, relates to endothelial dysfunction. Microalbuminuria also may be caused by altered endothelial pathophysiology in the insulin-resistant state.

Polycystic ovary syndrome

PCOS is highly associated with the metabolic syndrome, with a prevalence between 40 and 50%. Women with PCOS are 2–4 times more likely to have the metabolic syndrome than are women without PCOS.

Obstructive sleep apnea

OSA is commonly associated with obesity, hypertension, increased circulating cytokines, IGT, and insulin resistance. With these associations, it is not surprising that the metabolic syndrome is frequently present. Moreover, when biomarkers of insulin resistance are compared between patients with OSA and weight-matched controls, insulin resistance is more severe in patients with OSA. Continuous positive airway pressure (CPAP) treatment in OSA patients improves insulin sensitivity.

DIAGNOSIS

The diagnosis of the metabolic syndrome relies on satisfying the criteria listed in Table 60-1 by using tools at the bedside and in the laboratory. The medical history should include evaluation of symptoms for OSA in all patients and PCOS in premenopausal women. Family history will help determine risk for CVD and DM. Blood pressure and waist circumference measurements provide information necessary for the diagnosis.

Laboratory tests

Fasting lipids and glucose are needed to determine if the metabolic syndrome is present. The measurement of additional biomarkers associated with insulin resistance can be individualized. Such tests might include apoB, high-sensitivity CRP, fibrinogen, uric acid, urinary microalbumin, and liver function tests. A sleep study should be performed if symptoms of OSA are present. If PCOS is suspected on the basis of clinical features and anovulation, testosterone, luteinizing hormone, and follicle-stimulating hormone should be measured.

TREATMENT	The Metabolic Syndrome

LIFESTYLE (See also Chap. 58) Obesity is the driving force behind the metabolic syndrome. Thus, weight reduction is the primary approach to the disorder. With weight reduction, the improvement in insulin sensitivity is often accompanied by favorable modifications in many components of the metabolic syndrome. In general, recommendations for weight loss include a combination of caloric restriction, increased physical activity, and behavior modification. For weight reduction, caloric restriction is the most important component, whereas increases in physical activity are important for maintenance of weight loss. Some, but not all, evidence suggests that the addition of exercise to caloric restriction may promote relatively greater weight loss from the visceral depot. The tendency for weight regain after successful weight reduction underscores the need for long-lasting behavioral changes.

Diet Before prescribing a weight-loss diet, it is important to emphasize that it takes a long time for a patient to achieve an expanded fat mass; thus, the correction need not occur quickly. On the basis of ~3500 kcal = 1 lb of fat, ~500 kcal restriction daily equates to weight reduction of 1 lb per week. Diets restricted in carbohydrate typically provide a rapid initial weight loss.

However, after 1 year, the amount of weight reduction is usually unchanged. Thus, adherence to the diet is more important than which diet is chosen. Moreover, there is concern about diets enriched in saturated fat, particularly for patients at risk for CVD. Therefore, a high-quality diet—i.e., enriched in fruits, vegetables, whole grains, lean poultry, and fish—should be encouraged to provide the maximum overall health benefit.

Physical Activity Before a physical activity recommendation is provided to patients with the metabolic syndrome, it is important to ensure that the increased activity does not incur risk. Some high-risk patients should undergo formal cardiovascular evaluation before initiating an exercise program. For an inactive participant, gradual increases in physical activity should be encouraged to enhance adherence and avoid injury. Although increases in physical activity can lead to modest weight reduction, 60–90 min of daily activity is required to achieve this goal. Even if an overweight or obese adult is unable to achieve this level of activity, he or she will still derive a significant health benefit from at least 30 min of moderate-intensity daily activity. The caloric value of 30 min of a variety of activities can be found at *http://www.americanheart.org/presenter.jhtml?identifier=3040364*. Of note, a variety of routine activities, such as gardening, walking, and housecleaning, require moderate caloric expenditure. Thus, physical activity need not be defined solely in terms of formal exercise such as jogging, swimming, or tennis.

Obesity (See also Chap. 58) In some patients with the metabolic syndrome, treatment options need to extend beyond lifestyle intervention. Weight-loss drugs come in two major classes: appetite suppressants and absorption inhibitors. Appetite suppressants approved by the U.S. Food and Drug Administration include phentermine (for short-term use only, 3 months) and sibutramine. Orlistat inhibits fat absorption by ~30% and is moderately effective compared to placebo (~5% weight loss). Orlistat has been shown to reduce the incidence of type 2 diabetes, an effect that was especially evident in patients with baseline IGT.

Bariatric surgery is an option for patients with the metabolic syndrome who have a body mass index (BMI) >40 kg/m^2 or >35 kg/m^2 with comorbidities. Gastric bypass results in a dramatic weight reduction and improvement in the features of metabolic syndrome. A survival benefit has also been realized.

LDL CHOLESTEROL The rationale for the NCEP:ATPIII panel to develop criteria for the metabolic syndrome was to go beyond LDL cholesterol in identifying and reducing risk for CVD. The working assumption by the panel was that LDL cholesterol goals had already been achieved, and increasing evidence supports a linear reduction in CVD events with progressive lowering of LDL cholesterol. For patients with the metabolic syndrome and diabetes, LDL cholesterol should be reduced to <100 mg/dL and perhaps further in patients with a history of CVD events. For patients with the metabolic syndrome without diabetes, the Framingham risk score may predict a 10-year CVD risk that exceeds 20%. In these subjects, LDL cholesterol should also be reduced to <100 mg/dL. With a 10-year risk of <20%, however, the targeted LDL cholesterol goal is <130 mg/dL.

Diets restricted in saturated fats (<7% of calories), *trans*-fats (as few as possible), and cholesterol (<200 mg daily) should be applied aggressively. If LDL cholesterol remains above goal, pharmacologic intervention is needed. Statins (HMG-CoA reductase inhibitors), which produce a 20–60% lowering of LDL cholesterol, are generally the first choice for medication intervention. Of note, for each doubling of the statin dose, there is only ~6% additional lowering of LDL cholesterol. Side effects are rare and include an increase in hepatic transaminases and/or myopathy. The cholesterol absorption inhibitor ezetimibe is well tolerated and should be the second choice. Ezetimibe typically reduces LDL cholesterol by 15–20%. The bile acid sequestrants cholestyramine and colestipol are more effective than ezetimibe but must be used with caution in patients with the metabolic syndrome because they can increase triglycerides. In general, bile sequestrants should not be administered when fasting triglycerides are >200 mg/dL. Side effects include gastrointestinal symptoms (palatability, bloating, belching, constipation, anal irritation). Nicotinic acid has modest LDL cholesterol–lowering capabilities (<20%). Fibrates are best employed to lower LDL cholesterol when both LDL cholesterol and triglycerides are elevated. Fenofibrate may be more effective than gemfibrozil in this group.

TRIGLYCERIDES The NCEP:ATPIII has focused on non-HDL cholesterol rather than triglycerides. However, a fasting triglyceride value of <150 mg/dL is recommended. In general, the response of fasting triglycerides relates to the amount of weight reduction achieved. A weight reduction of >10% is necessary to lower fasting triglycerides.

A fibrate (gemfibrozil or fenofibrate) is the drug of choice to lower fasting triglycerides and typically achieve a 35–50% reduction. Concomitant administration with drugs metabolized by the 3A4 cytochrome P450 system (including some statins) greatly increases the risk of myopathy. In these cases, fenofibrate may be preferable to gemfibrozil. In the Veterans Affairs HDL Intervention Trial (VA-HIT), gemfibrozil was administered to men with known CHD and levels of HDL cholesterol <40 mg/dL. A coronary disease event and mortality rate benefit was experienced predominantly in men with hyperinsulinemia and/or diabetes, many of whom retrospectively were identified as having the metabolic syndrome. Of note, the amount of triglyceride lowering in the VA-HIT did not predict benefit. Although levels of LDL cholesterol did not change, a decrease in LDL particle number correlated with benefit. Although several additional clinical trials have been performed, they have not shown clear evidence that fibrates reduce CVD risk as a consequence of triglyceride lowering.

Other drugs that lower triglycerides include statins, nicotinic acid, and high doses of omega-3 fatty acids. In choosing a statin for this purpose, the dose must be high for the "less potent" statins (lovastatin, pravastatin, fluvastatin) or intermediate for the "more potent" statins (simvastatin, atorvastatin, rosuvastatin). The effect of nicotinic acid on fasting triglycerides is dose-related and less than that of fibrates (~20–40%). In patients with the metabolic syndrome and diabetes, nicotinic acid may increase fasting glucose. Omega-3 fatty acid preparations that include high doses of docosahexaenoic acid and eicosapentaenoic acid (~3.0–4.5 g daily) lower fasting triglycerides by ~40%. No interactions with fibrates or statins occur, and the main side effect is eructation with a fishy taste. This can be partially blocked by ingestion of the nutraceutical after freezing. Clinical trials of nicotinic acid or high-dose omega-3 fatty acids in patients with the metabolic syndrome have not been reported.

HDL CHOLESTEROL Beyond weight reduction, there are very few lipid-modifying compounds that increase HDL cholesterol. Statins, fibrates, and bile acid sequestrants have modest effects (5–10%), and there is no effect on HDL cholesterol with ezetimibe or omega-3 fatty acids. Nicotinic acid is the only currently available drug with predictable HDL cholesterol-raising properties. The response is dose-related and can increase HDL cholesterol ~30% above baseline. There is limited evidence at present that raising HDL has a benefit on CVD events independent of lowering LDL cholesterol, particularly in patients with the metabolic syndrome.

BLOOD PRESSURE The direct relationship between blood pressure and all-cause mortality rate has been well established, including patients with hypertension (>140/90) versus prehypertension (>120/80 but <140/90) versus individuals with normal blood pressure (<120/80). In patients with the metabolic syndrome without diabetes, the best choice for the first antihypertensive should usually be an angiotensin-converting enzyme (ACE) inhibitor or an angiotensin II receptor blocker, as these two classes of drugs appear to reduce the incidence of new-onset type 2 diabetes. In all patients with hypertension, a sodium-restricted diet enriched in fruits and vegetables and low-fat dairy products should be advocated. Home monitoring of blood pressure may assist in maintaining good blood pressure control.

IMPAIRED FASTING GLUCOSE In patients with the metabolic syndrome and type 2 diabetes, aggressive glycemic control may favorably modify fasting triglycerides and/or HDL cholesterol. In patients with IFG without a diagnosis of diabetes, a lifestyle intervention that includes weight reduction, dietary fat restriction, and increased physical activity has been shown to reduce the incidence of type 2 diabetes. Metformin has also been shown to reduce the incidence of diabetes, although the effect was less than that seen with lifestyle intervention.

INSULIN RESISTANCE Several drug classes (biguanides, thiazolidinediones [TZDs]) increase insulin sensitivity. Because insulin resistance is the primary pathophysiologic mechanism for the metabolic syndrome, representative drugs in these classes reduce its prevalence. Both metformin and TZDs enhance insulin action in the liver and suppress endogenous glucose production. TZDs, but not metformin, also improve insulin-mediated glucose uptake in muscle and adipose tissue. Benefits of both drugs have also been seen in patients with NAFLD and PCOS, and the drugs have been shown to reduce markers of inflammation and small dense LDL.

CHAPTER 60 The Metabolic Syndrome

APPENDIX

LABORATORY VALUES OF CLINICAL IMPORTANCE

Alexander Kratz ■ Michael A. Pesce ■ Robert C. Basner ■ Andrew J. Einstein

This Appendix contains tables of reference values for laboratory tests, special analytes, and special function tests. A variety of factors can influence reference values. Such variables include the population studied, the duration and means of specimen transport, laboratory methods and instrumentation, and even the type of container used for the collection of the specimen. The reference or "normal" ranges given in this appendix may therefore not be appropriate for all laboratories, and these values should only be used as general guidelines. Whenever possible, reference values provided by the laboratory performing the testing should be utilized in the interpretation of laboratory data. Values supplied in this Appendix reflect typical reference ranges in adults. Pediatric reference ranges may vary significantly from adult values.

In preparing the Appendix, the authors have taken into account the fact that the system of international units (SI, système international d'unités) is used in most countries and in some medical journals. However, clinical laboratories may continue to report values in "traditional" or conventional units. Therefore, both systems are provided in the Appendix. The dual system is also used in the text except for (1) those instances in which the numbers remain the same but only the terminology is changed (mmol/L for meq/L or IU/L for mIU/mL), when only the SI units are given; and (2) most pressure measurements (e.g., blood and cerebrospinal fluid pressures), when the traditional units (mmHg, mmH$_2$O) are used. In all other instances in the text the SI unit is followed by the traditional unit in parentheses.

REFERENCE VALUES FOR LABORATORY TESTS

TABLE 1

HEMATOLOGY AND COAGULATION

ANALYTE	SPECIMEN	SI UNITS	CONVENTIONAL UNITS
Activated clotting time	WB	70–180 s	70–180 s
Activated protein C resistance (factor V Leiden)	P	Not applicable	Ratio >2.1
ADAMTS13 activity	P	≥0.67	≥67%
ADAMTS13 inhibitor activity	P	Not applicable	≤0.4 U
ADAMTS13 antibody	P	Not applicable	≤18 U
Alpha$_2$ antiplasmin	P	0.87–1.55	87–155%
Antiphospholipid antibody panel			
PTT-LA (lupus anticoagulant screen)	P	Negative	Negative
Platelet neutralization procedure	P	Negative	Negative
Dilute viper venom screen	P	Negative	Negative
Anticardiolipin antibody	S		
IgG		0–15 arbitrary units	0–15 GPL
IgM		0–15 arbitrary units	0–15 MPL

(continued)

TABLE 1

HEMATOLOGY AND COAGULATION (*CONTINUED*)

ANALYTE	SPECIMEN	SI UNITS	CONVENTIONAL UNITS
Antithrombin III	P		
Antigenic		220–390 mg/L	22–39 mg/dL
Functional		0.7–1.30 U/L	70–130%
Anti-Xa assay (heparin assay)	P		
Unfractionated heparin		0.3–0.7 kIU/L	0.3–0.7 IU/mL
Low-molecular-weight heparin		0.5–1.0 kIU/L	0.5–1.0 IU/mL
Danaparoid (Orgaran)		0.5–0.8 kIU/L	0.5–0.8 IU/mL
Autohemolysis test	WB	0.004–0.045	0.4–4.50%
Autohemolysis test with glucose	WB	0.003–0.007	0.3–0.7%
Bleeding time (adult)		<7.1 min	<7.1 min
Bone marrow: See Table 7			
Clot retraction	WB	0.50–1.00/2 h	50–100%/2 h
Cryofibrinogen	P	Negative	Negative
D-dimer	P	220–740 ng/mL FEU	220–740 ng/mL FEU
Differential blood count	WB		
Relative counts:			
Neutrophils		0.40–0.70	40–70%
Bands		0.0–0.05	0–5%
Lymphocytes		0.20–0.50	20–50%
Monocytes		0.04–0.08	4–8%
Eosinophils		0.0–0.6	0–6%
Basophils		0.0–0.02	0–2%
Absolute counts:			
Neutrophils		$1.42–6.34 \times 10^9$/L	1420–6340/mm^3
Bands		$0–0.45 \times 10^9$/L	0–450/mm^3
Lymphocytes		$0.71–4.53 \times 10^9$/L	710–4530/mm^3
Monocytes		$0.14–0.72 \times 10^9$/L	140–720/mm^3
Eosinophils		$0–0.54 \times 10^9$/L	0–540/mm^3
Basophils		$0–0.18 \times 10^9$/L	0–180/mm^3
Erythrocyte count	WB		
Adult males		$4.30–5.60 \times 10^{12}$/L	$4.30–5.60 \times 10^6$/mm^3
Adult females		$4.00–5.20 \times 10^{12}$/L	$4.00–5.20 \times 10^6$/mm^3
Erythrocyte life span	WB		
Normal survival		120 days	120 days
Chromium labeled, half-life ($t_{1/2}$)		25–35 days	25–35 days
Erythrocyte sedimentation rate	WB		
Females		0–20 mm/h	0–20 mm/h
Males		0–15 mm/h	0–15 mm/h
Euglobulin lysis time	P	7200–14400 s	120–240 min
Factor II, prothrombin	P	0.50–1.50	50–150%
Factor V	P	0.50–1.50	50–150%
Factor VII	P	0.50–1.50	50–150%
Factor VIII	P	0.50–1.50	50–150%
Factor IX	P	0.50–1.50	50–150%
Factor X	P	0.50–1.50	50–150%
Factor XI	P	0.50–1.50	50–150%
Factor XII	P	0.50–1.50	50–150 %
Factor XIII screen	P	Not applicable	Present
Factor inhibitor assay	P	<0.5 Bethesda Units	<0.5 Bethesda Units
Fibrin(ogen) degradation products	P	0–1 mg/L	0–1 μg/mL
Fibrinogen	P	2.33–4.96 g/L	233–496 mg/dL
Glucose-6-phosphate dehydrogenase (erythrocyte)	WB	<2400 s	<40 min
Ham's test (acid serum)	WB	Negative	Negative

(continued)

TABLE 1

66

HEMATOLOGY AND COAGULATION (*CONTINUED*)

ANALYTE	SPECIMEN	SI UNITS	CONVENTIONAL UNITS
Hematocrit	WB		
Adult males		0.388–0.464	38.8–46.4
Adult females		0.354–0.444	35.4–44.4
Hemoglobin			
Plasma	P	6–50 mg/L	0.6–5.0 mg/dL
Whole blood:	WB		
Adult males		133–162 g/L	13.3–16.2 g/dL
Adult females		120–158 g/L	12.0–15.8 g/dL
Hemoglobin electrophoresis	WB		
Hemoglobin A		0.95–0.98	95–98%
Hemoglobin A$_2$		0.015–0.031	1.5–3.1%
Hemoglobin F		0–0.02	0–2.0%
Hemoglobins other than A, A$_2$, or F		Absent	Absent
Heparin-induced thrombocytopenia antibody	P	Negative	Negative
Immature platelet fraction (IPF)	WB	0.011–0.061	1.1–6.1%
Joint fluid crystal	JF	Not applicable	No crystals seen
Joint fluid mucin	JF	Not applicable	Only type I mucin present
Leukocytes			
Alkaline phosphatase (LAP)	WB	0.2–1.6 μkat/L	13–100 μ/L
Count (WBC)	WB	3.54–9.06 × 10^9/L	3.54–9.06 × 10^3/mm^3
Mean corpuscular hemoglobin (MCH)	WB	26.7–31.9 pg/cell	26.7–31.9 pg/cell
Mean corpuscular hemoglobin concentration (MCHC)	WB	323–359 g/L	32.3–35.9 g/dL
Mean corpuscular hemoglobin of reticulocytes (CH)	WB	24–36 pg	24–36 pg
Mean corpuscular volume (MCV)	WB	79–93.3 fL	79–93.3 μm^3
Mean platelet volume (MPV)	WB	9.00–12.95 fL	9.00–12.95
Osmotic fragility of erythrocytes	WB		
Direct		0.0035–0.0045	0.35–0.45%
Indirect		0.0030–0.0065	0.30–0.65%
Partial thromboplastin time, activated	P	26.3–39.4 s	26.3–39.4 s
Plasminogen	P		
Antigen		84–140 mg/L	8.4–14.0 mg/dL
Functional		0.70–1.30	70–130%
Plasminogen activator inhibitor 1	P	4–43 μg/L	4–43 ng/mL
Platelet aggregation	PRP	Not applicable	>65% aggregation in response to adenosine diphosphate, epinephrine, collagen, ristocetin, and arachidonic acid
Platelet count	WB	165–415 × 10^9/L	165–415 × 10^3/mm^3
Platelet, mean volume	WB	6.4–11 fL	6.4–11.0 μm^3
Prekallikrein assay	P	0.50–1.5	50–150%
Prekallikrein screen	P		No deficiency detected
Protein C	P		
Total antigen		0.70–1.40	70–140%
Functional		0.70–1.30	70–130%
Protein S	P		
Total antigen		0.70–1.40	70–140%
Functional		0.65–1.40	65–140%
Free antigen		0.70–1.40	70–140%
Prothrombin gene mutation G20210A	WB	Not applicable	Not present
Prothrombin time	P	12.7–15.4 s	12.7–15.4 s

(continued)

TABLE 1

HEMATOLOGY AND COAGULATION (*CONTINUED*)			
ANALYTE	SPECIMEN	SI UNITS	CONVENTIONAL UNITS
Protoporphyrin, free erythrocyte	WB	0.28–0.64 μmol/L of red blood cells	16–36 μg/dL of red blood cells
Red cell distribution width	WB	<0.145	<14.5%
Reptilase time	P	16–23.6 s	16–23.6 s
Reticulocyte count	WB		
Adult males		0.008–0.023 red cells	0.8–2.3% red cells
Adult females		0.008–0.020 red cells	0.8–2.0% red cells
Reticulocyte hemoglobin content	WB	>26 pg/cell	>26 pg/cell
Ristocetin cofactor (functional von Willebrand factor)	P		
Blood group O		0.75 mean of normal	75% mean of normal
Blood group A		1.05 mean of normal	105% mean of normal
Blood group B		1.15 mean of normal	115% mean of normal
Blood group AB		1.25 mean of normal	125% mean of normal
Serotonin release assay	S	<0.2 release	<20% release
Sickle cell test	WB	Negative	Negative
Sucrose hemolysis	WB	<0.1	<10% hemolysis
Thrombin time	P	15.3–18.5 s	15.3–18.5 s
Total eosinophils	WB	$150–300 \times 10^6$/L	150–300/mm^3
Transferrin receptor	S, P	9.6–29.6 nmol/L	9.6–29.6 nmol/L
Viscosity			
Plasma	P	1.7–2.1	1.7–2.1
Serum	S	1.4–1.8	1.4–1.8
von Willebrand factor (vWF) antigen (factor VIII:R antigen)			
Blood group O		0.75 mean of normal	75% mean of normal
Blood group A		1.05 mean of normal	105% mean of normal
Blood group B		1.15 mean of normal	115% mean of normal
Blood group AB		1.25 mean of normal	125% mean of normal
von Willebrand factor multimers	P	Normal distribution	Normal distribution
White blood cells: see "Leukocytes"			

Abbreviations: JF, joint fluid; P, plasma; PRP, platelet-rich plasma; S, serum; WB, whole blood.

TABLE 2

CLINICAL CHEMISTRY AND IMMUNOLOGY			
ANALYTE	SPECIMEN	SI UNITS	CONVENTIONAL UNITS
Acetoacetate	P	49–294 μmol/L	0.5–3.0 mg/dL
Adrenocorticotropin (ACTH)	P	1.3–16.7 pmol/L	6.0–76.0 pg/mL
Alanine aminotransferase (ALT, SGPT)	S	0.12–0.70 μkat/L	7–41 U/L
Albumin	S	40–50 g/L	4.0–5.0 mg/dL
Aldolase	S	26–138 nkat/L	1.5–8.1 U/L
Aldosterone (adult)			
Supine, normal sodium diet	S, P	<443 pmol/L	<16 ng/dL
Upright, normal	S, P	111–858 pmol/L	4–31 ng/dL
Alpha fetoprotein (adult)	S	0–8.5 μg/L	0–8.5 ng/mL
Alpha$_1$ antitrypsin	S	1.0–2.0 g/L	100–200 mg/dL
Ammonia, as NH$_3$	P	11–35 μmol/L	19–60 μg/dL
Amylase (method dependent)	S	0.34–1.6 μkat/L	20–96 U/L

(continued)

TABLE 2

CLINICAL CHEMISTRY AND IMMUNOLOGY (CONTINUED)

ANALYTE	SPECIMEN	SI UNITS	CONVENTIONAL UNITS
Androstendione (adult)	S		
Males		0.81–3.1 nmol/L	23–89 ng/dL
Females			
Premenopausal		0.91–7.5 nmol/L	26–214 ng/dL
Postmenopausal		0.46–2.9 nmol/L	13–82 ng/dL
Angiotensin-converting enzyme (ACE)	S	0.15–1.1 μkat/L	9–67 U/L
Anion gap	S	7–16 mmol/L	7–16 mmol/L
Apolipoprotein A-1	S		
Male		0.94–1.78 g/L	94–178 mg/dL
Female		1.01–1.99 g/L	101–199 mg/dL
Apolipoprotein B	S		
Male		0.55–1.40 g/L	55–140 mg/dL
Female		0.55–1.25 g/L	55–125 mg/dL
Arterial blood gases	WB		
[HCO_3^-]		22–30 mmol/L	22–30 meq/L
P_{CO_2}		4.3–6.0 kPa	32–45 mmHg
pH		7.35–7.45	7.35–7.45
P_{O_2}		9.6–13.8 kPa	72–104 mmHg
Aspartate aminotransferase (AST, SGOT)	S	0.20–0.65 μkat/L	12–38 U/L
Autoantibodies	S		
Anti-centromere antibody IgG		≤29 AU/mL	≤29 AU/mL
Anti-double-strand (native) DNA		<25 IU/L	<25 IU/L
Anti-glomerular basement membrane antibodies			
Qualitative IgG, IgA		Negative	Negative
Quantitative IgG antibody		≤19 AU/mL	≤19 AU/mL
Anti-histone antibodies		<1.0 U	<1.0 U
Anti-Jo-1 antibody		≤29 AU/mL	≤29 AU/mL
Anti-mitochondrial antibody		Not applicable	<20 Units
Anti-neutrophil cytoplasmic autoantibodies		Not applicable	<1:20
Serine proteinase 3 antibodies		≤19 AU/mL	≤19 AU/mL
Myeloperoxidase antibodies		≤19 AU/mL	≤19 AU/mL
Antinuclear antibody		Not applicable	Negative at 1:40
Anti-parietal cell antibody		Not applicable	None detected
Anti-RNP antibody		Not applicable	<1.0 U
Anti-Scl 70 antibody		Not applicable	<1.0 U
Anti-Smith antibody		Not applicable	<1.0 U
Anti–smooth muscle antibody		Not applicable	<1.0 U
Anti-SSA antibody		Not applicable	<1.0 U
Anti-SSB antibody		Not applicable	Negative
Anti-thyroglobulin antibody		<40 kIU/L	<40 IU/mL
Anti-thyroid peroxidase antibody		<35 kIU/L	<35 IU/mL
B-type natriuretic peptide (BNP)	P	Age and gender specific: <100 ng/L	Age and gender specific: <100 pg/mL
Bence Jones protein, serum qualitative	S	Not applicable	None detected
Bence Jones protein, serum quantitative	S		
Free kappa		3.3–19.4 mg/L	0.33–1.94 mg/dL
Free lambda		5.7–26.3 mg/L	0.57–2.63 mg/dL
K/L ratio		0.26–1.65	0.26–1.65
Beta-2-microglobulin	S	1.1–2.4 mg/L	1.1–2.4 mg/L
Bilirubin	S		
Total		5.1–22 μmol/L	0.3–1.3 mg/dL
Direct		1.7–6.8 μmol/L	0.1–0.4 mg/dL
Indirect		3.4–15.2 μmol/L	0.2–0.9 mg/dL

(continued)

TABLE 2

CLINICAL CHEMISTRY AND IMMUNOLOGY (*CONTINUED*)

ANALYTE	SPECIMEN	SI UNITS	CONVENTIONAL UNITS
C peptide	S	0.27–1.19 nmol/L	0.8–3.5 ng/mL
C1-esterase-inhibitor protein	S	210–390 mg/L	21–39 mg/dL
CA 125	S	<35 kU/L	<35 U/mL
CA 19-9	S	<37 kU/L	<37 U/mL
CA 15-3	S	<33 kU/L	<33 U/mL
CA 27-29	S	0–40 kU/L	0–40 U/mL
Calcitonin	S		
Male		0–7.5 ng/L	0–7.5 pg/mL
Female		0–5.1 ng/L	0–5.1 pg/mL
Calcium	S	2.2–2.6 mmol/L	8.7–10.2 mg/dL
Calcium, ionized	WB	1.12–1.32 mmol/L	4.5–5.3 mg/dL
Carbon dioxide content (TCO$_2$)	P (sea level)	22–30 mmol/L	22–30 meq/L
Carboxyhemoglobin (carbon monoxide content)	WB		
Nonsmokers		0.0–0.015	0–1.5%
Smokers		0.04–0.09	4–9%
Loss of consciousness and death		>0.50	>50%
Carcinoembryonic antigen (CEA)	S		
Nonsmokers		0.0–3.0 μg/L	0.0–3.0 ng/mL
Smokers		0.0–5.0 μg/L	0.0–5.0 ng/mL
Ceruloplasmin	S	250–630 mg/L	25–63 mg/dL
Chloride	S	102–109 mmol/L	102–109 meq/L
Cholesterol: see Table 5			
Cholinesterase	S	5–12 kU/L	5–12 U/mL
Chromogranin A	S	0–50 μg/L	0–50 ng/mL
Complement	S		
C3		0.83–1.77 g/L	83–177 mg/dL
C4		0.16–0.47 g/L	16–47 mg/dL
Complement total		60–144 CAE units	60–144 CAE units
Cortisol			
Fasting, 8 A.M.–12 noon	S	138–690 nmol/L	5–25 μg/dL
12 noon–8 P.M.		138–414 nmol/L	5–15 μg/dL
8 P.M.–8 A.M.		0–276 nmol/L	0–10 μg/dL
C-reactive protein	S	<10 mg/L	<10 mg/L

C-reactive protein, high sensitivity	S	Cardiac risk
		  Low: <1.0 mg/L
		  Average: 1.0–3.0 mg/L
		  High: >3.0 mg/L
			Cardiac risk
			  Low: <1.0 mg/L
			  Average: 1.0–3.0 mg/L
			  High: >3.0 mg/L

Creatine kinase (total)	S		
Females		0.66–4.0 μkat/L	39–238 U/L
Males		0.87–5.0 μkat/L	51–294 U/L
Creatine kinase-MB	S		
Mass		0.0–5.5 μg/L	0.0–5.5 ng/mL
Fraction of total activity (by electrophoresis)		0–0.04	0–4.0%
Creatinine	S		
Female		44–80 μmol/L	0.5–0.9 mg/dL
Male		53–106 μmol/L	0.6–1.2 mg/dL
Cryoglobulins	S	Not applicable	None detected
Cystatin C	S	0.5–1.0 mg/L	0.5–1.0 mg/L

(continued)

TABLE 2

CLINICAL CHEMISTRY AND IMMUNOLOGY (*CONTINUED*)

ANALYTE	SPECIMEN	SI UNITS	CONVENTIONAL UNITS
Dehydroepiandrosterone (DHEA) (adult)			
Male	S	6.2–43.4 nmol/L	180–1250 ng/dL
Female		4.5–34.0 nmol/L	130–980 ng/dL
Dehydroepiandrosterone (DHEA) sulfate	S		
Male (adult)		100–6190 µg/L	10–619 µg/dL
Female (adult, premenopausal)		120–5350 µg/L	12–535 µg/dL
Female (adult, postmenopausal)		300–2600 µg/L	30–260 µg/dL
11-Deoxycortisol (adult) (compound S)	S	0.34–4.56 nmol/L	12–158 ng/dL
Dihydrotestosterone			
Male	S, P	1.03–2.92 nmol/L	30–85 ng/dL
Female		0.14–0.76 nmol/L	4–22 ng/dL
Dopamine	P	0–130 pmol/L	0–20 pg/mL
Epinephrine	P		
Supine (30 min)		<273 pmol/L	<50 pg/mL
Sitting		<328 pmol/L	<60 pg/mL
Standing (30 min)		<491 pmol/L	<90 pg/mL
Erythropoietin	S	4–27 U/L	4–27 U/L
Estradiol	S, P		
Female			
Menstruating:			
Follicular phase		74–532 pmol/L	<20–145 pg/mL
Midcycle peak		411–1626 pmol/L	112–443 pg/mL
Luteal phase		74–885 pmol/L	<20–241 pg/mL
Postmenopausal		217 pmol/L	<59 pg/mL
Male		74 pmol/L	<20 pg/mL
Estrone	S, P		
Female			
Menstruating:			
Follicular phase		<555 pmol/L	<150 pg/mL
Luteal phase		<740 pmol/L	<200 pg/mL
Postmenopausal		11–118 pmol/L	3–32 pg/mL
Male		33–133 pmol/L	9–36 pg/mL
Fatty acids, free (nonesterified)	P	0.1–0.6 mmol/L	2.8–16.8 mg/dL
Ferritin	S		
Female		10–150 µg/L	10–150 ng/mL
Male		29–248 µg/L	29–248 ng/mL
Follicle-stimulating hormone (FSH)	S, P		
Female			
Menstruating			
Follicular phase		3.0–20.0 IU/L	3.0–20.0 mIU/mL
Ovulatory phase		9.0–26.0 IU/L	9.0–26.0 mIU/mL
Luteal phase		1.0–12.0 IU/L	1.0–12.0 mIU/mL
Postmenopausal		18.0–153.0 IU/L	18.0–153.0 mIU/mL
Male		1.0–12.0 IU/L	1.0–12.0 mIU/mL
Fructosamine	S	<285 umol/L	<285 umol/L
Gamma glutamyltransferase	S	0.15–0.99 µkat/L	9–58 U/L
Gastrin	S	<100 ng/L	<100 pg/mL
Glucagon	P	40–130 ng/L	40–130 pg/mL

(continued)

66.

APPENDIX Laboratory Values of Clinical Importance

TABLE 2

CLINICAL CHEMISTRY AND IMMUNOLOGY (*CONTINUED*)

ANALYTE	SPECIMEN	SI UNITS	CONVENTIONAL UNITS
Glucose	WB	3.6–5.3 mmol/L	65–95 mg/dL
Glucose (fasting)	P		
Normal		4.2–5.6 mmol/L	75–100 mg/dL
Increased risk for diabetes		5.6–6.9 mmol/L	100–125 mg/dL
Diabetes mellitus		Fasting >7.0 mmol/L	Fasting >126 mg/dL
		A 2-hour level of >11.1 mmol/L during an oral glucose tolerance test	A 2-hour level of ≥200 mg/dL during an oral glucose tolerance test
		A random glucose level of ≥11.1 mmol/L in patients with symptoms of hyper-glycemia	A random glucose level of ≥200 mg/dL in patients with symptoms of hyperglycemia
Growth hormone	S	0–5 μg/L	0–5 ng/mL
Hemoglobin A_{1c}	WB	0.04–0.06 HgB fraction	4.0–5.6%
Pre-diabetes		0.057–0.064 HgB fraction	5.7–6.4%
Diabetes mellitus		A hemoglobin A_{1c} level of ≥0.065 Hgb fraction as suggested by the American Diabetes Association	A hemoglobin A_{1c} level of ≥6.5% as suggested by the American Diabetes Association
Hemoglobin A_{1c} with estimated average glucose (eAg)	WB	eAg (mmoL/L) = 1.59 × HbA$_{1c}$ − 2.59	eAg (mg/dL) = 28.7 × HbA$_{1c}$ − 46.7
High-density lipoprotein (HDL) (see Table 5)			
Homocysteine	P	4.4–10.8 μmol/L	4.4–10.8 μmol/L
Human chorionic gonadotropin (HCG)	S		
Nonpregnant female		<5 IU/L	<5 mIU/mL
1–2 weeks postconception		9–130 IU/L	9–130 mIU/mL
2–3 weeks postconception		75–2600 IU/L	75–2600 mIU/mL
3–4 weeks postconception		850–20,800 IU/L	850–20,800 mIU/mL
4–5 weeks postconception		4000–100,200 IU/L	4000–100,200 mIU/mL
5–10 weeks postconception		11,500–289,000 IU/L	11,500–289,000 mIU/mL
10–14 weeks post conception		18,300–137,000 IU/L	18,300–137,000 mIU/mL
Second trimester		1400–53,000 IU/L	1400–53,000 mIU/mL
Third trimester		940–60,000 IU/L	940–60,000 mIU/mL
β-Hydroxybutyrate	P	60–170 μmol/L	0.6–1.8 mg/dL
17-Hydroxyprogesterone (adult)	S		
Male		<4.17 nmol/L	<139 ng/dL
Female			
Follicular phase		0.45–2.1 nmol/L	15–70 ng/dL
Luteal phase		1.05–8.7 nmol/L	35–290 ng/dL
Immunofixation	S	Not applicable	No bands detected
Immunoglobulin, quantitation (adult)			
IgA	S	0.70–3.50 g/L	70–350 mg/dL
IgD	S	0–140 mg/L	0–14 mg/dL
IgE	S	1–87 kIU/L	1–87 IU/mL
IgG	S	7.0–17.0 g/L	700–1700 mg/dL
IgG_1	S	2.7–17.4 g/L	270–1740 mg/dL
IgG_2	S	0.3–6.3 g/L	30–630 mg/dL
IgG_3	S	0.13–3.2 g/L	13–320 mg/dL
IgG_4	S	0.11–6.2 g/L	11–620 mg/dL
IgM	S	0.50–3.0 g/L	50–300 mg/dL
Insulin	S, P	14.35–143.5 pmol/L	2–20 μU/mL
Iron	S	7–25 μmol/L	41–141 μg/dL

(continued)

TABLE 2

CLINICAL CHEMISTRY AND IMMUNOLOGY (*CONTINUED*)

ANALYTE	SPECIMEN	SI UNITS	CONVENTIONAL UNITS
66–70 years		69–200 µg/L	69–200 ng/mL
71–75 years		64–188 µg/L	64–188 ng/mL
76–80 years		59–177 µg/L	59–177 ng/mL
81–85 years		55–166 µg/L	55–166 ng/mL
Somatostatin	P	<25 ng/L	<25 pg/mL
Testosterone, free			
Female, adult	S	10.4–65.9 pmol/L	3–19 pg/mL
Male, adult		312–1041 pmol/L	90–300 pg/mL
Testosterone, total,	S		
Female		0.21–2.98 nmol/L	6–86 ng/dL
Male		9.36–37.10 nmol/L	270–1070 ng/dL
Thyroglobulin	S	1.3–31.8 µg/L	1.3–31.8 ng/mL
Thyroid-binding globulin	S	13–30 mg/L	1.3–3.0 mg/dL
Thyroid-stimulating hormone	S	0.34–4.25 mIU/L	0.34–4.25 µIU/mL
Thyroxine, free (fT4)	S	9.0–16 pmol/L	0.7–1.24 ng/dL
Thyroxine, total (T4)	S	70–151 nmol/L	5.4–11.7 µg/dL
Thyroxine index (free)	S	6.7–10.9	6.7–10.9
Transferrin	S	2.0–4.0 g/L	200–400 mg/dL
Triglycerides (see Table 5)	S	0.34–2.26 mmol/L	30–200 mg/dL
Triiodothyronine, free (fT3)	S	3.7–6.5 pmol/L	2.4–4.2 pg/mL
Triiodothyronine, total (T3)	S	1.2–2.1 nmol/L	77–135 ng/dL
Troponin I (method dependent)	S, P		
99th percentile of a healthy population		0–0.04 µg/L	0–0.04 ng/mL
Troponin T	S, P		
99th percentile of a healthy population		0–0.01 µg/L	0–0.01 ng/mL
Urea nitrogen	S	2.5–7.1 mmol/L	7–20 mg/dL
Uric acid	S		
Females		0.15–0.33 mmol/L	2.5–5.6 mg/dL
Males		0.18–0.41 mmol/L	3.1–7.0 mg/dL
Vasoactive intestinal polypeptide	P	0–60 ng/L	0–60 pg/mL
Zinc protoporphyrin	WB	0–400 µg/L	0–40 µg/dL
Zinc protoporphyrin (ZPP)-to-heme ratio	WB	0–69 µmol ZPP/mol heme	0–69 µmol ZPP/mol heme

Abbreviations: P, plasma; S, serum; WB, whole blood.

TABLE 3

TOXICOLOGY AND THERAPEUTIC DRUG MONITORING

DRUG	THERAPEUTIC RANGE		TOXIC LEVEL	
	SI UNITS	CONVENTIONAL UNITS	SI UNITS	CONVENTIONAL UNITS
Acetaminophen	66–199 μmol/L	10–30 μg/mL	>1320 μmol/L	>200 μg/mL
Amikacin				
Peak	34–51 μmol/L	20–30 μg/mL	>60 μmol/L	>35 μg/mL
Trough	0–17 μmol/L	0–10 μg/mL	>17 μmol/L	>10 μg/mL
Amitriptyline/nortriptyline (total drug)	430–900 nmol/L	120–250 ng/mL	>1800 nmol/L	>500 ng/mL
Amphetamine	150–220 nmol/L	20–30 ng/mL	>1500 nmol/L	>200 ng/mL
Bromide	9.4–18.7 mmol/L	75–150 mg/dL	>18.8 mmol/L	>150 mg/dL
Mild toxicity			6.4–18.8 mmol/L	51–150 mg/dL
Severe toxicity			>18.8 mmol/L	>150 mg/dL
Lethal			>37.5 mmol/L	>300 mg/dL
Caffeine	25.8–103 μmol/L	5–20 μg/mL	>206 μmol/L	>40 μg/mL
Carbamazepine	17–42 μmol/L	4–10 μg/mL	>85 μmol/L	>20 μg/mL
Chloramphenicol				
Peak	31–62 μmol/L	10–20 μg/mL	>77 μmol/L	>25 μg/mL
Trough	15–31 μmol/L	5–10 μg/mL	>46 μmol/L	>15 μg/mL
Chlordiazepoxide	1.7–10 μmol/L	0.5–3.0 μg/mL	>17μmol/L	>5.0 μg/mL
Clonazepam	32–240 nmol/L	10–75 ng/mL	>320 nmol/L	>100 ng/mL
Clozapine	0.6–2.1 μmol/L	200–700 ng/mL	>3.7 μmol/L	>1200 ng/mL
Cocaine			>3.3 μmol/L	>1.0 μg/mL
Codeine	43–110 nmol/mL	13–33 ng/mL	>3700 nmol/mL	>1100 ng/mL (lethal)
Cyclosporine				
Renal transplant				
0–6 months	208–312 nmol/L	250–375 ng/mL	>312 nmol/L	>375 ng/mL
6–12 months after transplant	166–250 nmol/L	200–300 ng/mL	>250 nmol/L	>300 ng/mL
>12 months	83–125 nmol/L	100–150 ng/mL	>125 nmol/L	>150 ng/mL
Cardiac transplant				
0–6 months	208–291 nmol/L	250–350 ng/mL	>291 nmol/L	>350 ng/mL
6–12 months after transplant	125–208 nmol/L	150–250 ng/mL	>208 nmol/L	>250 ng/mL
>12 months	83–125 nmol/L	100–150 ng/mL	>125 nmol/L	150 ng/mL
Lung transplant				
0–6 months	250–374 nmol/L	300–450 ng/mL	>374 nmol/L	>450 ng/mL
Liver transplant				
Initiation	208–291 nmol/L	250–350 ng/mL	>291 nmol/L	>350 ng/mL
Maintenance	83–166 nmol/L	100–200 ng/mL	>166 nmol/L	>200 ng/mL
Desipramine	375–1130 nmol/L	100–300 ng/mL	>1880 nmol/L	>500 ng/mL
Diazepam (and metabolite)				
Diazepam	0.7–3.5 μmol/L	0.2–1.0 μg/mL	>7.0 μmol/L	>2.0 μg/mL
Nordiazepam	0.4–6.6 μmol/L	0.1–1.8 μg/mL	>9.2 μmol/L	>2.5 μg/mL
Digoxin	0.64–2.6 nmol/L	0.5–2.0 ng/mL	>5.0 nmol/L	>3.9 ng/mL
Disopyramide	5.3–14.7 μmol/L	2–5 μg/mL	>20.6 μmol/L	>7 μg/mL
Doxepin and nordoxepin				
Doxepin	0.36–0.98 μmol/L	101–274 ng/mL	>1.8 μmol/L	>503 ng/mL
Nordoxepin	0.38–1.04 μmol/L	106–291 ng/mL	>1.9 μmol/L	>531 ng/mL
Ethanol				
Behavioral changes			>4.3 mmol/L	>20 mg/dL
Legal limit			≥17 mmol/L	≥80 mg/dL
Critical with acute exposure			>54 mmol/L	>250 mg/dL
Ethylene glycol				
Toxic			>2 mmol/L	>12 mg/dL
Lethal			>20 mmol/L	>120 mg/dL

(continued)

TABLE 3

TOXICOLOGY AND THERAPEUTIC DRUG MONITORING (*CONTINUED*)

DRUG	THERAPEUTIC RANGE		TOXIC LEVEL	
	SI UNITS	CONVENTIONAL UNITS	SI UNITS	CONVENTIONAL UNITS
Ethosuximide	280–700 μmol/L	40–100 μg/mL	>700 μmol/L	>100 μg/mL
Everolimus	3.13–8.35 nmol/L	3–8 ng/mL	>12.5 nmol/L	>12 ng/mL
Flecainide	0.5–2.4 μmol/L	0.2–1.0 μg/mL	>3.6 μmol/L	>1.5 μg/mL
Gentamicin				
Peak	10–21 μmol/mL	5–10 μg/mL	>25 μmol/mL	>12 μg/mL
Trough	0–4.2 μmol/mL	0–2 μg/mL	>4.2 μmol/mL	>2 μg/mL
Heroin (diacetyl morphine)			>700 μmol/L	>200 ng/mL (as morphine)
Ibuprofen	49–243 μmol/L	10–50 μg/mL	>970 μmol/L	>200 μg/mL
Imipramine (and metabolite)				
Desimipramine	375–1130 nmol/L	100–300 ng/mL	>1880 nmol/L	>500 ng/mL
Total imipramine + desimipramine	563–1130 nmol/L	150–300 ng/mL	>1880 nmol/L	>500 ng/mL
Lamotrigine	11.7–54.7 μmol/L	3–14 μg/mL	>58.7 μmol/L	>15 μg/mL
Lidocaine	5.1–21.3 μmol/L	1.2–5.0 μg/mL	>38.4 μmol/L	>9.0 μg/mL
Lithium	0.5–1.3 mmol/L	0.5–1.3 meq/L	>2 mmol/L	>2 meq/L
Methadone	1.0–3.2 μmol/L	0.3–1.0 μg/mL	>6.5 μmol/L	>2 μg/mL
Methamphetamine	0.07–0.34 μmol/L	0.01–0.05 μg/mL	>3.35 μmol/L	>0.5 μg/mL
Methanol			>6 mmol/L	>20 mg/dL
Methotrexate				
Low-dose	0.01–0.1 μmol/L	0.01–0.1 μmol/L	>0.1 mmol/L	>0.1 mmol/L
High-dose (24h)	<5.0 μmol/L	<5.0 μmol/L	>5.0 μmol/L	>5.0 μmol/L
High-dose (48h)	<0.50 μmol/L	<0.50 μmol/L	>0.5 μmol/L	>0.5 μmol/L
High-dose (72h)	<0.10 μmol/L	<0.10 μmol/L	>0.1 μmol/L	>0.1 μmol/L
Morphine	232–286 μmol/L	65–80 ng/mL	>720 μmol/L	>200 ng/mL
Mycophenolic acid	3.1–10.9 μmol/L	1.0–3.5 ng/mL	>37 μmol/L	>12 ng/mL
Nitroprusside (as thiocyanate)	103–499 μmol/L	6–29 μg/mL	860 μmol/L	>50 μg/mL
Nortriptyline	190–569 nmol/L	50–150 ng/mL	>1900 nmol/L	>500 ng/mL
Phenobarbital	65–172 μmol/L	15–40 μg/mL	>258 μmol/L	>60 μg/mL
Phenytoin	40–79 μmol/L	10–20 μg/mL	>158 μmol/L	>40 μg/mL
Phenytoin, free	4.0–7.9 μg/mL	1–2 μg/mL	>13.9 μg/mL	>3.5 μg/mL
% Free	0.08–0.14	8–14%		
Primidone and metabolite				
Primidone	23–55 μmol/L	5–12 μg/mL	>69 μmol/L	>15 μg/mL
Phenobarbital	65–172 μmol/L	15–40 μg/mL	>215 μmol/L	>50 μg/mL
Procainamide				
Procainamide	17–42 μmol/L	4–10 μg/mL	>43 μmol/L	>10 μg/mL
NAPA (*N*-acetylprocainamide)	22–72 μmol/L	6–20μg/mL	>126 μmol/L	>35 μg/mL
Quinidine	6.2–15.4 μmol/L	2.0–5.0 μg/mL	>19 μmol/L	>6 μg/mL
Salicylates	145–2100 μmol/L	2–29 mg/dL	>2900 μmol/L	>40 mg/dL
Sirolimus (trough level)				
Kidney transplant	4.4–15.4 nmol/L	4–14 ng/mL	>16 nmol/L	>15 ng/mL
Tacrolimus (FK506) (trough)				
Kidney and liver				
Initiation	12–19 nmol/L	10–15 ng/mL	>25 nmol/L	>20 ng/mL
Maintenance	6–12 nmol/L	5–10 ng/mL	>25 nmol/L	>20 ng/mL
Heart				
Initiation	19–25 nmol/L	15–20 ng/mL		
Maintenance	6–12 nmol/L	5–10 ng/mL		

(continued)

TABLE 3

TOXICOLOGY AND THERAPEUTIC DRUG MONITORING (*CONTINUED*)

DRUG	THERAPEUTIC RANGE		TOXIC LEVEL	
	SI UNITS	CONVENTIONAL UNITS	SI UNITS	CONVENTIONAL UNITS
Theophylline	56–111 µg/mL	10–20 µg/mL	>168 µg/mL	>30 µg/mL
Thiocyanate				
After nitroprusside infusion	103–499 µmol/L	6–29 µg/mL	860 µmol/L	>50 µg/mL
Nonsmoker	17–69 µmol/L	1–4 µg/mL		
Smoker	52–206 µmol/L	3–12 µg/mL		
Tobramycin				
Peak	11–22 µg/L	5–10 µg/mL	>26 µg/L	>12 µg/mL
Trough	0–4.3 µg/L	0–2 µg/mL	>4.3 µg/L	>2 µg/mL
Valproic acid	346–693 µmol/L	50–100 µg/mL	>693 µmol/L	>100 µg/mL
Vancomycin				
Peak	14–28 µmol/L	20–40 µg/mL	>55 µmol/L	>80 µg/mL
Trough	3.5–10.4 µmol/L	5–15 µg/mL	>14 µmol/L	>20 µg/mL

TABLE 4

VITAMINS AND SELECTED TRACE MINERALS

SPECIMEN	ANALYTE	REFERENCE RANGE	
		SI UNITS	CONVENTIONAL UNITS
Aluminum	S	<0.2 µmol/L	<5.41 µg/L
Arsenic	WB	0.03–0.31 µmol/L	2–23 µg/L
Cadmium	WB	<44.5 nmol/L	<5.0 µg/L
Coenzyme Q10 (ubiquinone)	P	433–1532 µg/L	433–1532 µg/L
β-Carotene	S	0.07–1.43 µmol/L	4–77 µg/dL
Copper	S	11–22 µmol/L	70–140 µg/dL
Folic acid	RC	340–1020 nmol/L cells	150–450 ng/mL cells
Folic acid	S	12.2–40.8 nmol/L	5.4–18.0 ng/mL
Lead (adult)	S	<0.5 µmol/L	<10 µg/dL
Mercury	WB	3.0–294 nmol/L	0.6–59 µg/L
Selenium	S	0.8–2.0 umol/L	63–160 µg/L
Vitamin A	S	0.7–3.5 µmol/L	20–100 µg/dL
Vitamin B$_1$ (thiamine)	S	0–75 nmol/L	0–2 µg/dL
Vitamin B$_2$ (riboflavin)	S	106–638 nmol/L	4–24 µg/dL
Vitamin B$_6$	P	20–121 nmol/L	5–30 ng/mL
Vitamin B$_{12}$	S	206–735 pmol/L	279–996 pg/mL
Vitamin C (ascorbic acid)	S	23–57 µmol/L	0.4–1.0 mg/dL
Vitamin D$_3$,1,25-dihydroxy, total	S, P	36–180 pmol/L	15–75 pg/mL
Vitamin D$_3$, 25-hydroxy, total	P	75–250 nmol/L	30–100 ng/mL
Vitamin E	S	12–42 µmol/L	5–18 µg/mL
Vitamin K	S	0.29–2.64 nmol/L	0.13–1.19 ng/mL
Zinc	S	11.5–18.4 µmol/L	75–120 µg/dL

Abbreviations: P, plasma; RC, red cells; S, serum; WB, whole blood.

TABLE 5

CLASSIFICATION OF LDL, TOTAL, AND HDL CHOLESTEROL

LDL Cholesterol

<70 mg/dL	Therapeutic option for very high risk patients
<100 mg/dL	Optimal
100–129 mg/dL	Near optimal/above optimal
130–159 mg/dL	Borderline high
160–189 mg/dL	High
≥190 mg/dL	Very high

Total Cholesterol

<200 mg/dL	Desirable
200–239 mg/dL	Borderline high
≥240 mg/dL	High

HDL Cholesterol

<40 mg/dL	Low
≥60 mg/dL	High

Abbreviations: LDL, low-density lipoprotein; HDL, high-density lipoprotein.

Source: Executive summary of the third report of the National Cholesterol Education Program (NCEP) expert panel on detection, evaluation, and treatment of high blood cholesterol in adults (adult treatment panel III). JAMA 2001; 285:2486–97. Implications of Recent Clinical Trials for the National Cholesterol Education Program Adult Treatment Panel III Guidelines. SM Grundy et al for the Coordinating Committee of the National Cholesterol Education Program: Circulation 110:227, 2004.

REFERENCE VALUES FOR SPECIFIC ANALYTES

TABLE 6

CEREBROSPINAL FLUID[a]

	REFERENCE RANGE	
CONSTITUENT	**SI UNITS**	**CONVENTIONAL UNITS**
Osmolarity	292–297 mmol/kg water	292–297 mOsm/L
Electrolytes		
Sodium	137–145 mmol/L	137–145 meq/L
Potassium	2.7–3.9 mmol/L	2.7–3.9 meq/L
Calcium	1.0–1.5 mmol/L	2.1–3.0 meq/L
Magnesium	1.0–1.2 mmol/L	2.0–2.5 meq/L
Chloride	116–122 mmol/L	116–122 meq/L
CO_2 content	20–24 mmol/L	20–24 meq/L
P_{CO_2}	6–7 kPa	45–49 mmHg
pH	7.31–7.34	
Glucose	2.22–3.89 mmol/L	40–70 mg/dL
Lactate	1–2 mmol/L	10–20 mg/dL
Total protein:		
Lumbar	0.15–0.5 g/L	15–50 mg/dL
Cisternal	0.15–0.25 g/L	15–25 mg/dL
Ventricular	0.06–0.15 g/L	6–15 mg/dL
Albumin	0.066–0.442 g/L	6.6–44.2 mg/dL
IgG	0.009–0.057 g/L	0.9–5.7 mg/dL
IgG index[b]	0.29–0.59	
Oligoclonal bands (OGB)	<2 bands not present in matched serum sample	
Ammonia	15–47 μmol/L	25–80 μg/dL
Creatinine	44–168 μmol/L	0.5–1.9 mg/dL
Myelin basic protein	<4 μg/L	
CSF pressure		50–180 mmH₂O
CSF volume (adult)	~150 mL	
Red blood cells	0	0
Leukocytes		
Total	0–5 mononuclear cells per μL	
Differential		
Lymphocytes	60–70%	
Monocytes	30–50%	
Neutrophils	None	

[a]Since cerebrospinal fluid concentrations are equilibrium values, measurements of the same parameters in blood plasma obtained at the same time are recommended. However, there is a time lag in attainment of equilibrium, and cerebrospinal levels of plasma constituents that can fluctuate rapidly (such as plasma glucose) may not achieve stable values until after a significant lag phase.

[b]IgG index = CSF IgG (mg/dL) × serum albumin (g/dL)/serum IgG (g/dL) × CSF albumin (mg/dL).

APPENDIX

Laboratory Values of Clinical Importance

674

APPENDIX — Laboratory Values of Clinical Importance

TABLE 7A

DIFFERENTIAL NUCLEATED CELL COUNTS OF BONE MARROW ASPIRATES[a]

	OBSERVED RANGE (%)	95% RANGE (%)	MEAN (%)
Blast cells	0–3.2	0–3.0	1.4
Promyelocytes	3.6–13.2	3.2–12.4	7.8
Neutrophil myelocytes	4–21.4	3.7–10.0	7.6
Eosinophil myelocytes	0–5.0	0–2.8	1.3
Metamyelocytes	1–7.0	2.3–5.9	4.1
Neutrophils			
Males	21.0–45.6	21.9–42.3	32.1
Females	29.6–46.6	28.8–45.9	37.4
Eosinophils	0.4–4.2	0.3–4.2	2.2
Eosinophils plus eosinophil myelocytes	0.9–7.4	0.7–6.3	3.5
Basophils	0–0.8	0–0.4	0.1
Erythroblasts			
Male	18.0–39.4	16.2–40.1	28.1
Females	14.0–31.8	13.0–32.0	22.5
Lymphocytes	4.6–22.6	6.0–20.0	13.1
Plasma cells	0–1.4	0–1.2	0.6
Monocytes	0–3.2	0–2.6	1.3
Macrophages	0–1.8	0–1.3	0.4
M:E ratio			
Males	1.1–4.0	1.1–4.1	2.1
Females	1.6–5.4	1.6–5.2	2.8

[a]Based on bone marrow aspirate from 50 healthy volunteers (30 men, 20 women).

Abbreviation: M:E, myeloid to erythroid ratio.
Source: BJ Bain: Br J Haematol 94:206, 1996.

TABLE 7B

BONE MARROW CELLULARITY

AGE	OBSERVED RANGE	95% RANGE	MEAN
Under 10 years	59.0–95.1%	72.9–84.7%	78.8%
10–19 years	41.5–86.6%	59.2–69.4%	64.3%
20–29 years	32.0–83.7%	54.1–61.9%	58.0%
30–39 years	30.3–81.3%	41.1–54.1%	47.6%
40–49 years	16.3–75.1%	43.5–52.9%	48.2%
50–59 years	19.7–73.6%	41.2–51.4%	46.3%
60–69 years	16.3–65.7%	40.8–50.6%	45.7%
70–79 years	11.3–47.1%	22.6–35.2%	28.9%

Source: From RJ Hartsock et al: Am J Clin Pathol 1965; 43:326, 1965.

TABLE 8

STOOL ANALYSIS

	REFERENCE RANGE	
	SI UNITS	CONVENTIONAL UNITS
Alpha-1-antitrypsin	≤540 mg/L	≤54 mg/dL
Amount	0.1–0.2 kg/d	100–200 g/24 h
Coproporphyrin	611–1832 nmol/d	400–1200 µg/24 h
Fat		
Adult		<7 g/d
Adult on fat-free diet		<4 g/d
Fatty acids	0–21 mmol/d	0–6 g/24 h
Leukocytes	None	None
Nitrogen	<178 mmol/d	<2.5 g/24 h
pH	7.0–7.5	
Potassium	14–102 mmol/L	14–102 mmol/L
Occult blood	Negative	Negative
Osmolality	280–325 mosmol/kg	280–325 mosmol/kg
Sodium	7–72 mmol/L	7–72 mmol/L
Trypsin		20–95 U/g
Urobilinogen	85–510 µmol/d	50–300 mg/24 h
Uroporphyrins	12–48 nmol/d	10–40 µg/24 h
Water	<0.75	<75%

Source: Modified from: FT Fishbach, MB Dunning III: *A Manual of Laboratory and Diagnostic Tests*, 7th ed. Philadelphia, Lippincott Williams & Wilkins, 2004.

TABLE 9

675

URINE ANALYSIS AND RENAL FUNCTION TESTS

	REFERENCE RANGE	
	SI UNITS	CONVENTIONAL UNITS
Acidity, titratable	20–40 mmol/d	20–40 meq/d
Aldosterone	Normal diet: 6–25 µg/d	Normal diet: 6–25 µg/d
	Low-salt diet: 17–44 µg/d	Low-salt diet: 17–44 µg/d
	High-salt diet: 0–6 µg/d	High-salt diet: 0–6 µg/d
Aluminum	0.19–1.11 µmol/L	5–30 µg/L
Ammonia	30–50 mmol/d	30–50 meq/d
Amylase		4–400 U/L
Amylase/creatinine clearance ratio $[(Cl_{am}/Cl_{cr}) \times 100]$	1–5	1–5
Arsenic	0.07–0.67 µmol/d	5–50 µg/d
Bence Jones protein, urine, qualitative	Not applicable	None detected
Bence Jones protein, urine, quantitative		
Free Kappa	1.4–24.2 mg/L	0.14–2.42 mg/dL
Free Lambda	0.2–6.7 mg/L	0.02–0.67 mg/dL
K/L ratio	2.04–10.37	2.04–10.37
Calcium (10 meq/d or 200 mg/d dietary calcium)	<7.5 mmol/d	<300 mg/d
Chloride	140–250 mmol/d	140–250 mmol/d
Citrate	320–1240 mg/d	320–1240 mg/d
Copper	<0.95 µmol/d	<60 µg/d
Coproporphyrins (types I and III)	0–20 µmol/mol creatinine	0–20 µmol/mol creatinine
Cortisol, free	55–193 nmol/d	20–70 µg/d
Creatine, as creatinine		
Female	<760 µmol/d	<100 mg/d
Male	<380 µmol/d	<50 mg/d
Creatinine	8.8–14 mmol/d	1.0–1.6 g/d
Dopamine	392–2876 nmol/d	60–440 µg/d
Eosinophils	<100 eosinophils/mL	<100 eosinophils/mL
Epinephrine	0–109 nmol/d	0–20 µg/d
Glomerular filtration rate	>60 mL/min/1.73 m²	>60 mL/min/1.73 m²
	For African Americans multiply the result by 1.21	For African Americans multiply the result by 1.21
Glucose (glucose oxidase method)	0.3–1.7 mmol/d	50–300 mg/d
5-Hydroindoleacetic acid [5-HIAA]	0–78.8 µmol/d	0–15 mg/d
Hydroxyproline	53–328 µmol/d	53–328 µmol/d
Iodine, spot urine		
WHO classification of iodine deficiency:		
Not iodine deficient	>100 µg/L	>100 µg/L
Mild iodine deficiency	50–100 µg/L	50–100 µg/L
Moderate iodine deficiency	20–49 µg/L	20–49 µg/L
Severe iodine deficiency	<20 µg/L	<20 µg/L
Ketone (acetone)	Negative	Negative
17 Ketosteroids	3–12 mg/d	3–12 mg/d
Metanephrines		
Metanephrine	30–350 µg/d	30–350 µg/d
Normetanephrine	50–650 µg/d	50–650 µg/d

(continued)

TABLE 9

URINE ANALYSIS AND RENAL FUNCTION TESTS (*CONTINUED*)

	REFERENCE RANGE	
	SI UNITS	CONVENTIONAL UNITS
Microalbumin		
Normal	0.0–0.03 g/d	0–30 mg/d
Microalbuminuria	0.03–0.30 g/d	30–300 mg/d
Clinical albuminuria	>0.3 g/d	>300 mg/d
Microalbumin/creatinine ratio		
Normal	0–3.4 g/mol creatinine	0–30 μg/mg creatinine
Microalbuminuria	3.4–34 g/mol creatinine	30–300 μg/mg creatinine
Clinical albuminuria	>34 g/mol creatinine	>300 μg/mg creatinine
β_2-Microglobulin	0–160 μg/L	0–160 μg/L
Norepinephrine	89–473 nmol/d	15–80 μg/d
N-telopeptide (cross-linked), NTx		
Female, premenopausal	17–94 nmol BCE/mmol creatinine	17–94 nmol BCE/mmol creatinine
Female, postmenopausal	26–124 nmol BCE/mmol creatinine	26–124 nmol BCE/mmol creatinine
Male	21–83 nmol BCE/mmol creatinine	21–83 nmol BCE/mmol creatinine
BCE = bone collagen equivalent		
Osmolality	100–800 mosm/kg	100–800 mosm/kg
Oxalate		
Male	80–500 μmol/d	7–44 mg/d
Female	45–350 μmol/d	4–31 mg/d
pH	5.0–9.0	5.0–9.0
Phosphate (phosphorus) (varies with intake)	12.9–42.0 mmol/d	400–1300 mg/d
Porphobilinogen	None	None
Potassium (varies with intake)	25–100 mmol/d	25–100 meq/d
Protein	<0.15 g/d	<150 mg/d
Protein/creatinine ratio	Male: 15–68 mg/g Female: 10–107 mg/g	Male: 15–68 mg/g Female: 10–107 mg/g
Sediment		
Red blood cells	0–2/high-power field	
White blood cells	0–2/high-power field	
Bacteria	None	
Crystals	None	
Bladder cells	None	
Squamous cells	None	
Tubular cells	None	
Broad casts	None	
Epithelial cell casts	None	
Granular casts	None	
Hyaline casts	0–5/low-power field	
Red blood cell casts	None	
Waxy casts	None	
White cell casts	None	
Sodium (varies with intake)	100–260 mmol/d	100–260 meq/d
Specific gravity:		
After 12-h fluid restriction	>1.025	>1.025
After 12-h deliberate water intake	≤1.003	≤1.003
Tubular reabsorption, phosphorus	0.79–0.94 of filtered load	79–94% of filtered load
Urea nitrogen	214–607 mmol/d	6–17 g/d
Uric acid (normal diet)	1.49–4.76 mmol/d	250–800 mg/d
Vanillylmandelic acid (VMA)	<30 μmol/d	<6 mg/d

TABLE 10

NORMAL PRESSURES IN HEART AND GREAT VESSELS

PRESSURE (mmHg)	AVERAGE	RANGE
Right Atrium		
Mean	2.8	1–5
a wave	5.6	2.5–7
c wave	3.8	1.5–6
x wave	1.7	0–5
v wave	4.6	2–7.5
y wave	2.4	0–6
Right Ventricle		
Peak systolic	25	17–32
End-diastolic	4	1–7
Pulmonary Artery		
Mean	15	9–19
Peak systolic	25	17–32
End-diastolic	9	4–13
Pulmonary Artery Wedge		
Mean	9	4.5–13
Left Atrium		
Mean	7.9	2–12
a wave	10.4	4–16
v wave	12.8	6–21
Left Ventricle		
Peak systolic	130	90–140
End-diastolic	8.7	5–12
Brachial Artery		
Mean	85	70–105
Peak systolic	130	90–140
End-diastolic	70	60–90

Source: Reproduced from: MJ Kern *The Cardiac Catheterization Handbook*, 4th ed. Philadelphia, Mosby, 2003.

TABLE 11

CIRCULATORY FUNCTION TESTS

	RESULTS: REFERENCE RANGE	
TEST	SI UNITS (RANGE)	CONVENTIONAL UNITS (RANGE)
Arteriovenous oxygen difference	30–50 mL/L	30–50 mL/L
Cardiac output (Fick)	2.5–3.6 L/m^2 of body surface area per min	2.5–3.6 L/m^2 of body surface area per min
Contractility indexes		
Max. left ventricular dp/dt (dp/dt)	220 kPa/s (176–250 kPa/s)	1650 mmHg/s (1320–1880 mmHg/s)
DP when DP = 5.3 kPa	(37.6 ± 12.2)/s	(37.6 ± 12.2)/s
(40 mmHg) (DP, developed LV pressure)	3.32 ± 0.84 end-diastolic volumes per second	3.32 ± 0.84 end-diastolic volumes per second
Mean normalized systolic ejection rate (angiography)	1.83 ± 0.56 circumferences per second	1.83 ± 0.56 circumferences per second
Mean velocity of circumferential fiber shortening (angiography)		
Ejection fraction: stroke volume/ end-diastolic volume (SV/EDV)	0.67 ± 0.08 (0.55–0.78)	0.67 ± 0.08 (0.55–0.78)
End-diastolic volume	70 ± 20.0 mL/m^2 (60–88 mL/m^2)	70 ± 20.0 mL/m^2 (60–88 mL/m^2)
End-systolic volume	25 ± 5.0 mL/m^2 (20–33 mL/m^2)	25 ± 5.0 mL/m^2 (20–33 mL/m^2)
Left ventricular work		
Stroke work index	50 ± 20.0 (g·m)/m^2 (30–110)	50 ± 20.0 (g·m)/m^2 (30–110)
Left ventricular minute work index	1.8–6.6 [(kg·m)/m^2]/min	1.8–6.6 [(kg·m)/m^2]/min
Oxygen consumption index	110–150 mL	110–150 mL
Maximum oxygen uptake	35 mL/min (20–60 mL/min)	35 mL/min (20–60 mL/min)
Pulmonary vascular resistance	2–12 (kPa·s)/L	20–130 (dyn·s)/cm^5
Systemic vascular resistance	77–150 (kPa·s)/L	770–1600 (dyn·s)/cm^5

Source: E Braunwald et al: *Heart Disease*, 6th ed. Philadelphia, W.B. Saunders Co., 2001.

TABLE 12

NORMAL ECHOCARDIOGRAPHIC REFERENCE LIMITS AND PARTITION VALUES IN ADULTS

	WOMEN REFERENCE RANGE	MILDLY ABNORMAL	MODERATELY ABNORMAL	SEVERELY ABNORMAL	MEN REFERENCE RANGE	MILDLY ABNORMAL	MODERATELY ABNORMAL	SEVERELY ABNORMAL
Left ventricular dimensions								
Septal thickness, cm	0.6–0.9	1.0–1.2	1.3–1.5	≥1.6	0.6–1.0	1.1–1.3	1.4–1.6	≥1.7
Posterior wall thickness, cm	0.6–0.9	1.0–1.2	1.3–1.5	≥1.6	0.6–1.0	1.1–1.3	1.4–1.6	≥1.7
Diastolic diameter, cm	3.9–5.3	5.4–5.7	5.8–6.1	≥6.2	4.2–5.9	6.0–6.3	6.4–6.8	≥6.9
Diastolic diameter/BSA, cm/m²	2.4–3.2	3.3–3.4	3.5–3.7	≥3.8	2.2–3.1	3.2–3.4	3.5–3.6	≥3.7
Diastolic diameter/height, cm/m	2.5–3.2	3.3–3.4	3.5–3.6	≥3.7	2.4–3.3	3.4–3.5	3.6–3.7	≥3.8
Left ventricular volumes								
Diastolic, mL	56–104	105–117	118–130	≥131	67–155	156–178	179–201	≥202
Diastolic/BSA, mL/m²	35–75	76–86	87–96	≥97	35–75	76–86	87–96	≥97
Systolic, mL	19–49	50–59	60–69	≥70	22–58	59–70	71–82	≥83
Systolic/BSA, mL/m²	12–30	31–36	37–42	≥43	12–30	31–36	37–42	≥43
Left ventricular mass, 2D method								
Mass, g	66–150	151–171	172–182	≥183	96–200	201–227	228–254	≥255
Mass/BSA, g/m²	44–88	89–100	101–112	≥113	50–102	103–116	117–130	≥131
Left ventricular function								
Endocardial fractional shortening (%)	27–45	22–26	17–21	≤16	25–43	20–24	15–19	≤14
Midwall fractional shortening (%)	15–23	13–14	11–12	≤10	14–22	12–13	10–11	≤9
Ejection fraction, 2D method (%)	≥55	45–54	30–44	≤29	≥55	45–54	30–44	≤29
Right heart dimensions (cm)								
Basal RV diameter	2.0–2.8	2.9–3.3	3.4–3.8	≥3.9	2.0–2.8	2.9–3.3	3.4–3.8	≥3.9
Mid-RV diameter	2.7–3.3	3.4–3.7	3.8–4.1	≥4.2	2.7–3.3	3.4–3.7	3.8–4.1	≥4.2
Base-to-apex length	7.1–7.9	8.0–8.5	8.6–9.1	≥9.2	7.1–7.9	8.0–8.5	8.6–9.1	≥9.2
RVOT diameter above aortic valve	2.5–2.9	3.0–3.2	3.3–3.5	≥3.6	2.5–2.9	3.0–3.2	3.3–3.5	≥3.6
RVOT diameter above pulmonic valve	1.7–2.3	2.4–2.7	2.8–3.1	≥3.2	1.7–2.3	2.4–2.7	2.8–3.1	≥3.2
Pulmonary artery diameter below pulmonic valve	1.5–2.1	2.2–2.5	2.6–2.9	≥3.0	1.5–2.1	2.2–2.5	2.6–2.9	≥3.0
Right ventricular size and function in 4-chamber view								
Diastolic area, cm²	11–28	29–32	33–37	≥38	11–28	29–32	33–37	≥38
Systolic area, cm²	7.5–16	17–19	20–22	≥23	7.5–16	17–19	20–22	≥23
Fractional area change, %	32–60	25–31	18–24	≤17	32–60	25–31	18–24	≤17
Atrial sizes								
LA diameter, cm	2.7–3.8	3.9–4.2	4.3–4.6	≥4.7	3.0–4.0	4.1–4.6	4.7–5.2	≥5.3
LA diameter/BSA, cm/m²	1.5–2.3	2.4–2.6	2.7–2.9	≥3.0	1.5–2.3	2.4–2.6	2.7–2.9	≥3.0
RA minor axis, cm	2.9–4.5	4.6–4.9	5.0–5.4	≥5.5	2.9–4.5	4.6–4.9	5.0–5.4	≥5.5
RA minor axis/BSA, cm/m²	1.7–2.5	2.6–2.8	2.9–3.1	≥3.2	1.7–2.5	2.6–2.8	2.9–3.1	≥3.2

(continued)

TABLE 12

NORMAL ECHOCARDIOGRAPHIC REFERENCE LIMITS AND PARTITION VALUES IN ADULTS (CONTINUED)

	WOMEN REFERENCE RANGE	MILDLY ABNORMAL	MODERATELY ABNORMAL	SEVERELY ABNORMAL	MEN REFERENCE RANGE	MILDLY ABNORMAL	MODERATELY ABNORMAL	SEVERELY ABNORMAL
LA area, cm²	<20	20–30	30–40	≥41	<20	20–30	30–40	≥41
LA volume, mL	22–52	53–62	63–72	≥73	18–58	59–68	69–78	≥79
LA volume/BSA, mL/m²	16–28	29–33	34–39	≥40	16–28	29–33	34–39	≥40
Aortic stenosis, classification of severity								
Aortic jet velocity, m/s		2.6–2.9	3.0–4.0	>4.0		2.6–2.9	3.0–4.0	>4.0
Mean gradient, mmHg		<20	20–40	>40		<20	20–40	>40
Valve area, cm²		>1.5	1.0–1.5	<1.0		>1.5	1.0–1.5	<1.0
Indexed valve area, cm²/m²		>0.85	0.60–0.85	<0.6		>0.85	0.60–0.85	<0.6
Velocity ratio		>0.50	0.25–0.50	<0.25		>0.50	0.25–0.50	<0.25
Mitral stenosis, classification of severity								
Valve area, cm²		>1.5	1.0–1.5	<1.0		>1.5	1.0–1.5	<1.0
Mean gradient, mmHg		<5	5–10	>10		<5	5–10	>10
Pulmonary artery pressure, mmHg		<30	30–50	>50		<30	30–50	>50
Aortic regurgitation, indices of severity								
Vena contracta width, cm		<0.30	0.30–0.60	≥0.60		<0.30	0.30–0.60	≥0.60
Jet width/LVOT width, %		<25	25–64	≥65		<25	25–64	≥65
Jet CSA/LVOT CSA, %		<5	5–59	≥60		<5	5–59	≥60
Regurgitant volume, mL/beat		<30	30–59	≥60		<30	30–59	≥60
Regurgitant fraction, %		<30	30–49	≥50		<30	30–49	≥50
Effective regurgitant orifice area, cm²		<0.10	0.10–0.29	≥0.30		<0.10	0.10–0.29	≥0.30
Mitral regurgitation, indices of severity								
Vena contracta width, cm		<0.30	0.30–0.69	≥0.70		<0.30	0.30–0.69	≥0.70
Regurgitant volume, mL/beat		<30	30–59	≥60		<30	30–59	≥60
Regurgitant fraction, %		<30	30–49	≥50		<30	30–49	≥50
Effective regurgitant orifice area, cm²		<0.20	0.20–0.39	≥0.40		<0.20	0.20–0.39	≥0.40

Abbreviations: BSA, body surface area; CSA, cross-sectional area; LA, left atrium; LVOT, left ventricular outflow tract; RA, right atrium; RV, right ventricle; RVOT, right ventricular outflow tract; 2D, 2-dimensional.

Source: Values adapted from: American Society of Echocardiography, Guidelines and Standards. http://www.asecho.org/i4a/pages/index.cfm?pageid=3317. Accessed Feb 23, 2010.

TABLE 13

SUMMARY OF VALUES USEFUL IN PULMONARY PHYSIOLOGY

	SYMBOL	TYPICAL VALUES	
		MAN AGED 40, 75 kg, 175 cm TALL	WOMAN AGED 40, 60 kg, 160 cm TALL
Pulmonary Mechanics			
Spirometry—volume-time curves			
Forced vital capacity	FVC	5.0 L	3.4 L
Forced expiratory volume in 1 s	FEV_1	4.0 L	2.8 L
FEV_1/FVC	FEV_1%	80%	78%
Maximal midexpiratory flow rate	MMEF (FEF 25–75)	4.1 L/s	3.2 L/s
Maximal expiratory flow rate	MEFR (FEF 200–1200)	9.0 L/s	6.7 L/s
Spirometry—flow-volume curves			
Maximal expiratory flow at 50% of expired vital capacity	V_{max} 50 (FEF 50%)	5.0 L/s	4.0 L/s
Maximal expiratory flow at 75% of expired vital capacity	V_{max} 75 (FEF 75%)	2.1 L/s	2.0 L/s
Resistance to airflow:			
Pulmonary resistance	RL (R_L)	<3.0 (cmH_2O/s)/L	
Airway resistance	Raw	<2.5 (cmH_2O/s)/L	
Specific conductance	SGaw	>0.13 cmH_2O/s	
Pulmonary compliance			
Static recoil pressure at total lung capacity	Pst TLC	25 ± 5 cmH_2O	
Compliance of lungs (static)	CL	0.2 L cmH_2O	
Compliance of lungs and thorax	C(L + T)	0.1 L cmH_2O	
Dynamic compliance of 20 breaths per minute	C dyn 20	0.25 ± 0.05 L/cmH_2O	
Maximal static respiratory pressures:			
Maximal inspiratory pressure	MIP	>110 cmH_2O	>70 cmH_2O
Maximal expiratory pressure	MEP	>200 cmH_2O	>140 cmH_2O
Lung Volumes			
Total lung capacity	TLC	6.9 L	4.9 L
Functional residual capacity	FRC	3.3 L	2.6 L
Residual volume	RV	1.9 L	1.5 L
Inspiratory capacity	IC	3.7 L	2.3 L
Expiratory reserve volume	ERV	1.4 L	1.1 L
Vital capacity	VC	5.0 L	3.4 L
Gas Exchange (Sea Level)			
Arterial O_2 tension	Pa_{O_2}	12.7 ± 0.7 kPa (95 ± 5 mmHg)	
Arterial CO_2 tension	Pa_{CO_2}	5.3 ± 0.3 kPa (40 ± 2 mmHg)	
Arterial O_2 saturation	Sa_{O_2}	0.97 ± 0.02 (97 ± 2%)	
Arterial blood pH	pH	7.40 ± 0.02	
Arterial bicarbonate	HCO_3^-	24 + 2 meq/L	
Base excess	BE	0 ± 2 meq/L	
Diffusing capacity for carbon monoxide (single breath)	DL_{CO}	37 mL CO/min/mmHg	27 mL CO/min/mmHg
Dead space volume	V_D	2 mL/kg body wt	
Physiologic dead space; dead space-tidal volume ratio	V_D/V_T		
Rest		≤35% V_T	
Exercise		≤20% V_T	
Alveolar-arterial difference for O_2	P(A − a)$_{O_2}$	≤2.7 kPa ≤20 kPa (≤24 mmHg)	

Source: Based on: AH Morris et al: *Clinical Pulmonary Function Testing. A Manual of Uniform Laboratory Procedures*, 2nd ed. Salt Lake City, Utah, Intermountain Thoracic Society, 1984.

TABLE 14

GASTROINTESTINAL TESTS

TEST	RESULTS	
	SI UNITS	CONVENTIONAL UNITS
Absorption tests		
D-Xylose: after overnight fast, 25 g xylose given in oral aqueous solution		
Urine, collected for following 5 h	25% of ingested dose	25% of ingested dose
Serum, 2 h after dose	2.0–3.5 mmol/L	30–52 mg/dL
Vitamin A: a fasting blood specimen is obtained and 200,000 units of vitamin A in oil is given orally	Serum level should rise to twice fasting level in 3–5 h	Serum level should rise to twice fasting level in 3–5 h
Bentiromide test (pancreatic function): 500 mg bentiromide (chymex) orally; *p*-aminobenzoic acid (PABA) measured		
Plasma		>3.6 (±1.1) μg/mL at 90 min
Urine	>50% recovered in 6 h	>50% recovered in 6 h
Gastric juice		
Volume		
24 h	2–3 L	2–3 L
Nocturnal	600–700 mL	600–700 mL
Basal, fasting	30–70 mL/h	30–70 mL/h
Reaction		
pH	1.6–1.8	1.6–1.8
Titratable acidity of fasting juice	4–9 μmol/s	15–35 meq/h
Acid output		
Basal		
Females (mean ± 1 SD)	0.6 ± 0.5 μmol/s	2.0 ± 1.8 meq/h
Males (mean ± 1 SD)	0.8 ± 0.6 μmol/s	3.0 ± 2.0 meq/h
Maximal (after SC histamine acid phosphate, 0.004 mg/kg body weight, and preceded by 50 mg promethazine, or after betazole, 1.7 mg/kg body weight, or pentagastrin, 6 μg/kg body weight)		
Females (mean ± 1 SD)	4.4 ± 1.4 μmol/s	16 ± 5 meq/h
Males (mean ± 1 SD)	6.4 ± 1.4 μmol/s	23 ± 5 meq/h
Basal acid output/maximal acid output ratio	≤0.6	≤0.6
Gastrin, serum	0–200 μg/L	0–200 pg/mL
Secretin test (pancreatic exocrine function): 1 unit/kg body weight, IV		
Volume (pancreatic juice) in 80 min	>2.0 mL/kg	>2.0 mL/kg
Bicarbonate concentration	>80 mmol/L	>80 meq/L
Bicarbonate output in 30 min	>10 mmol	>10 meq

MISCELLANEOUS

TABLE 15

BODY FLUIDS AND OTHER MASS DATA

	REFERENCE RANGE	
	SI UNITS	CONVENTIONAL UNITS
Ascitic fluid: See Chap. 9		
Body fluid		
Total volume (lean) of body weight	50% (in obese) to 70%	
Intracellular	30-40% of body weight	
Extracellular	20-30% of body weight	
Blood		
Total volume		
Males	69 mL/kg body weight	
Females	65 mL/kg body weight	
Plasma volume		
Males	39 mL/kg body weight	
Females	40 mL/kg body weight	
Red blood cell volume		
Males	30 mL/kg body weight	$1.15–1.21$ L/m^2 of body surface area
Females	25 mL/kg body weight	$0.95–1.00$ L/m^2 of body surface area
Body mass index	$18.5–24.9$ kg/m^2	$18.5–24.9$ kg/m^2

TABLE 16

RADIATION-DERIVED UNITS

QUANTITY	MEASURES	OLD UNIT	SI UNIT	SPECIAL NAME FOR SI UNIT (ABBREVIATION)	CONVERSION
Activity	Rate of radioactive decay	curie (Ci)	Disintegrations per second (dps)	becquerel (Bq)	1 Ci $= 3.7 \times 10^{10}$ Bq 1 mCi $=$ 37 MBq 1 Bq $= 2.703 \times 10^{-11}$ Ci
Exposure	Amount of ionizations produced in dry air by x-rays or gamma rays, per unit of mass	roentgen (R)	Coulomb per kilogram (C/kg)	none	1 C/kg $=$ 3876 R 1 R $= 2.58 \times 10^{-4}$ C/kg 1 mR $=$ 258 pC/kg
Air kerma	Sum of initial energies of charged particles liberated by ionizing radiation in air, per unit of mass	rad	Joule per kilogram (J/kg)	gray (Gy)	1 Gy $=$ 100 rad 1 rad $=$ 0.01 Gy 1 mrad $=$ 10 μGy
Absorbed dose	Energy deposited per unit of mass in a medium, e.g., an organ/tissue	rad	Joule per kilogram (J/kg)	gray (Gy)	1 Gy $=$ 100 rad 1 rad $=$ 0.01 Gy 1 mrad $=$ 10 μGy
Equivalent dose	Energy deposited per unit of mass in a medium, e.g., an organ/tissue, weighted to reflect type(s) of radiation	rem	Joule per kilogram (J/kg)	sievert (Sv)	1 Sv $=$ 100 rem 1 rem $=$ 0.01 Sv 1 mrem $=$ 10 μSv
Effective dose	Energy deposited per unit of mass in a reference individual, doubly weighted to reflect type(s) of radiation and organ(s) irradiated	rem	Joule per kilogram (J/kg)	sievert (Sv)	1 Sv $=$ 100 rem 1 rem $=$ 0.01 Sv 1 mrem $=$ 10 μSv

ACKNOWLEDGMENTS

The contributions of Drs. Daniel J. Fink, Patrick M. Sluss, James L. Januzzi, and Kent B. Lewandrowski to this chapter in previous editions of Harrison's Principles of Internal Medicine are gratefully acknowledged. We also express our gratitude to Drs. Amudha Palanisamy and Scott Fink for careful review of tables and helpful suggestions.

APPENDIX

Laboratory Values of Clinical Importance

REVIEW AND SELF-ASSESSMENT[a]

Charles Wiener ∎ Cynthia D. Brown ∎ Anna R. Hemnes

QUESTIONS

DIRECTIONS: Choose the **one best** response to each question.

1. A 41-year-old female presents to your clinic with a week of jaundice. She notes pruritus, icterus, and dark urine. She denies fever, abdominal pain, or weight loss. The examination is unremarkable except for yellow discoloration of the skin. Total bilirubin is 6.0 mg/dL, and direct bilirubin is 5.1 mg/dL. AST is 84 U/L, and ALT is 92 U/L. Alkaline phosphatase is 662 U/L. CT scan of the abdomen is unremarkable. Right upper quadrant ultrasound shows a normal gallbladder but does not visualize the common bile duct. What is the most appropriate next management step?

   A. Antibiotics and observation
   B. Endoscopic retrograde cholangiopancreatography (ERCP)
   C. Hepatitis serologies
   D. HIDA scan
   E. Serologies for antimitochondrial antibodies

2. A 61-year-old male is admitted to your service for swelling of the abdomen. You detect ascites on clinical examination and perform a paracentesis. The results show a white blood cell count of 300 leukocytes/μL with 35% polymorphonuclear cells. The peritoneal albumin level is 1.2 g/dL, protein is 2.0 g/dL, and triglycerides are 320 mg/dL. Peritoneal cultures are pending. Serum albumin is 2.6 g/dL. Which of the following is the most likely diagnosis?

   A. Congestive heart failure
   B. Peritoneal tuberculosis
   C. Peritoneal carcinomatosis
   D. Chylous ascites
   E. Bacterial peritonitis

3. An 80-year-old woman is evaluated for a complaint of involuntary weight loss. Her baseline weight at her clinic visit 6 months ago was 67 kg. She reports that her appetite began to decrease about 2 months ago

3. (*Continued*)
   when she noticed that food no longer had the same taste. Her daughter accompanies her to the visit and reports that her mother seems increasingly listless and withdrawn. Her daughter also notes that her mother seems more forgetful, and her home has become disorganized. The patient has a history of hypertension and peripheral vascular disease. She had a transient ischemic attack 6 years ago, but has never had a stroke. There have been no recent changes to any medications. Her weight in the clinic today is 60 kg. What is the appropriate approach for the evaluation of this patient's weight loss?

   A. Ask the patient to return to the clinic in 1 month for repeat weight evaluation.
   B. Order thyroid function tests.
   C. Perform a Mini-Mental State Examination.
   D. Reassure the patient and her daughter that this degree of weight loss is not abnormal.
   E. Both B and C are correct.

4. The advantages of endoscopy over barium radiography in the evaluation of dysphagia include all of the following EXCEPT:

   A. Ability to intervene as well as diagnose
   B. Ability to obtain biopsy specimens
   C. Increased sensitivity for the detection of abnormalities identified by color, e.g., Barrett's metaplasia
   D. Increased sensitivity for the detection of mucosal lesions
   E. No meaningful risk to procedure

5. A 47-year-old man is evaluated in the emergency department for chest pain that developed at a restaurant after swallowing a piece of steak. He reports intermittent episodes of meat getting stuck in his lower chest over the past 3 years, but none as severe as this event. He denies food regurgitation outside of these episodes or heartburn symptoms. He is able to swallow liquids without difficulty and has not had any weight loss. Which of the following is the most likely diagnosis?

[a]Questions and answers were taken from Wiener C et al (eds): *Harrison's Principles of Internal Medicine Self-Assessment and Board Review*, 18th ed. New York: McGraw-Hill, 2012.

5. (*Continued*)
  A. Achalasia
  B. Adenocarcinoma of the esophagus
  C. Esophageal diverticula
  D. Plummer-Vinson syndrome
  E. Schatzki's ring

6. Which of the following has a well-established association with gastroesophageal reflux?

  A. Chronic sinusitis
  B. Dental erosion
  C. Pulmonary fibrosis
  D. Recurrent aspiration pneumonia
  E. Sleep apnea

7. A 36-year-old female with AIDS and a CD4 count of $35/mm^3$ presents with odynophagia and progressive dysphagia. The patient reports daily fevers and a 20-lb weight loss. She has been treated with clotrimazole troches without relief. On physical examination the patient is cachectic with a body mass index (BMI) of 16 and a weight of 86 lb. She has a temperature of 38.2°C (100.8°F) and is noted to be orthostatic by blood pressure and pulse. Examination of the oropharynx reveals no evidence of thrush. The patient undergoes esophagogastroduodenoscopy (EGD), which reveals serpiginous ulcers in the distal esophagus without vesicles. No yellow plaques are noted. Multiple biopsies are taken that show intranuclear and intracytoplasmic inclusions in large endothelial cells and fibroblasts. What is the best treatment for this patient's esophagitis?

  A. Ganciclovir
  B. Glucocorticoids
  C. Fluconazole
  D. Foscarnet
  E. Thalidomide

8. A 57-year-old man is evaluated with an esophagogastroduodenoscopy after an episode of hematemesis. The patient reports a history of tobacco use and hypercholesterolemia, but is otherwise healthy. He has had lower back pain for the past month and has been intermittently using acetaminophen 1000 mg for relief. His endoscopy shows a 3-cm duodenal ulcer. Which of the following statements is correct regarding this finding?

  A. The lesion should be biopsied as duodenal ulcers have an elevated risk of being due to carcinoma.
  B. First-line therapy should be discontinuation of acetaminophen use.

8. (*Continued*)
  C. The patient is not at risk for any associated cancers.
  D. Poor socioeconomic status is a risk factor for development of this condition.
  E. Antral gastritis is rarely found with this condition.

9. A 58-year-old man is evaluated for abdominal pain by his primary care physician. He reports severe stress at his job for the last 3 months and has since noted that he has epigastric pain that is relieved by eating and drinking milk. He has not had food regurgitation, dysphagia, or bloody emesis or bowel movements. He denies any symptoms in his chest. Peptic ulcer disease is suspected. Which of the following statements regarding noninvasive testing for *Helicobacter pylori* is true?

  A. There is no reliable noninvasive method to detect *H. pylori*.
  B. Stool antigen testing is appropriate for both diagnosis of and proof of cure after therapy for *H. pylori*.
  C. Plasma antibodies to *H. pylori* offer the greatest sensitivity for diagnosis of infection.
  D. Exposure to low-dose radiation is a limitation to the urea breath test.
  E. False-negative testing using the urea breath test may occur with recent use of NSAIDs.

10. A 44-year-old woman complains of 6 months of epigastric pain that is worst between meals. She also reports symptoms of heartburn. The pain is typically relieved by over-the-counter antacid medications. She comes to the clinic after noting her stools darkening. She has no significant past medical history and takes no medications. Her physical examination is normal except for diffuse mid-epigastric pain. Her stools are heme positive. She undergoes EGD, which demonstrates a well-circumscribed 2-cm duodenal ulcer that is positive for *H. pylori*. Which of the following is recommended initial therapy given these findings?

  A. Lansoprazole plus clarithromycin plus amoxicillin for 14 days
  B. Pantoprazole plus amoxicillin for 21 days
  C. Pantoprazole plus clarithromycin for 14 days
  D. Omeprazole plus bismuth plus tetracycline plus metronidazole for 14 days
  E. Omeprazole plus metronidazole plus clarithromycin for 7 days

11. A 57-year-old man with peptic ulcer disease experiences transient improvement with *Helicobacter pylori* eradication. However, 3 months later symptoms

11. (*Continued*)

recur despite acid–suppressing therapy. He does not take nonsteroidal anti–inflammatory agents. Stool analysis for *H. pylori* antigen is negative. Upper GI endoscopy reveals prominent gastric folds together with the persistent ulceration in the duodenal bulb previously detected and the beginning of a new ulceration 4 cm proximal to the initial ulcer. Fasting gastrin levels are elevated and basal acid secretion is 15 meq/h. What is the best test to perform to make the diagnosis?

A. No additional testing is necessary.
B. Blood sampling for gastrin levels following a meal.
C. Blood sampling for gastrin levels following secretin administration.
D. Endoscopic ultrasonography of the pancreas.
E. Genetic testing for mutations in the MEN1 gene.

12. A 23-year-old woman is evaluated by her primary care physician for diffuse, crampy abdominal pain. She reports that she has had abdominal pain for the last several years, but it is getting worse and is now associated with intermittent diarrhea without flatulence. This does not waken her at night. Stools do not float and are not hard to flush. She has not noted any worsening with specific foods, but she does have occasional rashes on her lower legs. She has lost about 5 kg over the last year. She is otherwise healthy and takes no medications. Which of the following is the most appropriate recommendation at this point?

A. Increased dietary fiber intake
B. Measurement of antiendomysial antibody
C. Measurement of 24-hour fecal fat
D. Referral to gastroenterologist for endoscopy
E. Trial of lactose-free diet

13. All of the following are direct complications of short bowel syndrome EXCEPT:

A. Cholesterol gallstones
B. Coronary artery disease
C. Gastric acid hypersecretion
D. Renal calcium oxalate calculi
E. Steatorrhea

14. A 54-year-old man is evaluated by a gastroenterologist for diarrhea that has been present for approximately 1 month. He reports stools that float and are difficult to flush down the toilet; these can occur at any time of day or night, but seem worsened by fatty meals. In addition, he reports pain in many

14. (*Continued*)

joints that lasts days to weeks and is not relieved by ibuprofen. His wife notes that the patient has had difficulty with memory for the last few months. He has lost 30 pounds and reports intermittent low-grade fevers. He takes no medications and is otherwise healthy. Endoscopy is recommended. Which of the following is the most likely finding on small-bowel biopsy?

A. Dilated lymphatics
B. Flat villi with crypt hyperplasia
C. Mononuclear cell infiltrate in the lamina propria
D. Normal small-bowel biopsy
E. PAS-positive macrophages containing small bacilli

15. A 54-year-old male presents with 1 month of diarrhea. He states that he has 8–10 loose bowel movements a day. He has lost 4 kg during this time. Vital signs and physical examination are normal. Serum laboratory studies are normal. A 24-hour stool collection reveals 500 g of stool with a measured stool osmolality of 200 mosmol/L and a calculated stool osmolality of 210 mosmol/L. Based on these findings, what is the most likely cause of this patient's diarrhea?

A. Celiac sprue
B. Chronic pancreatitis
C. Lactase deficiency
D. Vasoactive intestinal peptide tumor
E. Whipple's disease

16. Cobalamin absorption may occur in all of the following diseases EXCEPT:

A. Bacterial overgrowth syndrome
B. Chronic pancreatitis
C. Crohn's disease
D. Pernicious anemia
E. Ulcerative colitis

17. Which of the following statements regarding the epidemiology of inflammatory bowel disease is correct?

A. Monozygotic twins are highly concordant for ulcerative colitis.
B. Oral contraceptive use decreases the incidence of Crohn's disease.
C. Persons of Asian descent have the highest rates of ulcerative colitis and Crohn's disease.
D. Smoking may decrease the incidence of ulcerative colitis.
E. Typical age of onset for Crohn's disease is 40–50 years old.

18. A 24-year-old woman is admitted to the hospital with a 1-year history of severe abdominal pain and chronic diarrhea, which has been bloody for the past 2 months. She reports a 20-lb weight loss, frequent fevers, and night sweats. She denies vomiting. Her abdominal pain is crampy and primarily involves her right lower quadrant. She is otherwise healthy. Examination is concerning for an acute abdomen with rebound and guarding present. CT shows free air in the peritoneum. She is urgently taken to the operating room for surgical exploration, where she is found to have multiple strictures and a perforation of her bowel in the terminal ileum. The rectum was spared and a fissure from the duodenum to the jejunum is found. The perforated area is resected and adhesions lysed. Which of the following findings on pathology of her resected area confirms her diagnosis?

A. Crypt abscesses
B. Flat villi
C. Noncaseating granuloma throughout the bowel wall
D. Special stain for *Clostridium difficile* toxin
E. Transmural acute and chronic inflammation

19. A 45-year-old man with ulcerative colitis has been treated for the past 5 years with infliximab with excellent resolution of his bowel symptoms and endoscopic evidence of normal colonic mucosa. He is otherwise healthy. He is evaluated by a dermatologist for a lesion that initially was a pustule over his right lower extremity but has since progressed in size with ulceration. The ulcer is moderately painful. He does not recall any trauma to the area. On examination the ulcer measures 15 cm by 7 cm and central necrosis is present. The edges of the ulcer are violaceous. No other lesions are identified. Which of the following is the most likely diagnosis?

A. Erythema nodosum
B. Metastatic Crohn's disease
C. Psoriasis
D. Pyoderma gangrenosum
E. Pyoderma vegetans

20. Inflammatory bowel disease (IBD) may be caused by exogenous factors. Gastrointestinal flora may promote an inflammatory response or may inhibit inflammation. Probiotics have been used to treat IBD. Which of the following organisms has been used in the treatment of IBD?

A. *Campylobacter* spp.
B. *Clostridium difficile*

20. (*Continued*)
C. *Escherichia* spp.
D. *Lactobacillus* spp.
E. *Shigella* spp.

21. Your 33-year-old patient with Crohn's disease (CD) has had a disappointing disease response to glucocorticoids and 5-ASA agents. He is interested in steroid-sparing agents. He has no liver or renal disease. You prescribe once-weekly methotrexate injections. In addition to monitoring hepatic function and complete blood count, what other complication of methotrexate therapy do you advise the patient of?

A. Disseminated histoplasmosis
B. Lymphoma
C. Pancreatitis
D. Pneumonitis
E. Primary sclerosing cholangitis

22. Which of the following patients requires no further testing before making the diagnosis of irritable bowel syndrome and initiating treatment?

A. A 76-year-old woman with 6 months of intermittent crampy abdominal pain that is worse with stress and associated with bloating and diarrhea.
B. A 25-year-old woman with 6 months of abdominal pain, bloating, and diarrhea that has worsened steadily and now awakes her from sleep at night to move her bowels.
C. A 30-year-old man with 6 months of lower abdominal crampy pain relieved with bowel movements, usually loose. Symptoms are worse during the daytime at work and better on the weekend. Weight loss is not present.
D. A 19-year-old female college student with 2 months of diarrhea and worsening abdominal pain with occasional blood in her stool.
E. A 27-year-old woman with 6 months of intermittent abdominal pain, bloating, and diarrhea without associated weight loss. Crampy pain and diarrhea persist after a 48-hour fast.

23. A 29-year-old woman comes to see you in the clinic because of abdominal discomfort. She feels abdominal discomfort on most days of the week, and the pain varies in location and intensity. She notes constipation as well as diarrhea, but diarrhea predominates. In comparison to 6 months ago, she has more bloating and flatulence than she has had before. She identifies eating and stress as aggravating factors, and her pain is relieved by defecation. You suspect irritable bowel syndrome (IBS).

23. (*Continued*)
Laboratory data include white blood cell (WBC) count 8000/μL, hematocrit 32%, platelets 210,000/μL, and erythrocyte sedimentation rate (ESR) of 44 mm/h. Stool studies show the presence of lactoferrin but no blood. Which intervention is appropriate at this time?

A. Antidepressants
B. Ciprofloxacin
C. Colonoscopy
D. Reassurance and patient counseling
E. Stool bulking agents

24. After a careful history and physical, and a cost-effective workup, you have diagnosed a 24-year-old female patient with irritable bowel syndrome. What other condition would you reasonably expect to find in this patient?

A. Abnormal brain anatomy
B. Autoimmune disease
C. History of sexually transmitted diseases
D. Psychiatric diagnosis
E. Sensory hypersensitivity to peripheral stimuli

25. A 78-year-old woman is admitted to the hospital with fever, loss of appetite, and left lower quadrant pain. She is not constipated, but has not moved her bowels recently. Laboratory examination is notable for an elevated WBC count. These symptoms began approximately 3 days ago and have steadily worsened. Which of the following statements regarding the use of radiologic imaging to evaluate her condition is true?

A. Air-fluid levels are commonly seen on plain abdominal films.
B. Barium enema should not be performed because of the risk of perforation.
C. Lower gastrointestinal bleeding will likely be visualized on CT angiography.
D. A thickened colonic wall is not required on CT for the diagnosis of her likely condition.
E. Ultrasound of the pelvis is the best modality to visualize the likely pathologic process.

26. Which of the following patients is *MOST* appropriate for surgical management of their acute diverticulitis?

A. A 45-year-old woman with rheumatoid arthritis treated with infliximab and prednisone.
B. A 63-year-old woman with diverticulitis in the descending colon and a distal stricture.

26. (*Continued*)
C. A 70-year-old woman with end-stage renal disease with colonic wall thickening of 8 mm on CT scan.
D. A 77-year-old man with two episodes of diverticulitis in the past 2 years.
E. None of the above patients requires surgical management.

27. A 67-year-old man is evaluated in the emergency department for blood in the toilet bowl after moving his bowels. Blood was also present on the toilet paper after wiping. He reports straining and recent constipation. He has a history of systemic hypertension and hyperlipidemia. Vital signs are normal and he is not orthostatic. Anoscopy shows external hemorrhoids. Hematocrit is normal and bleeding does not recur during his 6-hour emergency department stay. Which of the following is the most appropriate management?

A. Ciprofloxacin and metronidazole
B. Cortisone suppositories, fiber supplementation
C. Hemorrhoidal banding
D. Operative hemorrhoidectomy
E. Upper endoscopy

28. Which of the following statements regarding anorectal abscess is true?

A. Anorectal abscess is more common in diabetic patients.
B. Anorectal abscess is more common in women.
C. Difficulty voiding is uncommon and should prompt further evaluation of anorectal abscess.
D. Examination in the operating room under anesthesia is required for adequate exploration in most cases.
E. The peak incidence is the seventh decade of life.

29. An 88-year-old woman is brought to your clinic by her family because she has become increasingly socially withdrawn. The patient lives alone and has been reluctant to visit or be visited by her family. Family members, including seven children, also note a foul odor in her apartment and on her person. She has not had any weight loss. Alone in the examining room, she only complains of hemorrhoids. On mental status examination, she has signs of depression. Which of the following interventions is most appropriate at this time?

A. Head CT scan
B. Initiate treatment with an antidepressant medication
C. Physical examination including genitourinary and rectal examination

29. (*Continued*)
   D. Screening for occult malignancy
   E. Serum thyroid-stimulating hormone

30. A 37-year-old woman presents with abdominal pain, anorexia, and fever of 4 days' duration. The abdominal pain is mostly in the left lower quadrant. Her past medical history is significant for irritable bowel syndrome, diverticulitis treated 6 months ago, and status post-appendectomy. Since her last bout of diverticulitis she has increased her fiber intake and avoids nuts and popcorn. Review of systems is positive for weight loss, daily chills and sweats, and "bubbles" in her urinary stream. Her temperature is 39.6°C. A limited CT scan shows thickened colonic wall (5 mm) and inflammation with pericolic fat stranding. She is admitted with a presumptive diagnosis of diverticulitis. What is the most appropriate management for this patient?

   A. A trial of rifaximin and a high-fiber diet
   B. Bowel rest, ciprofloxacin, metronidazole, and ampicillin
   C. Examination of the urine sediment
   D. Measurement of 24-hour urine protein
   E. Surgical removal of the affected colon and exploration

31. An 85-year-old woman is brought to a local emergency department by her family. She has been complaining of abdominal pain off and on for several days, but this morning states that this is the worst pain of her life. She is able to describe a sharp, stabbing pain in her abdomen. Her family reports that she has not been eating and seems to have no appetite. She has a past medical history of atrial fibrillation and hypercholesterolemia. She has had two episodes of vomiting and in the ER experiences diarrhea that is hemoccult positive. On examination she is afebrile, with a heart rate of 105 beats/min and blood pressure of 111/69 mmHg. Her abdomen is mildly distended and she has hypoactive bowel sounds. She does not exhibit rebound tenderness or guarding. She is admitted for further management. Several hours after admission she becomes unresponsive. Blood pressure is difficult to obtain and at best approximation is 60/40 mmHg. She has a rigid abdomen. Surgery is called and the patient is taken for emergent laparotomy. She is found to have acute mesenteric ischemia. Which of the following is true regarding this diagnosis?

   A. Mortality for this condition is greater than 50%.
   B. Risk factors include low-fiber diet and obesity.
   C. The "gold standard" for diagnosis is CT scan of the abdomen.

31. (*Continued*)
   D. The lack of acute abdominal signs in this case is unusual for mesenteric ischemia.
   E. The splanchnic circulation is poorly collateralized.

32. All of the following are potential causes of appendix obstruction and appendicitis EXCEPT:

   A. Ascaris infection
   B. Carcinoid tumor
   C. Cholelithiasis
   D. Fecalith
   E. Measles infection

33. Which of the following organisms is most likely to be causative in acute appendicitis?

   A. *Clostridium* species
   B. *Escherichia coli*
   C. *Mycobacterium tuberculosis*
   D. *Staphylococcus aureus*
   E. *Yersinia enterocolitica*

34. A 32-year-old woman is evaluated in the emergency department for abdominal pain. She reports a vague loss of appetite for the past day and has had progressively severe abdominal pain, initially at her umbilicus, but now localized to her right lower quadrant. The pain is crampy. She has not moved her bowels or vomited. She reports that she is otherwise healthy and has had no sick contact. Exam is notable for a temperature of 100.7°F, heart rate of 105 beats/min, and otherwise normal vital signs. Her abdomen is tender in the right lower quadrant and pelvic examination is normal. Urine pregnancy test is negative. Which of the following imaging modalities is most likely to confirm her diagnosis?

   A. CT of the abdomen without contrast
   B. Colonoscopy
   C. Pelvic ultrasound
   D. Plain film of the abdomen
   E. Ultrasound of the abdomen

35. A 38-year-old male is seen in the urgent care center with several hours of severe abdominal pain. His symptoms began suddenly, but he reports several months of pain in the epigastrium after eating, with a resultant 10-lb weight loss. He takes no medications besides over-the-counter antacids and has no other medical problems or habits. On physical examination temperature is 38.0°C (100.4°F), pulse 130 beats/min, respiratory rate 24 breaths/min, and blood pressure 110/50 mmHg. His abdomen has

35. (*Continued*)

absent bowel sounds and is rigid with involuntary guarding diffusely. A plain film of the abdomen is obtained and shows free air under the diaphragm. Which of the following is most likely to be found in the operating room?

A. Necrotic bowel
B. Necrotic pancreas
C. Perforated duodenal ulcer
D. Perforated gallbladder
E. Perforated gastric ulcer

36. Which of the following is the source of the peritonitis of the patient in question 35?

A. Bile
B. Blood
C. Foreign body
D. Gastric contents
E. Pancreatic enzymes

37. Enteric pathogens can produce diarrheal illness through a variety of mechanisms that lead to specific clinical characteristics. All of the following are characteristics of diarrhea caused by *Vibrio cholerae* EXCEPT:

A. Disease localized to the proximal small intestine
B. Fecal leukocytes
C. Fecal lactoferrin
D. Toxin production
E. Watery diarrhea

38. A 46-year-old woman travels to a rural area of Guatemala. Three days after arrival, she develops watery diarrhea with severe abdominal cramping. She reports two unformed stools daily for the past 2 days. She has noticed no blood in the stool and has not experienced a fever. What is the most likely cause of the patient's illness?

A. *Campylobacter jejuni*
B. Enterotoxigenic *Escherichia coli*
C. *Giardia lamblia*
D. Norovirus
E. *Shigella* spp.

39. For the case above, which of the following treatments would you recommend?

A. Azithromycin 10 mg/kg on day 1 with 5 mg/kg on days 2 and 3 if the diarrhea persists
B. Ciprofloxacin 500 mg three times daily for 5 days
C. Ciprofloxacin 750 mg once

39. (*Continued*)

D. Loperamide 4 mg once followed by 2 mg after passage of each unformed stool
E. Oral rehydration therapy only

40. Two hours after attending a company picnic, many individuals who attended the picnic develop an acute gastrointestinal illness. Food poisoning caused by *Staphylococcus aureus* is suspected. All of the following characteristics would be a common feature of food poisoning due to this organism EXCEPT:

A. Abdominal cramping
B. Diarrhea
C. Fever
D. Vomiting

41. You are the on-call physician practicing in a suburban community. You receive a call from a 28-year-old woman with a past medical history significant for sarcoidosis who is currently taking no medications. She is complaining of an acute onset of crampy diffuse abdominal pain and multiple episodes of emesis that are nonbloody. She has not had any lightheadedness with standing or loss of consciousness. When questioned further, the patient states that her last meal was 5 hours previously, when she joined her friends for lunch at a local Chinese restaurant. She ate from the buffet, which included multiple poultry dishes and fried rice. What should you do for this patient?

A. Ask the patient to go to the nearest emergency department for resuscitation with IV fluids.
B. Initiate antibiotic therapy with azithromycin.
C. Reassure the patient that her illness is self-limited and no further treatment is necessary if she can maintain adequate hydration.
D. Refer the patient for CT to assess for appendicitis.
E. Refer the patient for admission for IV vancomycin and ceftriaxone because of her immunocompromised state resulting from sarcoidosis.

42. Which of the following is a common manifestation of *Clostridium difficile* infection?

A. Fever
B. Nonbloody diarrhea
C. Adynamic ileus
D. Recurrence after therapy
E. All of the above

43. All of the following patients should be treated for *Clostridium difficile* infection EXCEPT:

43. *(Continued)*

    A. A 57-year-old nursing home resident with diarrhea for 2 weeks and pseudomembranes found on colonoscopy with no evidence of toxin A or B in the stool

    B. A 63-year-old woman with fever, leukocytosis, adynamic ileus, and a positive PCR for *C. difficile* in the stool

    C. A 68-year-old woman with recent course of antibiotics admitted to the medical intensive care unit after presentation to the emergency department with abdominal pain and diarrhea. She was found to have severe abdominal tenderness with absent bowel sounds, systemic hypotension, and colonic wall thickening on CT of the abdomen.

    D. A 75-year-old woman who received recent therapy with amoxicillin for an upper respiratory tract infection and now has two loose bowel movements per day for the past 3 days

44. A 78-year-old woman with dementia has been living in a nursing home for 5 years. She was been seen by her primary care provider for evaluation of diarrhea 4 weeks ago. At that time, a stool sample was positive by PCR for *Clostridium difficile*, and she was treated with oral metronidazole with some improvement in her symptoms. However, she has had five loose bowel movements per day starting 4 days ago and now has abdominal tenderness. Stool PCR remains positive. Which of the following is the most appropriate therapy?

    A. Fecal transplantation
    B. IV immunoglobulin
    C. Oral metronidazole
    D. Oral nitazoxanide
    E. Oral vancomycin

45. Which of the following antibiotics has the weakest association with the development of *Clostridium difficile*–associated disease?

    A. Ceftriaxone
    B. Ciprofloxacin
    C. Clindamycin
    D. Moxifloxacin
    E. Piperacillin/tazobactam

46. A 45-year-old man with a history of alcoholism and presumed cirrhosis is brought to the emergency department by his friend complaining of 2 to 3 days of increasing lethargy and confusion. He has not consumed alcohol in the past 2 years. He currently takes no medications and works at home as a video game designer. He has no risk factors for HIV.

46. *(Continued)*

He was referred by his primary care physician for a liver transplant evaluation and is scheduled to begin his evaluation next month. His vital signs included blood pressure of 90/60 mmHg, heart rate of 105 beats/min, temperature of 38.5°C, and respiratory rate of 10 breaths/min with O_2 saturation of 97% on room air. He is somnolent but is able to answer questions accurately. His skin is notable for many spider telangiectasias and palmar erythema. He has a distended diffusely tender abdomen with a positive fluid wave. Paracentesis reveals slightly cloudy fluid with WBC 1000/μL and 40% neutrophils. His blood pressure increases to 100/65 mmHg, and his heart rate decreases to 95 beats/min after 1 L of intravenous fluids. Which of the following statements regarding his condition and treatment is true?

    A. Fever is present in more than 50% of cases.
    B. Initial empiric therapy should include metronidazole or clindamycin for anaerobes.
    C. The diagnosis of primary (spontaneous) bacterial peritonitis is not confirmed because the percentage of neutrophils in the peritoneal fluid is less than 50%.
    D. The mostly causative organism for his condition is *Enterococcus*.
    E. The yield of peritoneal fluid cultures for diagnosis is greater than 90%.

47. A 48-year-old woman with a history of end-stage renal disease caused by diabetic renal disease is admitted to the hospital with 1 day of abdominal pain and fever. She has been on continuous ambulatory peritoneal dialysis (CAPD) for the past 6 months. She reports that for the past day she has had poor return of dialysate and is feeling bloated. She has had complications from her diabetes, including retinopathy and peripheral neuropathy. She is uncomfortable but not toxic. Her vital signs include a temperature of 38.8°C, blood pressure of 130/65 mmHg, heart rate of 105 beats/min, and respiratory rate of 15 breaths/min with room air O_2 saturation of 98%. Her abdomen is slightly distended and diffusely tender with rebound tenderness. A sample of dialysate reveals WBC 400/μL with 80% neutrophils. Empiric intraperitoneal antibiotic therapy should include:

    A. Cefoxitin
    B. Fluconazole
    C. Metronidazole
    D. Vancomycin
    E. Voriconazole

48. A 77-year-old man presents to the hospital with 1 week of fever, chills, nausea, and right upper quadrant pain. His temperature is 39°C, and he appears toxic. His blood pressure is 110/70 mmHg, heart rate is 110 beats/min, and respiratory rate is 22 breaths/min with room air O_2 saturation 92%. He has diminished breath sounds at the right base and diffuse tenderness in the right upper quadrant. He has a history of cholelithiasis but has declined elective cholecystectomy. His CT scan of the abdomen is shown in **Figure 48**. Which of the following statements regarding his condition or therapy is true?

FIGURE 48

A. Concomitant bacteremia is rare (<10%).

B. He should receive empiric antibiotics targeting *Candida* species.

C. He should receive empiric antibiotics targeting anaerobic organisms.

D. He should undergo percutaneous drainage.

E. His serum alkaline phosphatase is most likely normal.

49. A 41-year-old man with hepatitis C–associated ascites presents with acute abdominal pain. Physical examination is notable for temperature of 38.3°C, heart rate of 115 beats/min, blood pressure of 88/48 mmHg, respiratory rate of 16 breaths/min, and oxygen saturation of 99% on room air. The patient is in moderate discomfort and is lying still. He is alert and oriented. His lungs are clear. Cardiac examination is unremarkable. His abdomen is diffusely tender with distant bowel sounds, mild guarding, and no rebound tenderness. Laboratory studies reveal a leukocyte count of 11,630/μL with 94% neutrophils, hematocrit of 29%, and platelet count of 24,000/μL. Paracentesis reveals 658 PMNs/μL, total protein of 1.2 g/dL, and glucose of 24 mg/dL and Gram stain showing gram-negative rods, gram-positive cocci in chains, gram-positive rods, and yeast forms. All of the following are indicated EXCEPT:

49. (*Continued*)

A. Abdominal radiograph

B. Broad-spectrum antibiotics

C. Drotrecogin alfa

D. Intravenous fluid

E. Surgical consultation

50. *Helicobacter pylori* colonization increases the odds ratio of developing all of the following conditions EXCEPT:

A. Duodenal ulcer disease

B. Esophageal adenocarcinoma

C. Gastric adenocarcinoma

D. Gastric mucosa-associated lymphoid tissue (MALT) lymphoma

E. Peptic ulcer disease

51. One month after receiving a 14-day course of omeprazole, clarithromycin, and amoxicillin for *Helicobacter pylori*–associated gastric ulcer disease, a 44-year-old woman still has mild dyspepsia and pain after meals. What is the appropriate next step in management?

A. Empirical long-term proton pump inhibitor therapy

B. Endoscopy with biopsy to rule out gastric adeno-carcinoma

C. *H. pylori* serology testing

D. Second-line therapy for *H. pylori* with omeprazole, bismuth subsalicylate, tetracycline, and metronidazole

E. Urea breath test

52. In the developed world, seroprevalence of *Helicobacter pylori* infection is currently

A. Decreasing

B. Increasing

C. Staying the same

D. Unknown

53. A 42-year-old man with heme-positive stools and a history of epigastric pain is found to have a duodenal ulcer that is biopsy-proven positive for *H. pylori*. All of the following are effective eradication regimens EXCEPT:

A. Amoxicillin and levofloxacin for 10 days

B. Omeprazole, clarithromycin, and metronidazole for 14 days

C. Omeprazole, clarithromycin, and amoxicillin for 14 days

D. Omeprazole, bismuth, tetracycline, and metronidazole for 14 days

E. Omeprazole and amoxicillin for 5 days followed by omeprazole, clarithromycin, and tinidazole for 5 days

54. Five healthy college roommates develop a rapid (<8 hours) onset of abdominal pain, cramping, fever to 38.5°C, vomiting, and copious nonbloody diarrhea while camping. They immediately return for hydration and diagnosis. A stool culture grows *Salmonella enteritidis*. All of the statements regarding their clinical syndrome are true EXCEPT:

A. Antibiotic therapy is not indicated.
B. Bacteremia occurs in fewer than 10% of cases.
C. The most likely source was undercooked eggs.
D. There is no vaccine available for this illness.
E. They have enteric (typhoid) fever.

55. Two days after returning from a trip to Thailand, a 36-year-old woman develops severe crampy abdominal pain, fever to 40°C, nausea, and malaise. The next day, she begins having bloody mucopurulent diarrhea with worsening abdominal pain and continued fever. She reports she was in Bangkok during monsoonal flooding and ate fresh food from stalls. A stool examination shows many neutrophils, and culture grows *Shigella flexneri*. Which of the following statements regarding her clinical syndrome is true?

A. An effective vaccine for travelers is available.
B. Antibiotic therapy prolongs the carrier state and should not be administered unless she develops bacteremia.
C. Antimotility agents are effective in reducing the risk of dehydration.
D. Ciprofloxacin is recommended therapy.
E. Her disease can be distinguished from illness caused by *Campylobacter jejuni* on clinical grounds by the presence of fever.

56. A previously healthy 32-year-old graduate student at the University of Wisconsin describes 1 to 2 days of fever, myalgia, and headache followed by abdominal pain and diarrhea. He has experienced up to 10 bowel movements over the past day. He has noted mucus and blood in the stool. The patient notes that 3 days ago, he was at a church barbecue, where several people contracted a diarrheal illness. He has not traveled in more than 6 months and has no history of GI illness. Physical examination is unremarkable except for a temperature of 38.8°C and diffuse abdominal tenderness. Laboratory findings are notable only for a slightly elevated leukocyte count and an elevated erythrocyte sedimentation rate. Wright's stain of a fecal sample reveals the presence of neutrophils. Colonoscopy reveals inflamed mucosa. Biopsy of an affected area discloses mucosal

56. (*Continued*)
infiltration with neutrophils, monocytes, and eosinophils; epithelial damage, including loss of mucus; glandular degeneration; and crypt abscesses. Which of the following microbial pathogens is most likely to be responsible for his illness?

A. *Campylobacter*
B. *Escherichia coli*
C. Norwalk agent
D. Rotavirus
E. *Staphylococcus aureus*

57. In the patient described in question 56, which of the following is recommended therapy?

A. Azithromycin
B. Ceftriaxone
C. Lomotil only for symptoms
D. Metronidazole
E. Tinidazole

58. While working for a relief mission in Haiti, you are asked to see a 19-year-old patient with profuse watery diarrhea as shown in **Figure 58**. The patient is mildly hypotensive and tachycardic and is afebrile. There is no abdominal tenderness. All of the statements regarding this patient's illness are true EXCEPT:

FIGURE 58

58. (*Continued*)
Antibiotic therapy shortens the duration of disease and hastens clearance of the organism from stool.
A. Morbidity or death is mediated by bacteremia and multiorgan failure.
B. Point of care antigen testing is available.
C. The diarrhea is toxin mediated.
D. Vaccines with moderate efficacy are available outside the United States.

59. All of the following statements regarding Norwalk virus gastroenteritis are true EXCEPT:

A. Fever is common.
B. Incubation period is typically 5 to 7 days.
C. Infection is common worldwide.
D. It is a major cause of nonbacterial diarrhea outbreaks in the United States.
E. Transmission is typically fecal–oral.

60. All of the following statements regarding rotavirus gastroenteritis are true EXCEPT:

A. Fever occurs in more than 25% of cases.
B. Inflammatory diarrhea distinguishes rotaviral illness from Norwalk agent gastroenteritis.
C. It is a major cause of diarrheal death among children in the developing world.
D. Nausea is common.
E. Vaccination is recommended for all children in the United States.

61. A 45-year-old migrant worker originally from Mexico is evaluated for right upper quadrant pain, fever, and hepatic tenderness. He reports no diarrhea or bloody stool. He is found to have a large hepatic abscess on CT scan of the abdomen. Of note, he has been in the United States for approximately 10 years and was well until approximately 10 days ago. Which of the following tests can be used to confirm the diagnosis?

A. Examination of stool for trophozoites
B. Liver biopsy
C. PCR of stool for *Campylobacter* spp.
D. Response to empiric trial of iodoquinol
E. Serologic test for antibody to *E. histolytica*

62. Which of the following intestinal protozoal infections can be diagnosed with stool ova and parasite examination?

A. *Cryptosporidium* spp.
B. *Cyclospora* spp.
C. *Giardia* spp.

62. (*Continued*)
D. *Isospora* spp.
E. *Microsporidia* spp.
F. All of the above

63. A 17-year-old woman presents to the clinic complaining of vaginal itchiness and malodorous discharge. She is sexually active with multiple partners, and she is interested in getting tested for sexually transmitted diseases. A wet-mount microscopic examination is performed, and trichomonal parasites are identified. Which of the following statements regarding trichomoniasis is true?

A. A majority of women are asymptomatic.
B. No treatment is necessary because the disease is self-limited.
C. The patient's sexual partner need not be treated.
D. Trichomoniasis can only be spread sexually.
E. Trichomoniasis is 100% sensitive to metronidazole

64. A 19-year-old college student presents to the emergency department with crampy abdominal pain and watery diarrhea that has worsened over 3 days. He recently returned from a volunteer trip to Mexico. He has no past medical history and felt well throughout the trip. Stool examination shows small cysts containing four nuclei, and stool antigen immunoassay is positive for *Giardia* spp. Which of the following is a recommend treatment regimen for this patient?

A. Albendazole
B. Clindamycin
C. Giardiasis is self-limited and requires no antibiotic therapy
D. Paromomycin
E. Tinidazole

65. A 28-year-old woman is brought to the hospital because of abdominal pain, weight loss, and dehydration. She has been diagnosed with HIV/AIDS for the past 2 years with a history of oral candidiasis and pneumocystis pneumonia. She reports voluminous watery diarrhea over the past 2 weeks. Because of medical nonadherence, she has not taken any antiretroviral therapy. Routine stool ova and parasite examination is normal, but stool antigen testing reveals *Cryptosporidium* spp. Which of the following is the recommended therapy?

A. Metronidazole
B. Nitazoxanide
C. No therapy recommended because the diarrhea is self-limited.

65. (*Continued*)

    D. No effective specific therapy is available.

    E. Tinidazole

66. While attending the University of Georgia, a group of friends go on a 5-day canoeing and camping trip in rural southern Georgia. A few weeks later, one of the campers develops a serpiginous, raised, pruritic, erythematous eruption on the buttocks. *Strongyloides* larvae are found in his stool. Three of his companions, who are asymptomatic, are also found to have *Strongyloides* larvae in their stool. Which of the following is indicated in the asymptomatic carriers?

    A. Fluconazole

    B. Ivermectin

    C. Mebendazole

    D. Mefloquine

    E. Treatment only for symptomatic illness

67. All of the following are clinical manifestations of *Ascaris lumbricoides* infection EXCEPT:

    A. Asymptomatic carriage

    B. Fever, headache, photophobia, nuchal rigidity, and eosinophilia

    C. Nonproductive cough and pleurisy with eosinophilia

    D. Right upper quadrant pain and fever

    E. Small bowel obstruction

68. A 21-year-old college student in Mississippi comes to student health to ask advice about treatment for *Ascaris* infection. He is an education major and works 1 day a week in an elementary school, where a number of the students were recently diagnosed with ascariasis over the past 3 months. He feels well and reports being asymptomatic. A stool O&P reveals characteristic *Ascaris* eggs. Which of the following should you recommend?

    A. Albendazole

    B. Diethylcarbamazine (DEC)

    C. Fluconazole

    D. Metronidazole

    E. Vancomycin

69. A 38-year-old woman presents to the emergency department with severe abdominal pain. She has no past medical or surgical history. She recalls no recent history of abdominal discomfort, diarrhea, melena, bright red blood per rectum, nausea, or vomiting before this acute episode. She ate ceviche (lime-marinated raw fish) at a Peruvian restaurant 3 hours before presentation. On examination,

69. (*Continued*)

she is in terrible distress and has dry heaves. Her temperature is 37.6°C, heart rate is 128 beats/min, and blood pressure is 174/92 mmHg. Examination is notable for an extremely tender abdomen with guarding and rebound tenderness. Bowel sounds are present and hyperactive. Rectal examination findings are normal, and Guaiac test result is negative. The pelvic examination is unremarkable. The white blood cell count is 6738/μL and hematocrit is 42%. A complete metabolic panel and lipase and amylase levels are all within normal limits. CT of the abdomen shows no abnormality. What is the next step in her management?

    A. CT angiogram of the abdomen

    B. Pelvic ultrasonography

    C. Proton pump inhibitor therapy and observation

    D. Right upper quadrant ultrasonography

    E. Upper endoscopy

70. Which of the following is the most common symptom or sign of liver disease?

    A. Fatigue

    B. Itching

    C. Jaundice

    D. Nausea

    E. Right upper quadrant pain

71. In women, what is the average amount of reported daily alcohol intake that is associated with the development of chronic liver disease?

    A. 1 drink

    B. 2 drinks

    C. 3 drinks

    D. 6 drinks

    E. 12 drinks

72. Elevations in all of the following laboratory studies would be indicative of liver disease EXCEPT:

    A. 5′-Nucleotidase

    B. Aspartate aminotransferase

    C. Conjugated bilirubin

    D. Unconjugated bilirubin

    E. Urine bilirubin

73. A 26-year-old male resident is noticed by his attending physician to have yellow eyes after his 24-hour call period. When asked, the resident states he has no medical history, but on occasion he has thought he might have mild jaundice when he is stressed or has more than 4–5 alcoholic drinks. He never

73. (*Continued*)

sought medical treatment because he was uncertain, and his eyes would return fully to normal within 2 days. He denies nausea, abdominal pain, dark urine, light-colored stools, pruritus, or weight loss. On examination he has a body mass index of 20.1 kg/m², and his vital signs are normal. Scleral icterus is present. There are no stigmata of chronic liver disease. The patient's abdomen is soft and nontender. The liver span is 8 cm to percussion. The liver edge is smooth and palpable only with deep inspiration. The spleen is not palpable. Laboratory examinations are normal except for a total bilirubin of 3.0 mg/dL. Direct bilirubin is 0.2 mg/dL. Aspartate aminotransferase (AST), alanine aminotransferase (ALT), and alkaline phosphatase are normal. Hematocrit, lactate dehydrogenase (LDH), and haptoglobin are normal. Which of the following is the most likely diagnosis?

A. Autoimmune hemolytic anemia
B. Crigler-Najjar syndrome type 1
C. Choledocholithiasis
D. Dubin-Johnson syndrome
E. Gilbert's syndrome

74. What is the next step in the evaluation and management of the patient in question 73?

A. Genotype studies
B. Peripheral blood smear
C. Prednisone
D. Reassurance
E. Right upper quadrant ultrasound

75. A 34-year-old man presents to the physician complaining of yellow eyes. For the past week, he has felt ill with decreased oral intake, low-grade fevers (~100°F), fatigue, nausea, and occasional vomiting. With the onset of jaundice, he has noticed pain in his right upper quadrant. He currently uses marijuana and ecstasy, and has a prior history of injection drug use with cocaine. He has no other past medical history, but he was unable to donate blood 4 years previously for reasons that he cannot recall. His social history is remarkable for working as a veterinary assistant. On sexual history, he reports five male sexual partners over the past 6 months. He does not consistently use condoms. On physical examination, he appears ill and has obvious jaundice with scleral icterus. His liver is 15 cm to percussion and is palpable 6 cm below the right costal margin. The edge is smooth and tender to palpation. The spleen is not enlarged. There are no stigmata

75. (*Continued*)

of chronic liver disease. His AST is 1232 U/L, ALT is 1560 U/L, alkaline phosphatase is 394 U/L, total bilirubin is 13.4 mg/dL, and direct bilirubin is 12.2 mg/dL. His INR is 2.3, and aPTT is 52 seconds. Hepatitis serologies are sent and reveal the following:

Hepatitis A IgM negative
Hepatitis A IgG negative
Hepatitis B core IgM positive
Hepatitis B core IgG negative
Hepatitis B surface antigen positive
Hepatitis B surface antibody negative
Hepatitis B e antigen positive
Hepatitis B e antibody negative
Hepatitis C antibody positive

What is the cause of the patient's current clinical presentation?

A. Acute hepatitis A infection
B. Acute hepatitis B infection
C. Acute hepatitis C infection
D. Chronic hepatitis B infection
E. Drug-induced hepatitis

76. In the scenario described in question 75, what would be the best approach to prevent development of chronic hepatitis?

A. Administration of anti-hepatitis A virus IgG.
B. Administration of lamivudine.
C. Administration of pegylated interferon α plus ribavirin.
D. Administration of prednisone beginning at a dose of 1 mg/kg daily.
E. Do nothing and observe, as 99% of individuals with this disease recover.

77. Which of the following viral causes of acute hepatitis is most likely to cause fulminant hepatitis in a pregnant woman?

A. Hepatitis A
B. Hepatitis B
C. Hepatitis C
D. Hepatitis D
E. Hepatitis E

78. A 16-year-old woman had visited your clinic 1 month ago with jaundice, vomiting, malaise, and anorexia. Two other family members were ill with similar symptoms. Based on viral serologies, including a positive anti-hepatitis A virus (HAV) IgM, a diagnosis of hepatitis A was made. The patient was

78. (*Continued*)

treated conservatively, and 1 week after first presenting, she appeared to have made a full recovery. She returns to your clinic today complaining of the same symptoms she had 1 month ago. She is jaundiced, and an initial panel of laboratory tests returns elevated transaminases. Which of the following offers the best explanation of what has occurred in this patient?

A. Coinfection with hepatitis C
B. Inappropriate treatment of initial infection
C. Incorrect initial diagnosis; this patient likely has hepatitis B
D. Reinfection with hepatitis A
E. Relapse of hepatitis A

79. A 26-year-old woman presents to your clinic and is interested in getting pregnant. She seeks your advice regarding vaccines she should obtain, and in particular asks about the hepatitis B vaccine. She works as a receptionist for a local business, denies alcohol or illicit drug use, and is in a monogamous relationship. Which of the following is true regarding hepatitis B vaccination?

A. Hepatitis B vaccine consists of two IM doses 1 month apart.
B. Only patients with defined risk factors need to be vaccinated.
C. Pregnancy is not a contraindication to the hepatitis B vaccine.
D. This patient's hepatitis serologies should be checked before vaccination.
E. Vaccination should not be administered to children under 2 years old.

80. An 18-year-old man presents to a rural clinic with nausea, vomiting, anorexia, abdominal discomfort, myalgias, and jaundice. He describes occasional alcohol use and is sexually active. He describes using heroin and cocaine "a few times in the past." He works as a short-order cook in a local restaurant. He has lost 15.5 kg since his last visit to the clinic and appears emaciated and ill. On examination he is noted to have icteric sclerae and a palpable, tender liver below the right costal margin. In regard to acute hepatitis, which of the following is true?

A. A distinction between viral etiologies cannot be made using clinical criteria alone.
B. Based on age and risk factors, he is likely to have hepatitis B infection.
C. He does not have hepatitis E virus, as this infects only pregnant women.

80. (*Continued*)

D. This patient cannot have hepatitis C because his presentation is too acute.
E. This patient does not have hepatitis A because his presentation is too fulminant.

81. A 36-year-old male presents with fatigue and tea-colored urine for 5 days. Physical examination reveals jaundice and tender hepatomegaly, but is otherwise unremarkable. Laboratories are remarkable for an aspartate aminotransferase (AST) of 2400 U/L and an alanine aminotransferase (ALT) of 2640 U/L. Alkaline phosphatase is 210 U/L. Total bilirubin is 8.6 mg/dL. Which of the following diagnoses is least likely to cause this clinical picture and these laboratory abnormalities?

A. Acute hepatitis A infection
B. Acute hepatitis B infection
C. Acute hepatitis C infection
D. Acetaminophen ingestion
E. Budd-Chiari syndrome

82. Which of the following drugs has a direct toxic effect on hepatocytes?

A. Acetaminophen
B. Chlorpromazine
C. Halothane
D. Isoniazid
E. Rosuvastatin

83. A 32-year-old woman is admitted to the intensive care unit following an overdose of acetaminophen with coingestion of alcohol. She was known to be alert and interactive about 4 hours before her presentation when she had a fight with her boyfriend who then left the home. When he returned 6 hours later, he found an empty bottle of acetaminophen 500 mg capsules as well as an empty vodka bottle. The exact number of pills in the bottle is unknown but the full bottle held as much as 50 capsules. The patient was unresponsive and had vomited, so her boyfriend called 911. Upon arrival to the emergency department, the patient is stuporous. Her vital signs are as follows: pulse 109 beats/min, respiratory rate 20 breaths/min, blood pressure 96/52 mmHg, and oxygen saturation 95% on room air. Her examination shows mild nonspecific abdominal pain with palpation. The liver is not enlarged. Her initial laboratory values show a normal CBC, and normal electrolytes and kidney function. The AST is 68 U/L, ALT is 46 U/L, alkaline phosphatase is 110 U/L, and total bilirubin is 1.2 mg/dL. Glucose and

83. (*Continued*)

coagulation studies are normal. The serum alcohol level is 210 g/dL. The acetaminophen level is 350 μg/mL. What is the most appropriate next step in the treatment of this patient?

A. Administration of activated charcoal or cholestyramine.
B. Administration of N-acetylcysteine 140 mg/kg followed by 70 mg/kg every 4 hours for a total of 15–20 doses.
C. Continued monitoring of liver function, glucose, and coagulation studies every 4 hours with administration of N-acetylcysteine if these begin to change.
D. Do nothing as normal liver function tests and coagulation studies are indicative of only a minor ingestion.
E. Initiate hemodialysis for toxin clearance.

84. A 38-year-old woman is evaluated for elevated transaminase levels that were identified during routine laboratory testing for life insurance. She is originally from Thailand and immigrated to the United States 10 years previously. She has been married to an American for the past 12 years, having met him while he was living abroad for business. She previously worked in Thailand as a deputy tourism minister for the government, but is not currently employed. She has no significant past medical history. She had one uncomplicated pregnancy at the age of 22. When queried about risk factors for liver disease, she denies alcohol intake or drug abuse. She has never had a blood transfusion. She recalls an episode of jaundice that she did not seek evaluation for about 15 years ago. It resolved spontaneously. She currently feels well, and her husband wished to have her added to his life insurance policy. There are no stigmata of chronic liver disease. Her laboratory studies reveal an AST of 346 U/L, ALT of 412 U/L, alkaline phosphatase of 98 U/L, and total bilirubin of 1.5 mg/dL. Further workup includes the following viral studies: hepatitis A IgG +, hepatitis B surface antigen +, hepatitis B e antigen +, anti-HBV core IgG +, and hepatitis C IgG negative. The HBV DNA level is 4.8×10^4 IU/mL. What treatment do you recommend for this patient?

A. Entecavir.
B. Pegylated interferon.
C. Pegylated interferon plus entecavir.
D. No treatment is necessary.
E. Either A or C.

85. A 46-year-old man is known to have chronic hepatitis C virus (HCV) infection. He is a former IV drug user for more than 20 years who has been

85. (*Continued*)

abstinent from drug use for 1 year. He is asking whether he should receive treatment for his HCV infection. He has a prior history of hepatitis B virus (HBV) and has positive antibody to HBV surface antigen. He was treated for tricuspid valve endocarditis 3 years previously. He has no other medical history. He does not know when he acquired HCV. His laboratory studies show a positive HCV IgG antibody with a viral load of greater than 1 million copies. The virus is genotype 1. His AST is 62 U/L, and his ALT is 54 U/L. He undergoes liver biopsy, which demonstrates a moderate degree of bridging fibrosis. What do you tell him regarding his likelihood of progression and possibilities regarding treatment?

A. As he is infected with genotype 1, the likelihood of response to pegylated interferon and ribavirin is less than 40%.
B. Following 12 weeks of treatment, the expected viral load should be undetectable.
C. Given his normal liver enzymes on laboratory testing, he is unlikely to develop progressive liver injury.
D. If the patient elects to undergo treatment, the best regimen for individuals with genotype 1 disease is pegylated interferon and ribavirin for 24 weeks.
E. The presence of bridging fibrosis on liver biopsy is the most predictive factor of the development of cirrhosis over the next 10–20 years.

86. A 34-year-old woman is evaluated for fatigue, malaise, arthralgias, and a 10-lb weight loss over the past 6–8 weeks. She has no past medical history. Since feeling poorly, she has taken approximately one or two tablets of acetaminophen 500 mg daily. On physical examination, her temperature is 100.2°F, respiratory rate is 18 breaths/min, blood pressure is 100/48 mmHg, heart rate is 92 beats/min, and oxygen saturation is 96% on room air. She has scleral icterus. Her liver edge is palpable 3 cm below the right costal margin. It is smooth and tender. The spleen is not enlarged. She has mild synovitis in the small joints of her hands. Her AST is 542 U/L, ALT is 657 U/L, alkaline phosphatase is 102 U/L, total bilirubin is 5.3 mg/dL, and direct bilirubin is 4.8 mg/dL. Which of the following tests would be LEAST likely to be positive in this diagnosis?

A. Antinuclear antibodies in a homogeneous pattern
B. Anti-liver/kidney microsomal antibodies
C. Antimitochondrial antibodies
D. Hypergammaglobulinemia
E. Rheumatoid factor

87. In chronic hepatitis B virus (HBV) infection, the presence of hepatitis B e antigen (HBeAg) signifies which of the following?

   A. Development of liver fibrosis leading to cirrhosis.
   B. Dominant viral population is less virulent and less transmissible.
   C. Increased likelihood of an acute flare in the next 1–2 weeks.
   D. Ongoing viral replication.
   E. Resolving infection.

88. A 32-year-old woman is admitted to the hospital with fever, abdominal pain, and jaundice. She drinks approximately 6 beers daily and has recently increased her alcohol intake to more than 12 beers daily. She has no other substance abuse history and has no history of alcoholic liver disease or pancreatitis. She is not taking any medications. On physical examination, she appears ill and disheveled with a fruity odor to her breath. Her vital signs are as follows: heart rate 122 beats/min, blood pressure 95/56 mmHg, respiratory rate 22 breaths/min, temperature 101.2°F, and oxygen saturation 98% on room air. She has scleral icterus, and spider angiomata are present on the trunk. The liver edge is palpable 10 cm below the right costal margin. It is smooth and tender to palpation. The spleen is not palpable. No ascites or lower extremity edema is present. Laboratory studies demonstrate an AST of 431 U/L, ALT of 198 U/L, bilirubin of 8.6 mg/dL, alkaline phosphatase of 201 U/L, amylase of 88 U/L, and lipase of 50 U/L. Total protein is 6.2 g/dL, and albumin is 2.8 g/dL. The prothrombin time is 28.9 seconds. What is the best approach to treatment of this patient?

   A. Administer IV fluids, thiamine, and folate, and observe for improvement in laboratory tests and clinical condition.
   B. Administer IV fluids, thiamine, folate, and imipenem while awaiting blood culture results.
   C. Administer prednisone 40 mg daily for 4 weeks before beginning a taper.
   D. Consult surgery for management of acute cholecystitis.
   E. Perform an abdominal CT with IV contrast to assess for necrotizing pancreatitis.

89. A 48-year-old woman presents complaining of fatigue and itching. She has been tired for the past 6 months and has recently developed diffuse itching. It is worse in the evening hours, but it is intermittent. She does not note it to be worse following hot baths or showers. Her past medical history is significant only for hypothyroidism for which she takes

89. (Continued)
levothyroxine 125 µg daily. On physical examination, she has mild jaundice and scleral icterus. The liver is enlarged to 15 cm on palpation and is palpable 5 cm below the right costal margin. Xanthomas are seen on both elbows. Hyperpigmentation is noticeable on the trunk and arms where the patient has excoriations. Laboratory studies demonstrate the following: WBC 8900/µL, hemoglobin 13.3 g/dL, hematocrit 41.6%, and platelets 160,000/µL. The creatinine is 1.2 mg/dL. The AST is 52 U/L, ALT is 62 U/L, alkaline phosphatase is 216 U/L, total bilirubin is 3.2 mg/dL, and direct bilirubin is 2.9 mg/dL. The total protein is 8.2 g/dL, and albumin is 3.9 U/L. The thyroid-stimulating hormone is 4.5 U/mL. Antimitochondrial antibodies are positive. P-ANCA and C-ANCA are negative. What is the most likely cause of the patient's symptoms?

   A. Lymphoma
   B. Polycythemia vera
   C. Primary biliary cirrhosis
   D. Primary sclerosis cholangitis
   E. Uncontrolled hypothyroidism

90. A 63-year-old man presents to the emergency department complaining of hematemesis. The vomiting began abruptly and was not preceded by any abdominal pain or other symptoms. He describes the vomiting as about 500 mL of bright red blood. He has not had melena or bright red blood per rectum. He has known alcoholic cirrhosis and continues to drink at least 12 beers daily. He does not seek regular medical care, and he has not previously had an endoscopy to screen for varices. When he is initially evaluated in the emergency department, he is noted to be tachycardic with a heart rate of 125 beats/min and a blood pressure of 76/40. After 1 L of IV saline, his blood pressure increases to 92/56. He has an additional 300 mL of hematemesis upon arriving in the emergency department. The initial hematocrit is 32%. All of the following should be a part of the initial management of this patient EXCEPT:

   A. Administration of octreotide 100 µg/h by continuous IV infusion
   B. Administration of propranolol 10 mg four times daily
   C. Emergent GI consult for upper endoscopy
   D. Ongoing volume resuscitation with saline and packed red blood cells as needed to maintain adequate blood pressure
   E. Placement of large-bore IV access in the antecubital fossae or large central vein

91. A 42-year-old man with cirrhosis related to hepatitis C and alcohol abuse has ascites requiring frequent large-volume paracentesis. All of the following therapies would be indicated for this patient EXCEPT:

A. Fluid restriction to less than 2 L daily
B. Furosemide 40 mg daily
C. Sodium restriction to less than 2 g daily
D. Spironolactone 100 mg daily
E. Transjugular intrahepatic portosystemic shunt if medical therapy fails

92. Which of the following statements about cardiac cirrhosis is TRUE?

A. AST and ALT levels may mimic the very high levels seen in acute viral hepatitis.
B. Budd-Chiari syndrome cannot be distinguished clinically from cardiac cirrhosis.
C. Echocardiography is the gold standard for diagnosing constrictive pericarditis as a cause of cirrhosis.
D. Prolonged passive congestion from right-sided heart failure results first in congestion and necrosis of portal triads, resulting in subsequent fibrosis.
E. Venoocclusive disease can be confused with cardiac cirrhosis and is a major cause of morbidity and mortality in patients undergoing liver transplantation.

93. You are asked to consult on a 62-year-old white female with pruritus for 4 months. She has noted progressive fatigue and a 5-lb weight loss. She has intermittent nausea but no vomiting and denies changes in her bowel habits. There is no history of prior alcohol use, blood transfusions, or illicit drug use. The patient is widowed and had two heterosexual partners in her lifetime. Her past medical history is significant only for hypothyroidism, for which she takes levothyroxine. Her family history is unremarkable. On examination she is mildly icteric. She has spider angiomata on her torso. You palpate a nodular liver edge 2 cm below the right costal margin. The remainder of the examination is unremarkable. A right upper quadrant ultrasound confirms your suspicion of cirrhosis. You order a complete blood count and a comprehensive metabolic panel. What is the most appropriate next test?

A. 24-hour urine copper
B. Antimitochondrial antibodies (AMA)
C. Endoscopic retrograde cholangiopancreatography (ERCP)
D. Hepatitis B serologies
E. Serum ferritin

94. A 58-year-old man is evaluated for a new diagnosis of cirrhosis. The patient has a medical history of diabetes mellitus, hypertriglyceridemia, and hypertension. He takes pioglitazone, rosuvastatin, lisinopril, and atenolol. He is a lifetime nonsmoker and has never used IV drugs. He drinks about one glass of wine weekly. For about 4–8 years in his 20s, he admits to binge drinking as much as 12–18 beers on the weekends, but has not drunk more than two glasses of wine weekly for many years. He has never had a blood transfusion and has been in a monogamous sexual relationship for 30 years. He has no family history of liver disease. He works as a machinist in a factory making airplane engines. He denies chemical exposures. His physical examination is notable for a body mass index of 45.9 kg/m². He has stigmata of chronic liver disease including spider angiomata and caput medusa. Moderate ascites is present. Workup has shown no evidence of viral hepatitis, hemochromatosis, Wilson's disease, autoimmune hepatitis, or α_1 antitrypsin deficiency. He undergoes liver biopsy, which shows fibrosis in a perivenular and perisinusoidal distribution. Which of the following statements is TRUE regarding the cause of the patient's cirrhosis?

A. As opposed to individuals with metabolic syndrome alone, these individuals do not show significant insulin resistance.
B. The aspartate aminotransferase is commonly elevated to more than twice the alanine aminotransferase level.
C. The lack of steatohepatitis on liver biopsy rules out nonalcoholic fatty liver disease as a cause of the patient's cirrhosis.
D. The prevalence of the milder form of this disorder is between 10 and 20% in the United States and Europe, with as much as 10–15% of affected individuals developing cirrhosis in some series.
E. Treatment with ursodeoxycholic acid and HMG-CoA reductase inhibitors has been demonstrated to improve outcomes in this disorder.

95. A 44-year-old woman is evaluated for complaints of abdominal pain. She describes the pain as a postprandial burning pain. It is worse with spicy or fatty foods and is relieved with antacids. She is diagnosed with a gastric ulcer and is treated appropriately for *Helicobacter pylori*. During the course of her evaluation for her abdominal pain, the patient had a right upper quadrant ultrasound that demonstrated the presence of gallstones. Following treatment of *H. pylori,* her symptoms have resolved. She is requesting your opinion regarding whether treatment is

95. (*Continued*)

required for the finding of gallstone disease. Upon review of the ultrasound report, there were numerous stones in the gallbladder, including in the neck of the gallbladder. The largest stone measures 2.8 cm. What is your advice to the patient regarding the risk of complications and the need for definitive treatment?

A. Given the size and number of stones, prophylactic cholecystectomy is recommended.

B. No treatment is necessary unless the patient develops symptoms of biliary colic frequently and severely enough to interfere with the patient's life.

C. The only reason to proceed with cholecystectomy is the development of gallstone pancreatitis or cholangitis.

D. The risk of developing acute cholecystitis is about 5–10% per year.

E. Ursodeoxycholic acid should be given at a dose of 10–15 mg/kg daily for a minimum of 6 months to dissolve the stones.

96. A 62-year-old man has been hospitalized in intensive care for the past 3 weeks following an automobile accident resulting in multiple long-bone fractures and acute respiratory distress syndrome. He has been slowly improving, but remains on mechanical ventilation. He is now febrile and hypotensive, requiring vasopressors. He is being treated empirically with cefepime and vancomycin. Multiple blood cultures are negative. He has no new infiltrates or increasing secretions on chest radiograph. His laboratory studies demonstrated a rise in his liver function tests, bilirubin, and alkaline phosphatase. Amylase and lipase are normal. A right upper quadrant ultrasound shows sludge in the gallbladder, but no stones. The bile duct is not dilated. What is the next best step in the evaluation and treatment of this patient?

A. Discontinue cefepime.

B. Initiate treatment with clindamycin.

C. Initiate treatment with metronidazole.

D. Perform hepatobiliary scintigraphy.

E. Refer for exploratory laparotomy.

97. All of the following are associated with an increased risk for cholelithiasis EXCEPT:

A. Chronic hemolytic anemia

B. Female sex

C. High-protein diet

D. Obesity

E. Pregnancy

98. Which of the following statements regarding liver transplantation is TRUE?

A. Individuals with cholangiocarcinoma should be referred early for consideration of liver transplantation.

B. Living donor transplantation is only performed in children.

C. Reinfection with hepatitis B typically occurs in 35% or more of patients with liver transplantation.

D. The 5-year survival rate for orthotopic liver transplantation is about 50%.

E. The most common indication for liver transplantation is chronic hepatitis B infection.

99. A 55-year-old male with cirrhosis is seen in the clinic for follow-up of a recent hospitalization for spontaneous bacterial peritonitis. He is doing well and finishing his course of antibiotics. He is taking propranolol and lactulose. Besides complications of end-stage liver disease, he has well-controlled diabetes mellitus and had a basal cell carcinoma resected 5 years ago. The cirrhosis is thought to be due to alcohol abuse, and his last drink of alcohol was 2 weeks ago. He and his wife ask if he is a liver transplant candidate. He can be counseled in which of the following ways?

A. Because he had a skin cancer he is not a transplant candidate.

B. Because he has diabetes mellitus he is not a transplant candidate.

C. He is appropriate for liver transplantation and should be referred immediately.

D. He is not a transplant candidate as he has a history of alcohol dependence.

E. He is not a transplant candidate now, but may be after a sustained period of proven abstinence from alcohol.

100. A 27-year-old woman is admitted to the hospital with acute-onset severe right upper quadrant pain that radiates to the back. The pain is constant and not relieved with eating or bowel movements. Her labs show a marked elevation in amylase and lipase, and acute pancreatitis is diagnosed. Which of the following is the best first test to demonstrate the etiology of her pancreatitis?

A. Right upper quadrant ultrasound

B. Serum alcohol level

C. Serum triglyceride level

D. Technetium HIDA scan

E. Urine drug screen

101. A 58-year-old man with severe alcoholism is admitted to the hospital with acute pancreatitis. His symptoms have been present for 3 days and he has continued to drink heavily. He now has persistent vomiting and feels dizzy upon standing. On examination he has severe epigastric and right upper quadrant tenderness and decreased bowel sounds, and appears uncomfortable. A faint blue discoloration is present around the umbilicus. What is the significance of this finding?

A. A CT of the abdomen is likely to show severe necrotizing pancreatitis.
B. Abdominal plain film is likely to show pancreatic calcification.
C. Concomitant appendicitis should be ruled out.
D. He likely has a pancreatico-aortic fistula.
E. Pancreatic pseudocyst is likely present.

102. A 36-year-old man is admitted to the hospital with acute pancreatitis. In order to determine the severity of disease and risk of mortality, the BISAP (Bedside Index of Severity in Acute Pancreatitis) is calculated. All of the following variables are used to calculate this score EXCEPT:

A. Age greater than 60 years
B. BUN greater than 35
C. Impaired mental status
D. Pleural effusion
E. White blood cell count greater than 15,000 leukocytes/μL

103. A 54-year-old man is admitted to the intensive care unit with severe pancreatitis. His BMI is 30 or above and he has a prior history of diabetes mellitus. A CT of the abdomen is obtained and shows severe necrotizing pancreatitis. He is presently afebrile. Which of the following medications has been shown to be effective in the treatment of acute necrotizing pancreatitis?

A. Calcitonin
B. Cimetidine
C. Glucagon
D. Imipenem
E. None of the above

104. Which of the following statements is true regarding enteral feeding in acute pancreatitis?

A. A patient with persistent evidence of pancreatic necrosis on CT 2 weeks after acute presentation should be maintained on bowel rest.

104. (*Continued*)
B. All patients with elevations of amylase and lipase and CT evidence of pancreatitis should be fasted until amylase and lipase normalize.
C. Enteral feeding with a nasojejunal tube has been demonstrated to have fewer infectious complications than total parenteral nutrition in the management of patients with acute pancreatitis.
D. Patients requiring surgical removal of infected pancreatic pseudocysts should be treated with total parental nutrition.
E. Total parenteral nutrition has been shown to maintain integrity of the intestinal tract in acute pancreatitis.

105. A 47-year-old woman presents to the emergency department with severe mid-abdominal pain radiating to her back. The pain began acutely and is sharp. She denies cramping or flatulence. She has had two episodes of emesis of bilious material since the pain began, but this has not lessened the pain. She currently rates the pain as a 10 out of 10 and feels the pain is worse in the supine position. For the past few months, she has had intermittent episodes of right upper and mid-epigastric pain that occurs after eating but subsides over a few hours. This is associated with a feeling of excess gas. She denies any history of alcohol abuse. She has no medical history of hypertension or hyperlipidemia. On physical examination, she is writhing in distress and slightly diaphoretic. Vital signs are as follows: heart rate 127 beats/min, blood pressure 92/50 mmHg, respiratory rate 20 breaths/min, temperature 37.9°C, and 88% oxygen saturation on room air. Her body mass index is 29 kg/m^2. The cardiovascular examination reveals a regular tachycardia. The chest examination shows dullness to percussion at bilateral bases with a few scattered crackles. On abdominal examination, bowel sounds are hypoactive. There is no rash or bruising evident on inspection of the abdomen. There is voluntary guarding on palpation. The pain with palpation is greatest in the periumbilical and epigastric areas without rebound tenderness. There is no evidence of jaundice, and the liver span is about 10 cm to percussion. Amylase level is 750 IU/L, and lipase level is 1129 IU/L. Other laboratory values include aspartate aminotransferase (AST) 168 U/L, alanine aminotransferase (ALT) 196 U/L, total bilirubin 2.3 mg/dL, alkaline phosphatase level 268 U/L, lactate dehydrogenase (LDH) 300 U/L, and creatinine 1.9 mg/dL. The hematocrit is 43%, and white blood cell (WBC) count is 11,500/μL with 89% neutrophils. An arterial blood gas shows a pH of 7.32, PCO$_2$ of 32 mmHg, and a PO$_2$ of 56 mmHg. An ultrasound confirms a dilated

105. *(Continued)*

common bile duct with evidence of pancreatitis manifested as an edematous and enlarged pancreas. A CT scan shows no evidence of necrosis. After 3 L of normal saline, her blood pressure comes up to 110/60 mmHg with a heart rate of 105 beats/min. Which of the following statements best describes the pathophysiology of this disease?

A. Intrapancreatic activation of digestive enzymes with autodigestion and acinar cell injury
B. Chemoattraction of neutrophils with subsequent infiltration and inflammation
C. Distant organ involvement and systemic inflammatory response syndrome related to release of activated pancreatic enzymes and cytokines
D. All of the above

106. A 25-year-old female with cystic fibrosis is diagnosed with chronic pancreatitis. She is at risk for all of the following complications EXCEPT:

A. Vitamin B_{12} deficiency
B. Vitamin A deficiency
C. Pancreatic carcinoma
D. Niacin deficiency
E. Steatorrhea

107. A 64-year-old man seeks evaluation from his primary care physician because of chronic diarrhea. He reports that he has two or three large loose bowel movements daily. He describes them as markedly foul smelling, and they often leave an oily ring in the toilet. He also notes that the bowel movements often follow heavy meals, but if he fasts or eats low-fat foods, the stools are more formed. Over the past 6 months, he has lost about 18 kg. In this setting, he reports intermittent episodes of abdominal pain that can be quite severe. He describes the pain as sharp and in a mid-epigastric location. He has not sought evaluation

107. *(Continued)*

of the pain previously, but when it occurs he will limit his oral intake and treat the pain with non-steroidal anti-inflammatory drugs. He notes the pain has not lasted for more than 48 hours and is not associated with meals. His past medical history is remarkable for peripheral vascular disease and tobacco use. He currently smokes one pack of cigarettes daily. In addition, he drinks 2–6 beers daily. He has stopped all alcohol intake for up to a week at a time in the past without withdrawal symptoms. His current medications are aspirin 81 mg daily and albuterol metered dose inhaler (MDI) on an as-needed basis. On physical examination, the patient is thin but appears well. His body mass index is 18.2 kg/m². Vital signs are normal. Cardiac and pulmonary examinations are normal. The abdominal examination shows mild epigastric tenderness without rebound or guarding. The liver span is 12 cm to percussion and palpable 2 cm below the right costal margin. There is no splenomegaly or ascites present. There are decreased pulses in the lower extremities bilaterally. An abdominal radiograph demonstrates calcifications in the epigastric area, and CT scan confirms that these calcifications are located within the body of the pancreas. No pancreatic ductal dilatation is noted. Amylase level is 32 U/L, and lipase level is 22 U/L. What is the next most appropriate step in diagnosing and managing this patient's primary complaint?

A. Advise the patient to stop all alcohol use and prescribe pancreatic enzymes.
B. Advise the patient to stop all alcohol use and prescribe narcotic analgesia and pancreatic enzymes.
C. Perform angiography to assess for ischemic bowel disease.
D. Prescribe prokinetic agents to improve gastric emptying.
E. Refer the patient for endoscopic retrograde cholangiopancreatography (ERCP) for sphincterotomy.

ANSWERS

1. The answer is B.
(Chaps. 8 and 45) The clinical presentation is consistent with a cholestatic picture. Painless jaundice always requires an extensive workup, as many of the underlying pathologies are ominous and early detection and intervention often offers the only hope for a good outcome. The gallbladder showed no evidence of stones and the patient shows no evidence of clinical cholecystitis, and so a hepatobiliary iminodiacetic acid (HIDA) scan is not indicated. Similarly, antibiotics are not necessary at this point. The cholestatic picture without significant elevation of the transaminases on the liver function tests makes acute hepatitis unlikely. Antimitochondrial antibodies are elevated in cases of primary biliary cirrhosis (PBC), which may present in a similar fashion. However, PBC is far more common in women than in men, and the average age of onset is the fifth or sixth decade. The lack of an obvious lesion on CT scan does not rule out a source of the cholestasis in the biliary tree. Malignant causes such as cholangiocarcinoma and tumor of the ampulla of Vater, and nonmalignant causes such

as sclerosing cholangitis and Caroli's disease may be detected only by direct visualization with endoscopic retrograde cholangiopancreatography (ERCP). ERCP is useful both diagnostically and therapeutically, as stenting procedures may be done to alleviate the obstruction.

2. The answer is A.
(Chaps. 9 and 36) Diagnostic paracentesis is part of the routine evaluation in a patient with ascites. Fluid should be examined for its gross appearance, protein content, cell count and differential, and albumin. Cytologic and culture studies should be performed when one suspects infection or malignancy. The serum–ascites albumin gradient (SAG) offers the best correlation with portal pressure. A high gradient (>1.1 g/dL) is characteristic of uncomplicated cirrhotic ascites and differentiates ascites caused by portal hypertension from ascites not caused by portal hypertension in more than 95% of cases. Conditions that cause a low gradient include more "exudative" processes such as infection, malignancy, and inflammatory processes. Similarly, congestive heart failure and nephrotic syndrome cause high gradients. In this patient the SAG is 1.5 g/dL, indicating a high gradient. The low number of leukocytes and polymorphonuclear cells makes bacterial or tubercular infection unlikely. Chylous ascites often is characterized by an opaque milky fluid with a triglyceride level greater than 1000 mg/dL in addition to a low SAG.

3. The answer is E.
(Chap. 10) Involuntary weight loss (IWL) is a frequent finding in older individuals, affecting more than 25% of frail individuals older than 65 years. Clinically important weight loss is defined as a loss of more than 5% of body weight or more than 5 kg over the course of 6–12 months. In older individuals, weight loss is associated with hip fracture, pressure ulcers, decreased functional status, and death. There are many causes of IWL, with the most common categories being malignancy, chronic inflammatory or infectious disease, metabolic disorders, and psychiatric disorders. In older individuals, it is also important to consider neurologic disorders, including stroke leading to dysphagia, progressive vision loss, and dementia. IWL can be one of the earliest manifestations of Alzheimer's disease. An under-recognized cause of IWL is lack of access to food or inability to pay for food. When evaluating an individual for IWL, a complete physical examination, including a dental examination, should be performed to assess for obvious physical causes that would lead to weight loss. Medications may also lead to changes in appetite or weight loss. Patients should undergo age-appropriate cancer screening. In older individuals, a Mini-Mental State Examination, Mini-Nutritional Assessment, and assessment of performance of activities of daily living may be helpful. It may also be useful to observe the patient's eating. Depression

in the elderly may also present with loss of appetite and should be assessed. Laboratory studies could include a complete blood count, comprehensive metabolic panel, thyroid function tests, and erythrocyte sedimentation rate and C-reactive protein. HIV testing is indicated if risk factors are identified.

4. The answer is E.
(Chap. 13) Endoscopy, also known as esophagogastroduodenoscopy (EGD), is the best test for the evaluation of the proximal gastrointestinal tract. Because of high-quality images, disorders of color such as Barrett's metaplasia, and mucosal irregularities are easily demonstrated. The sensitivity of endoscopy is superior to that of barium radiography for mucosal lesions. Because the endoscope has an instrumentation channel, biopsy specimens are easily obtained and dilation of strictures can also be performed. The only advantage that barium radiography confers is the absence of the requirement for sedation, which, in some populations at risk for conscious sedation, is an important consideration.

5. The answer is E.
(Chap. 13) Intermittent solid food dysphagia is a classic symptom in Schatzki's ring in which a distal esophageal ring occurs at the squamocolumnar mucosal junction. The origin of these rings is unknown, and smaller rings with a lumen of greater than 13 mm are common in the general population (up to 15%). When the lumen is less than 13 mm, dysphagia may occur. Schatzki's rings typically occur in persons older than 40 years and often cause "steakhouse syndrome" from meat getting stuck at the ring. The rings are easily treated with dilation. Plummer-Vinson syndrome also includes esophageal rings, but typically the rings occur in the proximal esophagus, are associated with iron-deficiency anemia, and occur in middle-aged women. Achalasia involves both solid and liquid dysphagia often with regurgitation. Adenocarcinoma often includes solid and liquid dysphagia at later stages. Most esophageal diverticulae are asymptomatic.

6. The answer is B.
(Chap. 13) Aside from the discomfort and local complications of gastroesophageal reflux disease (GERD), a number of other non-GI–related sites may have a complication related to it. Syndromes with a well-established association with GERD include chronic cough, laryngitis, asthma, and dental erosions. Other diseases have implicated GERD as potentially contributory, but the role of GERD is less well established. These include pharyngitis, pulmonary fibrosis, chronic sinusitis, cardiac arrhythmias, sleep apnea, and recurrent aspiration pneumonia.

7. The answer is A.
(Chap. 13) This patient has symptoms of esophagitis. In patients with HIV, various infections can cause this

disease, including herpes simplex virus (HSV), cytomegalovirus (CMV), varicella–zoster virus (VZV), *Candida*, and HIV itself. The lack of thrush does not rule out *Candida* as a cause of esophagitis, and EGD is necessary for diagnosis. CMV classically causes serpiginous ulcers in the distal esophagus that may coalesce to form giant ulcers. Brushings alone are insufficient for diagnosis, and biopsies must be performed. Biopsies reveal intranuclear and intracytoplasmic inclusions with enlarged nuclei in large fibroblasts and endothelial cells. Given her notable swallowing symptoms, IV ganciclovir is the treatment of choice. Valganciclovir is an effective oral preparation. Foscarnet is useful in treating ganciclovir-resistant CMV. Herpes simplex virus manifests as vesicles and punched-out lesions in the esophagus, with the characteristic finding on biopsy of ballooning degeneration with ground-glass changes in the nuclei. It can be treated with acyclovir or foscarnet in resistant cases. Candida esophagitis has the appearance of yellow nodular plaques with surrounding erythema. Treatment usually requires fluconazole therapy. Finally, HIV alone can cause esophagitis that can be quite resistant to therapy. On EGD these ulcers appear deep and linear. Treatment with thalidomide or oral glucocorticoids is employed, and highly active antiretroviral therapy should be considered.

8. The answer is D.

(Chap. 13) The patient has a duodenal ulcer, which is almost universally due to *H. pylori* infection, although in a minority of cases NSAID use may either facilitate development or be the only identified cause. The patient was taking acetaminophen and not a traditional NSAID, making *H. pylori*–associated peptic ulcer disease the most likely cause of the findings. *H. pylori* infection is closely correlated with advancing age, low socioeconomic status, and low education levels. After initial infection, antral gastritis is very common, and in a portion of cases, duodenal or gastric ulcers form. Associated with these conditions is the development of gastric cancer or MALT lymphoma. Duodenal ulcers are rarely cancerous, although this is a not an uncommon finding in gastric cancers. After discovery of the ulcer, first-line therapy is eradication of *H. pylori* in addition to acid suppression.

9. The answer is D.

(Chap. 14) Noninvasive testing for *H. pylori* infection is recommended in patients with suggestive symptoms and no other indication for endoscopy, e.g., GI bleeding, atypical symptoms. Several tests have good sensitivity and specificity, including plasma serology for *H. pylori*, ^{14}C- or ^{13}C-urea breath test, and the fecal *H. pylori* antigen test. Sensitivity and specificity are greater than 80% and greater than 90%, respectively, for serology, while the urea breath test and fecal antigen testing are greater than 90% for both. Serology is not useful for early follow-up after therapy completion, as antibody titers will take

several weeks to months to fall. The urea breath test, which relies on the presence of urease secreted by *H. pylori* to digest the swallowed radioactive urea and liberate ^{14}C or ^{13}C as part of ammonia, is simple and rapid. It is useful for early follow-up, as it requires living bacteria to secrete urease and produce a positive test. The limitations to the test include the requirement for ingestion of radioactive materials, albeit low dose, and false-negative results with recent use of PPI, antibiotics, or bismuth compounds. Stool antigen testing is cheap and convenient, but is not established for proof of eradication.

10. The answer is A.

(Chap. 14) *H. pylori* should be eradicated in patients with documented peptic ulcer disease no matter the number of episodes, severity, presence of confounding factors (e.g., NSAID ingestion), or symptomatic status. Documented eradication of *H. pylori* is associated with substantially lower recurrence rates and symptom improvement. Treating patients with GERD who require long-term acid reduction therapy and the role of *H. pylori* eradication to prevent gastric cancer are controversial. Fourteen-day regimens are most effective. Shorter duration of therapy with current agents available has high recurrence rates. Dual-therapy regimens are not recommended because of eradication rates of less than 80%. A number of combinations are available (Table 14-4). Triple-therapy regimens (one antacid plus two antibiotics) for 14 days have an eradication rate of 85–90%. Antibiotic resistance is the most common cause of failure to eradicate in compliant patients. Unfortunately, there is no currently available test for *H. pylori* sensitivity to direct therapy. Quadruple therapy should be reserved for patients with failure to eradicate after an effective initial course.

11. The answer is C.

(Chap. 14) Fasting gastrin levels can be elevated in a variety of conditions including atrophic gastritis with or without pernicious anemia, G-cell hyperplasia, and acid suppressive therapy (gastrin levels increase as a consequence of loss of negative feedback). The diagnostic concern in a patient with persistent ulcers following optimal therapy is Zollinger-Ellison syndrome (ZES). The result is not sufficient to make a diagnosis because gastrin levels may be elevated in a variety of conditions. Elevated basal acid secretion also is consistent with ZES, but up to 12% of patients with peptic ulcer disease may have basal acid secretion as high as 15 meq/h. Thus, additional testing is necessary. Gastrin levels may go up with a meal (>200%), but this test does not distinguish G-cell hyperfunction from ZES. The best test in this setting is the secretin stimulation test. An increase in gastrin levels greater than 200 pg within 15 minutes of administering 2 µg/kg of secretin by IV bolus has a sensitivity and specificity of greater than 90% for ZES. Endoscopic

ultrasonography is useful in locating the gastrin-secreting tumor once the positive secretin test is obtained. Genetic testing for mutations in the gene that encodes the menin protein can detect the fraction of patients with gastrinomas that are a manifestation of multiple endocrine neoplasia type I (Wermer's syndrome). Gastrinoma is the second most common tumor in this syndrome following parathyroid adenoma, but its peak incidence is generally in the third decade.

12. The answer is B.

(*Chap. 15*) The patient presents with nonspecific gastrointestinal symptoms, but the presence of weight loss suggests malabsorption syndrome. Patients with lactose intolerance are usually able to relate symptoms to consumption of milk-based products and also report a strong history of crampy pain and flatulence. Therefore, a lactose-free diet is unlikely to be helpful. The patient does not have nocturnal diarrhea, which is commonly a feature of steatorrhea along with floating stools. In the absence of symptoms suggesting fat malabsorption, the first test should not be fecal fat measurement. As the patient has weight loss, irritable bowel syndrome is less likely, and an increase dietary fiber is unlikely to be useful. Finally, her symptoms may be consistent with celiac disease. The widespread availability of antibodies to gliadin, endomysial, and tTG can be easily measured in peripheral blood. Antiendomysial antibody has a 90–95% sensitivity and equal specificity, making it a reasonable first test in symptomatic individuals. The presence of the antibody is not diagnostic, however, and duodenal biopsy is recommended. Duodenal biopsy will show villous atrophy, absence or reduced height of villi, cuboidal appearance of surface epithelial cells, and increased lymphocytes and plasma cells in the lamina propria. These changes regress with complete removal of gluten from the diet.

13. The answer is B.

(*Chap. 15*) Short bowel syndrome is a descriptive term referring to the many clinical complications that may occur after resection of varying lengths of the small bowel. Rarely, these complications may be due to congenital abnormalities of the small bowel. Most commonly in adults, short bowel syndrome occurs in mesenteric vascular disease, primary mucosal or submucosal disease (Crohn's disease), and operations without preexisting small bowel disease such as trauma. Multiple factors contribute to diarrhea and steatorrhea including gastric acid hypersecretion, increased bile acids in the colon due to absent or decreased reabsorption in the small bowel, and lactose intolerance due to increased gastric acid secretion. Nonintestinal symptoms may include renal calcium oxalate calculi due to an increase in oxalate absorption by the large intestine with subsequent hyperoxaluria. This may be due to increased fatty acids in the colon that bind calcium, and thus calcium in the gut is not free to bind

oxalate and free oxalate is absorbed in the large intestine. Increased bile acid pool size results in the generation of cholesterol gallstones from supersaturating in gallbladder bile. Gastric hypersecretion of acid is well described and thought to be due to loss of inhibition of gastric acid secretion because of absent short bowel to secrete inhibitory hormones. Coronary artery disease is not described as a complication of short bowel syndrome.

14. The answer is E.

(*Chap. 15*) The patient presents with symptoms suggestive of Whipple's disease with a chronic multisystem disease often including diarrhea/steatorrhea, migratory arthralgias, weight loss, and CNS or cardiac problems. Generally the presentation is of insidious onset, and dementia is a late finding and poor prognostic sign. The disease primarily occurs in middle-aged white males. The diagnosis requires small bowel biopsy and demonstration of PAS-positive macrophages within the small bowel. Small bacilli are often present and suggest the diagnosis of Whipple's disease. Similar macrophages may be found in other affected organs, e.g., the CNS. Dilated lymphatics are present in patients with intestinal lymphangiectasia. Mononuclear cell infiltrate in the lamina propria is often demonstrated in patients with tropical sprue, and flat villi with crypt hyperplasia are the hallmark of celiac disease.

15. The answer is D.

(*Chap. 15*) This patient has a stool osmolality gap (measured stool osmolality - calculated stool osmolality) of less than 50 mosmol/L, suggesting a secretory rather than an osmotic cause for diarrhea. Secretory causes of diarrhea include toxin-mediated diarrhea (cholera, enterotoxigenic *Escherichia coli*) and intestinal peptide–mediated diarrhea in which the major pathophysiology is a luminal or circulating secretagogue. The distinction between secretory diarrhea and osmotic diarrhea aids in forming a differential diagnosis. Secretory diarrhea will not decrease substantially during a fast and has a low osmolality gap. Osmotic diarrhea will generally decrease during a fast and has a high (>50 mosmol/L) osmolality gap. Celiac sprue, chronic pancreatitis, lactase deficiency, and Whipple's disease all cause an osmotic diarrhea.

16. The answer is E.

(*Chaps. 15 and 16*) Cobalamin malabsorption may occur due to disease at multiple anatomic sites extending from the stomach to the ileum. In the past, the Schilling test was utilized to assess cobalamin absorption, but this test is not currently commercially available. Cobalamin is primarily present in meat, but dietary deficiency is rare except in strict vegans. Dietary cobalamin is bound in the stomach to R-binder protein that is synthesized in salivary glands and stomach. The cobalamin–R binder complex requires an acid medium. Therefore, achlorhydria of any cause may result in the inability for splitting of cobalamin from food and binding to R-binder protein. Cobalamin absorption has an absolute requirement for intrinsic factor, which allows uptake by specific receptors in the ileum. Intrinsic factor is produced and released by gastric parietal cells. Thus pernicious anemia, the autoimmune atrophy of parietal cells, is a cause of cobalamin malabsorption. Pancreatic protease enzymes lyse the cobalamin–R binder protein complex to release cobalamin in the proximal intestine where it is bound to intrinsic factor for ileal absorption. Thus a deficiency of pancreatic enzymes, such as in chronic pancreatitis, can lead to cobalamin malabsorption. Finally, cobalamin-intrinsic factor is absorbed via an intact epithelium in the ileum. Inflammation (Crohn's disease) or absence (surgical removal) of ileum will cause cobalamin malabsorption. The large intestine is not involved in cobalamin absorption; thus ulcerative colitis confined to the large intestine will not cause malabsorption.

17. The answer is D.

(Chap. 17) The incidence of inflammatory bowel disease is highly influenced by ethnicity, location, and environmental factors. Both conditions have their highest incidence in the United Kingdom and North America, and the peak incidence has a bimodal distribution of age of presentation: 15–30 years and 60–80 years. The incidence of both ulcerative colitis and Crohn's disease is highest among persons of the Ashkenazi Jewish population. Prevalence decreases progressively in non-Jewish white, African-American, Hispanic, and Asian populations. Cigarette smoking is associated with a decreased incidence of ulcerative colitis, but may cause Crohn's disease. Oral contraceptive use is associated with a slightly higher incidence of Crohn's disease, but not ulcerative colitis. Monozygotic twins are highly concordant for Crohn's disease, but not ulcerative colitis.

18. The answer is C.

(Chap. 17) Chronic bloody diarrhea associated with weight loss and systemic symptoms in a young person is highly suggestive of inflammatory bowel disease. Her surgical findings suggest discontinuous lesions, which is typical of Crohn's disease. Ulcerative colitis, in contrast, typically affects the rectum and proceeds caudally from there without normal mucosa until the area of inflammation terminates. The presence of strictures and fissures further supports the diagnosis of Crohn's disease, as these are not features of ulcerative colitis. Microscopically, both ulcerative colitis and Crohn's disease may have crypt abscess and, although Crohn's disease is more often transmural, full thickness disease may be present in ulcerative colitis. The hallmark of Crohn's disease is granulomas that may be present throughout the bowel wall and involve the lymph nodes, mesentery, peritoneum, liver, and pancreas. Although pathognomonic for Crohn's disease,

granulomas are only found in about half of surgical resections. Flat villi are not always present in either disease and are more commonly found in isolation with celiac disease.

19. The answer is D.

(Chap. 17) There are a number of dermatologic manifestations of inflammatory bowel disease (IBD), and each type of IBD has a particular predilection for different dermatologic conditions. This patient has pyoderma gangrenosum. Pyoderma gangrenosum can occur in up to 12% of patients with ulcerative colitis and is characterized by a lesion that begins as a pustule and progresses concentrically to surrounding normal skin. The lesions ulcerate with violaceous, heaped margins and surrounding erythema. They are typically found on the lower extremities. Often the lesions are difficult to treat and respond poorly to colectomy; similarly, pyoderma gangrenosum is not prevented by colectomy. Treatment commonly includes IV antibiotics, glucocorticoids, dapsone, infliximab, and other immunomodulatory agents. Erythema nodosum is more common in Crohn's disease, and attacks correlate with bowel symptoms. The lesions are typically multiple red hot, tender nodules measuring 1–5 cm and are found on the lower legs and arms. Psoriasis is more common in ulcerative colitis. Finally, pyoderma vegetans is a rare disorder in intertriginous areas reported to be a manifestation of inflammatory bowel disease in the skin.

20. The answer is D.

(Chap. 17, Cochrane Database Syst Rev 2007 Oct 17; [4]) Despite being described as a clinical entity for over a century, the etiology of IBD remains cryptic. Current theory is related to an interplay between inflammatory stimuli in genetically predisposed individuals. Recent studies have identified a group of genes or polymorphisms that confer risk of IBD. Multiple microbiologic agents, including some that reside as "normal" flora, may initiate IBD by triggering an inflammatory response. Anaerobic organisms (e.g., *Bacteroides* and *Clostridia* spp.) may be responsible for the induction of inflammation. Other organisms, for unclear reasons, may have the opposite effect. These "probiotic" organisms include *Lactobacillus* spp., *Bifidobacterium* spp., *Taenia suis*, and *Saccharomyces boulardii*. *Shigella*, *Escherichia*, and *Campylobacter* spp. are known to promote inflammation. Studies of probiotic therapy in adults and children with IBD have shown potential benefit for reducing disease activity.

21. The answer is D.

(Chap. 17) Methotrexate, azathioprine, cyclosporine, tacrolimus, and anti-tumor necrosis factor (TNF) antibody are reasonable options for patients with CD, depending on the extent of macroscopic disease. Pneumonitis is a rare but serious complication of methotrexate therapy.

Primary sclerosing cholangitis is an extraintestinal manifestation of inflammatory bowel disease (IBD). Pancreatitis is an uncommon complication of azathioprine, and IBD patients treated with azathioprine are at a fourfold increased risk of developing a lymphoma. Anti–TNF antibody therapy is associated with an increased risk of tuberculosis, disseminated histoplasmosis, and a number of other infections.

22. The answer is C.

(Chap. 18) Irritable bowel syndrome is characterized by the following: recurrence of lower abdominal pain with altered bowel habits over a period of time without progressive deterioration, onset of symptoms during periods of stress or emotional upset, absence of other systemic symptoms such as fever and weight loss, and small-volume stool without evidence of blood. Warning signs that the symptoms may be due to something other than irritable bowel syndrome include presentation for the first time in old age, progressive course from the time of onset, persistent diarrhea after a 48-hour fast, and presence of nocturnal diarrhea or steatorrheal stools. Each patient, except for patient C, has "warning" symptoms that should prompt further evaluation.

23. The answer is C.

(Chap. 18) Although this patient has signs and symptoms consistent with IBS, the differential diagnosis is large. Few tests are required for patients who have typical IBS symptoms and no alarm features. In this patient, alarm features include anemia, an elevated ESR, and evidence of WBCs in the stool. Alarm features warrant further investigation to rule out other gastrointestinal disorders such as colonic pathology including diverticular disease or inflammatory bowel disease. In this case, colonoscopy to evaluate for luminal lesions and mucosal characteristics would be the logical first step. At this point, with the warning signs, empiric therapy for IBS is premature. Reassurance, stool bulking agents, and antidepressants are all therapies to consider if a patient does indeed have IBS.

24. The answer is D.

(Chap. 18) Up to 80% of patients with irritable bowel syndrome (IBS) also have abnormal psychiatric features; however, no single psychiatric diagnosis predominates. The mechanism is not well understood but may involve altered pain thresholds. Although these patients are hypersensitive to colonic stimuli, this does not carry over to the peripheral nervous system. Functional brain imaging shows disparate activation in, for example, the mid-cingulate cortex, but brain anatomy does not discriminate IBS patients from those without IBS. An association between a history of sexual abuse and IBS has been reported. There is no reported association with sexually transmitted diseases. Patients with IBS do not have an increased risk of autoimmunity.

25. The answer is B.

(Chap. 19) The patient presents with classic signs of diverticulitis with fever, abdominal pain that is usually left lower quadrant, anorexia or obstipation, and leukocytosis. This most commonly occurs in older individuals. Patients may present with acute abdomen due to perforation, though this occurs in less than 25% of cases. Plain radiographs of the abdomen are seldom helpful, but may rarely show the presence of an air–fluid level in the left lower quadrant indicating a giant diverticulum with impending perforation. CT with oral contrast is the diagnostic modality of choice with the following findings: sigmoid diverticula, thickened colonic wall greater than 4 mm, and inflammation within the pericolic space with or without the collection of contrast material or fluid. Abscesses, if present, will also be demonstrated on CT. Barium enema and colonoscopy should be avoided in acute diverticulitis because the insufflation of air or contrast material may lead to perforation. Although diverticular disease may result in hematochezia, these are generally not temporally linked to diverticulitis.

26. The answer is B.

(Chap. 19) Medical management is appropriate for many patients with uncomplicated diverticular disease. Uncomplicated disease has fever, abdominal pain, leukocytosis, and anorexia/obstipation, while complicated disease includes that with abscess formation, perforation, strictures, or fistulae. Uncomplicated disease accounts for at least 75% of cases. Medical therapy generally involves bowel rest and antibiotics, usually trimethoprim/sulfamethoxazole or ciprofloxacin and metronidazole targeting aerobic gram-negative rods and anaerobic bacteria. Patients with more than two attacks of diverticulitis were previously thought to require surgical therapy, but newer data suggest that these patients do not have an increased risk of perforation and can continue medical management. Patients with immunosuppressive therapy, chronic renal failure, or collagen vascular disease have a fivefold higher risk of perforation during recurrent attacks. Surgical therapy is indicated for surgical low-risk patients with complicated disease.

27. The answer is B.

(Chap. 19) Hemorrhoids can be internal or external; however, they are normally internal and may prolapse to the external position. Hemorrhoids are staged in the following manner: stage I, enlargement with bleeding; stage II, protrusion with spontaneous reduction; stage III, protrusion requiring manual reduction; stage IV, irreducible protrusion. Stage I, which this patient has, is treated with fiber supplementation, cortisone suppositories, and/or sclerotherapy. Stage II is treated with fiber and cortisone suppositories. Stage III patients are offered the prior three therapies and banding or operative hemorrhoidectomy. Stage IV patients benefit from fiber and cortisone therapy as well as operative hemorrhoidectomy. While substantial upper GI bleeding may result in hematochezia, the absence of suggestive signs/symptoms and the consistent findings of hemorrhoids do not indicate the need for upper endoscopy.

28. The answer is A.

(Chap. 19) An anorectal abscess is an abnormal fluid-containing cavity in the anorectal region. Anorectal abscess results from an infection involving the glands surrounding the anorectal canal. The disease is more common in males with a peak incidence in the third to fifth decades. Patients with diabetes, inflammatory bowel disease, or who are immunocompromised are at increased risk for this condition. Perianal pain with defecation and fever are common presenting symptoms.

29. The answer is C.

(Chap. 19) This patient has symptoms (social isolation), signs (foul odor), and risk factors (multiparity) for procidentia (rectal prolapse) and fecal incontinence. Procidentia is far more common in women than men and is often associated with pelvic floor disorders. It is not uncommon for these patients to become socially withdrawn and suffer from depression because of the associated fecal incontinence. The foul odor is a result of poor perianal hygiene due to the prolapsed rectum. Although depression in the elderly is an important medical problem, it is too premature in the evaluation of this patient to initiate medical therapy for depression. Occult malignancy and thyroid abnormalities may cause fecal incontinence and depression, but a physical examination would be diagnostic and avoid costly tests. Often patients are concerned that they have a rectal mass or carcinoma. Examination after an enema often makes the prolapse apparent. Medical therapy is limited to stool bulking agents or fiber. Surgical correction is the mainstay of therapy.

30. The answer is E.

(Chap. 19) Surgical therapy is indicated in all low-risk surgical patients with complicated diverticular disease. Patients with at least two episodes of diverticulitis requiring hospitalization, with disease that does not respond to medical therapy, or who develop intraabdominal complications are considered to have complicated disease. Complicating this patient's relapse of diverticulitis is probably an enterovesicular fistula causing pneumaturia. Studies indicate that younger patients (<50 years) may experience a more aggressive form of the disease than older patients, and therefore waiting for more than two attacks before considering surgery is not recommended. Rifaximin is a poorly absorbed broad-spectrum antibiotic that, when combined with a fiber-rich diet, is associated with less frequent symptoms in patients with uncomplicated diverticular disease. Pneumaturia represents a potential surgical urgency and should not be confused with proteinuria.

31. The answer is A.

(Chap. 20) Mesenteric ischemia is a relatively uncommon and highly morbid illness. Acute mesenteric ischemia is usually due to arterial embolus (usually from the heart) or from thrombosis in a diseased vascular bed. Major risk factors include age, atrial fibrillation, valvular disease, recent arterial catheterization, and recent myocardial infarction. Ischemia occurs when the intestines are inadequately perfused by the splanchnic circulation. This blood supply has extensive collateralization and can receive up to 30% of the cardiac output, making poor perfusion an uncommon event. Patients with acute mesenteric ischemia will frequently present with pain out of proportion to their initial physical examination. As ischemia persists, peritoneal signs and cardiovascular collapse will follow. Mortality is greater than 50%. While radiographic imaging can suggest ischemia, the gold standard for diagnosis is laparotomy.

32. The answer is C.

(Chap. 22) Obstruction of the appendiceal lumen is believed to typically result in appendicitis. Although obstruction is most commonly caused by fecalith, which results from accumulation and inspissation of fecal matter around vegetable fibers, other causes have been described. These other potential causes include enlarged lymphoid follicles associated with viral infection (e.g., measles), inspissated barium, worms (e.g., pinworms, *Ascaris* and *Taenia*), and tumors such as carcinoma or carcinoid. Cholelithiasis is a common cause of acute pancreatitis.

33. The answer is E.

(Chap. 22) Infection with *Yersinia* organisms may potentially cause acute appendicitis after obstruction occurs. High complement fixation antibody titers have been found in up to 30% of proven cases of acute appendicitis. Chronic appendicitis is quite rare, but may occur due to tuberculosis, amebiasis, and actinomycosis.

34. The answer is A.

(Chap. 22) The patient presents with classic findings for acute appendicitis with anorexia, progressing to vague periumbilical pain, followed by localization to the right lower quadrant. Low-grade fever and leukocytosis are frequently present. Although acute appendicitis is primarily a clinical diagnosis, imaging modalities are frequently employed as the symptoms are not always classic. Plain radiographs are rarely helpful except when an opaque fecalith is found in the right lower quadrant (<5% of cases). Ultrasound may demonstrate an enlarged appendix with a thick wall, but is most useful to rule out ovarian pathology, tuboovarian abscess, or ectopic pregnancy. Recently both nonenhanced and contrasted CT have been shown be superior to ultrasound or plain radiograph in the diagnosis of acute appendicitis, with a positive predictive value of 95–97% and overall accuracy

of 90–97%. Findings often include a thickened appendix with periappendiceal stranding and often the presence of a fecalith. Free air is uncommon, even in the case of a perforated appendix. Nonvisualization of the appendix on CT is associated with surgical findings of a normal appendix 98% of the time. Colonoscopy has no role in the diagnosis of acute appendicitis.

35 and 36. The answers are C and D, respectively.

(Chap. 22) The patient presents with several months of epigastric abdominal pain that is worse after eating. His symptoms are highly suggestive of peptic ulcer disease, with the worsening pain after eating suggesting a duodenal ulcer. The current presentation with acute abdomen and free air under the diaphragm diagnoses perforated viscus. Perforated gallbladder is less likely in light of the duration of symptoms and the absence of the significant systemic symptoms that often accompany this condition. As the patient is relatively young with no risk factors for mesenteric ischemia, necrotic bowel from an infarction is highly unlikely. Pancreatitis can have a similar presentation, but a pancreas cannot perforate and liberate free air. Peritonitis is most commonly associated with bacterial infection, but it can be caused by the abnormal presence of physiologic fluids, for example, gastric contents, bile, pancreatic enzymes, blood, or urine, or by foreign bodies. In this case peritonitis most likely is due to the presence of gastric juice in the peritoneal cavity after perforation of a duodenal ulcer has allowed these juices to leave the gut lumen.

37. The answer is B.

(Chap. 23) Acute infectious diarrhea remains a leading cause of death worldwide, especially among children younger than 5 years of age. The major categories of acute diarrheal illness include noninflammatory, inflammatory, and penetrating diarrhea. Vibrio cholerae causes diarrhea through production of an enterotoxin, which is characteristic of noninflammatory diarrhea. After ingestion of a large volume (10^5–10^6) of organisms, V. cholerae attaches to the brush border of the small intestinal enterocytes and produces cholera toxin. The primary clinical characteristic of diarrheal illness caused by toxin production is profuse watery diarrhea that is not bloody. Fecal leukocytes are typically not present in noninflammatory diarrhea. However, a mild increase in fecal lactoferrin can be seen because this test is more sensitive for the presence of mild inflammation. Other pathogens that are common causes of noninflammatory diarrhea are enterotoxigenic Escherichia coli, Bacillus cereus, Staphylococcus aureus, and viral diarrhea, among others.

The site of inflammation in inflammatory diarrhea is typically the colon or distal small bowel. In inflammatory diarrhea, there is invasion of leukocytes into the wall of the intestines. The prototypical pathogen of inflammatory diarrhea is Shigella dysenteriae. Bloody stools are common, and the stool contains large quantities of fecal leukocytes and fecal lactoferrin. Other pathogens that cause inflammatory diarrhea are most Salmonella species, Campylobacter jejuni, enterohemorrhagic Escherichia coli, and Clostridium difficile.

Penetrating diarrhea is caused by either Salmonella typhi or Yersinia enterocolitica. The site of inflammation in penetrating diarrhea is the distal small bowel. In penetrating diarrhea, these organisms penetrate the intestinal wall and multiply within Peyer's patches and intestinal lymph nodes before disseminating into the bloodstream. Clinically, penetrating diarrhea presents as enteric fever with fever, relative bradycardia, abdominal pain, leukopenia, and splenomegaly.

38 and 39. The answers are B and D, respectively.

(Chap. 23) Traveler's diarrhea is common among individuals traveling to Asia, Africa, and Central and South America, affecting 25 to 50% of travelers to these areas. Most traveler's diarrhea begins within 3 to 5 days after arrival and is self-limited, lasting 1 to 5 days. Most individuals acquire traveler's diarrhea after consuming contaminated food or water. Although some organisms have a geographic association, enterotoxigenic and enteroaggregative Escherichia coli are found worldwide and are the most common causes of traveler's diarrhea. In Asia, Campylobacter jejuni is also common. This presentation would be uncommon for Shigella spp. because it most frequently causes bloody diarrhea. Norovirus is associated with a more profuse diarrhea. It has been the causative organism in large outbreaks on cruise ships. Giardia lamblia is a parasite that is responsible for 5% or less of traveler's diarrhea. The approach to treatment of traveler's diarrhea should be tailored to the severity of the patient's symptoms. In general, most cases are self-limited. As long as an individual is able to maintain adequate fluid intake, no specific therapy may be required if there are no more than one or two unformed stools daily without distressing abdominal symptoms, bloody stools, or fever. In this scenario, the patient is not having a large number of stools, but in the presence of distressing abdominal symptoms, use of bismuth subsalicylate or loperamide is recommended. If loperamide is used, an initial dose of 4 mg is given followed by 2 mg after passage of each unformed stool. Antibacterial therapy is only recommended if there is evidence of inflammatory diarrhea (bloody stools or fever) or there are more than two unformed stools daily. The antibacterial agent of choice is usually a fluoroquinolone. Ciprofloxacin given as a single dose of 750 mg or 500 mg three times daily for 3 days is typically effective. In Thailand, Campylobacter jejuni is a common agent and has a high degree of fluoroquinolone resistance. For travelers to Thailand who require antibiotics, azithromycin is recommended with an initial dose of 10 mg/kg on the first day followed by 5 mg/kg on days 2 and 3 if diarrhea persists.

40. The answer is C.

(Chap. 23) Acute bacterial food poisoning occurring 1 to 6 hours after ingestion of contaminated food is most commonly caused by infection with *Staphylococcus aureus* or *Bacillus cereus*. *S. aureus* is associated with ingestion of ham, poultry, potato or egg salad, mayonnaise, or cream pastries that have been allowed to remain at room temperature after cooking. *B. cereus* is classically associated with contaminated fried rice. The symptoms of bacterial food poisoning begin abruptly with nausea, vomiting, abdominal cramping, and diarrhea. However, fever is not a common finding and should cause one to consider other etiologies of vomiting and diarrhea.

41. The answer is C.

(Chap. 23) The patient most likely has food poisoning caused by contamination of the fried rice with *Bacillus cereus*. This toxin-mediated disease occurs when heat-resistant spores germinate after boiling. Frying before serving may not destroy the preformed toxin. The emetic form of illness occurs within 6 hours of eating and is self-limited. No therapy is necessary unless the patient develops severe dehydration. This patient currently has no symptoms consistent with volume depletion; therefore, she does not need intravenous fluids at present. Sarcoidosis does not predispose patients to infectious diseases.

42. The answer is E.

(Chap. 24) Although frequent nonbloody diarrheal illness is commonly associated with *Clostridium difficile* infection, other presentations are well described, including fever in 28% of cases, abdominal pain, and leukocytosis. Adynamic ileus is often seen with *C. difficile* infection, and leukocytosis in this condition should be a clue that *C. difficile* is at play. Recurrent infection after therapy has been described in 15 to 30% of cases.

43. The answer is D.

(Chap. 24) *Clostridium difficile* infection is diagnosed by the following means: diarrhea of three or more stools per day for 2 or more days with no other cause plus (1) demonstration of toxin A or B in the stool, (2) polymerase chain reaction for toxin-producing *C. difficile* of the stool, or (3) demonstration of pseudomembranes on colonoscopy. Although many tests are available, none has adequate sensitivity to definitively rule out *C. difficile* infection. Thus, empiric therapy is appropriate in a patient (such as patient C) with a high likelihood of *C. difficile* infection.

44. The answer is C.

(Chap. 24) The patient has evidence of recurrent *Clostridium difficile* infection, which occurs in up to 30% of treated patients. Because there is no evidence that she has severe infection and this is her first recurrence, the recommended therapy is to retreat with oral metronidazole.

Vancomycin is reserved for patients with severe infection either initially or with recurrence. Fecal transplantation, intravenous immunoglobulin, and oral nitazoxanide are all potential therapies for patients with multiple recurrences.

45. The answer is E.

(Chap. 24) Clindamycin, ampicillin, and cephalosporins (including ceftriaxone) were the first antibiotics associated with *Clostridium difficile*–associated disease and still are. More recently, broad-spectrum fluoroquinolones, including moxifloxacin and ciprofloxacin, have been associated with outbreaks of *C. difficile*, including outbreaks in some locations of a more virulent strain that has caused severe disease among elderly outpatients. For unclear reasons, β-lactams other than the later generation cephalosporins appear to carry a lesser risk of disease. Penicillin–β-lactamase combination antibiotics appear to have lower risk of *C. difficile*–associated disease than the other agents mentioned. Cases have even been reported associated with metronidazole and vancomycin administration. Nevertheless, all patients initiating antibiotics should be warned to seek care if they develop diarrhea that is severe or persists for more than 1 day because all antibiotics carry some risk for *C. difficile*–associated disease.

46. The answer is A.

(Chap. 25) Primary (spontaneous) bacterial peritonitis (PBP) occurs when the peritoneal cavity becomes infected without an apparent source of contamination. PBP occurs most often in patients with cirrhosis, usually with preexisting ascites. The bacterial likely invade the peritoneal fluid because of poor hepatic filtration in cirrhosis. Although fever is present in up to 80% of cases, abdominal pain, acute onset, and peritoneal signs are often absent. Patients may present with nonspecific findings such as malaise or worsening encephalopathy. A neutrophil count in peritoneal fluid of greater than 250/μL is diagnostic; there is no % neutrophil differential threshold. Diagnosis is often difficult because peritoneal culture findings are often negative. Blood cultures may reveal the causative organism. The most common organisms are enteric gram-negative bacilli, but gram-positive cocci are often found. Anaerobes are not common (in contrast to secondary bacterial peritonitis), and empiric antibiotics targeting them are not necessary if PBP is suspected. Third-generation cephalosporins or piperacillin–tazobactam are reasonable initial empiric therapy. Diagnosis requires exclusion of a primary intraabdominal source of peritonitis.

47. The answer is D.

(Chap. 25) This patient has continuous ambulatory peritoneal dialysis (CAPD)–associated peritonitis. Unlike primary or secondary bacterial peritonitis, this infection

is usually caused by skin organisms, most commonly *Staphylococcus* spp. The organisms migrate into the peritoneal fluid via the device. There may not be a tunnel or exit-site infection. Peritonitis is the most common reason for discontinuing CAPD. Y-connectors and diligent technique decrease the risk of CAPD. In contrast to PBP and similar to spontaneous bacterial peritonitis (SBP), the onset of symptoms is usually acute with diffuse pain and peritoneal signs. The dialysate will be cloudy with greater than 100 WBC/µL and greater than 50% neutrophils. Dialysate should be placed in blood culture media and often is often positive with one organism. Finding more than one organism in culture should prompt an evaluation for SBP. Empirical intraperitoneal coverage for CAPD peritonitis should be directed against staphylococcal species based on local epidemiology. If the patient is severely ill, intravenous antibiotics should be added. If the patient does not respond within 4 days, catheter removal should be considered.

48. The answer is D.

(Chap. 25) The computed tomography scan shows a large complex liver abscess in the right lobe. Liver abscesses may arise from hematogenous spread, biliary disease (most common currently), pylephlebitis, or contiguous infection in the peritoneal cavity. Fever is the only common physical finding in liver abscess. Up to 50% of patients may not have symptoms or signs to direct attention to the liver. Nonspecific symptoms are common, and liver abscess is an important cause of fever of unexplained origin in elderly patients. The only reliably abnormal serum studies are elevated alkaline phosphatase or WBC in 70% of patients. Liver abscess may be suggested by an elevated hemidiaphragm on chest radiograph. The most common causative organisms in presumed biliary disease are gram-negative bacilli. Anaerobes are not common unless pelvic or other enteric sources are suspected. Fungal liver abscesses occur after fungemia in immunocompromised patients receiving chemotherapy, often presenting symptomatically with neutrophil reconstitution. Drainage, usually percutaneous, is the mainstay of therapy and is useful initially diagnostically (Figure 25-3).

49. The answer is C.

(Chap. 25) It is important to distinguish between primary (spontaneous) and secondary peritonitis. Primary peritonitis is a result of long-standing ascites, usually as a result of cirrhosis. The pathogenesis is poorly understood but may involve bacteremic spread or translocation across the gut wall of usually only a single species of pathogenic bacteria. Secondary peritonitis is caused by rupture of a hollow viscous or irritation of the peritoneum caused by a contiguous abscess or pyogenic infection. It typically presents with peritoneal signs and in most cases represents a surgical emergency. Secondary peritonitis in a patient with cirrhosis is difficult to distinguish on clinical

grounds from primary (spontaneous) peritonitis. It is often overlooked because classic peritoneal signs are almost always lacking, and it is uniformly fatal in the absence of surgery. Suspicion for this diagnosis should occur when ascites shows a protein greater than 1 g/dL, lactate dehydrogenase (LDH) greater than serum LDH, glucose level below 50 mg/dL, or a polymicrobial Gram stain. When this diagnosis is suspected, abdominal radiography is indicated to rule out free air, and prompt surgical consultation is warranted. Unlike with primary (spontaneous) bacterial peritonitis, in cases of secondary peritonitis, antibiotics should include anaerobic coverage and often antifungal agents. This patient requires intravenous fluid because he has hypotension and tachycardia caused by sepsis. Drotrecogin alfa has been shown to reduce mortality in patients with sepsis, but it is not indicated in patients with thrombocytopenia, cirrhosis, and ascites.

50. The answer is B.

(Chap. 26) *Helicobacter pylori* is thought to colonize about 50% (30% in developed countries and >80% in developing countries) of the world's population. The organism induces a direct tissue response in the stomach, with evidence of mononuclear and polymorphonuclear infiltrates in all of those with colonization regardless of whether or not symptoms are present. Gastric ulceration and adenocarcinoma of the stomach arise in association with this gastritis. MALT is specific to *H. pylori* infection and because of prolonged B-cell activation in the stomach. Although *H. pylori* does not directly infect the intestine, it does diminish somatostatin production, indirectly contributing to the development of duodenal ulcers. Gastroesophageal reflux disease is not caused by *H. pylori* colonization. Recent studies have demonstrated that colonization by some strains of *H. pylori* may be protective for the development of adenocarcinoma of the esophagus and premalignant lesions such as Barrett's esophagus (odds ratio, 0.2–0.6).

51. The answer is E.

(Chap. 26) It is impossible to know whether the patient's continued dyspepsia is attributable to persistent *Helicobacter pylori* as a result of treatment failure or to some other cause. A quick noninvasive test to look for the presence of *H. pylori* is a urea breath test. This test can be done as an outpatient and gives a rapid, accurate response. Patients should not have received any proton pump inhibitors or antimicrobials in the meantime. Stool antigen test is another good option if urea breath testing is not available. If the urea breath test is positive more than 1 month after completion of first-line therapy, second-line therapy with a proton pump inhibitor, bismuth subsalicylate, tetracycline, and metronidazole may be indicated. If the urea breath test result is negative, the remaining symptoms are unlikely attributable to persistent *H. pylori* infection. Serology is useful only for

diagnosing infection initially, but it can remain positive and therefore misleading in those who have cleared *H. pylori*. Endoscopy is a consideration to rule out ulcer or upper gastrointestinal malignancy but is generally preferred after two failed attempts to eradicate *H. pylori*. Figure 26-2 outlines the algorithm for management of *H. pylori* infection.

52. The answer is A.
(Chap. 26) Helicobacter pylori is a disease of overcrowding. Transmission has therefore decreased in the United States as the standard of living has increased. It is predicated that the percentage of duodenal ulcers caused by factors other than *H. pylori* (e.g., use of nonsteroidal anti-inflammatory drugs) will increase over the upcoming decades. Controversial but increasing evidence suggests that *H. pylori* colonization may provide some protection from recent emerging gastrointestinal disorders, such as gastroesophageal reflux disease (and its complication, esophageal carcinoma). Therefore, the health implications of *H. pylori* eradication may not be simple.

53. The answer is A.
(Chap. 26) In vitro, *Helicobacter pylori* is susceptible to a wide variety of antibiotics. However, monotherapy is no longer recommended because of inadequate antibiotic delivery to the colonization niche and the development of resistance. All current regimens include a proton pump inhibitor (omeprazole or equivalent), H_2 blocker (ranitidine or equivalent), and/or bismuth. Regimens including quinolones may not be advisable because of common resistance and the risk of developing *Clostridium difficile* colitis. Current regimens have an eradication rate of 75 to 80%. (See Table 26-2.)

54. The answer is E.
(Chap. 27) Salmonella enteritidis is one of the causes of nontyphoidal salmonellosis (NTS) along with *Salmonella typhimurium* and other strains. Enteric (typhoid) fever is caused by *Salmonella typhi* or *Salmonella paratyphi*. Recent cases of gastroenteritis caused by NTS have been associated with undercooked or raw eggs. In contrast to *S. typhi* and *S. paratyphi*, which only have human reservoirs, the NTS can colonize livestock accounting for outbreaks related to contaminated water (fresh produce, undercooked ground meat, dairy products). The gastroenteritis caused by NTS is indistinguishable clinically for other enteric pathogens. The diarrhea is nonbloody and may be copious. The disease is typically self-limited in healthy hosts, and antibiotic therapy is not recommended because it does not change the course of disease and promotes resistance. Therapy may be necessary for neonates or debilitated elderly patients who are more likely to develop bacteremia. Bacteremia occurs in fewer than 10% of cases. Metastatic infections of bone, joint, and endovascular devices may occur. There is no vaccine for NTS. Oral and parenteral vaccines for *S. typhi* are available.

55. The answer is D.
(Chap. 28) Shigellosis remains a cause of dysentery in the developing world and sporadic cases caused by fecal–oral contamination occur in the developing and developed world. The human intestinal tract is the most prevalent reservoir for the bacteria. Clinical illness from *Shigella* infection can be caused by a very small inoculum. Shigellosis typically evolves through four phases: incubation, watery diarrhea, dysentery, and the postinfectious phase. The incubation period is usually 1 to 4 days, and the dysentery follows within hours to days. The dysentery syndrome is indistinguishable from other invasive enteropathogens (including *Campylobacter* spp.), and inflammatory bowel disease is also in the differential diagnosis. Because the organism is enteroinvasive, antibiotic therapy is indicated. Ciprofloxacin is generally recommended unless there is no or proven resistance. Ceftriaxone, azithromycin, pivmecillinam, and some recent quinolones are also effective. *Shigella* infection typically does not cause life-threatening dehydration. Antimotility agents are not recommended because they are thought to prolong the systemic symptoms and may increase the risk of toxic megacolon and hemolytic uremic syndrome. There is currently no commercially available vaccine for *Shigella* infection.

56. The answer is A.
(Chap. 29) Campylobacter spp. are motile, curved gram-negative rods. The principal diarrheal pathogen is *Campylobacter jejuni*. This organism is found in the gastrointestinal tract of many animals used for food production and is usually transmitted to humans in raw or undercooked food products or through direct contact with infected animals. More than half of cases are caused by insufficiently cooked contaminated poultry. *Campylobacter* infection a common cause of diarrheal disease in the United States. The illness usually occurs within 2 to 4 days after exposure to the organism in food or water. Biopsy of an affected patient's jejunum, ileum, or colon reveals findings indistinguishable from those of Crohn's disease and ulcerative colitis. Although the diarrheal illness is usually self-limited, it may be associated with constitutional symptoms, lasts more than 1 week, and recurs in 5 to 10% of untreated patients. Complications include pancreatitis, cystitis, arthritis, meningitis, and Guillain-Barré syndrome. The symptoms of *Campylobacter* enteritis are similar to those resulting from infection with *Salmonella typhi*, *Shigella* spp., and *Yersinia* spp.; all of these agents cause fever and the presence of fecal leukocytes. The diagnosis is made by isolating *Campylobacter* organisms from the stool, which requires selective media. *Escherichia coli* (enterotoxigenic), Norwalk agent, and rotavirus are generally not associated with the finding of fecal leukocytes. About 5 to 10% of untreated patients with *Campylobacter* enteritis develop recurrences that may be clinically and pathologically confused with inflammatory bowel disease.

57. The answer is A.

(Chap. 29) As is true with all acute diarrheal diseases, adequate volume resuscitation is central to treatment. Many patients with mild *Campylobacter* enteritis will resolve spontaneously, and not all patients clearly benefit from therapy. In the presence of high or persistent fever, bloody diarrhea, severe diarrhea, worsening symptoms, or symptoms persisting for more than 1 week, antibiotics are recommended. A 5- to 7-day course of erythromycin, azithromycin (and other macrolides), or ciprofloxacin is effective. Drug resistance to fluoroquinolones and tetracycline is increasing. Antimotility agents are not recommended because they have been associated with the development of serious complications, including toxic megacolon and hemolytic uremic syndrome. Tinidazole and metronidazole are used to treat a variety of nonbacterial diarrhea syndromes, including giardiasis and amoebiasis. Metronidazole is also used for *Clostridium difficile*–associated colitis.

58. The answer is B.

(Chap. 30) Cholera remains a worldwide problem with sporadic cases usually related to contact with fecally contaminated water or seafood. Humans are the only known reservoir of *Vibrio cholera*. Most cases are reported in Africa or Asia. After a century, cholera returned to Haiti after recent natural disasters and breakdown of public health measures. The watery diarrhea of cholera is mediated by a specific cholera toxin that binds to small intestine epithelium to cause profuse fluid secretion. The diarrhea of cholera is painless, nonbloody, and watery with mucus and few inflammatory cells. The term "rice-water" diarrhea refers to the appearance of water after soaking rice. Morbidity and mortality from cholera are from profound volume depletion. Rehydration is essential to therapy. Major improvements in care came from the development of oral rehydration solutions that take advantage of glucose–sodium co-transport in the small intestine. These solutions allowed effective rehydration in resource limited settings where intravenous rehydration was not practical. Diagnosis is by culture or point-of-care antigen detection dipstick assay. Antibiotics are not necessary for cure, but they diminish the duration and volume of fluid loss and hasten the clearance of the organism from stool. A single dose of doxycycline is effective in adults in areas where there is not resistance. Ciprofloxacin or azithromycin may be alternatives.

59. The answer is B.

(Chap. 31) The Norwalk virus is the prototype calicivirus that causes human disease. The calicivirus family, many of which cause gastroenteritis and diarrhea, particularly in children, includes norovirus and sapovirus. Most adults worldwide have antibodies to these viruses. However, they are a major cause of morbidity throughout the world and a frequent cause of nonbacterial diarrhea outbreaks in the United States. They spread via fecal–oral spread and have a low inoculum necessary for disease. In temperate regions, they tend to occur in cold weather months. The incubation period is less than 3 days, typically 24 hours. The onset of disease is rapid. Fever, myalgias, and headache are common. The diarrhea is nonbloody without fecal leukocytes. The disease is self-limited, and therapy is supportive.

60. The answer is B.

(Chap. 31) Nearly all children worldwide are infected with rotavirus by age 5 years. In the developing world, it remains a major cause of diarrheal death caused by volume depletion. Repeated infections occur with each subsequent episode of lesser severity. Therefore, severe disease is uncommon in adolescents and adults who may develop disease, particularly after contact with ill children. The disease typically has an abrupt onset with vomiting usually preceding diarrhea. Fever occurs in approximately one-third of cases. Stools usually do not contain blood, mucus, or inflammatory material. The disease is usually self-limited in 3 to 7 days. Because rotavirus is a major cause of childhood hospitalization and morbidity in the United States, vaccination is recommended for all U.S. children. Vaccination has less efficacy in the developing world because of a higher frequency of malnutrition, co-infection, and comorbidities, but is recommended by the World Health Organization for all children worldwide.

61. The answer is E.

(Chap. 32) Entamoeba histolytica is a common pathogen in areas of the world with poor sanitation and crowding. Transmission is oral–fecal, and the primary manifestation is colitis, often heme positive. Liver abscess is a common complication, occurring after the organism crosses the colonic border and travels through the portal circulation, subsequently lodging in the liver. At the time of presentation with liver abscess, the primary gastrointestinal infection has usually cleared, and organisms cannot be identified in the stool. Suggestive imaging with a positive serologic test result for *E. histolytica* is diagnostic. When a patient has a diagnostic imaging procedure, a positive amebic serology result is highly sensitive (>94%) and highly specific (>95%) for diagnosis of amebic liver abscess. Treatment for amebic liver abscess is generally with metronidazole. Luminal infection can be treated with paromomycin or iodoquinol. *Campylobacter* is a major cause of foodborne infectious diarrhea. Although usually self-limited, it may cause serious enteritis and inflammatory diarrhea but not liver abscess.

62. The answer is C.

(Chap. 33) Of the listed protozoa, only *Giardia* infection can be diagnosed with stool ova and parasite examination. Stool antigen immunoassay can be used to diagnose

Giardia and *Cryptosporidium* spp. Fecal acid-fast testing may be used to diagnose *Cryptosporidium*, *Isospora*, and *Cyclospora* spp. Microsporidia require special fecal stains or tissue biopsy for diagnosis.

63. The answer is D.

(Chap. 33) Trichomoniasis is transmitted via sexual contact with an infected partner. Many men are asymptomatic but may have symptoms of urethritis, epididymitis, or prostatitis. Most women have symptoms of infection that include vaginal itching, dyspareunia, and malodorous discharge. These symptoms do not distinguish *Trichomonas* infection from other forms of vaginitis, such as bacterial vaginosis. Trichomoniasis is not a self-limited infection and should be treated for symptomatic and public health reasons. Wet-mount examination for motile trichomonads has a sensitivity of 50 to 60% in routine examination. Direct immunofluorescent antibody staining of secretions is more sensitive and can also be performed immediately. Culture is not widely available and takes 3 to 7 days. Treatment should consist of metronidazole either as a single 2-g dose or 500-mg doses twice daily for 7 days; all sexual partners should be treated. Trichomoniasis resistant to metronidazole has been reported and is managed with increased doses of metronidazole or with tinidazole.

64. The answer is E.

(Chap. 33) Giardiasis is diagnosed by detection of parasite antigens in the feces or by visualizing cysts or trophozoites in feces or small intestine. There is no reliable serum test for this disease. Because a wide variety of pathogens are responsible for diarrheal illness, some degree of diagnostic testing beyond the history and physical examination is required for definitive diagnosis. Colonoscopy does not have a role in diagnosing *Giardia* infection. Giardiasis can persist in symptomatic patients and should be treated. Severe symptoms such as malabsorption, weight loss, growth retardation, and dehydration may occur in prolonged cases. Additionally, extraintestinal manifestations such as urticarial, anterior uveitis, and arthritis have been associated with potential giardiasis. A single oral 2-g dose of tinidazole is reportedly more effective than a 5-day course of metronidazole with cure rates above 90% for both. Paromomycin, an oral poorly absorbed aminoglycoside, can be used for symptomatic patients during pregnancy, but its efficacy for eradicating infection is not known. Clindamycin and albendazole do not have a role in treatment of giardiasis. Refractory disease with persistent infection can be treated with a longer duration of metronidazole.

65. The answer is D.

(Chap. 33) Cryptosporidium typically causes a self-limited diarrheal illness in immunocompetent patients but may cause severe debilitating disease in patients with severe immunodeficiency, such as advanced HIV infection. Outbreaks in immunocompetent hosts are caused by ingestion of oocysts. Infectious oocysts are excreted in human feces, causing human-to-human transmission. Waterborne transmission of oocysts accounts for disease in travelers and common-source outbreaks. Oocysts resist killing by routine chlorination of drinking and recreational water sources. Infection may be asymptomatic in immunocompetent and immunosuppressed hosts. Diarrhea is typically watery and nonbloody and may be associated with abdominal pain, nausea, fever, and anorexia. In immunocompetent hosts, symptoms usually subside in 1 to 2 weeks without therapy. In advanced AIDS with CD4 counts below $100/\mu L$, severe symptoms may develop, leading to significant electrolyte and volume loss. Nitazoxanide is approved for treatment of *Cryptosporidium* but to date has not been shown to be effective in HIV-infected patients. The best available therapy for these patients is antiretroviral therapy to reduce immune suppression. Tinidazole and metronidazole are used to treat giardiasis and trichomoniasis, not cryptosporidiosis.

66. The answer is B.

(Chap. 34) Strongyloides is the only helminth that can replicate in the human host, allowing autoinfection. Humans acquire *Strongyloides* when larvae in fecally contaminated soil penetrate the skin or mucous membranes. The larvae migrate to the lungs via the bloodstream; break through the alveolar spaces; ascend the respiratory airways; and are swallowed to reach the small intestine, where they mature into adult worms. Adult worms may penetrate the mucosa of the small intestine. Strongyloides is endemic in Southeast Asia, sub-Saharan Africa, Brazil, and the Southern United States. Many patients with *Strongyloides* are asymptomatic or have mild gastrointestinal symptoms or the characteristic cutaneous eruption, larval currens, as described in this case. Small bowel obstruction may occur with early heavy infection. Eosinophilia is common with all clinical manifestations. In patients with impaired immunity, particularly glucocorticoid therapy, hyperinfection or dissemination may occur. This may lead to colitis, enteritis, meningitis, peritonitis, and acute renal failure. Bacteremia or gram-negative sepsis may develop because of bacterial translocation through disrupted enteric mucosa. Because of the risk of hyperinfection, all patients with *Strongyloides* infection, even asymptomatic carriers, should be treated with ivermectin, which is more effective than albendazole. Fluconazole is used to treat candidal infections. Mebendazole is used to treat trichuriasis, enterobiasis (pinworm), ascariasis, and hookworm. Mefloquine is used for malaria prophylaxis.

67. The answer is B.

(Chap. 34) Ascaris lumbricoides is the longest nematode (15–40 cm) parasite of humans. It resides in tropical

and subtropical regions. In the United States, it is found mostly in the rural Southeast. Transmission is through fecally contaminated soil. Most commonly, the worm burden is low, and it causes no symptoms. Clinical disease is related to larval migration to the lungs or to adult worms in the gastrointestinal tract. The most common complications occur because of a high gastrointestinal adult worm burden, leading to small bowel obstruction (most often in children with a narrow-caliber small bowel lumen) or migration leading to obstructive complications such as cholangitis, pancreatitis, or appendicitis. Rarely, adult worms can migrate to the esophagus and be orally expelled. During the lung phase of larval migration (9–12 days after egg ingestion), patients may develop a nonproductive cough, fever, eosinophilia, and pleuritic chest pain. Eosinophilic pneumonia syndrome (Löffler's syndrome) is characterized by symptoms and lung infiltrates. Meningitis is not a known complication of ascariasis but can occur with disseminated strongyloidiasis in an immunocompromised host.

68. The answer is A.
(Chap. 34) Ascariasis should always be treated, even in asymptomatic cases, to prevent serious intestinal complications. Albendazole, mebendazole, and ivermectin are effective. These agents should not be administered to pregnant women. Pyrantel is safe in pregnancy. Metronidazole is used for anaerobic bacterial and *Trichomonas* infections. Fluconazole is mostly used to treat *Candida* infections. Diethylcarbamazine (DEC) is first-line therapy for active lymphatic filariasis. Vancomycin has no effect on nematodes.

69. The answer is E.
(Chap. 34) This patient's most likely diagnosis is anisakiasis. This is a nematode infection in which humans are an accidental host. It occurs hours to days after ingesting eggs that previously settled into the muscles of fish. The main risk factor for infection is eating raw fish. Presentation mimics an acute abdomen. History is critical because upper endoscopy is both diagnostic and curative. The implicated nematodes burrow into the mucosa of the stomach, causing intense pain, and must be manually removed by endoscope or, on rare occasion, surgery. There is no medical agent known to cure anisakiasis.

70. The answer is A.
(Chap. 35) The most common and most characteristic symptom of liver disease is fatigue. Unfortunately, it is also very nonspecific with little specific diagnostic utility. The fatigue in liver disease seems to improve in the morning and worsen throughout the day, but it can be intermittent. Jaundice is the hallmark of liver disease and is much more specific. Jaundice, however, is typically a sign of more advanced disease. Itching is also typically a symptom of more advanced disease and is more common

in cholestatic causes of liver disease. Nausea often occurs in severe disease and can be accompanied by vomiting. Right upper quadrant pain is a less common symptom and indicates stretching of the liver capsule.

71. The answer is B.
(Chap. 35) Women are more susceptible to the effects of alcohol on the liver. On average, drinking about two drinks daily can lead to chronic liver disease in women, whereas in men it is about three drinks daily. In individuals with alcoholic cirrhosis, the average daily alcohol intake is usually much higher, however, and heavy drinking for more than 10 years is typical before the onset of liver disease.

72. The answer is D.
(Chap. 36) It is important to understand the patterns of laboratory abnormalities that indicate liver disease is present. One way to consider laboratory evaluation of liver disease is to consider three general categories of tests: tests based on excretory function of the liver, tests of biosynthetic activity of the liver, and coagulation factors. The most common tests of liver function fall under the category of tests based on the detoxification and excretory function of the liver. These include serum bilirubin, urine bilirubin, ammonia, and enzyme levels. Bilirubin can exist as a conjugated and an unconjugated form. The unconjugated form is often referred to as the indirect fraction. Elevations in the unconjugated form of bilirubin are not related to liver disease, but are most commonly seen in hemolysis and a number of benign genetic conditions such as Gilbert's syndrome. In contrast, conjugated hyperbilirubinemia almost always indicates disease of the liver or biliary tract. Conjugated bilirubin is water soluble and is excreted in the urine, but unconjugated bilirubin is not. Rather, it binds to albumin in the blood. Therefore, bilirubinuria implies liver disease as well. Among the serum enzymes, it is useful to consider those that are associated with hepatocellular injury or those that reflect cholestasis. Alanine and aspartate aminotransferases are the primary enzymes that indicate hepatocyte injury. Alkaline phosphatase is the most common enzyme elevated in cholestasis, but bone disease also causes increased alkaline phosphatase. In some cases, one needs additional information to determine if the alkaline phosphatase is liver or bone in origin. Other tests that would be elevated in cholestatic liver disease are 5′-nucleotidase and γ-glutamyl transferase. The primary test of synthetic function is measurement of serum albumin. Coagulation factors can be directly measured, but impaired production of coagulation factors in liver disease is primarily inferred from elevations in prothrombin time.

73 and 74. The answers are E and D, respectively.
(Chap. 37) This patient is presenting with an asymptomatic and mild elevation in unconjugated hyperbilirubinemia

that has occurred during a time of increased stress, fatigue, and likely decreased caloric intake. This presentation is characteristic of Gilbert's syndrome (option E), an inherited disorder of bilirubin conjugation. In Gilbert's syndrome, there is a mutation of the *UGT1A1* gene that encodes bilirubin UDP-glucuronosyltransferase that leads to a reduction in activity on the enzyme to 10–35% of normal. This enzyme is of critical importance in the conjugation of bilirubin. Most of the time, there is no apparent jaundice, as the reduced ability to conjugate bilirubin is not reduced to a degree that leads to an elevation of bilirubin. However, during times of stress, fatigue, alcohol use, decreased caloric intake, or intercurrent illness, the enzyme can become overwhelmed, leading to a mild hyperbilirubinemia. Typical bilirubin levels are less than 4.0 mg/dL unless the individual is ill or fasting. Diagnosis usually occurs during young adulthood, and episodes are self-limited and benign. If a liver biopsy were to be performed, hepatic histology would be normal. No treatment is necessary as there are no long-term consequences of Gilbert's syndrome, and patient reassurance is recommended. Other inherited disorders of bilirubin conjugation are Crigler-Najjar syndrome types I and II. Crigler-Najjar syndrome type I is a congenital disease characterized by more dramatic elevations in bilirubin as high as 20–45 mg/dL that is first diagnosed in the neonatal period and is present throughout life. This rare disorder was once fatal in early childhood due to the development of kernicterus. However, with phototherapy, individuals are now able to survive into adulthood, although neurologic deficits are common. Crigler-Najjar syndrome type II is similar to type I, but the elevations in bilirubin are less. Kernicterus is rare. This is due to the fact that there is some residual function of the bilirubin UDP-glucuronosyltransferase enzyme (<10%), which is totally absent in type I disease. Hemolysis is another frequent cause of elevated unconjugated bilirubin. Hemolysis can be caused by many factors including medications, autoimmune disorders, and inherited disorders, among others. However, the normal hematocrit, LDH, and haptoglobin eliminate hemolysis as a possibility. Dubin-Johnson syndrome is another congenital hyperbilirubinemia. However, it is a predominantly conjugated hyperbilirubinemia caused by a defect in biliary excretion from hepatocytes. Obstructive choledocholithiasis is characterized by right upper quadrant pain that is often exacerbated by fatty meals. The absence of symptoms or elevation in other liver function tests, especially alkaline phosphatase, also makes this diagnosis unlikely.

75. The answer is B.
(Chap. 38) This patient presents with acute hepatitis, which has numerous etiologies. These include viruses, toxins/drugs, autoimmune diseases, metabolic disease, alcohol, ischemia, pregnancy, and other infectious etiologies including rickettsial diseases and leptospirosis. In this clinical scenario,

the patient has risk factors for hepatitis A, B, and C infection, including having had sex with men and a prior history of injection drug use. All acute viral hepatitis presents with a similar clinical pattern, although incubation periods vary after exposure. The most common initial symptoms are fatigue, anorexia, nausea, vomiting, myalgias, and headache. These symptoms precede the onset of jaundice by about 1–2 weeks. Once jaundice develops, the prodromal symptoms regress. On physical examination, there is usually obvious icterus with an enlarged and tender liver. Splenomegaly can occur. AST and ALT are elevated with peak levels that are quite variable between 400–4000 U/L, and alkaline phosphatase levels are increased to a much lesser degree. Hyperbilirubinemia (levels from 5 to 20 mg/dL) occurs with primarily increased levels of conjugated bilirubin. Thus, it is important to recognize the patterns of antibody production in the viral hepatitides. Hepatitis A is an RNA virus that presents with acute hepatitis and is transmitted by the fecal-oral route. In the acute state, the IgM would be elevated, which is not seen in this scenario. Hepatitis B virus is a DNA virus with three common antigens that are tested serologically to determine the time course of the illness. These antigens are the surface antigen, the core antigen, and the e antigen, which is a nucleocapsid protein produced from the same gene as the core antigen but is immunologically distinct. Several distinct patterns can be observed. In acute hepatitis B, the core IgM, surface antigen, and e antigens are all positive, which is what is seen in this case. At this point, the patient is highly infectious with viral shedding in body fluids, including saliva. In a late acute infection, core IgG may be positive at the same time as surface- and e-antigen positivity. In chronic hepatitis B, this same pattern of serologies is seen. If a patient has a prior infection without development of chronic hepatitis, the core IgG and surface antibody is positive. However, when immunity is obtained via vaccination, only the surface antibody (SAb) is positive; the e antigen and surface antigen will be negative since the patient was never infected. The variety of antigen-antibody positivities that can result are outlined in Table 38-5. Acute hepatitis C often is detectable with contemporary immunoassays early in the disease when the aminotransferases are positive. Thus, a positive HCV antibody could indicate acute hepatitis C in this individual. However, given his clinical history of prior injection drug use and inability to donate blood, this likely indicates chronic hepatitis C infection. In some instances, ecstasy has been reported to cause drug-induced hepatitis, but given the viral serologies in this patient, this would be unlikely.

76. The answer is E.
(Chap. 38) No treatment is recommended for acute hepatitis B in most individuals because 99% of infected individual recover without assistance. Therefore, it would not be expected that an individual would derive any particular benefit from treatment. In severe acute

hepatitis B, nucleoside analogues, including lamivudine, have been used successfully, although there are no clinical trial data to support such an approach. For acute hepatitis C, however, there is a growing body of literature to support the use of interferon α therapy to prevent the development of chronic hepatitis C. In a study of 44 patients, 98% had a sustained virologic response after 3 months, and therapy was continued for a total of 24 weeks. Many experts are now recommending that pegylated interferon α plus ribavirin be used as an alternative treatment for acute hepatitis C, although clinical trial data to support this approach is also lacking. Hepatitis A is an acute and self-limited illness that does not progress to chronic liver disease. Thus, no treatment is required. Anti–hepatitis A virus immunoglobulin can be given prophylactically following a known exposure to prevent the development of disease, but it is not helpful in established disease. There is no role for oral or IV corticosteroids in the treatment of acute viral hepatitis of any etiology. It has demonstrated no clinical benefit and may increase the risk of developing chronic disease.

77. The answer is E.

(Chap. 38) In most instances, patients with any form of acute viral hepatitis do not succumb to fulminant liver failure. However, pregnant women are highly susceptible to fulminant hepatic failure in the setting of acute hepatitis E infection. This RNA virus is an enteric virus that is endemic in India, Asia, Africa, the Middle East, and Central America, and is spread via contaminated water supplies. Person-to-person spread is rare. Generally, the clinical course of hepatitis E infection is mild, and the rate of fulminant hepatitis is only 1–2%. However, in pregnant women, this is as high as 10–20%. For hepatitis A and C, the rate of fulminant hepatic failure is about 0.1% or less. It is slightly higher for hepatitis B at around 0.1–1%. Hepatitis D occurs as a coinfection with hepatitis B virus. When the two viruses are acquired simultaneously, the rate of fulminant hepatitis is about 5% or less. When hepatitis D is acquired in the setting of chronic hepatitis B infection, this number rises to 20%.

78. The answer is E.

(Chap. 38) Hepatitis A is an acute, self-limited virus that is acquired almost exclusively via the fecal-oral route. It is classically a disease of poor hygiene and overcrowding. Outbreaks have been traced to contaminated water, milk, frozen raspberries and strawberries, green onions, and shellfish. Infection occurs mostly in children and young adults. It almost invariably resolves spontaneously and results in lifelong immunity. Fulminant disease occurs in 0.1% or less of cases, and there is no chronic form (in contrast to hepatitis B and C). Diagnosis is made by demonstrating a positive IgM antibody to HAV, as described in the case for this question. An IgG antibody to HAV

indicates immunity that has been obtained by previous infection or vaccination. A small proportion of patients will experience relapsing hepatitis weeks to months after a full recovery from HAV infection. This too is self-limited. There is no approved antiviral therapy for hepatitis A disease. An inactivated vaccine has decreased the incidence of the disease, and it is recommended for all U.S. children, high-risk adults, and travelers to endemic areas. Passive immunization with immune globulin is also available, and it is effective in preventing clinical disease before exposure or during the early incubation period.

79. The answer is C.

(Chap. 38) The current hepatitis B vaccine is a recombinant vaccine consisting of yeast-derived hepatitis B surface antigen particles. A strategy of vaccinating only high-risk individuals in the United States has been shown to be ineffective, and universal vaccination against hepatitis B is now recommended. Pregnancy is not a contraindication to vaccination. Vaccination should ideally be performed in infancy. Routine evaluation of hepatitis serologies is not cost-effective and is not recommended. The vaccine is given in three divided IM doses at 0, 1, and 6 months.

80. The answer is A.

(Chap. 38) A clear distinction between viral etiologies of acute hepatitis cannot be made on clinical or epidemiologic features alone. This patient is at risk for many forms of hepatitis due to his lifestyle. Given his occupation in food services, from a public health perspective it is important to make an accurate diagnosis. Serologies must be obtained to make a diagnosis. While hepatitis C virus typically does not present as an acute hepatitis, this is not absolute. Hepatitis E virus infects men and women equally and resembles hepatitis A virus in clinical presentation. This patient should be questioned regarding IV drug use, and in addition to hepatitis serologies, an HIV test should be performed.

81. The answer is C.

(Chaps. 36 and 38) Causes of extreme elevations in serum transaminases generally fall into a few major categories, including viral infections, toxic ingestions, and vascular/hemodynamic causes. Both acute hepatitis A and hepatitis B infections may be characterized by high transaminases. Fulminant hepatic failure may occur, particularly in situations in which acute hepatitis A occurs on top of chronic hepatitis C infection, or if hepatitis B and hepatitis D are cotransmitted. Most cases of acute hepatitis A or B infection in adults are self-limited. Hepatitis C is an RNA virus that does not typically cause acute hepatitis. However, it is associated with a high probability of chronic infection. Therefore, progression to cirrhosis and hepatoma is increased in patients with chronic hepatitis C infection. Extreme transaminitis is highly unlikely with acute hepatitis C infection. Acetaminophen remains one of the major causes of fulminant hepatic failure and is managed by prompt administration of N-acetylcysteine. Budd–Chiari syndrome is characterized by posthepatic thrombus formation. It often presents with jaundice, painful hepatomegaly, ascites, and elevated transaminases.

82. The answer is A.

(Chap. 39) The liver is the primary site for the metabolism of many drugs and as such is susceptible to injury related to drugs and toxins. Indeed, the most common cause of acute hepatic failure is drug-induced liver injury. In general, it is useful to think of chemical hepatotoxicity within two broad categories: direct toxic effects and idiosyncratic reactions. Drugs or toxins that cause a direct toxic effect on the liver are either poisons themselves or are metabolized to toxic substances. With agents that cause a direct toxic effect on hepatocytes, there is a predictable, dose-related pattern of injury, and the time to effect is relatively short. The most common drug or toxin causing direct hepatocyte toxicity is acetaminophen. In therapeutic doses, acetaminophen does not cause liver injury. However, in higher doses, one of the metabolites of acetaminophen, N-acetyl-p-benzoquinone-imine (NAPQI), can overwhelm the glutathione stores of the liver that are necessary to convert NAPQI to a nontoxic metabolite and lead to hepatocyte necrosis. Other medications or toxins that cause direct hepatocyte injury are carbon tetrachloride, trichloroethylene, tetracycline, and the Amanita phalloides mushroom. More commonly known as the deathcap mushroom, ingestion of a single mushroom can contain enough hepatotoxin to be lethal. Idiosyncratic reactions are infrequent and unpredictable. There is no dose dependency, and the timing of hepatic injury has little association with the duration of drug treatment. Many drugs produce idiosyncratic reactions, and often it is difficult to known when an idiosyncratic reaction will lead to more serious liver failure. Often, mild increases in transaminase levels will occur, but over time adaptation leads to a return of liver enzymes to normal levels. In other instances, idiosyncratic reactions can lead to fulminant hepatic failure. Although rare, serious hepatic reactions can lead to medications being removed from the market. It is now recognized that many idiosyncratic reactions are related to metabolites leading to liver injury. However, it is likely that individual genetic variations in liver metabolism are the primary cause, and these are not predictable effects of the drug given our current state of knowledge. Common medications that can lead to idiosyncratic drug reactions include halothane, isothane, isoniazid, HMG-CoA reductase inhibitors, and chlorpromazine.

83. The answer is B.

(Chap. 39) Acetaminophen overdose is the most common cause of acute liver failure and drug-induced liver failure that leads to transplantation. Acetaminophen is metabolized in the liver through two pathways. The primary pathway is a phase II reaction that produces nontoxic sulfate and glucuronide metabolites. The minor pathway occurs through a phase I reaction leading to the production of N-acetyl-p-benzoquinone-imine (NAPQI). This metabolite is directly toxic to liver cells and can lead to hepatocyte necrosis. With therapeutic use of acetaminophen, glutathione in the liver rapidly converts NAPQI to a nontoxic metabolite that is excreted in the urine. However, glutathione stores can become depleted in the setting of a large acute ingestion, chronic alcoholism, or the chronic ingestion of increased acetaminophen. In addition, because alcohol upregulates the first enzyme in the metabolic pathway, NAPQI accumulates more quickly in alcoholics. Given the known hepatotoxicity of acetaminophen, the U.S. Food and Drug Administration has recommended a maximum daily dose of no more than 3.25 g, with lower doses in individuals who use alcohol chronically. Acute ingestions of 10–15 g of acetaminophen is sufficient to cause clinical evidence of liver injury, and doses higher than 25 g can lead to fatal hepatic necrosis. The course of illness with acute acetaminophen ingestion follows a predictable pattern. Nausea, vomiting, abdominal pain, and shock occur within 4–12 hours after ingestion. Liver enzymes and synthetic function are normal during this time. Within 24–48 hours, these symptoms subside and are followed by evidence of hepatic injury. Maximal levels of aminotransferases can reach more than 10,000 U/L and may not occur until 4–6 days after ingestion. These patients must be followed carefully for fulminant hepatic failure with serious complications including encephalopathy, cerebral edema, marked coagulopathy, renal failure, metabolic acidosis, electrolyte abnormalities, and refractory shock. Levels of acetaminophen are predictive of the development of hepatotoxicity. The first level should be measured no sooner than 4 hours after a known ingestion. Levels should be plotted on a nomogram that relates acetaminophen levels to the time after ingestion. If at 4 hours the acetaminophen level is greater than 300 µg/mL, significant hepatotoxicity is likely. In the setting of overdose, it may be difficult to know the exact quantity and timing of the ingestion. For the patient presenting in the clinical scenario in this question, her acetaminophen level of greater than 300 µg/mL is quite concerning for a large ingestion, and treatment should be initiated immediately. The primary treatment for acetaminophen overdose is N-acetylcysteine. N-acetylcysteine acts to replete glutathione levels in the liver and also provides a reservoir of sulfhydryl groups to bind to the toxic metabolites. The typical dose of N-acetylcysteine is 140 mg/kg given as a loading dose, followed by 70 mg/kg every 4 hours for a total of 15–20 doses. This drug can also be given by continuous infusion. Activated charcoal or cholestyramine should only be given if the patient presents within

30 minutes after ingestion. Hemodialysis will not accelerate clearance of acetaminophen and will not protect the liver. Most patients with fulminant hepatic failure develop acute renal failure, often requiring hemodialysis. If a patient survives an acetaminophen overdose, there is usually no chronic liver injury.

84. The answer is E.
(Chap. 40) The patient in this scenario has evidence of chronic active hepatitis B virus (HBV) infection. The presence of hepatitis B e antigen (HBeAg) is indicative of ongoing viral replication, and individuals with HBeAg positivity typically have high levels of HBV DNA on testing. The spectrum of clinical infection in chronic hepatitis B is quite variable, and often individuals are asymptomatic with elevated liver enzymes identified on testing for other reasons. Thus, the decision to treat chronic HBV infection should not be based on clinical features. Most experts recommend treatment of HBeAg-positive chronic HBV infection with HBV DNA levels above 2 $\times$ 10^4 IU/mL if the ALT is elevated greater than twice the upper limit of normal. At present, many treatment options are available for the treatment of HBV infection and fall broadly into two categories: nucleoside analogues and interferons. While lamivudine and interferon were the first drugs used for the treatment of chronic HBV infection, these drugs have largely been supplanted by entecavir, tenofovir, and pegylated interferon as first-line therapy. When choosing among these agents, treatment can be tailored to specific patient preferences. Pegylated interferon achieves more rapid clearance of HBeAg and does not contribute to viral mutations. However, it is associated with systemic side effects that many find intolerable and requires weekly SC injections. In contrast, the oral agents often require a longer duration of therapy, are very well tolerated, and yield a more profound suppression of HBV DNA. However, mutations can occur with the use of these medications. Combination therapy does not appear to be more effective than single-drug therapy. The patient's husband should also be screened for hepatitis B given the continued viremia.

85. The answer is E.
(Chap. 40) Much information has been gained in recent decades about the progression and treatment of chronic hepatitis C virus (HCV) infection. Chronic hepatitis develops in about 85% of all individuals affected with HCV, and 20–25% of these individuals will progress to cirrhosis over about 20 years. Among those infected with HCV, about one-third of individuals will have normal or near–normal levels of aminotransferases, although liver biopsy demonstrates active hepatitis in as much as one-half of patients. Moreover, about 25% of individuals with normal aminotransferase levels at one point in time will develop elevations in these enzymes later, which can lead to progressive liver disease. Thus, normal aminotransferase

levels at a single point in time do not definitively rule out the possibility that cirrhosis can develop. Progression to end-stage liver disease in individuals with chronic HCV hepatitis is more likely in older individuals and in those with a longer duration of infection, advanced histologic stage and grade, genotype 1 infection, more complex quasi-species diversity, concomitant other liver disease, HIV infection, and obesity. Among these factors, the best prognostic indicator for the development of progressive liver disease is liver histology. Specifically, patients who have moderate to severe inflammation or necrosis including septal or bridging fibrosis have the greatest risk of developing cirrhosis over the course of 10–20 years. Indications for therapy in those with HCV include detectable levels of HCV RNA, portal or bridging fibrosis on liver biopsy, or moderate to severe hepatitis on liver biopsy. Contraindications to treatment are age greater than 60 years, mild hepatitis on liver biopsy, and severe renal insufficiency. Standard therapy for HCV infection is pegylated interferon plus ribavirin. While genotypes 1 and 4 are less responsive to therapy than genotypes 2 and 3, the current research demonstrates a response rate of at least 40% for genotypes 1 and 4. Interestingly, even in individuals who fail to show a virologic or biochemical response, 75% will have histologic improvement on liver biopsy. The treatment course for genotypes 1 and 4 is a minimum of 48 weeks, whereas genotypes 2 and 3 can be treated for as little as 24 weeks. Once treatment has been started, a repeat HCV viral load should be assessed at 12 weeks. At this point, a 2-log drop in viral load is expected. Failure to achieve this level of response suggests that a sustained virologic response is unlikely to occur. With a drop of this magnitude, however, the likelihood of a sustained virologic response is about 66% at the end of therapy, and if the viral load is undetectable at 12 weeks, the chances of a sustained virologic response is more than 80%.

86. The answer is C.
(Chap. 40) Three types of autoimmune hepatitis have been identified based on clinical and laboratory characteristics. Type I autoimmune hepatitis is a disorder typically seen in young women. The clinical characteristics can be variable from those of chronic hepatitis to fulminant hepatic failure, and many of the features are difficult to distinguish from other causes of chronic hepatitis. In some individuals, extrahepatic manifestations including fatigue, malaise, weight loss, anorexia, and arthralgias can be quite prominent. Liver enzymes are elevated but may not correlate with the clinical severity of disease. In more severe cases, elevations in serum bilirubin between 3 and 10 mg/dL can be seen. Hypoalbuminemia occurs in advanced disease, and hypergammaglobulinemia (>2.5 g/dL) is very common. The circulating antibody profile in autoimmune hepatitis depends to some extent on the type of hepatitis. Antinuclear antibodies are positive in a

homogeneous staining pattern almost invariably in the disease, and rheumatoid factor is also common. Perinuclear antineutrophilic cytoplasmic antibody may be positive, but in an atypical fashion. Anti–smooth muscle antibodies and anti–liver/kidney microsomal antibodies are frequently seen, but these are nonspecific as other causes of chronic hepatitis can lead to positivity of these enzymes. Because of the lack of a specific autoimmune profile, the diagnostic criteria for autoimmune hepatitis incorporate a variety of clinical and laboratory features. Specific features that argue against this diagnosis include prominent alkaline phosphatase elevation, presence of mitochondrial antibodies, markers of viral hepatitis, history of hepatotoxic drugs or excess alcohol intake, and histologic evidence of bile duct injury or atypical biopsy features including excess hepatic iron, fatty infiltration, and viral inclusions. Antimitochondrial antibodies are typically seen in primary biliary cirrhosis.

87. The answer is D.

(Chap. 40) In the course of acute hepatitis B, HBeAg positivity is common and usually transient. Persistence of HBeAg in the serum for 3 months or longer indicates an increased likelihood of development of chronic hepatitis B. In chronic hepatitis B, the presence of HBeAg in the serum indicates ongoing viral replication and increased infectivity. It is also a surrogate for inflammatory liver injury but not fibrosis. The development of antibody to HBeAg (anti-HBe) is indicative of the nonreplicative phase of HBV infection. During this phase, intact virions do not circulate and infectivity is less. Currently, quantification of HBV DNA with polymerase chain reaction allows risk stratification as fewer than 103 virions/μL is the approximate threshold for liver injury and infectivity.

88. The answer is C.

(Chap. 41) This patient presents with severe acute alcoholic hepatitis. In its earliest form, alcoholic liver disease is marked by fatty infiltration of the liver. In more acute alcoholic hepatitis, there is hepatocyte injury with balloon degeneration and necrosis. Many cases of alcoholic hepatitis are asymptomatic. However, as in this case, the severe manifestations can include fever, jaundice, spider nevi, and abdominal pain that can mimic an acute abdomen in its severity. On laboratory examination, the AST is typically elevated more than the ALT, although the total transaminase levels are rarely greater than 400 U/L. Hyperbilirubinemia can be quite marked, with lesser elevation in alkaline phosphatase. Hypoalbuminemia and coagulopathy are poor prognostic indicators. A discriminate function (DF) can be calculated as (4.6 × the prolongation of prothrombin time above control) + serum bilirubin. A DF greater than 32 is associated with a poor prognosis and is an indication for the treatment of acute alcoholic hepatitis. The Model for End-Stage Liver Disease (MELD) score can also be used for prognostication in acute alcoholic

hepatitis, with a score greater than 21 being an indication for treatment as well. This patient has a discriminate function of 73, indicating very severe disease and a poor prognosis. Complete abstinence from alcohol is imperative. Treatment with prednisone 40 mg daily (or prednisolone 32 mg daily) for 4 weeks should be initiated. Following the initial period, a taper should be achieved over a period of 4 weeks. Alternatively, pentoxifylline 400 mg three times daily for 4 weeks can also be used.

89. The answer is C.

(Chap. 42) The clinical presentation is consistent with a cholestatic picture, which can present with painless jaundice and pruritus. The pruritus can be prominent and is present in 50% of individuals at the time of diagnosis. The pruritus is typically intermittent and worse in the evening. There is no other prominent association such as following hot baths or showers, which occurs in polycythemia vera. Other causes of pruritus outside of cholestasis include lymphoma and uncontrolled hypo- or hyperthyroidism. However, the laboratory studies in this patient clearly represent cholestasis with an elevation in alkaline phosphatase and bilirubin. The clinical characteristics are more commonly seen in primary biliary cirrhosis compared to primary sclerosis cholangitis, as the patient is a middle-aged female with positive antimitochondrial antibodies. In contrast, primary sclerosing cholangitis is associated with positive perinuclear antineutrophil cytoplasmic antibodies in 65% of patients, and 50% of individuals with primary sclerosing cholangitis have a history of ulcerative colitis.

90. The answer is B.

(Chap. 42) Esophageal varices develop in the setting of portal hypertension associated most commonly with cirrhotic liver disease. In recent years, patients with cirrhosis have been commonly screened for varices by endoscopy, as about 33% will have varices on examination. Moreover, it is estimated that one-third of individuals with varices will develop bleeding. As this patient does not have medical care, it is unknown whether he has varices, but with the large volume of bleeding the patient has experienced, the treating physician should assume that the patient has variceal bleeding and act accordingly. The first step in the treatment of any individual with acute gastrointestinal bleeding is to ensure appropriate large-bore IV access, preferably in a large central vein or the antecubital fossae, and begin volume resuscitation. Volume resuscitation should be initiated with normal saline, and blood products should be administered when available. Once volume resuscitation has been initiated, emergent consultation with GI for endoscopic evaluation should be obtained. Endoscopic treatment should include esophageal band ligation, but in the acute setting, sclerotherapy may be used to control local bleeding with band ligation occurring at a future point in time.

If emergent endoscopy is not an option, placement of a Sengstaken-Blakemore or Minnesota tube to tamponade bleeding should be employed. In addition, vasoconstricting agents are used to decrease splanchnic blood flow. While vasopressin was initially the agent of choice, cardiovascular ischemia can occur with the high doses used in GI bleeding. The currently preferred agents are octreotide or somatostatin by continuous infusion. Nonspecific beta blockers such as propranolol or nadolol are used for the primary or secondary prevention of variceal bleeding, but are not prescribed in the acute setting as these agents could worsen hypotension.

91. The answer is A.

(Chap. 42) The cornerstone of the management of ascites is sodium restriction to less than 2 g daily. A common misconception is to institute a fluid restriction as well. However, this is neither effective nor necessary. With a sodium restriction to 2 g daily, most mild ascites can be managed quite well. If sodium restriction alone fails to correct ascites, then initiation of diuretics is required. Spironolactone at a dose of 100–200 mg daily is the initial diuretic used for ascites and can be titrated as high as 400–600 mg daily if tolerated. Loop diuretics can be added to spironolactone. The typical agent is furosemide beginning at 40–80 mg daily with the maximum doses being about 120–160 mg daily. Care must be taken to avoid renal dysfunction with loop diuretics, and higher doses may not be tolerated. If ascites is refractory to these treatments, transjugular intrahepatic portosystemic shunts (TIPS) can be considered. This procedure creates a portocaval shunt be introducing an expandable metal stent from the hepatic veins through the substance of the liver into the portal veins, creating a direct portocaval shunt. Thus, TIPS decreases portal pressures to decrease ascites and the risk of variceal bleeding. However, hepatic encephalopathy typically worsens following TIPS.

92. The answer is A.

(Chap. 42) Severe right-sided heart failure may lead to chronic liver injury and cardiac cirrhosis. Elevated venous pressure leads to congestion of the hepatic sinusoids and of the central vein and centrilobular hepatocytes. Centrilobular fibrosis develops, and fibrosis extends outward from the central vein, not the portal triads. Gross examination of the liver shows a pattern of "nutmeg liver." Although transaminases are typically mildly elevated, severe congestion, particularly associated with hypotension, may result in dramatic elevation of AST and ALT 50- to 100-fold above normal. Budd-Chiari syndrome, or occlusion of the hepatic veins or inferior vena cava, may be confused with congestive hepatopathy. However, the signs and symptoms of congestive heart failure are absent in patients with Budd-Chiari syndrome, and these patients can be easily distinguished clinically from those with heart failure. Venoocclusive disease may result

from hepatic irradiation and high-dose chemotherapy in preparation for hematopoietic stem cell transplantation. It is not a typical complication of liver transplantation. Although echocardiography is a useful tool for assessing left and right ventricular function, findings may be unimpressive in patients with constrictive pericarditis. A high index of suspicion for constrictive pericarditis (e.g., prior episodes of pericarditis, mediastinal irradiation) should lead to a right-sided heart catheterization with demonstration of "square root sign," which is the limitation of right heart filling pressure in diastole that is suggestive of restrictive cardiomyopathy. Cardiac magnetic resonance imaging may also be helpful in determining which patients should proceed to cardiac surgery.

93. The answer is B.

(Chap. 42) The presence of cirrhosis in an elderly woman with no prior risk factors for viral or alcoholic cirrhosis should raise the possibility of primary biliary cirrhosis (PBC). It is characterized by chronic inflammation and fibrous obliteration of intrahepatic ductules. The cause is unknown, but autoimmunity is assumed, as there is an association with other autoimmune disorders, such as autoimmune thyroiditis, CREST syndrome, and the sicca syndrome. The vast majority of patients with symptomatic disease are women. The antimitochondrial antibody test (AMA) is positive in over 90% of patients with PBC and only rarely is positive in other conditions. This makes it the most useful initial test in the diagnosis of PBC. Since there are false positives, if AMA is positive a liver biopsy is performed to confirm the diagnosis. The 24-hour urine copper collection is useful in the diagnosis of Wilson's disease. Hepatic failure from Wilson's disease typically occurs before age 50. Hemochromatosis may result in cirrhosis. It is associated with lethargy, fatigue, loss of libido, discoloration of the skin, arthralgias, diabetes, and cardiomyopathy. Ferritin levels are usually increased, and the most suggestive laboratory abnormality is an elevated transferrin saturation percentage. Although hemochromatosis is a possible diagnosis in this case, PBC is more likely in light of the clinical scenario. Although chronic hepatitis B and hepatitis C are certainly in the differential diagnosis and must be ruled out, they are unlikely because of the patient's history and lack of risk factors.

94. The answer is D.

(Chap. 44) This patient presents with nonalcoholic fatty liver disease (NAFLD) that has progressed to cirrhosis. It is now commonly thought that many individuals previously identified as having cryptogenic cirrhosis had NAFLD as a cause of end-stage liver disease. With the rising prevalence of obesity in the United States and Europe, NAFLD is expected to continue to rise. At present, the prevalence of NAFLD is estimated between to be 14–20%. Of these individuals, 30–40% with nonalcoholic steatohepatitis will develop advanced fibrosis and 10–15%

will develop outright cirrhosis. Most patients diagnosed with NAFLD are asymptomatic with incident note of elevated liver enzymes found on testing for other reasons. The ALT is typically slightly higher than the AST, and both enzymes are only mildly elevated. In most instances the ALT and AST are only 1.5–2 times the upper limit of normal. NAFLD often accompanies other components of the metabolic syndrome, with insulin resistance being a common link between these disorders. The diagnosis of NAFLD requires a careful history and examination to rule out other disorders. Alcohol intake should be less than 20 g/d. Comprehensive testing should include serologies for viral hepatitis, iron studies, ceruloplasmin, α_1 antitrypsin levels, and autoimmune serologies. Liver biopsy most commonly shows macrovesicular steatosis with a mixed inflammatory infiltrate in a lobular distribution. The fibrosis that occurs has a characteristic perivenular and perisinusoidal distribution. In cirrhotic patients, steatosis may not be seen, but can recur following transplant. The only known effective treatment for NAFLD is weight loss and exercise. Thiazolidinediones are currently being studied given their effects on insulin resistance. In addition, ongoing research into statins and ursodeoxycholic acid is being undertaken, but no specific medication can be recommended at this point for patients with NAFLD.

95. The answer is B.

(Chap. 45) In the National Health and Nutrition Examination Survey, the prevalence of gallstone disease in the United States was 7.9% in men and 16.6% in women. While the disease is quite prevalent, not all patients with gallstone disease require cholecystectomy. It is estimated that 1–2% of patients with asymptomatic gallstone disease will develop complications that will require surgery yearly. Therefore, it is important to know which patients with asymptomatic gallstones require referral for surgery. The first factor to consider is whether the patient has symptoms that are caused by gallstones and whether they are frequent enough and severe enough to necessitate surgery. Commonly called biliary colic, the classic symptoms of gallstone disease are right upper quadrant pain and fullness that begins suddenly and can last as long as 5 hours. Nausea and vomiting can accompany the episode. Vague symptoms of epigastric fullness, dyspepsia, and bloating following meals should not be considered biliary colic. A second factor that would be considered in recommending a patient for cholecystectomy is whether the patient has a prior history of complications of gallstone disease such as pancreatitis or acute cholecystitis. A final factor that would lead to the recommendation for cholecystectomy is the presence of anatomical factors that would increase the likelihood of complications such as a porcelain gallbladder or congenital abnormalities of the biliary tract. Individuals with very large stones (>3 cm) would also need to be considered carefully for cholecystectomy.

Ursodeoxycholic acid can be used in some instances to dissolve gallstones. It acts to decrease the cholesterol saturation of bile and also allows the dispersion of cholesterol from stones by producing a lamellar crystalline phase. It is only effective, however, in individuals with radiolucent stones measuring less than 10 mm.

96. The answer is D.

(Chap. 45) A practitioner needs to have a high index of suspicion for acalculous cholecystitis in critically ill patients who develop decompensation during the course of treatment for the underlying disease and have no other apparent source of infection. Some predisposing conditions for the development of acalculous cholecystitis include serious trauma or burns, postpartum following prolonged labor, prolonged parenteral hyperalimentation, and the postoperative period following orthopedic and other major surgical procedures. The clinical manifestations of acalculous cholecystitis are identical to calculous disease, but the disease is more difficult to diagnose. Ultrasonography and CT scanning typically only show biliary sludge, but they may demonstrate large and tense gallbladders. Hepatobiliary scintigraphy often shows delayed or absent gallbladder emptying. Successful management relies on accurate and early diagnosis. In critically ill patients, a percutaneous cholecystostomy may be the safest immediate procedure to decompress an infected gallbladder. Once the patient is stabilized, early elective cholecystectomy should be considered. Metronidazole to provide anaerobic coverage should be added, but this would not elucidate or adequately treat the underlying condition.

97. The answer is C.

(Chap. 45) Gallstones are very common, particularly in Western countries. Cholesterol stones are responsible for 80% of cases of cholelithiasis; pigment stones account for the remaining 20%. Cholesterol is essentially water insoluble. Stone formation occurs in the setting of factors that upset cholesterol balance. Obesity, cholesterol-rich diets, high-calorie diets, and certain medications affect the biliary secretion of cholesterol. Intrinsic genetic mutations in certain populations may affect the processing and secretion of cholesterol in the liver. Pregnancy results in both an increase in cholesterol saturation during the third trimester and changes in gallbladder contractility. Pigment stones are increased in patients with chronic hemolysis, cirrhosis, Gilbert's syndrome, and disruptions in the enterohepatic circulation. Although rapid weight loss and low-calorie diets are associated with gallstones, there is no evidence that a high-protein diet confers an added risk of cholelithiasis.

98. The answer is C.

(Chap. 46) In the United States, over 6000 individuals undergo liver transplants yearly. However, the demand for organs far outpaces the supply with a waiting list of over 16,000 individuals. The most common reasons for liver transplant are alcoholic cirrhosis and chronic hepatitis C infection. When evaluating someone for liver transplantation, it is important to ensure that the patient is an appropriate candidate. For individuals with alcoholic cirrhosis, sustained abstinence and recovery need to be demonstrated, although the recidivism rate is as high as 25% after transplantation. Absolute contraindications to liver transplant include uncontrolled infection, active substance or alcohol abuse, extrahepatobiliary malignancy (excluding nonmelanoma skin cancer), metastatic malignancy to the liver, AIDS, or life-threatening or advance systemic disease. Cholangiocarcinoma almost invariably recurs following liver transplantation. Thus, it is now considered a contraindication to transplant. While primarily performed in children, living donor transplantation is increasingly being considered in adults given the poor availability of cadaveric organs. In living donor transplantation, typically the right lobe of the liver is taken from a suitable healthy donor. Currently, living donor transplantation accounts for 4% of all liver transplants. It is certainly not without risk. The average healthy donor will be medically disabled for at least 10 weeks, and the risk of death for the donor is 0.2–0.4%. Individuals receiving all forms of liver transplant have demonstrated increasing survival over the past decades. The current 5-year survival rate is more than 60%. Following transplantation, however, rejection, infection, and recurrence of primary disease can occur. For chronic hepatitis B infection, reinfection of the transplant frequently occurs, but this may be reduced to as little as 35% with post-transplantation treatment with hepatitis B immunoglobulin. For hepatitis C, reinfection is universal and is associated with the development of allograft cirrhosis in 20–30% of patients within 5 years. Autoimmune diseases can also recur in the transplanted liver, although it can be difficult to differentiate between the autoimmune disease and rejection. Wilson's disease and α_1 antitrypsin deficiency, however, do not recur following transplantation.

99. The answer is E.

(Chap. 46) The patient has advanced cirrhosis with a high risk of mortality, as evidenced by his episode of spontaneous bacterial peritonitis. His diabetes and remote skin cancer (since it was a basal cell carcinoma, not melanoma) are not absolute contraindications for liver transplantation, but active alcohol abuse is. The other absolute contraindications to transplantation are life-threatening systemic disease, uncontrolled infections, preexisting advanced cardiac or pulmonary disease, metastatic malignancy, and life-threatening congenital malignancies. Ongoing drug or alcohol abuse is an absolute contraindication, and patients who would otherwise be suitable candidates should immediately be referred to appropriate counseling centers to achieve abstinence. Once that is

achieved for an acceptable period of time, transplantation can be considered. Indeed, alcoholic cirrhosis accounts for a substantial proportion of the patients who undergo liver transplantation.

100. The answer is A.

(Chap. 48) The most common cause of acute pancreatitis in the United States is gallstones causing common bile duct obstruction. Although bile duct obstruction may be demonstrated on technetium HIDA scan, right upper quadrant ultrasound is preferred for ease, demonstration of gallstones in the gallbladder, and demonstration of obstructed bile duct. Alcohol is the second most common cause, followed by complications of endoscopic retrograde cholangiopancreatography (ERCP). Hypertriglyceridemia accounts for 1–4% of cases with triglyceride levels usually greater than 1000 mg/dL. Other potential causes of pancreatitis include trauma, postoperative states, drugs such as valproic acid, anti-HIV medications, estrogens, and sphincter of Oddi dysfunction. Additionally, there are a number of rare causes that have been described. The most judicious first step in evaluation is to test for gallstones and pursue more rare causes after the most common cause has been ruled out.

101. The answer is A.

(Chap. 48) Physical examination in acute pancreatitis commonly shows an uncomfortable patient often with low-grade fever, tachycardia, and hypotension. Abdominal tenderness and muscle rigidity are often present to varying degrees. Cullen's sign is a faint blue discoloration around the umbilicus that may occur as the result of hemoperitoneum. Turner's sign is blue-red-purple or green-brown discoloration of the flanks from tissue catabolism of hemoglobin. Both of these signs indicate the presence of severe necrotizing pancreatitis.

102. The answer is E.

(Chap. 48) The BISAP (Bedside Index of Severity in Acute Pancreatitis) score has recently replaced Ranson's criteria and APACHE II severity scores as the recommended modality to assess the severity of pancreatitis due to the cumbersome nature of the prior scores and the requirement of prior scores to collect large amounts of clinical and laboratory data over time. Furthermore, the APACHE II and Ranson's scoring mechanisms did not have acceptable positive and negative predictive values in predicting severe acute pancreatitis. The BISAP score incorporates five variables in determining severity: BUN greater than 35 mg/dL, impaired mental status, presence of SIRS, age above 60 years, and pleural effusion on radiography. The presence of three or more of these factors is associated with substantially increased risk for in-hospital mortality. Additional risk factors initially predicting severity include BMI of 30 or above and comorbid disease.

103. The answer is E.

(Chap. 48) Several trials over the last several decades have demonstrated that there is no role for prophylactic antibiotics in the management of either interstitial or necrotizing pancreatitis. Antibiotics are recommended for only patients who appear septic at presentation while awaiting the results of culture data. If cultures are negative, antibiotics should be discontinued to decrease the risk of the development of fungal superinfection. Similarly, several drugs have been evaluated in the treatment of acute pancreatitis and found to be of no benefit. These drugs include H_2 blockers, glucagon, protease inhibitors such as aprotinin, glucocorticoids, calcitonin, nonsteroidal anti-inflammatory drugs, and lexipafant, a platelet-activating factor inhibitor. A recent meta-analysis of somatostatin, octreotide, and the antiprotease gabexate mesylate in the therapy of acute pancreatitis suggested a reduced mortality rate but no change in complications with octreotide, and no effect on mortality but reduced pancreatic damage with gabexate.

104. The answer is C.

(Chap. 48) Persistent inflammatory changes in the pancreas may remain for weeks to months after an episode of acute pancreatitis. Similarly, there may be prolonged elevation of amylase and lipase. In this regard, persistent changes on CT or persistent pancreatic enzyme elevation should not discourage clinicians from feeding hungry patients with acute pancreatitis. Although there had been prior concern that feeding patients with pancreatitis may exacerbate pancreatic inflammation, this has not been borne out. Similarly, enteral feeding with a nasojejunal tube in patients with acute pancreatitis has been demonstrated to have fewer infectious complications than feeding with total parenteral nutrition. Because of this, nasogastric feeding is the preferred method of nutritional support in acute pancreatitis. Enteral feeding also helps to maintain the integrity of the intestinal tract in acute pancreatitis.

105. The answer is D.

(Chap. 48) The pathophysiology of acute pancreatitis evolves in three phases. During the initial phase, pancreatic injury leads to intrapancreatic activation of digestive enzymes with subsequent autodigestion and acinar cell injury. Acinar injury is primarily attributed to activation of zymogens (proenzymes), particularly trypsinogen, by lysosomal hydrolases. Once trypsinogen is converted to trypsin, the activated trypsin further perpetuates the process by activating other zymogens to further autodigestion. The inflammation initiated by intrapancreatic activation of zymogens leads to the second phase of acute pancreatitis, with local production of chemokines that causes activation and sequestration of neutrophils in the pancreas. Experimental evidence suggests that neutrophilic inflammation can also cause further activation

of trypsinogen, leading to a cascade of increasing acinar injury. The third phase of acute pancreatitis reflects the systemic processes that are caused by release of inflammatory cytokines and activated proenzymes into the systemic circulation. This process can lead to the systemic inflammatory response syndrome with acute respiratory distress syndrome, extensive third-spacing of fluids, and multiorgan failure.

106. The answer is D.

(Chap. 48) Chronic pancreatitis is a common disorder in any patient population with relapsing acute pancreatitis, especially patients with alcohol dependence, pancreas divisum, and cystic fibrosis. The disorder is notable for both endocrine and exocrine dysfunction of the pancreas. Often diabetes ensues as a result of loss of islet cell function; though insulin-dependent, it is generally not as prone to diabetic ketoacidosis or coma as are other forms of diabetes mellitus. As pancreatic enzymes are essential to fat digestion, their absence leads to fat malabsorption and steatorrhea. In addition, the fat-soluble vitamins, A, D, E, and K, are not absorbed. Vitamin A deficiency can lead to neuropathy. Vitamin B_{12}, or cobalamin, is often deficient. This deficiency is hypothesized to be due to excessive binding of cobalamin by cobalamin-binding proteins other than intrinsic factor that are normally digested by pancreatic enzymes. Replacement of pancreatic enzymes orally with meals will correct the vitamin deficiencies and steatorrhea. The incidence of pancreatic adenocarcinoma is increased in patients with chronic pancreatitis, with a 20-year cumulative incidence of 4%. Chronic abdominal pain is nearly ubiquitous in this disorder, and narcotic dependence is common. Niacin is a water-soluble vitamin, and absorption is not affected by pancreatic exocrine dysfunction.

107. The answer is A.

(Chap. 48) This patient likely has chronic pancreatitis related to long-standing alcohol use, which is the most common cause of chronic pancreatitis in adults in the United States. Chronic pancreatitis can develop in individuals who consume as little as 50 g of alcohol daily (equivalent to ~30–40 ounces of beer). The patient's description of his loose stools is consistent with steatorrhea, and the recurrent bouts of abdominal pain are likely related to his pancreatitis. In most patients, abdominal pain is the most prominent symptom. However, up to 20% of individuals with chronic pancreatitis present with symptoms of maldigestion alone. The evaluation for chronic pancreatitis should allow one to characterize the pancreatitis as large- vs. small-duct disease. Large-duct disease is more common in men and is more likely to be associated with steatorrhea. In addition, large-duct disease is associated with the appearance of pancreatic calcifications and abnormal tests of pancreatic exocrine function. Women are more likely to have small-duct disease, with normal tests of pancreatic exocrine function and normal abdominal radiography. In small-duct disease, the progression to steatorrhea is rare, and the pain is responsive to treatment with pancreatic enzymes. The characteristic findings on CT and abdominal radiograph of this patient are characteristic of chronic pancreatitis, and no further workup should delay treatment with pancreatic enzymes. Treatment with pancreatic enzymes orally will improve maldigestion and lead to weight gain, but they are unlikely to fully resolve maldigestive symptoms. Narcotic dependence can frequently develop in individuals with chronic pancreatitis due to recurrent and severe bouts of pain. However, as this individual's pain is mild, it is not necessary to prescribe narcotics at this point in time. An ERCP or magnetic resonance cholangiopancreatography (MRCP) may be considered to evaluate for a possible stricture that is amenable to therapy. However, sphincterotomy is a procedure performed via ERCP that may be useful in treating pain related to chronic pancreatitis and is not indicated in the patient. Angiography to assess for ischemic bowel disease is not indicated as the patient's symptoms are not consistent with intestinal angina. Certainly, weight loss can occur in this setting, but the patient usually presents with complaints of abdominal pain after eating and pain that is out of proportion with the clinical examination. Prokinetic agents would likely only worsen the patient's malabsorptive symptoms and are not indicated.

Bold numbers indicate the start of the main discussion of the topic; numbers with "f" and "t" refer to figure and table pages, respectively.